Human Radiation Injury

Human Radiation Injury

DENNIS C. SHRIEVE, MD, PhD

Rudolph S. and Edna Reese Research Professor and Chair
Department of Radiation Oncology
University of Utah School of Medicine
Huntsman Cancer Hospital
Salt Lake City, Utah

JAY S. LOEFFLER, MD, FACR, FASTRO

Herman and Joan Suit Professor
Department of Radiation Oncology
Harvard Medical School
Chair, Department of Radiation Oncology
Massachusetts General Hospital
Boston, Massachusetts

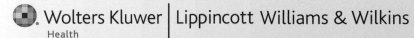

Health

Philadelphia · Baltimore · New York · London
Buenos Aires · Hong Kong · Sydney · Tokyo

Senior Executive Editor: Jonathan W. Pine, Jr.
Senior Product Manager: Emilie Moyer
Senior Manufacturing Manager: Benjamin Rivera
Senior Marketing Manager: Angela Panetta
Creative Services Director: Doug Smock
Production Service: SPi Technologies

Printed in China

Library of Congress Cataloging-in-Publication Data

Human radiation injury/[edited by] Dennis C. Shrieve, Jay S. Loeffler.—1st ed.
   p. ; cm.
Includes bibliographical references and index.
ISBN 978-1-60547-011-5 (alk. paper)
1. Radiation injuries.   I. Shrieve, Dennis C.   II. Loeffler, Jay S.
[DNLM: 1. Radiation Injuries—pathology.   2. Dose-Response Relationship, Radiation.
3. Radiation Effects.   4. Radiation Injuries—therapy.   WN 620 H918 2011]

RC93.H86   2011
616.9'897—dc22

                                                                              2010025903

To purchase additional copies of this book, call our customer service department at (800) 638-3030 or fax orders to (301) 223-2320. International customers should call (301) 223-2300.

Visit Lippincott Williams & Wilkins on the Internet: at LWW.com. Lippincott Williams & Wilkins customer service representatives are available from 8:30 am to 6 pm, EST.

                                          10 9 8 7 6 5 4 3 2 1

To all those who have been injured by radiation, in the hope that this body of knowledge will reduce the probability of others suffering a similar fate.

Contributing Authors

May Abdel-Wahab, MD, PhD
Associate Professor of Radiation Oncology
Department of Radiation Oncology
University of Miami
Miller School of Medicine
Miami, Florida

Christopher Anker, MD
Assistant Professor
Department of Radiation Oncology
University of Utah School of Medicine
Salt Lake City, Utah

Judith M. Bader, MD
Radiation Research Program
Division of Cancer Treatment and Diagnosis
National Cancer Institute, Bethesda, Maryland
Office of the Assistant Secretary for Preparedness and Response
Department of Health and Human Services,
Washington, District of Columbia

Igor J. Barani, MD
Assistant Professor of Clinical Radiation Oncology
Department of Radiation Oncology
University of California, San Francisco
San Francisco, California

Niranjan Bhandare, MS
Medical Physicist
Department of Radiation Oncology
University of Florida
Gainesville, Florida

M. Tariq Bhatti, MD
Associate Professor
Service Chief, Neuro-Ophthalmology
Department of Ophthalmology
Duke University
Durham, North Carolina

Michael Brada, BSc, FRCP, FRCR
Professor of Oncology
Department of Academic Radiotherapy
Institute of Cancer Research
Sutton, Surrey, United Kingdom
Professor of Oncology
Department of Neuro-Oncology and Lung
The Royal Marsden National Health Services Foundation Trust
London, United Kingdom
Surrey, United Kingdom

David J. Brenner PhD, DSc
Higgins Professor of Radiation Biophysics
Center for Radiological Research
Department of Radiation Oncology
Columbia University Medical Center
New York, New York

Paul D. Brown, MD
Professor
Department of Radiation Oncology
Mayo Clinic College of Medicine
Rochester, Minnesota

Michael D. Chan MD
Assistant Professor
Department of Radiation Oncology
Wake Forest University
Winston-Salem, North Carolina

Yen-Lin Evelyn Chen, MD
Instructor
Department of Radiation Oncology
Massachusetts General Hospital
Harvard Medical School
Boston, Massachusetts

Eric P. Cohen, MD
Professor
Department of Medicine
Medical College of Wisconsin
Chief
Department of Nephrology Section
Zablocki Veterans Affairs Medical Center
Milwaukee, Wisconsin

C. Norman Coleman, MD
Radiation Research Program
Division of Cancer Treatment and Diagnosis
National Cancer Institute, Bethesda, Maryland
Office of the Assistant Secretary for Preparedness and Response
Department of Health and Human Services,
Washington, District of Columbia

Ellen Cooke, MD
Resident
Department of Radiation Oncology
University of Utah School of Medicine
Salt Lake City, Utah

Jean-Marc Cosset, MD
Radiotherapy Department
Institut Curie
Paris, France

Francis A. Cucinotta, PhD
Chief Scientist
Space Radiation Program
National Aeronautics and Space Administration Johnson Space Center
Houston, Texas

Brian G. Czito, MD
Associate Professor
Department of Radiation Oncology
Duke University Medical Center
Durham, North Carolina

Marco de Santis, MD
Telefono Rosso-Teratology Information Service
Department of Obstetrics and Gynecology
Catholic University of the Sacred Heart
Rome, Italy

J. Debus, MD
Chair
Department of Radiation Oncology
University of Heidelberg
Heidelberg, Germany

Thomas F. Delaney
Associate Professor
Department of Radiation Oncology
Massachusetts General Hospital
Harvard Medical School
Boston, Massachusetts

James W. Denham, MD
Professor of Radiation Oncology
Newcastle Mater Hospital
Newcastle, New South Wales, Australia

Peter C. Ferguson, MD, MSc, FRCSC
Assistant Professor
Department of Surgery
Department of Surgical Oncology
Princess Margaret Hospital
Toronto, Ontario, Canada

John C. Flickinger, MD
Professor of Radiation Oncology
and Neurosurgery
University of Pittsburgh School of Medicine
Pittsburgh, Pennsylvania

Robert L. Foote, MD
Professor and Chair
Department of Radiation Oncology
Mayo Clinic College of Medicine
Rochester, Minnesota

Saeko Fujiwara, MD
Departments of Clinical Studies
Radiation Effects Research Foundation
Nagasaki and Hiroshima, Japan

David K. Gaffney, MD, PhD
Professor and Vice-Chair
Department of Radiation Oncology
Huntsman Cancer Hospital
University of Utah School of Medicine
Salt Lake City, Utah

Leo E. Gerweck, PhD
Associate Professor
Department of Radiation Oncology
Massachusetts General Hospital
Harvard Medical School
Boston, Massachusetts

Philippe Giraud, MD, PhD
Professor
Department of Radiation Oncology
Paris Descartes University (Paris V)
Associate Chief
Department of Radiation Oncology
European Georges Pompidou Hospital
Paris, France

Daniel Gomez, MD
Assistant Professor
Department of Radiation Oncology
M.D. Anderson Cancer Center
Houston, Texas

Victor J. Gonzalez, MD
Assistant Professor of Radiation Oncology
University of Arizona School of Medicine
Tucson, Arkansas

Paul M. Harari, MD
Professor and Chairman
Department of Human Oncology
University of Wisconsin
Madison, Wisconsin

Martin Hauer-Jensen, MD, PhD
Professor of Surgery and Pathology
University of Arkansas for Medical Sciences
Little Rock, Arkansas

Lisa Hazard, MD
Assistant Professor
Department of Radiation Oncology
Huntsman Cancer Hospital
University of Utah School of Medicine
Salt Lake City, Utah

Kathryn D. Held, PhD
Associate Professor
Department of Radiation Oncology
Massachusetts General Hospital
Harvard Medical School
Boston, Massachusetts

Mehdi Henni, MD
Department of Radiation Oncology
European Georges Pompidou Hospital
Paris, France

Frank J.P. Hoebers, MD, PhD
Radiation Oncologist
Department of Radiation Oncology
Netherlands Cancer Institute
Amsterdam, The Netherlands

Theodore S. Hong, MD
Assistant Professor
Massachusetts General Hospital
Harvard Medical School
Boston, Massachusetts

Nils Hovdenak, MD, PhD
Division of Gastroenterology
Section of Oncology
Haukeland University Hospital
University of Bergen
Bergen, Norway

Amy K. Huser, BA
Department of Radiation Oncology
James P. Wilmot Cancer Center
University of Rochester School of Medicine
Rochester, New York

Reshma Jagsi, MD, D.Phil
Assistant Professor
Department of Radiation Oncology
University of Michigan
Ann Arbor, Michigan

Peter A.S. Johnstone, MD, FACR
William A. Mitchell Professor and Chair
Department of Radiation Oncology
Indiana University School of Medicine
Indianapolis, Indiana

Josephine Kang, MD, PhD
Resident
Harvard Radiation Oncology Program
Boston, Massachusetts

Andrew Kee, MD
Department of Radiation Oncology
Legacy Good Samaritan Hospital
Portland, Oregon

Susan J. Knox, MD, PhD
Professor of Radiation Oncology
Stanford University School of Medicine
Stanford, California

Kevin R. Kozak, MD, PhD
Assistant Professor
Department of Human Oncology
University of Wisconsin School of Medicine and Public Health
Madison, Wisconsin

K. Sree Kumar, PhD
Assistant Professor
Uniformed Services University of the Health Sciences
Department of Radiation Biology
Bethesda, Maryland

Nadia N. Issa Laack, MD, MS
Assistant Professor
Department of Radiation Oncology
Mayo Clinic
Rochester, Minnesota

Brian D. Lawenda, MD
Adjunct Assistant Professor
Department of Radiation Oncology
Indiana University School of Medicine
Indianapolis, Indiana
Clinical Director
Department of Radiation Oncology
Naval Medical Center San Diego
San Diego, California

Colleen A. Lawton, MD
Professor
Department of Radiation Oncology
Medical College of Wisconsin
Milwaukee, Wisconsin

Ting Liu, MD
Assistant Professor
Department of Pathology
University of Utah School of Medicine
Salt Lake City, Utah

Jay S. Loeffler, MD, FACR, FASTRO
Herman and Joan Suit Professor of Radiation Oncology
Harvard Medical School
Chair, Department of Radiation Oncology
Massachusetts General Hospital
Boston, Massachusetts

Kiyohiko Mabuchi, MD, Dr PH
Senior Scientist
Department of Radiation Epidemiology Branch
National Cancer Institute
Bethesda, Maryland

Roger M. Macklis, MD
Professor and Chair Emeritus
Department of Radiation Oncology
Cleveland Clinic Foundation
Cleveland, Ohio

William M. Mendenhall, MD
Professor
Department of Radiation Oncology
University of Florida College of Medicine
Gainesville, Florida

Ruby F. Meredith, MD, PhD
Professor
Department of Radiation Oncology
University of Alabama at Birmingham
Birmingham, Alabama

Lynn Million, MD
Associate Professor
Department of Radiation Oncology
Huntsman Cancer Hospital
University of Utah School of Medicine
Salt Lake City, Utah

Bruce Minsky, MD
Associate Dean and Professor
Department of Radiation and Cellular Oncology
University of Chicago Medical Center
Chicago, Illinois

John E. Moulder, PhD
Professor
Department of Radiation Oncology
Medical College of Wisconsin
Milwaukee, Wisconsin

Nori Nakamura, PhD
Departments of Genetics and Radiation Effects
Research Foundation
Hiroshima, Japan

Carsten Nieder, MD
Professor
Institute of Clinical Medicine
University of Tromsø
Tromsø, Norway
Chief
Department of Radiation Oncology Unit
Nordland Hospital
Bodø, Norway

Paul Okunieff, MD
Director
University of Florida Cancer Center
Chair, Department of Radiation Oncology
University of Florida School of Medicine
Gainsville, Florida

Brian O'Sullivan, MD, FRCPC, FFRRCSI (Hon)
Professor
Department of Radiation Oncology
University of Toronto
Toronto, Ontario, Canada

Harald Paganetti, PhD
Associate Professor
Department of Radiation Oncology
Massachusetts General Hospital
Harvard Medical School
Boston, Massachusetts

James T. Parsons, MD
Department of Radiation Oncology
Bethesda Memorial Hospital
Boynton Beach, Florida

Alan Pollack, MD, PhD
Professor and Chair
Department of Radiation Oncology
University of Miami School of Medicine
Miami, Florida

Abram Recht, MD, FASTRO
Professor and Deputy Chief
Department of Radiation Oncology
Beth Israel Deaconess Hospital
Harvard Medical School
Boston, Massachusetts

Stefan Reiken, MD
Department of Radiation Oncology
University of Heidelberg
Heidelberg, Germany

Mike E. Robbins, PhD
Professor and Section Head, Radiation Biology
Department of Radiation Oncology
Wake Forest University School of Medicine
Winston-Salem, North Carolina

Nicola A. Rosenfelder, MBBS, MRCP, FRCP
Department of Medicine
MRC Clinical Sciences Centre
Faculty of Medicine
Hammersmith Hospital
Imperial College
London, United Kingdom

Kenneth Rosenzweig, MD
Professor and Chair
Department of Radiation Oncology
Mount Sinai School of Medicine
New York, New York

Arjun Sahgal, MD
Staff Radiation Oncologist
Department of Radiation Oncology
Odette Cancer Centre at Sunnybrook Health Sciences Centre
Associate Staff
Department of Radiation Oncology
Princess Margaret Hospital, Toronto, Ontario, Canada

Brenda Shank, MD, PhD, FASTRO, FACR
Division Director
Department of Radiation Oncology
J.C. Robinson, MD Regional Cancer Center
Doctors Medical Center
San Pablo, California

Edward G. Shaw, MD, MA
Professor
Department of Radiation Oncology
Wake Forest University
Baptist Medical Center
Winston-Salem, North Carolina

Helen A. Shih, MD
Assistant Professor
Department of Radiation Oncology
Massachusetts General Hospital
Harvard Medical School
Boston, Massachusetts

Yukiko Shimizu, PhD
Department of Epidemiology
Radiation Effects Research Foundation
Hiroshima, Japan

Roy E. Shore, PhD, DPH
Vice Chairman and Chief of Research
Radiation Effects Research Foundation
Hiroshima, Japan

Dennis C. Shrieve, MD, PhD
Rudolph S. and Edna Reese Research Professor and Chair
Department of Radiation Oncology
University of Utah School of Medicine
Huntsman Cancer Hospital
Salt Lake City, Utah

Patricia "Penny" Sneed, MD
Professor of Radiation Oncology
University of California, San Francisco
San Francisco, California

Fiona Stewart, BSc, PhD
Group Leader
Division of Experimental Therapy
The Netherlands Cancer Institute
Amsterdam, The Netherlands

Gianluca Straface, MD
Telefono Rosso-Teratology Information Service
Department of Obstetrics and Gynecology
Catholic University of the Sacred Heart
Rome, Italy

Herman D. Suit, MD, D.Phil
Andreas Soriano Distinguished Professor
Department of Radiation Oncology
Massachusetts General Hospital
Harvard Medical School
Boston, Massachusetts

Alphonse Taghian, MD, PhD
Associate Professor
Department of Radiation Oncology
Massachusetts General Hospital
Harvard Medical School
Boston, Massachusetts

Nancy J. Tarbell, MD
Dean for Academic and Clinical Affairs
C.C. Wang Professor of Radiation Oncology
Harvard Medical School
Department of Radiation Oncology
Massachusetts General Hospital
Boston, Massachusetts

Alexei Trofimov, PhD
Assistant Professor
Department of Radiation Oncology
Massachusetts General Hospital
Harvard Medical School
Boston, Massachusetts

Jonathan D. Tward, MD, PhD
Assistant Professor
Department of Radiation Oncology
Huntsman Cancer Hospital
University of Utah
Salt Lake City, Utah

Albert J. van der Kogel, PhD
Professor of Radiation Oncology
Academisch Ziekenhuis
Nijmegen, Holland

Kenneth D. Westover, MD, PhD
Resident
Harvard Radiation Oncology Program
Boston, Massachusetts

Henning Willers, MD
Assistant Professor
Department of Radiation Oncology
Massachusetts General Hospital
Harvard Medical School
Boston, Massachusetts

Christopher G. Willett, MD
Leonard Prosnitz Professor and Chairman
Department of Radiation Oncology
Duke University Medical Center
Durham, North Carolina

C. Shun Wong, MD
Department of Radiation Oncology
Sunnybrook and Women's College Health Sciences Center
University of Toronto
Toronto, Ontario, Canada

Michael Yassa, MD
Department of Radiation Oncology
European Georges Pompidou Hospital
Paris, France

Torunn Yock, MD
Assistant Professor of Radiation Oncology
Massachusetts General Hospital
Harvard Medical School
Boston, Massachusetts

Anthony L. Zietman, MD
William and Jenoit Shipley Professor of Radiation Oncology
Department of Radiation Oncology
Massachusetts General Hospital
Harvard Medical School
Boston, Massachusetts

Foreword

Fundamental dichotomies are consistent phenomena in medicine. Nowhere is this more clearly demonstrated than in considering radiation exposure. These begin with the Manichaean dualities seen when considering medical treatments in general: the scalpel used in surgery as compared to a dagger or sword, the chemical compound used as a therapeutic agent as compared to a poison, and radiation used in diagnosis and treatment as compared to excessive or unwanted radiation exposure either locally or systemically. These basic instruments of medicine are not completely beneficent; all have some instances of unwanted effects, but none with the aura of fear and loathing associated with radiation. X-rays and other ionizing radiations were heralded initially as medical miracles when first discovered by Roentgen, Marie and Pierre Curie and others, but after time, the unwanted consequences became apparent, as exemplified by such radiation martyrs as Marie Curie, her daughter Irene and son-in-law Frederick Joliot-Curie. All of these Nobel Laureates—Marie was honored twice, and the others once each—most probably died as a consequence of radiation exposure. As was true for many other radiation-related maladies, these occurred long after the exposure. Thus, in the use of medical radiation, the benefits appear early and many of the untoward consequences appear later. This leads to initial enthusiasm followed by profound disillusionment and a belief that with radiation, despite initial benefit, there persists a Damoclean Sword of risk over the head of the exposed person. Of course, this ominous concern was greatly accentuated in the mind of the public by the use of atomic weapons at the end of World War II and the radiation accidents such as at Three Mile Island and Chernobyl. This fear can only be ameliorated by accurate information about the causes, frequency, severity and the prevention or treatment of these radiation-associated conditions. This book provides the current state of knowledge applicable to human radiation injury and should help replace irrational fear with clear, quantifiable information.

Other dichotomies illustrated in radiation injury include the separation between acute and late radiation damage; locally applied as contrasted to systemic or total body exposure; one or a few radiation exposures versus fractionated radiation exposures; and preventive or ameliorating agents applied before exposure in contrast to postexposure treatment. Each of these is important to our understanding of the effective, appropriate use of radiation as a therapy, and each forms the subject of this volume. The book is divided by anatomic site and these various dichotomies are discussed as appropriate to the specific organs or treatments being considered. The volume begins with a section devoted to understanding the basic principles of radiation effect. Systemic exposure is then discussed with specific considerations of radiation exposure due to atomic bomb use, nuclear power plant operation and possible nuclear terrorism. Organ-specific effects are then detailed as appropriate to understanding, minimizing and managing radiation injuries.

The volume thus is appropriate to both health professionals involved in radiation use and a more general public interested in peaceful and wartime use of radiation. Specific to radiation treatment are methods to prevent or minimize injury such as organ-specific tolerance, treatment planning and the various types of technology used. Concern with systemic radiation exposure has a much wider application for health workers and the general public. This broad consideration of the deleterious effects of ionizing radiation, as well as the breadth of contributors, makes this book useful to a broad constituency.

With regard to radiation therapy, it would serve us well while reading this volume to see the parallels to the other major modalities. Drug overdose or inappropriate use is the malevolent aspect of pharmaceutical use. The very term "drug" can refer to either a therapeutic agent or narcotic abuse or trafficking. To the Greeks "pharmakos" meant both remedy and poison. The expected and unavoidable consequences of surgical procedures, such as limb amputation or organ removal, result in predictable, immediate unwanted effects. All of medicine attempts to maximize the benefit while limiting the harm of the treatment modality. Radiation use is no different: the Manichaean dichotomy is an essential characteristic of all of the current healing methods.

Samuel Hellman, MD

Preface

Never in our history has the potential for exposure to ionizing radiation—intentional or unintentional—been greater. The use of medical radiation, both diagnostic and therapeutic, is on the rise. The benefits of nuclear power production are to be balanced with the fear of human exposure to the radioactive core elements and environmental concerns. Fear of malevolent uses of radioactivity by terrorists, the ever present danger of existing and newly developed nuclear weapons, and the limitations and risks imposed on space travel by cosmic radiation are examples of current radiation-related concerns. Public awareness of the risks associated with ionizing radiation has never been greater. It is extremely important that those involved in the use of ionizing radiation and those with the responsibility to protect the public from radiation exposure be well informed of the real risks involved.

Human Radiation Injury was initially conceived as a reference book on normal tissue effects of radiation for radiation oncologists. From this idea emerged a text with broader scope and application. Along with chapters focused on the biologic mechanisms of radiation injury to individual organs are included chapters on special topics such as: biologic mechanisms of radiation damage; radiation carcinogenesis; response to terrorism involving radioactivity; the risks associated with nuclear power production; effects on the unborn; effects on atomic bomb survivors; and risks associated with space travel. While the book remains a source of information for radiation oncologists, it is also intended as a reference for all involved in the study and use of ionizing radiation and for those involved in policy making affecting medical, industrial or military uses of ionizing radiation.

A text like *Human Radiation Injury* is a collaboration involving the time and effort of many. Our goal was to have recognized experts author chapters in their particular area of interest and expertise. We wish to thank all the authors for their willingness to contribute their time and expertise and for their diligence in writing chapters containing the most up-to-date information. We also wish to thank Lippincott William & Wilkins and especially Jonathan Pine and Emilie Moyer for supporting this project.

Contents

SECTION I: Radiobiology and Pathology or Irradiated Normal Tissues

SECTION II: Whole Body Effects of Radiation

SECTION III: Organ-Specific Effects of Radiation

Human Radiation Injury

Kathryn D. Held
Henning Willers

Molecular and Cellular Basis of Radiation Injury

All normal tissue damage from ionizing radiation results from the initial energy deposition in tissue. Ionizing radiation, by definition, is electromagnetic radiation with sufficient energy to eject an orbital electron from an atom, that is, to ionize the atom or molecule. The physical processes initiated by traversal of radiation through matter involve ionizations and excitations, followed by radiation chemical events including free radical formation and reactions, then biochemistry including enzymatic processes, and ultimately the biological and physiological changes that are the topics of this book. These processes occur over varying timescales from 10^{-18} seconds to many years, as summarized in Figure 1.1. This chapter briefly reviews relevant aspects of radiation physics and radiation chemistry and then provides an overview of the major molecular and cellular radiation biology thought to underpin the expression of radiation damage in normal tissues.

OVERVIEW OF RADIATION PHYSICS AND RADIATION CHEMISTRY

TYPES OF IONIZING RADIATION: PHOTONS AND PARTICLES

X-rays and γ-rays are the most familiar forms of ionizing radiation. These electromagnetic radiations range in energy from 100 eV to over 1 GeV. X-rays and γ-rays have similar properties except for the ways in which they are produced. Most commonly, x-rays are produced in a machine that accelerates electrons onto a metal target, with the kinetic energy of the

electron being converted into x-rays, that is, photons produced extranuclearly, generally having a range of energies, depending on the energy of the incoming electrons and the target material. Gamma-rays are emitted during decay of radioactive nuclei, such as ^{60}Co. Because γ-rays result from discrete nuclear disintegrations, they have specific energies, for example, photons of 1.17 and 1.33 MeV are produced by ^{60}Co. As these radiations traverse matter, there is a continual loss of energy, and hence decrease in relative dose with depth, beyond an initial slight increase in dose, depending on the energy of the incident photons (Fig. 1.2).

Other ionizing radiations are particulate in nature. These include electrons, protons, α-particles, neutrons, and heavy charged particles. The small, negatively charged electrons can be accelerated to high energies in a linear accelerator in a manner that is useful in radiation therapy. Positively charged protons are of much greater mass, requiring more complex equipment to accelerate them, but have unique physical and dose deposition characteristics that make them useful in radiation oncology. As protons or any heavy charged particles traverse matter, their rate of energy loss changes such that the peak energy loss occurs over a very small region near the end of the particle range, producing the Bragg peak. In the Bragg peak, the relative ionization is significantly higher than that during the entrance into the material or tissue (Fig. 1.2). Importantly, on the distal side of the Bragg peak, the dose drops sharply to near zero. The depth of the Bragg peak in matter depends on the energy of the incident particle. In clinical use of proton beams, the narrow Bragg peak is spread to conform to the depth and diameter of the tumor being irradiated, resulting in

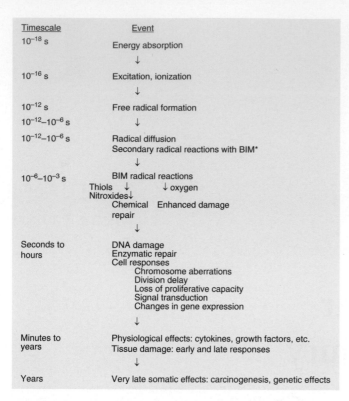

Figure 1.1. Sequence of events from the initial deposition of ionizing radiation energy in cells or tissue through events occurring days to years later. BIM, biologically important molecules (e.g., DNA).

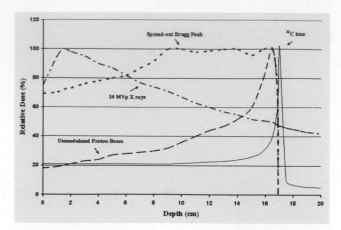

Figure 1.2. Depth-dose curves shown schematically for three types of ionizing radiation: 10-MV x-rays; a 160-MeV proton beam, with curves for both unmodulated and spread-out Bragg peak included; and an unmodulated 300-MeV beam of carbon ions. Note that all curves have been normalized, so the maximal dose for each is given as 100%.

somewhat increased entrance dose to relevant normal tissues, but maintaining the sharp decline in dose distal to the peak (Fig. 1.2).

X-rays, γ-rays, electrons, and high-energy protons (50–250 MeV) as used in radiation oncology are considered sparsely ionizing or low linear energy transfer (LET) radiations, reflecting the fact that the ionizations produced by these radiations are well separated in space, on a nanometer scale. Some particulate radiations are high LET or densely ionizing. Neutrons are produced by accelerating a charged particle such as a deuteron onto an appropriate target material, are emitted during fission of heavy radioactive atoms, or are components of space radiation. Alpha particles (nuclei of helium atoms) and heavy charged particles (nuclei of elements such as carbon, neon, and iron) are positively charged and hence can be accelerated. Carbon ions, in particular, are of interest for use in radiation therapy,[1] because of the dose localization possible with a Bragg peak (Fig. 1.2), as well as their greater biological effectiveness (see below). However, very large and expensive equipment is required to generate and use such ions clinically, so only a few heavy ion clinical facilities exist worldwide. Ionizing particles also are found in space, so further understanding of their biological properties is important to NASA.[2]

INTERACTIONS OF IONIZING RADIATION WITH CELLS

When ionizing radiation traverses biological material, some energy depositions occur directly in biologically important molecules, that is, DNA, causing ionizations. This is referred to as the *direct action of ionizing radiation*. However, much of a cell or tissue is water. Ionizing radiation energy deposited in water produces a positive ion, H_2O^+, and a free electron. These unstable ions undergo a series of reactions that lead to production of free radicals, molecular species with unpaired electrons in the outer shell. The water-derived free radicals include the hydroxyl radical ($\cdot OH$); the hydrogen radical ($\cdot H$); and the hydrated, or aqueous, electron (e^-_{aq}). These primary radicals can undergo recombination to produce the two molecular species, H_2O_2 and H_2. Thus, the radiolysis of water to produce the five primary species is summarized as[3]

$$H_2O \rightarrow \cdot OH, \cdot H, e^-_{aq}, H_2O_2, H_2$$

The water-derived free radicals are highly reactive, and their reactions with biologically important molecules such as DNA result in the indirect action of radiation. Numerous studies, for example, using chemical agents that selectively scavenge particular free radicals, have shown that $\cdot OH$ is the primary species that produces biologically important damage such as DNA strand breaks and cell killing. Consistent with cells and tissue being about 70% water, about 70% of the effect of low LET radiation in cells is due to the indirect action. With increasing ionizing density of radiation, for example, with alpha particles or heavy charged ions, the proportion of direct action increases and the resulting effect is likely to be more damaging on a per unit dose basis.

UNITS OF DOSE

Dose of ionizing radiations can be measured with great accuracy. The unit of exposure, Roentgen (R), characterizes the amount of radiation directed at a material. The more useful unit is that of absorbed dose, defined in SI units as the gray (Gy), which equals 1 J/kg. Some types of radiation, such as neutrons or densely ionizing particles, have greater biological effectiveness, as will be discussed briefly below. In order to take this into account, a unit of dose equivalence, called the sievert (Sv), is used, with an appropriate radiation weighting factor being

TABLE 1.1	International System of Radiation Units			
Quantity	*SI Unit*	*Other SI Units*	*Old Unit*	*Conversion*
Exposure	—	C/kg	roentgen (R)	1 C/kg = 3,876 R
Absorbed dose	Gray (Gy)	J/kg	rad (rad)	1 Gy = 100 rad
Dose equivalent	Sievert (Sv)	J/kg	rem (rem)	1 Sv = 100 rem
Activity	Becquerel (Bq)	s^{-1}	curie (Ci)	1 Bq – 2.7 × 10⁻¹¹ Ci

C, Coulomb

TABLE 1.2	Types of Radiation-Induced DNA Lesions and their Yields
Lesion	*Number per cell per Gy[a]*
DSBs	25–40
SSBs	1,000
Base damages	2,000–3,000
Sugar damages	1,000
DNA-DNA crosslinks	30
DNA-protein crosslinks	150
Abasic sites	200–300
Clustered lesions	~150[b]
Ionizations per cell nucleus	100,000

[a]Approximate number after irradiation with sparsely ionizing radiation such as x- or γ-rays, without enzymatic repair. Modified from Ward JF. DNA damage produced by ionizing radiation in mammalian cells: identities, mechanisms of formation, and reparability. *Prog Nucleic Acid Res Mol Biol.* 1988;35:95–125 and Goodhead DT. Initial events in the cellular effects of ionizing radiations: clustered damage in DNA. *Int J Radiat Biol.* 1994;65:7–17.

[b]Calculated from Sutherland BM, Bennett PV, Sidorkina O, et al. Clustered DNA damages induced in isolated DNA and in human cells by low doses of ionizing radiation. *Proc Natl Sci.* 2000;97: 103–108, where the ratio of clustered lesions to DSBs was about 4:1.

applied. For conventional x-rays, 1 Gy = 1 Sv, but for some radiations, for example, high LET radiations, the sievert dose can be much higher. The units of radiation dose are summarized in Table 1.1

MOLECULAR ASPECTS OF RADIATION EFFECTS ON CELLS

TYPES OF DNA DAMAGES

When the ·OH radical reacts with DNA, it produces radicals on both the sugar and the base components, with these DNA radicals reacting to produce a multitude of DNA products that are converted into the types of DNA lesions typically measured, including single-strand breaks (SSBs), damaged bases, and abasic sites. These lesions and their yields in cells irradiated with sparsely ionizing radiation are given in Table 1.2. Although SSB and base modifications are produced in highest yields, substantial data have indicated that DNA double-strand breaks (DSBs) correlate best with endpoints such as loss of clonogenic survival, chromosome aberrations, and mutagenesis (e.g., Ref. 4). However, more recently, it has come to be appreciated that clustered DNA lesions (also called *multiply damaged sites*) are probably most relevant for leading to those cellular endpoints.[5,6] As ionizing radiation traverses matter, the density of ionizations produced is not homogeneous on a nanometer scale, resulting in

regions of high and low ionization density. If one of the higher density regions occurs near a DNA molecule, the number of lesions caused in a small region of the DNA could be much greater than would occur with random, isolated ionizations (Fig. 1.3). The smallest of these regions of high densities of energy depositions are called *spurs* and may contain up to five ion pairs within about 4 nm (approximately the diameter of a DNA molecule). The resulting multiply damaged sites contain two or more DNA lesions clustered within one turn of the helix, such as two or more oxidized purines or pyrimidines, abasic sites, or strand breaks on opposing strands within a span of up to approximately 20 bp. As will be discussed also below, these clusters of lesions are expected to be more difficult for a cell to repair accurately than an isolated lesion. In fact, the clustering

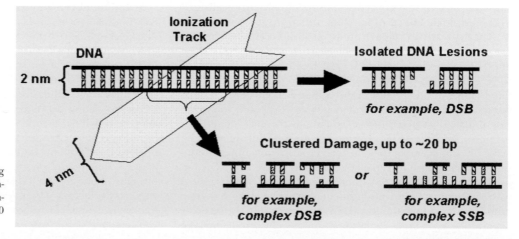

Figure 1.3. Schematic illustrating an isolated DNA lesion, such as a simple DSB, and clustered damages composed of multiple lesions within 2 to 20 bp on the DNA helix.

of lesions, producing damages that are less easily and accurately repaired, is thought to explain why ionizing radiation is much more efficient at killing cells per number of lesions produced than many other toxic agents, such as UV light, hydrogen peroxide, and aflatoxin.[5]

DNA REPAIR

It is widely accepted that DSBs produced by ionizing radiation represent the principal lesion that, if not repaired appropriately, can lead to cell death via the generation of lethal chromosomal aberrations or the induction of apoptosis.[7,8] Alternatively, an inaccurately repaired or unrepaired DSB may result in mutations or genomic rearrangements in a surviving cell, thereby causing genomic instability and contributing to malignant cell transformation. To protect cells from the potentially deleterious effects of DSB, complex damage response and repair pathways have evolved and are evolutionarily conserved.[9,10] These pathways remove endogenous DSB that may arise indirectly from two closely located SSB or during the repair of base damage produced by reactive oxygen species (ROS). Endogenous DSB may also arise at sites of collapse of DNA replication forks or result from topoisomerase II cleavage, thermal fluctuations, or spontaneous hydrolysis. It has been estimated that the spontaneous rate of DSB may be as high as 50 breaks per cell per cell cycle.[11] Two principal DSB repair pathways have been recognized, homologous recombination (HR) and nonhomologous end-joining (NHEJ), which employ largely separate but also overlapping protein complexes.[12–14] Briefly, DSB repair by HR requires an undamaged template molecule that contains a homologous DNA sequence, typically on the sister chromatid in the S and G2 phases of the cell cycle. In contrast, nonhomologous rejoining of two double-stranded DNA ends, which may occur in all cell-cycle phases, does not require an undamaged partner and does not rely on extensive homologies between the recombining ends. DSB repair is closely integrated with cell-cycle checkpoints that function to halt cell-cycle progression to allow repair.[10] How a cell chooses to attempt repair versus initiating apoptosis is the subject of intense research efforts.

There appears to be significant overlap in the pathways that remove endogenous versus ionizing radiation-induced DSB.[15] However, important differences likely exist. For example, while DSB arising during replication are primarily repaired by HR, radiation-induced breaks are mainly rejoined by NHEJ. Accordingly, cells with defective NHEJ, such as caused by loss of Ku80 or XRCC4 function, are hypersensitive to the cytotoxic effects of ionizing radiation. In contrast, loss of XRCC4 leads to a much more pronounced repair defect for endonuclease-induced DSB, which may resemble endogenous breaks, compared to loss of Ku80.[16] Lastly, it remains to be established whether our knowledge of the repair of isolated DSB can be applied to the removal of clustered lesions containing DSB. Clustered damages are expected to constitute poorly reparable lesions, which may produce mutations, induce inaccurate transcription, or persist during the cell cycle.[17,18] It is possible that clustered lesions are subject to the same processing and repair pathways as frank DSB. On the other hand, adjacent SSBs and base damage may interfere with DSB repair, and attempts at repairing clustered base damage can induce de novo DSBs that are difficult to repair accurately.[19,20] Thus, radiation-induced clustered damage may engage combinations of different repair pathway components. While an in-depth review of this topic is beyond the scope of this chapter, it is clear that data for human cells and tissues are limited and that it will be extremely important to gain a more detailed understanding on how clustered DNA damage is processed and repaired.

DNA REPAIR AND NORMAL TISSUE INJURY

A discussion of the potential effects of DNA repair on normal tissue injury requires a brief introduction of the concept of acute and late occurring normal tissue toxicity, which is discussed further below. Acute toxicity typically becomes manifest during a course of fractionated radiation therapy over several weeks and includes transient effects such as erythema, mucositis, or diarrhea. In contrast, late toxicity is expressed after latent periods of months to years following completion of radiation and includes typically irreversible effects such as radiation fibrosis, atrophy, vascular damage, neural damage and a range of endocrine and growth-related effects (reviewed in Ref. 21). Injury to acutely responding normal tissues, such as skin and mucosa, is best understood as the effect of radiation on the proliferative capacity of epithelial target cells. Thus, variations in the intrinsic radiation sensitivity of these cells are expected to affect the degree of acute tissue toxicity. For example, individuals suffering from rare autosomal recessive syndromes, such as ataxia telangiectasia, Nijmegen breakage syndrome, or Fanconi anemia, typically are hypersensitive to the cytotoxic effects of ionizing radiation, and cells derived from these individuals exhibit defects in the response to and repair of radiation-induced DNA damage.[22,23] Therefore, there likely exist a significant number of individuals in the general population with heterozygous mutations or single nucleotide polymorphisms (SNPs) that are associated with increased acute normal tissue toxicity. However, the evidence in support of such a relationship is not consistent to date and the subject of active investigation (reviewed in Refs. 21, 24–26). The impact of a given mutation or SNP on DNA repair capacity and cellular radiation sensitivity is often unknown, complicating the interpretation of correlative clinical studies. Testing the radiation sensitivity of cells from patients with specific SNPs or mutations is also not straightforward as the cell type under investigation (such as fibroblasts versus lymphocytes) and assay type (such as chromosomal versus DNA repair versus cell survival assay) affect study outcome. It has been proposed that a correlation between cellular and clinical radiation sensitivity (i.e., commonly encountered grade 2/3 toxicity by EORTC/RTOG scoring criteria) is most likely to be revealed by scoring radiation-induced chromosomal aberrations in lymphocytes,[27] which requires validation in future studies. It is also important to appreciate that even small variations in the cellular DNA repair capacity that could be difficult to detect with a given assay may affect cellular sensitivity to radiation.[28]

An association between cellular DNA repair capacity or radiation sensitivity and injury to late responding normal tissues is even less clear than for acute toxicity, as elegantly discussed by Bentzen.[21] Rather, the expression of late radiation damage appears dependent on an orchestrated biological response brought about by the release of proinflammatory cytokines and growth factors. The pathological progression of radiation toxicity in many late responding normal tissues seems to be a consequence of an early inflammatory phase followed by late stromal alterations. In the lung, for example, radiation-induced pneumonitis is followed by fibrosis (reviewed in Refs. 21, 29, and 30).

CHROMOSOME ABERRATIONS

Chromosome abberations represent a readily visible type of DNA damage caused by ionizing radiation that is readily observable microscopically during mitosis after cell irradiation. Types of aberrations commonly induced by radiation include dicentrics, rings, acentric fragments, deletions, translocations, and anaphase bridges. It is generally assumed that chromosome aberrations arise from unrepaired (or inaccurately repaired) DSB, and increases in aberrations generally correlate well with decreases in cell survival.[31] The frequency of aberrations is radiation dose dependent and in normal tissues with significant proportions of mitotically active cells (e.g., bone marrow, intestinal crypts) can be used as an indication of dose received under some conditions. In recent years, there has been considerable interest in using chromosome aberrations in lymphocytes, isolated from an irradiated individual and stimulated to divide in culture, as a biodosimeter, for example, in astronauts[32] or potentially in individuals exposed to radiation in an accident or terrorist event.[33] It is important to keep in mind that the aberrations reflect the induction of the underlying DNA damage, the repair (or attempts to repair) of the damage, and the removal/death of cells in which the damage is not compatible with cell survival (i.e., loss of critical genetic material); hence, the yield and complexity of the aberrations can change with time after the radiation exposure.[34]

The potential importance of chromosomal aberrations for acute normal tissue toxicity derives from its relation to cellular DSB repair mechanisms, as discussed above. In addition, lymphocyte radiation sensitivity has been correlated with late toxicity in some studies,[35] perhaps representing "consequential" late effects, that is, resulting from preceding severe acute injury. However, other studies have not detected a correlation between lymphocyte radiation sensitivity and late effects, which likely reflects the fact that DNA repair mechanisms have little obvious relevance for the expression of late normal tissue injury and furthermore is consistent with the notion that chromosomal aberrations are less relevant in tissues that consist of mostly noncycling cells. It is therefore questionable whether the sensitivity of late responding normal tissues to fractionated radiation can be explained by the occurrence of interacting DSB leading to chromosomal aberrations.[36]

BASIC CELLULAR RADIATION BIOLOGY

LOSS OF REPRODUCTIVE CAPACITY

The most extensively used approach to study radiation effects on cells in culture has been the clonogenic assay, that is, measurement of the ability of a single cell to proliferate indefinitely, thereby forming a clone or colony. It should be kept in mind that following radiation exposure, the loss of the ability to form a colony can result from any of a number of different processes that either decrease cell proliferative ability or cause cell death. Decreased proliferative ability can result from induction of cell-cycle arrest, quiescence, senescence, or terminal differentiation. Radiation-induced cell-cycle arrest has

been studied extensively and shown to be a radiation dose-dependent phenomenon in which cells transiting the mitotic cycle can be temporarily arrested in the G1, G2, or S phases of the cell cycle (reviewed, e.g., in Refs. 37 and 38). In some cell types, depending on the dose, the temporary arrest may become permanent. The cell-cycle arrest is controlled by checkpoint genes such as ATM, p53, and RB (e.g., Ref. 38). Arrest in G2 is the most commonly observed, and in most cases appears to be p53-independent, although this is controversial. G1 arrest requires a wild-type p53 pathway, although most normal cells/tissues (excluding those from individuals with Li Fraumeni syndrome) will have wild-type p53 function. Quiescence is generally thought to be a reversible, physiological process whereby cells are arrested in a G0-like state, before the restriction point, so the molecular characteristics of the cells may differ from those in "G1 arrest," although much less is known about the molecular biology of quiescent cells. Senescence, on the other hand, is considered to be an irreversible process, a permanent arrest in G1, involving genes such as p16INK4a and pRB, and characterized by expression of the marker SA-β-gal (senescence-activated β-galactosidase).[39] Terminal differentiation is an irreversible, physiological process. Because it appears to be highly relevant in cancer cells, radiation-induced cell-cycle arrest has received the most attention, but radiation-induced quiescence, senescence, and differentiation may all be relevant in cellular responses of some normal tissues.

Radiation-induced cell death can take multiple forms. The predominant form of cell death is mitotic death/catastrophe in which cells die when they are unable to go through mitosis, generally as a result of chromosome loss or damage or problems with spindle formation.[40] Mitotic catastrophe is often delayed (hours to days) after irradiation because cells have to progress through the cell cycle to mitosis. Not infrequently, cells divide one or more times after irradiation prior to the progeny undergoing death.[41,42] The actual manifestation of cell death can occur as necrosis, apoptosis, or autophagy, depending on type of cells/tissue and, in some cases, radiation dose. Necrosis is considered a nonphysiological cell death in which cells lose plasma membrane integrity and ion homeostasis, swell and burst. The cellular DNA is randomly fragmented, and the release of cell contents can evoke inflammation and immune reactions in the tissue. In contrast, apoptosis, or programmed cell death, is an active, gene-directed process of cellular self-destruction with characteristic changes in cell morphology and a distinctive pattern of DNA fragmentation.[43,44] Although apoptosis has been much more extensively studied in tumors than in normal tissues following ionizing radiation, apoptosis is prominent in hematopoietic cells such as lymphocytes and thymocytes and has been observed in normal cells such as keratinocytes and endothelial cells as well as in normal tissues including gastrointestinal tract, hippocampus (in both oligodendrocytes and neural precursors), thyroid, and salivary gland. The pathways involved in radiation-induced apoptosis are numerous, complex and involve a great deal of crosstalk; discussion of the molecular mechanisms is beyond the scope of this chapter, and the reader is referred to several reviews (e.g., Refs. 45–47). Autophagy, or type II programmed cell death, is a regulated process whereby cellular organelles and other components are sequestered in autophagosomes that then fuse with lysosomes leading to self-destruction.[44] To date, there has been limited study of radiation-induced autophagy, so its relevance in normal tissues is not clear.[48]

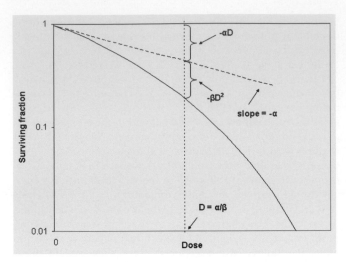

Figure 1.4. Schematic of the LQ model for radiation cell survival curves. The continuously bending curve is fitted by the expression $SF = e^{-(\alpha D + \beta D^2)}$, where SF is the surviving fraction, D is the dose, and α and β are the coefficients for the linear and the quadratic components, respectively.

CELL SURVIVAL CURVES

Cell survival curves have typically been used to express the relationship between the radiation dose and the proportion of cells that survive (form a colony) any given dose. Survival after a single dose of radiation is a probability function, with survival curves typically having a region at low doses where cell killing is less efficient per unit dose than at higher doses where the curves become steeper or continuously bending, as illustrated in Figure 1.4. The curvature of the curve is ascribed to the ability of irradiated cells to accumulate and repair sublethal damage, with lethality resulting from the interaction of two or more sublethal events (reviewed in Ref. 49). Several mathematical models have been developed to describe the shapes of cell survival curves, but the most commonly used model currently is the linear-quadratic (LQ) formula

$$SF = e^{-(\alpha D + \beta D^2)}$$

where SF is the surviving fraction, D is dose, and α and β are coefficients. The α term is related to the initial low dose component that is linear with dose and β is related to the higher dose component that has a quadratic dependence on dose. The α/β ratio is the dose at which overall killing by the two components is equal and thus is a useful descriptor of the relative contributions of the two components to cell killing and the effect of dose fractionation on them, as will be discussed below. It is relatively easy to obtain survival curves with cells that can readily be cultured in vitro, for example, many tumor cells, but only a limited number of cell types derived from normal tissues can be cultured. In a few instances, survival curves have been determined for cells from selected normal tissues in which cells can be removed from irradiated tissues and cultured back in vivo, for example, hematopoietic cells growing in spleen or mammary cells injected into a fat pad. The range of radiation sensitivities that have been seen in survival curves with normal tissues is about two- to threefold, although there can be quite significant differences in the size of the initial low dose shoulders on the curves.[36] The shape of cell survival curves, and in

particular the width of the shoulder, is useful for understanding differences between responses of early and late responding normal tissues and the impact of fractionation, as will be discussed shortly.

MODIFICATION OF RADIATION RESPONSE BY BIOLOGICAL FACTORS

Responses of cells and normal tissues to radiation can be modified by biological, chemical, and physical factors. One of the most important biological factors is cellular repair. Two types of repair expressed at the cellular level have been recognized, based on the operational way in which the processes are studied. Potentially lethal damage repair (PLDR) is the repair that occurs after irradiation, depending on the post–irradiation conditions of the cells.[50] If cells are held in conditions that are unfavorable to cell growth, such as in confluent culture (density inhibition), or without nutrients, they can repair damage and clonogenic survival increases. However, for cells stimulated to progress through the cell cycle after irradiation, PLDR does not occur or is reduced and clonogenic survival is decreased. PLDR has been demonstrated in experimental tumors by showing increased cell survival when cells are allowed to remain in a tumor for several hours after irradiation prior to undergoing explant and culture in vitro compared to cells explanted and cultured immediately after irradiation.[50] PLDR has also been shown to occur in a few normal tissues where such assays can be conducted. However, the relevance of PLDR in most normal tissues is unclear, although one assumes it occurs to some degree since most cells in normal tissues are in a quiescent state.

The second type of cellular repair is sublethal damage repair (SLDR), which is thought to be a critical repair process in tissues because it is responsible for the "sparing" of radiation response with dose fractionation or low dose rate exposures. SLDR is defined as the repair that occurs between fractions when a radiation exposure is divided into two or more fractions.[36] The cellular repair is seen as an increase in clonogenic survival when any given dose is split into two or more exposures, with repair being maximal within 2 to 6 hours, depending on cells or tissue.[51] If one looks at survival curves, the repair of SLD is seen as the reappearance of the low dose shoulder region of the survival curve, and this can occur repeatedly with each dose fraction, if sufficient time is allowed between fractions for full repair. When radiation exposure occurs at low dose rate (e.g., <10 cGy/min), SLDR occurs during the irradiation, and the subsequent dose response curve can be thought of as a reflection of the continuous reiteration of the low dose shoulder, yielding the so-called effective dose curve. When all repair occurs during the exposure at low dose rate, the survival curve will become purely linear (on the semi–log scale) with the slope equivalent to the α component of the single-dose curve, assuming no cell division has occurred to increase the apparent cell survival even more.

Unfortunately, at this time, it is not clear whether mechanistically or molecularly, SLDR and PLDR are actually separate processes, nor is it possible to relate the cellular-level PLDR and SLDR to specific DNA damage repair processes.

A second biologically based factor that can affect cellular response to radiation is the cell-cycle phase in which cells are located at the time of irradiation. Cells are most sensitive to loss of clonogenicity from radiation exposure when they are in the G2/M phase of the cell cycle at the time of irradiation, and most resistant when irradiated in the late S phase.[52] If cells have a sufficiently long G1 phase, a period of increased resistance can also be demonstrated in early G1. From looking at clonogenic survival curves generated from cells irradiated in various cell-cycle phases, it is clear that the primary differences are in the shoulder regions of the curves: the survival curves for radiation sensitive G2/M phase cells have nearly exponential shape with little shoulder, that is, little ability to repair damage between fractions, while the survival curves for resistant late S phase cells show greater shoulders, or greater repair capacity (summarized in Ref. 36).

An additional complexity to the cell-cycle phase sensitivity differences is the ability of radiation to induce cell-cycle arrest. In theory, at least, an initial dose of radiation in a fractionated exposure, or dose given at a low dose rate, could alter the cell-cycle progression by inducing a G2, G1, or S phase arrest and, thus, resynchronizing the cells, potentially in a different phase of the cell cycle. However, in vivo, such effects cannot currently be demonstrated.

One could debate the relevance of these cell-cycle sensitivity differences to many normal tissues where the bulk of the cells are well differentiated or quiescent. However, there may be some relevance in early responding tissues, such as bone marrow and gastrointestinal tract, where the stem cell and/or early progenitor components may be in active cell cycle.

MODIFICATION OF RADIATION RESPONSE BY CHEMICAL OR PHARMACOLOGIC FACTORS

Numerous chemical and pharmacological factors can alter the response of cells and tissues to radiation. The best known, most general, and most effective of these factors is oxygen. Cells that are radiobiologically hypoxic (usually taken to be cells at 100 ppm oxygen or less) are typically about three times more resistant to damage by sparsely ionizing radiation than are well-aerated cells (summarized in Ref. 36). In other words, oxygen is a very effective radiation sensitizer, or, conversely, hypoxia is a potent radiation protector. The presence of hypoxic cells in some types of human tumors and their role in limiting curability of some tumors is well established.[53] Since most normal tissues are well oxygenated, one assumes there is limited relevance of the oxygen effect there. However, since it has been shown recently that bone marrow stem cells may reside in a hypoxic niche,[54] one could speculate that hypoxia may play a role in radioresistance of that particular stem cell type in vivo.

There are chemical and pharmacologic agents that are radiation sensitizers. In radiation oncology, the primary interest has been in attempting to exploit such agents to achieve a therapeutic gain through causing greater tumor cell killing than normal tissue damage. However, one should be aware that these agents may also increase radiosensitivity of normal tissues via any of a number of different mechanisms. For example, hydroxyurea can increase radiation damage by preferentially killing cells in S phase and blocking surviving cells in the relatively radiosensitive late G1 phase. The synergistic effects of adriamycin, an antibiotic that can act by inhibiting topoisomerase II and/or via free radical mechanisms, with radiation are well known, particularly with regard to induction of heart damage. Other chemotherapy agents that can interact with radiation to increase normal tissue damage include cis-platin, 5-fluorouracil, and taxanes.

Interest in agents that decrease damage from radiation in normal tissues has increased substantially in recent years due to concerns about radiological or nuclear terrorism or accidents. In this context, it is important to distinguish radiation protectors, mitigators, and treatment: radioprotectors are generally taken to be agents that alter the initial radiation chemical events, and, hence, must be present at the time of irradiation to alter the effects of the exposure; mitigators are agents given after the radiation exposure but before symptoms appear in order to prevent or reduce progression of normal tissue damage; and treatments are applied when symptoms appear in order to facilitate recovery.[55,56] The most extensively studied and, to date, the most effective radiation protectors are thiols, or sulfhydryl-containing compounds. In clonogenic assays, under appropriate conditions, thiols can protect cells by factors of 2–3, although in vivo the protection factors are generally much less.[36] Simplistically, thiols are thought to act via a "chemical repair" process, whereby they donate a hydrogen atom to a free radical in DNA to restitute the original DNA molecule. Amifostine (ethyol, WR2721), a phosphorothiate prodrug that is converted into a free thiol in the body, has been shown in animal studies to give substantial protection to bone marrow and lesser protection to selected other tissues. It is the only thiol in clinical use and is FDA approved for use against xerostomia in patients undergoing radiation therapy for head and neck cancer. Other small molecule antioxidants such as the nitroxide Tempol are effective radioprotectors in cells and animals and are being studied for use in humans.[57] Also, it has been shown that some thiol-containing compounds upregulate the antioxidant enzyme manganese superoxide dismutase (SOD2; MnSOD), via an NF-κB-mediated pathway, that leads to a delayed radioprotective effect.[58]

In recent years, development of radiation protectors and mitigators has centered largely on two classes of agents: cytokines/growth factors or antioxidants/anti-inflammatory drugs. As discussed below, irradiated cells or tissues produce a number of different cytokines and growth factors.[29,59] These endogenously produced agents, as well as exogenously applied ones, can be radiation protectors/mitigators or sensitizers, depending on the specific agent, its concentration, cell or tissue type, and timing. Growth factors such as granulocyte colony–stimulating factor or keratinocyte growth factor (palifermin) act when given after irradiation by stimulating proliferation of their target stem or early progenitor cells so that tissue regeneration is enhanced.

It has become clear that the responses of many tissues to radiation involve oxidative stress and/or inflammatory processes that can occur acutely and also persist for many months after the radiation exposure.[56,60] Hence, approaches using antioxidants and anti-inflammatory agents are under development. Increasing superoxide dismutase (SOD) activity in cells or tissues by overexpressing SOD, using an MnSOD transgene/liposome delivery vehicle or using an SOD-catalase mimetic, Eukarion-189, has been shown in animal studies to radioprotect various tissues.[61–64] In most cases, the treatments were started prior to radiation, so the modulations may have been radioprotective in the classic sense, as well as mitigative. However, it has been reported in both pigs and humans that treatment of radiation-induced fibrosis with liposomal SOD is effective.[65,66] Recent studies have also suggested that pentoxifylline plus α-tocopherol (vitamin E) is effective at attenuating radiation-induced fibrosis.[65,67]

IMPORTANCE OF RADIATION QUALITY FOR BIOLOGIC RESPONSE

Radiation quality is an important determinant of the impact of radiation on cells and tissues. When cells are exposed to radiations that are more densely ionizing, that is, of higher LET, the shouldered, or continuously bending, survival curves generally seen with cells irradiated with x- or γ-rays give way to survival curves that become steeper and more purely exponential, that is, the shoulder decreases. Typically, increasing biological effect of densely ionizing radiations is expressed in terms of relative biological effect (RBE), the ratio of dose of the reference low LET radiation to the dose of high LET radiation for any given biological effect. The reference radiation historically has been 250 kVp x-rays but is now frequently ^{60}Co γ-rays. In general, the relative effectiveness of radiation increases with increasing LET to a maximum, which, for example occurs at about 100 keV/μm when the endpoint is clonogenic survival, then decreases at very high LET values. The absolute values of RBE at any given LET, however, depend greatly on type of cells or tissue, endpoint, radiation dose, and dose rate or fractionation.[68] It was recognized in the 1940s that use of high LET radiations (initially neutrons) might yield therapeutic advantages for cancer treatment because the densely ionizing radiations should result in reduced cellular repair, reduced cell-cycle differential, and lower oxygen effect in tumors. However, what was not appreciated at the time was the differential dependence on fractionation for late responding tissues compared to tumors or early responding tissues treated with low LET radiation (see below). Hence, disastrous late normal tissue complications ensued. In recent years, interest in radiation oncology use of high LET radiations has been revived, principally in the form of carbon ions. In addition to the biological advantages of increased effectiveness and reduced oxygen effect in tumors, heavy charged ions have the physical advantages of dose localization with increased relative dose at the Bragg peak and a sharp dose drop-off on the distal side of the peak (Fig. 1.2). Clinical studies with 290 MeV carbon ions (LET approximately 13 keV/μm) have been conducted in Japan and Germany and have indicated good efficacy in several tumor types, with minimal normal tissue toxicity.[1] It is important to remember that energetic protons, as used in radiation oncology (i.e., 65–250 MeV), have the important physical advantage of the increased relative dose in the Bragg peak, but are sparsely ionizing radiation with biological properties similar to those of x- and γ-rays.

Galactic cosmic rays (GCRs) and, to a much lesser extent, solar particle events contain heavy ions. Since astronauts outside the earth's protective magnetic fields, that is, on the moon or in transit to Mars, will be exposed to the heavy ions in GCRs, NASA also has considerable interest in the biological effects of these ionizing species on normal tissues.[2]

INTRACELLULAR AND INTERCELLULAR SIGNALING

The classic descriptions of radiation-induced damage in cells, as just discussed, are based on responses triggered by DNA damage in the cells exposed to radiation. In the past 15 years, there has been increasing acceptance that so-called nontargeted effects can also occur in which biological responses are not directly related to the amount of energy deposited in the DNA of the cells traversed by the radiation, but can result from non–DNA-damage-initiated events and can be seen in nonirradiated cells. The effects include induction of signaling pathways that are independent of DNA damage, bystander effects, adaptive responses, and genomic instability.

RADIATION-INDUCED INTRACELLULAR SIGNAL TRANSDUCTION PATHWAYS

Substantial advances have been made in understanding how radiation triggers signal transduction pathways within individual cells and between cells, thus causing or altering cellular responses. Some of these signaling pathways may be initiated by events at the plasma membrane or in mitochondria.[69,70] Although different intracellular signaling pathways may be activated to varying degrees in different cell types or contexts, ionizing radiation can regulate expression of early response genes such as c-fos, c-jun, and early growth response-1, and a number of intracellular signaling pathways have been shown to be activated by radiation, including RAS-ERK1/2 or PI3K-AKT-mTOR prosurvival pathways and Rho-JNK or p38 MAPK prodeath pathways. It is beyond the scope of this chapter to discuss these radiation-induced signaling processes in detail; the reader is referred to several reviews.[69,70]

In addition to the free radicals and ROS produced by ionizing radiation on submillisecond time scales after the deposition of energy, it has become clear that irradiated cells, and even their unirradiated neighbors and progeny (more on that below), can exhibit persistent and prolonged increases in ROS and reactive nitrogen species for minutes or days after irradiation (e.g., Refs. 71 and 72). A primary site of generation of some of these reactive species appears to be mitochondria, and the ROS appear to be involved in intracellular signaling processes. Importantly, these cell-based findings may be paralleled in vivo, where increased oxidative stress after radiation exposure has also been documented and may play a role in radiation-induced late effects (reviewed in Refs. 56 and 60), particularly in concert with activation of cytokines.[66]

"NONTARGETED" EFFECTS OF RADIATION— INTERCELLULAR COMMUNICATION

Bystander effects, genomic instability, and adaptive responses are considered to be "nontargeted" effects of radiation and involve intracellular and, particularly, intercellular signaling. These three effects and their potential relevance to normal tissue radiation biology will be described briefly here.

Radiation-induced bystander effects are cellular responses occurring in unirradiated cells that are near to or sharing medium with irradiated cells (reviewed in Refs. 73–75). The responses seen in bystander cells include decreased clonogenic survival, mutagenesis, changes in gene expression, DNA damage, and increased ROS. A number of studies have shown that bystander responses occur after low radiation doses, then saturate as dose increases, often in the 10 to 30 cGy dose range.[76,77] Furthermore, microbeam studies have indicated that bystander responses can be seen after irradiation of a single cell in a population of hundreds of cells[78,79] even if the cell is irradiated with particles that do not traverse the nucleus.[79,80] This has led to suggestions that at low doses, cellular responses might be dominated by bystander effects[75,81,82] and concerns that in some clinical situations where larger volumes of normal tissue could be exposed to smaller doses (e.g., intensity-modulated radiation therapy [IMRT]), there could be increased incidences of treatment-induced cancer.[83] Although the molecular mechanisms underlying the bystander effect are not yet clear, it is evident that signaling, or intercellular communication, from the irradiated cells to the unirradiated cells is involved. The signal may be diffusible through medium[77,84] or transmitted via gap junctions.[85,86] At this time, the molecular nature of the signal is not clear, although there is evidence for roles of ROS,[77,87] nitric oxide,[88] or calcium,[89,90] as well as cytokines such as interleukin-8 (IL-8)[91] and transforming growth factor β (TGFβ; TGFB).[92,93] Other studies have suggested involvement of oxidative enzymes such as Cox-2 or NADPH oxidase,[94,95] the transcription factor NF-κB,[96] and mitochondria.[79,96] A model unifying many of these potential mechanisms has been proposed.[82] Several studies with 3D tissue models have also demonstrated bystander responses,[97] and these responses can occur over significant distances (e.g., up to 1 mm)[98] and for times up to 48 hours.[99]

It has long been recognized that radiation can produce clastogenic factors in plasma of irradiated individuals.[100–102] Abscopal effects, defined as effects at sites distant from the locally irradiated site,[103] have also been described in the clinical literature for years. Although originally, the abscopal effect was described as regression of an unirradiated tumor when a tumor in a different anatomic location was irradiated, the term now is often used more broadly to describe biological responses in tumors or normal tissues that are distant from the site of irradiation of a tumor or normal tissue.[104] Some work suggests that abscopal effects are an immune system response[105] and that they are triggered by death or stress in tumor cells.[104] Although it is not clear whether the same molecular mechanism(s) apply to both the bystander effects described for cells in culture and to the in vivo "out of field" effects, suggestions that oxidative stress and cytokines/growth factors are involved in both the in vitro and the in vivo responses suggest there may be some commonalities.

Genomic instability is the increase in chromosomal instability, mutations, apoptosis, or other deleterious effects in the progeny of irradiated cells, often many generations after the radiation exposure.[73,106,107] The high frequency of genomic instability in progeny of irradiated cells of normal tissue origin is not consistent with a mutational mechanism, although the underlying mechanisms are poorly understood. Genomic instability has also been demonstrated in progeny of unirradiated bystander cells. Observations of roles for ROS and/or various cytokines in both genomic instability and bystander responses have led to suggestions that the two responses may be interrelated.[73] However, it is clear that the interactions and radiation-induced signaling are quite complex, since, for example, radiation can activate cell-mediated inflammatory processes that cause DNA damage in stem cells[108,109] or radiation-induced signals from fibroblasts can induce apoptosis in transformed epithelial cells.[110]

The radiation-induced adaptive response was originally described as the decrease in frequency of chromosome aberrations in irradiated human lymphocytes when the cells were treated with a low "priming" dose prior to a larger "challenge" dose.[111] Since then, the observations have been reported in numerous labs with a variety of test systems (e.g., Refs. 11 and 113). Typically, adaptation is most effectively induced by doses around 10 cGy, and about 4 hours is needed after the priming dose for maximal induction of adaptation. The mechanism(s) underlying adaptation is/are unclear, although it is often

thought that important mediators are DNA repair and cell-cycle regulatory systems (reviewed in Ref. 114). There is, however, increasing evidence that adaptation and bystander effects may be interrelated, and that reactive oxygen and nitrogen species may play roles.[114–116]

In summary, the "nontargeted" cellular responses (bystander effects, genomic instability, and adaptive effects) may all have in common involvement of oxidative stress, inflammatory-like response pathways, and induction of cytokines/growth factors. Although these effects have generally been considered in terms of relevance to carcinogenesis, late-appearing adverse chronic side effects in irradiated normal tissues may be associated with similar oxidative and inflammatory effects,[109,117] suggesting these phenomena could, in some cases, play roles in the mechanisms of normal tissue damage.

CYTOKINES AND CYTOKINE CASCADES IN NORMAL TISSUES

Cytokines are soluble proteins that regulate various cell and tissue interactions and processes including cell death, senescence, proliferation, angiogenesis, inflammation and genomic instability, fibrosis, and immune reactions. They are very potent and generally are produced only transiently in response to stimuli, initiating cascades that may involve multiple cytokines and cytokine receptors. Radiation activates "danger" signals that induce expression of numerous cytokines and cytokine receptors in cells and animals (reviewed in Ref. 117). Cytokines may cause either radiation protection or sensitization, depending on the particular cytokine and the target cell or tissue. Classic examples are the radiation protection afforded to bone marrow by tumor necrosis factor, TNF α (TNFA) or IL-1[118] or of endothelial cells and lung tissue in some mouse strains by bFGF.[119,120] In contrast, TGFβ can radiosensitize bone marrow[118] while IL-12 radiosensitizes gut, but radioprotects bone marrow.[121]

Cytokines also clearly play roles in pathogenesis of radiation-induced normal tissue damage, with a good example being TNF-α; in the brain TNF-α is thought to mediate vascular and immune responses that lead to edema and breakdown of the blood-brain barrier, as well as gliosis and oligodendrocyte cell death.[122] In some tissues, the cytokine signals may come in "waves," with early inflammatory responses resolving rapidly, but later signals being reactivated days, weeks, or months later as a result of dysregulated processes and leading to a perpetual cytokine cascade (reviewed in Ref. 117 and 123).

One of the most widely studied radiation-induced cytokines is TGFβ. This profibrotic cytokine is activated by radiation-induced proteolytic cleavage extracellularly and causes fibroblast differentiation and senescence as well as stimulating collagen formation,[124] which contribute to the fibrosis. Levels of this cytokine in patients' serum before irradiation have been associated with higher risk of developing pneumonitis, and increased levels after radiotherapy predict for lung injury (reviewed in Refs. 123 and 125). Interestingly, in cell studies, radiation activation of TGFβ has been shown to selectively induce cell death in transformed or genetically unstable cells,[110,126] suggesting that in some situations it may act in an anticarcinogenesis fashion.

In summary, although cytokines and cytokine receptors are involved in cell and tissue responses to radiation, the effects of any given cytokine can depend on the cell type, level of cytokine, radiation dose, and tissue context. In some scenarios, the induction of certain cytokines can be protective (e.g., radioprotective or anticarcinogenic), but in many cases, the induction is detrimental, leading to inflammation and fibrosis. Interactions between cytokines and intracellular signaling pathways, for example, involving NFκB, are areas of intense research interest, as are possible roles of cytokines in bystander signaling.

GENERAL CONCEPTS OF NORMAL TISSUE DAMAGE FROM RADIATION

In 1906, Bergonie and Tribondeau proposed that tissues are more radiation sensitive if they contain cells that are mitotically active, normally undergo many divisions, and are undifferentiated.[127] However, it is now recognized that this relationship is a vast oversimplification,[49] as for example nonproliferating or slowly proliferating tissues such as the kidneys are highly radiosensitive. In fact, responses of normal tissues to radiation depend on a complex interplay between (a) the inherent radiation sensitivity of cells in the tissue (especially stem cells, but also vascular and maybe other stromal cells), (b) kinetics of the cell populations in the tissue, and (c) the organization of the tissue. Some of these concepts are reviewed below.

PROBABILITY OF NORMAL TISSUE COMPLICATIONS

The Normal Tissue Complication Probability (NTCP) after radiation exposure is a function of radiation dose and generally exhibits a sigmoid shape. If one compares data from studies that have determined dose response curves for various normal tissues based on lethality in animals after single-dose, localized irradiation to the tissue of interest, it is clear that bone marrow is the most radiation sensitive tissue, consistent with clonogenic cell survival curves where bone marrow stem cells are the most radiosensitive normal tissue cells. Such normal tissue complication curves also show that lung, a late responding tissue, is relatively sensitive, particularly in the situation where the whole thorax is irradiated. Although comparison of NTCP curves highlights the quite different radiation sensitivities of various tissues, it should be realized that NTCP depends not only on the dose and tissue, but also on dose fractionation schedule, tissue volume irradiated, toxicity endpoint, time of assessment of complications, and acceptable risk or tolerance.

LATENCY AND TOLERANCE

In clinical radiation oncology, tissue tolerance doses (TDs) in humans are often expressed as TD5/5, that is, the dose likely to produce normal tissue complications in 5% of patients within 5 years of radiation exposure. Although a 5-year time frame is used for expression of TDs, it should be appreciated that different normal tissues show very different latent times between radiation exposure and occurrence of tissue damage, depending on the kinetics of the cell populations in the tissue, and latency is not necessarily an indicator of radiation sensitivity. Early, or acutely, responding normal tissues such as hematopoietic system, gastrointestinal tract, and skin contain functional mature epithelial cells of limited, short, life spans. When these mature cells are lost by normal cell turnover, stem cells are required to replace them; however, since the stem cells in these tissues are sensitive to killing by radiation, the tissue damage is

expressed when the mature cells are lost, for example, within 30 to 60 days for circulating blood cells such as white blood cells and platelets or within 7 to 10 days for mature intestinal epithelial cells on the villi. In contrast, late damage occurs in tissues that show only slow or little cell turnover, such as lung, kidney, CNS, although some late responding tissues are moderately radiation sensitive.

NORMAL TISSUE ORGANIZATION

Radiation sensitivity of normal tissues depends not only on intrinsic cellular sensitivity and population kinetics, but also on the tissue organization. Functional subunits (FSUs) reflect the structural organization of tissues.[36,128] FSUs can be discrete anatomic units, such as the kidney nephron, or volumes of tissue, as in skin, and are thought to contain a limited number of clonogenic cells, such that survival of at least one clonogen is required for the FSU to survive and regenerate the tissue. FSUs can be arranged in either series or parallel, and the arrangement can explain some of the importance of radiation volume for tissue responses.[128] For tissues where FSUs are arranged in series, for example, spinal cord, the complication dose response curve is relatively shallow and shifted to higher doses when only a small volume is irradiated, but steepens and shifts to lower doses as volume increases. In other words, a low dose to a large volume may cause little damage, but a high dose to a small volume may be highly deleterious because loss of a single FSU can result in overt damage. In tissues where FSUs are arranged in parallel, such as lung or kidney, a low dose to a large volume can be hazardous, although a high dose to a small volume can be well tolerated because maintenance of function depends on the amount of tissue that is not damaged.

ACUTE VERSUS LATE RESPONDING TISSUES; FRACTIONATION

Fractionation means that the total dose of radiation given to a patient is divided into a number of daily treatments of a specific size. Over the past 100 years, fractionation with five daily treatments per week, employing 1.8 to 2 Gy per fraction, has evolved empirically.[129,130] Compared to delivering the entire radiation treatment in a single setting, fractionation was discovered to spare late responding normal tissues relative to tumors, thereby allowing the delivery of tumoricidal doses of radiation. Radiobiologically, the sparing of normal tissues by fractionation can be described by the recovery of cells from damage between fractions, as described above.

Importantly, there is a consistent difference between early and late responding normal tissues in their sensitivity to changes in fractionation. Late responding tissues exhibit a greater ability to recover during fractionated exposure than do early responding tissues, which is illustrated in Figure 1.5. The response of early responding tissues to single-dose irradiation versus fractionation using examples of 2 or 4 Gy per fraction is shown in the upper panel. Dividing the total dose of 12 Gy into six 2-Gy fractions yields a higher relative survival rate than dividing it into three 4-Gy fractions. The difference between these fractionation schemes is more pronounced for late responding tissues, shown in the lower panel, because the β component of the survival curve is larger than for early responding tissues. Of note, for this display, it is assumed that the fractionation sensitivity of late responding normal tissues is related to the survival of

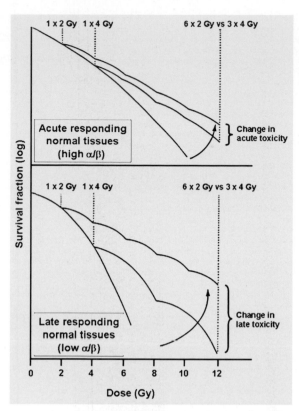

Figure 1.5. Illustration of fractionation effects due to split dose recovery emphasizing the importance of dose per fraction in early- versus late-responding normal tissues.

a putative target cell population (on the *y*-axis), which is likely an oversimplification, but useful for illustration purposes.

The different fractionation effect on acute and late responding tissues can be described using the ratio of the linear to quadratic components of the survival curves, that is, the α/β ratio. α/β ratios for normal tissues have been compiled by Thames et al.[129,131] Generally, for acute responding tissues the α/β is high, about 8 to 20 Gy, with 10 Gy commonly used as a typical value. In contrast, late responding tissues have α/β values of approximately 1 to 5 Gy, reflecting a greater contribution of the β component. Thus, α/β ratios can be used to quantify and compare the effects of fractionation.

Clinical applicability may be illustrated with a sample calculation. A radiation treatment that delivers 45 Gy at 1.8 Gy per fraction to the spinal cord is not expected to cause transverse myelitis.[132,133] If the fractionation is changed to 2.5 Gy per fraction, the total dose must be reduced by how much to maintain the same spinal cord tolerance (assuming an α/β of 1.5 Gy for the spinal cord)? We use the following formula:

$$D_{\text{new}} = D_{\text{old}} \times \frac{(\alpha/\beta) + d_{\text{old}}}{(\alpha/\beta) + d_{\text{new}}},$$

where D = total dose and d = dose per fraction.

Thus, $D_{\text{new}} = 45\,\text{Gy} \times (1.5 + 1.8)/(1.5 + 2.5) = 37\,\text{Gy}$. Therefore, the new fractionation scheme may only deliver 14 to 15 fractions of 2.5 Gy for a total dose of 35 to 37.5 Gy for the same low probability of late cord injury as seen with 45 Gy at 1.8 Gy per fraction. By contrast, for acute responding tissues with an α/β of 10 Gy, the difference would be much smaller:

$D_{\text{new}} = 45\,\text{Gy} \times (10 + 1.8)/(10 + 2.5) = 42.5\,\text{Gy}$. Thus, the total dose would need to be reduced by only a small amount to maintain an isoeffect in terms of acute normal tissues complications.

For estimates of fractionation sensitivity of normal tissues, it is important to realize that critical organs such as spinal cord may or may not be exposed to tumor prescription doses entailing daily fractions of 1.8 to 2 Gy. For example, for the irradiation of lung cancers, traditional treatment arrangements have used anterior and posterior opposed portals that treat the cord to the maximum TD of approximately 45 to 50 Gy at approximately 2 Gy fractions, which is followed by a boost phase utilizing entirely off-cord beam angles, thereby only delivering additional scatter dose to the cord. In contrast, modern radiation treatments utilize multiple-field arrangements including off-cord beams or the use of IMRT. In these settings, the dose per fraction given to the spinal cord will be much lower than 1.8 to 2 Gy. For example, assuming a tumor prescription dose of 70 Gy at 2 Gy/fraction over 35 fractions using IMRT, the cord may be exposed to 45 Gy at dose fractions of approximately 1.3 Gy (45/35 Gy). This resulting reduction in fraction size would be predicted to be associated with sparing of late responding tissues, thereby potentially allowing a compensatory increase in total dose for isoeffect. It would be therefore important to know whether the LQ model remains valid at fraction sizes of <2 Gy. However, there are only limited data on the tolerance of late responding tissues to doses of <2 Gy per fraction. Interestingly, experiments on kidney and skin actually suggest an increased radiation sensitivity when fraction size was decreased below 1 Gy.[134] In these studies, tissue tolerance was observed to decrease by a factor of 2 over a narrow dose range. In contrast, for spinal cord, no increase in radiation sensitivity was observed at <1 Gy per fraction.

Conversely, the increasing clinical use of stereotactic radiosurgery (SRS) and body radiation therapy with doses per fraction of up to approximately 20 Gy has redirected interest to the question of whether the LQ model is accurate for doses >8 to 10 Gy and for a number of fractions as small as 1 to 3.[135,136] Likely, the sensitivity of individual cells to radiation becomes less and less important with increasing doses and acute and late toxicity will be dictated by more complex tissue responses. Much additional research will be needed to understand the potentially fundamentally different radiation biology underlying the effects of ablative radiation doses up to 20 Gy per fraction.

SUMMARY

In recent years, dramatic advances have been made in understanding the molecular and cellular process underlying radiation sensitivity of normal tissues. Although it is clear that the radiation sensitivity of individual cells, particularly stem and/ or progenitor cells, and their kinetics are important determinants of tissue response to radiation, it is also increasingly evident that "no cell is an island." The complex interactions and signaling between cells in a given tissue and even between different tissues and organs in a whole organism are also critical to determining response of the tissues and organs to the stresses imposed by radiation exposure. Much is yet to be learned at the cellular and molecular level that will enhance our ability to tailor fractionation patterns and modify cell and tissue responses to improve outcomes of radiation therapy by reducing normal tissue effects.

REFERENCES

1. Schulz-Ertner D, Tsujii H. Particle radiation therapy using proton and heavier ion beams. *J Clin Oncol.* 2007;25:953–964.
2. Durante M, Cucinotta FA. Heavy ion carcinogenesis and human space exploration. *Nat Rev Cancer.* 2008;8:465–472.
3. Spinks JWT, Woods RJ. *Introduction to Radiation Chemistry.* 3rd ed. New York, NY: John Wiley & Sons, Inc.; 1990.
4. Radford IR. The level of induced DNA double-strand breakage correlates with cell killing after X-irradiation. *Int J Radiat Biol.* 1985;48:45–54.
5. Ward JF. DNA damage produced by ionizing radiation in mammalian cells: identities, mechanisms of formation, and reparability. *Prog Nucleic Acid Res Mol Biol.* 1988;35:95–125.
6. Goodhead DT. Initial events in the cellular effects of ionizing radiations: clustered damage in DNA. *Int J Radiat Biol.* 1994;65:7–17.
7. Helleday T, Lo J, van Gent DC, et al. DNA double-strand break repair: from mechanistic understanding to cancer treatment. *DNA Repair (Amst).* 2007;6:923–935.
8. Willers H, Dahm-Daphi J, Powell SN. Repair of radiation damage to DNA. *Br J Cancer.* 2004;90:1297–1301.
9. Lisby M, Rothstein R. Choreography of recombination proteins during the DNA damage response. *DNA Repair (Amst).* 2009;8:1068–1076.
10. Su TT. Cellular responses to DNA damage: one signal, multiple choices. *Annu Rev Genet.* 2006;40:187–208.
11. Vilenchik MM, Knudson AG. Endogenous DNA double strand breaks: production, fidelity of repair, and induction of cancer. *Proc Natl Sci.* 2003;100:12871–12876.
12. Mahaney BL, Meek K, Lees-Miller SP. Repair of ionizing radiation-induced DNA double-strand breaks by non-homologous end-joining. *Biochem J.* 2009;417:639–650.
13. Li X, Heyer WD. Homologous recombination in DNA repair and DNA damage tolerance. *Cell Res.* 2008;18:99–113.
14. Shrivastav M, De Haro LP, Nickoloff JA. Regulation of DNA double-strand break repair pathway choice. *Cell Res.* 2008;18:134–147.
15. Jackson SP, Bartek J. The DNA-damage response in human biology and disease. *Nature.* 2009;461:1071–1078.
16. Schulte-Uentrop L, El-Awady RA, Schliecker L, et al. Distinct roles of XRCC4 and Ku80 in homologous end-joining of endonuclease- and ionizing radiation-induced DNA double-strand breaks. *Nucleic Acid Res.* 2008;36:2561–2569.
17. Sutherland BM, Bennett PV, Sidorkina O, et al. Clustered damages and total lesions induced in DNA by ionizing radiation: oxidized bases and strand breaks. *Biochemistry.* 2000;39:8026–8031.
18. Sutherland BM, Bennett PV, Sidorkina O, et al. Clustered DNA damages induced in isolated DNA and in human cells by low doses of ionizing radiation. *Proc Natl Sci.* 2000;97:103–108.
19. Gulston M, de Lara C, Davis E, et al. Processing of clustered DNA damage generates additional double-strand breaks in mammalian cells post-irradiation. *Nucleic Acid Res.* 2004;32:1602–1609.
20. Neijenhuis S, Verwijs-Janssen M, Kasten-Pisula U, et al. Mechanism of cell killing after ionizing radiation by a dominant negative DNA polymerase beta. *DNA Repair (Amst).* 2009;8:336–346.
21. Bentzen SM. Preventing or reducing late side effects of radiation therapy: radiobiology meets molecular pathology. *Nat Rev Cancer.* 2006;6:702–713.
22. Alter B. Radiosensitivity in Fanconi's anemia patients. *Radiother Oncol.* 2002;62:345–347.
23. Pollard JA, Gatti RA. Clinical radiosensitivity with DNA repair disorders: an overview. *Int J Radiat Oncol Biol Phys.* 2009;74:1323–1331.
24. Alsner J, Andreassen CN, Overgaard J. Genetic markers for prediction of normal tissue toxicity after radiotherapy. *Semin Radiat Oncol.* 2008;18:126–135.
25. Andreassen CN, Alsner J, Overgaard J, et al. TGFB1 polymorphisms are associated with risk of late normal tissue complications in the breast after radiotherapy for early breast cancer. *Radiother Oncol.* 2005;75:18–21.
26. Chistiakov DA, Voronova NV, Chistiakov PA. Genetic variations in DNA repair genes, radio-sensitivity to cancer and susceptibility to acute tissue reactions in radiotherapy-treated cancer patients. 2008;47:809–824.
27. Borgmann K, Hoeller U, Nowack S, et al. Individual radiosensitivity measured with lymphocytes may predict the risk of acute reaction after radiotherapy. *Int J Radiat Oncol Biol Phys.* 2008;71:256–264.
28. Kasten-Pisula U, Tastan H, Dikomey E. Huge differences in cellular radiosensitivity due to only very small variations in double-strand break repair capacity. *Int J Radiat Biol.* 2005;81:409–419.
29. Rodemann HP, Blaese MA. Responses of normal cells to ionizing radiation. *Semin Radiat Oncol.* 2007;17:81–88.
30. Kong FM, Ten Haken R, Eisbruch A, et al. Non-small cell lung cancer therapy-related pulmonary toxicity: an update on radiation pneumonitis and fibrosis. *Semin Oncol.* 2005;32:S42–S54.
31. Cornforth MN, Bedford JS. A quantitative comparison of potentially lethal damage repair and the rejoining of interphase chromosome breaks in low passage normal human fibroblasts. *Radiat Res.* 1987;111:385–405.
32. George K, Durante M, Wu H, et al. Chromosome aberrations in the blood lymphocytes of astronauts after space flight. *Radiat Res.* 2001;156:731–738.
33. Vaurijoux A, Gruel G, Pouzoulet F, et al. Strategy for population triage based on dicentric analysis. *Radiat Res.* 2009;171:541–548.
34. George K, Willingham V, Cucinotta FA. Stability of chromosome aberrations in the blood lymphocytes of astronauts measured after space flight by FISH chromosome painting. *Radiat Res.* 2005;164:474–480.
35. Borgmann K, Roper B, El-Awady RA, et al. Indicators of late normal tissue response after radiotherapy for head and neck cancer: fibroblasts, lymphocytes, genetics, DNA repair, and chromosome aberrations. *Radiother Oncol.* 2002;64:141–152.
36. Hall EJ, Giaccia AJ. *Radiobiology for the Radiologist.* 6th ed. New York, NY: Lippincott Williams & Wilkins; 2005.
37. Zhou BB, Elledge SJ. The DNA damage response: putting checkpoints in perspective. *Nature.* 2000;408:433–439.
38. Lobrich M, Jeggo PA. The impact of a negligent G2/M checkpoint on genomic instability and cancer induction. *Nat Rev Cancer.* 2007;7:861–869.
39. Campisi J, di Fagagna F. Cellular senescence: when bad things happen to good cells. *Nat Rev Mol Cell Biol.* 2007;8:729–740.
40. Vakifahmetoglu H, Olsson M, Zhivotovsky B. Death through tragedy: mitotic catastrophe. *Cell Death Differ.* 2008;15:1153–1162.
41. Thompson LH, Suit HD. Proliferation kinetics of X-irradiated mouse L cells studied with time lapse photography. II. *Int J Radiat Biol.* 1969;15:347–362.
42. Chu K, Teele N, Dewey MW, et al. Computerized video time lapse study of cell cycle delay and arrest, mitotic catastrophe, apoptosis and clonogenic survival in irradiated 14-3-3σ and CDKN1A (p21) knockout cell lines. *Radiat Res.* 2004;162:270–286.
43. Kerr JFR, Winterford CM, Harmon BV. Apoptosis. Its significance in cancer and cancer therapy. *Cancer.* 1994;73:2013–2026.
44. Hotchkiss RS, Strasser A, McDunn JE, et al. Cell death. *N Engl J Med.* 2009;361:1570–1583.
45. Held KD. Radiation-induced apoptosis and its relationship to loss of clonogenic survival. *Apoptosis.* 1997;2:265–282.
46. Kolesnick R, Fuks Z. Radiation and ceramide-induced apoptosis. *Oncogene.* 2003;22:5897–5906.
47. Belka C, Jendrossek V, Pruschy M, et al. Apoptosis-modulating agents in combination with radiotherapy – current status and outlook. *Int J Radiat Oncol Biol Phys.* 2004;58:542–554.
48. Zois CE, Koukourakis MI. Radiation-induced autophagy in normal and cancer cells. Towards novel cytoprotection and radio-sensitization policies. *Autophagy.* 2009;5:442–450.
49. Willers H, Held KD. Introduction to Clinical Radiation Biology. *Hematol Oncol Clin North Am.* 2006;20:1–24.
50. Little JB, Hahn GM, Frindel E, et al. Repair of potentially lethal damage in vitro and in vivo. *Radiology.* 1973;106:689–694.
51. Elkind MM, Sutton-Gilbert H, Moses WB, et al. Radiation response of mammalian cells in culture. V. Temperature dependence of the repair of X-ray damage in surviving cells (aerobic and hypoxic). *Radiat Res.* 1965;25:359–377.
52. Sinclair WK, Morton RA. X-ray sensitivity during the cell generation cycle of cultured Chinese hamster cells. *Radiat Res.* 1966;29:450–479.
53. Brown JM, Wilson WR. Exploiting tumour hypoxia in cancer treatment. *Nat Rev Cancer.* 2004;4:437–447.
54. Parmar K, Mauch P, Vergilio J-A, et al. Distribution of hematopoietic stem cells in the bone marrow according to regional hypoxia. *Proc Natl Sci.* 2007;104:5431–5436.
55. Stone HB, Moulder JE, Coleman CN, et al. Models for evaluating agents intended for the prophylaxis, mitigation and treatment of radiation injuries: Report of an NCI Workshop, December 3–4, 2003. *Radiat Res.* 2004;162:711–728.
56. Moulder JE, Cohen EP. Future strategies for mitigation and treatment of chronic radiation-induced normal tissue injury. *Semin Radiat Oncol.* 2007;17:141–148.
57. Soule BP, Hyodo F, Matsumoto K, et al. The chemistry and biology of nitroxide compounds. *Free Radic Biol Med.* 2007;42:1632–1650.
58. Murley JS, Kataoka Y, Weydert CJ, et al. Delayed cytoprotection after enhancement of Sod2 (MnSOD) gene expression in SA-NH mouse sarcoma cells exposed to WR-1065, the active metabolite of amifostine. *Radiat Res.* 2002;158:101–109.
59. Brush J, Lipnick SL, Phillips T, et al. Molecular mechanisms of late normal tissue injury. *Semin Radiat Oncol.* 2007;17:121–130.
60. Robbins MEC, Zhao W. Chronic oxidative stress and radiation-induced late normal tissue injury: a review. *Int J Radiat Biol.* 2004;80:251–259.
61. Epperly MW, Dixon T, Wang H, et al. Modulation of radiation-induced life shortening by systemic intravenous MnSOD-plasmid liposome gene therapy. *Radiat Res.* 2008;170:437–443.
62. Rabbani ZN, Anscher MS, Folz RJ. Overexpression of extracellular superoxide dismutase reduces acute radiation induced lung toxicity. *BMC Cancer.* 2005;5:59.
63. Langan AR, Kahn MA, Yeung IWT. Partial volume rat lung irradiation: the protective/mitigating effects of Eukarion-189, a superoxide dismutase-catalase mimetic. *Radiother Oncol.* 2006;92:231–238.
64. Greenberger JS, Epperly MW. Review. Antioxidant gene therapeutic approaches to normal tissue radioprotection and tumor radiosensitization. *In Vivo.* 2007;21(2):141–146.
65. Delanian S, Lefaix J-L. Current management for late normal tissue injury: radiation-induced fibrosis and necrosis. *Semin Radiat Oncol.* 2007;17:99–197.
66. Delanian S, Lefaix J-L. The radiation-induced fibroatrophic process: therapeutic perspective via the antioxidant pathway. *Radiother Oncol.* 2004;73:119–131.
67. Chiao TB, Lee AJ. Role of pentoxifylline and vitamin E in attenuation of radiation-induced fibrosis. *Ann Pharmacother.* 2005;39:516–522.
68. Skarsgard LD. Radiobiology with heavy charged particles: a historical review. *Phys Med.* 1998;14(Suppl. 1):1–19.
69. Dent P, Yacoub A, Fisher PB, et al. MAPK pathways in radiation responses. *Oncogene.* 2003;22:5885–5896.
70. Valerie K, Yacoup A, Hagan MP, et al. Radiation-induced cell signaling: inside-out and outside-in. *Mol Cancer Ther.* 2007;6:789–801.
71. Giedzinski E, Rola R, Fike JR, et al. Efficient production of reactive oxygen species in neural precursor cells after exposure to 250 MeV protons. *Radiat Res.* 2005;164:540–544.
72. Dayal D, Martin SM, Limoli CL, et al. Hydrogen peroxide mediates the radiation-induced mutator phenotype in mammalian cells. *Biochem J.* 2008;413:185–191.
73. Morgan WF. Non-targeted and delayed effects of exposure to ionizing radiation: I. Radiation-induced genomic instability and bystander effects in vitro. *Radiat Res.* 2003;159:567–580.
74. Morgan WF. Non-targeted and delayed effects of exposure to ionizing radiation: II. Radiation-induced genomic instability and bystander effects in vivo, clastogenic factors and transgenerational effects. *Radiat Res.* 2003;159:581–596.
75. Prise KM, Schettino G, Folkard M, et al. New insights on cell death from radiation exposure. *Lancet Oncol.* 2005;6:520–528.

76. Schettino G, Folkard M, Michael BD, et al. Low-dose binary behavior of bystander cell killing after microbeam irradiation of a single cell with focused Ck X rays. *Radiat Res.* 2005;163:332–336.

77. Yang H, Asaad N, Held KD. Medium-mediated intercellular communication is involved in bystander responses of X-irradiated normal human fibroblasts. *Oncogene.* 2005;24: 2096–2103.

78. Shao C, Furusawa Y, Kobayashi Y, et al. Bystander effect induced by counted high-LET particles in confluent human fibroblasts: a mechanistic study. *FASEB J.* 2003;17:1422–1427.

79. Tartier L, Gilchrist S, Burdak-Rothkamm S, et al. Cytoplasmic irradiation induces mitochondrial-dependent 53BP1 protein relocalization in irradiated and bystander cells. *Cancer Res.* 2007;67:5872–5879.

80. Shao C, Folkard M, Michael BD, et al. Targeted cytoplasmic irradiation induces bystander responses. *Proc Natl Sci.* 2004;101:13495–13500.

81. Brenner DJ, Little JB, Sachs RK. The bystander effect in radiation oncogenesis: II. A quantitative model. *Radiat Res.* 2001;155:402–408.

82. Hei TK, Zhou H, Ivanov VN, et al. Mechanism of radiation-induced bystander effects: a unifying model. *J Pharm Pharmacol.* 2008;60:943–950.

83. Hall EJ, Wuu C-S. Radiation-induced second cancers: the impact of 3D-CRT and IMRT. *Int J Radiat Oncol Biol Phys.* 2003;56:83–88.

84. Mothersill C, Seymour C. Medium from irradiated human epithelial cells but not human fibroblasts reduces the clonogenic survival of unirradiated cells. *Int J Radiat Biol.* 1997;71:421–427.

85. Azzam EI, de Toledo SM, Gooding T, et al. Intercellular communication is involved in the bystander regulation of gene expression in human cells exposed to very low fluences of alpha particles. *Radiat Res.* 1998;150:497–504.

86. Azzam EI, de Toledo SM, Little JB. Oxidative metabolism, gap junctions and the ionizing radiation-induced bystander effect. *Oncogene.* 2003;22:7050–7057.

87. Narayanan PK, Goodwin EH, Lehnert BE. Alpha particles initiate biological production of superoxide anions and hydrogen peroxide in human cells. *Cancer Res.* 1997;57:3963–3971.

88. Shao C, Furusawa Y, Aoki M, et al. Nitric oxide-mediated bystander effect induced by heavy-ions in human salivary gland tumor cells. *Int J Radiat Biol.* 2002;78:837–844.

89. Lyng F, Maguire P, McClean B, et al. The involvement of calcium and MAP kinase signaling pathways in the production of radiation-induced bystander effects. *Radiat Res.* 2006;165:400–409.

90. Shao C, Lyng FM, Folkard M, et al. Calcium fluxes modulate the radiation-induced bystander responses in targeted glioma and fibroblast cells. *Radiat Res.* 2006;166:479–487.

91. Narayanan PK, LaRue KEA, Goodwin EH, et al. Alpha particles induce the production of interleukin-8 by human cells. *Radiat Res.* 1999;152:57–63.

92. Iyer R, Lehnert BE. Factors underlying the cell growth-related bystander responses to α particles. *Cancer Res.* 2000;60:1290–1298.

93. Shao C, Folkard M, Prise KM. Role of TGF-beta1 and nitric oxide in the bystander response of irradiated glioma cells. *Oncogene.* 2008;27:434–440.

94. Zhou H, Ivanov VN, Gillespie J, et al. Mechanism of radiation-induced bystander effect: role of the cyclooxygenase-2 signaling pathway. *Proc Natl Sci.* 2005;102:14641–14646.

95. Azzam EI, de Toledo SM, Spitz DR, et al. Oxidative metabolism modulates signal transduction and micronucleus formation in bystander cells from α-particle-irradiated normal human fibroblast cultures. *Cancer Res.* 2002;62:5436–5442.

96. Zhou H, Ivanov VN, Lien Y-C, D, et al. Mitochondrial function and nuclear factor-kB mediated signaling in radiation-induced bystander effects. *Cancer Res.* 2008;68:2233–2240.

97. Belyakov OV, Folkard M, Mothersill C, et al. A proliferation-dependent bystander effect in primary porcine and human urothelial explants in response to targeted irradiation. *Br J Cancer.* 2003;88:767–774.

98. Belyakov OV, Mitchell SA, Parikh D, et al. Biological effects in unirradiated human tissue induced by radiation damage up to 1 mm away. *Proc Natl Sci.* 2005;102:14203–1428.

99. Sedelnikova OA, Nakamura A, Kovalchuk O, et al. DNA double-strand breaks form in bystander cells after microbeam irradiation of three-dimensional human tissue models. *Cancer Res.* 2007;67:4295–4302.

100. Hollowell JG, Littlefield LG. Chromosome damage induced by plasma of X-rayed patients: an indirect effect of X-rays. *Proc Soc Exp Biol Med.* 1968;129:240–244.

101. Goh K-O, Sumner H. Breaks in normal human chromosomes: are they induced by a transferable substance in the plasma of persons exposed to total-body irradiation? *Radiat Res.* 1968;35:171–181.

102. Emerit I. Reactive oxygen species, chromosome mutation, and cancer: possible role of clastogenic factors in carcinogenesis. *Free Radic Biol Med.* 1993;16:99–109.

103. Mole RJ. Whole body irradiation—radiology or medicine? *Br J Radiol.* 1953;26:234–241.

104. Formenti SC, Demaria S. System effects of local radiotherapy. *Lancet Oncol.* 2009;10:718–726.

105. Demaria S, Ng B, Devitt ML, et al. Ionizing radiation inhibition of distant untreated tumors (abscopal effect) is immune mediated. *Int J Radiat Oncol Biol Phys.* 2004;58:862–870.

106. Little JB. Genomic instability and bystander effects: a historical perspective. *Oncogene.* 2003;22:6978–6987.

107. Wright EG, Coates PJ. Untargeted effects of ionizing radiation: implications for radiation pathology. *Oncogene.* 2006;597:119–132.

108. Coates PJ, Lorimore SA, Wright EG. Damaging and protective cell signalling in the untargeted effects of ionizing radiation. *Mutat Res.* 2004;568:5–20.

109. Lorimore SA, Chrystal JA, Robinson JI, et al. Chromosomal instability in unirradiated hematopoietic cells induced by macrophages exposed in vivo to ionizing radiation. *Cancer Res.* 2008;68:8122–8126.

110. Portess DI, Bauer G, Hill MA, et al. Low-dose irradiation of nontransformed cells stimulates the selective removal of precancerous cells via intercellular induction of apoptosis. *Cancer Res.* 2007;67:1246–1253.

111. Olivieri G, Bodycote Y, Wolff S. Adaptive response of human lymphocytes to low concentrations of radioactive thymidine. *Science.* 1984;223:594–597.

112. Wolff S. The adaptive response in radiobiology: evolving insights and implications. *Environ Health Perspect* 1998;106(Suppl. 1):277–283.

113. Kadhim MA. Role of genetic background in induced instability. *Oncogene.* 2003;22:6994–6999.

114. Matsumoto H, Tomita M, Otsuka K, et al. A new paradigm in radioadaptive response developing from microbeam research. *J Radiat Res.* 2009;50(Suppl.):A67–A79.

115. Kadhim MA, Moore SR, Goodwin EH. Interrelationship amongst radiation-induced genomic instability, bystander effect, and the adaptive response. *Mutat Res.* 2004; 568:21–32.

116. Zhang Y, Zhou J, Baldwin J, et al. Ionizing radiation-induced bystander mutagenesis and adaptation: quantitative and temporal aspects. *Mutat Res.* 2009;671:20–25.

117. McBride WH, Chiang C-S, Olson JL, et al. Failla Memorial Lecture: a sense of danger from radiation. *Radiat Res.* 2004;162:1–19.

118. Neta R. Modulation with cytokines of radiation injury: suggested mechanisms of action. *Environ Health Perspect.* 1997;105 (Suppl 6):1462–1465.

119. Haimovitz-Friedman A, Vlodavsky I, Chaudhuri A, et al. Autocrine effects of fibroblast growth factor in repair of radiation damage in endothelial cells. *Cancer Res.* 1991;51:2552–2558.

120. Fuks Z, Alfieri A, Haimovitz-Friedman A, et al. Intravenous basic fibroblast growth factor protects the lung but not the mediastinal organs against radiation-induced apoptosis in vivo. *Cancer J.* 1995;1:62–72.

121. Neta R, Stiefel SM, Ali M. In lethally irradiated mice interleukin-12 protects bone marrow but sensitizes intestinal tract to damage from ionizing radiation. *Ann N Y Acad Sci.* 1995;762:274–280.

122. Daigle JL, Hong J-H, Chiang C-S, et al. The role of tumor necrosis factor signaling pathways in the response of murine brain to irradiation. *Cancer Res.* 2001;61:8859–8865.

123. Stone HB, Coleman CN, Anscher MS, et al. Effects of radiation on normal tissues: consequences and mechanisms. *Lancet Oncol.* 2003;4:529–536.

124. Barcellos-Hoff MH. How do tissues respond to damage at the cellular level? The role of cytokines in irradiated tissues. *Radiat Res.* 1998;150:S109–S120.

125. Anscher MS, Vujaskovic Z. Mechanisms and potential targets for prevention and treatment of normal tissue injury after radiation therapy. *Semin Oncol.* 2005;32(Suppl. 3):S86–S91.

126. Maxwell CA, Fleisch MC, Costes SV, et al. Targeted and nontargeted effects of ionizing radiation that impact genomic instability. *Cancer Res.* 2008;68:8304–8311.

127. Bergonie J, Tribondeau L. Interpretation of some results of radiotherapy and an attempt at determining a logical technique of treatment. *Radiat Res.* 1959;11:587–588.

128. Withers HR, Taylor JMG, Maciejewski B. Treatment volume and tissue tolerance. *Int J Radiat Oncol Biol Phys.* 1988;14:751–759.

129. Thames HD, Hendry JH. *Fractionation in Radiotherapy.* New York, NY: Taylor & Francis; 1987.

130. Willers H, Heilmann HP, Beck-Bornholdt HP. One hundred years of radiotherapy. Historical origins and development of fractionated irradiation in German speaking countries. *Strahlenther Onkol.* 1998;174:53–63.

131. Thames HD, Bentzen SM, Turesson I, et al. Time-dose factors in radiotherapy: a review of the human data. *Radiother Oncol.* 1990;19:219–235.

132. Baumann M, Budach V, Appold S. Radiation tolerance of the human spinal cord [in German]. *Strahlenther Onkol.* 1994;170:131–139.

133. Schultheiss TE. The radiation dose-response of the human spinal cord. *Int J Radiat Oncol Biol Phys.* 2008;71:1455–1459.

134. Beck-Bornholdt HP, Dubben HH, Liertz-Peterson C, et al. Hyperfractionation: where do we stand? *Radiother Oncol.* 1997;43:1–21.

135. Brenner DJ. The linear-quadratic model is an appropriate methodology for determining isoeffective doses at large doses per fraction. *Semin Radiat Oncol.* 2008;18:234–239.

136. Kirkpatrick JP, Meyer JJ, Marks LB. The linear-quadratic model is inappropriate to model high dose per fraction effects in radiosurgery. *Semin Radiat Oncol.* 2008;18:240–243.

Ting Liu
Lynn Million

Pathology of Radiation Injury

The histologic effects induced by ionizing radiation were reported soon after the discovery of x-rays by Conrad Roentgen in December 1895. Emil Grubbe, a medical student at that time, reported "severe itching on the back of his hand followed shortly by swelling, inflammation, pain, blistering, loss of hair, and eventually breaking down of the skin" after experimenting with the "new" x-rays. The potential effectiveness of ionizing radiation causing similar damage in cancer cells was realized and the therapeutic use of ionizing irradiation was begun in 1896.[1]

Over the past century, therapeutic radiation has improved cure rates for most types of cancers. However, potentially damage-inducing morphologic alterations in normal tissues are known to develop immediately and continue to progress long after exposure to therapeutic radiation. As a result, two major classifications of radiation injury have emerged: acute (hours or days after radiation exposure) and delayed (months or years after radiation exposure). Delayed radiation injury is the most common observation encountered by surgical pathologists.[2]

"Sensitivity" of an organ is one of the most important factors determining the degree of susceptibility of human tissues to radiation injury. Organs that exhibit high mitotic activity and rapid proliferative rates have a greater chance of expressing cellular damage and morphologic alterations after radiation exposure as compared with organs that display low mitotic activity and low proliferative rates. The gonads and bone marrow are organs considered to be more radiation sensitive, while adult bone, myocardium, smooth muscle, and cartilage are organs considered to be more radiation resistant.[3–7]

No single pathognomonic or specific morphologic feature characterizes radiation injury. Therefore, it is important for the surgical pathologist to have knowledge of prior radiation exposure to accurately interpret histologic specimens. Total radiation dose, daily radiation dose (fractionation), type of ionizing radiation utilized (orthovoltage, megavoltage, electrons, protons, neutrons), field size, time for cancer treatment, and whether surgery or chemotherapy was included determine the extent of normal tissue injury. Pathologic changes seen in human tissues after radiation exposure can be broadly grouped into three categories: *epithelial* (parenchymal), *stromal* (mesenchymal), and *vascular*.

EPITHELIAL CHANGES AFTER RADIATION EXPOSURE

ATROPHY

Atrophy is one of the most common morphologic changes associated with radiation injury and is characterized by progressive loss of number and volume of epithelial cells.[2–8] Atrophic changes can be seen in any organ with an epithelial lining, including the skin, subcutaneous tissue, gastrointestinal system, genitourinary organs, respiratory tract, breast, and salivary glands. The distribution, degree, and extent of atrophy are focal and random. Severe atrophy is more commonly observed in radiation-sensitive organs, including the gastrointestinal system, genitourinary organs, and reproductive systems, whereas mild atrophy is more typical in organs that are considered radiation resistant, such as the liver and endocrine system.

Prostate glands exposed to radiation may show glandular atrophy characterized by a reduction in the number and size of acini. In benign irradiated prostate glands, the secretory epithelium is flat with scant eosinophilic cytoplasm. To distinguish residual or recurrent prostate carcinoma from benign glandular atrophy after radiation, architectural alteration is considered a more reliable feature than cytologic atypia.[9–11] Major and minor salivary gland atrophies are often severe but focal in distribution and can be associated with fibrous tissue replacement months after exposure.[6,12] Breast tissue that has been irradiated commonly shows epithelial atrophy in the epidermis, sweat glands, and sebaceous glands. Mammary lobular unit atrophy is a prominent morphologic feature characteristic of delayed radiation injury (Fig. 2.1).[13,14]

NECROSIS AND ULCERATION

Necrosis and ulceration often coexist and generally precede the atrophic stage.

Specimens from the upper and lower gastrointestinal tracts obtained shortly after radiation often show sharply demarcated mucosal ulcers, for example, after intraluminal brachytherapy boosts for esophageal/gastroesophageal junction carcinoma (Fig. 2.2A). The ulcerated areas exhibit mucosal necrosis and denudation of the epithelium with an ulcer base consisting of

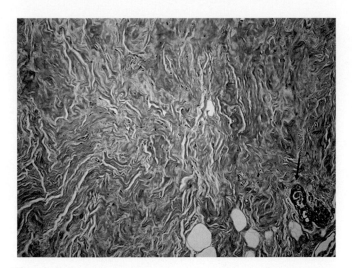

Figure 2.1. H&E-stained section. A low-power view demonstrating postradiation breast tissue with significant hyalinizing stromal fibrosis and marked mammary lobular unit atrophy (*arrow*, H&E, magnification 40×).

mixed inflammatory cells, necrotic debris, and granulation tissue, extending to the submucosa (Fig. 2.2B). Adjacent to the ulcer, submucosal fibrosis may result in thickening of the adjacent tissues, such as esophageal or rectal wall.[5,12,15,16] Necrosis without ulceration is an uncommon manifestation of delayed radiation injury, except in the central nervous system where it can be seen in the white matter of the cerebral hemispheres (see Chapter 24).[17,18]

METAPLASIA

By definition, metaplasia is the reversible replacement of a differentiated cell with another mature differentiated cell type. Squamous metaplasia of benign prostatic ducts and urothelium is a common finding after radiation therapy.[3,7,8,12]

EPITHELIAL ATYPIA

Cytologic atypia has been identified in most irradiated organs and can be misinterpreted as malignant disease.[3,12] To discern whether the morphologic features are consistent with radiation-associated atypia versus carcinoma, the following features should be considered: significantly enlarged nuclei with dense "smudgy" appearance, cells with normal to low nuclear/cytoplasm ratio, and well-preserved tissue architecture, despite cellular pleomorphism.[12] Interpretation of intraoperative frozen section is difficult when ruling out recurrent or residual malignancy as radiation-associated epithelial atypia is often observed in prostate, breast, bladder, lungs, salivary glands, and squamous mucosa of the head and neck region.

Irradiated benign prostatic glands demonstrate enlarged and pyknotic nuclei of the secretory cells, often adjacent to normal-appearing cells (Fig. 2.3). Irradiated prostatic glands harboring carcinoma usually show less epithelial atypia than irradiated benign glands and, if present, show minimal change in the histologic features of the high-grade prostatic intraepithelial neoplasm component.[9] Irradiated prostatic carcinoma cells exhibit abundant vacuolated or foamy cytoplasm with hyperchromatic nuclei arranged in small glands, nests, or single cells (Fig. 2.4A, B). Additional helpful features to distinguish irradiated prostatic carcinoma from benign irradiated glands include the presence of blue-tinged mucin, an infiltrative growth pattern, and perineural invasion.[10,11] In addition, lack of a basal cell layer in malignant glands detected by immunostaining with high molecular-weight cytokeratins (34βE12) and P63 favors malignancy.

Specimens of irradiated gastrointestinal tissue examined after radiation therapy frequently demonstrate atypia often in conjunction with residual carcinomas as seen in the gastroesophageal junction specimen of Figure 2.5.[19,20] Giant tumor cells show marked nuclear enlargement with smudgy nuclei and prominent nucleoli. These radiation-induced morphologic changes rarely cause diagnostic problems except when grading tumors for differentiation. In benign epithelium, the presence of cytologic atypia can be diagnostically challenging, especially

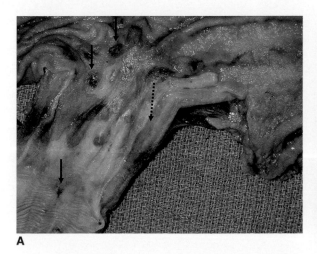

A

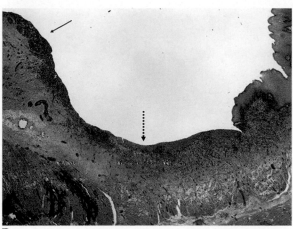

B

Figure 2.2. **A:** An esophagogastrectomy specimen shortly after radiation for lower esophageal adenocarcinoma showing superficial mucosal ulcers (*solid arrows*) and submucosal fibrosis (*dashed arrow*) with indistinct gastroesophageal junction. **B:** A low magnification (H&E, 20×) reveals a mucosal ulcer in an irradiated esophagus. The esophageal epithelium shows erosion and denudation within an ulcer base located in the submucosa (*dashed arrow*). Residual adenocarcinoma is illustrated adjacent to the ulcer (*arrow*).

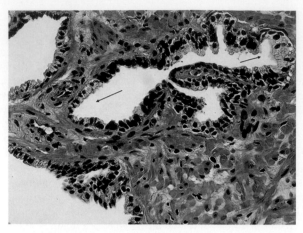

Figure 2.3. Benign prostate glands (H&E, high magnification, 400×) showing morphologic features after radiation exposure: within the same gland, there is normal-appearing glandular epithelium (*arrows*) admixed with highly atypical hyperchromatic epithelium secondary to radiation effect.

during intraoperative consultations, in distinguishing malignant from nonmalignant cells.

In irradiated mammary glands, cytological atypia of the benign terminal duct-lobular unit epithelium is characterized by enlarged hyperchromatic nuclei, prominent nucleoli, and eosinophilic and vacuolated cytoplasm. Irradiated breast carcinoma, however, shows little or no appreciable morphological changes, often resembling the original cancer.[14]

DYSPLASIA

Dysplasia is considered a premalignant alteration and is characterized by increased nucleus-to-cytoplasm ratio, hyperchromasia,

irregular nuclear contours, prominent nucleoli, and, occasionally, atypical mitoses. The loss of normal tissue architecture is an important diagnostic feature. Radiation-induced dysplasia occurs in squamous epithelium but rarely in tissues with non-squamous lining. Dysplasia may have an appearance similar to that of reactive atypia, a benign reparative process.

STROMAL CHANGES AFTER RADIATION EXPOSURE

FIBROSIS

Stromal fibrosis is one of the most consistent findings in delayed radiation injury. Head and neck regions, breast, genitourinary, and gastrointestinal tissues are frequent sites of stromal fibrosis seen after radiation exposure. Some organs rarely develop fibrosis after radiation exposure, most notably the lens and central nervous system. The bone marrow responds to irradiation with serous atrophy and fatty replacement but fibrosis is very rare. Additionally, irradiated liver and bone will demonstrate necrosis but not fibrosis or hyalinization, except in areas where tumor was previously present.

The presence of postradiation stromal fibrosis is dependent on the radiation dose and time from exposure and is usually confined within the radiation field. Morphologically, stromal fibrosis appears unevenly distributed within the tissues, showing hyalinizing, acellular acidophilic collagen (Fig. 2.6).[2–8,12] Although, these features are not pathognomonic, they are characteristic of delayed radiation injury. In the upper gastrointestinal tract, one of the more common histologic findings is extensive submucosal and, occasionally, transmural fibrosis. Scattered fibroblasts with variable degree of cytological atypia are frequently found. Circumferential submucosal fibrosis with thickened walls can lead to luminal narrowing and increase the risk for obstruction.[12]

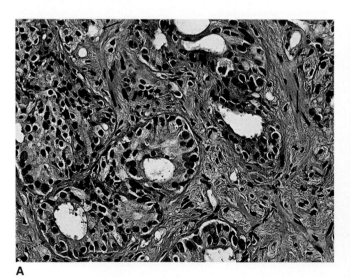

A

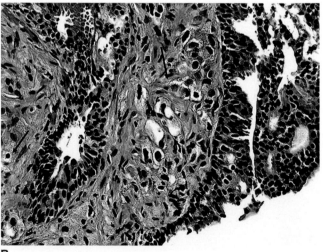

B

Figure 2.4. **A:** Postirradiated prostate shows atypical basal cell hyperplasia (H&E, 200×) with hyperchromatic nuclei and prominent nucleoli (*dashed arrow*). Adjacent to and between the benign glands is residual carcinoma (*arrows*). The tumor cells are arranged in small nests or singly distributed with abundant foamy cytoplasm and hyperchromatic nuclei. **B:** A high-power view (H&E, 400×) of radiation-associated cytologic atypia in residual prostatic carcinoma. The neoplastic cells are arranged in nests or singly distributed with voluminous vacuolated/foamy cytoplasm and hyperchromatic nuclei (*arrows*).

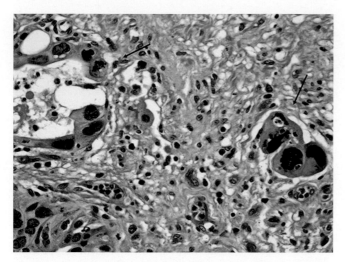

Figure 2.5. A high magnification (H&E, 400×) view of radiation-related cytologic atypia in residual carcinoma at gastroesophageal junction. The tumor cells exhibit marked atypia with enlarged hyperchromatic nuclei, prominent nucleoli, and atypical mitosis (*arrows*).

In the setting of early breast cancer, limited surgery (lumpectomy) followed by radiation therapy is often recommended for breast preservation with the goal of optimizing cosmesis. Subcutaneous radiation-induced breast fibrosis can lead to scarring and a contracted breast, occurring most frequently in areas of prior surgery, such as the surgical incision. Morphologically, mammary stromal fibrosis exhibits hyalinizing, inhomogeneous, acellular, and eosinophilic collagen deposition superimposed on mammary lobular unit atrophy (Fig. 2.1).[13,14,21]

Fibrinous exudate, a delayed radiation injury, can be seen in the dermis of overlying skin and in the submucosa of gastrointestinal and genitourinary organs and pericardium. Fibrinous exudates are characterized in hematoxylin and eosin (H&E) sections by a delicate irregular, reticular, often basophilic acellular material. Special stains, such as Fraser-Lendrum, can help further characterize the exudate.

ATYPICAL FIBROBLASTS

Atypical fibroblasts (AFs), also called radiation fibroblasts, are a characteristic histologic alteration noted after radiation therapy. They are frequently observed in the gastrointestinal submucosa, respiratory tract, urinary system, skin, soft tissue, and breast. They are rarely identified in organs such as liver, kidney, heart, lung, or brain.[2,3,6–8,12] Morphologically, the AFs are randomly distributed depicting markedly angulated basophilic cytoplasm ("swallow tail"), enlarged and hyperchromatic nuclei with no mitotic activity.[3,12] AFs are thought to represent a reactive and benign reparative phenomenon and therefore have also been observed in association with acute and chronic inflammation. AFs in the lamina propria of the urinary bladder have been described after treatment with bacillus Calmette-Guérin. Since AFs are a nonspecific finding, their presence can represent diagnostic challenges, particularly when distinguishing AFs in irradiated soft tissue sarcoma specimens from residual sarcoma (Fig. 2.7A, B).

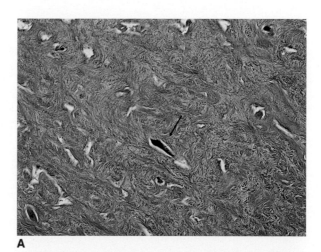

A

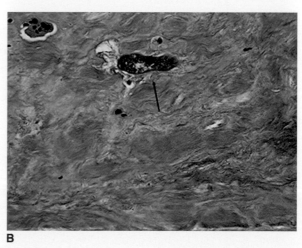

B

Figure 2.7. **A:** A high-power view (H&E, 400×) of AFs seen in postradiation tissue. For this case, an AF is identified in fibrotic tissue after radiation therapy for a soft tissue sarcoma. The AF is significantly enlarged with a hyperchromatic and smudgy nucleus and a "shallow tail" (*arrow*). **B:** A large AF (H&E, high-power view, 400×) is observed in irradiated soft tissue. The degree of atypia is striking with significant cytomegaly and marked enlarged nucleus. The nucleus is hyperchromatic with prominent nucleoli (*arrow*).

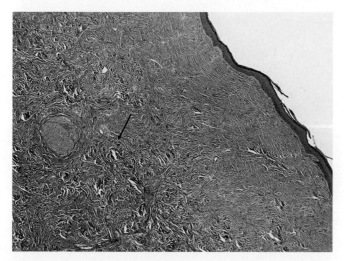

Figure 2.6. A low-power view (H&E, 20×) of subcutaneous fibrosis in elbow after radiation therapy for a soft tissue sarcoma. The section shows extensive fibrosis with paucity of cells and dense collagen (*arrow*).

STROMAL NECROSIS

Stromal necrosis is rare after radiation exposure and when present represents a delayed radiation injury. It can be found in any organ where stroma is present. Fat necrosis of the breast, whether caused by surgical trauma or by radiation, may mimic recurrent neoplasm.

VASCULAR CHANGES AFTER RADIATION EXPOSURE

Blood vessels play an important role in the pathogenesis of acute and delayed radiation injury. Late vascular injury contributes to secondary organ damage through decreased perfusion leading to tissue ischemia, necrosis, ulceration, and fibrosis. Endothelial cells are the most radiation-sensitive cell type comprising the vasculature. Blood vessel size also determines susceptibility to radiation injury. Common morphologic changes of blood vessels include endothelial damage, intimal hyperplasia, and vascular wall fibrosis.

CAPILLARIES

Capillaries are the most frequent blood vessel to be affected by irradiation as they are mainly composed of endothelial cells with radiation injury leading to thrombosis, obstruction, or capillary destruction. Clinical manifestations of capillary injury include telangiectasia seen as abnormal blood vessels on skin surfaces or as hematuria developing after irradiation of the bladder.

ARTERIOLES

Radiation injury in small arterioles commonly develops in the gastrointestinal tract, skin, and brain. Morphologically, swollen endothelial cells with hyperchromatic smudged nuclei, endothelial cell proliferation, and indistinct smooth muscle cell borders with thickening and hyalinization of the tunica media are described.

SMALL AND MEDIUM-SIZED ARTERIES

Alterations of medium-sized arteries are characterized by cytologic atypia in endothelial cells, including nuclear enlargement with hyperchromatic and pyknotic nuclei that protrude "hobnail-like" into the vascular lumen. Random medial wall necrosis and mural thickening with hyalinization can be seen on microscopic examination. Occasionally, foamy or vacuolated macrophages within the vascular wall of small arterioles are identified (Fig. 2.8A). The characteristic features of radiation injury in small to medium arteries include three distinct changes: intimal fibrosis, transmural healed necrosis, and intimal plaque formation with foamy macrophages. Intimal fibrosis may be concentric or eccentric with mild intimal cell atypia leading to vascular luminal narrowing and may result in significant vascular occlusion (Fig. 2.8B). Transmural necrosis can result in segmental wall fibrosis with organizing thrombus and prominent perivascular fibrosis frequently noted. Intimal plaques with foamy macrophages between endothelium and internal elastic are less common. Delayed, focal acute lymphocytic vasculitis is an uncommon but striking pathologic finding that has been detected in small arteries in a variety of human tissues including the breast and gastrointestinal tract and has been described in the epicardium of swine after endovascular brachytherapy.[22] Transmural fibrosis seen in small arteries may represent the healed stage of necrotizing vasculitis.

LARGE ARTERIES AND VEINS

Radiation-induced morphologic changes in large muscular and elastic arteries are not frequently observed. Fibrosis and atheromas are difficult to distinguish from spontaneous atherosclerosis. Rupture of irradiated arterial walls is rare and, if it occurs,

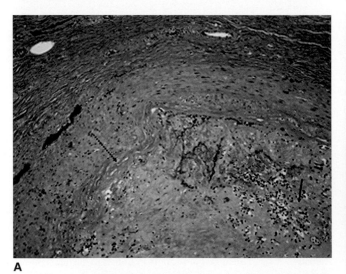

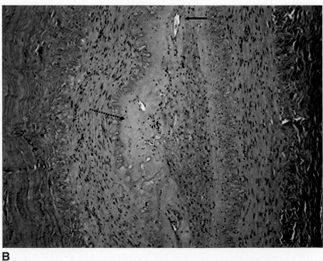

A

B

Figure 2.8. A: A low-power view (H&E, 100×) reveals postradiation histologic changes in a small artery. There is significant intimal proliferation, fibrosis (*dashed arrow*), and collections of macrophages (*arrow*). **B:** A low-power view of a cross section (H&E, 200×) of small artery shows postradiation vascular injury including marked intimal proliferation, fibrosis (*dashed arrow*), chronic inflammatory infiltration, and hyalinization with significant vascular luminal occlusion (*arrow*).

is usually a result of direct traumatic injury, such as surgery.[23] The venous segments of the vascular tree are the least affected by ionizing radiation

PATHOLOGIC FINDINGS IN SPECIFIC ORGANS

HEART AND GREAT VESSELS

Radiation-induced heart disease includes pericarditis, pericardial effusion, myocardial fibrosis, and coronary artery disease. Pericardial disease characterized by fibrosis and exudates was the most common delayed radiation injury to the heart but has now been surpassed by coronary artery disease. The histologic features of radiation-induced coronary artery disease are similar to those of atherosclerosis.[24–27]

LUNG

Radiation-induced lung disease is divided into two distinct entities: acute radiation pneumonitis (ARP) and pulmonary fibrosis (PF).[4,12,28,29] ARP is characterized by a markedly increased number of macrophages in alveolar spaces, mixed chronic inflammatory infiltration, fibroblasts in the alveolar septa, and type II pneumocyte hyperplasia with variable degree of associated atypia. Hyaline membranes (homogenous, acellular, and eosinophilic material) are identified lining the alveolar septa. The morphologic changes of ARP are identical to those of acute respiratory distress syndrome from diffuse alveolar injury.[15] Months or years after the development of ARP, irradiated lungs can progress to PF and show pathologic changes such as alveolar septa fibrosis, diffuse fibrotic areas, or scarred tissue replacing alveolar spaces and bronchiolitis obliterans. Unlike ARP, PF is observed as a sharply demarcated fibrous lesion within the previously irradiated site.

LIVER

Radiation-induced liver injury is characterized by a venoocclusive disease (VOD), which involves the central veins and afferent sinusoids of the lobules in the irradiated parenchyma. After irradiation, VOD is sharply limited to the exposed area, while after chemotherapy, a more diffuse VOD is seen.

KIDNEYS

Radiation-induced nephropathy is characterized by tubular atrophy, stromal fibrosis, diffuse glomerular sclerosis, vascular intimal proliferation with foamy cells, and arteriolar narrowing.[30–32]

NEOPLASIA

Radiation-induced malignancies include carcinomas, sarcomas, and hematopoietic malignancies.[12,33–35] When establishing a pathologic diagnosis of radiation-induced secondary malignancy, the tumor must develop within or adjacent to the radiation field. Radiation-induced carcinomas are most commonly observed in the following organs: thyroid, breast, lung, liver, skin, gastrointestinal tract, and ovary. Sarcomas are reported in the liver, uterus, breast, bone, and soft tissue. Benign and malignant tumors can develop in the central nervous system. Radiation-induced secondary malignancies look similar to their spontaneously arising malignancy. There are no distinguishing pathologic features that would suggest that these tumors arose in a previously irradiated organ or tissue. Radiation-induced carcinogenesis is discussed in detail in Chapter 7.

CONCLUSION

Radiation-induced morphologic alterations can be seen in nearly every organ and can be broadly categorized into injury of epithelial, stromal, and vascular tissues. Epithelial (parenchymal) postradiation changes commonly include atrophy, necrosis/ulceration, metaplasia, atypia, dysplasia, and neoplasia. Postradiation stromal (mesenchymal) changes include atypical fibroblastic cells, stromal fibrosis, fibrinous exudates, and stromal necrosis. Radiation-induced vascular changes include endothelial swelling, endothelial atypia, medial necrosis, medial hyalinizing/fibrosis, and microthrombus formation. None of these features are pathognomic in distinguishing radiation induced change from other disease processes, such as recurrent cancer. Knowledge of prior history of radiation exposure is essential for the examining pathologist to establish the correct diagnosis.

ACKNOWLEDGMENT

The authors would like to thank Luis F. Fajardo, MD, professor of Department of Pathology at Stanford University. Dr Fajardo has made numerous expert suggestions, modifications, and corrections during preparation of this chapter.

REFERENCES

1. Case JT. History of radiation therapy. *Prog Radiat Ther*. 1958;1:13–41.
2. Fajardo LF. Basic mechanisms and general morphology of radiation injury. *Semin Roentgenol*. 1993;28:297–302.
3. Fajardo LF. The pathology of ionizing radiation as defined by morphologic patterns. *Acta Oncol*. 2005;44:13–22.
4. Fajardo LF, Berthrong M. Radiation injury in surgical pathology. Part I. *Am J Surg Pathol*. 1978;2:159–199.
5. Berthrong M, Fajardo LF. Radiation injury in surgical pathology. Part II. Alimentary tract. *Am J Surg Pathol*. 1981;5:153–178.
6. Fajardo LF, Berthrong M. Radiation injury in surgical pathology. Part III. Salivary glands, pancreas and skin. *Am J Surg Pathol*. 1981;5:279–296.
7. Fajardo LF. Morphologic patterns of radiation injury. *Front Radiat Ther Oncol*. 1989;23:75–84.
8. Berthrong M. Pathologic changes secondary to radiation. *World J Surg*. 1986;10:155–170.
9. Bostwick DG, Egbert BM, Fajardo LF. Radiation injury of the normal and neoplastic prostate. *Am J Surg Pathol*. 1982;6:541–551.
10. Magi-Galluzzi C, Sanderson H, Epstein JI. Atypia in nonneoplastic prostate glands after radiotherapy for prostate cancer: duration of atypia and relation to type of radiotherapy. *Am J Surg Pathol*. 2003;27:206–212.
11. Bostwick DG, Meiers I. Diagnosis of prostatic carcinoma after therapy. *Arch Pathol Lab Med*. 2007;131:360–371.
12. Fajardo L, Berthong M, Anderson R. *Radiation Pathology*. Oxford: Oxford University Press; 2001.
13. Chaturvedi AK, Engels EA, Gilbert ES, et al. Second cancers among 104,760 survivors of cervical cancer: evaluation of long-term risk. *J Natl Cancer Inst*. 2007;99:1634–1643.
14. Ronckers CM, Erdmann CA, Land CE. Radiation and breast cancer: a review of current evidence. *Breast Cancer Res*. 2005;7:21–32.
15. DeMeester SR. Adenocarcinoma of the esophagus and cardia: a review of the disease and its treatment. *Ann Surg Oncol*. 2006;13:12–30.
16. Leupin N, Curschmann J, Kranzbuhler H, et al. Acute radiation colitis in patients treated with short-term preoperative radiotherapy for rectal cancer. *Am J Surg Pathol*. 2002;26:498–504.
17. Perry A, Schmidt RE. Cancer therapy-associated CNS neuropathology: an update and review of the literature. *Acta Neuropathol*. 2006;111:197–212.

20 *Section I • Radiobiology and Pathology or Irradiated Normal Tissues*

18. Nishioka H, Hirano A, Haraoka J, et al. Histological changes in the pituitary gland and adenomas following radiotherapy. *Neuropathology.* 2002;22:19–25.
19. Bindu L, Balaram P, Mathew A, et al. Radiation-induced changes in oral carcinoma cells—a multiparametric evaluation. *Cytopathology.* 2003;14:287–293.
20. Cupp JS, Koong AC, Fisher GA, et al. Tissue effects after stereotactic body radiotherapy using cyberknife for patients with abdominal malignancies. *Clin Oncol (R Coll Radiol).* 2008;20:69–75.
21. Schnitt SJ, Connolly JL, Khettry U, et al. Pathologic findings on re-excisions of the primary site in breast cancer patients considered for treatment by primary radiation therapy. *Cancer.* 1987;59:675–681.
22. Fajardo LF, Prionas SD, Kaluza GL, et al. Acute vasculitis after endovascular brachytherapy. *Int J Radiat Oncol Biol Phys.* 2002;53:714–719.
23. Fajardo LF, Lee A. Rupture of major vessels after radiation. *Cancer.* 1975;36:904–913.
24. Westerhof PW, van der Putte CJ. Radiation pericarditis and myocardial fibrosis. *Eur J Cardiol.* 1976;4:213–218.
25. Adams MJ, Lipshultz SE, Schwartz C, et al. Radiation-associated cardiovascular disease: manifestations and management. *Semin Radiat Oncol.* 2003;13:346–356.
26. Fajardo LF. Radiation-induced coronary artery disease. *Chest.* 1977;71:563–564.
27. Stewart JR, Fajardo LF, Gillette SM, et al. Radiation injury to the heart. *Int J Radiat Oncol Biol Phys.* 1995;31:1205–1211.
28. Katzenstein AL, Bloor CM, Leibow AA. Diffuse alveolar damage—the role of oxygen, shock, and related factors. A review. *Am J Pathol.* 1976;85:209–228.
29. Davis SD, Yankelevitz DF, Henschke CI. Radiation effects on the lung: clinical features, pathology, and imaging findings. *Am J Roentgenol.* 1992;159:1157–1164.
30. Cassady JR. Clinical radiation nephropathy. *Int J Radiat Oncol Biol Phys.* 1995;31:1249–1256.
31. Willett CG, Tepper JE, Orlow EL, et al. Renal complications secondary to radiation treatment of upper abdominal malignancies. *Int J Radiat Oncol Biol Phys.* 1986;12:1601–1604.
32. Zuelzer WW, Palmer HD, Newton WA Jr. Unusual glomerulonephritis in young children probably radiation nephritis. *Am J Pathol.* 1950;26:1019–1039.
33. Fajardo LF. Ionizing radiation and neoplasia. *Monogr Pathol.* 1986:97–125.
34. Belka C, Budach W, Kortmann RD, et al. Radiation induced CNS toxicity—molecular and cellular mechanisms. *Br J Cancer.* 2001;85:1233–1239.
35. Preston DL, Ron E, Tokuoka S, et al. Solid cancer incidence in atomic bomb survivors: 1958–1998. *Radiat Res.* 2007;168:1–64.

Normal Tissue Radiobiology: Animal Models of Radiation Injury

INTRODUCTION

The options for large-scale studies of the various aspects of exposure to ionizing radiation in humans are highly limited and, in many cases, ethically prohibited. On the other hand, many facets of the radiation response of living organisms cannot be studied in vitro cell or organ culture systems, as the latter lack the influence and integrated contribution of the whole organism to the development and expression of injury, as well as its modulation and repair. Therefore, animal models provide an invaluable resource for identifying and quantifying the wide range of effects of ionizing radiation at all levels of the response, that is, molecular, cellular, organ, and organism. Additionally, several models have been developed permitting the quantitative analyses of the relationship between dose, dose rate or fractionation, radiation quality, and other exposure scenarios and the various effects of the exposure on tissues and organisms. As pertains to in vitro studies, in vivo studies not only have shown that response is governed by physical factors such as radiation dose rate and quality but also have revealed pronounced differences in how specific tissues and organs respond to the exposure. This provides a precious basis for developing strategies to modulate response, which may then—after careful testing—be translated into similar approaches in humans exposed, accidentally, intentionally, or unavoidably, for example, during radiotherapy. Animal models also provide powerful tools for identifying the role of specific genes and gene products and their integration in pathogenetic networks in the development of injury. Information derived from experimental animal studies in rodents and larger mammals has significantly impacted the fields of radiation therapy, radiation risk estimates, and radiation protection.

The value and relevance of animal models for elucidating radiation injury in humans arise from the similarity of their responses to radiation at the cellular, tissue, and organism level, and the relatively short time over which radiation damage is manifest, especially in rodent models. In addition to the biologic similarities, economy favors the use of small animal models for studies of quantitative aspects of radiation injury and protection, especially those requiring very substantial numbers of test subjects.

Upon receiving whole-body irradiation (WBI), mice, rats, and other mammals, including humans, exhibit and eventually die of the same radiation syndromes: hematopoietic, gastrointestinal (GI), and cerebrovascular. In addition, either as a consequence of the failure of these systems or due to direct radiation damage, other organs or organ systems such as skin, mucocutaneous tissue, liver, kidney, respiratory, and the cardiovascular systems may exhibit severe changes and failure. This pertains to all mammalian species including humans.[1] Even at very low doses, some tissues may display clinically relevant changes, that is, the formation of cataract in the eye lens (reviewed in Ref. 2), or changes in the reproductive system.[3] These, however, are usually expressed at much later time points after irradiation.

The rank order of the threshold doses for eliciting the hematopoietic, GI, and cerebrovascular syndromes is the same across species, as are the sequence and relative time periods postirradiation for the development of injury and mortality from each syndrome. Mouse strains exhibiting varying responses to radiation are particularly useful for assessing and identifying the mechanisms and pathobiology of radiation injury. An increasing number of genetically modified rodent models, both knockout and transgenic, as well as options for the conditional knockout or activation of genes in the adult organism have more recently complemented these strain-specific differences. Larger animals including nonhuman primates will continue to be useful for validation of the efficacy of promising radioprotectors, mitigators, or therapeutics of injury, after such strategies have been developed and screened in rodent models.

This chapter briefly examines the use and the potential of animal models to characterize and quantitate radiation injury; the principles derived from these studies, and gives perspectives of how novel methodologies in biological research, physical administration of irradiation (e.g., high precision treatment facilities for small animals), and morphologic (small animal CT, MRI) and functional imaging (small animal PET, SPECT) will impact future radiobiological studies.

A LETHAL DOSE OF RADIATION: THE HEMATOPOIETIC SYNDROME

In the event of accidental or intentional whole-body exposure to ionizing radiation, severe radiation sickness and death via the hematopoietic syndrome occur at dose levels that do not sufficiently damage any other organ system to lead to death. At somewhat higher doses, damage to the epithelia of the GI tract (GI syndrome) may lead to significant morbidity and mortality at post-irradiation intervals before damage to the hematopoietic system becomes life threatening. At doses that markedly exceed the threshold doses for induction of the hematopoietic and GI syndromes, death may occur within a few to several hours due to cerebrovascular damage.

Radiation-induced bone marrow injury leads to hemorrhaging, leukopenia with consequent infection, and anemia. The biological basis is the reproductive sterilization of hematopoietic stem cells, which primarily reside in the bone marrow. These stem cells—by definition—retain the capacity to self-renew as well as to give rise to the progenitor cells of the lymphoid and myeloid series. Progenitors have only a limited proliferative capacity. Lymphoid progenitor cells produce T- and B-lymphocytes, and natural killer (NK) cells. They may also repopulate other lymphatic organs such as the spleen and lymph nodes. Myeloid progenitor cells produce granulocyte-macrophage progenitors and erythroid megakaryocyte progenitors. The latter progenitor gives rise to mature red blood cells and platelets; the former to neutrophils, eosinophils, basophils, and macrophages.

With the exception of the multipotent stem cells, all bone marrow progenitors are relatively sensitive to radiation, with the mature lymphocyte and its lymphocytic progenitor being especially sensitive. Unlike most other cell types, cells of the lymphocytic series die via an apoptotic process; a dose of 0.5 Gy or less leads to a measurable decrease in the circulating lymphocyte population. Following an LD_{50} dose of radiation (dose at which death is expected in 50% of the exposed individuals and approximately 7 Gy in several mouse strains), the numbers of circulating granulocytes, thrombocytes, and erythrocytes decrease at a rate that reflects their normal blood lifespan. Due to the relatively long lifespan of the mature red blood cells, anemia develops after leucopenia and thrombocytopenia, and may reach a minimum as the other circulating blood elements are returning to normal, due to the reconstitution of their surviving progenitor pools. Anemia may be exacerbated due to bleeding that along with infection is a common complication and cause of death.

Studies into the effects of radiation on the hematopoietic system were stimulated by observations of the symptoms and causes of death occurring several weeks to a few months following the atomic bombing at Hiroshima and Nagasaki. Soon following Hiroshima and Nagasaki, in the late 1940s it was shown that WBI of mice induces many of the same clinical symptoms and hematopoietic changes observed in humans,[4] including reduced blood white cell counts, infections, and bleeding. Additionally, animal experiments demonstrated that shielding of a bone or the spleen of rodents exposed to WBI substantially reduces the severity and lethality of WBI. Shortly thereafter, it was shown that injection of bone marrow from donor mice into lethally irradiated host mice led to donor repopulation of the host marrow and protected against the hematopoietic syndrome.[5]

In the early 1960s, McCulloch and Till[6,7] developed procedures for directly and quantitatively assessing the relationship between the clonogenic survival of bone marrow cells and radiation dose. These investigators irradiated recipient mice to a dose of radiation that would lead to death from the bone marrow syndrome approximately 15 days later, but which was below the dose that would lead to the more rapidly lethal GI syndrome. Following irradiation, the mice were tail vein injected with bone marrow cells obtained from nonirradiated donor mice. Approximately 8 to 12 days later, the recipient mice were killed, at which time a number of macroscopic bone marrow colonies were found on the surface of the spleen (colony-forming units—spleen, CFU-S). As the number of spleen colonies was directly dependent on the number of injected marrow cells, they were able to determine the fraction of proliferative marrow cells killed per unit dose of radiation. With the spleen colony formation assay, donor mice may be exposed to various whole-body doses of irradiation, the marrow removed, cells counted, and injected into the lethally irradiated recipient mice; alternatively, the marrow of donor mice may be removed, irradiated in vitro, and then injected into the recipient mice. The spleen colony assay is conceptually similar to other elegant in vivo to in vivo dose-response assays, such as the mammary gland and thyroid stem cell assays[8,9] and lung colony assay for assessing the sensitivity of tumor cells.[10]

In addition to these in vivo to in vivo stem cell transfer assays, several quantitative in situ assays have been developed for assessing the sensitivity of normal tissue stem cells by Withers and Withers et al.,[11–14] including spermatogenic, kidney tubule, epidermis, and jejunal crypt stem cells. Functional assays have been developed for assessing early and late damage to a variety of organs including skin,[15] lung,[16] spinal cord,[17] kidney,[18] Robbins and Hopewell,[19] and heart.[20,21] These assays have repeatedly been employed to evaluate the radiosensitivity of these organs to various types of radiation, for example, low and high linear energy transfer (LET) radiation, as well as various dose fractionation schemes and volume effect studies, and potential modulators of sensitivity. In general, the radiosensitivity parameters of a particular cell type differ little whether irradiated in vivo and assessed in vivo or in vitro, or irradiated in vitro and assessed in vitro or in vivo.

Figure 3.1 shows the relationship between the radiation dose and the survival of spleen colony-forming bone marrow cells.[7] Unlike several cell types, bone marrow–derived CFU-S have a limited ability to sustain sublethal radiation damage in the low-dose region, and as pertains to all cell types, at higher doses, cell killing increases exponentially with increasing dose. The D_0 dose, which is the dose that reduces the surviving fraction by a factor of "e" or approximately 63% in the exponential portion of the survival curve, is approximately 0.95 Gy. Table 3.1 shows the dose of radiation leading to 50% mortality (LD_{50}) in various species, and the estimated number of transplanted bone marrow cells required for rescue, per kg body-weight.[22] An inverse correlation is observed between the LD_{50} of a species and its body-weight. The data superficially suggest that, for example, human bone marrow may be more sensitive to radiation than mouse bone marrow. However, this interpretation is inconsistent with the number of transplanted bone marrow cells needed to rescue the various species from death following a lethal dose of radiation. Ten times more human bone marrow cells are required to rescue humans from lethality than to rescue mice, per kg body-weight, suggesting that the stem cell concentration is approximately ten times higher in the mice than humans per unit weight.

The role of bone marrow–derived spleen colony-forming cells in the development of and rescue from the hematopoietic syndrome has been directly demonstrated by the reinjection of a single spleen colony into a lethally irradiated recipient. The injected cells retain the capacity to produce sufficient functional

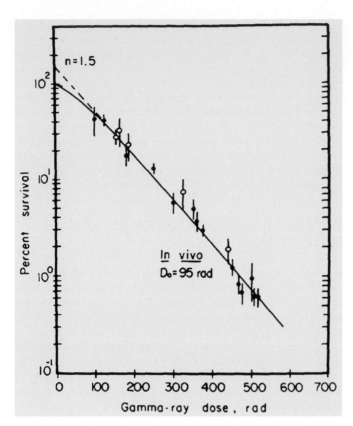

Figure 3.1. In vivo bone marrow cell survival curve. The bone marrow of mice exposed to various doses of WBI was removed and intravenously injected into lethally irradiated recipient mice. The recipient mice were killed 8 to 12 days later, prior to the onset of radiation-induced death, and the number of donor bone marrow colonies growing in the spleen was counted. Bone marrow progenitor cells exhibit a limited capacity to sustain radiation damage sublethally. From McCulloch JE, Till JE. The sensitivity of cells from normal mouse bone marrow to gamma radiation in vitro and in vivo. *Radiat Res.* 1962;16:822–832.

long-term engraftment. Jones et al.[23] transplanted male CFU-S cells and various bone marrow subtractions into lethally irradiated female mice. Survival and long-term engraftment of host marrow and other hematopoietic organs was evaluated with a Y chromosome–specific probe. These studies demonstrated that two classes of cells are required for long-term engraftment and survival, that is, committed progenitors that sustain the host through the initial aplasia, and more primitive stem cells with long-term multilineage repopulating ability, which give rise to long-term engraftment, few of which are found in 8 to 12 day old spleen colonies. Various marrow fractionation procedures such as magnetic enrichment of cells bound to iron-labeled antibodies to specific cell markers as well as cell sorting of fluorescent-labeled antibodies to specific markers or combinations of markers, have been developed to fractionate both bone marrow and peripheral blood into specific highly enriched cell subpopulations. This has facilitated the assessment of the hematopoietic hierarchy, the functions and interaction of the various lineages, and substantially contributed to the clinical application of hematopoietic rescue procedures in the treatment of diseases such as leukemia.

In the therapeutic use of WBI followed by donor rescue, irradiation is frequently given in a slightly protracted fractionation schedule over several days to minimize side effects of normal tissue damage to radiosensitive organs such as the lung, liver, kidney, and eye lens. However, for the same total dose, more relapses occur with fractionated versus single-dose schedules, along with increased rejection of allogeneic grafts. This has necessitated an increase in the WBI dose with associated increased normal tissue damage. A variety of in vitro and in vivo assays have been developed to assess the response of the more primitive stem cells compartment of bone marrow.[24–26] Down et al.[26] examined the single and fractionated dose radiation sensitivity of various subsets of bone marrow cells. Unlike the more differentiated bone marrow cells, the slowly proliferating stem cells exhibited a substantially greater radiation resistance and capacity to recover from sublethal radiation damage. The substantial capacity to sustain and recover sublethal radiation damage is a common feature of several late-reacting normal tissues.

The more differentiated and sensitive spleen colony–forming cells exhibit significant apoptotic death, which has been shown to involve a P53-dependent pathway. Westphal et al.[27] evaluated the radiation sensitivity of the latter cells, both in vitro and in vivo. P53 null mice were more resistant to lethal

myeloid and lymphoid cells to rescue the recipient mice from the acute phase of the hematopoietic syndrome. Nevertheless, even though spleen colony cells possess a significant regenerative and proliferative capacity, it is not unlimited. Several studies have established that an earlier multipotent stem cell that may not be present in the 8 to 12 day old spleen colony is required for

TABLE 3.1	Dose of Radiation Causing 50% Lethality the Hematopoietic Syndrome, and Number of Transplanted Bone Marrow Cells Required for Rescue		
Species	Body Weight (kg)	LD_{50} (Gy)	Rescue Dose (cells × 10⁻⁶/kg body weight)
Mouse	0.025	7	2
Rat	0.20	6.75	3
Rhesus monkey	2.8	5.25	7.5
Dog	12	3.7	17.5
Human	70	4	20

Modified from Vriesendorp HM, van Bekkum DW. Susceptibility to total body irradiation. In Broerse JJ, MacVittae T, eds. *Response to Total Body Irradiation in Different Species.* Amsterdam: Martinus Nijhoff, 1984.

doses of WBI than wild-type mice of the parental strain, likely due to reduced apoptosis.

Substantial mouse strain–dependent differences in response to radiation have been observed for a number of organs and tissues and have proven useful for identifying the critical target cell populations and mechanisms of variable radiation sensitivity. The dose leading to 50% lethality in 30 days, $LD_{50/30}$ (most deaths via the hematopoietic syndrome in mice occur in 10–30 days postradiation), is significantly lower for BALB/c mice than pertains to most mouse strains. In an analysis of the repair of radiation-induced DNA double-strand breaks, Okayasu et al.[28] found that DNA repair proficiency was reduced in BALB/c mice along with their $LD_{50/30}$ versus more resistant strains. Similarly, severe combined immuno-deficient (SCID) mice exhibit a pronounced defect in DNA double-strand break repair, and a markedly reduced ($LD_{50/30}$) following WBI. The repair deficiency in SCID mice arises from a mutation in the gene which codes for the DNA double-strand break repair protein DNA-PK_{CS}.

In addition to various strains of wild-type as well as knockout and transgenic mice, immunocompromised mice such as the SCID and Rag mouse strains are being developed and utilized to support the growth of the complete human hematopoietic system.[29,30] These chimeric models provide an additional resource for a more detailed understanding of the human hematopoietic system: its hierarchy, regulation, and function.

THE GASTROINTESTINAL AND THE MUCOCUTANEOUS SYNDROME

The epithelia of the GI tract, oral cavity, esophagus, and the skin are—similar to the bone marrow—turnover tissues, with tissue-specific stem cells, transit cells with a limited prolifera-tive capacity (similar to progenitor cells in the bone marrow), and postmitotic functional epithelial cells that differentiate and are eventually lost at the surface due to mechanical and chemical stress. However, a variety of animal experiments in various models as well as clinical observations demonstrated that despite a similar radiosensitivity, the clinical symptoms and their biological basis are largely different between the GI tract and other mucosa or the epidermis. This has recently led to a differentiation between the GI syndrome and the mucocutane-ous syndrome.[31,32]

Both syndromes develop after exposure of large volumes of intestine or significant areas of skin or mucosa to single doses in the range of >10 Gy. In the GI tract, the loss of epithelial function preceding epithelial cell loss primarily results in mal-absorption. The consequence is diarrhea as the lead symptom. In the later course, besides severe dehydration, infections are seen, also promoted by an impairment of immune function during the developing hematopoietic syndrome.

In contrast, in oral mucosa and epidermis, ulceration, that is, epithelial denudation, develops, which—depending on exposed area and dose—are associated with severe pain and fluid loss and are prone to infection, which can also progress into systemic septicemia.

Animal models for GI or mucocutaneous reactions to total or large-field partial body irradiation have been established as early as those for the hematopoietic syndrome. These include irradiation of pig and rodent skin, or abdominal or upper body irradiation of rodents. In many of these early studies, lethality

was used as an endpoint. Following total body or regional abdominal irradiation, LD_{50} values for death in mice via the GI syndrome are in the range of 10 to 13 Gy, depending on the quality of x-irradiation, that is, orthovoltage or megavoltage and the particular strain of mouse investigated. Goepp and Fitch[33] proved the relevance of oral mucositis for the survival of mice after irradiation of the head. For total head irradiation of mice including the oral cavity, LD_{50} values are 4 to 6 Gy higher, and death occurs 4 to 5 days later than pertains to the GI syndrome. Gross and microscopic changes observed in several organs were delayed by 5 days but otherwise similar to those found in mice following complete deprivation of food and water.

PATHOGENESIS OF NORMAL TISSUE RADIATION EFFECTS

It must be noted, that in general, most studies of the pathogen-esis of normal tissue radiation responses are based on irradia-tion of individual organs, in contrast to the above-mentioned investigations of large volume or total body irradiation. In the latter situation, the combined pathobiology eventually resulting in multiorgan involvement is different, particularly because of the contribution of radiation effects on the immune system. In consequence, the radiopathology, and also the radiobiological parameters, for example, the fractionation effect, are different from a scenario of single or even partial organ irradiation.

As pathogenetic investigations in humans are not easy to perform and are mainly restricted to patients receiving radio-therapy, most of our knowledge of radiation pathogenesis is based on studies of animal models. These investigations were not only used to characterize the pathogenesis of normal tissue effects, but also the radiobiological factors affecting these effects (fractionation, dose rate, radiation quality, time factor), and ways to modify the normal tissue response. The development of modern molecular techniques, the pathogenetic pathways, and the interaction between various pathogenetic networks can be described. This is the basis for specific biology-based inter-ventions to ameliorate radiation side effects. These, in return, have to be tested in suitable normal tissue animal models. More recently, with the assistance of progress in the precision of administration of radiation and the resolution of modern imag-ing techniques, animal models of partial organ irradiation have been developed for studies into the volume effect.

With regard to the time course of radiation effects in normal tissues, early (acute) and late (chronic) effects must be distin-guished. The former occur during or shortly after a course of radiotherapy or other radiation exposure. The latter, in con-trast, only become clinically visible after latent times of months to years, even in experimental animals. This classification is pri-marily based on the time of first diagnosis. However, early and late effects also have different general (radio)biological charac-teristics, which distinguish them.[34]

Early effects are usually found in tissues with permanent pro-liferation that counteracts ongoing physiological cell loss (turn-over tissues), such as bone marrow, epidermis, or mucosa of the upper and lower intestinal tract. They form the basis of the lead syndromes of the acute radiation disease, as described above. The manifestation of radiation effects is based on a radiation-induced reduction in cell proliferation due to the killing of stem cells, while cell loss, which is usually independent of the radiation exposure, continues at its physiological rate over a wide dose range. The consequence of this imbalance is a progressive cell depletion eventually resulting in complete loss of functional cells. Regularly, inflammatory changes accompany the response. Healing, which is usually complete after irradiation of smaller volumes/areas, like in radiotherapy, is based on the proliferation of surviving cells within the irradiated volume or migration of cells from unirradiated tissue and into the irradiated field. More recently, a role for circulating hematopoietic or mesenchymal stem cells has been identified.[35]

Late radiation side effects are essentially found in all organs. Their pathobiology is more complex compared to early effects. The dominating changes occur in the parenchyma of the organs, *that is*, in the tissue-specific compartments, and also in the connective and vascular tissues. Regularly, the immune system (macrophages, mast cells) contributes to the tissue reaction. Late radiation effects hence represent a multifaceted, orchestrated response with various components.[34] Late radiation sequelae, in contrast to early effects, with few exceptions, are irreversible and progressive, with increasing severity observed with longer follow-up times. Moreover, the latent time from irradiation to clinical manifestation is inversely dependent on dose. In general, early and late radiation effects are independent with regard to their pathogenesis, and conclusions from the severity of early reactions on the risk of late effects cannot be drawn. However, in some organ systems, interactions between the early and the chronic component of the radiation response can occur, resulting in *consequential late effects (CLEs)*. This is the case when the early-responding tissue compartments (e.g., epithelia) have a protective function against mechanical and/or chemical exposure. This barrier function is impaired during the acute radiation reaction due to cell depletion. In consequence, secondary trauma can impact on the target structures of the late sequelae (connective tissue, vasculature) in addition to the direct effects of radiation, which can then aggravate the late radiation response. CLEs have been demonstrated in animal models and patients for intestine, urinary tract, oral mucosa, and particularly stressed skin localizations.[34,36]

THE FRACTIONATION EFFECT —RECOVERY PHENOMENA

When clinical treatment plans were developed in the 1970s to alter the number of fractions per week, for example from 5 to 2, it was observed that although the early normal tissue effects were similar, there was a pronounced increase in late normal tissue morbidity. Concurrent with these clinical observations, a number of comprehensive experimental studies quantitatively examined the relationship between total dose, dose per fraction, and the manifestation of early and long-term normal tissue reactions in a variety of animal models for a variety of functional and morphological endpoints.[37]

The results obtained by various investigators in rodent models are summarized in Figure 3.2.[38,39] The solid lines in Figure 3.2 pertain to late endpoints, while the dashed lines show early responses. Changes in dose per fraction differentially affect the frequency or severity of early versus late normal tissue reactions. For tissues such as lung, kidney, spinal cord, and skin (fibrosis), a decrease in the dose per fraction allows for a markedly greater total dose to elicit the same response. For early-reacting tissues such as epidermis (skin desquamation), jejunum, or bone marrow, a substantially smaller increase in

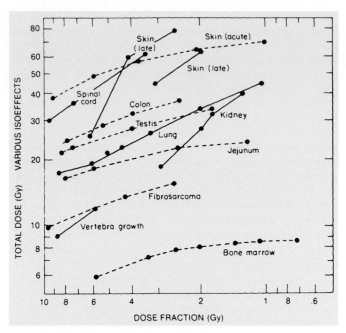

Figure 3.2. Total dose required to produce the same effect as a function of dose per fraction for various early (*dashed curve*) and late tissue reactions (*solid curve*). The possible influence of regeneration during the multifraction experiments was excluded by experimental design. For late tissue reactions, the increase in total dose with decreasing dose per fraction is more pronounced than pertains to early-reacting tissues and reactions. These results indicate the critical target cells for late tissue reactions exhibit a greater capacity to sustain and repair sublethal radiation damage with decreasing dose per fraction. From Withers HR. Biologic basis for altered fractionated schemes. *Cancer.* 1985;55:2086–2095, with permission.

total dose can elicit the same response, as the dose per fraction decreases. In other words, isoeffective total doses increase with a decrease in dose per fraction (equivalent to an increase in the number of fractions), and this increase is substantially more pronounced for late radiation effects.

As a consequence, when dose is administered in fewer large doses per fraction, and the total dose is adjusted to maintain the same acute morbidity, late-reacting tissue will exhibit substantially more damage. In cases where late normal tissue reactions limit dose, a reduction in dose per fraction thus may allow an increase in the biologically equivalent dose to the tumor, for the same level of late normal tissue damage. These observations, particularly in animal models where complete dose effect curves for various endpoints can be generated, have resulted in the development of mathematical models for the description of single and fractionated dose effects. The linear-quadratic model[40] is currently the accepted model for isoeffect calculations. Examples for the application of this model can be found in Hall and Giaccia,[41] Joiner and Bentzen,[37] and Bentzen and Joiner[42] and are further discussed in Chapter 4. In careful comparisons with results of the respective analyses of clinical data, it was demonstrated that the main parameter of this model, the α/β-ratio, can be quantitatively translated across species. For early normal tissue injuries, the value of α/β is in the range of 6 to 14 Gy. In contrast, for late normal tissue reactions, α/β values are in the range of 1.5 to 6 Gy.

Most experimental studies assessing the effect of variable-dose fractionation protocols have been performed with doses per fraction ranging from approximately 2 Gy to substantially larger doses per fraction. Results obtained from high dose per fraction data may not be appropriate for calculating the total dose required to achieve the same effect, when employing doses per fraction significantly <2 Gy, as it may underestimate the increasingly predominant effect of the alpha component with decreasing dose per fraction.[43,44] Tucker and Thames[45] reviewed experimental data for a variety of tissues, and the factors influencing the dose per fraction below which a sparing effect of fractionation was unlikely to be resolved. Due to statistical probabilities, tissue heterogeneity, and the number of subjects evaluated at each dose, they concluded that for the analyzed data, an additional sparing effect of decreasing dose per fraction would not likely be resolved when the dose per fraction decreased below $0.05 \times \alpha/\beta$. This again emphasizes the relatively greater sparing effect observed in low α/β versus high α/β tissue, with decreasing dose per fraction.

Linear-quadratic calculations are based on the assumption of complete recovery of the sublethal damage between fractions. Decades of experimental studies in animal models for a variety of endpoints have shown that recovery follows an exponential function. Repair data are well fit to a monoexponential function in most tissues, although a better fit to the data in a limited number of tissues is provided by a biexponential, which is described by either one (monoexponential) or two (biexponential) half-times of repair. In contrast to α/β values, which appear to be quantitatively transferable between species, comparison of experimental and clinical data indicates that halftimes of recovery are shorter in experimental animals, particularly rodents. Usually, halftimes are in the range of a few hours. As a rule of thumb, intervals between fractions in multiple-fractions-per-day protocols should be at least 6 hours in order to allow for complete recovery. For some tissues, such as spinal cord, even longer intervals would be desirable.

THE EFFECT OF OVERALL TREATMENT TIME—NORMAL TISSUE REPOPULATION

A prolongation of the overall treatment time in radiotherapy results in an increase in radiation tolerance of early-responding turnover tissues. This phenomenon is called *normal tissue repopulation*. The detailed quantitative description and the characterization of the underlying mechanisms are almost exclusively based on studies in animal models. In particular, mouse oral mucosa has been used as a model of oral mucositis in head-and-neck cancer patients, but further investigations have also been performed in mouse epidermis, rat epidermis, pig epidermis, and mouse lip mucosa.[46,47] A similar time course of changes in isoeffective doses with increasing overall treatment time was observed in all these tissues, as schematically displayed in Figure 3.3. Tolerance remained constant within the initial treatment period and subsequently increased almost linearly. The time of onset of this increase was tissue dependent, with 5 to 7 days in mouse oral mucosa and skin, and 20 to 30 days in rat and pig skin.[46] The capacity of repopulation, once these processes have started, was estimated by Dörr[47,48] in terms of the dose (number of 2 Gy-fractions) compensated per day. In human oral mucosa, 0.5 to 1 fractions are counteracted per day. Experimental data indicate similar numbers—close to

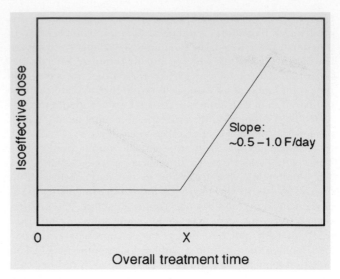

Figure 3.3. Schematic presentation of the time course of repopulation in turnover tissues. The dose required to induce a defined effect (isoeffective dose) remains constant over a certain time interval (0…X), which is tissue specific, but also dose dependent. Once repopulation becomes effective (time X), isoeffective doses increase constantly. The increase amounts to the equivalent of ca. 0.5 to 1 fractions of 2 Gy/day.

one fraction of 2 Gy/day—for all tissues studied with few exceptions. In some studies, where various weekly doses were applied, dependence of the repopulation rate on the dose intensity (Gy/week) was observed.[47]

In oral mucosa, changes in mucosal cell density and proliferation have been studied in detail (summarized in Ref. 49). A decrease in cell numbers to ca. 70% occurred during the first week of daily fractionated treatment. Subsequently, constant to increasing numbers were found, despite the continued irradiation at the same doses. In good agreement, mucosal proliferation was significantly suppressed during the first week and subsequently returned to subnormal to near normal values. Similar observations were made in other tissues.[50] In good accordance, in human oral mucosa, a reduction of cell production and consequently a steep decline in cell numbers were observed over the initial week of radiotherapy.[51] Subsequently, proliferation rates were partially restored and cell depletion occurred significantly slower.

With regard to the biological mechanisms underlying repopulation, three observations have been made accordingly in animal and clinical studies: (a) Dose is compensated with increasing overall treatment time once repopulation has become effective, indicating a net production of tissue stem cells, which define tissue tolerance. This must be based on the production of two new stem cells, rather than only one stem cell daughter, per stem cell division, that is, a loss of the division asymmetry. (b) The rate at which this compensation occurs is in the range of 5 × 2 Gy/week, indicating five symmetrical stem cell divisions per week, and hence accelerated stem cell proliferation. (c) The physiological loss of cells from the tissue is counteracted after the lag phase of repopulation, resulting in reduced but nearly constant cell numbers. This can only be explained by a residual proliferative activity (abortive divisions) of doomed cells. In general, the mechanisms of repopulation can be summarized as three A's: *a*symmetry loss, *a*cceleration of stem cell divisions, and *a*bortive divisions.[49,52]

The question of the regulation of these processes remains. It has been demonstrated that the lag time before repopulation is shorter, the higher the radiation dose is.[47,53] Hence, the stem cell depletion rate may regulate the onset of repopulation based on autoregulatory processes within the stem cell compartment. Acceleration of stem cell divisions may be caused by overall cell depletion and impairment of the epithelial barrier function, mediated via an increase in the signals that physiologically regulate proliferation. The stem cell proliferation rate then translates into the initial rate of abortive divisions of sterilized cells. However, the doomed cells may also directly respond to paracrine signals released due to tissue hypoplasia.[34]

INHOMOGENEOUS DOSE DISTRIBUTIONS—THE VOLUME EFFECT

Enormous progress in the precision of conformal administration of irradiation to the clinical tumor volume has mainly been based on developments in the technologies of computer-assisted diagnoses, treatment planning, and delivery. This resulted in a move from relatively simple geometries of the irradiated volumes, for example, four-field boxes, to highly complex geometries achieved with modern multiple-field irradiations or intensity-modulated radiotherapy. Even more recently, image-guided radiotherapy (IGRT), that is, adaptation of the dose distribution to (at least almost) real-time imaging and comparison with the planned distribution, has been introduced. These developments were associated with a move from more homogeneous distribution of the doses within total or large parts of normal tissues and organs to highly complex dose inhomogeneities. These are usually summarized by dose volume histograms (DVHs), and DVH parameters are frequently applied to estimate normal tissue complication probability (NTCP models). The validity of these NTCP models, however, has still to be demonstrated.[54]

One excellent option to improve the NTCP model parameters, and to improve the modeling strategies, is the use of animal models. Initially, due to experimental methods available, these volume studies of partial organ irradiation have been carried out in large animal models. Based on the recent development of experimental technologies for diagnostic procedures and administration of irradiation, with a slight delay compared to clinical developments, such studies can now also be performed in small animals. For example, intensive studies on the volume effect in spinal cord have been carried out with a high-precision proton beam (examples in Ref. 54). Moreover, detailed studies on the volume effect in mouse lung have been performed based on precise planning of the dose delivery based on CT scans.[55,56] High-precision photon therapy facilities for the irradiation of small animals, including options for IGRT, are already commercially available, allowing for even more precise and detailed animal studies into the volume effects in various organs. The latter particularly includes regional variations of radiosensitivity within the organs, which have been shown, for example, for lung[55,56] and CNS.[57] These are currently—among other factors—ignored by NTCP models.

BIOLOGICAL RESPONSE MODIFICATION

The effective modification of normal tissue radiation effects is closely connected with the characterization of the underlying pathobiology and pathophysiology. Options for interventions are given at any of the pathogenetic steps, from the very early induction of radicals to the delayed proliferative changes in early-reacting tissues or even the chronic fibrotic remodeling.[52] An essential prerequisite for the development and validation of such strategies is adequate animal models. Currently, the vast majority of approaches to modify normal tissue side effects is purely experimental and still has to be validated in clinical studies.

One major prerequisite for the reasonable application of normal tissue response modifiers is the association with a therapeutic gain. This can be either achieved by selectivity for normal tissues and hence exclusion of similar effects in tumors, or by an at least relatively higher effect on normal tissues compared to tumors.

Most of the (in vivo) studies on biological response modification in normal tissues have been performed with single-dose irradiation. Besides scenarios of radiological accidents or attacks, there are only few situations where this is relevant for radiation oncology. These include stereotactic radiotherapy, intraoperative irradiation, brachytherapy with few high dose fractions, and perhaps treatments given over short time periods, such as total body irradiation as a conditioning treatment for stem/progenitor cell transplantation.

For application to standard external radiotherapy, protection and mitigation strategies must be tested using experimental fractionation protocols as close to the clinical situation as possible, that is, comprising daily fractionation with doses in the clinical range, administered over several weeks. The latter is required, for example, in order to test for potential interactions, beneficial or counterproductive, with repopulation processes (see above). Modification approaches must also be tested for endpoints that are clinically relevant.

The experimental approaches that can be found in the literature have recently been summarized in Ref. 52. Approaches to induce systemic or local hypoxia, thus increasing cellular radiation tolerance, have been found effective. Data on the administration of radical scavengers (e.g., amifostine) or cellular detoxifiers (superoxide dismutase, selenium) are controversial. More recently, growth factors and inhibitors of growth factor receptors have become available for modulation of specific signaling pathways. A variety of growth factors has been studied for their potential to modulate normal tissue effects of radiotherapy. Most prominent examples are hematopoietic growth factors (granulocyte colony-stimulating factor [G-CSF], granulocyte–macrophage colony–stimulating factors [GM-CSF]) to ameliorate radiation effects in the bone marrow, but also in other tissues, such as oral mucosa. Keratinocyte growth factor (KGF) has been demonstrated to effectively ameliorate the radiation response of oral and other mucosal membranes.[48] In the central nervous system and the kidney, insulin-like growth factor-1 and platelet-derived growth factor have been suggested for the prevention of radiation-induced necrosis.

Several interleukins, as well as angiogenic growth factors, such as FGF-1 and FGF-2 and vascular endothelial growth factor, and others have been proposed for the modification of GI reactions to irradiation. Among the most prominent growth factor signaling cascades for which an upregulation in early-responding normal tissues after irradiation has been observed, are the epidermal growth factor pathway (upregulation of the receptor EGFR) and the tumor necrosis factor-α pathway (upregulation of the growth factor). For late-responding tissues, a significant stimulation of transforming growth factor β has been reported. These processes hence may be targeted in order to modify normal tissue radiation effects. The efficacy of such strategies, however, must be validated in animal studies (e.g., Ref. 58).

The severity of early radiation effects during fractionated irradiation is clearly connected to the efficacy of repopulation (see above). Therefore, stimulation of proliferation has been suggested to reduce early tissue injury. Besides the administration of growth factors such as KGF, removal of the superficial epithelial layers in order to increase the normal trigger for proliferation was tested. When fractionated irradiation was applied, stimulated proliferation translated into an increased radiation tolerance, which was attributed to an earlier onset of repopulation processes.[53] Alternatively, low-level laser treatment was successfully administered to oral mucosa in head-and-neck cancer patients to remove superficial material, as reviewed by Genot and Klastersky.[59] The angiotensin system appears to be involved in the development of fibrosis, at least in the lung and the kidney. Therefore, angiotensin-converting enzyme inhibitors and antagonists of the angiotensin II receptor were tested for their potential to mitigate or treat late radiation effects in rat models.[60,61] The drugs have been shown to be effective in the prevention and treatment of kidney sequelae of irradiation.[61]

A novel, potentially selective approach for the amelioration of normal tissue radiation effects is the treatment with (adult) stem cells. This includes the administration of bone marrow (i.e., hematopoietic plus mesenchymal stem cells) or mesenchymal stem cells, or the mobilization of autologous stem cells by growth factors, for example, G-CSF. These strategies have been tested in preclinical models of radiation injury in skin, salivary glands, intestine, and oral mucosa.[35]

In conclusion, a variety of approaches for prophylaxis, mitigation, or management of radiation side effects has been tested in animal models. Only a few of the strategies that have already been translated into clinical studies are described in the text above. It must be noted that many experimental studies have been carried out in combination with single-dose irradiation. This may reflect a clinical scenario of stereotactic irradiation, brachytherapy, or myeloablative conditioning for stem cell transplantation. However, it clearly lacks relevance for fractionated radiotherapy over several weeks where, for example, repopulation processes in early-responding tissues are a dominating factor of tissue radiation tolerance. Parallel studies with single and fractionated doses of radiation have clearly demonstrated that the results can be entirely contradictory. During fractionated irradiation, intervention at intervals before the onset of repopulation can result in effects that are different from later time points. In general, modification of normal tissue responses to radiation exposure requires thorough preclinical testing with appropriate in vivo (animal) models, analyzing clinically relevant endpoints after irradiation with adequate (fractionation) protocols. The mechanisms of action of effective interventions must be clarified in order to develop optimal clinical strategies.

In order to guarantee a clinical benefit, possible tumor effects of the normal tissue modification strategies must be assessed. This must be done under the same premises with regard to suitability of the in vivo models, relevance of treatment protocols, and endpoints. A therapeutic gain can only be expected, if an advantage of the normal tissue results over the tumor effects is demonstrated.

RADIATION CARCINOGENESIS

One dominating concern of many applications of radiation at doses, which are well below those that lead to acute, potentially lethal syndromes, or after local irradiation to individual organs, is radiation-induced carcinogenesis. Irradiation of the human population is often accidental, with attendant uncertainties in radiation quality, exposure dose, and duration and quality of postexposure observation. In addition, as controlled intentional exposures are unacceptable, much of our understanding of the risk of radiation-induced cancer has been obtained in animals. Beginning in 1947, Russell et al. performed studies involving the irradiation of millions of mice and measured the induction of mutations in their offspring.[62,63] This foundational study of mammalian radiation genetics showed that the genetic risk from radiation was small relative to the cancer risk.

In the roughly 60 years following Hiroshima and Nagasaki, studies in mice and other mammals have shown that the dose-response relationship for carcinogenesis cannot be defined by a single number characterizing risk per unit dose. These studies have shown that multiple factors determine risk, including dose, dose rate, overall exposure time, type and quality of radiation, gender, age at the time of exposure, and the particular tissue irradiated. Figure 3.4 illustrates a fundamental aspect of the relationship between dose and observed cancer incidence.[64] This study shows that following acute whole-body x-irradiation of RF male mice, over a dose range that is not immediately lethal, the incidence of myeloid leukemia per mouse increases with dose, and then plateaus and decreases. This study suggests that carcinogenesis per unit dose is thus likely dependent on the efficiency of transforming cells, and the efficiency of killing

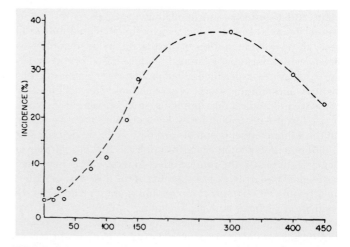

Figure 3.4. Incidence of myeloid leukemia in mice exposed to whole-body x-irradiation. The decrease in incidence at doses >300 rad (3 Gy) is suggestive of cell killing of transformed or potentially transformed cells. Reprinted with permission from Upton AC. The dose-response relationship in radiation induced cancer. *Cancer Res.* 1961;21:717–729.

TABLE 3.2	Relative Risk of Death from Various Neoplasms for Japanese Survivors and for Mice: Risk Values are for 1 Gy Absorbed Dose			
	Mice		*Japanese Survivors*	
Neoplasm	*Relative Risk*	*95% Confidence Interval*	*Relative Risk*	*90% Confidence Interval*
Ca lung	1.77	(1.48–2.17)	1.66	(1.38–2.00)
Ca female breast	2.00	(1.62–2.60)	1.86	(1.41–2.48)
Leukemia[a]	5.38	—	6.27	(4.89–8.07)
Liver tumors	3.60	(2.60–5.10)	1.74	(0.96–3.21)

[a]Relative risk for myeloid leukemia and thymic lymphoma were combined to obtain a value for "leukemia."
Reprinted with permission from Storer JB, Mitchell TJ, Fry RJM. Extrapolation of the relative risk of radiogenic neoplasms across mouse strains and to man. *Radiat Res.* 1988;114:331–353.

transformed and nontransformed cells. The balance between these two principal effects of ionizing radiation governs the shape of the dose cancer incidence curve, which may be linear, curvilinear, bell-shaped, or rise to a plateau, depending on the tissue and dose range examined.

As pertains to other aspects of radiation injury, the pertinent question is whether experimental results obtained in mice and other mammals can be extrapolated to man. This pertains not only to quantitative data, for example, cancer incidence per unit dose, but also to principles, for example, whether the effect of changing dose rate on cancer incidence, which is observed in mice, also pertains to man. In a detailed set of experiments and analyses, Storer et al.[65] examined whether cancer risk from single acute doses of x-irradiation could be extrapolated from mice to man. A total of total of 9,763 mice of four strains and both sexes in two strains were used in the study. All moribund and dead animals were autopsied and along with histological verification, the role of the tumor as being the cause of death, or incidental, was made. Ten-week old mice were exposed to 0, 0.50, 1.0, and 2.0 Gy ^{137}Cs irradiation. Significant and pronounced differences in life-shortening and the incidence of specific tumors were observed between the mouse strains. The incidence of some radiation-induced cancers types was insufficient to be of use for statistical analyses, and not all tumor types exhibited a linear increase in incidence with a linear increase in dose, over the same dose range. Employing tumors that exhibited a linear increase in incidence with dose, two interrelated questions were examined: Is the susceptibility to radiation-induced cancers related to the natural incidence (which varied appreciably among the mouse strains)? Is the incidence of cancer induction better described by an absolute or relative risk model? In the absolute risk model, the observed radiation-induced cancer risk is added to the spontaneous risk to achieve the total risk. In the relative risk model, the risk of radiation-induced cancer is directly related to the spontaneous risk, and radiation acts multiplicatively to yield the total risk. The results of the study showed that the relative risk model was significantly superior to the absolute model for predicting the observed incidence of radiation-induced cancer. That is, the total risk of inducing cancer of a specific histology by radiation per unit dose was a multiple the spontaneous risk, across mouse strains.

To determine if risk estimates could be extrapolated from mouse to man, the incidence of cancer in the atomic bomb survivors in Japan was compared to risk estimates for the same tumors in mice. Incidence data from Hiroshima and Nagasaki included all age groups over a 38-year post–irradiation exposure period and therefore did not include later-appearing radiation-induced tumors. The relative risk of the Japanese data was based on a linear extrapolation of the risk to a 1 Gy dose, based on T65DR dosimetry. Subsequent adjustments and refinements of the dose estimates do not appreciably alter the relative risk estimates.[66] Table 3.2 shows the relative cancer risk estimates in mouse and man for homologous tissues. For lung, breast, and leukemia, the estimates obtained in mice do not significantly differ between mouse and man. For all liver tumors, the relative risk was higher in mice than man. The authors noted that the predominant tumors in Japanese survivors were carcinomas of the liver and intrahepatic bile duct, whereas in mice hepatomas predominated. Considering only hepatocellular carcinomas in mice (for which the incidence was sufficiently high for use only in C3H male mice), the relative risk was similar in the two species.

In addition to an examination of the relationship between risk estimates across mouse strains and those among mice, non-human primates, and humans,[65,67] several other aspects of the relationship between dose and cancer incidence have been examined in detail in animal studies. Taken together, the major findings of these studies are that cancer incidence per unit dose is strain and gender dependent, is specific organ and tumor type dependent, and, for several tumor types, does not linearly increase with dose in the 0.5 to 2 Gy dose range. As recently reviewed in detail by Suit et al.,[68] these variant dose-response relationships have been confirmed or appear likely to pertain in rodents, canine, nonhuman primates, and humans.

It is of note that most radiation cancer risk estimates have been performed in the dose range ≥0.05 Gy. Experimentally based risk estimates, and the shape of the dose-response curve for substantially lower doses, for example, background to 200 mGy, are limited.[69,70] Di Majo et al.[69] evaluated life shortening and the incidence of solid neoplasms in two strains of mice exposed to high and low LET radiation from doses of 5 to 320 mGy. Their studies were interpreted as suggesting the existence of a region at low doses, where the incidence of solid neoplasm does not increase beyond the background incidence. However, as the estimation of incidence at very low doses of radiation requires the exposure of several thousand subjects, the study does not resolve whether a threshold dose for induction of solid cancers, or specific types of tumors exists, or fully resolve the shapes of the induction curves at very low doses.

Using the same models as are employed to evaluate dose-response relationships for x-ray and γ irradiation, studies in animals have established that cancer risk per unit dose is dependent upon the quality, for example, ionization density, of radiation. An example is the extensive studies performed to evaluate the carcinogenic effects of densely ionizing radiation such as neutrons.[69-71] These studies have clearly shown that the dose versus cancer risk relationships for densely ionizing radiations exhibit similar characteristics, but also substantial differences from the x-irradiation dose-response relationship. The risk of cancer for both radiations is dependent on the competitive effects of cell killing and radiation-induced transformation. Similarly, as pertains to x-rays, neutron carcinogenesis is tissue, dose, strain, and gender specific. However, there is generally little if any reduction in the efficiency of cancer induction as is observed with x-irradiation, when a dose above a few Gy is fractionated or protracted. Secondly, for x-irradiation, the efficiency of induction of some cancers appears to increase with the square of the dose (above a few Gy), whereas with high LET irradiations, cancer induction appears to increase linearly with a linear increase in dose. Thirdly, for many if not all specific cancers, the risk of cancer per unit dose is substantially higher following more densely ionizing irradiations than x- or γ-radiation.

CONCLUSION

Animal models provide substantial and significant knowledge relevant to normal tissue effects of radiation, and substantially supplement that which is available from the extant human experience. In many instances, such as the influence of radiation quality and the effect of dose fractionation and protraction on risk, animal studies have provided the bulk of the data and insight. Data from animal models are in many instances scientifically superior to that obtained from study of the exposed human population. The dose administered is known with greater accuracy and precision; normal tissue effects can be monitored over the lifetime of the animal, and pathological evaluation and confirmation of the specific cause of death are assessed in the great majority of cases.

REFERENCES

1. Fliedner TM, Dörr H, Meineke V. Multi-organ involvement as a pathogenetic principle of the radiation syndromes: a study involving 110 case histories documented in SEARCH and classified as the bases of haematopoietic indicators of effect. *BJR Suppl.* 2005;27:1–8.
2. Ainsbury EA, Bouffler SD, Dörr W, et al. Radiation cataractogenesis—a review of recent studies. *Radiat Res.* 2009;172:1–9.
3. Bezold G, Gottlober P, Gall H, et al. Accidental radiation exposure and azoospermia. *J Androl.* 2000;21:403–408.
4. Jacobsen LO, Marks EK, Gaston EO, et al. Effect of spleen protection on mortality following X-irradiation. *J Lab Clin Med.* 1949;34:1538–1543.
5. Lorenz E, Uphoff ED, Reid TR, et al. Modification of acute radiation injury in mice and guinea pigs by bone marrow injection. *Radiology.* 1951;58:863–877.
6. McCulloch EA, Till JE. The radiation sensitivity of normal mouse bone marrow cells, determined by quantitative marrow transplantation into irradiated mice. *Radiat Res.* 1960;13:115–125.
7. McCulloch JE, Till JE. The sensitivity of cells from normal mouse bone marrow to gamma radiation in vitro and in vivo. *Radiat Res.* 1962;16:822–832.
8. Gould MN, Clifton KH. Evidence of a unique in situ compnent of the repair of radiation damage. *Radiat Res.* 1979;77:149–155.
9. Mulcahy RT, Gould MN, Clifton KH. The survival of thyroid cells: in vivo irradiation and in situ repair. *Radiat Res.* 1980;84:523–528.
10. Hill RP, Bush RS. The effect of continuous or fractionated irradiation on a murine sarcoma. *Br J Radiol.* 1973;46:167–174.
11. Withers HR, Hunter N, Barkley HT Jr, et al. Radiation survival and regeneration characteristics of spermatogenic stem cells of mouse testis. *Radiat Res.* 1974;57:88–103.
12. Withers HR, Mason KA, Thames HD. Late radiation response of kidney assayed by tubule cell survival. *Br J Radiol.* 1986;59:587–595.
13. Withers HR. The dose-survival relationship for irradiation of epithelial cells of mouse skin. *Br J Radiol.* 1967;40:187–194.
14. Withers HR, Mason KA, Reid BO, et al. Response of mouse intestine to neutrons and gamma rays in relation to dose fractionation and division cycle. *Cancer.* 1974;34:39–47.
15. Fowler JR, Morgan RL, Silvester JA, et al. Experiments with fractionated treatment of the skin of pigs: 1. Fractionation up to 28 days. *Br J Radiol.* 1963;36:188–196.
16. Travis EL, Down JD, Holmes SJ, et al. Radiation pneumonitis and fibrosis in mouse lung assayed by respiratory frequency and histology. *Radiat Res.* 1980;84:133–142.
17. van der Kogel AJ. Central nervous system injury in small animal models. In: Guten PH, Leibel SA, Sheline GE, eds. *Radiation Injury to the Nervous System.* New York: Raven Press; 1991:91–112.
18. Stewart FA, Soranson JA, Alpen EL, et al. Radiation-induced renal damage: the effects of hyperfractionation. *Radiat Res.* 1984;98:407–420.
19. Robbins ME, Hopewell JW. Effect of single doses of X-rays on renal function in the pig after the irradiation of both kidneys. *Radiother Oncol.* 1988;11:253–262.
20. Yeung TK, Hopewell JW. Effects of single doses of radiation on cardiac function in the rat. *Radiother Oncol.* 1985;3:339–345.
21. Lauk S, Kiszel Z, Buschmann J, et al. Radiation-induced heart disease in rats. *Int J Radiat Oncol Biol Phys.* 1985;11:801–808.
22. Vriesendorp HM, van Bekkum DW. Response to total body irradiation in different species. In: Broerse JJ, MacVittie T, eds. *Susceptibility to Total-body Irradiation.* Amsterdam, The Netherlands: Martinus Nijoff; 1964.
23. Jones RJ, Wagner JE, Celano P, et al. Separation of pluripotent haematopoietic stem cells rom spleen colony-forming cells. *Nature.* 1990;347(6289):188–189.
24. Meijne EIM, van der Winden-Gronewegen RJM, Plomacher RE, et al. The effects of X-irradiation on hematopoietic stem cell compartments in the mouse. *Exp Hematol.* 1991;19:617–623.
25. Ploemacher RE, van Os R, Van Buerden CAJ, et al. Murine hematopoietic stem cells with long-term engraftment and marrow repopulating ability are less radiosensitive to gamma radiation than are spleen colony forming cells. *Int J Radiat Biol.* 1992;66:481–499.
26. Down JD, Boudewijn A, van Os R, et al. Variations in radiation sensitivity among different hematopoietic stem cell subsets following fractionated irradiation. *Blood.* 1995;86:122–127.
27. Westphal CH, Rowan S, Schmaltz C, et al. atm and p53 cooperate in apoptosis and suppression of tumorigenesis but not in resistance to acute radiation toxicity. *Nat Genet.* 1997;16(4):397–401.
28. Okayasu R, Suetomi K, Yu Y, et al. A deficiency in DNA repair and DNA-PKcs expression in the radiosensitive BALB/c mouse. *Cancer Res.* 2000;60:4342–4345.
29. Hiramatsu H, Nishikomori R, Heike T, et al. Complete reconstitution of human lymphocytes from cord blood CD34+ cells using NOD/SCID/gamma null mice model. *Blood.* 2003;102:873–882.
30. Traggiai E, Chicha L, Mazzucchelli L, et al. Development of a human adaptive immune system in cord cell-transplanted mice. *Science.* 2004;304:104–107.
31. Peter RU. Cutaneous radiation syndrome in multi-organ failure. *BJR Suppl.* 2005;27:180–184.
32. Peter RU, Gottlober P. Management of cutaneous radiation injuries: diagnostic principles of the cutaneous radiation syndrome. *Mil Med Suppl.* 2002;167:110–112.
33. Goepp R, Fitch F. Pathological study of oral radiation death in mice. *Radiat Res.* 1962;16:833–845.
34. Dörr W. Pathogenesis of normal tissue side effects. In: Joiner M, van der Kogel A, eds. *Basic Clinical Radiobiology.* London, UK: Hodder Arnold; 2009:169–190.
35. Coppes R, De Haan G, Dörr W, et al. Further improvement of radiotherapy through side effect reduction by stem cell transplantation. *Radiother Oncol.* 2006;81(suppl 1):S58.
36. Dörr W, Hendry JH. Consequential late effects in normal tissues. *Radiother Oncol.* 2001;61:369–379.
37. Joiner M, Bentzen SM. Fractionation: the linear-quadratic approach. In: Joiner M, van der Kogel A, eds. *Basic Clinical Radiobiology.* 4th ed. London, UK: Hodder Arnold; 2009:102–119.
38. Withers HR. Biologic basis for altered fractionated schemes. *Cancer.* 1985;55:2086–2095.
39. Thames HD, Withers HR, Peters LJ, et al. Changes in early and late radiation response with altered dose fractionation: implications for dose-survival relationships. *Int J Radiat Oncol Biol Phys.* 1982;8:219–226.
40. Thames HD Jr, Withers HR, Peters LJ. Tissue repair capacity and repair kinetics deduced from multifractionated or continuous irradiation regimens with incomplete repair. *Br J Cancer Suppl.* 1984;6:263–269.
41. Hall EJ, Giaccia AJ. *Radiobiology for the Radiologist.* 6th ed. Philadelphia, PA: Lippincott Williams and Wilkins; 2006.
42. Bentzen SM, Joiner M. The linear-quadratic approach in clinical practice. In: Joiner M, van der Kogel A, eds. *Basic Clinical Radiobiology.* 4th ed. London, UK: Hodder Arnold; 2009:120–134.
43. Wong CS, Hao Y, Hill RP. Response of rat spinal cord to very small doses per fraction: lack of enhanced radiosensitivity. *Radiother Oncol.* 1995;36:44–49.
44. Lavey RS, Taylor JMG, Tward JD, et al. The extent, time course, and fraction size dependence of mouse spinal cord recovery from radiation injury. *Int J Radiat Oncol Biol Phys.* 1994;30:609–617.
45. Tucker SL, Thames HD Jr. Flexure dose: the low-dose limit of effective fractionation. *Int J Radiat Oncol Biol Phys.* 1983;9:1373–1383.
46. Hopewell JW, Nyman J, Turesson I. Time factor for acute tissue reactions following fractionated irradiation: a balance between repopulation and enhanced radiosensitivity. *Int J Radiat Biol.* 2003;79:513–524.
47. Dörr W. Modulation of repopulation processes in oral mucosa: experimental results. *Int J Radiat Biol.* 2003;79:531–537.
48. Dörr W. Oral mucosa: response modification by keratinocyte growth factor. In: Nieder C, Milas L, Ang KK, eds. *Biological Modification of Radiation Response.* Berlin, Heidelberg-New York: Springer; 2003:113–122.
49. Dörr W. Three A's of repopulation during fractionated irradiation in squamous epithelia: asymmetry loss, acceleration of stem-cell divisions and abortive divisions. *Int J Radiat Biol.* 1997;72:635–643.

50. Shirazi A, Liu K, Trott KR. Epidermal morphology, cell proliferation and repopulation in mouse skin during daily fractionated irradiation. *Int J Radiat Biol.* 1995;68:215–222.
51. Dörr W, Hamilton CS, Boyd T, et al. Radiation-induced changes in cellularity and proliferation in human oral mucosa. *Int J Radiat Oncol Biol Phys.* 2002;52:911–917.
52. Dörr W. Biological response modifiers: normal tissues. In: Joiner M, van der Kogel A, eds. *Basic Clinical Radiobiology.* 4th ed. London, UK. Hodder Arnold; 2009:301–315.
53. Dörr W, Kummermehr J. Increased radiation tolerance of mouse tongue epithelium after local conditioning. *Int J Radiat Biol.* 1992;61:369–379.
54. Dörr W, van der Kogel AJ. The volume effect in radiotherapy. In: Joiner M, van der Kogel A, eds. *Clinical Radiobiology.* London, UK: Hodder Arnold; 2009:191–206.
55. Liao ZX, Travis EL, Tucker SL. Damage and morbidity from pneumonitis after irradiation of partial volumes of mouse lung. *Int J Radiat Oncol Biol Phys.* 1995;32:1359–1370.
56. Travis EL, Liao ZX, Tucker SL. Spatial heterogeneity of the volume effect for radiation pneumonitis in mouse lung. *Int J Radiat Oncol Biol Phys.* 1997;38:1045–1054.
57. Bijl HP, van Luijk P, Coopes RP, et al. Regional differences in radiosensitivity across the rat cervical spinal cord. *Int J Radiat Oncol Biol Phys.* 2005;61:543–551.
58. Haagen J, Krohn H, Rollig S, et al. Effect of selective inhibitors of inflammation on oral mucositis: preclinical studies. *Radiother Oncol.* 2009; [Epub in print].
59. Genot MT, Klastersky J. Low-level laser for prevention and therapy of oral mucositis induced by chemotherapy or radiotherapy. *Curr Opin Oncol.* 2005;17:236–240.
60. Molteni A, Moulder JE, Cohen EF, et al. Control of radiation-induced pneumopathy and lung fibrosis by angiotensin-converting enzyme inhibitors and an angiotensin II type 1 receptor blocker. *Int J Radiat Biol.* 2000;76:523–532.
61. Moulder JE, Fish BL, Cohen EP. Treatment of radiation nephropathy with ACE inhibitors and AII type-1 and type-2 receptor antagonists. *Curr Pharm Des.* 2007;13:1317–1325.
62. Russell WL, Russell LB, Grower JS, et al. Radiation dose rate and mutation frequency. *Science.* 1958;128(3358):1546–1550.
63. Russell LB, Russell WL. Frequency and nature of specific-locus mutations induced in female mice by radiation and chemicals: a review. *Mutat Res.* 1992;296(1–2):107–127.
64. Upton AC. The dose-response relationship in radiation induced cancer. *Cancer Res.* 1961;21:717–729.
65. Storer JB, Mitchell TJ, Fry RJM. Extrapolation of the relative risk of radiogenic neoplasm across mouse strains and to man. *Radiat Res.* 1988;114:331–353.
66. Preston DL, Pierce DA, Shimizu Y, et al. Effect of recent changes in atomic bomb survivor dosimetry on cancer mortality risk estimates. *Radiat Res.* 2004;162:377–389.
67. Carnes BA, Olshansky SJ, Grahn D. An interspecies prediction of the risk of radiation-induced mortality. *Radiat Res.* 1998;149:487–492.
68. Suit H, Goldberg S, Niemierko A, et al. Secondary carcinogenesis in patients treated with radiation: a review of data on radiation-induced cancers in humans, non-human primate, canine and rodent subjects. *Radiat Res.* 2007;167:12–42.
69. DiMajo V, Rebessi S, Pazzaglia A, et al. Carcinogenesis in laboratory mice after low doses of ionizing radiation. *Radiat Res.* 2003;159:102–108.
70. Heidenriech WF0, Carnes BA, Paretzke HG. Lung cancer risk in mice: analysis of fractionation effects and neutron RBE with a biologically motivated model. *Radiat Res.* 2006;166:794–809.
71. Elkind, M.M. Physical, biophysical, and cell-biological factors that can contribute to enhanced neoplastic transformation by fission-spectrum neutrons. Rad Res 128, S47–S52 (1991).

Radiation Dose Fractionation and Normal Tissue Injury

The differential effects of dividing a total dose of radiation into two or more "fractions" separated in time have been appreciated since early in the 20th century. Early experiments in animals demonstrated a sparing effect of dose fractionation, requiring higher total doses to achieve similar biological effects with several doses compared to a single dose. Rapidly growing tissues generally demonstrated less sparing than slowly proliferating tissues leading to the early practice of treating tumors with multiple smaller doses of radiation with the intent of limiting the effects on normal tissues. This continues to be standard practice in most clinical situations. However, the human population is exposed to radiation from a variety of sources and exposure may take place in seconds, as in an industrial accident, or over a lifetime, as with background radiation. This chapter provides a brief overview of our understanding of radiation dose fractionation with emphasis on effects in normal tissues.

EARLY EXPERIMENTS IN FRACTIONATION

Early radiobiological research in Europe included studies of the effects of fractionated doses compared to single doses of ionizing radiation. French physicians Bergonié and Tribondeau reported differential effects of fractionated radiation on neoplastic and normal tissues.[1] Building on this work, Regaud and Ferroux[2] published a landmark paper in 1927 entitled

> Discordance des éffets des rayons X, d'une part dans la peau, d'autre part dans le testicule, par fractionnement de la dose: diminution de l'efficacité dans la peau, maintien de l'efficacité dans le testicule.

These authors described a decrease in efficacy in terms of skin damage following radiation when the dose was divided into two to four fractions separated by several days compared to a single dose. No such decrease (or a much lesser one) in biological effectiveness was detected in the testicular epithelium. Such results led to the use of fractionated radiotherapy in clinical practice to treat tumors (rapidly proliferating, like seminal epithelium) in order to spare toxicity to the dose-limiting normal tissue, which in the day of superficial x-rays was skin necrosis. These results were taken together with the earlier work of Bergonié and Tribondeau to yield general principles regarding radiosensitivity and effects of dose fractionation based on tissue type, degree of cellular differentiation, mitotic activity, and mitotic "future." (Table 4.1)

Further studies in other systems as well as early clinical radiotherapy experience supported these early findings.[3–6] Virtually all tissues and biological systems studied were spared by dose fractionation. In other words, when dose was divided into two or more fractions, the total dose required to produce a given biological effect was increased. However, the magnitude of this effect varied depending on the tissue or system under study following the general guidelines outlined in Table 4.1 (Fig. 4.1).

EARLY CLINICAL EXPERIENCE

Early in the 20th century, there was controversy over the superiority of single-dose radiation therapy versus the delivery of divided doses or fractionated treatment. It was known, based on the early work of Bergonié and Tribondeau, that differences in radiosensitivity existed among different cell types depending on the extent of mitotic activity. Proponents of the single-dose methods based their preference on the incorrect supposition that rapidly proliferating tumor cells were able to repair radiation damage better than more slowly proliferating normal tissues, while those favoring the fractionated approach cited the higher probability with multiple daily dosing of irradiating cells in mitosis, a state believed (correctly) to confer greater radiosensitivity. The results and interpretation of the experiments by Regaud and Ferroux[2] led to the treatment of tonsillar and laryngeal carcinomas with daily low-dose radiotherapy sessions and judging the total dose by assessment of the skin and mucosal reaction. The series, reported by Coutard in 1929,[7] was the first demonstration of cure of deep-seated tumors with fractionated radiotherapy. Similar techniques continue to be used for the majority of cancer patients treated with radiotherapy today, although various fractionation schedules are being studied and compared.[8,9]

TABLE 4.1	General Principles of Radio-sensitivity Based on Early Experimental Work[1,2]		
Cell Type	*Radiosensitivity*	*Sparing by Fractionation*
Undifferentiated	High	Low
Rapidly proliferating		
High mitotic rate		
Long "mitotic future"		
Differentiated	Low	High
Slowly or nonproliferating		
Short or no mitotic future		

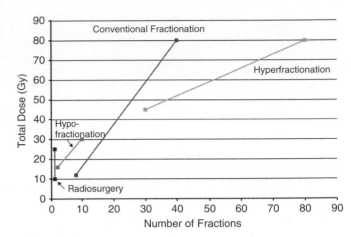

Figure 4.2. The range of total dose and number of fractions used in various fractionation schedules used in modern radiotherapy.

FRACTIONATION SCHEDULES USED IN MODERN RADIOTHERAPY

The term *standard fractionation* remains in use today to refer to the delivery of daily doses of 1.8 to 2.0 Gy, 5 days per week. However, single-dose treatments remain in use and the total number of treatments and the dose delivered with each fraction can vary considerably. Indeed, there is a trend in radiotherapy toward "nonstandard" fractionation for many indications: multiple daily fractions, hyperfraction-ation, hypofractionation, and single doses (Fig. 4.2). In addi-tion, continuous low-dose rate irradiation is also employed

in radiotherapy and is the major mode of irradiation from environmental and natural background sources. It has been the goal of considerable basic and clinical research to under-stand the biological basis of fractionated radiotherapy and to develop models to predict outcomes for various fractionation schedules.[10]

SURVIVAL CURVES AND SUBLETHAL DAMAGE REPAIR

A new era of radiobiology emerged with the development of tis-sue culture techniques that allowed for measurement of single cell survival following exposure to various doses of radiation.[11] The single-dose mammalian cell radiation survival curve has a typical shape consisting of a rapidly bending initial portion or "shoulder" region followed by an exponential or less curved portion (Fig. 4.3). Elkind and Sutton[12] used these methods to demonstrate that two doses of radiation, separated in time, led to less cell killing than the same total dose delivered all at once (Fig. 4.4). This was interpreted as repair of "sublethal damage" between the two doses. The time required for "com-plete" repair between fractions is tissue dependent. Animal experiments have demonstrated repair half-times between 0.45 and 1.5 hours.[10] Working in primate spinal cord, Ang et al. have demonstrated biexponential repair kinetics with half times of 0.7 and 3.8 hours for the fast and slow compo-nents, respectively. This work indicates that even a 6 to 8 hour interval will lead to accumulation of unrepaired sublethal damage and lower the tolerance dose of spinal cord.[13] This prediction has been supported by increased rates of myelopa-thy seen in patients treated for head and neck cancers with three fractions per day.[14] Based on these results, it is strongly recommended that when twice-daily fractionation is used the two fractions are separated in time by at least 6 hours, more when feasible.

Repair of sublethal radiation damage in normal tissues is one of the processes taking place between doses of fractionated radiotherapy. "Four Rs" are often discussed: Repair of sublethal damage, Reoxygenation of hypoxic regions, Redistribution of cells in the cell cycle, and Repopulation.[15] Of these factors,

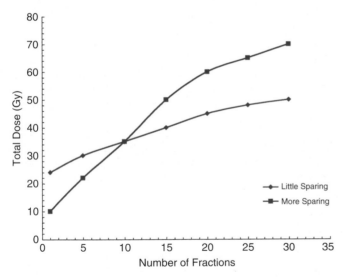

Figure 4.1. Schematic of the effect of dose fractionation on tis-sues. Nearly all tissues are spared by dose fractionation. The magni-tude of the effect is tissue dependent. Relatively little sparing may be demonstrated for rapidly proliferating, undifferentiated tissues, including most malignant tumors (red). Much greater sparing is com-monly seen in slowly, or nonproliferating, well-differentiated tissues (blue). The curves represent pairs of total dose and dose per fraction resulting in similar biological effect (isoeffect) for a particular tissue and endpoint. An example would be a high probability of tumor con-trol (red) and a low probability of a late toxicity of radiation (blue). The two curves may cross, indicating that for many situations dose fractionation is necessary in order to limit toxicity while maintaining tumor control.

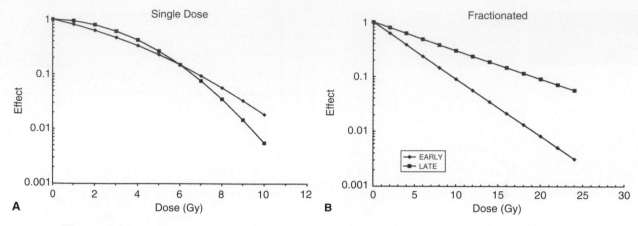

Figure 4.3. Comparison of single-dose effect curves (**A**) and fractionated dose-effect curves (**B**) for late-responding, low α/β tissues (blue) and early-responding, high α/β tissues (red). The small advantage seen in the low dose region sparing low α/β tissues (**A**) is amplified through dose fractionation (**B**).

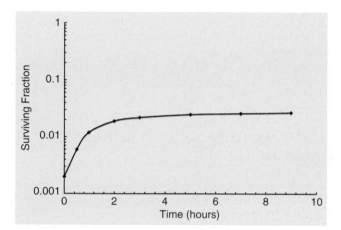

Figure 4.4. Schematic of the results of the first experiments demonstrating repair of sublethal damage between two doses of radiation. Cell survival increased with elapsed time between two equal doses of radiation.[12]

discussed in more detail in Chapter 1, only repair contributes significantly to effects of dose fractionation on normal tissues.

EARLY MODELS OF THE BIOLOGICAL EFFECTIVENESS OF DIFFERENT FRACTIONATION SCHEDULES

It has long been recognized that the biological effectiveness of a course of radiotherapy (or a series of doses in an experimental system) depends on the total dose and the manner in which the dose is delivered. Early attempts to correlate isoeffective regimens concentrated on the effect of the overall time taken to deliver the entire course of radiotherapy. Recovery factors were used in early radiotherapy to account for the loss of effect seen when total dose was fractionated. Multiplying the single dose required for a given effect by the recovery factor gave the equivalent dose to be given over a specific number of days to produce the same biological effect. Reisner and others published tables of recovery factors for erythema and dry desquamation in human skin.[16–18]

An early proposal by Strandqvist[19] used a simple exponential model relating dose to the overall time

$$D = kT^n$$

where D is the total dose to achieve a given effect (in normal tissue or tumor), T is the overall time in days to deliver the treatment course, and n is an exponent <1 effectively defining the slope of the line describing the pairs of total dose and overall time resulting in equivalent biological effects on a log-log plot (isoeffect line). k is the single dose required to produce the defined level of effect and in turn defining the set of doses and overall times predicted to achieve that effect. Working with skin, Strandqvist reported the same slope ($n = 0.22$) for isoeffective curves for various levels of skin reaction and tumor cure (Fig. 4.5). This predicted no advantage in therapeutic ratio for the various possible dose/time regimens. Strandqvist proposed that this slope was in good agreement with the recovery factor data of Reisner and MacComb and Quimby.[16,18]

However, later work by Cohen[20] estimated a slope for normal skin of 0.30 to 0.33 that was significantly different than the 0.22 predicted by Strandqvist for skin cancer. This implied different capacities for recovery from radiation damage in different

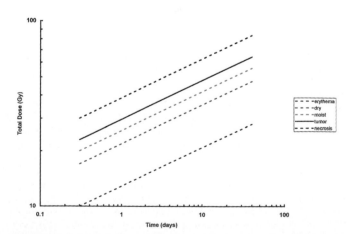

Figure 4.5. Isoeffect lines from the results of Strandqvist for various effects in skin and for local control of skin cancer. Redrawn from Strandqvist.[19]

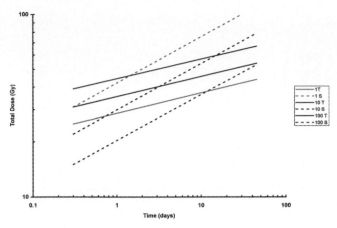

Figure 4.6. Isoeffective radiation schedules reported by von Essen to result in either 3% probability of skin necrosis (dotted lines) or a 99% probability of tumor regression (solid lines). The isoeffect lines are shown for different volumes (1, 10, or 100 cm³) of irradiated skin (S) or tumor (T). Note that each pair of curves for a particular volume cross at progressively longer times for larger volumes, implying the need for more prolonged fractionation schedules with larger volumes in order to maintain therapeutic efficacy without undue risk of late complication (redrawn with permission from von Essen[22]).

tissues, in this case normal skin and skin cancer. This differential recovery of normal tissues and tumor was taken to explain the superiority of fractionated radiotherapy in producing tumor cures without skin necrosis. In addition, this "advantage" in favor of the normal skin predicted an increasing therapeutic ratio with increased overall time (or number of fractions). Cohen, and later von Essen, also demonstrated that the volume of normal tissue irradiated was a significant factor in determining tolerance dose, with larger volumes demonstrating a given level of effect at lower doses compared to smaller volumes.[21,22] Conversely, larger tumors required higher doses than smaller ones to achieve the same probability of tumor control (Fig. 4.6).

In 1969, Ellis[23] published the Nominal Standard Dose model. This model used an exponent for fraction number (N) of 0.24, based on the Strandqvist model.[19] The exponent of time (T) was much lower at 0.11 and was derived from the previous work of Strandqvist and Cohen.[20,21,24]

$$\text{Total dose} = \text{NSD} \times N^{0.24} \times T^{0.11}$$

NSD is the tolerance in a single fraction, taken to be about 18 Gy for skin necrosis. Orton and Ellis[25] published time, dose, fractionation (TDF) tables for clinical use to calculate partial tolerance and equivalence of fractionation schedules for radiotherapy patients.

Early in the history of radiotherapy and radiobiology, the assumption that overall time was more important than number of fractions in determining the biological effectiveness of a total radiation dose was rarely challenged. Fowler et al.[26] tested this assumption in a series of experiments on pig skin and clearly established that, for the normal tissue reactions studied, number of fractions and dose per fraction were more important than overall time.

The results show clearly that for medium-term reactions the number (and size) of fractions is more important than the effect of slow tissue repair or repopulation over the period 5 to 28 days.

RADIOBIOLOGY OF FRACTIONATED RADIATION

Largely due to the notion that fraction size and total dose determined the probability of a late radiation-related injury, the linear-quadratic (LQ) formulation came into common usage in the late 1970s largely replacing the NSD model.[27] This model is based on simple assumptions, is useful in comparing fractionation schedules, and differentiates among tissues with different capacities for interfraction repair.[28]

It may be considered that DNA is the target molecule for cell killing by ionizing radiation and that a double-strand break in the DNA is necessary and sufficient to cause cell death. Double-strand breaks may be effectively produced by a single particle track in number proportional to D, or by the interaction of two single-strand breaks caused by separate particle tracks and occurring closely in space and time in number proportional to D^2 (Fig. 4.7). These two types of lethal lesions are variably produced at rates proportional to the coefficients $\alpha(\text{Gy}^{-1})$ and $\beta(\text{Gy}^{-2})$. Single-strand breaks alone may be repaired and therefore represent sublethal damage. Such a model is described by the LQ formula

$$\text{SF} = e^{-(\alpha D + \beta D^2)}$$

where SF is surviving fraction and D is dose of radiation in Gy.[29] α is the coefficient related to single event cell killing and β the coefficient related to cell killing through the interaction of sublethal events. The term $(\alpha D + \beta D^2)$ represents the average number of lethal lesions produced following a dose of D. α/β is the ratio of the relative contributions of these two components to overall cell kill. α/β is the *single dose* at which overall cell killing is equally due to these two components:

$$\alpha D = \beta D^2$$

or

$$D = \alpha/\beta$$

A spectrum of fractionation schedules are used to treat benign and malignant conditions with radiotherapy, ranging from single fraction radiosurgery to fully fractionated courses of radiotherapy. When radiation dose is divided into a number of small fractions separated by sufficient time to allow full (or nearly

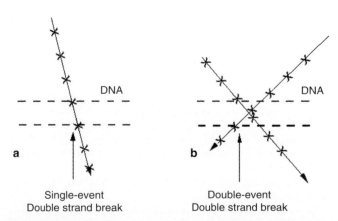

Figure 4.7. Schematic representation of double-strand break production by single events (proportional to αD) or interaction of events (proportional to βD^2).

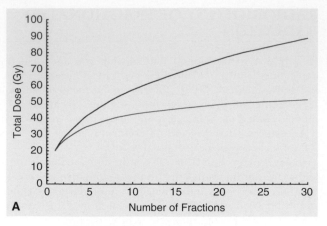
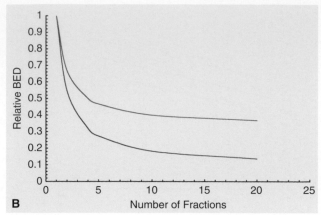

A — Number of Fractions

B — Number of Fractions

Figure 4.8. The effect of dose fractionation on the biological effectiveness of x-radiation for low α/β (blue) versus high α/β (red) tissues. **A:** Isoeffect curves show the increase in total dose required to maintain biological effectiveness with increasing number of fractions. **B:** Decreasing biological effectiveness with increasing fraction number while maintaining total dose.

full) repair, each fraction produces a similar biological effect (see Fig. 4.3B).

For multiple fractions, the effect of n fractions of dose per fraction d becomes

$$SF = (e^{-\alpha d - \beta d^2})^n$$

A basic principle of radiobiology and radiotherapy is that dose fractionation "spares" virtually all cell and tissue types. "Sparing" in this context means that, for a given total dose, there will always be less molecular damage and a lower level of biological effect associated with multiple fractions compared to a single dose, based on the principle of repair of sublethal damage following each fraction. As the number of fractions increases, the total dose ($n \times d$) required to achieve a certain level of biological effect also increases (Fig. 4.8). The magnitude of the sparing effect of dose fractionation varies, however, and depends on the ratio α/β. The biologically effective dose (BED) is represented by

$$BED(Gy_{\alpha/\beta}) = nd\left[1 + \frac{d}{\alpha/\beta}\right]$$

where BED is expressed in $Gy_{\alpha/\beta}$ to indicate that it should be used only to compare effects in tissues with the same α/β, n is the number of fractions of dose d, and nd is, therefore, the total dose (D). BED can be expressed as

$$BED(Gy_{\alpha/\beta}) = D \times F$$

where F is a "fractionation factor" or relative effectiveness,

$$F = \left[1 + \frac{d}{\alpha/\beta}\right]$$

F increases with increasing dose/fraction d but the effect is dampened by α/β, being greatest for lower α/β and may be negligible for very high α/β, since as α/β becomes large F approaches 1.

The LQ model is a means of estimating the effects of dose fractionation. Other factors, such as a rapid doubling time, may be accounted for by additional terms; however, these factors are not significant in late-responding normal tissues.[30]

Mechanistically, a larger α/β indicates relatively little contribution from interaction of sublethal events. A lower α/β indicates a greater contribution from this type of damage. Since sublethal damage may be repaired following a dose of radiation, cells with a lower α/β ratio are spared to a greater extent by fractionation than are cell types with a larger α/β (Fig. 4.8).

The importance of fraction size is clear when considering the impact of simultaneously increasing total dose and dose per fraction in therapeutic treatment planning. The effect is especially important when considering late-responding normal tissue effects (low α/β). Small spatial errors in dosimetry may place a normal structure in a higher isodose volume. This leads to an effect coined by Withers[31] as "double trouble," reference to the simultaneous increase in dose per fraction and total dose. While a change in total dose without a change in dose per fraction will lead to a linear increase in BED, a simultaneous increase in dose per fraction and total dose has much greater impact on BED. Such effects are particularly striking when considering single, high dose rate exposures (Fig. 4.9).

Even a modest increase in dose per fraction has been shown to result in increased toxicity. Michalski et al.[32] recently reported

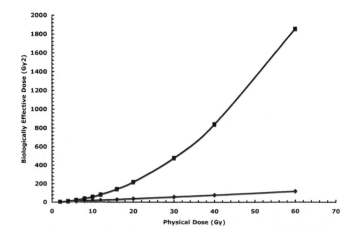

Figure 4.9. Comparison of physical dose versus BED for single fractions (red) and multiple fractions of 2 Gy (blue). A doubling of physical dose from 20 to 40 Gy doubles the BED for 2 Gy fractions but increases the BED nearly four-fold for the single fraction case (α/β = 2 Gy).

a significantly increased risk of Grade 2 or greater gastrointestinal and genitourinary toxicity in prostate cancer patients receiving doses of 78 Gy in 2 Gy fractions compared to 79.2 Gy in 1.8 Gy fractions.

Malignant tumors and other rapidly proliferating tissues (e.g., skin, mucosa, and bone marrow) demonstrate high α/β (8–12) and exhibit modest sparing through dose fractionation.[33] Some malignancies, for example prostate cancer, may exhibit the properties of a lower α/β.[34] Many normal tissues, including those of the CNS, have lower α/β (2–4) and demonstrate marked sparing with dose fractionation. This effect is demonstrated by comparing the total dose required to maintain BED or the BED for a given total dose delivered in various numbers of fractions (see Fig. 4.8). The magnitude of this effect of dose fractionation is quantitatively very different for low versus high α/β tissues. This forms the basis for simultaneously maintaining efficacy for tissues with high α/β while decreasing toxicity for tissues with low α/β through dose fractionation. α/β has been estimated for a number of normal tissue effects in experimental systems (Table 4.2).

While many α/β have been estimated in experimental systems, clinical data may also be used to estimate α/β based on isoeffective fractionation schedules. If two fractionation schedules result in an equivalent clinical effect, they may be assumed to have the same BED for that effect and the LQ model may be used to calculate the α/β.[35]

Since

$$\text{BED}(\text{Gy}_{\alpha/\beta}) = D\left[1 + \frac{d}{\alpha/\beta}\right]$$

by setting $\text{BED}_1 = \text{BED}_2$, the unknown α/β is calculated as follows:

$$\text{BED}_1 = \text{BED}_2$$

or

$$D_1\left[1 + \frac{d_1}{\alpha/\beta}\right] = D_2\left[1 + \frac{d_2}{\alpha/\beta}\right]$$

or

$$\alpha/\beta = \frac{(D_2 \times d_2) - (D_1 \times d_1)}{D_1 - D_2}$$

TABLE 4.2	Estimates of α/β in Experimental Systems		
Tissue	*Endpoint*	*α/β*	*Reference*
EARLY-RESPONDING TISSUES			
Skin	Desquamation	9.4	65
		10.5	66
	Epilation	6.5	67
Jejunum	Crypt cell survival	7.1	68
Colon	Crypt cell survival	8.4	69
Testis	"Stem" cell survival	13.9	70
LATE-RESPONDING TISSUES			
Spinal cord	Paralysis	2.0–2.3	13,71
Brain	Death	2.1	72
Lens	Cataract	1.2	73
Kidney	Frequency	1.6	74
Bladder	Frequency	7.2	75
Bowel	Stricture	4.0	76
Skin	Contracture	<2.4	77
Lung	LD/50	2.1–3.0	78–80

Adapted from Thames HD, Hendry JH. *Fractionation in Radiotherapy.* London: Taylor & Francis; 1987.

A more meaningful estimate may be derived from multiple fractionation schedules resulting in similar biological effects. An example is the treatment of benign schwannomas of the acoustic nerve (acoustic neuroma) with radiation. Historically, single fraction radiosurgery doses of 18 to 20 Gy were used, resulting in tumor control rates >90%, but high rates of cranial neuropathies, including hearing loss. Single doses used today are 12 to 13 Gy and continue to provide >90% tumor control, but with significant decrease in morbidity, including hearing loss, trigeminal and facial neuropathies.[36] Additionally, equivalent local control and levels of hearing preservation have been achieved with schedules using between 1 and 32 fractions without significant trigeminal or facial neuropathies.[37] Using these data, the α/β may be estimated using the reciprocal plot method of Douglas and Fowler (Fig. 4.10).[27] This involves rearrangement of the

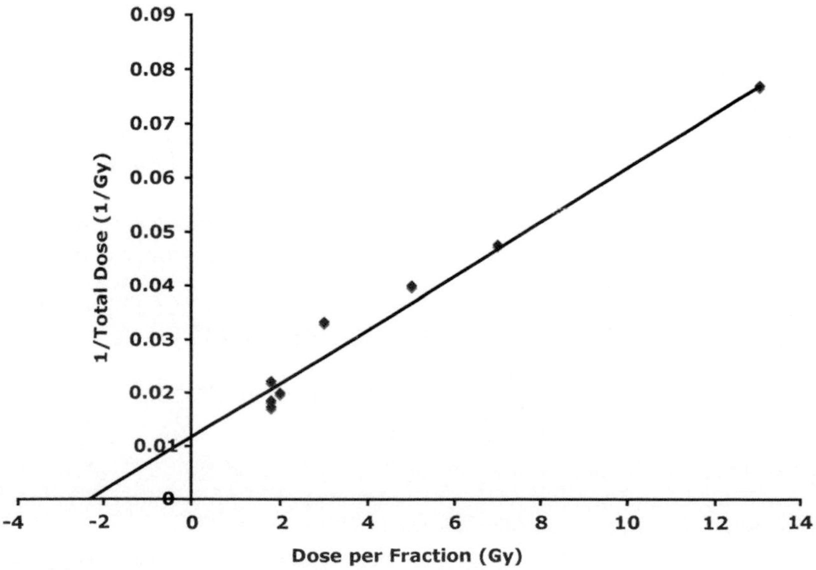

Figure 4.10. Inverse plot of clinical fractionation regimens that have resulted in similar rates of hearing loss following radiotherapy for acoustic schwannoma. The α/β is estimated from the x-intercept, in this case 2.3 Gy. The goodness of fit of the data points to a straight line ($R^2 = 0.9818$) indicates excellent conformity to the LQ model.

TABLE 4.3	Estimates of α/β Derived from Clinical Data		
Tissue	Endpoint	α/β	Reference
EARLY-RESPONDING TISSUES			
Skin	Erythema Desquamation	6.5–16	81,82
Lung	Pneumonitis	>8.8	83
LATE-RESPONDING TISSUES			
Spinal cord	Paralysis	0.87–3.3	84,85
Brain	Necrosis	2.1	51
Lens	Cataract	<1	86
Bowel	Grade 4	>2.2	87
Skin	Telangiectasia	2.7–4.5	88
Lung	Fibrosis	3.6	89

Adapted from Thames HD, Hendry JH. *Fractionation in Radiotherapy.* London: Taylor & Francis; 1987.

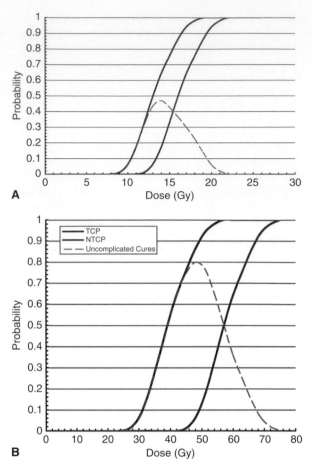

A

B

Figure 4.11. Curves schematically comparing the probability of tumor control (TCP) with the probability of a normal tissue complication (NTCP). **A:** For single doses, the curves are positioned relatively close to one another. Normal tissue complications may be avoided only by minimizing the dose to the critical normal structure. Such a situation may occur when a normal structure such as optic nerve lies adjacent to a tumor being treated with single-dose radiosurgery. **B:** Dose fractionation separates the TCP and the NTCP curves allowing for a higher probability of tumor control without significant risk of normal tissue complication. The "Uncomplicated Cure" curve is TCP-NTCP.

LQ equation so that inverse total dose $(1/D)$ may be plotted against dose per fraction (d):

$$\frac{1}{D} = \frac{\alpha}{SF} + \left[\frac{\beta}{SF}\right]d$$

This estimates an α/β of 2.3 Gy. This is consistent with the late-responding nature of cranial nerve VIII to radiation. The goodness of fit to linearity in this model is a measure of how well the LQ model estimates biological effectiveness of various schedules.[38] It should also be pointed out that none of these fractionation schedules appear to have a clear advantage in terms of therapeutic ratio. The estimated α/β for acoustic neuroma is similar and each fractionation schedule results in excellent tumor control and equivalent rates of preservation of useful hearing.[37] The decision to fractionate or use single-dose radiosurgery for acoustic neuromas is based on tumor size and volume effects on normal tissue risk for brain, brain stem, and cranial nerve.[39] In general, clinically estimated α/β are in good agreement with those derived from animal experiments (Table 4.3).[40]

THERAPEUTIC RATIO

The goal of altered fractionation should be to improve the *therapeutic ratio*. Therapeutic ratio is a concept inherent to all medical therapies. In its simplest form, it may be semiquantitatively expressed for cancer therapy as

Therapeutic ratio = TCP/NTCP

where TCP is the probability of tumor cure (or control) and NTCP is the probability of a normal tissue complication.

MODEL PREDICTING TUMOR CONTROL PROBABILITY BASED ON CELL SURVIVAL

The probability of tumor control (TCP) is a function of the likelihood of inactivating all tumor cells in a given tumor following Poisson statistics. If it is assumed that every tumor cell must be killed to control a tumor, TCP is given by

$$TCP = e^{-SF \times N}$$

where SF is the surviving fraction and N the total number of cells in the tumor. SF × N is then the average number of viable cells remaining in a tumor receiving a certain treatment. TCP is then the probability of no cells remaining viable under these conditions. TCP is a function of total dose and dose per fraction (BED), N (tumor bulk), and radiosensitivity of the tumor. This model leads to a sigmoid dose response curve for TCP (Fig. 4.11).

NORMAL TISSUE RADIOBIOLOGY

MODEL PREDICTING NORMAL TISSUE COMPLICATIONS

The probability of normal tissue complication (NTCP) following radiotherapy is, like tumor control probability, a function of dose and dose per fraction (BED), the tissue at risk (radiosensitivity) and the volume irradiated. NTCP has been shown

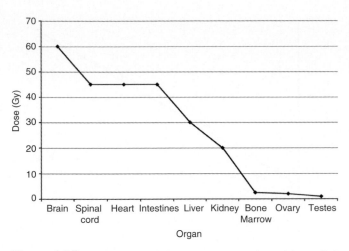

Figure 4.12. Tolerance doses for various organs derived from clinical practice.[90]

to be well represented by the model first described by Lyman and Wolbarst.[41] This is represented graphically as a sigmoid-shaped curve similar to that obtained for tumor cure (Fig. 4.11). Curves for a wide variety of normal tissue endpoints have been generated. Although each has a similar shape, the relative placement of these curves along the dose axis may be quite different. In other words, the tolerance of normal tissues to radiation is highly variable (Fig. 4.12). In clinical radiotherapy, the relative positions of the curves for tumor cure and normal tissue complication define what is known as the *therapeutic ratio*.

An ideal therapeutic ratio would be described by curves that allow 100% tumor cure without appreciable probability of normal tissue complication. The opposite extreme would be exemplified by a tumor requiring high dose radiation for cure located within a critical normal structure with a low tolerance to radiation. In practice, a regimen that maximizes the probability of an uncomplicated cure is optimal. For the situation where α/β for tumor is higher than that for critical normal tissue, dose fractionation will always serve to separate the

TCP and NTCP curves and increase the therapeutic ratio (Fig. 4.11).

DOSE RATE EFFECTS

Conventional fractionated radiotherapy is delivered at dose rates of 200 cGy/min or greater. Background, environmental radiation is received at much lower dose rates. It is well established that dose rate greatly influences the biological effects of ionizing radiation.[42] When dose rate is reduced below about 100 cGy/min, the total dose required to produce a specific biological effect is increased. It is generally accepted that this effect is due to repair of sublethal damage during the period of irradiation. As dose rate is lowered, a greater proportion of sublethally damaged sites are repaired before a second event can occur to combine and create a lethal lesion. At a dose rate of approximately 1 cGy/min, the mammalian dose-effect curve represented by the LQ model approaches the pure single-hit component of the curve represented by

$$E = e^{-\alpha D}.$$

In effect continuous, low-dose rate irradiation is an extreme form of fractionated radiotherapy (Fig. 4.13). With pure α component as a limit to the dose-rate effect, the extent of sparing due to low dose rate, like fractionation, is greatest in those tissues exhibiting the lowest α/β and more β-type reparable, sublethal damage.

Dose-rate effects have been demonstrated for a variety of normal tissues. Fu et al.[43] demonstrated a protection factor of >2 in jejunal crypt cell survival in mice when dose rate was lowered from 2.7 Gy/min to 0.3 Gy/h. Mazeron et al.[44] demonstrated that local control of oral cavity tumors did not fall significantly with the use of lower dose rate. However, in the same patients, the rate of late toxicity (necrosis) was about halved when dose rates of <0.05 Gy/h were used, compared to higher dose rates (Fig. 4.14).

The risk of brain necrosis in patients treated for brain tumors increases rapidly with single doses in excess of 15 to 20 Gy delivered at high dose rate (radiosurgery).[45–47] Similar rates of

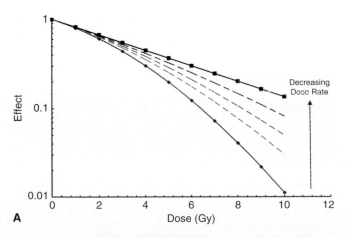

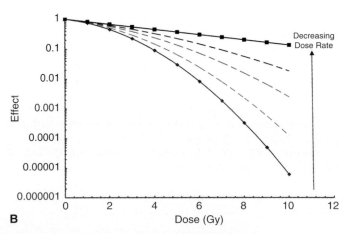

Figure 4.13. Dose-effect curves for low dose rate irradiation compared to high dose rate for tissues exhibiting high α/β (**A**) and low α/β (**B**). Tissues with low α/β are spared more by low dose rate radiation due to a larger component of sublethal damage that may be repaired during the protracted radiation time.

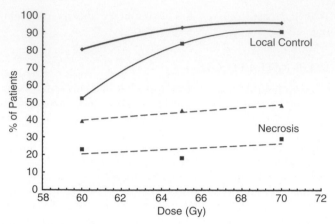

Figure 4.14. Results of a clinical study comparing local control of tumor (solid lines) and rates of radionecrosis (dashed lines) as a function of dose rate. Dose rates were ≥0.5 Gy/h (blue) or <0.5 Gy/h (red). When sufficient doses were used (≥65 Gy), there was an improvement in therapeutic ratio with the lower dose rate (redrawn with permission from Mazeron et al.[44]).

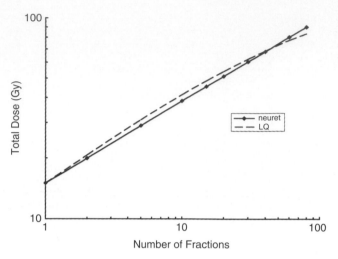

Figure 4.15. Data predicting low risk of radionecrosis comparing the model of Sheline et al.[51] to a fit of the data to the LQ model using an $\alpha/\beta = 2$ Gy.

brain necrosis result following doses >60 Gy of low dose-rate irradiation (brachytherapy).[45,48]

Mutation doubling rates have been shown to be substantially lower following low dose-rate irradiation, compared to high dose rate. As part of the "Megamouse Project" it was shown that the mutation doubling dose was about 30 cGy for acute exposures and about 100 cGy for low dose-rate exposure.[49] This is important since human germ line mutations may occur following continuous low dose-rate exposures, from occupational or environmental sources, or from an acute exposure from radiation therapy or an accident.

A final example of dose-rate effects is seen in the estimates of cancer risk following radiation exposure. For the entire population, including young children, the risk is estimated to be 10×10^{-2} per Sv and 5×10^{-2} per Sv for high and low dose-rate exposures, respectively.[50]

MODELS TO COMPARE BED OF DIFFERENT FRACTIONATION SCHEMES

It is important when investigating nonconventional fractionation schemes to have some basis for the choice of fraction size, total dose, and interval between fractions. If α/β were well established for all tumors and normal tissues, the LQ model would provide such a basis. Other models have been developed for specific normal tissues. Considering the difficulty of gathering clinical data to construct isoeffect curves for various fractionation schemes, most models are not inconsistent with the predictions of the LQ model.[38]

Sheline et al.[51] described a model for predicting the risk of brain necrosis as a function of total dose and number of fractions. The model defined an isoeffect line for total dose as a function of fraction number defining tolerance for various schedules. They defined the neuret, similar to BED,

$$\text{Neuret} = D \times N^{-0.41} \times T^{-0.03}$$

where D is the total dose in cGy, N the number of fractions, and T the overall time in days. This relationship demonstrated the

strong dependence on N, a surrogate for fraction size, and the very weak dependence on overall time, T. These data may also be well fit to the LQ model using an α/β of 2.0 without a time factor (Fig. 4.15).

The literature would indicate that the formula derived by Sheline et al. could approximate isoeffect curves for other CNS effects such as optic neuropathy and spinal cord injury[52–54] (Table 4.4). A common feature for these models is an exponent of N similar to that found by Sheline et al. and a nearly 0 exponent of time (T). This emphasizes the importance of the number of fractions, or fraction size, in determining the tolerance dose of normal tissues in the CNS. For most late-responding normal tissues, the overall time of treatment is relatively unimportant within the range normally encountered in a single radiation course.[53]

Attempts to model isoeffective dose regimens for the risk of optic neuropathy following fractionated radiotherapy have led to a similar model published by Goldsmith et al.[52] They defined the *optic ret* as

$$\text{Optic ret} = D \times N^{-0.53}$$

finding that attempts to fit clinical data to the LQ model resulted in possible negative α/β, a case that has no real meaning.

TABLE 4.4		Clinical Modeling of N and T for Various CNS Effects		
Author	*Reference*	*Site/Effect*	*Exponent of N*	*Exponent of T*
Sheline et al.	51	Brain/necrosis	−0.41	−0.03
Wara et al.	54	Spinal cord/ myelopathy	−0.38	−0.058
Van der Kogel	53	Spinal cord/ myelopathy	−0.4	0
Goldsmith et al.	52	Optic nerve/ neuropathy	−0.53	0

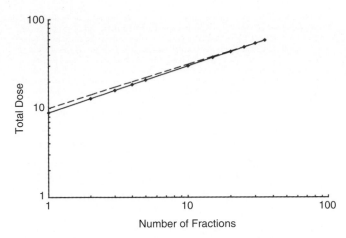

Figure 4.16. Comparison of prediction of low risk of optic neuropathy using the optic ret model of Goldsmith et al.[52] (blue) or the LQ model and an extremely low $\alpha/\beta = 0.1$ Gy (red).

They defined a threshold for optic neuropathy defining a "safe" regimen as one resulting in no more than 890 optic ret. This corresponds to 5,400 cGy in 30 fractions; 3,750 cGy in 15 fractions; and 3,000 cGy in 10 fractions, all commonly used fractionation schedules. Although not based on single fraction data, the optic ret model predicts that a single fraction of 8.9 Gy would be safe to the optic apparatus. This agrees very well with single fraction tolerance doses proposed in the literature, which range from 8 to 10 Gy.[55,56] The total dose predicted by the optic ret model to be safe may be calculated as

$$D\,(\text{Gy}) = \frac{8.9\,\text{Gy}}{N^{-0.53}}$$

This model emphasizes the well-established importance of fraction size in determining optic nerve tolerance to radiotherapy[57,58] and demonstrates a fractionation response consistent with an extremely low α/β (Fig. 4.16).

Other surrogates for BED are commonly used including equivalent doses. Using the LQ model, and substituting in the BED formula, equivalent dose in 2 Gy fractions may be calculated[59]:

$$\text{ED}(2\,\text{Gy}) = \frac{\alpha/\beta + d_1}{\alpha/\beta + 2}$$

Other models are not based on the LQ model. For example, the product $d \times D$ has been reported to correlate with the risk of brain necrosis.[60]

CURRENT CONTROVERSY IN THE RADIOBIOLOGY OF DOSE FRACTIONATION

It is generally agreed that at relatively low doses per fraction, that is, those used in conventionally fractionated radiotherapy, the LQ formula does a good job in predicting isoeffective regimens. However, question remains as to whether the model should be relied on to predict equivalent biological effectiveness when large doses per fraction are used, such as in stereotactic radiosurgery or stereotactic body radiotherapy. Park et al. proposed that at larger doses per fraction the LQ model overpredicted

biological effect, due to the continuously bending shape of the dose-response curve at high doses.[61] They recommended a linear response be added to the curve to maintain what they predicted was a more accurate prediction at high doses per fraction. Fowler[62] pointed out that a similar curve could result from an α/β of approximately 20 Gy. He felt that this was a more reasonable approach that did not require "throwing the α/β (model) baby out with the bath water."

An alternative analysis of the LQ model invoked an *increased* biological effectiveness at high doses per fraction due to effects on vasculature that only occur when dose per fraction exceeds approximately 10 to 12 Gy.[63,64] The additional tissue damage caused by the effects on vascular endothelial cells at high doses per fraction would cause the LQ model to underestimate the biological effect of such doses.

Brenner investigated the applicability of the LQ model to high doses per fraction and concluded that the LQ model provided "reasonable" prediction of results up to about 18 Gy. This was based on fitting in vivo experimental data of early and late normal tissue using the inverse plot of Douglas and Fowler and testing for goodness of fit.[27,38]

CONCLUSION

Dose fractionation, including effects of low dose-rate irradiation, greatly influences the biological effectiveness of ionizing radiation. These effects of fractionation extend from effects on mutation rates and carcinogenesis to applications in modern radiotherapy of cancer. The LQ model provides a means to predict these effects and has proved useful in the full range of radiobiological applications. Further understanding of the mechanisms by which radiation affects normal cell, tissue, and organ function is needed to more fully understand the effects of dose fractionation.

REFERENCES

1. Bergonie J, Tribondeau L. De quelques resultats de la radiotherapie et essai de fixation d'une technique rationale. *C R Acad Sci.* 1906;143:983–985.
2. Regaud C, Ferroux R. Discordance des effets des rayons X, d'une part dans la peau, d'autre part dans le testicule, par fractionnement de la dose: diminution de l'efficacite dans la peau, maintien de l'efficacite dans le testicule. *C R Soc Biol.* 1927;97:431–434.
3. Schwarz G. Über Desensibilisierung gegen Rontgen-und Radiumstrahlen. *Munch Med Wschr.* 1909;24:1–2.
4. Mohr, OL. Mikroskopische Untersuchung zu Experimenten über den Einfluss der Radiumstrahlen und der Kältewirkung auf die Chromatinreifung und das Heterchromosom bei Decticus verruccivorus. *Archiv für Mikroskopische Anatomie.* 1919;92(1): 300–368.
5. Nather K, Schinz HR. Teirexperimentielle Studien zum Krebsprobelm. I. Gibt es eine Reizdosis bei malignen tumoren? *Mitt Grenzgeb Med Chir.* 1923;36:620–660.
6. Thames HD. Early fractionation methods and the origins of the NSD concept. *Acta Oncol.* 1988;27:89–103.
7. Coutard H. Die Rontgenbehandlung der epithelialen Krebse der Tonsillengegend. *Stahlentherapie.* 1929;33:249–252.
8. Fowler JF. Non-standard fractionation in radiotherapy. *Int J Radiat Oncol Biol Phys.* 1984;10:755–759.
9. Fu KK, Pajak T, Trotti A, et al. A Radiation Therapy Oncology Group (RTOG) Phase III randomized study to compare hyperfractionation and two variants of accelerated fractionation to standard fractionation radiotherapy for head and neck squamous cell carcinomas: First report of RTOG 9003. *Int J Radiat Oncol Biol Phys.* 2000;48:7–16.
10. Thames HD, Hendry JH. *Fractionation in Radiotherapy.* London: Taylor & Francis; 1987.
11. Puck TT, Marcus PI. Action of x-rays on mammalian cells. *J Exp Med.* 1956;103:653–666.
12. Elkind MM, Sutton H. X-ray damage and recovery in mammalian cells in culture. *Nature.* 1959;184:1293–1295.
13. Ang KK, Jiang GL, Guttenberger R, et al. Impact of spinal cord repair kinetics on the practice of altered fractionation schedules. *Radiother Oncol.* 1992;25:287–294.
14. Dische S. Accelerated treatment and radiation myelitis (editorial). *Radiother Oncol.* 1991;20:1–2.
15. Withers HR. The 4 R's of radiotherapy. In: Lett JT, Adler H, eds. *Advances in Radiation Biology.* Vol 5. New York: Academic Press; 1975:241.
16. Reisner A. Hauterythem und Roentgenstrahlung. *Ergebrisse der Medizinischen Strahlenforschung.* 1933;6:1–60.

17. Duffy J, Arnesen AN, Edward LV. The rate of recuperation of human skin following irradiation. *Radiology.* 1934;23:486–490.

18. MacComb WS, Quimby EH. The rate of recovery of human skin from the effects of hard or soft Roentgen rays or gamma rays. *Radiology.* 1936;27:196–204.

19. Strandqvist M. Studien uber die kumulitive Wirkung der Rongtenstrahlen bei Fraktionerung. *Acta Radiol.* 1944;25(supp 55):1–300.

20. Cohen L. Clinical radiation dosage, Pt II. *Br J Radiol.* 1949;22:706–713.

21. Cohen BH. Clinical radiation dosage. *Br J Radiol.* 1949;22(255):160–163.

22. Von Essen CF. A spatial model of time-dose-area relationships in radiation therapy. *Radiology.* 1963;81:881–883.

23. Ellis F. Dose, time and fractionation: a clinical hypothesis. *Clin Radiol.* 1969;20:1–7.

24. Ellis F. Nominal standard dose and the ret. *Br J Radiol.* 1971;44:101–108.

25. Orton CG, Ellis F. Q simplification of the use of NSD concept in practical radiotherapy. *Br J Radiol.* 1973;46:529–537.

26. Fowler JF, Morgan RL, Silvester JA, et al. Experiments with fractionated X-ray treatment of the skin of pigs. *Br J Radiol.* 1963;36(423):188–196.

27. Douglas BG, Fowler JF. The effect of multiple small doses of X-rays on skin reactions in the mouse and a basic interpretation. *Radiat Res.* 1976;66:401–426.

28. Thames HD, Withers HR, Peters LJ, et al. Changes in early and late radiation responses with altered dose fractionation: implications for dose-survival relationships. *Int J Radiat Oncol Biol Phys.* 1982;8:219–226.

29. McBride WH, Withers HR. Biologic basis of radiation therapy. *Principles & Practice of Radiation Oncology.* 4th ed. Philadelphia, PA: Lippincott, Williams and Wilkins; 2004:96–136.

30. Brenner DJ. Correlations between a/b and T1/2: implications for clinical biological modelling. *Br J Radiol.* 1992;65:1051–1054.

31. Withers HR. Biologic Basis of radiation therapy. In: Perez CA, Brady LW, eds. *Principles and Practice of Radiation Oncology.* New York: J.B. Lippincott Company; 1992:64–96.

32. Michalski JM, Bae K, Roach M, et al. Long-term toxicity following D3D conformal radiation therapy for prostate cancer from the RTOG 9406 Phase I/II dose escalation study. *Int J Radiat Oncol Biol Phys.* 2010;76(1):14–22.

33. Fowler JF. What next in fractionation? *Br J Radiol.* 1984;49(supp):285–300.

34. Fowler JF. The radiobiology of prostate cancer including new aspects of fractionated radiotherapy. *Acta Oncol.* 2005;44:265–276.

35. Anker CJ, Shrieve DC. Basic Principles of Radiobiology Applied to Radiotherapy of Benign Skull Base Tumors. *Otolaryng Clinics N America.* 2009;42:601–621.

36. Chopra R, Kondziolka D, Niranjan A, et al. Long-term follow-up of acoustic schwannoma radiosurgery with marginal tumor doses of 12 to 13 Gy. *Int J Radiat Oncol Biol Phys.* 2007;68:845–851.

37. Anker CA, Shrieve DC. Basic principles of radiobiology applied to radiosurgery and radiotherapy of benign skull base tumors. *Otolaryngol Clin North Am.* 2009;42(4):601–621.

38. Brenner DJ. The linear-quadratic model is an appropriate methodology for determining isoeffective doses at large doses per fraction. *Semin Radiat Oncol.* 2008;18:234–239.

39. Chan AW, Black PM, Ojemann RG, et al. Stereotactic radiotherapy for vestibular schwannoma: favorable outcome with minimal toxicity. *Neurosurg.* 2005;57:60–70.

40. Thames HD, Bentzen SM, Turesson I, et al. Fractionation parameters for human tissues and tumors. *Int J Radiat Biol.* 1989;56:701–710.

41. Lyman JT, Wolbarst AB. Optimization of radiation therapy. III. A method of assessing complication probabilities from dose-volume histograms. *Int J Radiat Oncol Biol Phys.* 1987;13:103–109.

42. Hall EJ, Bedford JS. Dose rate: its effect on the survival of HeLa cells irradiated with gamma rays. *Radiat Res.* 1964;22:305.

43. Fu KK, Phillips TL, Kane LJ, et al. Tumor and normal tissue response to irradiation in vivo: variation with decreasing dose rates. *Radiol.* 1975;114(3):709–716.

44. Mazeron JJ, Simon JM, Le Pechoux C, et al. Effect of dose rate on local control and complications in definitive irradiation of T 1–2 squamous cell carcinomas of mobile tongue and floor of mouth with interstitial iridium-192. *Radiother Oncol.* 1991;21:39–47.

45. Shrieve DC, Alexander E III, Wen PY, et al. Comparison of stereotactic radiosurgery and brachytherapy in the treatment of recurrent glioblastoma multiforme. *Neurosurgery.* 1995;36:275–284.

46. Shrieve DC, Alexander EI, Black PM, et al. Treatment of patients with primary glioblastoma multiforme with standard postoperative radiotherapy and radiosurgical boost: prognostic factors and long-term outcome. *J Neurosurg.* 1999;90:72–77.

47. Shaw E, Scott C, Souhami L, et al. Single dose radiosurgical treatment of recurrent previously irradiated primary brain tumors and brain metastases: final report of RTOG protocol 90–05. *Int J Radiat Oncol Biol Phys.* 2000;47:291–298.

48. Scharfen CO, Sneed PK, Wara WM, et al. High activity iodine—125 interstitial implant for gliomas. *Int J Radiat Oncol Biol Phys.* 1992;24(4):583–591.

49. Russell WL, Kelly EM. Mutation frequencies in male mice and the estimation of genetic hazards of radiation in men. *Proc Natl Acad Sci USA.* 1982;79(542–544).

50. Protection ICoR. Recommendations. *Annals of the ICRP Publication 60.* Oxford: Pergamon Press; 1990.

51. Sheline GE, Wara WM, Smith V. Therapeutic irradiation and brain injury. *Int J Radiat Oncol Biol Phys.* 1980;6(9):1215–1228.

52. Goldsmith BJ, Rosenthal SA, Wara WM, et al. Optic neuropathy after irradiation of meningioma. *Radiology.* 1992;185:71–76.

53. van der Kogel AJ. Central nervous system radiation injury in small animals. In: Gutin PH, Leibel SA, Sheline GE, eds. *Radiation Injury in the Nervous System.* New York: Raven Press, Ltd.; 1991:91–111.

54. Wara WM, Phillips TL, Sheline GE, et al. Radiation tolerance of the spinal cord. *Cancer.* 1975;35:1558–1562.

55. Tishler RB, Loeffler JS, Lunsford LD, et al. Tolerance of cranial nerves of the cavernous sinus to radiosurgery. *Int J Radiat Oncol Biol Phys.* 1993;27(2):215–221.

56. Leber KA, Bergloff J, Pendl G. Dose-response tolerance of the visual pathways and cranial nerves of the cavernous sinus to stereotactic radiosurgery. *J Neurosurg.* 1998;88:43–50.

57. Harris JR, Levene MB. Visual complications following irradiation for pituitary adenomas and craniopharyngiomas. *Ther Radiol.* 1976;120:167–171.

58. Parsons JT, Bova FJ, Fitzgerald CR, et al. Radiation optic neuropathy after megavoltage external-beam irradiation: Analysis of time-dose factors. *Int J Radiat Oncol Biol Phys.* 1994;30(4):755–763.

59. Barton M. Tables of equivalent doses in 2 Gy fractions: simple application of the linear quadratic formula. *Int J Radiat Oncol Biol Phys.* 1995;31:371–378.

60. Lee AWM, Kwong DL, Leung S-F, et al. Factors affecting risk of symptomatic temporal lobe necrosis: significance of fractional dose and treatment time. *Int J Radiat Oncol Biol Phys.* 2002;53:75–85.

61. Park C, Papiez L, Zhang S, et al. Universal Survival curve and single fraction equivalent dose: useful tools in understanding potency of ablative radiotherapy. *Int J Radiat Oncol Biol Phys.* 2008;70:847–852.

62. Fowler JF. Linear quadratics is alive and well: In regard to Park et al. (*Int J Radiat Oncol Biol Phys.* 2008;70:847–852). *Int J Radiat Oncol Biol Phys.* 2008;72:957–959.

63. Kirkpatrick JP, Meyer JJ, Marks LB. The linear-quadratic model is inappropriate to model high dose per fraction effects in radiosurgery. *Semin Radiat Oncol.* 2008;18:240–243.

64. Garcia-Barros M, Paris F, Cordon-Cardo C, et al. Tumor response to radiotherapy regulated by endothelial cell apoptosis. *Science.* 2003;300:1155–1159.

65. Fowler JF, Denekamp J, Delapeyre C, et al. Skin reactions in mice after multifraction X-radiation. *Int J Radiat Biol.* 1974;25:213–223.

66. Joiner MC, Denekamp J, Maughan RL. The use of 'top-up' experiments to investigate the effect of very small doses per fraction in mouse skin. *Int J Radiat Biol.* 1986;49:565–580.

67. Vegesna V, Withers HR, Taylor JMG. The effect of depigmentation and multifractionated irradiation on resting hair follicles. *Radiat Res.* 1987;111:464–473.

68. Withers HR, Chu AM, Reid BO, et al. Response of mouse jejunum to multifraction radiation. *Int J Radiat Oncol Biol Phys.* 1975;1:41–52.

69. Tucker SL, Withers HR, Mason KA, et al. A dose-surviving fraction curve for colonic mucosa. *Eur J Cancer Clin Oncol.* 1983;19:433–437.

70. Thames HD, Withers HR. Test of equal effect per fraction and estimation of initial clonogen number in microcolony assays of survival after fractionated irradiation. *Br J Radiol.* 1980;53:1071–1077.

71. Ruifrok ACC, Kleiboer BJ, Van der Kogel AJ. Fractionation sensitivity of the rat cervical spinal cord during radiation treatment. *Radiother Oncol.* 1992;25:295–300.

72. Hornsey S, Morris CC, Myers R, et al. Relative biological effectiveness for damage to the central nervous system by neutrons. *Int J Radiat Oncol Biol Phys.* 1981;7:185–189.

73. Schenken LL, Hagemann RF. Time/dose relationships in experimental cataractogenesis. *Radiology.* 1975;117:193–198.

74. Williams MV, Denekamp J. Radiation induced renal damage in mice: influence of fraction size. *Int J Radiat Oncol Biol Phys.* 1984;10:885–894.

75. Stewart FA, Randhawa VS, Michael BD. Multifraction irradiation of mouse bladders. *Radiother Oncol.* 1984;2:131–140.

76. Terry NHA, Denekamp J. RBE values and repair characteristics for colo-rectal injury after caesium-137 gamma-ray and neutron irradiation. II. Fractionation up to ten doses *Br J Radiol.* 1984;57:617–629.

77. Withers HR, Thames HD, Flow BL, et al. The relationship of acute and late skin injury in 2 and 5 fraction/week g-ray therapy. *Int J Radiat Oncol Biol Phys.* 1978;4:595–601.

78. Hornsey S, Kutsutani Y, Field SB. Damage to mouse lung with fractionated neutrons and x-rays. *Radiology.* 1975;116:171–174.

79. Parkins CS, Fowler JF. Repair in mouse lung of multifraction x-rays and neutrons: extension to 40 fractions. *Br J Radiol.* 1985;58:1097–1103.

80. Wara WM, Phillips TL, Margolis LW, et al. Radiation pneumonitis: A new approach to the derivation of time-dose factors. *Cancer.* 1973;32(3):547–552.

81. Turesson I, Notter G. The influence of the overall treatment time in radiotherapy on the acute reaction: comparison of the effects of daily and twice-a-week fractionation on human skin. *Int J Radiat Oncol Biol Phys.* 1984;10:607–618.

82. Turesson I, Thames HD. Repair capacity and kinetics of human skin during fractionated radiotherapy: erythema, desquamation, and telangiectasia after 3 and 5 year's follow-up. *Radiother Oncol.* 1989;15:169–188.

83. Cox JD. Fractionation: a paradigm for clinical research in radiation oncology. *Int J Radiat Oncol Biol Phys.* 1987;13:1271–1281.

84. Dische S, Martin WMC, Anderson P. Radiation myelopathy in patients treated for carcinoma of the bronchus using a six fraction regime of radiotherapy. *Br J Radiol.* 1981;54:29–35.

85. Schultheiss TE. The radiation dose-response of the human spinal cord. *Int J Radiat Oncol Biol Phys.* 2008;71:1455–1459.

86. Belkacemi Y, Touboul E, Méric JB, et al. Cataracte radio-induite: aspects physiopathologiques, radiobiologiques et cliniques. *Cancer Radiother.* 2001;5:397–412.

87. Edsmyr F, Andersson L, Esposti PL, et al. Irradiation therapy with multiple small fractions per day in urinary bladder cancer. *Radiother Oncol.* 1985;4:197–203.

88. Turesson I, Notter G. The influence of fraction size in radiotherapy of the late normal tissue reaction—II: comparison of the effects of daily and twice-a-week fractionation on human skin. *Int J Radiat Oncol Biol Phys.* 1984;10:599–606.

89. Overgaard M. The clinical implication of non-standard fractionation. *Int J Radiat Oncol Biol Phys.* 1985;11:1225–1229.

90. Emami B, Lyman J, Brown A, et al. Tolerance of normal tissue to therapeutic irradiation. *Int J Radiat Oncol Biol Phys.* 1991;21(1):109–122.

CHAPTER

5

Kevin R. Kozak
Paul M. Harari

Agents Impacting Radiosensitivity

INTRODUCTION

The primary objectives for a course of therapeutic radiation include (a) durable local tumor control and (b) unaltered normal tissue function and cosmesis. These aims are inextricably linked and are often at odds with one another. A clear dose-response relationship for local tumor control has long been recognized, thus, "more dose, better control." However, with dose escalation, irradiated normal tissues are also more likely to be adversely affected. The goal of the radiation oncology team is therefore to strike the best balance between these competing aims: optimize tumor control probability and minimize normal tissue damage. Although ionizing radiation appears, on the surface, to be a "blunt instrument," radiation oncologists have several tools to aid them in achieving a more refined balance. The most widely recognized tools include straightforward physical approaches: conformal radiation delivery and fractionation. The former applies evolving technologies in radiation delivery and imaging science to limit radiation dose to uninvolved tissues, thereby minimizing normal tissue complication probability. The latter capitalizes on differences in growth kinetics and repair capacity between normal tissues and tumor tissue.

Additional strategies to enhance the utility of ionizing radiation involve combining it with agents that favorably alter radiation response. In general terms, such agents can be radiosensitizers that enhance radiation damage or radioprotectors that reduce radiation damage. The somewhat paradoxical assertion that both radiosensitizers and radioprotectors may improve the clinical outcomes of a course of radiation therapy demands a brief examination of an important general concept in cancer therapy: therapeutic index.

Therapeutic index, or therapeutic ratio, refers to the balance between tumor control and normal tissue complications and is best illustrated graphically (Fig. 5.1). In an optimal clinical scenario, the ratio of tumor control probability to normal tissue complication probability is high (i.e., the therapeutic index or ratio is high) and acceptable tumor control probabilities can be obtained with little to no risk to normal tissues (Fig. 5.1A). This scenario is rarely encountered. More generally, the dose-response curves for normal tissues and tumor tissue are less widely separated and some balance must be struck between tumor control and the risk of complications (Fig. 5.1B).

Radiosensitizers and radioprotectors permit modulation of both normal tissue and tumor dose-response curves. However, this modulation does not necessarily translate into clinical ben-

efit. For example, if a radiosensitizer is combined with ionizing radiation but enhances the radiosensitivity of both at-risk normal tissue and tumor tissue equally, no alteration of the therapeutic index, and thus no clinical gain, is achieved (Fig. 5.1C). Similarly, a radioprotector that reduces normal tissue sensitivity and also protects the tumor may not provide any benefit. In fact, in both these circumstances, the net clinical effect will almost always be negative as radiosensitizers and radioprotectors, like most systemic agents, have attendant toxicities distinct from their local effects (e.g., hypotension or nausea with a radioprotector). Even further degradation of the therapeutic index can occur if a radioprotector selectively protects tumor tissue or if a radiosensitizer selectively sensitizes normal tissue (Fig. 5.1D).

These critical concepts must be borne in mind when contemplating the use of an agent that impacts radiosensitivity. Importantly, these concepts must also be considered when reviewing the ever-expanding clinical and scientific literature focused on such agents. The literature is replete with reports of systemic agents that augment tumor responses to ionizing radiation. Unfortunately, it is uncommon for such reports to examine the impact of the studied agent on potentially at-risk normal tissues. It is even less common for such reports to rigorously assess the nature of the augmented response: does the agent have additive, subadditive, or supra-additive (synergistic) effects with radiation? These issues are crucial in determining the potential clinical utility of a specific radiation modifier.

Despite these and other challenges, significant efforts have been dedicated to the development of agents that favorably modify the therapeutic index. Much of the early work on radiation sensitivity modifiers emerged from the recognition that human solid tumors often contain significant regions of hypoxia, areas known to be less sensitive to low linear energy transfer radiation (e.g., photons), and this topic will be reviewed in some detail. Radiation protectors will comprise the second subset of agents discussed. Conventional cytotoxic therapies will then be reviewed with particular attention to the interaction of these agents with ionizing radiation. The evidence for the utility of combined modality therapy will be examined using specific tumor examples. More recently, molecularly targeted therapeutics, or biologicals, have emerged as important agents in the oncologic armamentarium, and early investigation of combination regimens with ionizing radiation has shown promise. The potential of these agents to beneficially alter the therapeutic index will be explored. Finally, a brief commentary will be offered on hyperthermia—a time-tested,

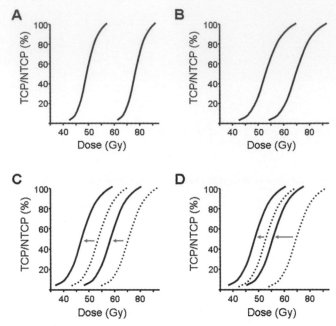

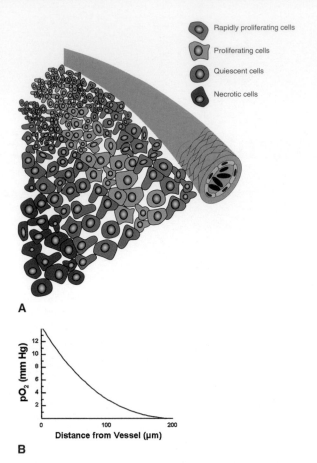

Figure 5.1. Therapeutic index. Tumor control probability (TCP, *blue*) and normal tissue complication probability (NTCP, *red*) are shown as a function of radiation dose. **A:** An idealized clinical setting with a high therapeutic index — high probability of tumor control with little risk of normal tissue complications. **B:** Realistic clinical setting where high probabilities of tumor control are associated with significant risks of normal tissue complication. **C:** Modification of TCP and NTCP by a radiosensitizer. With comparable radiosensitization of tumor and normal tissue, there is no therapeutic gain. **D:** Unfavorable modification of TCP and NTCP by a radiosensitizer that preferentially sensitizes normal tissue.

Figure 5.2. Hypoxia in tumors. **A:** Distribution of tumor cell subsets and (**B**) oxygen tension as a function of distance from a functional blood vessel.

but less frequently employed, physical modality that alters radiation dose-response characteristics.

HYPOXIA-RELATED RADIOSENSITIZERS

Normal tissue vascular architecture ensures that all reproductively intact, normal cells are located within approximately 200 μm of a blood capillary so that adequate levels of oxygen and other nutrients are obtainable *via* diffusion (Fig. 5.2A).[1] Tumor cells, like their normal counterparts, require oxygen and nutrients for survival and proliferation. In fact, both primary tumors and metastatic lesions appear to begin as small, avascular cellular aggregates that may remain dormant for extended periods until new blood vessels provide wider access to oxygen and nutrients.[2–4] This pathophysiologic process has been termed the *angiogenic switch* and permits tumor growth beyond a few cubic millimeters. However, in contrast to the orderly distribution of blood capillaries in normal tissues, tumor-driven angiogenesis results in structurally and functionally chaotic vascular beds. Tumor blood vessels tend to be dilated, saccular, tortuous, and anatomically disorganized resulting in marked heterogeneity in blood supply throughout a solid tumor.[5–11] These aberrancies, coupled with tumor overgrowth of supporting vessels, lead to areas of hypoxia and necrosis. Two forms of hypoxia are recognized. Chronic or diffusion-limited hypoxia is evidenced when tumor cells reside beyond the diffusion limits of oxygen (Fig. 5.2B). This form of hypoxia was first documented in the classic histopathologic experiments of Thomlinson and Gray[12] who identified "cords" of viable tumor cells along blood vessels in human lung cancers

accompanied by rims of necrotic cells beyond 180 μm. The second form of hypoxia, known as *acute* or *perfusion-limited hypoxia*, occurs during intermittent reductions in blood flow characteristic of the abnormal vasculature of solid tumors.

As these observations into tumor vascular biology and hypoxia were emerging, contemporaneous studies were identifying oxygen tension as a critical determinant in low linear energy transfer radiosensitivity. By the 1930s, the notion that oxygen may enhance tumor cell radiosensitivity was fairly well established.[13,14] By the 1950s, quantitative descriptions of the oxygen enhancement ratio (OER)—the ratio of hypoxic to oxic doses needed to achieve equivalent biological effects— were reported for a number of biological systems.[15–21] In most systems, the OER was found to be two- to threefold suggesting hypoxic cells may be profoundly radioresistant. The dual concepts of tumor hypoxia and hypoxic radioresistance met when Powers and Tolmach[22] reported a multicomponent tumor cell survival curve in a murine lymphosarcoma model. The biphasic radioresponse provided a key experimental demonstration of hypoxic cells in a solid tumor and simultaneously suggested that this minority population of relatively radioresistant cells may be crucial in determining tumor control (Fig. 5.3).

Subsequent investigations, particularly in animal models, have supported a potential role for hypoxic tumor cells in determining radiocurability. The role for hypoxia in determining radiocurability of human tumors subjected to fractionated radiation therapy, however, remains the subject of debate. Beyond its

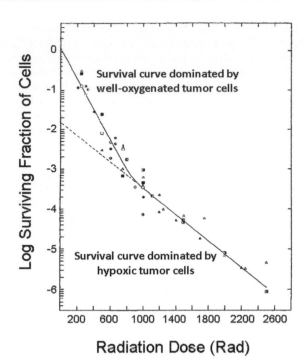

Figure 5.3. Multicomponent cell survival curve reflecting the significance of hypoxic cells in solid tumors treated with radiation. Survival of mouse lymphosarcoma (6*C3HED*) cells irradiated in vivo. (Reprinted with permission from Macmillan Publishers Ltd: Powers WE, Tolmach LJ. A multicomponent x-ray survival curve for mouse lymphosarcoma cells irradiated in vivo. *Nature.* 1963;197:710–711.)

impact on radiation sensitivity, hypoxia drives several other pathways affecting tumor (patho)physiology. For example, hypoxia has been shown to select for more malignant, more invasive, and genetically unstable cancer cells.[23–25] Thus, although worse outcomes have been associated with hypoxia in a number of human tumors treated with radiation therapy, it remains challenging to definitively attribute poorer outcomes to hypoxia-related radioresistance.[26–28] Nonetheless, based on the aforementioned observations coupled with the clear therapeutic index offered (normal tissue is rarely hypoxic in the adult), significant effort has been dedicated to overcoming tumor hypoxia to enhance radiosensitivity and, perhaps, radiocurability.

Among the most conceptually straightforward approaches to altering tumor oxygen tension involves increasing tumor oxygen supply by manipulating the composition of inspired gas. Early mouse studies evaluating oxygen or carbogen (95% O_2 + 5% CO_2) breathing were promising with significant reductions in tumor control doses compared to air breathing.[29–31] Importantly, mouse xenograft experiments have suggested a correlation between the change in tumor hypoxic fraction and tumor control doses lending credence to the presumed mechanism of action of oxygen breathing.[32] Further therapeutic gains were found to be achievable with hyperbaric gases[33,34]

Churchill-Davidson et al.[35–38] initiated clinical investigation on the value of high-oxygen-content gas breathing in the 1950s. The logistical complexity of delivering radiation therapy under these conditions resulted in the selection of unconventional, hypofractionated schemes confounding interpretation of results. However, radiation combined with hyperbaric oxygen appeared to offer a clinical advantage compared to radiation in air. These promising early results inspired a series of Medical Research Council (MRC) randomized trials of hyperbaric oxygen in head and neck, cervical, lung, and bladder cancer (Table 5.1). Significant local control and survival benefits were achieved in head and neck and cervical cancers. In contrast, no survival benefit was observed for bladder cancer and borderline improvements were observed in lung cancer at early timepoints.[39,40] Meta-analysis of 17 hyperbaric oxygen studies involving over 2,000 patients with a variety of primary lesions, demonstrated an absolute local control benefit of 6.6% (relative improvement, 14.6%).[41] Clinical attempts to minimize logistical complexities by substituting normobaric oxygen for hyperbaric oxygen met with less success.[42,43]

A potential limitation of high-oxygen-content breathing is that this manipulation addresses only chronic, or diffusion-limited, hypoxia. Acute hypoxia, produced by transient closure of tumor blood vessels, is not altered by oxygen inhalation. In fact, pure oxygen inspiration leads to physiologic vasoconstriction that can be avoided with the inclusion of 5% CO_2, hence the use of carbogen. Nonetheless, acute hypoxia remains a potential limitation of such approaches. Extensive preclinical investigation led to the identification of nicotinamide as an agent capable of inhibiting the transient closure of tumor blood vessels.[44–49] Thus, the combination of carbogen and nicotinamide offers the potential to relieve both chronic and acute tumor hypoxia. The intriguing combination of accelerated radiation therapy (to limit tumor cell proliferation) with carbogen breathing and nicotinamide (to limit tumor hypoxia) or ARCON has shown promise in early clinical trials and remains the subject of ongoing investigations.[50]

TABLE 5.1	MRC Randomized Trials of Hyperbaric Oxygen					
	4-year Local Control			*4-year Overall Survival*		
Anatomic Site and Study	*Hyperbaric*	*Air*	*p*	*Hyperbaric*	*Air*	*p*
HEAD AND NECK						
MRC I (*N* = 276)	55%	31%	<0.001	37%	37%	NS
MRC II (*N* = 127)	69%	41%	<0.01	62%	24%	0.001
BLADDER CANCER						
MRC (*N* = 236)	—	—	—	31%	35%	NS
BRONCHOGENIC CANCER						
MRC I (*N* = 78)	—	—	—	8%	8%	NS
MRC II (*N* = 197)	—	—	—	12%	2%	NS
CERVICAL CANCER						
MRC (*N* = 320)	66%	43%	0.001	40%	31%	0.032

Despite the sound rationale and documented efficacy of these techniques, hyperbaric oxygen and related treatment strategies have largely been abandoned due to logistical challenges and simpler alternatives to overcoming, or exploiting, tumor hypoxia. One investigative approach involves simply increasing oxygen delivery capacity by increasing red blood cell mass. Both red blood cell transfusion and exogenous erthropoietic agents have been examined as methods to overcome tumor hypoxia. Enthusiasm for these interventions developed as anemia was found to be a critical prognostic/predictive factor in a number of malignancies.[51] Enthusiasm was further supported by early studies suggesting improved outcomes with transfusion in anemic cervical cancer patients undergoing definitive radiotherapy.[52–54] However, careful analysis suggests that these studies are confounded by selection biases that preclude the conclusion that anemia correction by transfusion impacts outcome.[55–57] Similarly, erythropoietin (or analog) treatment showed promise in anemic lung cancer patients receiving chemotherapy and anemic cancer patients receiving nonplatinum chemotherapy.[58,59] However, subsequent trials in mainly nonanemic metastatic breast cancer patients and anemic head and neck cancer patients actually suggested outcomes may be impaired by erythropoietic agents.[60,61] There are a number of potential causes for the mixed results observed with such interventions and include the inability to increase tumor pO_2 as markedly as systemic pO_2,[62–64] the inability to increase pO_2 in all areas of a tumor to optimal levels due to abnormal vasculature,[65] and undesired "off-target" effects of interventions (e.g., immunosuppression with transfusion[66–68]). Furthermore, tumor reoxygenation during radiation therapy with standard fractionation may limit the impact of providing additional oxygen to tumor tissue.

In the 1950s and 1960s, as the radiosensitizing effects of oxygen were being explored both in the laboratory and the clinic, radiation chemists were simultaneously attempting to identify small molecules that might mimic oxygen as hypoxic cell radiosensitizers. At least two lines of reasoning inspired this effort. First, the complex logistics of high-oxygen-content breathing made a small molecule substitute, deliverable orally or intravenously, attractive. Second, a metabolically stable, small molecule oxygen mimic might potentially overcome the inherent pharmacologic lability of oxygen; as oxygen is "forced" into tumor tissue, viable tumor cells near blood vessels metabolize it limiting concentrations at distances. Theoretically, a metabolically stable oxygen mimic might diffuse widely through a solid tumor. In 1960, Bridges[60] reported that N-ethylmaleimide, when present during radiation, significantly reduced the colony-forming capacity of E. coli. Importantly, Bridges also demonstrated that this effect was more marked in an anaerobic environment.[69,70] In a medicinal/radiation chemistry tour de force, Adams et al.[71–75] identified nitroimidazoles as hypoxic cell radiosensitizers that fulfilled essential criteria for clinical utility: (a) selective sensitization of hypoxic cells, (b) metabolic stability, (c) appropriate lipophilicity to permit distant diffusion, and (d) sensitization at low radiation doses akin to those used in clinical fractionated radiation therapy (e.g., 2 Gy). The first candidate compound, misonidazole, was embraced and extensively studied.

In vitro, anoxic mammalian cells were found to be nearly as radiosensitive as identical cells cultured in an oxic environment when radiation was performed in the presence of low dose misonidazole (1–10 mM).[76–78] Furthermore, mouse models suggested misonidazole could shift tumor control probability curves with magnitudes consistent with a hypoxic cell sensitizing

mechanism (i.e., 1.8–2-fold).[79–82] Based on these encouraging data, misonidazole was introduced into clinical trials in a number of malignancies. Unfortunately, no significant advantage was observed with misonidazole among dozens of randomized controlled trials and neurotoxicity was evident.[83–92] Spurred by the preclinical promise of misonidazole and tantalizing suggestions from clinical trials that certain subsets of patients may benefit from its use, additional medicinal chemical efforts were directed at designing an improved nitroimidazole hypoxic cell sensitizer.[89]

These efforts led to development and testing of etanidazole, a significantly less neurotoxic nitroimidazole related to misonidazole.[93] Unfortunately, clinical trials with etanidazole failed to demonstrate a clinical benefit.[94,95] Subsequent investigations with another misonidazole derivative, nimorazole, were more promising. Overgaard and colleagues randomized 422 patients with pharynx or supraglottic larynx cancer to conventional, definitive radiation therapy with nimorazole or placebo. Nimorazole improved both locoregional control (49% vs. 33%) and 5-year disease-specific survival (52% vs. 41%); additionally, a trend toward improved overall survival with nimorazole was observed.[96] In efforts to clarify the magnitude of clinical benefit achievable with hypoxic cell radiosensitizers (and other modulators of hypoxia), Overgaard[97] recently updated a comprehensive meta-analysis including over 6,000 cancer patients treated with primary radiation therapy with curative intent and randomized to receive a nitroimidazole hypoxic sensitizer or placebo. The use of a hypoxic sensitizer improved locoregional control by 20% (OR: 0.80, 95% CI: 0.72–0.89). Despite this fairly dramatic benefit, nitroimidazole sensitization has not gained a significant foothold in practice. In Overgaard's[97] words, this apparent paradox "sadly indicates how difficult it is to advance even sound clinical concepts and shows that there is a long way to go before true evidenced-based medicine will get the platform it deserves." Despite the general lack of enthusiasm for hypoxic cell sensitizers in clinical practice, basic and clinical research continues and new agents, with improved pharmacokinetic and pharmacodynamic properties, appear regularly in the literature.[98–102]

A class of therapeutics related, in principle, to the nitroimidazoles deserves brief mention, namely, hypoxic cell cytotoxins. Although not necessarily modulators of the radiation response, these agents selectively kill hypoxic cells and thus are thematically related to hypoxic cell radiosensitizers. These agents include well known, and broadly used, chemotherapeutics that were found, only in hindsight, to be more toxic to hypoxic cells than aerated cells. Mitomycin C is the prototypical example. Discovered in 1958, mitomycin C was shown to have antitumor activity and used in the treatment of human cancers by 1959.[103–105] The observation that mitomycin C may require bioreductive transformation for activity was not made until 1963 and a full appreciation of the reductive mechanisms for mitomycin bioactivation required decades. Unfortunately, the hypoxic-to-oxic cytotoxicity ratio of mitomycin C is quite modest (≤5) and normal tissue toxicity is significant thereby limiting its utility as a directed hypoxic cytotoxin. In contrast, medicinal chemical efforts to improve the tolerance of nitroimidazoles in the 1980s gave rise to the benzotriazine di-N-oxides, a class of agents with hypoxic-to-oxic cytotoxicity ratios orders of magnitude higher than mitomycin C. Tirapazamine, the model benzotriazine di-N-oxide, has been shown to be up to 300-fold more selective for hypoxic cell killing.[106] The biochemical mechanism for this remarkable selectivity is both elegant and straightforward (Fig. 5.4); tirapazamine requires bioreductive activation, and

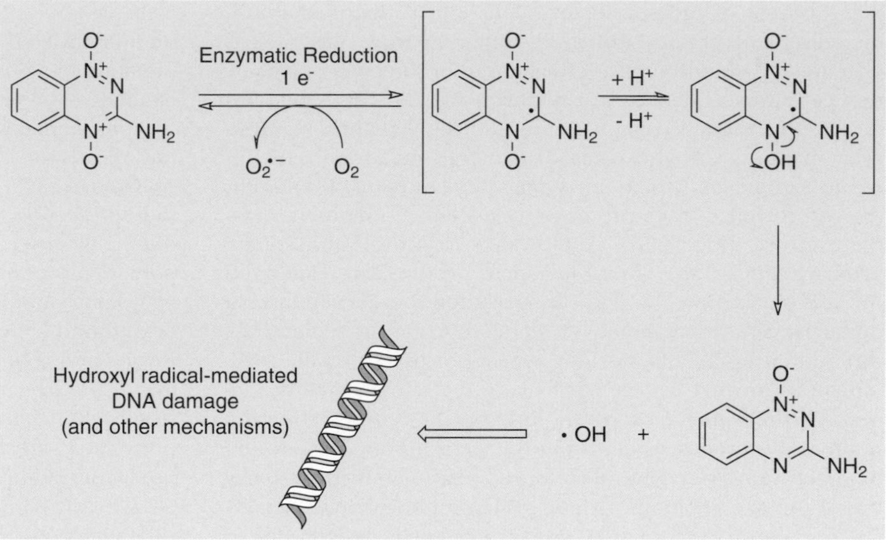

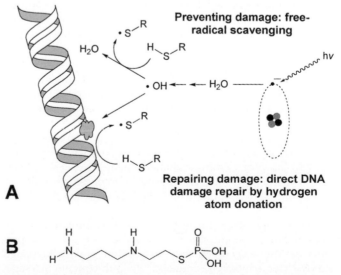

Figure 5.4. Tirapazamine reductive bioactivation, oxidative inactivation, and mechanism of action.

this process is readily reversible in the presence of molecular oxygen. Although incompletely explored, tirapazamine has shown promising activity in some clinical settings.[107] Unfortunately, recently completed randomized trials in locally advanced head and neck cancer that studied the addition of tirapazamine to conventional chemoradiation regimens do not identify an overall survival advantage with the addition of the hypoxic cytotoxin.[108] However, for the subset of patients in whom tumor hypoxia was identified on pretreatment imaging using [18F]-fluoromisonidazole positron emission tomography, there appeared to be a benefit for tirapazamine suggesting that the selection of patients with documented tumor hypoxia may be valuable to highlight the beneficial impact of tirapazamine.[109]

At the core of all investigations into hypoxia-related radiosensitization is the abnormal vascular architecture of solid tumors that gives rise to hypoxic tumor cells. Theoretically, then, one approach to radiosensitization would be to normalize the tumor vasculature permitting more homogeneous and effective oxygen delivery. This would lead to a reduction in the number of radioresistant, hypoxic tumor cells and increase tumor radiosensitivity and curability. Tumor vascular bed abnormalities arise from an underlying imbalance between proangiogenic and antiangiogenic factors, and emerging data suggest that pharmacologic manipulation of this balance, for example with vascular endothelial growth factor (VEGF) antagonists, may lead to more functional tumor vessels.[8] The resultant improvement in tumor oxygenation should enhance the efficacy of radiation therapy. This concept has been validated in preclinical models and is the subject of several ongoing clinical investigations (see "Targeted Therapy/Biologics" section of this chapter).[110] Alternatively, one could reduce the functional impact of tumor vascular bed abnormalities by altering the ability of red blood cells to traverse the tortuous and acutely narrowed tumor vessels. Pentoxifylline is a hemorrheologic methylxanthine derivative originally developed to improve circulation. It is known to alter red blood cell deformability and modify clotting responses. In preclinical models, pentoxifylline enhances tumor radioresponses, presumably by improving blood flow through abnormal tumor vessels, and thus, tumor oxygenation.[111–113] Early clinical investigations into the utility of pentoxifylline are thus far inconclusive.[114–116]

RADIOPROTECTORS

An alternative to selective tumor radiosensitization for improving the therapeutic ratio is selective normal tissue radioprotection. Several radioprotective approaches have been explored. Among the most intensively investigated strategies centers on the ability of certain compounds, particularly thiols, to interrupt the chain of chemical events that bridge radiation-induced ionization events with biological damage (Fig. 5.5A). In 1949, Patt et al.[117] reported that intravenous cysteine reduced the lethality of a single, high dose of radiation (800 R) in rats by 40% to 73% depending on cysteine dose and formulation. Importantly, they further showed that cysteine treatment *after* radiation and cystine, cysteine's oxidized counterpart, offered no radioprotection. Spurred by this observation and the keen appreciation for the potentially devastating effects of nuclear weapon–related radiotoxicity engendered by events in Nagasaki and Hiroshima, the United States military poured resources into the

Figure 5.5. A: Implicated mechanisms in thiol radioprotection. **B:** Structure of amifostine.

development of radioprotectors. This effort identified thiols, including endogenous sulfhydryl containing molecules such as cysteine and glutathione, as efficient radioprotectors that likely reduce radiation damage *via* both free-radical scavenging and direct DNA damage repair (among other mechanisms). However, this program also revealed that free sulfhydryl moieties led to significant toxicity in rodents and humans. Eventually, the prototypical radioprotector, amifostine, emerged from these efforts (Fig. 5.5B). Amifostine is a phosphorothionate prodrug with a more favorable toxicity profile than related thiols. It is bioactivated by dephosphorylation thereby unmasking the active sulfhydryl moiety. A therapeutic gain is achieved by differential uptake: amifostine appears to preferentially accumulate in normal tissues, particularly the salivary glands, kidneys, and intestine. In contrast, little uptake is observed in the brain and in tumor tissue. Brain uptake is minimal due to the blood-brain barrier. Several factors appear to contribute to low tumor uptake including lower alkaline phosphatase activity (potentially due to lower pH) and reduced drug delivery due to aberrant tumor vasculature.[118] Promising, though not entirely consistent, preclinical studies prompted clinical investigation of amifostine.

More than a dozen randomized, placebo-controlled trials have now been reported with concurrent amifostine and radiation therapy. Theoretically, radioprotector trials can be designed in two ways. First, a radioprotector, such as amifostine, can be used to reduce treatment toxicity; in this case, radiation doses are unaltered between the treatment and the placebo arms. A key element of this design is assuring that tumor radioprotection does not occur; otherwise, tumor control would be expected to decline. Second, a radioprotector can be used to enhance tumor control by escalating radiation doses and titrating toxicity to a common level in the treatment and the placebo arms. This latter design is of course very challenging; if normal tissue radioprotection is overestimated, unacceptable toxicity may result. The clinical studies conducted to date have generally used the former design employing amifostine with normal tissue radioprotection (i.e., treatment toxicity) as the primary endpoint. Even with comparable designs, clinical results have not been uniformly consistent. However, several common themes have emerged and have been succinctly captured in a recent meta-analysis of 14 randomized trials of radiotherapy with or without concurrent amifostine.[119] Amifostine use increased risks of grade 3 and 4 nausea and vomiting as well as hypotension. In contrast, amifostine reduced the risk of acute and late xerostomia, mucositis, esophagitis, dysphagia, acute pneumonitis, and cystitis by 62% to 85%. Importantly, no differences in overall response or relapse rates were detected between amifostine and placebo groups; complete response rates were actually superior in the amifostine group. The U.S. Food and Drug Administration has approved amifostine to reduce the incidence of xerostomia in head and neck cancer patients undergoing postoperative radiation therapy. Novel schedules, routes of administration, and dosing are under investigation to broaden the utility of this promising radioprotector.

The role of cytokines in modulating radiation responses has been appreciated for decades. The first hints that immunomodulating cytokines may act as radioprotectors were provided by the observation that bacterial endotoxins increased survival in irradiated animals.[120,121] Subsequent investigations have demonstrated that individual cytokines can rescue animals from radiation damage and lethality. For example,

Neta et al.[122] reported that pretreatment with recombinant interleukin-1 (IL-1) protected mice from the lethal effects of radiation in a dose-dependent manner. Moreover, treatment of irradiated mice with anti-IL-1 antibodies reduced 30-day survival by approximately 50% suggesting that IL-1 is an endogenous radioprotector.[123] Similar studies have shown that tumor necrosis factor-α,[123,124] and transforming growth factor-β[124–126] offer radioprotection in preclinical models. However, these models often rely on crude endpoints such as radiation lethality and obscure more subtle, yet clinically relevant, biological phenomena. For example, the radioprotection conferred by IL-1 has been found to be critically dependent on the model employed. Kovacs and colleagues demonstrated that mouse mortality following 7.5 to 9.5 Gy whole-body radiation was reduced in two strains of mice from 60% to 5% to 10% when the animals were pretreated with IL-1. However, if tumor-bearing animals were used, the radioprotective effects of an identical dose of IL-1 were nearly eliminated.[127] Hancock and colleagues confirmed the radioprotective effects of IL-1 on intestinal crypt cells when the cytokine was given 20 hours prior to radiation. However, they further demonstrated that IL-1 actually sensitized intestinal crypt cells to ionizing radiation when the cytokine was given 4 to 8 hours prior to radiation. Studies of the potential value of IL-12 as a radioprotector demonstrated, as expected, that IL-12 protected against hematopoietic failure. However, these same studies demonstrated intestinal radiosensitization and enhanced death due to the gastrointestinal syndrome.[128] In addition to these complexities, most cytokines possess a spectrum of inherent toxicities. Thus, translation into the human clinical environment has been quite slow. Ongoing efforts to refine cytokine-based radioprotective strategies may bridge the current translational gap.[129,130]

Several growth factors have been explored as radioprotectors including acidic and basic fibroblast growth factor,[131–134] VEGF,[134] hepatocyte growth factor,[135] epidermal growth factor (EGF),[136] granulocyte-macrophage colony stimulating factor (GM-CSF),[137,138] and keratinocyte growth factor. The latter two were sufficiently promising to merit assessment in phase II/III human studies. The Radiation Therapy Oncology Group reported a phase III study evaluating the impact of concurrent GM-CSF on radiation-induced mucositis in head and neck cancer patients with radiation ports encompassing >50% of the oral cavity and/or oropharynx.[139] GM-CSF failed to reduce acute mucositis compared to the placebo arm. Furthermore, nearly a quarter of the patients in the GM-CSF arm discontinued GM-CSF treatment due to toxicity (compared to 0% in the placebo arm). Recombinant keratinocyte growth factor, palifermin, is approved to decrease the incidence and the duration of severe oral mucositis in patients with hematologic malignancies receiving myelotoxic therapy requiring hematopoietic stem cell support. Based on promising results in this setting, palifermin has been subjected to evaluation in additional oncologic settings. In an initial phase I/II, randomized study in head and neck cancer patients receiving concurrent cisplatin, 5-fluorouracil and hyperfractionated radiation therapy, weekly intravenous palifermin was found to be well tolerated and appeared to reduce the duration of grade 3 and 4 mucositis and grade 2 to 4 acute xerostomia and dysphagia.[140] Unfortunately, a follow-on, multi-institutional, phase II randomized study in a comparable patient cohort failed to reproduce the radioprotective benefits of palifermin.[141] The interpretation of the latter was hindered by a number of study limitations including a premature cutoff for toxicity evaluation, nonstandardized toxicity evaluation, underestimations of dropout rates, altered radiation fractionation schemes compared to the phase I/II study, and a relatively low dose of palifermin. Despite the limitations, retrospective subset analyses did suggest palifermin benefits patients receiving hyperfractionated radiation therapy (approximately half of the patient cohort). Ongoing investigations are addressing a number of the aforementioned study limitations and may establish a niche for palifermin as a radioprotector.

Pharmacologic radioprotective approaches designed to eliminate or reduce the OER in normal tissues have also been investigated. Probably the best studied agents are the substituted benzaldehydes. These agents were originally designed to preferentially bind oxyhemoglobin imparting a left-shift in the oxygen dissociation curve; this shift increases the affinity of hemoglobin for oxygen and decreases the amount of oxygen available to tissues.[142,143] Originally envisaged as sickle cell anemia therapeutics, the substituted benzaldehydes have also been explored as potential radioprotectors. BW12C (5-[-2-formyl-3-hydroxyphenoxy] pentanoic acid), a prototypical substituted benzaldehyde, has been shown to protect some normal tissues from radiation damage; however, tumor radioprotection has also been documented.[144–151] Clinical trials of BW12C in cancer patients have been limited and, to date, have not involved combination therapy with radiation. However, in efforts to induce hypoxia and thereby enhance mitomycin C efficacy, the combination of mitomycin C and BW12C has been evaluated in patients with advanced gastrointestinal malignancies.[152,153] Unfortunately, this combination met with little clinical success. Alternative normal tissue hypoxia-inducing strategies have included carbon monoxide breathing,[154] systemic administration of the vasoconstrictor leukotriene C$_4$,[155] and the use of perfused deoxygenated dextran-hemoglobin.[156,157] Unfortunately, none of these strategies have proven useful in the clinical setting.

A number of other agents, with incompletely characterized mechanisms of action, have been studied as potential radioprotectors including prostagandins,[158–163] antioxidants,[164] angiotensin-converting enzyme inhibitors and angiotensin receptor blockers,[165–173] corticosteroids,[174] heavy metals,[175–179] various plant extracts,[180–189] and fatty acids.[190,191] To date, none of these strategies have significantly impacted routine clinical practice. In part, the disconnect between radioprotector development and clinical use rests on the central tenet of therapeutic index. For most studied agents, the relative protection for normal tissue and tumor tissue remains ill-defined, and clinicians have shown wise precaution in advancing a radioprotector into human trials until resoundingly positive evidence demonstrates tumor control will not be compromised.

Promising new strategies for radioprotection are evolving in parallel with increases in our understanding of the molecular mechanisms of radiation responses. Burdelya et al.[192] provide an elegant example of a molecularly targeted approach to radioprotection. Recognizing that (A) apoptosis represents a major mechanism of cell loss in radiosensitive tissues and (B) tumor cells often acquire resistance to apoptosis through constitutive activation of nuclear factor-κB (NF-κB), Burdelya et al. asked whether pharmacologic agents could be developed that activate NF-κB in radiosensitive normal tissue without inducing untoward acute inflammatory responses. Attention was focused on benign gut microflora known to activate NF-κB and play a protective role in the gastrointestinal tract. The bacterial

protein flagellin, the only known agonist of Toll-like receptor 5, was identified as a potential radioprotector. Flagellin proved to be a potent radioprotector improving survival of mice exposed to lethal doses of radiation. Serial modification of flagellin, to reduce immunogenicity and toxicity, yielded a polypeptide, CBLB502, containing the complete N- and C-terminal domains of flagellin separated by a flexible linker. This agent retained the NF-κB activating properties of flagellin, was exceptionally well tolerated, and proved to be a more potent radioprotector than amifostine in mice. CBLB502 was also shown to be an effective radioprotector in rhesus monkeys. Importantly, in mouse tumor models, no tumor protection was observed. Similar, though less mature, molecularly targeted radioprotective approaches are the subject of ongoing, intensive investigation.[193]

CYTOTOXIC CHEMOTHERAPY

Almost without exception, cytotoxic chemotherapeutics have the capacity to alter radiation responses. However, the type and magnitude of this alteration varies for each drug and detailed review of the interaction between ionizing radiation and each clinically used cytotoxic is well beyond the scope of this chapter. Nonetheless, several general principles can provide a framework for understanding the interaction of chemotherapy with ionizing radiation.

The impact of any chemotherapeutic on radiosensitivity can take on one of three forms. First, an agent may have no effect on radiosensitivity; in this case the effects of concurrent treatment are identical to the effects expected if the two treatments were given independently (i.e., sequentially). This lack of interaction is often referred to as *additivity*. Second, combined treatment may yield a net biological effect less than anticipated from the two treatments given independently; this interaction is commonly called *antagonism*. Third, combined treatment may yield a net biological effect greater than that expected if the two treatments were given independently and this is often referred to as a *synergistic* or *supra-additive interaction*. These simple concepts warrant definition as they are often misapplied to experimental and clinical data. For example, the observation that the combination of drug A and ionizing radiation produces an effect greater than that observed with radiation alone often leads to claims that drug A synergizes with radiation. In fact, such an experiment essentially states that A + B > B and provides no evidence of the interaction between drug A and ionizing radiation; antagonistic, additive, and synergistic interactions are all possible. Less obvious misapplications of these concepts are also widespread.[194] Second, misinterpretations of radiation and chemotherapy interactions can have profound clinical implications. For example, the choice between concurrent and sequential chemoradiotherapy critically depends on understanding the interactions of the two modalities. Several methods for rigorously defining the mode of cytotoxic agent interaction (including ionizing radiation) have been proposed including, most popularly, isobologram analysis[195,196] and median effect principle analysis.[197] When interpreting studies examining combined treatment with a cytotoxic agent and radiation, close attention to the methods used to define the interactions is essential.

Further complicating the evaluation of combined chemoradiotherapy in whole animals or humans is a tendency to reductionism. Defining the impact of a given chemotherapeutic on radiosensitivity is not as simple as determining tumor control. Individual cytotoxic agents may have unique, organ-specific toxicities and, consequently, may have organ-specific interactions with radiation. Furthermore, toxicity related to radiosensitization must be examined in clinical context. Increases in acute, transient toxicities do not have the same clinical implications as increases in late, permanent toxicities. For example, bleomycin has been widely explored in concurrent chemoradiation regimens for locally advanced head and neck cancer.[198–202] Although results are not entirely consistent, the addition of bleomycin to radiation appears to dramatically enhance acute toxicities (e.g., mucositis) without significantly increasing late toxicities.[199,203] In contrast, potentially fatal lung toxicity can develop with combinations of bleomycin and lung irradiation thus warranting exceptional caution in lung cancer chemoradiation regimens.[204–206]

The molecular mechanisms of chemotherapy-induced radiosensitization are nearly as diverse as the agents themselves. However, several general themes can be culled from available data. Mammalian cell radiosensitivity varies depending on their residence in particular cell cycle phases.[207–209] The magnitude of radiosensitivity differences between the most sensitive (M) and least sensitive (late S) phases is comparable to the OER (i.e., two- to threefold). Several chemotherapeutics appear to confer radiosensitization by shifting cells toward more radiosensitive cell cycle phases including 5-fluorouracil,[210] fludarabine,[211] and the taxanes.[212] Another commonly implicated mechanism of radiosensitization involves inhibition of radiation-induced DNA double-strand break repair. Hydroxyurea,[213,214] 5-fluorouracil,[215,216] cisplatin,[217–222] and vinorelbine,[223,224] among others, have been shown to radiosensitize, in part, through this mechanism. The halogenated thymidine analogs, 5-bromo-2′-deoxyuridine (BrdUrd) and 5-iodo-2′-deoxyuridine (IdUrd), increase the number of DNA double-strand breaks in addition to inhibiting their repair.[225–227] Reductions in base excision repair (fludarabine), increases in complementary DNA damage (gemcitabine), and modulation of growth factor signaling (gemcitabine) represent additional, less frequently invoked, molecular mechanisms of radiosensitization.[228–230] For a number of chemotherapeutics, the mechanisms of radiosensitization remain imperfectly defined.

The clinical utility of combining cytotoxic chemotherapy with radiotherapy may best be exemplified by the evolution of anal squamous cell carcinoma treatment. By 1970, radical surgery had largely supplanted definitive radiation therapy as the standard of care for anal cancer treatment. However, local failure rates remained quite high. In an effort to improve surgical results, Nigro et al. evaluated neoadjuvant chemoradiation with modest dose (30 Gy) radiation combined with 5-fluorouracil and mitomycin C. In 1974, Nigro et al.[231] reported their preliminary results with three patients undergoing this treatment regimen (or minor variations thereof). Two of the three patients proceeded to abdominoperineal resection and in neither case was viable tumor tissue detected. In the third patient, who refused surgery, there was no evidence of tumor recurrence over a year after chemoradiation. Further investigations with this regimen demonstrated high rates of pathologic complete response rates and led to the realization that surgical resection was not an essential component of anal cancer therapy.[232–234] Subsequent phase III trials demonstrated that concurrent mitomycin C and 5-fluorouracil with radiation was superior to radiation alone, radiation with 5-fluorouracil alone, and radiation with induction and concurrent 5-fluorouracil and cisplatin.[235–238]

The clinical success of the so-called Nigro regimen prompted preclinical studies of the mechanisms of radiosensitization. The complexities of connecting preclinical and clinical data are highlighted by the results of Dobrowsky et al.[239] who found that the mode of interaction between mitomycin C, 5-fluorouracil and ionizing radiation depended critically on the endpoint examined. Using plating efficiency as an endpoint, assessed at the 0.04 level, isobologram analyses suggested radiation interacted supradditively with 5-fluorouracil, mitomycin C, and the combination of drugs. However, when surviving viable cells were used as an endpoint, assessed at the 0.01 level, mitomycin C was found to interact additively with radiation and 5-fluorouracil and radiation were found to be antagonistic. Regardless of the exact mode of interaction, the Nigro regimen remains the standard of care for anal cancer therapy.

As with anal cancer, radiation therapy and surgery have traditionally served as the mainstays of glioblastoma treatment. Given dismal outcomes with median survival typically <1 year, extensive efforts have been directed at identifying effective cytotoxic chemotherapy. However, until recently, there were few convincing data that adjuvant chemotherapy provided a significant survival benefit compared to radiation therapy alone.[240] Trials initiated in the 1990s demonstrated that the oral alkylating agent, temozolomide, was active in recurrent glioblastoma.[241,242] This signal of activity led quickly to studies in the primary treatment setting. By 2002, phase 2 data were available suggesting concomitant temozolomide and radiation therapy followed by adjuvant temozolomide yielded superior survival rates compared to historical controls treated with radiation alone. By 2005, a joint European Organization for Research and Treatment of Cancer/National Cancer Institute of Canada multicenter, phase 3 trial provided unequivocal evidence that this combined temozolomide and radiation regimen was superior to radiation alone in the treatment of glioblastoma.[243] The addition of temozolomide to radiation therapy increased median survival from 12.1 months to 14.6 months and 2-year survival more than doubled from 10.4% to 25.6%. Importantly, the regimen was well tolerated with grade 3 or 4 hematologic toxicities in 7% of patients during the concurrent phase of treatment. Given the design of the phase 2 and 3 trials, the interaction of temozolomide with ionizing radiation in this population remains imperfectly defined. It is unclear whether the survival benefits observed are attributable to the concurrent temozolomide, the adjuvant temozolomide, or both. Mechanistically, it remains unclear whether the primary mechanism of action of temozolomide in this regimen is enhancement of radiation response (concurrent), independent cytotoxicity (adjuvant), or both. In an effort to dissect the relative contribution of altered radiation responses and independent cytotoxicity, Sher and colleagues retrospectively reviewed two cohorts of glioblastoma patients treated with either concurrent and adjuvant temozolomide or adjuvant temozolomide alone.[244] Patients who received concurrent and adjuvant temozolomide experienced 2-year overall survival of 51% compared to 36% for those treated with adjuvant temozolomide alone suggesting that radioresponse potentiation is an important factor contributing to the efficacy of temozolomide. In translational studies conducted in parallel with clinical trials, silencing of the *MGMT* gene encoding O[6]–methylguanine-DNA methyltransferase, a protein involved in the repair of temozolomide-induced DNA lesions, was found to be an independent favorable prognostic factor and predict clinical benefit from temozolomide treatment.[245] These findings raise the possibility that temozolomide use may best be guided by molecular studies.

In addition to anal cancer and glioblastoma, concurrent chemoradiation has emerged as a critical component in the standard management of cancers of the head and neck,[246–249] lung,[250,251] esophagus,[252,253] stomach,[254] pancreas,[255] rectum,[256] bladder,[257–260] and cervix.[261–265] Roles for chemoradiation are being explored in several other malignancies.

As discussed above, chemotherapy modulates radiosensitivity of both tumor and normal tissue. Extending the chemoradiation paradigm to additional malignancies requires careful design of regimens to achieve maximal tumor control while maintaining toxicity within clinically acceptable parameters. Failure to achieve this balance not only risks excessive toxicity but may compromise cure rates. For example, the Northern California Oncology Group tested concurrent radiation therapy and low-dose (5 mg) bleomycin twice weekly in a randomized trial involving 96 patients with stage III or IV inoperable head and neck cancer.[199] The addition of bleomycin increased 2-year locoregional control from 26% to 64% and doubled the 3-year relapse-free survival from 15% to 31%. These clinical benefits came at the cost of increased acute toxicity; however, this increase resulted in neither a prolongation of the treatment course nor a reduction in delivered radiation dose. Additionally, increased acute toxicity did not translate into a statistically significant increase in late toxicity. In stark contrast, the European Organization for Research and Treatment of Cancer conducted a similar study evaluating concurrent radiation therapy with higher-dose (15 mg) bleomycin twice weekly in a randomized trial of 199 patients with T2-4 squamous cell carcinoma of the oropharynx.[198] In this trial, the addition of bleomycin more than tripled acute toxicity over radiation alone (21% vs. 72%) but failed to improve primary tumor response 6 weeks after completion of radiation or 6-year survival rates. This discrepancy is likely, in part, explained by the prolongation of treatment time in 30% of patients receiving combined modality therapy. Thus, the toxicity of high-dose bleomycin (i.e., normal tissue radiosensitization) appears to negate the anticipated therapeutic gains of combined modality therapy. Undoubtedly,

novel and more refined chemoradiation regimens, founded both on the lessons learned from prior experiences like these and improvements in our understanding of the mechanisms of chemotherapeutic antitumor activity, will continue to improve our ability to cure cancer patients.

TARGETED THERAPY/BIOLOGICS

Dramatic improvements in our understanding of the molecular mechanisms of tumorigenesis and tumor progression have ushered in an era of targeted therapeutics. Although many signaling cascades have been explored for their anticancer potential, two particular targeted approaches that alter radiation responses will serve as examples of the promise of combined regimens incorporating targeted therapies and ionizing radiation.

In 1962, Cohen[266] reported the isolation of a heat-stable protein from male mouse submaxillary glands that elicited precocious tooth eruption and eyelid separation in newborn mice and rats. Subsequent investigations demonstrated that the isolated protein, now known as epidermal growth factor (EGF), orchestrates a complex program of biochemical and morphological events leading to, among other things, cell proliferation, differentiation, and migration.[267] The EGF receptor (EGFR) was isolated in 1980 and subsequently shown to consist of an extracellular ligand-binding domain, a transmembrane domain, and an intracellular tyrosine kinase domain.[268,269] Over the last three decades, characterization of the EGFR family has led to the identification of four receptors and an ever-expanding array of ligands (Fig. 5.6). Functionally, ligand binding induces dimerization of receptors (homo- or heterodimers). Dimerization results in tyrosine kinase activation and phosphorylation of key tyrosine residues within the intracellular domain. Phosphorylated tyrosines recruit scaffolding and signaling proteins to the receptor intracellular domain thus initiating downstream signaling. The specific signal transduced is a complex function of the ligand involved in receptor activation, the receptor pairs activated (including differences between homo- and heterodimers), the concentrations of both ligand and receptor, the duration of activation, and

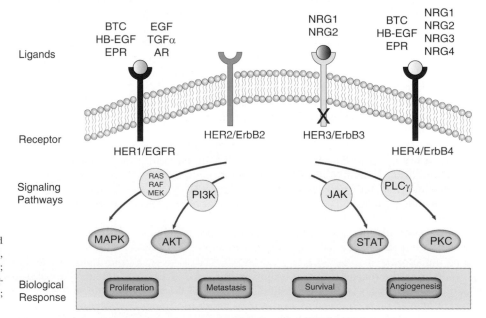

Figure 5.6. The EGFR family, ligands, and signaling pathways. AR, amphiregulin; BTC, betacellulin; EGF, epidermal growth factor; EPR, epiregulin; HB-EGF, heparin binding-epidermal growth factor; NRG, neuregulins; TGFα, transforming growth factor α.

the composition of downstream effectors present at the time of activation.

Just 4 years following isolation, EGFR was identified as a proto-oncogene due to its homology with the transforming protein encoded by the *v-erb-B* oncogene of avian erythroblastosis virus.[270] Since that time, the concept that inhibiting EGFR signaling may have antitumor activity has been extensively investigated and validated.[271-274] Specifically, several observations suggest EGFR inhibitors may favorably alter radiation responses. Balaban et al.[275] demonstrated that monoclonal antibodies to EGFR sensitized tumor epithelial cells to radiation by facilitating radiation-induced apoptosis. Ionizing radiation has been shown to induce EGFR autophosphorylation and downstream signaling. Moreover, Schmidt-Ullrich et al.[276] demonstrated that in a human squamous carcinoma cell line, radiation-induced proliferation was critically dependent on EGFR signaling. An inverse correlation of EGFR expression and radiosensitivity has been demonstrated in both murine and human tumors.[277-281] Based on these observations, a series of preclinical investigations was initiated and demonstrated the ability of EGFR inhibitors to enhance radiation responses in tumor model systems.[282-297] An array of mechanisms underlying radiation-response enhancement by EGFR inhibition have been identified including alterations in cell-cycle distribution, increased apoptosis and necrosis, attenuation of DNA damage repair, antiangiogenic effects, and inhibition of tumor cell motility.[283,284,286,287,295,298] Although the mechanistic studies failed to identify a single unifying mode of interaction for EGFR inhibitors and ionizing radiation, the diverse results likely reflect a complicated interaction that may, in reality, be dependent on multiple variables including the tumor type and location, EGFR inhibitor class, doses of both radiation and EGFR inhibitor, as well as host factors.

As preclinical data were evolving in support of concurrent radiation and EGFR inhibition, early clinical trials were initiated. A strong signal of clinical activity was provided by a phase I trial of the anti-EGFR antibody, cetuximab, in combination with radiation therapy in 16 patients with advanced squamous cell carcinoma of the head and neck.[299] Of 15 evaluable patients, 13 achieved a complete response and two achieved a partial response. Based on these promising results and the rich preclinical data supporting concurrent radiation and EGFR inhibition, a multinational, randomized study comparing radiotherapy alone with radiotherapy plus cetuximab in the treatment of locoregionally advanced head and neck cancer was launched in 1999.[300] The addition of cetuximab not only improved locoregional control (median duration of locoregional control: 24.4 vs. 14.9 months), but also improved overall survival by approximately 10%. For cetuximab-treated patients, median survival was 49.0 months compared to 29.3 months among patients treated with radiation alone. The 10% overall survival benefit has now been confirmed with 5-year median follow-up.[301] Importantly, the addition of cetuximab did not result in marked increases in toxicity. This study represents the first phase III trial to demonstrate a survival benefit attributable to a molecular-targeted agent delivered concurrently with high-dose radiation therapy. Undoubtedly, this study foreshadows additional successes for combined regimens of targeted therapies and ionizing radiation.

Following the recognition that tumors require neovascularization for growth beyond a few millimeters in size, the process of angiogenesis emerged as a promising target for cancer therapy. The original rationale for antiangiogenic therapy involved obliterating tumor vessels, thereby starving tumor cells of required oxygen and nutrients and preventing tumor growth (Fig. 5.7A). VEGF is among the most potent proangiogenic factors and, based on current evidence, appears to be the most critical angiogenic molecule in tumorigenesis. Over the past decade, multiple inhibitors of VEGF signaling have proven beneficial as monotherapy or in combination with cytotoxic chemotherapy.[302-307] Prompted by these successes, preclinical and early clinical investigation of regimens combining VEGF inhibition with ionizing radiation has been initiated.

As discussed above, low linear energy transfer radiation is most efficacious in an oxic environment. If an antiangiogenic agent trimmed tumor vessels, hypoxia may increase and, consequently, radiation sensitivity may decline. In fact, Murata et al.[308] confirmed this possibility in a murine mammary cancer model. Mice bearing mammary carcinomas were treated with 10 fractions of radiation alone or with concurrent TNP-470 (100 mg/kg), a synthetic antiangiogenic agent related to fumagillin. The 50% tumor control dose was found to increase from 67.4 to 77.3 Gy with the addition of TNP-470 demonstrating that concurrent antiangiogenic therapy may reduce radiocurability. Interestingly, when the same experiment was conducted under hypoxic conditions, no differences were observed between the two arms. In contrast, Teicher et al.,[309-312] in a series of murine model studies, reported that antiangiogenic agents, including TNP-470, paradoxically decreased tumor hypoxia and enhanced tumor responses to cytotoxins including radiation. Similar results have been reported in a number of other preclinical models.[110,313] In addition, early clinical studies suggest that antiangiogenics generally potentiate, rather than antagonize, the effects of radiation therapy.[314-321] Moreover, clinical experience shows that currently available antiangiogenic therapies are unable to achieve durable tumor control when used as monotherapy.[322] At least two distinct mechanisms of interaction between antiangiogenic agents and ionizing radiation may explain the deviation of these observations from the ideal tumor starvation model originally envisioned.

In 2001, Jain[323] hypothesized that the judicious application of antiangiogenic agents can "normalize" the abnormal tumor vasculature resulting in more efficient delivery of drugs and oxygen to tumor cells (Fig. 5.7B). The increase in oxygen would, theoretically, enhance radiosensitivity. Considerable evidence has now been generated in support of the normalization hypothesis. In an orthotopic glioma model, Winkler et al.[110] demonstrated that an inhibitor of VEGF signaling reduced tumor hypoxia over a well-defined time interval. The combination of radiation therapy and antiangiogenic agent was additive outside the "normalization window" but synergistic during the window when hypoxia was most markedly reduced. Additional metrics for normalization paralleled the changes in hypoxia and radiosensitivity; enhanced pericyte coverage of tumor vessels and a thinning of the abnormally thick tumor vessel basement membrane were observed. Importantly, support for the normalization hypothesis has also been obtained in humans (Fig. 5.8). In a phase I trial of neoadjuvant therapy in patients with locally advanced adenocarcinoma of the rectum, Willett et al.[319] examined a number of vascular parameters before and after treatment with the VEGF-specific antibody bevacizumab. This trial involved an induction phase (bevacizumab alone) followed by a combined modality phase (bevacizumab, 5-fluorouracil, radiation therapy) prior to definitive surgical

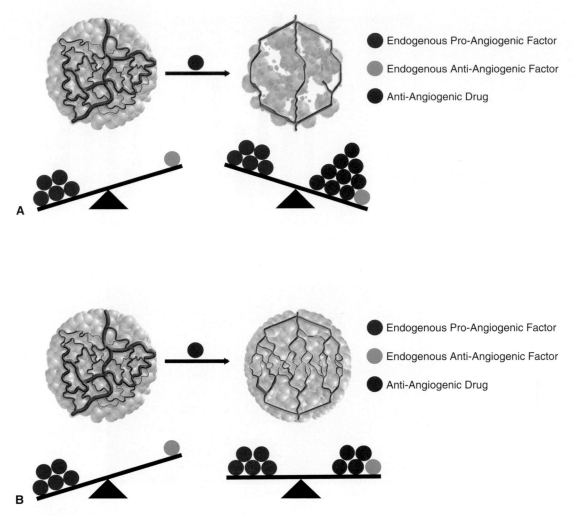

Figure 5.7. A: The unrealized ideal: antiangiogenic therapy dramatically and durably shifts the balance of pro- and antiangiogenic factors to starve a tumor of necessary nutrients and oxygen. **B:** Vascular normalization: judicious use of an antiangiogenic drug normalizes the abnormal tumor vasculature improving antineoplastic drug and oxygen delivery.

resection. Bevacizumab alone caused reductions in tumor blood perfusion and blood volume, and this was accompanied by a reduction in microvascular density. Despite the apparent antivascular effects, [^{18}F]-fluorodeoxyglucose positron emission tomography generally revealed no change in tumor uptake suggesting the efficiency of the remaining tumor blood vessels after bevacizumab treatment was improved. Further evidence for vascular normalization was provided by the observations that in the majority of patients tumor vessel pericyte coverage improved and the abnormally high pretreatment tumor interstitial fluid pressure declined after bevacizumab therapy. Promising pathological responses hinted that the observed vascular normalization may improve radioresponses. Vascular normalization has also been observed in recurrent glioblastoma patients treated with the VEGF receptor inhibitor, cediranib. After cediranib monotherapy, tumor vessel size and vascular permeability were sharply reduced leading to reductions in vasogenic edema. Ongoing investigations should provide necessary insights into the clinical utility of vascular normalization particularly in relation to its ability to alter radiation responses.

A second implicated mechanism for the radiosensitizing properties of antiangiogenic therapy involves complementary targeting of tumor vascular endothelium. Radiation-induced vascular damage may contribute to tumor control.[324] Furthermore, radiation itself induces expression of proangiogenic molecules including VEGF and VEGF receptors.[325,326] Thus, increased proangiogenic signaling may enhance endothelial cell survival after ionizing radiation.[327,328] Inhibition of this survival signaling may enhance radiation-induced vascular damage and, therefore, tumor control. For example, Mauceri et al.[329] examined the combined effects of ionizing radiation and angiostatin, an endogenous antiangiogenic molecule. Combined treatment of mice bearing four different tumor types resulted in supradditive growth inhibition compared to either angiostatin or radiation alone. Examination of tumor vasculature following treatment suggested significant interactive antivascular effects. In vitro assays with human endothelial cells demonstrated significant interactive cytotoxic effects of angiostatin and ionizing radiation. In contrast, no cytotoxic or radiosensitizing effects of angiostatin were observed when tumor cells were examined in vitro. Multiple mechanisms of

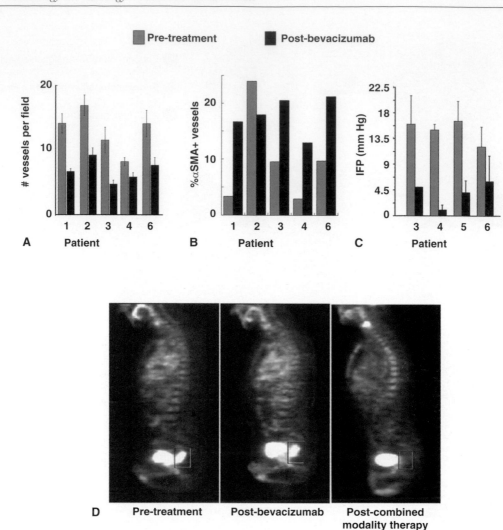

Figure 5.8. Vascular normalization in rectal cancer patients following treatment with the anti-VEGF antibody, bevacizumab. Tumor vessel normalization following a single injection of bevacizumab is suggested by the (**A**) reduced tumor microvessel density, (**B**) increased fraction of tumor vessels with pericyte coverage, and (**C**) reduced interstitial fluid pressure (IFP). (**D**) Positron emission tomography reveals no change in 18-fluorode-oxyglucose (FDG) uptake after a single dose of bevacizumab and complete resolution of FDG uptake following combined modality therapy (bevacizumab, 5-fluorouracil, pelvic external beam radiation therapy). The stability of FDG uptake following bevacizumab monotherapy, despite marked reductions in microvessel density, suggests the efficiency of persistent tumor blood vessels after bevacizumab treatment is improved. (Reprinted with permission from Macmillan Publishers Ltd: Willett CG, Boucher Y, di Tomaso E, et al. Direct evidence that the VEGF-specific antibody bevacizumab has antivascular effects in human rectal cancer. *Nat Med.* 2004;10:145–147.)

antiangiogenic radiosensitization may operate simultaneously and may lead to complex alterations in radioresponses. Nonetheless, antiangiogenics appear capable of favorably modulating radiation efficacy, and a strong rationale exists for continued evaluation of combined antiangiogenic and radiation regimens.

In part based on the clinical success of EGF and VEGF inhibitors, enormous effort is being dedicated to developing novel agents that target additional molecular pathways involved in tumor development, progression, and metastasis. As these agents emerge, testing in combination with radiation will provide insights into their ability to favorably alter radiation responses. In complementary work, as the biological underpinnings of the radiation response are better elucidated, novel targets will undoubtedly be identified that may permit the development of highly specific radiomodulators.

Among countless targets currently under investigation, histone deacetylase, NF-κB, insulin-like growth factor-1, heat-shock protein 90, phosphatidylinositol-3-kinase/mammalian target of rapamycin/akt, and farnesyltransferase all have shown promise.[330] It seems likely that the enormous potential of such targeted approaches will dramatically alter the practice of radiation oncology in the near future.

HYPERTHERMIA

The potential value of hyperthermia in cancer was first reported in 1866 when tumor regression was observed after a high fever due to erysipelas.[331] Subsequently, bacterial pyrogens were tested in cancer patients.[332] Hyperthermia was explored in conjunction with radiotherapy in the early 20th century; however, it was not until the 1970s that combinations of radiation and hyperthermia were intensely investigated.[333-337] These studies demonstrated that the addition of hyperthermia to ionizing radiation results in both complementary additive cytotoxicity and synergistic radiosensitization. The independent, additive effects of hyperthermia, in part, reflect cell-cycle-specific sensitivity to heat. As discussed, maximal radiosensitivity is seen in M-phase and maximal radioresistance in late S-phase. In contrast, late S-phase cells display maximal sensitivity to hyperthermia.[338] Furthermore, radioresistant hypoxic cells are similarly sensitive to hyperthermia when compared to well-oxygenated cells. In some systems, chronically hypoxic cells are actually more sensitive to hyperthermia probably due to the coexistence of an acidic, nutrient-poor environment, factors known to impact cell sensitivity to heat.[339,340]

In addition to these independent, complementary interactions, hyperthermia has clearly been shown to enhance radiosensitivity. Maximal radiosensitization, expressed as a thermal enhancement ratio or TER, occurs when the two modalities are used simultaneously.[336] The TER decreases markedly with increasing time intervals between the two treatments; when radiation precedes hyperthermia, the TER declines to 1 after a few hours. Similarly, if hyperthermia precedes radiation, the TER declines quickly with increasing time intervals though some sensitization may be detectable for several hours. Several mechanisms have been identified that may contribute to genuine thermal radiosensitization including inhibition of critical DNA repair pathways and alterations in blood flow and tumor oxygenation.

These observations prompted clinical evaluation of combined hyperthermia and ionizing radiation, and several phase III trials have been reported. The Radiation Therapy Oncology Group registered 307 patients with superficial measurable tumors, primarily head and neck and breast primaries, to a trial of radiation therapy (4 Gy twice weekly to a total dose of 32 Gy) with or without hyperthermia (42.5°C, 60 minutes immediately following radiation).[341] Although no difference in response rates was observed for the entire patient cohort, the addition of hyperthermia improved complete responses of tumors <3 cm in diameter. The failure of hyperthermia to yield a significant clinical benefit was attributed, in part, to the use of highly variable heating techniques and crude thermal dosimetry.[342] In contrast, two single institution randomized studies have demonstrated statistically significant improvements in complete response rates when hyperthermia is added to radiation therapy in the treatment of advanced head and neck cancer.[343,344] In one of these trials, improvements in local control translated into a 5-year overall survival benefit.[344] Randomized studies in patients with advanced pelvic tumors, metastatic melanoma, glioblastoma, breast cancer, and esophageal cancer have generally suggested hyperthermia adds to local control and may improve survival compared to radiation alone.[345-350] Despite these promising signals of efficacy, the clinical use of hyperthermia is restricted to a relatively small cohort of centers with established expertise. In parallel to the use of hypoxic cell sensitizers and hyperbaric oxygen, hyperthermia has largely been relegated to highly specialized centers due to profound technical challenges involved in delivering high-quality treatment. As dedicated teams of engineers, physicists, and physicians develop improved technologies for hyperthermia delivery, this radiosensitizing modality may experience a revival.

CONCLUSIONS

Ionizing radiation is a time-tested, curative treatment modality for a broad spectrum of malignancies. Despite ongoing advances and refinements, there remains ample room for improvement. An array of systemic agents that alter radiation response profiles is currently emerging for oncology practice. As our understanding of the complex molecular processes that influence radiation response expands, new promising radiomodulators will enter the therapeutic oncology armamentarium. Dedicated preclinical experimentation, clever translational studies, and well-designed clinical trials will be required to optimally incorporate existing and novel agents into contemporary radiation regimens. Fortunately, these efforts afford the potential to improve patient outcomes.

REFERENCES

1. Krogh A. *The Anatomy & Physiology of Capillaries.* New York, NY: Yale University Press; 1922.
2. Folkman J. Tumor angiogenesis: therapeutic implications. *N Engl J Med.* 1971;285:1182–1186.
3. Gao D, Nolan DJ, Mellick AS, et al. Endothelial progenitor cells control the angiogenic switch in mouse tumor metastasis. *Science.* 2008;319:195–198.
4. Holmgren L, O'Reilly MS, Folkman J. Dormancy of micrometastases: balanced proliferation and apoptosis in the presence of angiogenesis suppression. *Nat Med.* 1995;1:149–153.
5. Baish JW, Gazit Y, Berk DA, et al. Role of tumor vascular architecture in nutrient and drug delivery: an invasion percolation-based network model. *Microvasc Res.* 1996;51:327–346.
6. Baish JW, Jain RK. Cancer, angiogenesis and fractals. *Nat Med.* 1998;4:984.
7. Jain RK. Determinants of tumor blood flow: a review. *Cancer Res.* 1988;48:2641–2658.
8. Jain RK. Normalization of tumor vasculature: an emerging concept in antiangiogenic therapy. *Science.* 2005;307:58–62.
9. Less JR, Posner MC, Skalak TC, et al. Geometric resistance and microvascular network architecture of human colorectal carcinoma. *Microcirculation.* 1997;4:25–33.
10. Less JR, Skalak TC, Sevick EM, et al. Microvascular architecture in a mammary carcinoma: branching patterns and vessel dimensions. *Cancer Res.* 1991;51:265–273.
11. Less JR, Skalak TC, Sevick EM, et al. Microvascular network architecture in a mammary carcinoma. *EXS.* 1992;61:74–80.
12. Thomlinson RH, Gray LH. The histological structure of some human lung cancers and the possible implications for radiotherapy. *Br J Cancer.* 1955;9:539–549.
13. Crabtree HG, Cramer W. Action of radium on cancer cells: some factors affecting susceptibility of cancer cells to radium. *Proc R Soc Lond B Biol Sci.* 1933;113:238.
14. Mottram JC. Factor of importance in radiosensitivity of tumours. *Br J Radiol.* 1936;9:606–614.
15. Alper T, Howard-Flanders P. Role of oxygen in modifying the radiosensitivity of *E. coli* B. *Nature.* 1956;178:978–979.
16. Deschner EE, Gray LH. Influence of oxygen tension on x-ray-induced chromosomal damage in Ehrlich ascites tumor cells irradiated in vitro and in vivo. *Radiat Res.* 1959;11:115–146.
17. Gray LH, Conger AD, Ebert M, et al. The concentration of oxygen dissolved in tissues at the time of irradiation as a factor in radiotherapy. *Br J Radiol.* 1953;26:638–648.
18. Howard-Flanders P, Alper T. The sensitivity of microorganisms to irradiation under controlled gas conditions. *Radiat Res.* 1957;7:518–540.
19. Howard-Flanders P, Pirie A. The effect of breathing oxygen on the radiosensitivity of the rabbit lens and the use of oxygen in x-ray therapy. *Radiat Res.* 1957;7:357–364.
20. Howard-Flanders P, Scott OC. Tissue oxygen tension and radiotherapy. A review and bibliography based on a conference in Burlington, Vermont, August 1958. *Radiology.* 1960;74:956–963.
21. Howard-Flanders P, Wright EA. Effect of oxygen on the radiosensitivity of growing bone and a possible danger in the use of oxygen during radiotherapy. *Nature.* 1955;175:428–429.
22. Powers WE, Tolmach LJ. A multicomponent x-ray survival curve for mouse lymphosarcoma cells irradiated in vivo. *Nature.* 1963;197:710–711.
23. Brown JM, Giaccia AJ. The unique physiology of solid tumors: opportunities (and problems) for cancer therapy. *Cancer Res.* 1998;58:1408–1416.
24. Harris AL. Hypoxia—a key regulatory factor in tumour growth. *Nat Rev Cancer.* 2002;2:38–47.
25. Pouyssegur J, Dayan F, Mazure NM. Hypoxia signalling in cancer and approaches to enforce tumour regression. *Nature.* 2006;441:437–443.
26. Brizel DM, Scully SP, Harrelson JM, et al. Tumor oxygenation predicts for the likelihood of distant metastases in human soft tissue sarcoma. *Cancer Res.* 1996;56:941–943.
27. Hockel M, Schlenger K, Aral B, et al. Association between tumor hypoxia and malignant progression in advanced cancer of the uterine cervix. *Cancer Res.* 1996;56:4509–4515.
28. Nordsmark M, Bentzen SM, Rudat V, et al. Prognostic value of tumor oxygenation in 397 head and neck tumors after primary radiation therapy. An international multi-center study. *Radiother Oncol.* 2005;77:18–24.
29. Dusault LA. The effect of oxygen on the response of spontaneous tumours in mice to radiotherapy. *Br J Radiol.* 1963;36:749–754.
30. Dusault LA. Optimum O_2/CO_2 ratio in radiotherapy. *Radiology.* 1964;82:333.
31. Suit HD, Marshall N, Woerner D. Oxygen, oxygen plus carbon dioxide, and radiation therapy of a mouse mammary carcinoma. *Cancer.* 1972;30:1154–1158.

32. Grau C, Horsman MR, Overgaard J. Improving the radiation response in a C3H mouse mammary carcinoma by normobaric oxygen or carbogen breathing. *Int J Radiat Oncol Biol Phys.* 1992;22:415–419.
33. Perry PM, Nias AH. The optimum pressure of oxygen for radiotherapy of a mouse tumour. *Br J Radiol.* 1992;65:784–786.
34. Suit HD. Application of radiobiologic principles to radiation therapy. *Cancer.* 1968;22: 809–815.
35. Churchill-Davidson I. Oxygenation in radiotherapy. *J Obstet Gynaecol Br Emp.* 1959;66: 855–856.
36. Churchill-Davidson I, Foster CA, Thomlinson RH. High-pressure oxygen and radiotherapy. *Med World.* 1958;88:125–128.
37. Churchill-Davidson I, Sanger C, Thomlinson RH. High-pressure oxygen and radiotherapy. *Lancet.* 1955;268:1091–1095.
38. Churchill-Davidson I, Sanger C, Thomlinson RH. Oxygenation in radiotherapy. II. Clinical application. *Br J Radiol.* 1957;30:406–422.
39. Radiotherapy and hyperbaric oxygen. Report of a Medical Research Council Working Party. *Lancet.* 1978;2:881–884.
40. Dische S. Hyperbaric oxygen: the Medical Research Council trials and their clinical significance. *Br J Radiol.* 1978;51:888–894.
41. Saunders M, Dische S. Clinical results of hypoxic cell radiosensitisation from hyperbaric oxygen to accelerated radiotherapy, carbogen and nicotinamide. *Br J Cancer Suppl.* 1996;27:S271–S278.
42. Bergsjo P, Kolstad P. Clinical trial with atmospheric oxygen breathing during radiotherapy of cancer of the cervix. *Scand J Clin Lab Invest Suppl.* 1968;106:167–171.
43. Rubin P, Hanley J, Keys HM, et al. Carbogen breathing during radiation therapy-the Radiation Therapy Oncology Group Study. *Int J Radiat Oncol Biol Phys.* 1979;5:1963–1970.
44. Horsman MR. Nicotinamide and other benzamide analogs as agents for overcoming hypoxic cell radiation resistance in tumours. A review. *Acta Oncol.* 1995;34:571–587.
45. Horsman MR, Chaplin DJ, Overgaard J. Combination of nicotinamide and hyperthermia to eliminate radioresistant chronically and acutely hypoxic tumor cells. *Cancer Res.* 1990;50:7430–7436.
46. Horsman MR, Hansen PV, Overgaard J. Radiosensitization by nicotinamide in tumors and normal tissues: the importance of tissue oxygenation status. *Int J Radiat Oncol Biol Phys.* 1989;16:1273–1276.
47. Horsman MR, Overgaard J, Christensen KL, et al. Mechanism for the reduction of tumour hypoxia by nicotinamide and the clinical relevance for radiotherapy. *Biomed Biochim Acta.* 1989;48:S251–S254.
48. Horsman MR, Siemann DW, Chaplin DJ, et al. Nicotinamide as a radiosensitizer in tumours and normal tissues: the importance of drug dose and timing. *Radiother Oncol.* 1997;45:167–174.
49. Horsman MR, Wood PJ, Chaplin DJ, et al. The potentiation of radiation damage by nicotinamide in the SCCVII tumour in vivo. *Radiother Oncol.* 1990;18:49–57.
50. Kaanders JH, Bussink J, van der Kogel AJ. ARCON: a novel biology-based approach in radiotherapy. *Lancet Oncol.* 2002;3:728–737.
51. Varlotto J, Stevenson MA. Anemia, tumor hypoxemia, and the cancer patient. *Int J Radiat Oncol Biol Phys.* 2005;63:25–36.
52. Bush RS, Jenkin RD, Allt WE, et al. Definitive evidence for hypoxic cells influencing cure in cancer therapy. *Br J Cancer Suppl.* 1978;3:302–306.
53. Grogan M, Thomas GM, Melamed I, et al. The importance of hemoglobin levels during radiotherapy for carcinoma of the cervix. *Cancer.* 1999;86:1528–1536.
54. Kapp KS, Poschauko J, Geyer E, et al. Evaluation of the effect of routine packed red blood cell transfusion in anemic cervix cancer patients treated with radical radiotherapy. *Int J Radiat Oncol Biol Phys.* 2002;54:58–66.
55. Bush RS. Current status and treatment of localized disease and future aspects. *Int J Radiat Oncol Biol Phys.* 1984;10:1165–1174.
56. Bush RS. The significance of anemia in clinical radiation therapy. *Int J Radiat Oncol Biol Phys.* 1986;12:2047–2050.
57. Fyles AW, Milosevic M, Pintilie M, et al. Anemia, hypoxia and transfusion in patients with cervix cancer: a review. *Radiother Oncol.* 2000;57:13–19.
58. Littlewood TJ, Bajetta E, Nortier JW, et al. Effects of epoetin alfa on hematologic parameters and quality of life in cancer patients receiving nonplatinum chemotherapy: results of a randomized, double-blind, placebo-controlled trial. *J Clin Oncol.* 2001;19: 2865–2874.
59. Vansteenkiste J, Pirker R, Massuti B, et al. Double-blind, placebo-controlled, randomized phase III trial of darbepoetin alfa in lung cancer patients receiving chemotherapy. *J Natl Cancer Inst.* 2002;94:1211–1220.
60. Henke M, Laszig R, Rube C, et al. Erythropoietin to treat head and neck cancer patients with anaemia undergoing radiotherapy: randomised, double-blind, placebo-controlled trial. *Lancet.* 2003;362:1255–1260.
61. Leyland-Jones B, Semiglazov V, Pawlicki M, et al. Maintaining normal hemoglobin levels with epoetin alfa in mainly nonanemic patients with metastatic breast cancer receiving first-line chemotherapy: a survival study. *J Clin Oncol.* 2005;23:5960–5972.
62. Kelleher DK, Mattheinsen U, Thews O, et al. Blood flow, oxygenation, and bioenergetic status of tumors after erythropoietin treatment in normal and anemic rats. *Cancer Res.* 1996;56:4728–4734.
63. Kelleher DK, Matthiensen U, Thews O, et al. Tumor oxygenation in anemic rats: effects of erythropoietin treatment versus red blood cell transfusion. *Acta Oncol.* 1995;34:379–384.
64. Sundfor K, Lyng H, Kongsgard UL, et al. Polarographic measurement of pO_2 in cervix carcinoma. *Gynecol Oncol.* 1997;64:230–236.
65. Fukumura D, Jain RK. Tumor microenvironment abnormalities: causes, consequences, and strategies to normalize. *J Cell Biochem.* 2007;101:937–949.
66. Dzik S, Mincheff M, Puppo F. Apoptosis, transforming growth factor-beta, and the immunosuppressive effect of transfusion. *Transfusion.* 2002;42:1221–1223.
67. Gharehbaghian A, Haque KM, Truman C, et al. Effect of autologous salvaged blood on postoperative natural killer cell precursor frequency. *Lancet.* 2004;363:1025–1030.
68. Santin AD, Bellone S, Palmieri M, et al. Effect of blood transfusion during radiotherapy on the immune function of patients with cancer of the uterine cervix: role of interleukin-10. *Int J Radiat Oncol Biol Phys.* 2002;54:1345–1355.
69. Bridges BA. Sensitization of *Escherichia coli* to gamma radiation by *N*-ethylmaleimide. *Nature.* 1960;188:415.
70. Bridges BA. The chemical sensitization of *Pseudomonas* species to ionizing radiation. *Radiat Res.* 1962;16:232–242.
71. Adams GE, Ahmed I, Clarke ED, et al. Structure-activity relationships in the development of hypoxic cell radiosensitizers. III. Effects of basic substituents in nitroimidazole sidechains. *Int J Radiat Biol Relat Stud Phys Chem Med.* 1980;38:613–626.
72. Adams GE, Clarke ED, Flockhart IR, et al. Structure-activity relationships in the development of hypoxic cell radiosensitizers. I. Sensitization efficiency. *Int J Radiat Biol Relat Stud Phys Chem Med.* 1979;35:133–150.
73. Adams GE, Clarke ED, Gray P, et al. Structure-activity relationships in the development of hypoxic cell radiosensitizers. II. Cytotoxicity and therapeutic ratio. *Int J Radiat Biol Relat Stud Phys Chem Med.* 1979;35:151–160.
74. Adams GE, Cooke MS. Electron-affinic sensitization. I. A structural basis for chemical radiosensitizers in bacteria. *Int J Radiat Biol Relat Stud Phys Chem Med.* 1969;15:457–471.
75. Adams GE, Dewey DL. Hydrated electrons and radiobiological sensitisation. *Biochem Biophys Res Commun.* 1963;12:473–477.
76. Adams GE, Flockhart IR, Smithen CE, et al. Electron-affinic sensitization. VII. A correlation between structures, one-electron reduction potentials, and efficiencies of nitroimidazoles as hypoxic cell radiosensitizers. *Radiat Res.* 1976;67:9–20.
77. Asquith JC, Watts ME, Patel K, et al. Electron affinic sensitization. V. Radiosensitization of hypoxic bacteria and mammalian cells in vitro by some nitroimidazoles and nitropyrazoles. *Radiat Res.* 1974;60:108–118.
78. Moore BA, Palcic B, Skarsgard LD. Radiosensitizing and toxic effects on the 2-nitroimidazole Ro-07–0582 in hypoxic mammation cells. *Radiat Res.* 1976;67:459–473.
79. Hill SA, Fowler JF. Radiosensitizing and cytocidal effects on hypoxic cells of Ro-07-0582, and repair of x-ray injury, in an experimental mouse tumour. *Br J Cancer.* 1977;35:461–469.
80. Sheldon PW, Foster JL, Fowler JF. Radiosensitization of C3H mouse mammary tumours by a 2-nitroimidazole drug. *Br J Cancer.* 1974;30:560–565.
81. Sheldon PW, Fowler JF. Radiosensitization by misonidazole (Ro-07-0582) of fractionated X-rays in a murine tumour. *Br J Cancer Suppl.* 1978;3:242–245.
82. Sheldon PW, Hill SA, Foster JL, et al. Radiosensitization of C3H mouse mammary tumours using fractionated doses of x rays with the drug Ro-07–0582. *Br J Radiol.* 1976;49:76–80.
83. Abratt RP, Craighead P, Reddi VB, et al. A prospective randomised trial of radiation with or without oral and intravesical misonidazole for bladder cancer. *Br J Cancer.* 1991;64:968–970.
84. Grigsby PW, Winter K, Wasserman TH, et al. Irradiation with or without misonidazole for patients with stages IIIB and IVA carcinoma of the cervix: final results of RTOG 80-05. Radiation Therapy Oncology Group. *Int J Radiat Oncol Biol Phys.* 1999;44:513–517.
85. Huncharek M. Meta-analytic re-evaluation of misonidazole in the treatment of high grade astrocytoma. *Anticancer Res.* 1998;18:1935–1939.
86. Komarnicky LT, Phillips TL, Martz K, et al. A randomized phase III protocol for the evaluation of misonidazole combined with radiation in the treatment of patients with brain metastases (RTOG-7916). *Int J Radiat Oncol Biol Phys.* 1991;20:53–58.
87. Minsky BD, Leibel SA. The treatment of hepatic metastases from colorectal cancer with radiation therapy alone or combined with chemotherapy or misonidazole. *Cancer Treat Rev.* 1989;16:213–219.
88. Overgaard J, Bentzen SM, Kolstad P, et al. Misonidazole combined with radiotherapy in the treatment of carcinoma of the uterine cervix. *Int J Radiat Oncol Biol Phys.* 1989;16:1069–1072.
89. Overgaard J, Hansen HS, Andersen AP, et al. Misonidazole combined with split-course radiotherapy in the treatment of invasive carcinoma of larynx and pharynx: report from the DAHANCA 2 study. *Int J Radiat Oncol Biol Phys.* 1989;16:1065–1068.
90. Stehman FB, Bundy BN, Keys H, et al. A randomized trial of hydroxyurea versus misonidazole adjunct to radiation therapy in carcinoma of the cervix. A preliminary report of a Gynecologic Oncology Group study. *Am J Obstet Gynecol.* 1988;159:87–94.
91. Stehman FB, Bundy BN, Thomas G, et al. Hydroxyurea versus misonidazole with radiation in cervical carcinoma: long-term follow-up of a Gynecologic Oncology Group trial. *J Clin Oncol.* 1993;11:1523–1528.
92. Van den Bogaert W, van der Schueren E, Horiot JC, et al. The EORTC randomized trial on three fractions per day and misonidazole (trial no. 22811) in advanced head and neck cancer: long-term results and side effects. *Radiother Oncol.* 1995;35:91–99.
93. Brown JM, Yu NY, Brown DM, et al. SR-2508: a 2-nitroimidazole amide which should be superior to misonidazole as a radiosensitizer for clinical use. *Int J Radiat Oncol Biol Phys.* 1981;7:695–703.
94. Eschwege F, Sancho-Garnier H, Chassagne D, et al. Results of a European randomized trial of Etanidazole combined with radiotherapy in head and neck carcinomas. *Int J Radiat Oncol Biol Phys.* 1997;39:275–281.
95. Lee DJ, Cosmatos D, Marcial VA, et al. Results of an RTOG phase III trial (RTOG 85-27) comparing radiotherapy plus etanidazole with radiotherapy alone for locally advanced head and neck carcinomas. *Int J Radiat Oncol Biol Phys.* 1995;32:567–576.
96. Overgaard J, Hansen HS, Overgaard M, et al. A randomized double-blind phase III study of nimorazole as a hypoxic radiosensitizer of primary radiotherapy in supraglottic larynx and pharynx carcinoma. Results of the Danish Head and Neck Cancer Study (DAHANCA) Protocol 5-85. *Radiother Oncol.* 1998;46:135–146.
97. Overgaard J. Hypoxic radiosensitization: adored and ignored. *J Clin Oncol.* 2007;25:4066–4074.
98. Dobrowsky W, Huigol NG, Jayatilake RS, et al. AK-2123 (Sanazol) as a radiation sensitizer in the treatment of stage III cervical cancer: results of an IAEA multicentre randomised trial. *Radiother Oncol.* 2007;82:24–29.
99. Huilgol NG, Chatterjee N, Mehta AR. An overview of the initial experience with AK-2123 as a hypoxic cell sensitizer with radiation in the treatment of advanced head and neck cancers. *Int J Radiat Oncol Biol Phys.* 1996;34:1121–1124.

100. Okkan S, Atkovar G, Sahinler I, et al. A randomised study of ornidazole as a radiosensitiser in carcinoma of the cervix: long term results. *Br J Cancer Suppl.* 1996;27:S282–286.
101. Sunamura M, Karasawa K, Okamoto A, et al. Phase III trial of radiosensitizer PR-350 combined with intraoperative radiotherapy for the treatment of locally advanced pancreatic cancer. *Pancreas.* 2004;28:330–334.
102. Ullal SD, Shenoy KK, Pai MR, et al. Safety and radiosensitizing efficacy of sanazole (AK 2123) in oropharyngeal cancers: randomized controlled double blind clinical trial. *Indian J Cancer.* 2006;43:151–155.
103. Shiraha Y, Sakai K, Teranaka T. Clinical trials of mitomycin C, a new antitumor antibiotic; preliminary report of results obtained in 82 consecutive cases in the field of general surgery. *Antibiot Annu.* 1958;6:533–540.
104. Sugiura K. Studies in a tumor spectrum. VIII. The effect of mitomycin C on the growth of a variety of mouse, rat, and hamster tumors. *Cancer Res.* 1959;19:438–445.
105. Wakaki S. Recent advance in research on antitumor mitomycins. *Cancer Chemother Rep.* 1961;13:79–86.
106. Brown JM. The hypoxic cell: a target for selective cancer therapy—eighteenth Bruce F. Cain Memorial Award lecture. *Cancer Res.* 1999;59:5863–5870.
107. Rischin D, Peters L, Fisher R, et al. Tirapazamine, cisplatin, and radiation versus fluorouracil, cisplatin, and radiation in patients with locally advanced head and neck cancer: a randomized phase II trial of the Trans-Tasman Radiation Oncology Group (TROG 98.02). *J Clin Oncol.* 2005;23:79–87.
108. Rischin D, Peters B, O'Sullivan B, et al. Phase III study of tirapazamine, cisplatin and radiation versus cisplatin and radiation for advanced squamous cell carcinoma of the head and neck. *J Clin Oncol.* 2008;26:LBA6008.
109. Rischin D, Hicks RJ, Fisher R, et al. Prognostic significance of [^{18}F]-misonidazole positron emission tomography-detected tumor hypoxia in patients with advanced head and neck cancer randomly assigned to chemoradiation with or without tirapazamine: a substudy of Trans-Tasman Radiation Oncology Group Study 98.02. *J Clin Oncol.* 2006;24:2098–2104.
110. Winkler F, Kozin SV, Tong RT, et al. Kinetics of vascular normalization by VEGFR2 blockade governs brain tumor response to radiation: role of oxygenation, angiopoietin-1, and matrix metalloproteinases. *Cancer Cell.* 2004;6:553–563.
111. Collingridge DR, Rockwell S. Pentoxifylline improves the oxygenation and radiation response of BA1112 rat rhabdomyosarcomas and EMT6 mouse mammary carcinomas. *Int J Cancer.* 2000;90:256–264.
112. Lee I, Biaglow JE, Lee J, et al. Physiological mechanisms of radiation sensitization by pentoxifylline. *Anticancer Res.* 2000;20:4605–4609.
113. Zywietz F, Bohm L, Sagowski C, et al. Pentoxifylline enhances tumor oxygenation and radiosensitivity in rat rhabdomyosarcomas during continuous hyperfractionated irradiation. *Strahlenther Onkol.* 2004;180:306–314.
114. Johnson FE, Harrison BR, McKirgan LW, et al. A phase II evaluation of pentoxifylline combined with radiation in the treatment of brain metastases. *Int J Oncol.* 1998;13: 801–805.
115. Kwon HC, Kim SK, Chung WK, et al. Effect of pentoxifylline on radiation response of non-small cell lung cancer: a phase III randomized multicenter trial. *Radiother Oncol.* 2000;56:175–179.
116. Stewart DJ, Dahrouge S, Agboola O, et al. Cranial radiation and concomitant cisplatin and mitomycin-C plus resistance modulators for malignant gliomas. *J Neurooncol.* 1997;32: 161–168.
117. Patt HM, Tyree EB, Straube RL, et al. Cysteine protection against X irradiation. *Science.* 1949;110:213–214.
118. Andreassen CN, Grau C, Lindegaard JC. Chemical radioprotection: a critical review of amifostine as a cytoprotector in radiotherapy. *Semin Radiat Oncol.* 2003;13:62–72.
119. Sasse AD, Clark LG, Sasse EC, et al. Amifostine reduces side effects and improves complete response rate during radiotherapy: results of a meta-analysis. *Int J Radiat Oncol Biol Phys.* 2006;64:784–791.
120. Smith WW, Alderman IM, Gillespie RE. Increased survival in irradiated animals treated with bacterial endotoxins. *Am J Physiol.* 1957;191:124–130.
121. Smith WW, Alderman IM, Gillespie RE. Hematopoietic recovery induced by bacterial endotoxin in irradiated mice. *Am J Physiol.* 1958;192:549–556.
122. Neta R, Douches S, Oppenheim JJ. Interleukin 1 is a radioprotector. *J Immunol.* 1986;136:2483–2485.
123. Neta R, Oppenheim JJ, Schreiber RD, et al. Role of cytokines (interleukin 1, tumor necrosis factor, and transforming growth factor beta) in natural and lipopolysaccharide-enhanced radioresistance. *J Exp Med.* 1991;173:1177–1182.
124. Neta R, Oppenheim JJ, Douches SD. Interdependence of the radioprotective effects of human recombinant interleukin 1 alpha, tumor necrosis factor alpha, granulocyte colony-stimulating factor, and murine recombinant granulocyte-macrophage colony-stimulating factor. *J Immunol.* 1988;140:108–111.
125. Booth D, Haley JD, Bruskin AM, et al. Transforming growth factor-B3 protects murine small intestinal crypt stem cells and animal survival after irradiation, possibly by reducing stem-cell cycling. *Int J Cancer.* 2000;86:53–59.
126. Potten CS, Booth D, Haley JD. Pretreatment with transforming growth factor beta-3 protects small intestinal stem cells against radiation damage in vivo. *Br J Cancer.* 1997;75: 1454–1459.
127. Kovacs CJ, Gooya JM, Harrell JP, et al. Altered radioprotective properties of interleukin I alpha (IL-1) in non-hematologic tumor-bearing animals. *Int J Radiat Oncol Biol Phys.* 1991;20:307–310.
128. Neta R, Stiefel SM, Finkelman F, et al. IL-12 protects bone marrow from and sensitizes intestinal tract to ionizing radiation. *J Immunol.* 1994;153:4230–4237.
129. Frasca D, Baschieri S, Boraschi D, et al. Radiation protection and restoration by the synthetic 163–171 nonapeptide of human interleukin 1 beta. *Radiat Res.* 1991;128:43–47.
130. Singh VK, Srinivasan V, Seed TM, et al. Radioprotection by *N*-palmitoylated nonapeptide of human interleukin-1beta. *Peptides.* 2005;26:413–418.
131. Okunieff P, Abraham EH, Moini M, et al. Basic fibroblast growth factor radioprotects bone marrow and not RIF1 tumor. *Acta Oncol.* 1995;34:435–438.
132. Okunieff P, Li M, Liu W, et al. Keratinocyte growth factors radioprotect bowel and bone marrow but not KHT sarcoma. *Am J Clin Oncol.* 2001;24:491–495.
133. Okunieff P, Wang X, Rubin P, et al. Radiation-induced changes in bone perfusion and angiogenesis. *Int J Radiat Oncol Biol Phys.* 1998;42:885–889.
134. Okunieff P, Mester M, Wang J, et al. In vivo radioprotective effects of angiogenic growth factors on the small bowel of C3H mice. *Radiat Res.* 1998;150:204–211.
135. Fan S, Wang JA, Yuan RQ, et al. Scatter factor protects epithelial and carcinoma cells against apoptosis induced by DNA-damaging agents. *Oncogene.* 1998;17:131–141.
136. Epstein JB, Gorsky M, Guglietta A, et al. The correlation between epidermal growth factor levels in saliva and the severity of oral mucositis during oropharyngeal radiation therapy. *Cancer.* 2000;89:2258–2265.
137. Hendry JH. Biological response modifiers and normal tissue injury after irradiation. *Semin Radiat Oncol.* 1994;4:123–132.
138. Talmadge JE, Tribble H, Pennington R, et al. Protective, restorative, and therapeutic properties of recombinant colony-stimulating factors. *Blood.* 1989;73:2093–2103.
139. Ryu JK, Swann S, LeVeque F, et al. The impact of concurrent granulocyte macrophage-colony stimulating factor on radiation-induced mucositis in head and neck cancer patients: a double-blind placebo-controlled prospective phase III study by Radiation Therapy Oncology Group 9901. *Int J Radiat Oncol Biol Phys.* 2007;67:643–650.
140. Brizel DM, Herman T, Goffinet D, et al. A phase I/II trial of escalating doses of recombinant human keratinocyte growth factor (rHuKGF) in head & neck cancer (HNC) patients receiving radiotherapy (RT) with concurrent chemotherapy (CCT). *Int J Radiat Oncol Biol Phys.* 2001;51.
141. Brizel DM, Murphy BA, Rosenthal DI, et al. Phase II study of palifermin and concurrent chemoradiation in head and neck squamous cell carcinoma. *J Clin Oncol.* 2008;26: 2489–2496.
142. Beddell CR, Goodford PJ, Kneen G, et al. Substituted benzaldehydes designed to increase the oxygen affinity of human haemoglobin and inhibit the sickling of sickle erythrocytes. *Br J Pharmacol.* 1984;82:397–407.
143. Keidan AJ, Franklin IM, White RD, et al. Effect of BW12C on oxygen affinity of haemoglobin in sickle-cell disease. *Lancet.* 1986;1:831–834.
144. Adams GE, Barnes DW, du Boulay C, et al. Induction of hypoxia in normal and malignant tissues by changing the oxygen affinity of hemoglobin—implications for therapy. *Int J Radiat Oncol Biol Phys.* 1986;12:1299–1302.
145. Adams GE, Stratford IJ, Nethersell AB, et al. Induction of severe tumor hypoxia by modifiers of the oxygen affinity of hemoglobin. *Int J Radiat Oncol Biol Phys.* 1989;16: 1179–1182.
146. Cole S, Robbins L. Manipulation of oxygenation in a human tumour xenograft with BW12C or hydralazine: effects on responses to radiation and to the bioreductive cytotoxicity of misonidazole or RSU-1069. *Radiother Oncol.* 1989;16:235–243.
147. Honess DJ, Nethersell AB, Bleehen NM. In vitro and in vivo studies using BW12C: toxicity, haemoglobin modification and effects on the radiosensitivity of normal marrow and RIF-1 tumours in mice. *Int J Radiat Biol.* 1992;61:83–94.
148. Honess DJ, White RD, Nethersell AB, et al. Effect of the manipulation of oxyhemoglobin status by BW12C on tumor thermosensitivity and on blood flow in tumor and normal tissues in mice. *Int J Radiat Oncol Biol Phys.* 1989;16:1187–1190.
149. Kalra R, Bremner JC, Wood PJ, et al. 31P MRS to monitor the induction of tumor hypoxia by the modification of the oxygen affinity of hemoglobin using BW 589C. *Int J Radiat Oncol Biol Phys.* 1994;29:285–288.
150. Stevens G, Hill SA, Joiner MC, et al. The effect of BW12C on the radiosensitivity and necrosis of murine tissues and tumours. *Australas Radiol.* 1994;38:199–203.
151. van den Aardweg GJ, Hopewell JW, Barnes DW, et al. Modification of the radiation response of pig skin by manipulation of tissue oxygen tension using anesthetics and administration of BW12C. *Int J Radiat Oncol Biol Phys.* 1989;16:1191–1194.
152. Propper DJ, Levitt NC, O'Byrne K, et al. Phase II study of the oxygen saturation curve left shifting agent BW12C in combination with the hypoxia activated drug mitomycin C in advanced colorectal cancer. *Br J Cancer.* 2000;82:1776–1782.
153. Ramsay JR, Bleehen NM, Dennis I, et al. Phase I study of BW12C in combination with mitomycin C in patients with advanced gastrointestinal cancer. *Int J Radiat Oncol Biol Phys.* 1992;22:721–725.
154. Grau C, Nordsmark M, Khalil AA, et al. Effect of carbon monoxide breathing on hypoxia and radiation response in the SCCVII tumor in vivo. *Int J Radiat Oncol Biol Phys.* 1994;29:449–454.
155. Walden TL Jr. Leukotriene C4-induced radioprotection: the role of hypoxia. *Radiat Res.* 1992;132:359–367.
156. Hill RP, Porter LS, Ives SA, et al. Initial studies of hypoxic radioprotection by deoxygenated dextran-hemoglobin. *Int J Radiat Oncol Biol Phys.* 1984;10:369–373.
157. Wong JT, Hill RP. Biophysical basis of hypoxic radioprotection by deoxygenated dextran-hemoglobin. *Int J Radiat Oncol Biol Phys.* 1986;12:1303–1306.
158. Hanson WR, Houseman KA, Collins PW. Radiation protection in vivo by prostaglandins and related compounds of the arachidonic acid cascade. *Pharmacol Ther.* 1988;39: 347–356.
159. Hanson WR, Houseman KA, Nelson AK, et al. Radiation protection of the murine intestine by misoprostol, a prostaglandin E1 analogue, given alone or with WR-2721, is stereospecific. *Prostaglandins Leukot Essent Fatty Acids.* 1988;32:101–105.
160. Hanson WR, Zhen W, Geng L, et al. The prostaglandin E1 analog, misoprostol, a normal tissue protector, does not protect four murine tumors in vivo from radiation injury. *Radiat Res.* 1995;142:281–287.
161. van Buul PP, van Duyn-Goedhart A, Sankaranarayanan K. In vivo and in vitro radioprotective effects of the prostaglandin E1 analogue misoprostol in DNA repair-proficient and -deficient rodent cell systems. *Radiat Res.* 1999;152:398–403.
162. Walden TL Jr, Farzaneh NK. Radioprotection by 16,16 dimethyl prostaglandin E_2 is equally effective in male and female mice. *J Radiat Res (Tokyo).* 1995;36:1–7.
163. Walden TL Jr, Patchen M, Snyder SL. 16,16-Dimethyl prostaglandin E_2 increases survival in mice following irradiation. *Radiat Res.* 1987;109:440–448.

164. Lawenda BD, Kelly KM, Ladas EJ, et al. Should supplemental antioxidant administration be avoided during chemotherapy and radiation therapy? *J Natl Cancer Inst*. 2008;100: 773–783.
165. Cohen EP, Fish BL, Moulder JE. Angiotensin II infusion exacerbates radiation nephropathy. *J Lab Clin Med*. 1999;134:283–291.
166. Cohen EP, Fish BL, Sharma M, et al. Role of the angiotensin II type-2 receptor in radiation nephropathy. *Transl Res*. 2007;150:106–115.
167. Molteni A, Moulder JE, Cohen EF, et al. Control of radiation-induced pneumopathy and lung fibrosis by angiotensin-converting enzyme inhibitors and an angiotensin II type 1 receptor blocker. *Int J Radiat Biol*. 2000;76:523–532.
168. Molteni A, Moulder JE, Cohen EP, et al. Prevention of radiation-induced nephropathy and fibrosis in a model of bone marrow transplant by an angiotensin II receptor blocker. *Exp Biol Med (Maywood)*. 2001;226:1016–1023.
169. Moulder JE, Fish BL, Cohen EP. Angiotensin II receptor antagonists in the treatment and prevention of radiation nephropathy. *Int J Radiat Biol*. 1998;73:415–421.
170. Moulder JE, Fish BL, Cohen EP. Impact of angiotensin II type 2 receptor blockade on experimental radiation nephropathy. *Radiat Res*. 2004;161:312–317.
171. Moulder JE, Fish BL, Cohen EP, et al. Angiotensin II receptor antagonists in the prevention of radiation nephropathy. *Radiat Res*. 1996;146:106–110.
172. Moulder JE, Fish BL, Regner KR, et al. Angiotensin II blockade reduces radiation-induced proliferation in experimental radiation nephropathy. *Radiat Res*. 2002;157:393–401.
173. Ward WF, Lin PJ, Wong PS, et al. Radiation pneumonitis in rats and its modification by the angiotensin-converting enzyme inhibitor captopril evaluated by high-resolution computed tomography. *Radiat Res*. 1993;135:81–87.
174. Halnan KE. The effect of corticosteroids on the radiation skin reaction. A random trial to assess the value of local application of prednisolone and neomycin ointment after x-ray treatment of basal cell carcinoma. *Br J Radiol*. 1962;35:403–408.
175. Matsubara J, Tajima Y, Ikeda A, et al. A new perspective of radiation protection by metallothionein induction. *Pharmacol Ther*. 1988;39:331–333.
176. Matsubara J, Tajima Y, Karasawa M. Metallothionein induction as a potent means of radiation protection in mice. *Radiat Res*. 1987;111:267–275.
177. Miura N, Satoh M, Imura N, et al. Protective effect of bismuth nitrate against injury to the bone marrow by gamma-irradiation in mice: possible involvement of induction of metallothionein synthesis. *J Pharmacol Exp Ther*. 1998;286:1427–1430.
178. Renan MJ, Dowman PI. Increased radioresistance of tumor cells exposed to metallothionein-inducing agents. *Radiat Res*. 1989;120:442–455.
179. Satoh M, Miura N, Naganuma A, et al. Prevention of adverse effects of gamma-ray irradiation after metallothionein induction by bismuth subnitrate in mice. *Eur J Cancer Clin Oncol*. 1989;25:1727–1731.
180. Boloor KK, Kamat JP, Devasagayam TP. Chlorophyllin as a protector of mitochondrial membranes against gamma-radiation and photosensitization. *Toxicology*. 2000;155:63–71.
181. Devi PU, Ganasoundari A. Radioprotective effect of leaf extract of Indian medicinal plant Ocimum sanctum. *Indian J Exp Biol*. 1995;33:205–208.
182. Devi PU, Ganasoundari A. Modulation of glutathione and antioxidant enzymes by Ocimum sanctum and its role in protection against radiation injury. *Indian J Exp Biol*. 1999;37:262–268.
183. Ganasoundari A, Devi PU, Rao BS. Enhancement of bone marrow radioprotection and reduction of WR-2721 toxicity by Ocimum sanctum. *Mutat Res*. 1998;397:303–312.
184. Ganasoundari A, Devi PU, Rao MN. Protection against radiation-induced chromosome damage in mouse bone marrow by Ocimum sanctum. *Mutat Res*. 1997;373:271–276.
185. Ganasoundari A, Zare SM, Devi PU. Modification of bone marrow radiosensitivity by medicinal plant extracts. *Br J Radiol*. 1997;70:599–602.
186. Hsu HY, Yang JJ, Ho YH, et al. Difference in the effects of radioprotection between aerial and root parts of Lycium chinense. *J Ethnopharmacol*. 1999;64:101–108.
187. Hsu HY, Yang JJ, Lin SY, et al. Comparisons of geniposidic acid and geniposide on antitumor and radioprotection after sublethal irradiation. *Cancer Lett*. 1997;113:31–37.
188. Kamat JP, Boloor KK, Devasagayam TP, et al. Antioxidant properties of Asparagus racemosus against damage induced by gamma-radiation in rat liver mitochondria. *J Ethnopharmacol*. 2000;71:425–435.
189. Kumar P, Kuttan R, Kuttan G. Radioprotective effects of Rasayanas. *Indian J Exp Biol*. 1996;34:848–850.
190. Hopewell JW, Robbins ME, van den Aardweg GJ, et al. The modulation of radiation-induced damage to pig skin by essential fatty acids. *Br J Cancer*. 1993;68:1–7.
191. Hopewell JW, van den Aardweg GJ, Morris GM, et al. Amelioration of both early and late radiation-induced damage to pig skin by essential fatty acids. *Int J Radiat Oncol Biol Phys*. 1994;30:1119–1125.
192. Burdelya LG, Krivokrysenko VI, Tallant TC, et al. An agonist of toll-like receptor 5 has radioprotective activity in mouse and primate models. *Science*. 2008;320:226–230.
193. Deng X, Yin X, Allan R, et al. Ceramide biogenesis is required for radiation-induced apoptosis in the germ line of C. elegans. *Science*. 2008;322:110–115.
194. Chou TC. Theoretical basis, experimental design, and computerized simulation of synergism and antagonism in drug combination studies. *Pharmacol Rev*. 2006;58:621–681.
195. Loewe S. Antagonisms and antagonists. *Pharmacol Rev*. 1957;9:237–242.
196. Steel GG, Peckham MJ. Exploitable mechanisms in combined radiotherapy-chemotherapy: the concept of additivity. *Int J Radiat Oncol Biol Phys*. 1979;5:85–91.
197. Chou TC, Talalay P. Quantitative analysis of dose-effect relationships: the combined effects of multiple drugs or enzyme inhibitors. *Adv Enzyme Regul*. 1984;22:27–55.
198. Eschwege F, Sancho-Garnier H, Gerard JP, et al. Ten-year results of randomized trial comparing radiotherapy and concomitant bleomycin to radiotherapy alone in epidermoid carcinomas of the oropharynx: experience of the European Organization for Research and Treatment of Cancer. *NCI Monogr*. 1988:275–278.
199. Fu KK, Phillips TL, Silverberg IJ, et al. Combined radiotherapy and chemotherapy with bleomycin and methotrexate for advanced inoperable head and neck cancer: update of a Northern California Oncology Group randomized trial. *J Clin Oncol*. 1987;5: 1410–1418.
200. Shanta V, Krishnamurthi S. Combined bleomycin and radiotherapy in oral cancer. *Clin Radiol*. 1980;31:617–620.
201. Vermund H, Kaalhus O, Winther F, et al. Bleomycin and radiation therapy in squamous cell carcinoma of the upper aero-digestive tract: a phase III clinical trial. *Int J Radiat Oncol Biol Phys*. 1985;11:1877–1886.
202. Zakotnik B, Smid L, Budihna M, et al. Concomitant radiotherapy with mitomycin C and bleomycin compared with radiotherapy alone in inoperable head and neck cancer: final report. *Int J Radiat Oncol Biol Phys*. 1998;41:1121–1127.
203. Zakotnik B, Budihna M, Smid L, et al. Patterns of failure in patients with locally advanced head and neck cancer treated postoperatively with irradiation or concomitant irradiation with Mitomycin C and Bleomycin. *Int J Radiat Oncol Biol Phys*. 2007;67:685–690.
204. Catane R, Schwade JG, Turrisi AT III, et al. Pulmonary toxicity after radiation and bleomycin: a review. *Int J Radiat Oncol Biol Phys*. 1979;5:1513–1518.
205. Nygaard K, Smith-Erichsen N, Hatlevoll R, et al. Pulmonary complications after bleomycin, irradiation and surgery for esophageal cancer. *Cancer*. 1978;41:17–22.
206. Samuels ML, Johnson DE, Holoye PY, et al. Large-dose bleomycin therapy and pulmonary toxicity. A possible role of prior radiotherapy. *JAMA*. 1976;235:1117–1120.
207. Sinclair WK, Morton RA. Variations in X-ray response during the division cycle of partially synchronized Chinese hamster cells in culture. *Nature*. 1963;199:1158–1160.
208. Sinclair WK, Morton RA. X-ray and ultraviolet sensitivity of synchronized Chinese hamster cells at various stages of the cell cycle. *Biophys J*. 1965;5:1–25.
209. Sinclair WK, Morton RA. X-ray sensitivity during the cell generation cycle of cultured Chinese hamster cells. *Radiat Res*. 1966;29:450–474.
210. Hwang HS, Davis TW, Houghton JA, et al. Radiosensitivity of thymidylate synthase-deficient human tumor cells is affected by progression through the G1 restriction point into S-phase: implications for fluoropyrimidine radiosensitization. *Cancer Res*. 2000;60: 92–100.
211. Gregoire V, Van NT, Stephens LC, et al. The role of fludarabine-induced apoptosis and cell cycle synchronization in enhanced murine tumor radiation response in vivo. *Cancer Res*. 1994;54:6201–6209.
212. Milas L, Milas MM, Mason KA. Combination of taxanes with radiation: preclinical studies. *Semin Radiat Oncol*. 1999;9:12–26.
213. Sinclair WK. Hydroxyurea: effects on Chinese hamster cells grown in culture. *Cancer Res*. 1967;27:297–308.
214. Sinclair WK. The combined effect of hydroxyurea and x-rays on Chinese hamster cells in vitro. *Cancer Res*. 1968;28:198–206.
215. Bruso CE, Shewach DS, Lawrence TS. Fluorodeoxyuridine-induced radiosensitization and inhibition of DNA double strand break repair in human colon cancer cells. *Int J Radiat Oncol Biol Phys*. 1990;19:1411–1417.
216. Hughes LL, Luengas J, Rich TA, et al. Radiosensitization of cultured human colon adenocarcinoma cells by 5-fluorouracil: effects on cell survival, DNA repair, and cell recovery. *Int J Radiat Oncol Biol Phys*. 1992;23:983–991.
217. Dolling JA, Boreham DR, Brown DL, et al. Modulation of radiation-induced strand break repair by cisplatin in mammalian cells. *Int J Radiat Biol*. 1998;74:61–69.
218. Dolling JA, Boreham DR, Brown DL, et al. Cisplatin-modification of DNA repair and ionizing radiation lethality in yeast, Saccharomyces cerevisiae. *Mutat Res*. 1999;433:127–136.
219. Frit P, Canitrot Y, Muller C, et al. Cross-resistance to ionizing radiation in a murine leukemic cell line resistant to cis-dichlorodiammineplatinum(II): role of Ku autoantigen. *Mol Pharmacol*. 1999;56:141–146.
220. Haveman J, Castro Kreder N, Rodermond HM, et al. Cellular response of X-ray sensitive hamster mutant cell lines to gemcitabine, cisplatin and 5-fluorouracil. *Oncol Rep*. 2004;12:187–192.
221. Myint WK, Ng C, Raaphorst GP. Examining the non-homologous repair process following cisplatin and radiation treatments. *Int J Radiat Biol*. 2002;78:417–424.
222. Turchi JJ, Henkels KM, Zhou Y. Cisplatin-DNA adducts inhibit translocation of the Ku subunits of DNA-PK. *Nucleic Acids Res*. 2000;28:4634–4641.
223. Fukuoka K, Arioka H, Iwamoto Y, et al. Mechanism of vinorelbine-induced radiosensitization of human small cell lung cancer cells. *Cancer Chemother Pharmacol*. 2002;49:385–390.
224. Fukuoka K, Arioka H, Iwamoto Y, et al. Mechanism of the radiosensitization induced by vinorelbine in human non-small cell lung cancer cells. *Lung Cancer*. 2001;34:451–460.
225. Iliakis G, Kurtzman S, Pantelias G, et al. Mechanism of radiosensitization by halogenated pyrimidines: effect of BrdU on radiation induction of DNA and chromosome damage and its correlation with cell killing. *Radiat Res*. 1989;119:286–304.
226. Jones GD, Ward JF, Limoli CL, et al. Mechanisms of radiosensitization in iododeoxyuridine-substituted cells. *Int J Radiat Biol*. 1995;67:647–653.
227. Webb CF, Jones GD, Ward JF, et al. Mechanisms of radiosensitization in bromodeoxyuridine-substituted cells. *Int J Radiat Biol*. 1993;64:695–705.
228. Chun PY, Feng FY, Scheurer AM, et al. Synergistic effects of gemcitabine and gefitinib in the treatment of head and neck carcinoma. *Cancer Res*. 2006;66:981–988.
229. Feng FY, Varambally S, Tomlins SA, et al. Role of epidermal growth factor receptor degradation in gemcitabine-mediated cytotoxicity. *Oncogene*. 2007;26:3431–3439.
230. Yamauchi T, Nowak BJ, Keating MJ, et al. DNA repair initiated in chronic lymphocytic leukemia lymphocytes by 4-hydroperoxycyclophosphamide is inhibited by fludarabine and clofarabine. *Clin Cancer Res*. 2001;7:3580–3589.
231. Nigro ND, Vaitkevicius VK, Considine B Jr. Combined therapy for cancer of the anal canal: a preliminary report. *Dis Colon Rectum*. 1974;17:354–356.
232. Leichman L, Nigro N, Vaitkevicius VK, et al. Cancer of the anal canal. Model for preoperative adjuvant combined modality therapy. *Am J Med*. 1985;78:211–215.
233. Nigro ND. Multidisciplinary management of cancer of the anus. *World J Surg*. 1987;11: 446–451.
234. Sischy B, Doggett RL, Krall JM, et al. Definitive irradiation and chemotherapy for radiosensitization in management of anal carcinoma: interim report on Radiation Therapy Oncology Group study no. 8314. *J Natl Cancer Inst*. 1989;81:850–856.
235. UKCCCR Anal Cancer Trial Working Party. Epidermoid anal cancer: results from the UKCCCR randomised trial of radiotherapy alone versus radiotherapy, 5-fluorouracil,

and mitomycin. UK Co-ordinating Committee on Cancer Research. *Lancet.* 1996;348: 1049–1054.

236. Ajani JA, Winter KA, Gunderson LL, et al. Fluorouracil, mitomycin, and radiotherapy vs fluorouracil, cisplatin, and radiotherapy for carcinoma of the anal canal: a randomized controlled trial. *JAMA.* 2008;299:1914–1921.

237. Bartelink H, Roelofsen F, Eschwege F, et al. Concomitant radiotherapy and chemotherapy is superior to radiotherapy alone in the treatment of locally advanced anal cancer: results of a phase III randomized trial of the European Organization for Research and Treatment of Cancer Radiotherapy and Gastrointestinal Cooperative Groups. *J Clin Oncol.* 1997;15:2040–2049.

238. Flam M, John M, Pajak TF, et al. Role of mitomycin in combination with fluorouracil and radiotherapy, and of salvage chemoradiation in the definitive nonsurgical treatment of epidermoid carcinoma of the anal canal: results of a phase III randomized intergroup study. *J Clin Oncol.* 1996;14:2527–2539.

239. Dobrowsky W, Dobrowsky E, Rauth AM. Mode of interaction of 5-fluorouracil, radiation, and mitomycin C: in vitro studies. *Int J Radiat Oncol Biol Phys.* 1992;22:875–880.

240. Stewart LA. Chemotherapy in adult high-grade glioma: a systematic review and meta-analysis of individual patient data from 12 randomised trials. *Lancet.* 2002;359:1011–1018.

241. Brada M, Hoang-Xuan K, Rampling R, et al. Multicenter phase II trial of temozolomide in patients with glioblastoma multiforme at first relapse. *Ann Oncol.* 2001;12:259–266.

242. Yung WK, Albright RE, Olson J, et al. A phase II study of temozolomide vs. procarbazine in patients with glioblastoma multiforme at first relapse. *Br J Cancer.* 2000;83:588–593.

243. Stupp R, Mason WP, van den Bent MJ, et al. Radiotherapy plus concomitant and adjuvant temozolomide for glioblastoma. *N Engl J Med.* 2005;352:987–996.

244. Sher DJ, Henson JW, Avutu B, et al. The added value of concurrently administered temozolomide versus adjuvant temozolomide alone in newly diagnosed glioblastoma. *J Neurooncol.* 2008;88:43–50.

245. Hegi ME, Diserens AC, Gorlia T, et al. MGMT gene silencing and benefit from temozolomide in glioblastoma. *N Engl J Med.* 2005;352:997–1003.

246. Bernier J, Domenge C, Ozsahin M, et al. Postoperative irradiation with or without concomitant chemotherapy for locally advanced head and neck cancer. *N Engl J Med.* 2004;350:1945–1952.

247. Brizel DM, Albers ME, Fisher SR, et al. Hyperfractionated irradiation with or without concurrent chemotherapy for locally advanced head and neck cancer. *N Engl J Med.* 1998;338:1798–1804.

248. Cooper JS, Pajak TF, Forastiere AA, et al. Postoperative concurrent radiotherapy and chemotherapy for high-risk squamous-cell carcinoma of the head and neck. *N Engl J Med.* 2004;350:1937–1944.

249. Forastiere AA, Goepfert H, Maor M, et al. Concurrent chemotherapy and radiotherapy for organ preservation in advanced laryngeal cancer. *N Engl J Med.* 2003;349:2091–2098.

250. Blackstock AW, Govindan R. Definitive chemoradiation for the treatment of locally advanced non small-cell lung cancer. *J Clin Oncol.* 2007;25:4146–4152.

251. Turrisi AT III, Kim K, Blum R, et al. Twice-daily compared with once-daily thoracic radiotherapy in limited small-cell lung cancer treated concurrently with cisplatin and etoposide. *N Engl J Med.* 1999;340:265–271.

252. Herskovic A, Martz K, al-Sarraf M, et al. Combined chemotherapy and radiotherapy compared with radiotherapy alone in patients with cancer of the esophagus. *N Engl J Med.* 1992;326:1593–1598.

253. Tepper J, Krasna MJ, Niedzwiecki D, et al. Phase III trial of trimodality therapy with cisplatin, fluorouracil, radiotherapy, and surgery compared with surgery alone for esophageal cancer: CALGB 9781. *J Clin Oncol.* 2008;26:1086–1092.

254. Macdonald JS, Smalley SR, Benedetti J, et al. Chemoradiotherapy after surgery compared with surgery alone for adenocarcinoma of the stomach or gastroesophageal junction. *N Engl J Med.* 2001;345:725–730.

255. Willett CG, Czito BG, Bendell JC, et al. Locally advanced pancreatic cancer. *J Clin Oncol.* 2005;23:4538–4544.

256. Sauer R, Becker H, Hohenberger W, et al. Preoperative versus postoperative chemoradiotherapy for rectal cancer. *N Engl J Med.* 2004;351:1731–1740.

257. Kachnic LA, Kaufman DS, Heney NM, et al. Bladder preservation by combined modality therapy for invasive bladder cancer. *J Clin Oncol.* 1997;15:1022–1029.

258. Kaufman DS, Shipley WU, Griffin PP, et al. Selective bladder preservation by combination treatment of invasive bladder cancer. *N Engl J Med.* 1993;329:1377–1382.

259. Shipley WU, Winter KA, Kaufman DS, et al. Phase III trial of neoadjuvant chemotherapy in patients with invasive bladder cancer treated with selective bladder preservation by combined radiation therapy and chemotherapy: initial results of Radiation Therapy Oncology Group 89-03. *J Clin Oncol.* 1998;16:3576–3583.

260. Tester W, Caplan R, Heaney J, et al. Neoadjuvant combined modality program with selective organ preservation for invasive bladder cancer: results of Radiation Therapy Oncology Group phase II trial 8802. *J Clin Oncol.* 1996;14:119–126.

261. Keys HM, Bundy BN, Stehman FB, et al. Cisplatin, radiation, and adjuvant hysterectomy compared with radiation and adjuvant hysterectomy for bulky stage IB cervical carcinoma. *N Engl J Med.* 1999;340:1154–1161.

262. Morris M, Eifel PJ, Lu J, et al. Pelvic radiation with concurrent chemotherapy compared with pelvic and para-aortic radiation for high-risk cervical cancer. *N Engl J Med.* 1999;340:1137–1143.

263. Peters WA III, Liu PY, Barrett RJ II, et al. Concurrent chemotherapy and pelvic radiation therapy compared with pelvic radiation therapy alone as adjuvant therapy after radical surgery in high-risk early-stage cancer of the cervix. *J Clin Oncol.* 2000;18:1606–1613.

264. Rose PG, Bundy BN, Watkins EB, et al. Concurrent cisplatin-based radiotherapy and chemotherapy for locally advanced cervical cancer. *N Engl J Med.* 1999;340:1144–1153.

265. Whitney CW, Sause W, Bundy BN, et al. Randomized comparison of fluorouracil plus cisplatin versus hydroxyurea as an adjunct to radiation therapy in stage IIB-IVA carcinoma of the cervix with negative para-aortic lymph nodes: a Gynecologic Oncology Group and Southwest Oncology Group study. *J Clin Oncol.* 1999;17:1339–1348.

266. Cohen S. Isolation of a mouse submaxillary gland protein accelerating incisor eruption and eyelid opening in the new-born animal. *J Biol Chem.* 1962;237:1555–1562.

267. Carpenter G, Cohen S. Epidermal growth factor. *Annu Rev Biochem.* 1979;48:193–216.

268. Carpenter G, King L Jr, Cohen S. Epidermal growth factor stimulates phosphorylation in membrane preparations in vitro. *Nature.* 1978;276:409–410.

269. Cohen S, Carpenter G, King L Jr. Epidermal growth factor-receptor-protein kinase interactions. Co-purification of receptor and epidermal growth factor-enhanced phosphorylation activity. *J Biol Chem.* 1980;255:4834–4842.

270. Downward J, Yarden Y, Mayes E, et al. Close similarity of epidermal growth factor receptor and v-erb-B oncogene protein sequences. *Nature.* 1984;307:521–527.

271. Masui H, Kawamoto T, Sato JD, et al. Growth inhibition of human tumor cells in athymic mice by anti-epidermal growth factor receptor monoclonal antibodies. *Cancer Res.* 1984;44:1002–1007.

272. Mendelsohn J. Targeting the epidermal growth factor receptor for cancer therapy. *J Clin Oncol.* 2002;20:1S-13S.

273. Mendelsohn J, Baselga J. Status of epidermal growth factor receptor antagonists in the biology and treatment of cancer. *J Clin Oncol.* 2003;21:2787–2799.

274. Mendelsohn J, Baselga J. Epidermal growth factor receptor targeting in cancer. *Semin Oncol.* 2006;33:369–385.

275. Balaban N, Moni J, Shannon M, et al. The effect of ionizing radiation on signal transduction: antibodies to EGF receptor sensitize A431 cells to radiation. *Biochim Biophys Acta.* 1996;1314:147–156.

276. Schmidt-Ullrich RK, Mikkelsen RB, Dent P, et al. Radiation-induced proliferation of the human A431 squamous carcinoma cells is dependent on EGFR tyrosine phosphorylation. *Oncogene.* 1997;15:1191–1197.

277. Akimoto T, Hunter NR, Buchmiller L, et al. Inverse relationship between epidermal growth factor receptor expression and radiocurability of murine carcinomas. *Clin Cancer Res.* 1999;5:2884–2890.

278. Ang KK, Berkey BA, Tu X, et al. Impact of epidermal growth factor receptor expression on survival and pattern of relapse in patients with advanced head and neck carcinoma. *Cancer Res.* 2002;62:7350–7356.

279. Dassonville O, Formento JL, Francoual M, et al. Expression of epidermal growth factor receptor and survival in upper aerodigestive tract cancer. *J Clin Oncol.* 1993;11: 1873–1878.

280. Rubin Grandis J, Melhem MF, Gooding WE, et al. Levels of TGF-alpha and EGFR protein in head and neck squamous cell carcinoma and patient survival. *J Natl Cancer Inst.* 1998;90:824–832.

281. Sheridan MT, O'Dwyer T, Seymour CB, et al. Potential indicators of radiosensitivity in squamous cell carcinoma of the head and neck. *Radiat Oncol Investig.* 1997;5:180–186.

282. Bianco C, Bianco R, Tortora G, et al. Antitumor activity of combined treatment of human cancer cells with ionizing radiation and anti-epidermal growth factor receptor monoclonal antibody C225 plus type I protein kinase A antisense oligonucleotide. *Clin Cancer Res.* 2000;6:4343–4350.

283. Bianco C, Tortora G, Bianco R, et al. Enhancement of antitumor activity of ionizing radiation by combined treatment with the selective epidermal growth factor receptor-tyrosine kinase inhibitor ZD1839 (Iressa). *Clin Cancer Res.* 2002;8:3250–3258.

284. Chinnaiyan P, Huang S, Vallabhaneni G, et al. Mechanisms of enhanced radiation response following epidermal growth factor receptor signaling inhibition by erlotinib (Tarceva). *Cancer Res.* 2005;65:3328–3335.

285. Huang SM, Bock JM, Harari PM. Epidermal growth factor receptor blockade with C225 modulates proliferation, apoptosis, and radiosensitivity in squamous cell carcinomas of the head and neck. *Cancer Res.* 1999;59:1935–1940.

286. Huang SM, Harari PM. Modulation of radiation response after epidermal growth factor receptor blockade in squamous cell carcinomas: inhibition of damage repair, cell cycle kinetics, and tumor angiogenesis. *Clin Cancer Res.* 2000;6:2166–2174.

287. Huang SM, Li J, Armstrong EA, et al. Modulation of radiation response and tumor-induced angiogenesis after epidermal growth factor receptor inhibition by ZD1839 (Iressa). *Cancer Res.* 2002;62:4300–4306.

288. Milas L, Mason K, Hunter N, et al. In vivo enhancement of tumor radioresponse by C225 antiepidermal growth factor receptor antibody. *Clin Cancer Res.* 2000;6:701–708.

289. Nasu S, Ang KK, Fan Z, et al. C225 antiepidermal growth factor receptor antibody enhances tumor radiocurability. *Int J Radiat Oncol Biol Phys.* 2001;51:474–477.

290. Nyati MK, Maheshwari D, Hanasoge S, et al. Radiosensitization by pan ErbB inhibitor CI-1033 in vitro and in vivo. *Clin Cancer Res.* 2004;10:691–700.

291. Rao GS, Murray S, Ethier SP. Radiosensitization of human breast cancer cells by a novel ErbB family receptor tyrosine kinase inhibitor. *Int J Radiat Oncol Biol Phys.* 2000;48: 1519–1528.

292. Saleh MN, Raisch KP, Stackhouse MA, et al. Combined modality therapy of A431 human epidermoid cancer using anti EGFr antibody C225 and radiation. *Cancer Biother Radiopharm.* 1999;14:451–463.

293. She Y, Lee F, Chen J, et al. The epidermal growth factor receptor tyrosine kinase inhibitor ZD1839 selectively potentiates radiation response of human tumors in nude mice, with a marked improvement in therapeutic index. *Clin Cancer Res.* 2003;9:3773–3778.

294. Shintani S, Li C, Mihara M, et al. Enhancement of tumor radioresponse by combined treatment with gefitinib (Iressa, ZD1839), an epidermal growth factor receptor tyrosine kinase inhibitor, is accompanied by inhibition of DNA damage repair and cell growth in oral cancer. *Int J Cancer.* 2003;107:1030–1037.

295. Solomon B, Hagekyriakou J, Trivett MK, et al. EGFR blockade with ZD1839 ("Iressa") potentiates the antitumor effects of single and multiple fractions of ionizing radiation in human A431 squamous cell carcinoma. Epidermal growth factor receptor. *Int J Radiat Oncol Biol Phys.* 2003;55:713–723.

296. Williams KJ, Telfer BA, Stratford IJ, et al. ZD1839 ('Iressa'), a specific oral epidermal growth factor receptor-tyrosine kinase inhibitor, potentiates radiotherapy in a human colorectal cancer xenograft model. *Br J Cancer.* 2002;86:1157–1161.

297. Zhou H, Kim YS, Peletier A, et al. Effects of the EGFR/HER2 kinase inhibitor GW572016 on EGFR- and HER2-overexpressing breast cancer cell line proliferation, radiosensitization, and resistance. *Int J Radiat Oncol Biol Phys.* 2004;58:344–352.

298. Huang SM, Li J, Harari PM. Molecular inhibition of angiogenesis and metastatic potential in human squamous cell carcinomas after epidermal growth factor receptor blockade. *Mol Cancer Ther.* 2002;1:507–514.

299. Robert F, Ezekiel MP, Spencer SA, et al. Phase I study of anti-epidermal growth factor receptor antibody cetuximab in combination with radiation therapy in patients with advanced head and neck cancer. *J Clin Oncol.* 2001;19:3234–3243.

300. Bonner JA, Harari PM, Giralt J, et al. Radiotherapy plus cetuximab for squamous-cell carcinoma of the head and neck. *N Engl J Med.* 2006;354:567–578.

301. Bonner JA, Harari PM, Giralt J, et al. Prolongation of survival with the addition of cetuximab to radiation in patients with locoregionally advanced head and neck cancer (SCCHN): five year results from a randomized trial. *Int J Radiat Oncol Biol Phys.* 2008;72:e2–e23.

302. Escudier B, Eisen T, Stadler WM, et al. Sorafenib in advanced clear-cell renal-cell carcinoma. *N Engl J Med.* 2007;356:125–134.

303. Hurwitz H, Fehrenbacher L, Novotny W, et al. Bevacizumab plus irinotecan, fluorouracil, and leucovorin for metastatic colorectal cancer. *N Engl J Med.* 2004;350:2335–2342.

304. Miller K, Wang M, Gralow J, et al. Paclitaxel plus bevacizumab versus paclitaxel alone for metastatic breast cancer. *N Engl J Med.* 2007;357:2666–2676.

305. Motzer RJ, Hutson TE, Tomczak P, et al. Sunitinib versus interferon alfa in metastatic renal-cell carcinoma. *N Engl J Med.* 2007;356:115–124.

306. Sandler A, Gray R, Perry MC, et al. Paclitaxel-carboplatin alone or with bevacizumab for non-small-cell lung cancer. *N Engl J Med.* 2006;355:2542–2550.

307. Yang JC, Haworth L, Sherry RM, et al. A randomized trial of bevacizumab, an anti-vascular endothelial growth factor antibody, for metastatic renal cancer. *N Engl J Med.* 2003;349:427–434.

308. Murata R, Nishimura Y, Hiraoka M. An antiangiogenic agent (TNP-470) inhibited reoxygenation during fractionated radiotherapy of murine mammary carcinoma. *Int J Radiat Oncol Biol Phys.* 1997;37:1107–1113.

309. Teicher BA, Dupuis NP, Robinson MF, et al. Antiangiogenic treatment (TNP-470/minocycline) increases tissue levels of anticancer drugs in mice bearing Lewis lung carcinoma. *Oncol Res.* 1995;7:237–243.

310. Teicher BA, Holden SA, Ara G, et al. Influence of an anti-angiogenic treatment on 9L gliosarcoma: oxygenation and response to cytotoxic therapy. *Int J Cancer.* 1995;61:732–737.

311. Teicher BA, Holden SA, Ara G, et al. Potentiation of cytotoxic cancer therapies by TNP-470 alone and with other anti-angiogenic agents. *Int J Cancer.* 1994;57:920–925.

312. Teicher BA, Holden SA, Dupuis NP, et al. Potentiation of cytotoxic therapies by TNP-470 and minocycline in mice bearing EMT-6 mammary carcinoma. *Breast Cancer Res Treat.* 1995;36:227–236.

313. Ansiaux R, Baudelet C, Jordan BF, et al. Thalidomide radiosensitizes tumors through early changes in the tumor microenvironment. *Clin Cancer Res.* 2005;11:743–750.

314. Crane CH, Ellis LM, Abbruzzese JL, et al. Phase I trial evaluating the safety of bevacizumab with concurrent radiotherapy and capecitabine in locally advanced pancreatic cancer. *J Clin Oncol.* 2006;24:1145–1151.

315. Czito BG, Bendell JC, Willett CG, et al. Bevacizumab, oxaliplatin, and capecitabine with radiation therapy in rectal cancer: phase I trial results. *Int J Radiat Oncol Biol Phys.* 2007;68:472–478.

316. Lai A, Filka E, McGibbon B, et al. Phase II pilot study of bevacizumab in combination with temozolomide and regional radiation therapy for up-front treatment of patients with newly diagnosed glioblastoma multiforme: interim analysis of safety and tolerability. *Int J Radiat Oncol Biol Phys.* 2008;71:1372–1380.

317. Nieder C, Wiedenmann N, Andratschke NH, et al. Radiation therapy plus angiogenesis inhibition with bevacizumab: rationale and initial experience. *Rev Recent Clin Trials.* 2007;2:163–168.

318. Seiwert TY, Haraf DJ, Cohen EE, et al. Phase I study of bevacizumab added to fluorouracil- and hydroxyurea-based concomitant chemoradiotherapy for poor-prognosis head and neck cancer. *J Clin Oncol.* 2008;26:1732–1741.

319. Willett CG, Boucher Y, di Tomaso E, et al. Direct evidence that the VEGF-specific antibody bevacizumab has antivascular effects in human rectal cancer. *Nat Med.* 2004;10:145–147.

320. Willett CG, Boucher Y, Duda DG, et al. Surrogate markers for antiangiogenic therapy and dose-limiting toxicities for bevacizumab with radiation and chemotherapy: continued experience of a phase I trial in rectal cancer patients. *J Clin Oncol.* 2005;23:8136–8139.

321. Willett CG, Duda DG, di Tomaso E, et al. Complete pathological response to bevacizumab and chemoradiation in advanced rectal cancer. *Nat Clin Pract Oncol.* 2007;4:316–321.

322. Jain RK, Duda DG, Clark JW, et al. Lessons from phase III clinical trials on anti-VEGF therapy for cancer. *Nat Clin Pract Oncol.* 2006;3:24–40.

323. Jain RK. Normalizing tumor vasculature with anti-angiogenic therapy: a new paradigm for combination therapy. *Nat Med.* 2001;7:987–989.

324. Garcia-Barros M, Paris F, Cordon-Cardo C, et al. Tumor response to radiotherapy regulated by endothelial cell apoptosis. *Science.* 2003;300:1155–1159.

325. Gorski DH, Beckett MA, Jaskowiak NT, et al. Blockage of the vascular endothelial growth factor stress response increases the antitumor effects of ionizing radiation. *Cancer Res.* 1999;59:3374–3378.

326. Kermani P, Leclerc G, Martel R, et al. Effect of ionizing radiation on thymidine uptake, differentiation, and VEGFR2 receptor expression in endothelial cells: the role of VEGF(165). *Int J Radiat Oncol Biol Phys.* 2001;50:213–220.

327. Gupta VK, Jaskowiak NT, Beckett MA, et al. Vascular endothelial growth factor enhances endothelial cell survival and tumor radioresistance. *Cancer J.* 2002;8:47–54.

328. Hess C, Vuong V, Hegyi I, et al. Effect of VEGF receptor inhibitor PTK787/ZK222584 [correction of ZK222548] combined with ionizing radiation on endothelial cells and tumour growth. *Br J Cancer.* 2001;85:2010–2016.

329. Mauceri HJ, Hanna NN, Beckett MA, et al. Combined effects of angiostatin and ionizing radiation in antitumour therapy. *Nature.* 1998;394:287–291.

330. Chinnaiyan P, Allen GW, Harari PM. Radiation and new molecular agents, part II: targeting HDAC, HSP90, IGF-1R, PI3K, and Ras. *Semin Radiat Oncol.* 2006;16:59–64.

331. Busch W. Uber den Einfluss, welchen heftigere Erysipelen zuweilig auf organisierte Neubildungen ausuben. *Verhandlugen des naturhistorischen Vereines der preussischen Rheinlande und Westphalens.* 1866;23:28.

332. Coley WB. The treatment of malignant tumors by repeated inoculations of erysipelas: with a report of ten original cases. *Am J Med Sci.* 1893;105:486.

333. Dewey WC, Hopwood LE, Sapareto SA, et al. Cellular responses to combinations of hyperthermia and radiation. *Radiology.* 1977;123:463–474.

334. Dewey WC, Thrall DE, Gillette EL. Hyperthermia and radiation—a selective thermal effect on chronically hypoxic tumor cells in vivo. *Int J Radiat Oncol Biol Phys.* 1977;2:99–103.

335. Overgaard J. The effect of sequence and time intervals of combined hyperthermia and radiation treatment. *Br J Radiol.* 1977;50:763–765.

336. Sapareto SA, Hopwood LE, Dewey WC. Combined effects of X irradiation and hyperthermia on CHO cells for various temperatures and orders of application. *Radiat Res.* 1978;73:221–233.

337. Sapareto SA, Raaphorst GP, Dewey WC. Cell killing and the sequencing of hyperthermia and radiation. *Int J Radiat Oncol Biol Phys.* 1979;5:343–347.

338. Westra A, Dewey WC. Variation in sensitivity to heat shock during the cell-cycle of Chinese hamster cells in vitro. *Int J Radiat Biol Relat Stud Phys Chem Med.* 1971;19:467–477.

339. Gerweck LE, Nygaard TG, Burlett M. Response of cells to hyperthermia under acute and chronic hypoxic conditions. *Cancer Res.* 1979;39:966–972.

340. Koutcher JA, Barnett D, Kornblith AB, et al. Relationship of changes in pH and energy status to hypoxic cell fraction and hyperthermia sensitivity. *Int J Radiat Oncol Biol Phys.* 1990;18:1429–1435.

341. Perez CA, Pajak T, Emami B, et al. Randomized phase III study comparing irradiation and hyperthermia with irradiation alone in superficial measurable tumors. Final report by the Radiation Therapy Oncology Group. *Am J Clin Oncol.* 1991;14:133–141.

342. Perez CA, Gillespie B, Pajak T, et al. Quality assurance problems in clinical hyperthermia and their impact on therapeutic outcome: a Report by the Radiation Therapy Oncology Group. *Int J Radiat Oncol Biol Phys.* 1989;16:551–558.

343. Datta NR, Bose AK, Kapoor HK, et al. Head and neck cancers: results of thermoradiotherapy versus radiotherapy. *Int J Hyperthermia.* 1990;6:479–486.

344. Valdagni R, Amichetti M. Report of long-term follow-up in a randomized trial comparing radiation therapy and radiation therapy plus hyperthermia to metastatic lymph nodes in stage IV head and neck patients. *Int J Radiat Oncol Biol Phys.* 1994;28:163–169.

345. Overgaard J, Gonzalez Gonzalez D, Hulshof MC, et al. Randomised trial of hyperthermia as adjuvant to radiotherapy for recurrent or metastatic malignant melanoma. European Society for Hyperthermic Oncology. *Lancet.* 1995;345:540–543.

346. Overgaard J, Gonzalez Gonzalez D, Hulshof MC, et al. Hyperthermia as an adjuvant to radiation therapy of recurrent or metastatic malignant melanoma. A multicentre randomized trial by the European Society for Hyperthermic Oncology. *Int J Hyperthermia.* 1996;12:3–20.

347. Sneed PK, Stauffer PR, McDermott MW, et al. Survival benefit of hyperthermia in a prospective randomized trial of brachytherapy boost ± hyperthermia for glioblastoma multiforme. *Int J Radiat Oncol Biol Phys.* 1998;40:287–295.

348. Sugimachi K, Kuwano H, Ide H, et al. Chemotherapy combined with or without hyperthermia for patients with oesophageal carcinoma: a prospective randomized trial. *Int J Hyperthermia.* 1994;10:485–493.

349. van der Zee J, Gonzalez Gonzalez D, van Rhoon GC, et al. Comparison of radiotherapy alone with radiotherapy plus hyperthermia in locally advanced pelvic tumours: a prospective, randomised, multicentre trial. Dutch Deep Hyperthermia Group. *Lancet.* 2000;355:1119–1125.

350. Vernon CC, Hand JW, Field SB, et al. Radiotherapy with or without hyperthermia in the treatment of superficial localized breast cancer: results from five randomized controlled trials. International Collaborative Hyperthermia Group. *Int J Radiat Oncol Biol Phys.* 1996;35:731–744.

6

Comorbidities Impacting Radiosensitivity

INTRODUCTION

The importance of a multidisciplinary approach in the treatment of cancer is becoming increasingly evident. The collaboration among surgical oncology, medical oncology, and radiation oncology is essential in providing optimal care to patients with various malignancies. The treatment of early-stage breast cancer is just one example which eloquently illustrates this collaborative effort with standard treatment often including breast-conserving surgery, adjuvant radiation, and evaluation for further systemic therapies, including chemotherapy and hormonal agents. With the integration of multidisciplinary cancer care for patients with increasingly complex medical histories and comorbid conditions, it is important to gain an understanding of how different patient factors and different patient comorbidities may affect treatment using these three distinct modalities. This chapter will review the relevant published literature regarding comorbidities that may potentially impact radiosensitivity, including collagen vascular disease (CVD), inflammatory bowel disease (IBD), multiple sclerosis (MS), HIV infection, diabetes, hypertension, and hereditary radiosensitivity syndromes.

COLLAGEN VASCULAR DISEASE

The role of radiation therapy in patients with CVDs has long been controversial. Initial case reports of severe radiation-induced toxicity in the setting of CVD were published in the 1970s.[1,2] Since then, several larger case reports have been published further addressing this issue.[3–8] Due to these case reports, in 1992, the American College of Radiology published guidelines stating that "a history of collagen vascular disease is a relative contraindication to breast conservation treatment because published reports indicate that such patients tolerate irradiation poorly.[9]" Since this report, several large retrospective studies have been published with conflicting results.[10–13] To date, more than 300 cases have been published evaluating the potential risks of acute and late toxicities for patients with CVD.

Additionally, there are recent studies that suggest an increased incidence of malignancies in patients with autoimmune connective tissue diseases.[14–17] Hematologic malignancies, in particular non-Hodgkin lymphoma, have been found at a greater incidence in patients with rheumatoid arthritis (RA)[14] and Sjögren disease.[17] Patients with systemic sclerosis may have up to a twofold risk of development of cancer,[15] especially lung

cancer in patients with underlying pulmonary fibrosis.[16,18] Although controversial, some studies have also suggested an increase in the prevalence of breast cancer in patients with systemic sclerosis compared to the general population.[15] Patients with CVDs may therefore be at greater risk for developing malignancies that require radiation as part of a comprehensive treatment plan.

Patients with early-stage breast cancer in the setting of quiescent CVD are often recommended to undergo a mastectomy to avoid possible acute and late effects associated with radiation. The determination of whether to treat patients in the setting of CVD with irradiation for either curative or palliative intent has yet to be definitely established. One recent study has suggested that radiation therapy may be inappropriately withheld from lupus patients with cancer for fear of severe late complications.[19]

Classification of Collagen Vascular Disease

The classification of CVD encompasses a heterogeneous group of disorders, which is categorized by alterations in immunoregulatory mechanisms, leading to the production of autoantibodies and abnormalities in cell-mediated immunity. These autoantibodies are directed toward elements of the extracellular matrix, including collagen and elastin, which act as structural and functional support to different organs. Clinical manifestations of CVDs commonly include skin rash, fibrosis, and arthritis due to inflammation of the skin and joints. In more severe cases, CVDs may also involve systemic organs, which lead to the disease related sequelae of pleuritis, pericarditis, and nephropathy. Most of the published case reports have evaluated RA, systemic lupus erythematosus (SLE), dermatomyositis, scleroderma, and mixed connective tissue diseases in the setting of therapeutic radiation. Table 6.1 reviews general characteristics of these most common collagen vascular disorders.

Initial Case Reports

Prior to the late 1980s, anecdotal reports circulated of excessive toxicity from radiation in patients with CVD.[1,2] In 1989, Teo et al.[6] published one of the initial case reports evaluating radiation-induced toxicity in 10 patients diagnosed with nasopharyngeal carcinoma and dermatomyositis. Eight of nine patients developed acute confluent mucositis necessitating treatment break. With a mean follow-up of 51.8 months, nine patients

TABLE 6.1	Summary of Clinical Features of Common CVDs		
Disorder	*Demographics*	*Clinical Presentation*	*Associated Antibodies*
RA	Most common diagnosis of CVD.	Autoimmune, inflammatory disorder affecting synovial joints. Classic: AM stiffness improved with use, symmetric joint involvement, systemic symptoms (fever, fatigue, pleuritis, pericarditis)	80% with +RF (anti-IgG Ab)
SLE	90% Female, between ages 14 and 45.	Clinical Presentation: fever, fatigue, weight loss, joint pain, malar rash, photosensitivity. Associated with endocarditis, Raynaud phenomenon, and nephrotic syndrome.	Anti-ANA-sensitive Anti-dsDNA-specific Anti-Smith-specific
Scleroderma	75% females.	Excessive fibrosis and collagen deposit throughout body 1. Diffuse—widespread skin involvement, early visceral involvement, rapid progression 2. CREST-calcinosis, Raynaud phenomenon, esophageal dysmotility, sclerodactyly, telangiectasias Limited skin involvement. More benign.	Diffuse: Anti Scl-70 CREST: Anti-centromere
Dermatomyositis	Females: males—2:1. Bimodality peak, in children 5–10, adult peak age 50.	Clinical presentation: Pruritis, scaly rash, proximal muscle weakness and tenderness, arthralgias, heliotrope rash.	Anti-ANA Anti-tRNA transferase
Sjogren syndrome	Predominantly in females, age 40–60.	Classic triad: Dry eyes, dry mouth, arthritis. Associated with parotid gland enlargement, increased risk of B cell lymphomas.	Anti-SSB and anti-SSA.
MCTD	Predominantly women. Peak onset: 20–30s.	Most common: Raynaud phenomenon, puffy hands, arthralgias, myalgias, and fatigue.	Anti-U$_1$ RNP

Source: Wo J, Taghian AG. Radiotherapy in setting of collagen vascular disease. *Int J Radiat Oncol Biol Phys.* 2007;69(5):1347–1353.

developed subcutaneous fibrosis and complete xerostomia lasting variable intervals posttreatment. Two patients suffered radiation skin necrosis with ulceration and another patient developed CN VI and XII palsies 10 years after radiotherapy.

Shortly after, Fleck et al.[3] published a case report of the MD Anderson experience with breast irradiation, treated to 40 to 50 Gy via ^{60}Co photons with variable doses of electron boosts, in nine patients with CVDs. Of four with preexisting CVD, three developed severe complications. One patient developed exaggerated moist desquamation requiring early treatment termination at 40 Gy and symptoms of brachial plexopathy. A second patient received a dose reduction to 55 Gy, but nevertheless, developed severe soft tissue necrosis requiring chest wall resection and reconstruction, radiation-induced rib fractures, and radiation-induced pulmonary fibrosis. The last patient developed severe soft tissue necrosis and subsequent complications of bronchopleural-cutaneous fistula and osteoradionecrosis of the clavicle, sternum, and rib cage. Of the five patients who developed CVD after radiation therapy, none developed complications related to the radiation treatment. These findings suggest that patients with preexisting diagnoses of CVD may be at greater risk of radiation toxicity than those subsequently diagnosed with CVD.

In 1991, Varga et al.[5] described four patients with stable systemic sclerosis and limited skin involvement who developed exaggerated cutaneous, subcutaneous, and visceral fibrotic reactions in the irradiated areas. This was the first published report of fibrosis extending beyond the radiation fields leading to fibrous encapsulation of internal organs. All patients had clinically stable scleroderma for at least 6 months prior to radiation treatment, but subsequently developed severe acute skin toxicities within the treatment fields despite aggressive treatment with penicillamine, an antifibrotic agent shown to improve

skin involvement and survival in scleroderma.[20,21] Three patients (75%) subsequently developed fatal complications due to recurrent small bowel obstructions from extensive visceral fibrosis and cachexia ($n = 2$) and recurrent aspiration pneumonia from esophageal strictures requiring G-tube placement ($n = 1$).

Due to these initial case reports, in 1992, the American College of Radiology published guidelines stating a "history of collagen vascular disease is a relative contraindication to breast conservation treatment because published reports indicate that such patients tolerate irradiation poorly.[9]" These initial reports sparked an interest in evaluating these findings in a matched controlled setting.

Total Lymphoid Irradiation

In the 1970s, total lymphoid irradiation (TLI) was considered as an acceptable alternative treatment for intractable RA.[22,23] A feasibility study published in the *NEJM* reported TLI to a total dose of 20 Gy resulted in significant joint tenderness relief and improvement of function 6 months after treatment.[22] Although initially promising, with longer follow-up, the toxicities outweighed the clinical benefits and the treatment eventually fell out of favor. Hart[24] reported on the alarming rates of radiation-induced complications seen in this subset of patients compared to Hodgkin's patients who were treated with higher doses. Radiation-related side effects reported in two early trials included xerostomia, hypothyroidism, severe transient leukopenia, skin irritation, and dysphagia.[22,23,25,26] Long-term follow-up studies involving 32 patients treated with TLI reported two deaths due to respiratory failure complicating rheumatoid lung disease.[27] Despite the relatively small numbers, these findings appear to support previous findings that even modest doses of radiation may sensitize treated tissues to increased risk of toxicities.

Retrospective Studies

Four matched case-controlled studies[10–12,28] and one single-institution retrospective study have been published to date.[13] The majority of studies have evaluated radiation-induced toxicity in all malignancies,[10,12,13,28,29] but one recent study focused on early-stage breast cancer patients treated with partial mastectomy and radiation.[11] These studies are summarized in Table 6.2. Ross et al.[10] published the first matched-pair case-control study performed at the University of Iowa that investigated whether 61 patients with CVD were at increased risk for radiation-induced treatment complications. With a median follow-up of 16 months among patients treated definitively, there was no significant difference between the CVD and the control groups in terms of acute (11% vs. 7%, $p = 0.375$) or late (10% vs. 7%, $p = 0.69$) complications. There was, however, a trend toward increased incidence of fatal complications in patients with CVD versus the matched control group (5% vs. 0%, $p = 0.25$). These fatal complications included radiation-induced bowel necrosis, small bowel obstruction with bladder necrosis, and radiation-induced chronic pericarditis. Additionally, RA was associated with a trend toward increased late complications (24% vs. 5%, $p = 0.125$), whereas SLE was associated with a trend toward increased acute toxicities (36% vs. 18%, $p = 0.5$). Therefore, the first published single large case-matched study found that differences in acute and late toxicities were less than expected and not statistically significant. However, this series was criticized for short follow-up time, which could potentially bias against differences in late complications.[10]

In 1997, Morris and Powell[13] published the largest retrospective review to date of 209 cancer patients treated with radiotherapy at Massachusetts General Hospital with documented CVD. Of the 209 cases, a majority of patients were diagnosed with RA (64%), followed by SLE (12%), polymyositis/dermatomyositis (8%), scleroderma (8%), and a smaller representation by ankylosing spondylitis, juvenile RA, discoid lupus erythematosus, and mixed connective tissue disorder (MCTD). With a median dose of 45 Gy (range: 10–87.6 Gy), significant acute toxicity was reported in 10% of irradiated sites. With a median follow-up of 6 years, 5-year late complication rates were significantly associated with development of acute reactions (29% vs. 9%) and with diagnosis of non-RA CVDs (21% vs. 6%, $p = 0.0002$). NSAID use at time of irradiation also was found to predict for a statistically lower risk of late complications compared to patients not taking NSAIDs (6% vs. 14%, $p = 0.04$). A similar trend was noted in other medications that modify CVD activity including steroids, but these differences were not statistically significant. Among patients treated with radiation to multiple sites, when the initial site of treatment was not associated with significant late toxicity, the subsequent risk of late toxicity was low for additional sites of treatment. Morris and Powell[13] concluded that while RA did not appear to increase the risk of late toxicity, patients who developed severe acute reactions and patients with non-RA CVD were at significantly higher rates of long-term toxicity. Due to their findings, they recommended evaluation of radiation therapy for these patients on a case-by-case nature.

Since that time, two additional matched control studies have been published. In 2003, Phan et al.[12] reported the results of 38 patients with documented CVD. Due to the lack of effect of RA in the study by Morris and Powell,[13] patients with RA were excluded from this study. With a median follow-up of 35 months, there was no difference in the incidence of either acute or late complications between the two groups. A subset analysis of patients with scleroderma revealed slightly higher rates of acute and late complications compared to controls; however, there were only two patients with scleroderma in this series. Thus, the major drawback of this study is the small number of cases, especially when the cases are further divided by subset analysis according to diagnosis. This study, as well as other prior studies, lacked the statistical power to conclusively establish the effect of CVD on radiation complications.

Most recently, Lin et al. published the largest single institution matched retrospective series of 73 patients with CVD treated at the University of Michigan from 1985 to 2005. With a median follow-up of 1.3 years, they reported a significantly higher risk of late toxicity in patients with CVD compared to controls (29.1% vs. 14%, $p = 0.001$) and a trend toward increased severe late toxicity (9.3% vs. 3.7%, $p = 0.079$). In contrast, acute toxicity was not found to be significantly higher in patients with CVD. Use of oral cytotoxic rheumatologic agents was found to be associated with decreased risk of acute toxicity ($p = 0.0263$), whereas concurrent infusional chemotherapy was associated with an increased risk of any ($p = 0.009$) or severe late toxicity ($p = 0.009$). In particular, by crude analysis, the subset of patients receiving pelvic irradiation or with CVD diagnoses of SLE or scleroderma were found to be at greater risk of severe toxicity; however, definitive conclusions are limited by insufficient power with subset analysis. Thus, the authors concluded that although radiation therapy was generally well tolerated, RT in the setting of CVD may be associated with higher rate of late toxicity.[28]

TABLE 6.2			**Summary of Retrospective Series Evaluating the Risk of Acute and Late Toxicities Among Patients with CVD**						
				Grade 3+ Acute Toxicities			*Grade 3+ Late Toxicities*		
Author	*Year*	*No. of Patients*	*Median Follow-Up*	*CVD (%)*	*Control (%)*	*p*	*CVD (%)*	*Control (%)*	*p*
Ross et al.[10]	1993	61	16 months	11	7	0.375	10	7	0.69
Morris and Powell[13]	1997	209	6 years	10			23		
Phan et al.[12]	2003	38	35 months	7	7		7	7	
Chen et al.[11]	2001	36	12.5 years	14	8	0.40	17	3	0.0095
Lin et al.[28]	2008	73	1.3 years	10.5	10.4	0.075	9.30	3.70	0.079

Source: Wo J, Taghian AG. Radiotherapy in setting of collagen vascular disease. *Int J Radiat Oncol Biol Phys.* 2007;69(5):1347–1353.

Breast Conservation Therapy

The ability to achieve good cosmesis is important in determining which breast cancer patients are optimal candidates for lumpectomy and radiotherapy versus mastectomy. Long-term cosmesis has been reported to be good to excellent results in 57% to 88% of patients treated with breast-conserving therapy. Other potential long-term complications including rib fractures, radiation pneumonitis, brachial plexopathy, and lymphedema from whole breast irradiation have also been rarely reported after breast irradiation.[30-33] However, if breast irradiation was found to cause excessive fibrosis or increased late morbidity in patients with CVD, then the benefit of breast-conserving therapy would be lost in this group of patients. Ransom and Cameron[2] were the first to publish a case report on pronounced fibrosis and shoulder stiffness in an irradiated patient with scleroderma. As previously described, Fleck et al.[3] would later report three patients with preexisting CVD who developed exaggerated acute and late toxicities. Robertson et al.[4] subsequently published a case report of two patients with CVD who developed extremely poor cosmetic results secondary to fibrosis after breast irradiation. One patient with RA required simple mastectomy after 11 months, and a second patient with scleroderma developed new manifestations of scleroderma, including esophageal fibrosis and pectoralis muscle fibrosis, causing limited range of motion in her left arm. Due to the acceleration of systemic disease, the authors recommended that breast irradiation should be avoided in all patients with scleroderma. Similarly, Mayr et al.[34] published the first case report of a patient with MCTD who developed exaggerated acute and late complications with significant compromise in breast cosmesis. Given these findings, there has been reluctance by some oncologists to recommend breast conservation in this setting.

Even with modern-day techniques that limit dose to normal tissues with beam arrangement optimization, reports of severe acute toxicity still persist. Recently, Hernandez et al.[35] reported severe confluent radiation-induced dermatitis and radiation pneumonitis in a woman with RA, Sjogren syndrome, and stage IV primary biliary cirrhosis treated with whole breast radiotherapy (refer to Fig. 6.1). Three-dimensional (3D) planning was used, with intensity-modulated radiation therapy (IMRT) to limit dose inhomogeneity to no >1.1% above prescribed doses.

Despite modern techniques, this case demonstrates that there still are incidences of increased radiation-induced toxicity in the setting of CVD.

To date, Chen et al.[11] have published the only matched case-control study of 36 patients investigating breast-conserving therapy in the setting of CVD. Compared to prior matched controlled studies, Chen et al. included only patients with active disease at the time of radiation. With a median follow-up time of 12.5 years, similar to prior published studies, there was no significant difference noted between CVD patients and control groups with respect to acute complications (14% vs. 8%, $p = 0.40$). However, this study reported a statistically increased risk of late complications between the two groups (17% vs. 3%, $p = 0.0095$). On subset analysis based on CVD diagnosis, only the diagnosis of scleroderma was found to predict for late complications (75% vs. 0%, $p = 0.00052$). Again, this study was limited by small sample size and statistical power.[11] These findings again suggest that patients with scleroderma may be at greater risk for radiation-induced late toxicities, thereby impairing the cosmetic results achieved with breast-conserving therapy.

Scleroderma

Although the results of the retrospective studies described above have been variable, many of the studies have suggested an increased risk of radiation-related toxicity in patients with scleroderma. Due to these findings, Gold et al.[36] published the Mayo Clinic experience of 20 patients with scleroderma treated with radiation between 1980 and 2003. With a median follow-up of 4.7 years, grade 3 or higher acute toxicity was reported in only three patients (15%), which were felt to be consistent with historical controls (refer to Fig. 6.2). Treatment intent, which the authors used as a surrogate for treatment dose, and the extent of sclerodermal organ involvement were the only factors found to predict for acute complications. In addition, only three patients (15%) were found with grade 3 or higher late toxicities. Therefore, the authors concluded that in general, patients tolerated treatment well with lower-than-anticipated rates of acute and chronic toxicities. The major limitation of this study, however, was limited follow-up and small number of cases. Five of 15 patients treated with curative intent died within 1 year of completion of radiation therapy, thereby limiting the

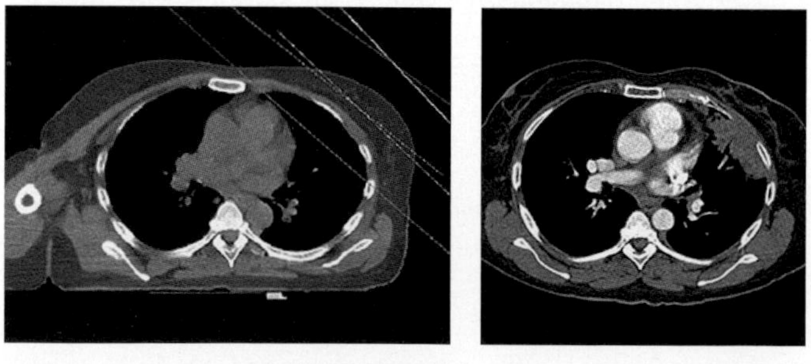

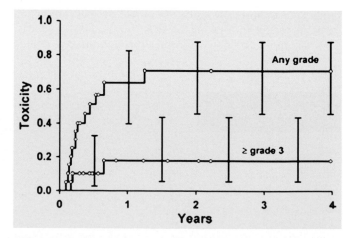

Figure 6.1. Comparison of tangential fields (**left**) with computed tomography scan at 2 months postradiotherapy for a 55-year-old female with history of RA, Sjogren syndrome, and stage IV primary biliary cirrhosis treated with adjuvant radiation therapy after breast-conserving surgery for invasive breast cancer (**right**). Nonanatomic distribution of consolidation is noted, corresponding to treated fields. Reprinted with permission from Hernandez S, et al. Severe acute toxicity from whole breast radiotherapy in the setting of collagen vascular disease. *Am J Clin Oncol.* 2006;29(6):647–648.

Figure 6.2. Rates of chronic toxicity in 20 patients with scleroderma treated with radiation. Reprinted with permission from Gold DG, et al. Radiotherapy for malignancy in patients with scleroderma: The Mayo Clinic experience. *Int J Radiat Oncol Biol Phys.* 2007;67(2):559–567.

follow-up for longer-term toxicities.[36] Due to their findings, the authors suggested that scleroderma may not be an absolute contraindication to radiotherapy.

In an attempt to minimize possible acute and late toxicities, Delanian et al.[37] treated three patients with scleroderma with deliberately reduced doses from 65 Gy to 40 to 45 Gy in 1.8-Gy fractions. Despite the dose reduction, treatment was complicated by fatal hemorrhagic alveolitis, compatible with underlying sclerodermal pulmonary involvement, femoral artery thrombosis, and skin necrosis. The authors concluded that a reduction in both the dose and the volume treated should be recommended to minimize potential for acute and longer-term complications. Some have postulated that a reduction in the dose per fraction may be more beneficial, since dose per fraction has been found to determine late radiation damage.[38]

Systemic Lupus Erythematosus

With regard to the diagnosis of SLE, the published results are controversial. Although some studies have suggested that SLE may confer an increased risk of acute and late toxicities,[10,13] subset analyses of CVD diagnosis have failed to identify increased rates of early and late complications associated with SLE.[11,12] There has even been the suggestion more recently that radiation therapy may be inappropriately withheld from patients with SLE.[19] Only one study to date has specifically addressed the potential complication rate in patients with SLE treated with radiotherapy. Pinn et al. retrospectively evaluated 21 patients with SLE treated with 34 courses of external beam radiotherapy (EBRT) and one low dose rate (LDR) prostate implant. With a median follow-up of 5.6 years, 21% developed grade 3+ acute toxicity. The 5- and 10-year actuarial rates of grade 3+ late toxicity were 28% and 40%, respectively. Univariate predictors of severe late toxicity were found to be absence of photosensitivity, absence of arthritis, and presence of a malar rash. The presence of a malar rash may simply be a surrogate for more severe SLE; however, the association of chronic toxicity with an absence of photosensitivity and arthritis was less interpretable. The authors thus concluded that the risk of acute and late toxicity in patients with SLE was moderate but should not deter clinicians from providing radiotherapy.[29] Despite these findings, however, many clinicians would likely still consider active lupus erythematosus an absolute or relative contraindication.[9]

Hypotheses of Pathophysiologic Mechanisms

Different mechanisms have been proposed to explain the observations of increased late toxicities in patients with CVD. Some have postulated that microvascular damage caused by radiation and CVD may be additive.[7] However, Ross et al.[10] in their study failed to show any increased risk of late toxicity in the presence of other concurrent vascular insults including diabetes, hypertension, or symptomatic atherosclerosis. Interference with normal tissue repair mechanisms has also been postulated to potentiate radiation-induced damages seen within the radiation portal fields.[39] In addition, it has been hypothesized that localized radiation may lead to damage of vascular endothelial cells. In turn, damage to endothelial cells is thought to expose the basement membrane and release possible antigenic factors systemically. The subsequent formation of autoantibodies against basement membrane and systemic antigens leads to inflammation of irradiated tissues. Cytokine

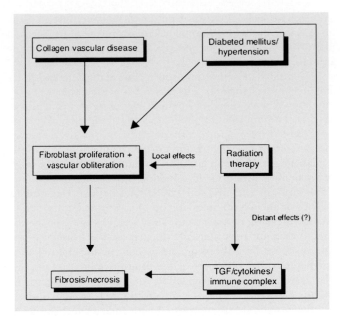

Figure 6.3. Potential mechanism for radiation-induced toxicity in collagen vascular disorder, diabetes mellitus, and hypertension. Reprinted with permission from Chon BH, Loeffler JS. The effect of nonmalignant systemic disease on tolerance to radiation therapy. *Oncologist.* 2002;7:136–143.

production and release are stimulated, which induce fibroblast proliferation, collagen synthesis, and ultimately fibrosis (Ref. 4, refer to Fig. 6.3). Recent in vitro studies supporting this hypothesis have shown increased production of transforming growth factor-beta (TGF-β) and macrophage-derived fibroblast growth factors in irradiated cell cultures.[40–43] The release of TGF-β can in turn lead to an increase in collagen gene transcription and, ultimately, tissue fibrosis.[44]

CONCLUSION

Although numerous case reports have been published to suggest an increased risk of acute and late toxicities in patients with CVD treated with radiation, the results from large retrospective series remain controversial. None of the four published matched controlled studies to date have shown a statistically significant increase in acute toxicities in this patient population.[11–13] In addition, only one of these matched controlled studies has been able to demonstrate a statistically significant increase in the risk of severe late complications in patients with CVD.[10] This statistical significance disappeared with subset analysis by disease in all patients but scleroderma.[10] In contrast, the largest published retrospective series by Morris and Powell[13] reported that non-RA patients, including patients with scleroderma and SLE, are at significantly increased risk for developing late toxicities.

Subset analyses of these trials, however, allow for general conclusions to be drawn regarding specific diagnoses. A majority of published studies have suggested that a diagnosis of scleroderma may increase the risk of developing both acute and late toxicities,[11–13] although perhaps not as much as previously anticipated.[36] Although there are limited data at this time, patients with RA are unlikely to be at significantly increased risk of acute or late radiation-induced complications.[13] Due to small number of cases, especially with subset analysis by disease, these prior studies have lacked statistical power to be conclusive. A large prospective, multi-institutional trial may provide more clarity in identifying patients at highest risk for radiation-induced acute and late toxicities.

It is important to interpret these clinical findings and translate them into changes in daily practice that will improve patient outcome. When evaluating a patient who presents with a history of CVD, it is important to obtain a complete rheumatologic history. Close involvement of a rheumatologist to actively manage the patient's disease before and during treatment may be useful to manage symptoms. In addition, initiation of NSAIDs or other cytotoxic therapies prior to initiation of treatment may confer a lower risk of late effects.[13] The effect of concurrent chemotherapy on the development of complications has not been well established, although a recent study suggests that concurrent chemoradiation may increase the risk of late complications. There should be a thorough discussion among the radiation oncologist, other members of the multidisciplinary team, and the patient with regard to possible increased risk of acute and late toxicities from radiation and alternative treatment options. All patients should be monitored with long-term follow-up to evaluate for late toxicity. Techniques to reduce the volume treated, total treatment dose, and daily dose fractionation scheme have been suggested to minimize these risks. Finally, treatment decisions should be made in conjunction with the patient and should be evaluated on an individual basis.

INFLAMMATORY BOWEL DISEASE

IBD is a family of gastrointestinal (GI) disorders marked by inflammation of the bowel, and most notably includes Crohn disease and ulcerative colitis. IBD typically presents with relapsing and remitting symptoms of abdominal pain, emesis, diarrhea, hematochezia, and weight loss. IBD has also been associated with extraintestinal and systemic manifestations including ankylosing spondylitis, pyoderma gangrenosum, and primary sclerosing cholangitis. Table 6.3 highlights the classic clinical and pathologic distinguishing characteristics of Crohn disease and ulcerative colitis.

Numerous studies have established the association between IBD and subsequent development of colorectal cancer. In 1925, Crohn and Rosenberg[45] documented the first case of colorectal cancer occurring in association with ulcerative colitis. By the 1960s, numerous studies reported the increased incidence of colorectal cancer among patients with Crohn disease.[46,47] More

recently published literature have estimated a 30-fold higher risk of colon cancer in patients with IBD compared to age- and sex-matched controls from the same population,[48] with estimated 5- and 20-year actuarial rates of developing colorectal cancer of 5% and 15%, respectively.[48,49]

In the 1980s, several small case series reported that abdominal or pelvic irradiation may exacerbate the symptoms of IBD and suggested that IBD be established as a relative contraindication to pelvic irradiation.[50–53] Schofield et al.[50] were the first to report severe exacerbations of IBD requiring surgical intervention in a patient treated with pelvic irradiation in the setting of ulcerative colitis. Subsequently, Hoffman et al.[51] reported requirement for treatment cessation due to exacerbation of IBD in a young female patient treated with cervical cancer. However, contrary to these findings, Tiersten and Saltz[52] found no severe acute complications among five patients with IBD treated with pelvic irradiation and usually with concurrent 5-fluorouracil for GI malignancies. These studies, however, have been criticized for small number of patients, each ranging from one to five patients.[50–53] The lack of long-term follow-up and specific details regarding radiation treatment delivery was also limitations of these studies.

Retrospective Studies of External Beam Radiotherapy

Radiation therapy has been established as an integral component to optimal multimodality care in numerous pelvic and GI malignancies. Several large randomized controlled trials have reported decreased locoregional recurrence and improved disease-free survival and overall survival in patients with locally advanced rectal carcinoma treated with preoperative and postoperative chemoradiation.[54–56] Additionally, definitive chemoradiation with concurrent cisplatin has now been established as standard of care for patients with locally advanced cervical cancer.[57,58] Despite the published benefit of radiation therapy in treatment of these malignancies, clinicians are often hesitant to administer pelvic irradiation in the setting of IBD due to concerns for increased acute and late toxicity and poor radiation tolerance.

In 1999, Green et al. sought to determine the effect and tolerance of pelvic irradiation among patients with IBD diagnosed with rectal cancer. They published the largest retrospective review to date of 47 patients (35 with Crohn disease, 12 with ulcerative colitis) with IBD and rectal cancer treated between 1960 and 1994 at Mount Sinai Hospital.[59] In total, 15 patients received pelvic irradiation as a component of their treatment including 2 patients treated with preoperative radiation therapy, 12 treated with postoperative chemoradiation, and 1 patient treated with definitive chemoradiation for unresectable disease. Patients were treated with conventional 2D plans to a median dose of 50.4 Gy (range: 5–55.8 Gy). After a median follow-up of 24 months, the authors reported an acute complication rate, deemed as Radiation Therapy Oncology Group (RTOG) grade 3 or higher toxicity, of 20% amongst patients receiving pelvic irradiation. Two patients developed grade 3 skin reactions, and one patient developed grade 4 GI toxicity, requiring a 4-week treatment break and a short hospitalization for management of dehydration. Two patients (13%) developed small bowel obstructions postirradiation; however, they resolved spontaneously with conservative management. Additionally, the authors reported no long-term complications within irradiated patients. By comparing toxicity rates in this series to historical controls,[55,56,60] the authors concluded that the complication

TABLE 6.3	Differences Between Crohn Disease and Ulcerative Colitis		
Clinical and Pathologic Features	Crohn Disease	Ulcerative Colitis
Involvement of upper GI	Yes	No
Hematochezia	No	Yes
Fistula formation and perianal disease	Common	No
Transmural inflammation	Yes	No
Granuloma formation	Yes	No
Fissures and skip lesions	Common	Rare
Distorted crypt architecture	Less common	Yes

rates among IBD patients compared favorably to the general population. Due to poor survival outcomes noted in high-risk groups, many of whom were not treated with radiation therapy, the authors argued that aggressive adjuvant therapy, including pelvic irradiation with or without chemotherapy, should be recommended to IBD-associated rectal cancer patients. Two main limitations of this study, however, include the small patient numbers treated with radiation therapy within this study and the comparison of results to historical controls.[59]

In 2000, Willett et al. published the largest study to date evaluating acute and late toxicity in patients with IBD treated with abdominal or pelvic irradiation at Massachusetts General Hospital. They identified 28 patients with IBD (10 with Crohn disease, 18 with ulcerative colitis) treated with abdominal or pelvic radiation from 1970 to 1999. All patients were treated with a curative intent with planned delivery of >40 Gy for diagnoses of various GI, genitourinary (GU), or gynecologic malignancies. The authors categorized patients as being treated with either specialized radiation treatment techniques ($n = 16$) including smaller radiation fields, treatment in the decubitus position, proton radiotherapy, or scheduled treatment breaks in an attempt to minimize radiation toxicity, or with more conventional approaches ($n = 12$).[53] With a follow-up of 32 months, the overall incidence of severe toxicity was 46%, including one grade 5 late complication. Twenty-one percent of patients required treatment cessation due to severe acute toxicity at doses ranging from 12.4 to 64.8 Gy. Additionally, after a mean follow-up of 12 months posttreatment, 29% (8/28) of patients required hospitalization or surgical intervention due to late toxicity. Although there was no difference in rates of severe acute toxicity by irradiation technique, the 5-year actuarial rate of late toxicity was statistically higher at 73% for patients treated by conventional approaches compared to 23% for patients treated by specialized treatment techniques ($p = 0.02$, Fig. 6.4). Acute toxicity did not appear to portend late toxicity, as only one patient with acute toxicity subsequently developed late toxicity (17%). Although a higher rate of late complications was observed in patients with ulcerative colitis compared to Crohn disease, these findings were confounded by higher rates of conventional radiation techniques in patients with ulcerative colitis.[53] Thus, contrary to findings by Green et al.,[59] the authors concluded that judicious use of radiation therapy should be employed. Due to its retrospective nature, however, this study is limited potentially by selection bias.[53]

Song et al.[61] similarly explored the incidence of GI complications in 24 patients with IBD treated with radiotherapy between 1979 and 1990 at Johns Hopkins University. Within this cohort, 15 patients were diagnosed with Crohn disease, 7 were diagnosed with ulcerative colitis, and 2 with IBD not otherwise specified. In contrast to prior studies that were site specific, this study included patients treated to a variety of sites including head and neck ($n = 2$), chest ($n = 8$), TBI ($n = 1$), and abdomen/pelvis ($n = 17$) with some patients treated to more than one site. Patients received a median dose of 45 Gy (range: 9–70.2 Gy) and 15 patients were treated with concurrent chemotherapy. All patients were treated with conventional techniques, although occasionally, more conservative blocking was employed. With a median follow-up of 11 months, 21% of patients experienced grade 3 or higher acute GI toxicity, all of whom received concurrent chemotherapy. Although most patients completed their planned course of radiation, one patient undergoing prostate irradiation developed severe radiation enteritis and IBD exacerbation at 28.8 Gy, ultimately requiring a diverting ileostomy. In addition, two patients (8%), both treated with pelvic irradiation for rectal cancer, reported grade 3 or higher late GI toxicity requiring surgical intervention for small bowel obstruction 6 months posttreatment. In the subset of patients treated with either abdominopelvic irradiation or total body irradiation, the crude rates of acute and late toxicity were 19% and 13%, respectively.[61] Similar to prior published studies, Song et al.[61] found that IBD diagnosis, prior history of IBD related surgeries, use of IBD medications at time of RT, and pretreatment status of IBD were not associated with an increased risk of acute or severe late toxicity. However, the authors suggested that concurrent chemotherapy potentially may exacerbate the risk of acute grade 3 or 4 complications, as all severe acute toxicity occurred in the setting of concurrent chemoradiation.[61]

One of the main limitations of all these studies is the difficulty in differentiating late morbidity secondary to radiation treatment from natural history of IBD itself. Surgical intervention has been reported up to 78% of Crohn disease patients within 20 years of diagnosis,[62] with a reoperation rate of 75% to 90% of patients for recurrent IBD.[62,63] Although postirradiation surgical intervention is often attributed to late toxicity radiation therapy, the natural progression of IBD is a potential confounder of these effects. Thus, the risk of acute and late complications attributable to radiation therapy may in fact be lower than published rates in existing literature. Table 6.4 summarizes the results found within the existing published literature regarding rate of acute and late toxicity in this subset of patients.

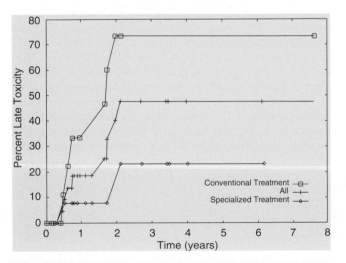

Figure 6.4. Actuarial rate of severe toxicity among patients with IBD undergoing EBRT for abdominal or pelvic malignancies stratified by radiation treatment method. Reprinted with permission from Willett CG, et al. Acute and late toxicity of patients with inflammatory bowel disease undergoing irradiation for abdominal and pelvic neoplasms. *Int J Radiat Oncol Biol Phys.* 2000;46(4):995–998.

Prostate Brachytherapy

To date, there has been only one published study evaluating the role of prostate brachytherapy in patients with IBD. Grann and Wallner[64] published their experience of six patients with IBD treated at MSKCC with prostate brachytherapy. Due to

TABLE 6.4		Summary of Existing Published Literature in Crohn Disease					
	Year	*n*	*Sites Irradiated*	*Radiation Modality*	*Follow-Up (months)*	*Acute Toxicity Rate*	*Late Toxicity Rate*
Willett et al.[53]	2000	28	Pelvis	EBRT	32	21%	29%
Green et al.[59]	1999	15	Pelvis	EBRT	24	20%	13%
Song et al.[61]	2001	24	Various	EBRT	11	21%	8%
Grann and Wallner[64]	1998	6	Prostate	Brachytherapy	42	0%	0%

concerns for potential increased toxicity with external beam radiotherapy, prostate cancer patients within their institution had been generally advised to undergo brachytherapy as an alternative, in order to decrease the amount of rectal surface area receiving radiation. Treatment plans were designed to treat the preimplant prostatic margin to a dose of 150 Gy, without special considerations for minimizing rectal surface dose. With a median follow-up of 3.7 years, none of the patients experienced significant acute or late GI complications following implantation. Two patients developed mild rectal urgency and mild hematochezia that resolved spontaneously. Thus, the authors concluded that prostate brachytherapy is safe for patients with a history of IBD.[64]

Hypotheses of Pathophysiologic Mechanisms

Although the exact pathophysiologic cause of IBD has not been fully elucidated, dysregulation of the immune response has long been implicated as part of the pathogenesis of this disease entity. One theory is that IBD may result from an abnormal mucosal immune system, or specific defects in cellular or humoral immunity, which is directed against typical luminal bacteria.[65] A second theory is that IBD may result from an appropriate immune response to normal intestinal organisms that typically do not elicit a response due to alterations within the mucosal barrier function.[65] Histologically, Crohn disease has been characterized by transmural nodular lymphoid aggregates, proliferative changes within the muscularis mucosa, endothelial edema, and excess collagen deposition that all contribute to development of transmural fibrosis. In contrast, although there is typically less fibrosis noted in ulcerative colitis, chronic perivascular inflammatory infiltrate within the mucosa and submucosa can be quite appreciable.

The potential mechanism by which radiation therapy is thought to exacerbate IBD is similar to those described for CVD. Preexisting free radicals from chronic states of inflammation have been proposed to increase the effects of radiation.[66] Additionally, it has been hypothesized that patients with chronic ulcerative colitis may have deficient DNA repair mechanism, thereby increasing the sensitivity to radiation and chemotherapy.[67] Moreover, it has been hypothesized that patients with IBD may also be at increased risk of late radiation-induced toxicity due to prior histories of abdominal or pelvic surgeries, due to increased volume of small bowel falling into the treatment field postoperatively.[61]

CONCLUSION

Prior to initiating radiation treatment, a firm understanding of sites of IBD involvement and current state of IBD activity

should be obtained. For those patients in whom radiation therapy is deemed appropriate, radiation therapy techniques should be employed, when possible, to maximally spare normal tissues.[53] In addition, for patients undergoing surgery, placement of surgical clips for precise tumor localization and surgical mesh placement for bowel mobilization out of the radiation field should be considered. Many recent concurrent chemoradiation protocols have demonstrated increased local control and/or survival at the cost of increased toxicity.[55–58] In this subset of patients, the use of concurrent chemotherapy should be considered judiciously when appropriate, as it has been associated with a significant increase in the rates of acute complications. Due to the limitations of the currently available reports, however, further studies would be helpful to validate findings in the current existing literature and to further draw a distinction between radiation-related toxicities and the natural course of IBD.

MULTIPLE SCLEROSIS

MS is an inflammatory autoimmune disorder that targets the central nervous system. Although the exact mechanisms are not entirely understood, MS is thought to be mediated by autoreactive T-cells directed against components of myelin, altered cellular function, and even cell death.[68,69] Patients with MS can present with a myriad of neurologic symptoms including paresthesia of the limb and face, visual loss, subacute motor degeneration, diplopia, gait disturbance, and vertigo. Clinical neurologic deficits are attributed to loss of nerve insulation from compact myelin, diminished efficacy of nerve conduction, and axonal degeneration. MS is characterized by a chronic inflammatory state with a relapsing and remitting course in 80% of patients. This eventually leads to plaque formation within the central nervous system, and subsequent worsening neurologic functional status.[70] The theory of an underlying autoimmune disorder as the primary etiology of MS is supported by numerous studies that have suggested an increased incidence of other autoimmune disorders among these patients, including autoimmune thyroid disease, type I diabetes mellitus, and IBD in these patients.[71–74]

External Beam Radiotherapy: Potential Cause of MS Exacerbation?

In the early 1900s, fractionated EBRT was hypothesized to be a potentially effective treatment for MS.[75] However, in 1959, Lampert et al.[76] published the first case series documenting significant, potentially fatal neurotoxicity complications, in patients with MS treated with EBRT to the brain due to accelerated demyelination. McMeekin et al.[77] subsequently published

TABLE 6.5		Summary of Retrospective Case Series of EBRT Toxicity Among Patients with MS			
Series	Year	Number of Cases	Tumor Location	RT Dose (Gy)	Time to Symptoms (months)
Lampert et al.[76]	1959	1/1	EAC[a]	57.5	2
McMeekin et al.[77]	1969	1/1	Base of skull and EAC	53.5	2
Nahser et al.[79]	1986	1/2	Frontal lobe	60	8
Peterson et al.[80]	1993	4/5	Frontal and parietal lobes	40–60	0.1–24
Murphy et al.[78]	2003	1/1	Parotid gland	50	1
Pakos et al.[81]	2005	1/1	Frontal lobes	60	2

[a]EAC, external auditory canal.

a case report of a patient with autopsy-confirmed demyelinating plaques located in the prior radiation field within the brainstem and cerebellar white matter, which were felt to be temporally related to radiation treatment. More recently, in 2003, Murphy et al. reported acute clinical and radiographic exacerbation of MS symptoms in a patient treated with parotid irradiation for adenoid cystic carcinoma. Posttreatment magnetic resonance imaging (MRI) demonstrated new hyperintense lesions in the cerebellum, corresponding to the localization of the patient's symptoms and the region defined by the 50% isodose line.[78] Numerous other studies have published findings supporting an increased incidence of neurotoxicity in MS patients treated with external beam radiation.[78–81] Table 6.5 summarizes published literature regarding demyelinating injury after fractionated EBRT in patients with MS.

Not all studies, however, have demonstrated MS exacerbations and increased risk of treatment-related neurotoxicity among MS patients treated with external beam radiotherapy. Contrary to prior case reports, in 1980, Tourtellotte et al.[82] reported that a review of published literature demonstrated no evidence of MS exacerbation among 344 patients treated with CNS irradiation from 1903 to 1970. Nevertheless, radiation oncologists are often hesitant to treat patients with MS with EBRT to the brain due to concerns of fatal or disabling neurotoxicity.[76]

In 2006, Miller et al. published the largest modern retrospective study accessing the incidence of neurotoxicity among patients with MS treated with external beam radiotherapy. Between 1976 and 2004, the authors identified 15 consecutively treated patients with MS who were treated with external beam radiotherapy to the brain at the Mayo Clinic. The majority of the patients carried diagnoses of primary brain tumors (60%), with a minority of patients treated for brain metastases. Due to clinical ambiguity in defining MS, patients with probable or possible diagnosis of MS were excluded from the analysis. Using the Common Terminology Criteria for Adverse Effects (CTC) v.3.0, a team of radiation oncologists and neurologists defined toxicity as the appearance of neurologic symptoms that were attributable to lesions within the irradiated field. Clinical and radiographic evaluation was performed to exclude the presence of tumor progression as a possible explanation to the onset of symptoms. With a median follow-up of 6.0 years, although no severe acute MS exacerbations were reported during treatment, six patients experienced grade 4 or greater neurotoxicity with a median of 1.0 year (range: 0.2–4.3 years). Actuarial 1- and 5-year rate of grade 4 neurologic toxicity reported to be 25% and 57%, respectively, after radiation therapy. Neurotoxicity

was noted to develop at a median dose of 50 Gy, with a range of 37.5 to 54 Gy. On univariate analysis, opposed field irradiation encompassing the temporal lobes, central white matter, and brainstem was found to be associated with an increased risk of neurotoxicity ($p < 0.04$). Thus, the authors concluded that patients with MS may be at higher risk of neurotoxicity after radiotherapy to the brain compared to normal controls.[83]

Determining the risk of neurotoxicity after EBRT to the brain is extremely difficult and is subject to numerous limitations. Limited statistical power from small case series, difficulty in defining MS as a clinical entity, and competing causes of neurological decline in these patients are all significant limitations in these studies. Moreover, the vast majority of patients were treated in the era before routine use of MRI. Thus, the detection of tumor recurrence or tumor progression that may have contributed to neurological progression may have been missed by less sensitive forms of imaging. Lastly, these studies are all limited by their retrospective nature and outdated radiation techniques and dose fractionation schema. Even in the most recent study by Miller et al.,[83] only half of the patients were treated after 1986. Consequently, these studies do not adequately address the risk of modern radiotherapy and, in particular, the risk of intracranial stereotactic fractionated radiotherapy and radiosurgery, which may reduce the amount of white matter receiving radiation dose, in patients in MS. Some studies, discussed in a later section, however seem to suggest that radiosurgery may be safe and effective in patients with MS.[84] Prospective data, however, are extremely difficult to obtain due to the low prevalence of MS among those treated with radiation therapy.

Hypothesis of Pathophysiologic Mechanisms

The mechanism by which radiation therapy is thought to potentially exacerbate demyelination and neurologic decline in patients with MS is not well elucidated. Some have hypothesized that radiation may have an effect on oligodendrocytes/type 2 astrocytes and their progenitor cells. Others have suggested that radiation may alter the cytokine environment, vasculature, and potentially disrupt the blood-brain barrier within the irradiated fields, leading to further injury.[85–87] More recently, Miller et al.[83] have suggested that MS patients may lack the ability of normal patients to repair radiation-induced demyelination of the CNS and other early delayed effects of radiation toxicity. Further studies will hopefully help elucidate the pathophysiologic mechanisms that may account for these clinical findings.

The Role of Radiosurgery for Multiple Sclerosis Tremor

Radiosurgical treatment of tremors for different movement disorders has been performed for more than 25 years. Numerous studies have reported successful tremor control with stereotactic surgery among patients diagnosed with a myriad of movement disorders, including Parkinson disease and essential tremor. Due to success in these movement disorders, palliation of MS tremor has been attempted more recently through neurosurgical intervention. Tremor is estimated to occur in approximately 25% of patients with MS and can be severely disabling in 6%.[88] Numerous medical therapies have been proposed, but often with disappointing results.[89] Additionally, invasive surgical procedures including stereotactic thalamotomy and thalamic deep brain stimulation have been found to offer clinical improvements, but often only temporarily.[89] As a result, several other recent studies have evaluated the efficacy of radiosurgical thalamotomy among patients with tremors refractory to medical intervention.[84]

Mathieu et al.[84] from the University of Pittsburgh recently published their experience of six patients with disabling MS tremors treated with Gamma Knife thalamotomy. All patients had medically refractory intention tremors with a median duration of 3 years. With a median follow-up of 27.5 months, the authors noted clinical improvement in tremor among all patients after a median latency period of 2.5 months. Four of six patients were noted by caregivers to demonstrate an improvement in their functional status, with the most significant improvement noted in the degree of tremor amplitude. Posttreatment, one patient developed transient contralateral hemiparesis that improved with steroids. In contrast to prior studies suggesting the potential of increased neurotoxicity in patients with MS treated with external beam radiotherapy, it has been postulated that due to smaller radiation field sizes and more rapid dose fall-off with radiosurgery, neurological treatment-related complications may be less.[84]

CONCLUSION

The effect of radiotherapy in patients with MS is currently controversial. Although several small retrospective case series have suggested that these patients may be at increased risk of neurotoxicity after fractionated EBRT to the brain,[76–80,83] these findings have not been consistently noted in published literature.[82] In many clinical scenarios, however, brain radiotherapy can be an important, if not integral, component of multidisciplinary care provided to these patients. In the setting of MS, the decision should be made on an individual case basis and the potential benefits and risks of radiotherapy should be carefully considered. Additionally, more recent literature may suggest a potential role for radiosurgery as treatment for refractory tremors and trigeminal neuralgia in patients with MS.[84] However, due to limited clinical experience with radiosurgical intervention in these patients, this is predominantly used only among patients with medically refractory and debilitating symptoms. Additional follow-up may help shed light on long-term efficacy and complications of these treatments.

HIV INFECTION

Since the discovery of HIV and AIDS in 1985,[90] more than 1 million people in the United States are estimated to be infected with HIV.[91] Patients with HIV infection have been found to be at increased risk for numerous malignancies.[92,93] A recent meta-analysis suggested that among HIV-infected patients, immunodeficiency may play a role in conferring a higher risk of infection-related malignancies.[94] Compared to the general population, Melbye and colleagues found that HIV-infected patients possess a 40- to 80-fold increased risk for developing HPV-related anal cancer.[95,96]

With the introduction of highly active antiretroviral therapy (HAART), an increase in CD4 counts and survival prolongation has been noted. With improving survival rates among HIV-infected patients treated with antiretroviral agents, prevention, effective treatment, and maintenance of treatment tolerability of HIV-related malignancies have become an increasingly important issue.

HIV Infection and Tolerance to Radiation Therapy

Numerous recent studies have emerged evaluating the tolerance of HIV patients to cancer-related treatments. The tolerance of HIV-patients to radiation therapy has been investigated in numerous different malignancies[97,98] but has been most thoroughly evaluated in the setting of anal cancer.[99–102] Standard treatment for squamous cell carcinoma of the anus in the general population has consisted of definitive concurrent chemoradiation, frequently with 5-fluorouracil and mitomycin C.[103–106] In the late 1980s, however, several published case series suggested that HIV-infected patients may experience increased treatment-related acute toxicities, either from radiation therapy administered alone or with concurrent chemotherapy.[97,98,107,108] Inherent cellular radiosensitivity[109] and glutathione deficiency[110] were proposed as possible explanations for increased radiosensitivity among AIDS patients. Among HIV-infected patients treated for anal carcinoma, numerous studies reported an increased requirement for treatment break, hospitalization, and chemotherapy dose reduction.[58,107] One study by Kim et al.[111] evaluated outcomes and toxicities among 13 HIV-positive patients treated with definitive chemoradiation and found a significantly higher rate of major acute treatment toxicity among HIV-positive patients (80% vs. 30%, $p < 0.005$). More recently in 2006, Edelman and Johnstone retrospectively reviewed 17 HIV-positive patients treated with definitive chemoradiation to a median dose of 54 Gy, and all but one patient received concurrent 5-FU and mitomycin C. With a median follow-up of 25.6 months, 47% and 56% of patients developed grade 3 acute dermatologic and hematologic toxicity, respectively.[100] Compared to historical controls, these rates were found to be greater than previously reported among the general population in randomized controlled trials.[105,112,113] The authors reported, however, no acute or late complications were documented in the only patient treated with concurrent 5-FU and cisplatin. The authors thus concluded that standard chemoradiation regimens yield significant acute complications.[100]

In 2008, Oehler-Janne published a multicentric cohort comparison of 40 HIV-positive patients with HAART and 81 HIV-negative patients treated with definitive chemoradiation for anal carcinoma. The authors found although there was no difference in median total radiation dose received, radiation therapy duration was significantly longer in HIV-positive patients. Additionally, HIV-positive patients were statistically less likely to receive inguinal irradiation or a brachytherapy boost than HIV-negative patients. Although there was no statistical difference in compliance with prescribed chemotherapeutic regimens, HIV patients were less likely to be prescribed mitomycin C compared to HIV-positive patients. Overall, 50% of HIV-positive patients developed grade 3+ toxicities, with HIV-infected patients more likely to develop grade 3+ dermatologic (35% vs. 17%, $p = 0.04$) and hematologic toxicities (33% vs. 12%, $p = 0.08$) compared to the HIV-negative cohort. The authors thus concluded that acute toxicity continues to represent a major clinical challenge in treatment of these patients.[114]

Despite these findings, numerous other published series have suggested that standard combined modality therapy may be safely provided.[115,116] Cleator et al. reported on 12 HIV-infected patients treated with definitive radiation therapy administered with concurrent 5-FU and mitomycin C. In this series, Cleator et al. modified standard treatment regimens by administering a single dose of mitomycin C, and requiring a 4 to 6 week break prior to a perineal boost. Although a majority of patients experienced some mild degree of toxicity, the overall rates of grade 3+ hematologic, dermatologic, and GI toxicity were 25%, 8%, and 17%, respectively, which were comparable to historical controls. Due to the acceptable tolerability of HIV-positive patients in their series, the authors recommended that HIV-positive patients should be treated with standard combined modality therapy regimens.[115]

Additionally, Chiao et al. published a large retrospective cohort study evaluating 1,184 patients (1,009 HIV negative, 175 HIV positive) diagnosed with squamous cell carcinoma of the anus between 1998 and 2004. In this study, the authors found that HIV-positive individuals were as likely as HIV-negative patients to receive treatment, and both groups had similar 2-year survival rates. As a result, the authors concluded that treatment should not be withheld or deintensified based on HIV status. However, this study had numerous limitations including the inability to evaluate specific treatment modalities (i.e., chemotherapy agent provided, radiation dose delivered) and lack of treatment-related toxicity data.[116]

Due to concerns for higher complication rates among HIV-positive patients, numerous treatment alterations have been suggested, including use of cisplatin instead of mitomycin C, use of lower radiation doses, smaller radiation treatment fields, and use of IMRT.[99,100,117] Cisplatin-based regimens have resulted in lower treatment-related acute hematologic complication rates compared to mitomycin C.[100-102] Thus, some studies have suggested that for these patients, cisplatin may be a more

tolerable, and thus, appropriate choice.[102] However, a recently published RTOG randomized controlled trial comparing concurrent chemoradiation with 5-FU/mitomycin to 5-FU/cisplatin found that cisplatin-based therapy resulted in a significantly higher colostomy rate within the general population. The results of this trial suggest that cisplatin-based regimens may yield inferior clinical outcomes to mitomycin-based regimens. With these new findings, cisplatin-based regimens should be avoided in the general population and should be considered only in patients in whom mitomycin C would not be tolerable.[106]

Due to concerns for radiation-related treatment toxicities, Peddada et al.[99] evaluated acute and late toxicities among HIV-positive patients treated to a lower radiation dose of 30 Gy and reported acceptable toxicity. However, a recent study of concurrent chemoradiation with cisplatin-based chemotherapy and high dose radiation to 60 to 70 Gy was well tolerated with acute grade 3+ dermatologic and GI complication rates of 44% and 0%, respectively. These findings suggest that lowering radiation dose in order to minimize treatment-related toxicities may not be necessary.[101]

Additionally, newer 3D-treatment planning and newer radiation treatment techniques, including 3D conformal RT and IMRT, may potentially minimize radiation toxicity by dose sparing while maximizing target volume dose to involved areas. A recent study by Salama et al. demonstrated the patient tolerability of IMRT in conjunction with concurrent chemotherapy for anal carcinoma. In this multicenter trial, 53 patients, including 8 HIV-positive patients, received IMRT and concurrent chemotherapy. Grade 3 or higher dermatologic and GI acute toxicities were noted in 38% and 17% of patients, respectively, with 42% of patients requiring a treatment break.[117] The Radiation Therapy Oncology Group is currently running a multi-institutional phase II trial to confirm these results. Table 6.6 summarizes treatment-related acute toxicities reported by selected published case series.

The Effect of CD4 Count on Treatment Tolerance

The relationship of CD4 count and treatment tolerance has been addressed in several small observational studies. Hoffman et al. evaluated the significance of pretreatment CD4 count on treatment tolerance among 17 HIV-positive patients diagnosed with anal carcinoma. All patients were treated with curative intent, either receiving definitive chemoradiation

TABLE 6.6		**Summary of Selected Case Series of Acute Treatment-Related Toxicities Among HIV-Positive Patients with Anal Carcinoma**				
				Grade 3+ Acute Complication Rates (%)		
Series	*No.*	*RT Dose*	*Chemotherapy*	*Hematologic (%)*	*Dermatologic (%)*	*GI (%)*
Edelman and Johnstone[100]	17	50.4–60.4	5-FU + MMC	56	47	24
Cleator et al.[115]	12	38–51	5-FU + MMC	25	8	17
Blazy et al.[102]	9	60–70	5-FU + Cis	44	44	0
Kim et al.[111]	13	50–54	5-FU + MMC	23	38	23
Chadha et al.[195]	9	50	5-FU + MMC	22	78	0
Oehler-Janne et al.[114]	40	52–60	Varied	33	35	10
Peddada et al.[99]	8	30	5-FU + MMC	38	50	13
Wexler et al.[102]	32	45–61	5-FU + MMC	69	25	28

MMC, mitomycin C.

(n = 16) or radiation therapy alone (n = 1). Patients were categorized by CD4 counts as patients with CD4 counts ≤200 (n = 8) or patients with CD4 counts ≥200 (n = 9). With a median follow-up of 17 months, among patients with CD4 counts ≤200, 88% developed severe treatment-related toxicities including moist desquamation (n = 5) and neutropenia (n = 2), requiring treatment breaks of 1 to 4 weeks. Additionally, 25% required early termination of radiation treatment and 50% required hospitalization for treatment-related complications. In contrast, among patients with CD4 counts ≥200, 44% of patients required a 2-week treatment break secondary to moist desquamation; however, none required hospitalization. As a result, the authors concluded that patients with CD4 count ≤200 had markedly increased likelihood of developing treatment-related morbidity and, thus, should be treated cautiously.[118] Place et al.[119] subsequently published a series of 14 HIV-positive patients supporting an increased toxicity among patients treated with CD4 counts ≤200. Numerous other studies, however, have not identified CD4 count as a significant predictive factor in determination of acute or late toxicity.[100,101]

CONCLUSION

Combined modality therapy in the treatment of squamous cell carcinoma of the anus among HIV-positive patients has been generally effective and tolerable. When possible, HIV-positive patients should be treated similar to the general population; however, individual treatment decisions should be made on a case-by-case basis, taking into account CD4 count, performance status, and HAART therapy use. All HIV-positive patients should be followed closely with an HIV infectious disease specialist throughout the duration of their oncologic treatment. Additionally, HIV-positive patients should be evaluated for and placed on HAART therapy if appropriate. Although some studies have previously suggested that HIV-positive patients may experience greater acute treatment-related toxicity, several studies have suggested that treatment-related toxicities may be greatest among patients with CD4 counts ≤200.[118] Dose reduction in chemotherapeutic regimens, consideration of chemotherapeutic alternatives to mitomycin C, and use of radiation alone can be considered in patients with active HIV/AIDS-related complications or with a history of opportunistic infections. Emerging radiation techniques in the treatment of anal carcinoma, including IMRT, may help further reduce dermatologic and GI treatment complications. Additional prospective studies and phase III trials will be needed to test new treatment strategies in HIV-infected patients with squamous cell cancer of the anus.

DIABETES AND HYPERTENSION

Diabetes mellitus is a growing epidemic within the United States, now afflicting more than 17 million people.[120] Chronic diabetes can lead to multiorgan complications, many of which stem from microvascular occlusive changes resulting in arteriolar obliteration, capillary obliteration, and atherosclerosis.[121,122] These changes can ultimately lead to decreased tissue perfusion, which in the setting of wound healing may inhibit normal tissue repair. As a clinical consequence of these pathophysiologic changes, numerous surgical series have reported increased wound complications among diabetic patients.[122,123] It has been proposed that diabetics may similarly experience impairments in normal tissue damage repair after radiation therapy.[124]

To date, there is little published literature regarding the effect of diabetes and hypertension on subsequent risk for radiation-induced normal tissue damage. In the 1970s, Maruyama et al. first addressed the potential correlation of diabetes status and radiation-induced toxicity. They retrospectively reviewed 271 patients treated at the University of Kentucky treated with radiotherapy for cervical cancer. Of nine patients who developed small bowel obstructions, seven patients (78%) were diabetic and three patients (34%) had concomitant diagnoses of hypertension. As a result, the authors concluded that diabetes predisposed cervical cancer patients treated with radiotherapy to developing small bowel obstructions.[125] In a follow-up study from the University of Kentucky, Van Nagell et al. demonstrated higher rates of severe bladder and rectal injuries among diabetic patients treated with radiotherapy for cervical cancer compared to the general population ($p < 0.002$). Of six patients who developed fistulas in the absence of local recurrence, all had preexisting diabetes and hypertension. In addition, among 15 pathologic specimens obtained from patients treated with surgery alone, patients with diabetes or hypertension were noted to have significant arteriolar narrowing in rectal or bladder vessels. Based on these findings, the authors argued that preexisting diabetes and hypertension may predispose patients to developing radiation-related treatment toxicity due to underlying microvascular disease.[121]

Subsequently, Harwood and Tierie published a series evaluating the effect of diabetes and hypertension on radiation normal tissue toxicity among 204 glottic cancer patients treated with definitive radiation. A preexisting condition of diabetes and/or hypertension was found to significantly increase the risk of subsequent development of late complications including laryngeal edema requiring tracheotomy, laryngeal stenosis, or laryngeal necrosis. The risk of major late complications was 67% among diabetic, hypertensive patients compared to 5% in control patients ($p = 0.01$). Likewise, the risk of major complications was 30% among diabetics compared to 6% in control patients ($p = 0.024$). These findings support prior studies that suggest increased radiotoxicity among patients with diabetes and hypertension.[126]

More recently, Herold et al. sought to determine whether diabetes mellitus was independently predictive of late radiation toxicity among prostate cancer patients treated with external beam radiotherapy. They identified 944 prostate cancer patients, including 121 patients with either type I or type II diabetes, treated at Fox Chase Cancer Center between 1989 and 1996 with 3D-CRT to a median dose of 72 Gy. With a median follow-up of 36 months, the rates of acute morbidity did not differ between diabetics and nondiabetics. However, diabetic patients were found to have a significantly higher rate of late grade 2 GI toxicities (27% vs. 17%, $p = 0.011$) and late grade 2 GU toxicities (14% vs. 6%, $p = 0.001$). Additionally, there was a trend toward increased late grade 3 and 4 GI complications among diabetic patients, but not grade 3 and 4 GU toxicities. Diabetics were also found to develop late GU complications significantly earlier than nondiabetics (median: 10 months vs. 24 months, $p = 0.02$). On multivariate regression, radiation dose, rectal blocking, diabetic status were all independently predictive of late grade 2 GI complications. However, in predicting grade 2 GU toxicity, only diabetic status remained independently significant. Thus, the authors concluded that diabetes status is a strong predictor of late GI and GU complications and may predict for earlier development of complications.[124] Similarly, Debus et al.[127] found that diabetes status was independently predictive of brainstem toxicity among 367 patients with chondromas and chondrosarcomas of the base of skull. Despite these findings, diabetes and hypertension have not been found to independent predictors of radiation toxicity in other published retrospective series.[128,129]

CONCLUSION

These studies suggest that preexisting comorbidities of diabetes mellitus and hypertension may potentiate development of late toxicity; however, due to the retrospective nature and limited power of these studies, it is difficult to draw any firm conclusions. With further investigation, we will hopefully gain a better understanding of the complex interplay between diabetes and normal tissue repair.

HEREDITARY SYNDROMES THAT IMPACT RADIOSENSITIVITY

The recognition and repair of DNA damage is an extremely complex process that involves an intricate interplay of numerous genes and their products.[38] During the last decade, an increasing number of published reports have suggested that individual genetic variations, which can alter the function of large multiprotein complexes responsible for detection of DNA damage, may impact radiosensitivity.[130–134] The identification of candidate radiosensitivity genes and the determination of their role in development of adverse radiation response are an active area of ongoing investigation.[133] Table 6.7 provides a summary of potential radiosensitivity disorders and their associated candidate genes. Several hereditary syndromes, including ataxia-telangiectasia (AT) and Fanconi anemia (FA), have emerged as syndromes that may affect radiosensitivity. Current efforts are now underway to develop predictive tests to determine an individual's risk for adverse radiation response, based on the possession of these specific genetic variants.[133]

Ataxia-Telangiectasia

AT is a rare autosomal recessive disorder with an estimated incidence of 1 in 20,000 to 100,000 live births.[135,136] Clinical symptoms associated with homozygous AT include progressive cerebellar ataxia, abnormal eye movement, and ocular telangiectaias.[137] Additionally, patients with AT have been found to be at increased risk for immunodeficiency, malignancy, radiation sensitivity, and diabetes mellitus.[138–141] AT patients have a poor prognosis with a median life expectancy of 25 years.[142,143] Currently, there is no specific treatment for the multiorgan effects of AT, with progressive pulmonary disease and cancer among the leading causes of mortality.[142,143] Heterozygous carriers of an ATM gene variant have a higher prevalence in the United States and may be present in up to 2.0% of Caucasians.[135,136] Heterozygous carriers of ATM gene variants do not typically express the classic clinical symptoms of AT.

The ATM gene, the defective gene in AT, has been mapped to chromosome 11q22.3 and is expressed in all tissues of the body.[144,145] ATM is part of a signaling cascade involved in detection of DNA double-strand breaks and cell-cycle checkpoint control.[146–150] The ATM gene product has been found to function as a protein kinase that phosphorylates serine or threonine in target proteins.[150,151] Many ATM substrates are cell-cycle regulators that are integral to normal cellular response

TABLE 6.7	Summary of Potential Radiosensitivity-Associated Disorders

Radiosensitivity-Associated Disorders

Syndrome	Gene	Localization
ADA-deficient SCID	ADA	20q13.11
AT	ATM	11q22.3–23.1
Breast cancer	BRCA2	13q12.3
Breast/ovarian cancer	BRCA1	17q21
DNA-PK deficiency	DNA-PKc	8q11
Fanconi A	FANCA	16q24.3
Fanconi B	FANCB	?
Fanconi C	FANCC	9q22.3
Fanconi D	FANCD	3p26–p22
Fanconi G (XRCC9)	FANCG	9p13
Ku70	KU70	22q13
Ku86 (XRCC5)	KU86	2q33–q35
Leukemia predisposition	Ligase IV	13q33–q34
CHK1 deficiency	CHK1	11q22–q24
Li-Fraumeni syndrome	CHK2	22q12.1
MRE11 deficiency (ATLD)	MRE11	11q21
Multiple endocrine neoplasia II	MEN2	10q21.1
NBS	NBS1	8q21
Rad50	RAD50	5q31
X-linked agammaglobulinemia	BTK	X21.3
XRCC4	XRCC4	5q13

Source: Gatti RA, et al. Localization of an ataxia-telangiectasia gene to chromosome 11q22–23. *Nature.* 1988;336(6199):577–580.

to DNA damage, including p53, breast-cancer-associated 1 (BRCA1), p53-binding protein (53BP1), and checkpoint kinase CHK2.[152] In the presence of DNA damage, the ATM kinase stalls the progression of the cell cycle by phosphorylating p53, a tumor suppressor gene.[145,146,149] In the absence of a functional ATM kinase, cells with DNA damage continue to cycle and may pass on DNA aberrations to their daughter cells. Over 60% to 70% of homozygous AT patients carry truncating mutations and thus produce no detectable ATM kinase.[153] In contrast, heterozygotes often carry a missense mutation of the ATM gene that exerts a dominant negative effect, resulting in disruption of normal protein function.[154] As a result, cells derived from heterozygous ATM gene mutation carriers often exhibit a radiosensitivity response between patients with homozygous ATM mutations and the general population.[155–159] With the accumulation of somatic mutations over time, these cells may undergo malignant transformation. Due to these processes, patients with AT have been found to be at higher risk of developing breast cancer and other malignancies.[136,143,160,161] Overall, 10% to 20% of patients with AT are predicted to be diagnosed with a malignancy, with majority of patients being diagnosed with leukemia or lymphoma.[140,143] Heterozygous carriers of ATM gene variants are more likely to develop solid tumors, with the most significant relative risks observed for female breast cancer.[135,136,140,160–163]

The ATM gene was first hypothesized to confer increased radiosensitivity more than 40 years ago, when AT patients were reported to experience significant radiation-related toxicity.[141,164] Several studies investigating ATM on the cellular level have confirmed enhanced radiosensitivity in cells from patients with heterozygous AT mutations.[165,166] Moreover, cells derived from patients with the heterozygous mutation for the ATM mutation exhibited a degree of radiosensitivity in between patients who carry the homozygous mutation and patients without the mutation.[155–159] However, subsequent studies failed to demonstrate a positive correlation between the presence of ATM mutation and greater normal tissue damage among breast cancer patients.[167–169] These initial studies were limited by use of protein truncation assays to detect ATM mutations. More recent studies have employed other techniques, including denaturing high-performance liquid chromatography to detect missense mutations, which are more prevalent among heterozygous carriers and cancer patients.[170,171]

Even more recently, possession of ATM genetic DNA variants has been found to possibly predict potential clinical adverse response to radiation therapy.[131,172–174] To date, several studies have attempted to determine the predictive value of ATM gene mutations to risk to development of adverse late radiation complications.[173–175] In 2002, Iannuzzi et al. screened 46 patients treated with breast-conserving surgery and adjuvant radiation therapy for sequence alterations in the ATM gene. By retrospectively evaluating acute and late radiation toxicity by RTOG criteria, the authors were able to compare rates of late toxicity among patients found with and without ATM sequence alterations. In their initial series, they identified nine ATM mutations in six patients. With a median follow-up of 3.2 years, the presence of an ATM mutation was found to predict for increased rate of grade 3 and 4 late subcutaneous toxicity ($p = 0.001$), but not acute toxicity ($p = 0.7$). All three of the patients who manifested grade 3 and 4 subcutaneous late toxicity possessed an ATM gene variant. In contrast, among the 43 patients without severe grade 3 and 4 late toxicity, only 3 (7%) of patients possessed an ATM gene variant. Thus, the authors concluded that possession of an ATM mutation may predict for an increase in subcutaneous late tissue toxicity after breast irradiation.[173]

Subsequently, Ho et al. screened 131 patients treated with breast-conserving surgery and adjuvant radiation therapy for sequence alterations in the ATM gene. Of the 131 screened patients, 51 patients were identified with 30 different ATM sequence alterations. Among patients with ATM sequence alterations, the rate of grade II toxicity was significantly higher at 41% compared to 23% among patients without ATM sequence alterations (OR: 2.4, 95% CI: 1.1–5.2). Additionally, the authors identified the particular G→A single nucleotide polymorphism at nucleotide 5557, which was found to predict for a statistically higher rates for grade II to IV late toxicity compared to patients without the mutation (53% vs. 27%, OR: 3.1). Thus, the authors concluded that sequence variants located in the ATM gene, in particular the 5557 G→A polymorphism, may predict for late adverse radiation responses in breast cancer patients.[175] These findings were recently confirmed by Andreassen et al.[134] who reported increased radiosensitivity among Danish breast cancer patients found with homozygous and heterozygous (AG) genotypes of the ATM 5557 G→A variant. A subsequent independent cohort of Danish breast cancer patients, however, failed to validate these findings.[172]

Cesaretti et al. demonstrated a positive correlation between the presence of a specific ATM codon 1853 polymorphism and the increased risk of developing radiation-induced proctitis after radiotherapy. Rectal bleeding was found to occur in 4 of 13 patients (31%) with an ATM variant compared to 1 of 23 (4%) without a genetic alteration among patients who had <0.7 cm³ of rectal tissue receiving the implant prescription dose ($p = 0.05$). This relationship persisted among patients with larger volumes of rectum receiving the implant prescription (36% vs. 5%, $p = 0.04$).[174] A follow-up study by Damaraju et al.[176] evaluating a Canadian cohort of prostate cancer patients, however, did not demonstrate a relationship between the ATM codon 1853 polymorphism and an increased risk of rectal or bladder toxicity. Additional large-scale cohort studies will be necessary to confirm the involvement of these genetic variants in predicting radiation-induced acute and late tissue responses.

Ataxia-Telangiectasia-Like Disorder

Ataxia-telangiectasia-like disorder (ATLD) is an autosomal recessive disorder caused by inheritance of MRE11 gene mutations, which disrupts DNA double-strand break recognition and repair.[177] This syndrome was only described recently within two families originally thought to have very mild forms of AT syndrome.[177] To date, ATLD has only been identified in a small number of individuals. Clinically, patients with ATLD may present with progressive ataxia without telangiectasias and often exhibit progressive neurologic degeneration, but often at a slower rate than AT patients.[178,179] Fibroblasts from these patients were found to be clearly radiosensitive, although not as strikingly as those from AT patients.[177] However, cells from ATLD patients were found to repair DNA double-strand breaks similar to wild-type levels, and thus the search for the mechanism of radiosensitivity is still ongoing.[38]

Nijmegen Breakage Syndrome

Nijmegen breakage syndrome (NBS) is a hereditary syndrome due to inheritance of a defective NBS gene. Patients with NBS clinically present with mental retardation and microcephaly.[180,181] NBS is a direct phosphorylation target of ATM and is an integral component of a multiprotein complex, necessary for DNA double-strand break repair. The mechanism of AT, ATLD1, and NBS sensitivity to ionizing radiation is likely similar, although additional studies will be necessary to elucidate these pathways.[38]

Fanconi Anemia

FA is an autosomal recessive or X-linked disorder thought to arise from genetic aberrations involving any one of at least twelve different FA genes.[182–187] Clinically, FA is characterized by multiple congenital abnormalities including short stature, skeletal anomalies, increased incidence of solid tumors and leukemias, bone marrow failure, and cellular sensitivity to DNA crosslinking agents.[188,189] Due to loss of genomic stability through defects within the FA pathway, patients with FA are predisposed to developing cancer.[190] In particular, FA patients are at increased risk for developing acute myeloid leukemia, and gynecologic or head and neck squamous cell carcinomas.[191] The proteins encoded by these FA genes are components of a common DNA repair pathway, referred to as the FA/BRCA pathway. Recent research has suggested that the FA pathway may have a specific role in coordinating at least three DNA repair pathways following DNA crosslinking damage.[192]

The risks of radiation therapy in patients with FA have not been thoroughly evaluated. Although some clinical reports have suggested that tumors from patients with FA demonstrate increased radiosensitivity, fibroblasts derived from individuals with mutated forms of the FA proteins did not always exhibit increased radiosensitivity.[193] Alter reviewed all published literature regarding

14 FA patients with cancer treated with radiotherapy and concluded that there was insufficient evidence to guide appropriate management of FA patients based on these individual cases.[194] Future clinical and radiobiologic studies will continue to shed light on these complex pathways and their clinical implications.

CONCLUSION

Significant advances have been achieved in determining the role of genetic variations within DNA repair genes in predicting clinical radiosensitivity. ATM-associated missense mutations and NBS1 truncated mutations are likely significant contributors to the increased risk of radiation-induced malignancy in the general population. To date, small series have suggested that heterozygous carriers of ATM gene variants may be at increased risk for early and late adverse radiation-related reactions. Additional, large cohort studies will be necessary to confirm these findings and further identify other genes candidates that may influence adverse response to radiotherapy. In the upcoming years, there will likely be variations in additional genes that are discovered, which may also play a role in the development of adverse radiation responses in normal tissues. Current efforts, including the Gene-PARE project, are now underway to develop predictive tests to determine an individual's risk for adverse radiation response, based on the possession of these specific genetic variants.[133] By improving these prediction tools, physicians will be able to tailor treatment recommendations to the individual patient and minimize treatment-related toxicities.

CHAPTER CONCLUSION

Radiation therapy is an important and integral component of cancer management, often conferring a survival benefit. However, the presence of comorbidities including CVD, IBD, MS, HIV infection, diabetes, hypertension, and hereditary radiosensitivity syndromes may predict for increased acute and late radiation toxicities. Due to the small, retrospective nature of many of these studies, the association of these comorbid conditions and radiation tolerance has not been fully elucidated. However, radiation oncologists should discuss the risk versus benefits of receiving radiation therapy with their patients on a case-by-case basis. Improving the ability to predict the risk of acute and late toxicity will aid in the clinical decision-making process. Future research will ideally aid in identification of further risk stratification for radiation toxicity among patients, both through a better understanding of genetic markers and other patient factors that may contribute.

REFERENCES

1. Urtasan RC. A complication of the use of radiation for malignant neoplasia in chronic discoid lupus erythematosus. *J Can Assoc Radiol.* 1971;22:168.
2. Ransom DT, Cameron FG. Scleroderma–a possible contra-indication to lumpectomy and radiotherapy in breast carcinoma. *Australas Radiol.* 1987;31:317–318.
3. Fleck R, McNeese MD, Ellerbroek NA, et al. Consequences of breast irradiation in patients with pre-existing collagen vascular diseases. *Int J Radiat Oncol Biol Phys.* 1989;17:829–833.
4. Robertson JM, Clarke DH, Pevzner MM, et al. Breast conservation therapy. Severe breast fibrosis after radiation therapy in patients with collagen vascular disease. *Cancer.* 1991;68:502–508.
5. Varga J, Haustein UF, Creech RH, et al. Exaggerated radiation-induced fibrosis in patients with systemic sclerosis. *JAMA.* 1991;265:3292–3295.
6. Teo P, Tai TH, Choy D. Nasopharyngeal carcinoma with dermatomyositis. *Int J Radiat Oncol Biol Phys.* 1989;16:471–474.
7. Abu-Shakra M, Lee P. Exaggerated fibrosis in patients with systemic sclerosis (scleroderma) following radiation therapy. *J Rheumatol.* 20:1601–1603.
8. Hareyama M, Nagakura H, Tamakawa M, et al. Severe reaction after chemoradiotherapy of nasopharyngeal carcinoma with collagen disease. *Int J Radiat Oncol Biol Phys.* 1995;33:971.
9. Winchester DP, Cox JD. Standards for diagnosis and management of invasive breast carcinoma. American College of Radiology. American College of Surgeons. College of American Pathologists. Society of Surgical Oncology. *CA Cancer J Clin.* 1998;48:83–107.
10. Ross JG, Hussey DH, Mayr NA, et al. Acute and late reactions to radiation therapy in patients with collagen vascular diseases. *Cancer.* 1993;71:3744–3752.
11. Chen AM, Obedian E, Haffty BG. Breast-conserving therapy in the setting of collagen vascular disease. *Cancer J.* 2001;7:480–491.
12. Phan C, Mindrum M, Silverman C, et al. Matched-control retrospective study of the acute and late complications in patients with collagen vascular diseases treated with radiation therapy. *Cancer J.* 2003;9:461–466.
13. Morris MM, Powell SN. Irradiation in the setting of collagen vascular disease: acute and late complications. *J Clin Oncol.* 15:2728–2735.
14. Georgescu L, Quinn GC, Schwartzman S, et al. Lymphoma in patients with rheumatoid arthritis: association with the disease state or methotrexate treatment. *Semin Arthritis Rheum.* 1997;26:794–804.
15. Abu-Shakra M, Guillemin F, Lee P. Cancer in systemic sclerosis. *Arthritis Rheum.* 1993;36:460–464.
16. Roumm AD, Medsger TA, Jr. Cancer and systemic sclerosis. An epidemiologic study. *Arthritis Rheum.* 1985;28:1336–1340.
17. Voulgarelis M, Dafni UG, Isenberg DA, et al. Malignant lymphoma in primary Sjogren's syndrome: a multicenter, retrospective, clinical study by the European Concerted Action on Sjogren's Syndrome. *Arthritis Rheum.* 1999;42:1765–72.
18. Rosenthal AK, McLaughlin JK, Gridley G, et al. Incidence of cancer among patients with systemic sclerosis. *Cancer.* 1995;76:910–914.
19. Benk V, Al-Herz A, Gladman D, et al. Role of radiation therapy in patients with a diagnosis of both systemic lupus erythematosus and cancer. *Arthritis Rheum.* 2005;53:67–72.
20. Steen VD, Medsger TA, Jr., Rodnan GP. D-Penicillamine therapy in progressive systemic sclerosis (scleroderma): a retrospective analysis. *Ann Intern Med.* 1982;97:652–659.
21. Jimenez SA, Sigal SH. A 15-year prospective study of treatment of rapidly progressive systemic sclerosis with D-penicillamine [see comment]. *J Rheumatol.* 1991;18:1496–1503.
22. Kotzin BL, Strober S, Engleman EG, et al. Treatment of intractable rheumatoid arthritis with total lymphoid irradiation. *N Engl J Med.* 1981;305:969–976.
23. Trentham DE, Belli JA, Anderson RJ, et al. Clinical and immunologic effects of fractionated total lymphoid irradiation in refractory rheumatoid arthritis. *N Engl J Med.* 1981;305:976–982.
24. Hart LE. Total lymphoid irradiation to treat rheumatoid arthritis? *CMAJ.* 1986;134:218–219.
25. Strober S, Tanay A, Field E, et al. Efficacy of total lymphoid irradiation in intractable rheumatoid arthritis. A double-blind, randomized trial. *Ann Intern Med.* 1985;102:441–449.
26. Field EH, Strober S, Hoppe RT, et al. Sustained improvement of intractable rheumatoid arthritis after total lymphoid irradiation. *Arthritis Rheum.* 1983;26:937–946.
27. Tanay A, Field EH, Hoppe RT, et al. Long-term followup of rheumatoid arthritis patients treated with total lymphoid irradiation. *Arthritis Rheum.* 1987;30:1–10.
28. Lin A, Abu-Isa E, Griffith KA, et al. Toxicity of radiotherapy in patients with collagen vascular disease. *Cancer.* 2008;113:648–653.
29. Pinn ME, Gold DG, Petersen IA, et al. Systemic lupus erythematosus, radiotherapy, and the risk of acute and chronic toxicity: the Mayo Clinic Experience. *Int J Radiat Oncol Biol Phys.* 2008;71:498–506.
30. Wazer DE, DiPetrillo T, Schmidt-Ullrich R, et al. Factors influencing cosmetic outcome and complication risk after conservative surgery and radiotherapy for early-stage breast carcinoma. *J Clin Oncol.* 1992;10:356–363.
31. Delouche G, Bachelot F, Premont M, et al. Conservation treatment of early breast cancer: long term results and complications. *Int J Radiat Oncol Biol Phys.* 1987;13:29–34.
32. Sneeuw KC, Aaronson NK, Yarnold JR, et al. Cosmetic and functional outcomes of breast conserving treatment for early stage breast cancer. 1. Comparison of patients' ratings, observers' ratings, and objective assessments. *Radiother Oncol.* 1992;25:153–159.
33. Sarin R, Dinshaw KA, Shrivastava SK, et al. Therapeutic factors influencing the cosmetic outcome and late complications in the conservative management of early breast cancer. *Int J Radiat Oncol Biol Phys.* 1993;27:285–292.
34. Mayr NA, Riggs CE, Jr., Saag KG, et al. Mixed connective tissue disease and radiation toxicity. A case report. *Cancer.* 1997;79:612–618.
35. Hernandez S, Evans SB, Wazer DE. Severe acute toxicity from whole breast radiotherapy in the setting of collagen vascular disease. *Am J Clin Oncol.* 2006;29:647–648.
36. Gold DG, Miller RC, Petersen IA, et al. Radiotherapy for malignancy in patients with scleroderma: The Mayo Clinic experience. *Int J Radiat Oncol Biol Phys.* 2007;67:559–567.
37. Delanian S, Maulard-Durdux C, Lefaix JL, et al. Major interactions between radiation therapy and systemic sclerosis: is there an optimal treatment? *Eur J Cancer.* 1996;32A:738–739.
38. Hall E. Radiobiology for the Radiologist. In: EJ H ed. 6th ed. Philadelphia, PA: Lippincott; 2006:211–229.
39. McCormick B. Selection criteria for breast conservation. The impact of young and old age and collagen vascular disease. *Cancer.* 1994;74:430–435.
40. Canney PA, Dean S. Transforming growth factor beta: a promotor of late connective tissue injury following radiotherapy? *Br J Radiol.* 1990;63:620–623.
41. Kureshi SA, Hofman FM, Schneider JH, et al. Cytokine expression in radiation-induced delayed cerebral injury. *Neurosurgery.* 1994;35:822–829; discussion 829–830.
42. Martin M, Remy J, Daburon F. In vitro growth potential of fibroblasts isolated from pigs with radiation-induced fibrosis. *Int J Radiat Biol Relat Stud Phys Chem Med.* 1986;49:821–828.
43. Thornton SC, Walsh BJ, Bennett S, et al. Both in vitro and in vivo irradiation are associated with induction of macrophage-derived fibroblast growth factors. *Clin Exp Immunol.* 1996;103:67–73.
44. Jimenez SA, Derk CT. Following the molecular pathways toward an understanding of the pathogenesis of systemic sclerosis. *Ann Intern Med.* 2004;140:37–50.
45. Crohn BB RH. The sigmoidoscopic picture of chronic ulcerative colitis (non-specific). *Am J Med Sci.* 1925;170:220–228.

46. Perrett AD, Truelove SC, Massarella GR. Crohn's disease and carcinoma of colon. *Br Med J.* 1968;2:466–468.
47. Davis A, Caley JP. Crobn's disease with carcinoma of the colon. *Postgrad Med J.* 1960;36:380–383.
48. Allan R. Cancer risk in ulcerative colitis and Crohn's disease. In: Lennard-Jones L TS, Corona AB, eds. *Inflammatory Bowel Disease.* London, UK: Churchill Livingstone; 1992.
49. Ohman U. Colorectal carcinoma in patients less than 40 years of age. *Dis Colon Rectum.* 1982;25:209–214.
50. Schofield PF, Holden D, Carr ND. Bowel disease after radiotherapy. *J R Soc Med.* 1983;76:463–466.
51. Hoffman M, Kalter C, Roberts WS, et al. Early cervical cancer coexistent with idiopathic inflammatory bowel disease. *South Med J.* 1989;82:905–906.
52. Tiersten A, Saltz LB. Influence of inflammatory bowel disease on the ability of patients to tolerate systemic fluorouracil-based chemotherapy. *J Clin Oncol.* 1996;14:2043–2046.
53. Willett CG, Ooi CJ, Zietman AL, et al. Acute and late toxicity of patients with inflammatory bowel disease undergoing irradiation for abdominal and pelvic neoplasms. *Int J Radiat Oncol Biol Phys.* 2000;46:995–998.
54. Gastrointestinal Tumor Study Group. Prolongation of the disease-free interval in surgically treated rectal carcinoma. *N Engl J Med.* 1985;312:1465–1472.
55. Douglass HO Jr, Moertel CG, Mayer RJ, et al. Survival after postoperative combination treatment of rectal cancer. *N Engl J Med.* 1986;315:1294–1295.
56. Folkesson J, Birgisson H, Pahlman L, et al. Swedish Rectal Cancer Trial: long lasting benefits from radiotherapy on survival and local recurrence rate. *J Clin Oncol.* 2005;23:5644–5650.
57. Rose PG, Bundy BN, Watkins EB, et al. Concurrent cisplatin-based radiotherapy and chemotherapy for locally advanced cervical cancer. *N Engl J Med.* 1999;340:1144–1153.
58. Morris M, Eifel PJ, Lu J, et al. Pelvic radiation with concurrent chemotherapy compared with pelvic and para-aortic radiation for high-risk cervical cancer. *N Engl J Med.* 1999;340:1137–1143.
59. Green S, Stock RG, Greenstein AJ. Rectal cancer and inflammatory bowel disease: natural history and implications for radiation therapy. *Int J Radiat Oncol Biol Phys.* 1999;44:835–840.
60. Fisher B, Wolmark N, Rockette H, et al. Postoperative adjuvant chemotherapy or radiation therapy for rectal cancer: results from NSABP protocol R-01. *J Natl Cancer Inst.* 1988;80:21–29.
61. Song DY, Lawrie WT, Abrams RA, et al. Acute and late radiotherapy toxicity in patients with inflammatory bowel disease. *Int J Radiat Oncol Biol Phys.* 2001;51:455–459.
62. Mekhjian HS, Switz DM, Watts HD, et al. National Cooperative Crohn's Disease Study: factors determining recurrence of Crohn's disease after surgery. *Gastroenterology.* 1979;77:907–913.
63. Greenstein AJ, Sachar DB, Pasternack BS, et al. Reoperation and recurrence in Crohn's colitis and ileocolitis Crude and cumulative rates. *N Engl J Med.* 1975;293:685–690.
64. Grann A, Wallner K. Prostate brachytherapy in patients with inflammatory bowel disease. *Int J Radiat Oncol Biol Phys.* 1998;40:135–138.
65. Xavier RJ, Podolsky DK. Unravelling the pathogenesis of inflammatory bowel disease. *Nature.* 2007;448:427–434.
66. Grisham MB. Oxidants and free radicals in inflammatory bowel disease. *Lancet.* 1994;344:859–861.
67. Sanford KK, Price FM, Brodeur C, et al. Deficient DNA repair in chronic ulcerative colitis. *Cancer Detect Prev.* 1997;21:540–545.
68. Weiner HL. Multiple sclerosis is an inflammatory T-cell-mediated autoimmune disease. *Arch Neurol.* 2004;61:1613–1615.
69. Roach ES. Is multiple sclerosis an autoimmune disorder? *Arch Neurol.* 2004;61:1615–1616.
70. Compston A, Coles A. Multiple sclerosis. *Lancet.* 2002;359:1221–1231.
71. Karni A, Abramsky O. Association of MS with thyroid disorders. *Neurology.* 1999;53:883–885.
72. Heinzlef O, Alamowitch S, Sazdovitch V, et al. Autoimmune diseases in families of French patients with multiple sclerosis. *Acta Neurol Scand.* 2000;101:36–40.
73. Gupta G, Gelfand JM, Lewis JD. Increased risk for demyelinating diseases in patients with inflammatory bowel disease. *Gastroenterology.* 2005;129:819–826.
74. Irizarry M. *Multiple Sclerosis.* Boston: Butterworth-Heinemann; 1997.
75. Duhain. Un cas de sclerosis en plaque, ameliore par la radiotherapie. *C Acad Sci Ref Arch Elec Med.* 1903.
76. Lampert P, Tom MI, Rider WD. Disseminated demyelination of the brain following Co60 (gamma) radiation. *Arch Pathol.* 1959;68:322–330.
77. McMeekin RR, Hardman JM, Kempe LG. Multiple sclerosis after x-radiation. Activation by treatment of metastatic glomus tumor. *Arch Otolaryngol.* 1969;90:617–621.
78. Murphy CB, Hashimoto SA, Graeb D, et al. Clinical exacerbation of multiple sclerosis following radiotherapy. *Arch Neurol.* 2003;60:273–275.
79. Nahser HC, Vieregge P, Nau HE, et al. Coincidence of multiple sclerosis and glioma. Clinical and radiological remarks on two cases. *Surg Neurol.* 1986;26:45–51.
80. Peterson K, Rosenblum MK, Powers JM, et al. Effect of brain irradiation on demyelinating lesions. *Neurology.* 1993;43:2105–2112.
81. Pakos EE, Tsekeris PG, Chatzidimou K, et al. Astrocytoma-like multiple sclerosis. *Clin Neurol Neurosurg.* 107:152–157.
82. Tourtellotte WW, Potvin AR, Baumhefner RW, et al. Multiple sclerosis de novo CNS IgG synthesis. Effect of CNS irradiation. *Arch Neurol.* 1980;37:620–624.
83. Miller RC, Lachance DH, Lucchinetti CF, et al. Multiple sclerosis, brain radiotherapy, and risk of neurotoxicity: the Mayo Clinic experience. *Int J Radiat Oncol Biol Phys.* 2006;66:1178–1186.
84. Mathieu D, Kondziolka D, Niranjan A, et al. Gamma knife thalamotomy for multiple sclerosis tremor. *Surg Neurol.* 2007;68:394–399.
85. Belka C, Budach W, Kortmann RD, et al. Radiation induced CNS toxicity–molecular and cellular mechanisms. *Br J Cancer.* 2001;85:1233–1239.
86. Behin A, Delattre JY. Complications of radiation therapy on the brain and spinal cord. *Semin Neurol.* 2004;24:405–417.
87. Schultheiss TE, Kun LE, Ang KK, et al. Radiation response of the central nervous system. *Int J Radiat Oncol Biol Phys.* 1995;31:1093–1112.
88. Pittock SJ, McClelland RL, Mayr WT, et al. Prevalence of tremor in multiple sclerosis and associated disability in the Olmsted County population. *Mov Disord.* 2004;19:1482–1485.
89. Alusi SH, Glickman S, Aziz TZ, et al. Tremor in multiple sclerosis. *J Neurol Neurosurg Psychiatry.* 1999;66:131–134.
90. Cooper DA, Gold J, Maclean P, et al. Acute AIDS retrovirus infection. Definition of a clinical illness associated with seroconversion. *Lancet.* 1985;1:537–540.
91. http://www.cdc.gov, 2008.
92. Ancelle-Park R. Expanded European AIDS case definition. *Lancet.* 1993;341:441.
93. Herida M, Mary-Krause M, Kaphan R, et al. Incidence of non-AIDS-defining cancers before and during the highly active antiretroviral therapy era in a cohort of human immunodeficiency virus-infected patients. *J Clin Oncol.* 2003;21:3447–3453.
94. Grulich AE, van Leeuwen MT, Falster MO, et al. Incidence of cancers in people with HIV/AIDS compared with immunosuppressed transplant recipients: a meta-analysis. *Lancet.* 2007;370:59–67.
95. Melbye M, Cote TR, Kessler L, et al. High incidence of anal cancer among AIDS patients. The AIDS/Cancer Working Group. *Lancet.* 1994;343:636–639.
96. Frisch M, Glimelius B, van den Brule AJ, et al. Sexually transmitted infection as a cause of anal cancer. *N Engl J Med.* 1997;337:1350–1358.
97. Watkins EB, Findlay P, Gelmann E, et al. Enhanced mucosal reactions in AIDS patients receiving oropharyngeal irradiation. *Int J Radiat Oncol Biol Phys.* 1987;13:1403–1408.
98. Gichangi P, Bwayo J, Estambale B, et al. HIV impact on acute morbidity and pelvic tumor control following radiotherapy for cervical cancer. *Gynecol Oncol.* 100:405–411.
99. Peddada AV, Smith DE, Rao AR, et al. Chemotherapy and low-dose radiotherapy in the treatment of HIV-infected patients with carcinoma of the anal canal. *Int J Radiat Oncol Biol Phys.* 1997;37:1101–1105.
100. Edelman S, Johnstone PA. Combined modality therapy for HIV-infected patients with squamous cell carcinoma of the anus: outcomes and toxicities. *Int J Radiat Oncol Biol Phys.* 2006;66:206–211.
101. Blazy A, Hennequin C, Gornet JM, et al. Anal carcinomas in HIV-positive patients: high-dose chemoradiotherapy is feasible in the era of highly active antiretroviral therapy. *Dis Colon Rectum.* 2005;48:1176–1181.
102. Wexler A, Berson AM, Goldstone SE, et al. Invasive anal squamous-cell carcinoma in the HIV-positive patient: outcome in the era of highly active antiretroviral therapy. *Dis Colon Rectum.* 2008;51:73–81.
103. Nigro ND, Seydel HG, Considine B, et al. Combined preoperative radiation and chemotherapy for squamous cell carcinoma of the anal canal. *Cancer.* 1983;51:1826–1829.
104. UKCCCR Anal Cancer Trial Working Party, UK Co-ordinating Committee on Cancer Research. Epidermoid anal cancer: results from the UKCCCR randomised trial of radiotherapy alone versus radiotherapy, 5-fluorouracil, and mitomycin. *Lancet.* 1996;348:1049–1054.
105. Bartelink H, Roelofsen F, Eschwege F, et al. Concomitant radiotherapy and chemotherapy is superior to radiotherapy alone in the treatment of locally advanced anal cancer: results of a phase III randomized trial of the European Organization for Research and Treatment of Cancer Radiotherapy and Gastrointestinal Cooperative Groups. *J Clin Oncol.* 1997;15:2040–2049.
106. Ajani JA, Winter KA, Gunderson LL, et al. Fluorouracil, mitomycin, and radiotherapy vs fluorouracil, cisplatin, and radiotherapy for carcinoma of the anal canal: a randomized controlled trial. *JAMA.* 2008;299:1914–1921.
107. Holland JM, Swift PS. Tolerance of patients with human immunodeficiency virus and anal carcinoma to treatment with combined chemotherapy and radiation therapy. *Radiology.* 1994;193:251–254.
108. Rotman M, Lange CS. Anal cancer: radiation and concomitant continuous infusion chemotherapy. *Int J Radiat Oncol Biol Phys.* 1991;21:1385–1387.
109. Formenti SC, Chak L, Gill P, et al. Increased radiosensitivity of normal tissue fibroblasts in patients with acquired immunodeficiency syndrome (AIDS) and with Kaposi's sarcoma. *Int J Radiat Biol.* 1995;68:411–412.
110. Vallis KA. Glutathione deficiency and radiosensitivity in AIDS patients. *Lancet.* 1991;337:918–919.
111. Kim JH, Sarani B, Orkin BA, et al. HIV-positive patients with anal carcinoma have poorer treatment tolerance and outcome than HIV-negative patients. *Dis Colon Rectum.* 2001;44:1496–1502.
112. Martenson JA, Lipsitz SR, Lefkopoulou M, et al. Results of combined modality therapy for patients with anal cancer (E7283). An Eastern Cooperative Oncology Group study. *Cancer.* 1995;76:1731–1736.
113. Bosset JF, Roelofsen F, Morgan DA, et al. Shortened irradiation scheme, continuous infusion of 5-fluorouracil and fractionation of mitomycin C in locally advanced anal carcinomas. Results of a phase II study of the European Organization for Research and Treatment of Cancer. Radiotherapy and Gastrointestinal Cooperative Groups. *Eur J Cancer.* 2003;39:45–51.
114. Oehler-Janne C, Huguet F, Provencher S, et al. HIV-specific differences in outcome of squamous cell carcinoma of the anal canal: a multicentric cohort study of HIV-positive patients receiving highly active antiretroviral therapy. *J Clin Oncol.* 2008;26:2550–2557.
115. Cleator S, Fife K, Nelson M, et al. Treatment of HIV-associated invasive anal cancer with combined chemoradiation. *Eur J Cancer.* 2000;36:754–748.
116. Chiao EY, Giordano TP, Richardson P, et al. Human immunodeficiency virus-associated squamous cell cancer of the anus: epidemiology and outcomes in the highly active antiretroviral therapy era. *J Clin Oncol.* 2008;26:474–479.
117. Salama JK, Mell LK, Schomas DA, et al. Concurrent chemotherapy and intensity-modulated radiation therapy for anal canal cancer patients: a multicenter experience. *J Clin Oncol.* 2007;25:4581–4586.
118. Hoffman R, Welton ML, Klencke B, et al. The significance of pretreatment CD4 count on the outcome and treatment tolerance of HIV-positive patients with anal cancer. *Int J Radiat Oncol Biol Phys.* 1999;44:127–131.
119. Place RJ, Gregorcyk SG, Huber PJ, et al. Outcome analysis of HIV-positive patients with anal squamous cell carcinoma. *Dis Colon Rectum.* 2001;44:506–512.
120. http://diabetes.niddk.nih.gov/dm/pubs/statistics/#allages.

121. van Nagell JR Jr, Parker JC Jr, Maruyama Y, et al. Bladder or rectal injury following radiation therapy for cervical cancer. *Am J Obstet Gynecol.* 1974;119:727–732.

122. Meyer JS. Diabetes and wound healing. *Crit Care Nurs Clin North Am.* 1996;8:195–201.

123. Morain WD, Colen LB. Wound healing in diabetes mellitus. *Clin Plast Surg.* 1990;17:493–501.

124. Herold DM, Hanlon AL, Hanks GE. Diabetes mellitus: a predictor for late radiation morbidity. *Int J Radiat Oncol Biol Phys.* 1999;43:475–479.

125. Maruyama Y, Van Nagell JR Jr, Utley J, et al. Radiation and small bowel complications in cervical carcinoma therapy. *Radiology.* 1974;112:699–703.

126. Harwood AR, Tierie A. Radiotherapy of early glottic cancer–II. *Int J Radiat Oncol Biol Phys.* 1979;5:477–482.

127. Debus J, Hug EB, Liebsch NJ, et al. Brainstem tolerance to conformal radiotherapy of skull base tumors. *Int J Radiat Oncol Biol Phys.* 1997;39:967–975.

128. Jereczek-Fossa BA, Badzio A, Jassem J. Factors determining acute normal tissue reactions during postoperative radiotherapy in endometrial cancer: analysis of 317 consecutive cases. *Radiother Oncol.* 2003;68:33–39.

129. Mayahara H, Murakami M, Kagawa K, et al. Acute morbidity of proton therapy for prostate cancer: the Hyogo Ion Beam Medical Center experience. *Int J Radiat Oncol Biol Phys.* 2007;69:434–443.

130. Safwat A, Bentzen SM, Turesson I, et al. Deterministic rather than stochastic factors explain most of the variation in the expression of skin telangiectasia after radiotherapy. *Int J Radiat Oncol Biol Phys.* 2002;52:198–204.

131. Fernet M, Hall J. Genetic biomarkers of therapeutic radiation sensitivity. *DNA Repair (Amst).* 2004;3:1237–1243.

132. Baumann M, Holscher T, Begg AC. Towards genetic prediction of radiation responses: ESTRO's GENEPI project. *Radiother Oncol.* 2003;69:121–125.

133. Ho AY, Atencio DP, Peters S, et al. Genetic predictors of adverse radiotherapy effects: the Gene-PARE project. *Int J Radiat Oncol Biol Phys.* 2006;65:646–655.

134. Andreassen CN, Overgaard J, Alsner J, et al. ATM sequence variants and risk of radiation-induced subcutaneous fibrosis after postmastectomy radiotherapy. *Int J Radiat Oncol Biol Phys.* 2006;64:776–783.

135. Swift M, Morrell D, Massey RB, et al. Incidence of cancer in 161 families affected by ataxia-telangiectasia. *N Engl J Med.* 1991;325:1831–1836.

136. Swift M, Reitnauer PJ, Morrell D, et al. Breast and other cancers in families with ataxia-telangiectasia. *N Engl J Med.* 1987;316:1289–1294.

137. Sedgwick RP BE. Ataxia-Telangiectasia. In: JMBV DJ ed. *Handbook of Clinical Neurology: Hereditary Neuropathies and Spinocerebellar Atrophies.* New York City: Elsevier Science Publishers; 1991:347.

138. Nowak-Wegrzyn A, Crawford TO, Winkelstein JA, et al. Immunodeficiency and infections in ataxia-telangiectasia. *J Pediatr.* 2004;144:505–511.

139. Bott L, Lebreton J, Thumerelle C, et al. Lung disease in ataxia-telangiectasia. *Acta Paediatr.* 2007;96:1021–1024.

140. Olsen JH, Hahnemann JM, Borresen-Dale AL, et al. Cancer in patients with ataxia-telangiectasia and in their relatives in the nordic countries. *J Natl Cancer Inst.* 2001;93:121–127.

141. Morgan JL, Holcomb TM, Morrissey RW. Radiation reaction in ataxia telangiectasia. *Am J Dis Child.* 1968;116:557–558.

142. Crawford TO, Skolasky RL, Fernandez R, et al. Survival probability in ataxia telangiectasia. *Arch Dis Child.* 2006;91:610–611.

143. Morrell D, Cromartie E, Swift M. Mortality and cancer incidence in 263 patients with ataxia-telangiectasia. *J Natl Cancer Inst.* 1986;77:89–92.

144. Gatti RA, Berkel I, Boder E, et al. Localization of an ataxia-telangiectasia gene to chromosome 11q22-23. *Nature.* 1988;336:577–580.

145. Savitsky K, Bar-Shira A, Gilad S, et al. A single ataxia telangiectasia gene with a product similar to PI-3 kinase. *Science.* 1995;268:1749–1753.

146. Canman CE, Lim DS. The role of ATM in DNA damage responses and cancer. *Oncogene.* 1998;17:3301–3308.

147. Savitsky K, Sfez S, Tagle DA, et al. The complete sequence of the coding region of the ATM gene reveals similarity to cell cycle regulators in different species. *Hum Mol Genet.* 1995;4:2025–2032.

148. Baskaran R, Wood LD, Whitaker LL, et al. Ataxia telangiectasia mutant protein activates c-Abl tyrosine kinase in response to ionizing radiation. *Nature.* 1997;387:516–519.

149. Rotman G, Shiloh Y. ATM: from gene to function. *Hum Mol Genet.* 1998;7:1555–1563.

150. Shiloh Y. ATM and related protein kinases: safeguarding genome integrity. *Nat Rev Cancer.* 2003;3:155–168.

151. Kastan MB, Lim DS. The many substrates and functions of ATM. *Nat Rev Mol Cell Biol.* 2000;1:179–186.

152. McKinnon PJ. ATM and ataxia telangiectasia. *EMBO Rep.* 2004;5:772–776.

153. Dork T, Bendix R, Bremer M, et al. Spectrum of ATM gene mutations in a hospital-based series of unselected breast cancer patients. *Cancer Res.* 2001;61:7608–7615.

154. Spring K, Ahangari F, Scott SP, et al. Mice heterozygous for mutation in Atm, the gene involved in ataxia-telangiectasia, have heightened susceptibility to cancer. *Nat Genet.* 2002;32:185–190.

155. Pandita TK, Hittelman WN. Increased initial levels of chromosome damage and heterogeneous chromosome repair in ataxia telangiectasia heterozygote cells. *Mutat Res.* 1994;310:1–13.

156. Sanford KK, Parshad R, Price FM, et al. Enhanced chromatid damage in blood lymphocytes after G2 phase x irradiation, a marker of the ataxia-telangiectasia gene. *J Natl Cancer Inst.* 1990;82:1050–1054.

157. Paterson MC, MacFarlane SJ, Gentner NE, et al. Cellular hypersensitivity to chronic gamma-radiation in cultured fibroblasts from ataxia-telangiectasia heterozygotes. *Kroc Found Ser.* 1985;19:73–87.

158. Weeks DE, Paterson MC, Lange K, et al. Assessment of chronic gamma radiosensitivity as an in vitro assay for heterozygote identification of ataxia-telangiectasia. *Radiat Res.* 1991;128:90–99.

159. Parshad R, Sanford KK, Jones GM, et al. G2 chromosomal radiosensitivity of ataxia-telangiectasia heterozygotes. *Cancer Genet Cytogenet.* 1985;14:163–168.

160. Athma P, Rappaport R, Swift M. Molecular genotyping shows that ataxia-telangiectasia heterozygotes are predisposed to breast cancer. *Cancer Genet Cytogenet.* 1996;92:130–134.

161. Olsen JH, Hahnemann JM, Borresen-Dale AL, et al. Breast and other cancers in 1445 blood relatives of 75 Nordic patients with ataxia telangiectasia. *Br J Cancer.* 2005;93:260–265.

162. Su Y, Swift M. Mortality rates among carriers of ataxia-telangiectasia mutant alleles. *Ann Intern Med.* 2000;133:770–778.

163. Renwick A, Thompson D, Seal S, et al. ATM mutations that cause ataxia-telangiectasia are breast cancer susceptibility alleles. *Nat Genet.* 2006;38:873–875.

164. Gotoff SP, Amirmokri E, Liebner EJ. Ataxia telangiectasia. Neoplasia, untoward response to x-irradiation, and tuberous sclerosis. *Am J Dis Child.* 1967;114:617–625.

165. DahlBerg WK, Little JB. Response of dermal fibroblast cultures from patients with unusually severe responses to radiotherapy and from ataxia telangiectasia heterozygotes to fractionated radiation. *Clin Cancer Res.* 1995;1:785–790.

166. Cole J, Arlett CF, Green MH, et al. Comparative human cellular radiosensitivity: II. The survival following gamma-irradiation of unstimulated (G0) T-lymphocytes, T-lymphocyte lines, lymphoblastoid cell lines and fibroblasts from normal donors, from ataxia-telangiectasia patients and from ataxia-telangiectasia heterozygotes. *Int J Radiat Biol.* 1988;54:929–943.

167. Clarke RA, Goozee GR, Birrell G, et al. Absence of ATM truncations in patients with severe acute radiation reactions. *Int J Radiat Oncol Biol Phys.* 1998;41:1021–1027.

168. Oppitz U, Bernthaler U, Schindler D, et al. Sequence analysis of the ATM gene in 20 patients with RTOG grade 3 or 4 acute and/or late tissue radiation side effects. *Int J Radiat Oncol Biol Phys.* 1999;44:981–988.

169. Weissberg JB, Huang DD, Swift M. Radiosensitivity of normal tissues in ataxia-telangiectasia heterozygotes. *Int J Radiat Oncol Biol Phys.* 1998;42:1133–1136.

170. Concannon P, Gatti RA. Diversity of ATM gene mutations detected in patients with ataxia-telangiectasia. *Hum Mutat.* 1997;10:100–107.

171. Telatar M, Teraoka S, Wang Z, et al. Ataxia-telangiectasia: identification and detection of founder-effect mutations in the ATM gene in ethnic populations. *Am J Hum Genet.* 1998;62:86–97.

172. Andreassen CN, Alsner J, Overgaard M, et al. Risk of radiation-induced subcutaneous fibrosis in relation to single nucleotide polymorphisms in TGFB1, SOD2, XRCC1, XRCC3, APEX and ATM–a study based on DNA from formalin fixed paraffin embedded tissue samples. *Int J Radiat Biol.* 2006;82:577–586.

173. Iannuzzi CM, Atencio DP, Green S, et al. ATM mutations in female breast cancer patients predict for an increase in radiation-induced late effects. *Int J Radiat Oncol Biol Phys.* 2002;52:606–613.

174. Cesaretti JA, Stock RG, Atencio DP, et al. A genetically determined dose-volume histogram predicts for rectal bleeding among patients treated with prostate brachytherapy. *Int J Radiat Oncol Biol Phys.* 2007;68:1410–1416.

175. Ho AY, Fan G, Atencio DP, et al. Possession of ATM sequence variants as predictor for late normal tissue responses in breast cancer patients treated with radiotherapy. *Int J Radiat Oncol Biol Phys.* 2007;69:677–684.

176. Damaraju S, Murray D, Dufour J, et al. Association of DNA repair and steroid metabolism gene polymorphisms with clinical late toxicity in patients treated with conformal radiotherapy for prostate cancer. *Clin Cancer Res.* 2006;12:2545–2554.

177. Stewart GS, Maser RS, Stankovic T, et al. The DNA double-strand break repair gene hMRE11 is mutated in individuals with an ataxia-telangiectasia-like disorder. *Cell.* 1999;99:577–587.

178. Hernandez D, McConville CM, Stacey M, et al. A family showing no evidence of linkage between the ataxia telangiectasia gene and chromosome 11q22-23. *J Med Genet.* 1993;30:135–140.

179. Klein C, Wenning GK, Quinn NP, et al. Ataxia without telangiectasia masquerading as benign hereditary chorea. *Mov Disord.* 1996;11:217–220.

180. Weemaes CM, Hustinx TW, Scheres JM, et al. A new chromosomal instability disorder: the Nijmegen breakage syndrome. *Acta Paediatr Scand.* 1981;70:557–564.

181. The International Nijmegen Breakage Syndrome Study Group. Nijmegen breakage syndrome. *Arch Dis Child.* 2000;82:400–406.

182. de Winter JP, Rooimans MA, van Der Weel L, et al. The Fanconi anaemia gene FANCF encodes a novel protein with homology to ROM. *Nat Genet.* 2000;24:15–16.

183. Joenje H, Levitus M, Waisfisz Q, et al. Complementation analysis in Fanconi anemia: assignment of the reference FA-H patient to group A. *Am J Hum Genet.* 2000;67:759–762.

184. Strathdee CA, Gavish H, Shannon WR, et al. Cloning of cDNAs for Fanconi's anaemia by functional complementation. *Nature.* 1992;356:763–737.

185. Lo Ten Foe JR, Rooimans MA, Bosnoyan-Collins L, et al. Expression cloning of a cDNA for the major Fanconi anaemia gene, FAA. *Nat Genet.* 1996;14:320–333.

186. de Winter JP, Leveille F, van Berkel CG, et al. Isolation of a cDNA representing the Fanconi anemia complementation group E gene. *Am J Hum Genet.* 2000;67:1306–1308.

187. de Winter JP, Waisfisz Q, Rooimans MA, et al. The Fanconi anaemia group G gene FANCG is identical with XRCC9. *Nat Genet.* 1998;20:281–283.

188. Auerbach AD, Wolman SR. Susceptibility of Fanconi's anaemia fibroblasts to chromosome damage by carcinogens. *Nature.* 1976;261:494–496.

189. German J, Schonberg S, Caskie S, et al. A test for Fanconi's anemia. *Blood.* 1987;69:1637–1641.

190. Kennedy RD, D'Andrea AD. The Fanconi Anemia/BRCA pathway: new faces in the crowd. *Genes Dev.* 2005;19:2925–2940.

191. D'Andrea AD, Grompe M. The Fanconi anaemia/BRCA pathway. *Nat Rev Cancer.* 2003;3:23–34.

192. Kennedy RD, D'Andrea AD. DNA repair pathways in clinical practice: lessons from pediatric cancer susceptibility syndromes. *J Clin Oncol.* 2006;24:3799–3808.

193. Marcou Y, D'Andrea A, Jeggo PA, et al. Normal cellular radiosensitivity in an adult Fanconi anaemia patient with marked clinical radiosensitivity. *Radiother Oncol.* 2001;60:75–79.

194. Alter BP. Radiosensitivity in Fanconi's anemia patients. *Radiother Oncol.* 2002;62:345–347.

195. Wo J, Taghian A. Radiotherapy in setting of collagen vascular disease. *Int J Radiat Oncol Biol Phys.* 2007;69:1347–1353.

196. Chadha M, Rosenblatt EA, Malamud S, et al. Squamous-cell carcinoma of the anus in HIV-positive patients. *Dis Colon Rectum.* 1994;37:861–865.

CHAPTER

7

David J. Brenner
Herman D. Suit

Radiation-Induced Oncogenesis at Low and High Doses

INTRODUCTION

There is little question that intermediate and high doses of ionizing radiation, say above 100 mSv, given acutely or over a prolonged period, produce deleterious consequences in humans including, but not exclusively, cancer. At much lower doses (<1 mSv, typical of most radiological examination other than CT), risk estimates require extrapolating risks from those estimated at higher doses. At much higher doses (>10 Gy), risk estimates are either extrapolated from those estimated at lower doses, or are estimated from radiotherapy-related second-cancer data.

Of course, the dose distribution in normal tissues after radiation therapy involves both high and low doses. As radiotherapeutic techniques have improved, smaller volumes of normal tissues are exposed to very high doses, but larger volumes of normal tissue are exposed to low and intermediate doses, for example with intensity-modulated x-ray therapy. The significance of this change depends, of course, on the nature of the dose-response relationship between radiation dose and, for example, cancer risk.

LOW-DOSE RADIATION RISK ESTIMATES IN HUMANS

Compared to higher doses, the risks of low doses of radiation are likely to be lower, and progressively larger epidemiological studies are required to quantify the risk to a useful degree of precision. For example, if the excess risk were proportional to the radiation dose, and if a sample size of 500 persons were

needed to quantify the effect of a 1,000 mSv dose, then a sample size of 50,000 would be needed for a 100-mSv dose, and about 5 million for a 10-mSv dose.[1,2] In other words, to maintain statistical precision and power, the necessary sample size increases approximately as the inverse square of the dose. This is because, as the dose goes down, the signal (radiation risk) to noise (natural background risk) ratio decreases.

We will focus here largely on epidemiological studies of exposed human populations though, as described subsequently in the chapter, much ancillary information can be obtained from animal studies and from *in vitro* studies.

ACUTE LOW-DOSE EXPOSURES

The epidemiological study with the highest statistical power for evaluating low-dose risks is the Life Span Study (LSS) cohort of more than 80,000 atomic-bomb survivors of the 1945 atomic explosions[3]—because the cohort is large, follow-up is both complete and very long, and the survivors were exposed to a wide range of reasonably well-characterized radiation doses. While the A-bomb survivor analyses have often been considered as high-dose studies, in fact the mean dose in the exposed group on the LSS cohort is only 200 mSv, with almost 50% of the exposed individuals in the cohort (>25,000 individuals) having doses below 50 mSv. Cancer incidence,[4,5] cancer mortality,[3] and non–cancer-related mortality[3] have been estimated, though almost half the exposed population—and a larger fraction of the individuals exposed as children—are still alive. Between 1950 and 1997, there were 9,335 deaths from solid cancer and 31,881 deaths from noncancer diseases. It is estimated that about 5% of the solid cancer deaths and 0.8% of the noncancer deaths were associated with the radiation exposure. Over the dose range on which estimates could be made, the radiation-related risks appear to increase linearly with dose. A typical risk estimate is that for an individual exposed at age 30, the solid cancer risk at age 70 was increased by 47%/Sv.[3]

In the LSS study, organ dose estimates are available for all individuals included in the analysis, and the results are presented in dose group categories; a comparison Japanese population is used that was sufficiently far from the explosions that the doses were <5 mSv. The individuals in the lowest dose category from 5 to 125 mSv (mean dose: 34 mSv) show a significant ($p = 0.025$) increase in solid-cancer related mortality.[3] There is the possibility of bias in these low-dose cancer mortality risk estimates; for example, individuals nearer the blast might be more likely to have cancer recorded on their death certificates, and also the stated cause of death was generally not based on autopsy findings. There is less potential for such bias in the cancer incidence studies[4,5]; here, the A-bomb survivors in the dose range from 5 to 100 mSv (mean dose: 29 mSv) show a significantly increased solid cancer incidence ($p = 0.05$) compared with the population who were exposed to <5 mSv.

The A-bomb survivor risks discussed represent an average of all exposed individuals. There is good evidence that there are subpopulations at greater or lower risk than the average, depending on age,[6] genetic status,[7] or other factors.[8] Radiation risks in children are expected to be higher due to the higher proportion of dividing cells in younger individuals, and also because of the longer lifespan available for a potential cancer to be expressed. Childhood cancer risks after prenatal x-ray exposure have been extensively studied: A detailed analysis of the many studies of childhood cancer risks from diagnostic *in utero* exposures concluded that a 10-mSv dose to the embryo and fetus does indeed cause a significant and quantifiable increase in the risk of childhood cancer[9]; Mole[10] has argued that the most reliable risk estimate from these studies comes from prenatal examinations in Britain during the period 1958 to 1961, for which the estimated mean fetal dose is 6 mSv and the odds ratio for childhood cancer deaths is 1.23 (95% CI: 1.04–1.48).

PROTRACTED LOW-DOSE EXPOSURES

Much attention has been given to studies of large numbers of radiation workers who were chronically exposed to low radiation doses. In a 15-country collaborative study,[11] 407,391 nuclear industry workers were monitored individually for external radiation, with 5.2 million person-years of follow-up. The overall average cumulative recorded dose was 19.4 mSv. A significant association was seen between radiation dose and all-cause mortality (excess relative risk [ERR] 0.42/Sv, 90% CI: 0.07, 0.79; 18,993 deaths). This was mainly attributable to a dose-related increase in all cancer mortality (ERR/Sv 0.97, 90% CI: 0.28, 1.77; 5,233 deaths). The interpretation of this large study has not been without controversy,[12] but the more recent publication[13] of an individual country study with more statistical power, from the UK National Registry for Radiation Workers, adds significant support to the 15-country worker risk estimates.[12]

As with the acute exposures, it is informative to examine childhood exposure, as the risks are expected to be higher and thus easier to quantify. The US scoliosis cohort study[14] of females exposed under age 20 to multiple diagnostic x-rays (mean breast dose 108 mSv in 25 exposures) demonstrated a statistically significant increased risk for breast cancer (relative risk, RR = 1.6, 95% CI: 1.1–2.6); the excess risk remained significant when the analysis was limited to individuals with breast doses between 10 and 90 mSv.

Ron et al.[15] studied children who received fractionated irradiation of the scalp as treatment for tinea capitis (five fractions, mean total thyroid dose: 62 mSv, dose range: 40–70 mSv); compared to matched, unirradiated comparison subjects, they showed a statistically significant increase in thyroid cancer risk (RR = 3.3, 95% CI: 1.6–6.7). Higher risks were seen when the age at exposure was limited to under 5 years (RR = 5.0, 95% CI: 2.7–10.3). A subsequent pooled analysis[16] of five cohort studies of thyroid cancer after childhood exposure to external radiation (four of these studies, including the scalp irradiation study described above, were of fractionated exposure) showed clear evidence of an increased risk of thyroid cancer (RR = 2.5, 95% CI: 2–4) at a mean dose to the thyroid of 50 mSv (dose range: 10–90 mSv).

LABORATORY-BASED ONCOGENESIS STUDIES AT LOW-DOSE AND INTERMEDIATE DOSES

Extensive studies of radiation transformation/carcinogenesis on mammalian cell lines *in vitro* and on experimental animals have established that the dose-response relationships are quite variable. It will be seen that the laboratory-based data are by no means definitive. For example, at low doses there is often considerable interlaboratory variability,[17] which is perhaps not surprising at doses when the signal-to-noise ratio is not advantageous, resulting in a strong dependence on background control rates. In animal studies, there are substantial variations in the dose-response relationships between species, between strains, and as a function of age and gender, as well as between organs of an individual animal.

Findings of quantitative investigations of malignant transformation of mammalian cells *in vitro*, and in laboratory animals are briefly reviewed. These data emphasize the complexity of the dose-response relationships for oncogenic transformation and radiation-induced cancer at low doses.

IN VITRO RADIATION-INDUCED ONCOGENIC TRANSFORMATION

In the first quantitative study of this kind, Borek and Hall[18] found that the increase in radiation-induced transformation frequency (TF) of hamster embryo cells with dose was linear from 0.1 to 2 Gy.

Han and Elkind[19] employed $C_3H_{10}T\frac{1}{2}$ cells (partially transformed mouse embryo derived cells) and irradiated with 50-kVp x-rays to determine transformation rates in vitro. The lowest dose investigated was approximately 0.8 Gy, at which the TF was approximately 8×10^{-5} surviving cells. This increased steeply and exponentially to 200×10^{-5} at approximately 3.5 Gy and then reached a plateau of approximately 350×10^{-5} at approximately 7 Gy. Thus, in this study, there was not an observed linear dose-response curve over the dose range approximately 0.8 to approximately 3.5 Gy. It may be noted here that if the TF is computed on the basis of the total number of cells irradiated rather than the number of surviving cells at each dose level, there is a steep increase in transformation yield up to 4 Gy and then a near comparably steep decline up to 12 Gy. The transformation frequencies were 1×10^{-3} at 4 Gy but only 6×10^{-6} at 12 Gy. Thus as the dose increases, there is a progressively smaller number of viable cells available to be transformed. Han et al.[20] also measured oncogenic transformation at γ-ray dose rates of approximately 1 mGy/min. The TF versus dose curve was similar at dose rates of 1,000 and 1 mGy/min. A plateau in transformation yield was reached at approximately 7 Gy for both dose rates, but at the frequency of approximately 50×10^{-5} for the low-dose rate compared with 350×10^{-5} for the high-dose rate irradiation.

Miller et al.[21] performed extensive measurements of *in vitro* transformation of $C_3H_{10}T\frac{1}{2}$ cells by 250-kVp x-rays and neutron irradiation. They used approximately 4×10^5 cells/25 cm^2 flask that were 48 hours into exponential growth. At 0, 0.5, 1, 2, 4, and 8 Gy, transformation frequencies were 4, 10, 10, 30, 68, and 225×10^{-5}, that is, a slightly upwardly curving dose-response relationship.

Heyes and Mill[22] determined *in vitro* TF of CGL1 cells for doses from 0.27 to 5.4 Gy. There was a linear increase in TF over that dose range.

By contrast, there are several reports of a lack of increase, or even a reduced oncogenic transformation rate, after doses below 50 mGy. Azzam et al.[23] irradiated $C_3H_{10}T\frac{1}{2}$ cells with γ rays in confluent cultures at 2.4 mGy/min, and incubated for 24 hours prior to replating. The total doses were 1, 10, and 100 mGy and at each dose, the transformation rate was less than observed for the control cultures. Elmore et al.[24] used 232-MeV proton beams to determine TF of CGL1 cells in subconfluent cultures at very low doses; the TF was less than that of the controls at 5 and 50 mGy but increased approximate linearly from 100 to 600 mGy. In a series of reports, Redpath et al.[25] have studied extensively the transformation of CGL1 cell line (a nontumorigenic HeLa × skin fibroblast cell) at these low-dose levels; they reported a reduced transformation rate compared to controls at 0.4, 1, and 4 mGy; at 180 and 360 mGy, the transformation rate increased.

In summary, from these *in vitro* studies of radiation-induced oncogenic transformation, a linear increase in risk is supported by experimental data for doses above 0.25 Gy. At lower doses, the results are highly variable, at least in part due to issues in variability in background control rates, even within the same cell line.[17]

CARCINOGENESIS IN WHOLE-BODY IRRADIATED EXPERIMENTAL ANIMALS

In an extensive series of studies, Ullrich et al.[26] examined radiation-induced cancer induction by single doses of γ rays, in whole-body irradiated (WBI) young female RFM mice. They employed 15,236 mice in this series of experiments in the determination of the incidence of eight tumor types in the control and irradiated mice. WBI doses were 0.0, 0.1, 0.25, 0.5, 1, 1.5, and 3 Gy. The mice were followed to end of life and autopsy examination performed. Thus, there were tumor frequency data for 56 dose and tumor types. Four of the eight tumors were less frequent after 0.25 Gy than in control mice, namely reticulum cell sarcoma, lung adenoma, and tumors of the uterus and breast. At 1.5 Gy, the frequency of reticulum cell sarcoma and lung adenoma was significantly less than in the control mice. However, the observed thymic lymphoma and Harderian tumor rates increased linearly with dose. Ullrich et al.[27] followed this

work with a similar study on induction of myeloid leukemia in 10-week-old male RFM mice. There was a lower frequency after 0.1 Gy than in the control mice. From 0.5 to 3 Gy, the increase in risk with dose was consistent with a linear back projection to zero dose.

Storer et al.[28] reported a comprehensive investigation of radiation carcinogenesis of 0.5, 1, and 2 Gy WBI based on female BALB/c Bd and RFM mice, and on female and male C3Hf/Bd and C57BL/6Bd mice. The mice were observed for duration of life and were examined by autopsy to determine the incidence of carcinoma of the lung, breast, liver, ovary, adrenal gland, Harderian gland, myeloid leukemia, thymic lymphoma, and reticulum cell sarcoma. There was a very wide range in the frequency of these tumors across strains and gender. For example, the incidence of liver cancer varied between 1% and 73.5% in male mice of the two strains studied. For female mice of four strains, the range was 0.1% and 10.7%. This experiment generated 50 data sets on incidence for the nine tumor types. From these data, of 50 dose-tumor slots, there was a near consistent trend for tumor incidence to increase with dose. This was not, however, invariable, in that the incidence of four tumors at 2 Gy was less than at 1 Gy in 23 possible tests. There were fewer cancers in the 0.5 Gy for two tumors than the control groups. In summary, there were examples of a nonlinear dose-response relationship over the range of 0 to 2 Gy for several specific tumors.

Thomson et al.[29] determined tumor frequency after γ ray WBI of 110-day-old female 1776 B6CF1 mice. Doses were 0, 0.225, 0.45, or 0.9 Gy. The incidence of all primary tumors and of epithelial, connective tissue, lymphoreticular, and lung tumors in control and irradiated mice is given in Table 7.1. Tumor incidence was increased only for the lung, at 0.225 and 0.45 Gy. Life span for control mice was 739 days and life shortening was 12, 6, and 34 days after 0.225, 0.45, and 0.9 Gy.

Maisin et al.[30] reported the tumor incidence in 2,907 male C57BL mice following single dose or ten fractions (24 hours between fractions) γ-ray WBI to 0.25, 0.5, 1, 2, 4, or 6 Gy. The mice were 12 weeks old at irradiation and were observed for their life span and then autopsied. Life span declined as the dose increased to 6 Gy, at a rate of 31 days/Gy for single dose, and 20 days/Gy for ten-fraction irradiation. Thus, for the end point of survival time, effectiveness decreased with the change from single to ten fractions. A surprising finding was that the incidence of carcinoma + sarcoma was less than in control mice, for all single acute dose levels, that is, 0.25 to 6 Gy. For leukemia and thymoma, the incidence increased quite sharply at the 4 and 6 Gy doses. For the ten equal dose irradiation assay, the lifetime

TABLE 7.1	Cumulative Risk of Tumor Death at 900 to 999 days, by Tumor Type and Dose[29]			
	Dose (mGy)			
Tumor Type	*0 mGy*	*225 mGy*	*450 mGy*	*900 mGy*
All primary tumors	0.63	0.67	0.62	0.70
Epithelial	0.22	0.23	0.22	0.36
Connective tissue	0.53	0.56	0.52	0.54
Lymphoreticular	0.47	0.50	0.44	0.48
Lung	0.13	0.25	0.28	0.29

incidence of carcinomas and sarcomas, or of all tumors, was generally slightly greater than that of the controls for doses of 0.25 to 6 Gy. That is, ten-fraction irradiation was of equal or moderately higher effectiveness than single dose irradiation for induction of cancer, but substantially less effective in shortening life span.

Single dose 250 kVp x-ray WBI was administered to 629 one-month old female BC3F1 mice and followed for the life span incidence of tumors by Di Majo et al.[31] Doses were 0.04, 0.08, 0.16, and 0.32 Gy. There was a nonlinear increase in tumors with dose to 0.16 and then an apparent decline at 0.32 Gy.

Covelli et al.[32] measured cancer incidence in 2,110 three-month-old male BC3F1 mice given 250 kVp WBI. Frequency of malignant lymphoma and solid tumors was not increased at 0.5 and 1 Gy.

To assess the risk of radiation-induced cancer in beagles, Benjamin et al.[33] delivered ^{60}Co whole-body irradiation to 1,343 beagles at ages from 8 days post coitus to 365 days post partum, and examined life span cancer incidence. The cumulative incidences of all malignancies after 0.16 and 0.83 Gy for all ages at irradiation were similar and higher than controls.

Wood[34] and Yochmowitz et al.[35] reported a 24-year follow-up study of WBI Macaca mullata, treated with γ rays or protons. Monkeys that received 0.2 to 2.8 Gy developed fewer malignant neoplasms than the control animals.

LIFE SHORTENING IN WHOLE-BODY IRRADIATED EXPERIMENTAL ANIMALS

Upton et al.[36] exposed 2,301 RF/Un 8 to 10 week old male mice to low-dose rate WBI γ rays and monitored for duration of life. The doses per days were 0.05, 0.15, and 0.77 Gy. The life span was increased slightly at 0.05, 0.15, and 0.77 Gy/d. As total dose was further increased, survival was reduced. The incidence of tumors was increased in all irradiated groups, but the increase with dose did not follow any obvious pattern. For the female mice, there was a progressive shortening of life span with dose. Tumor incidence was marginally lower at doses of 0.02 to 0.28 Gy in five of seven groups, that is, different from that found for male mice. At higher doses, the incidence was raised at all but a few dose levels.

Thomson et al.[37] gave fractionated WBI to male B6CF1 mice on a one fraction per week schedule of 0.07 or 0.32 Gy to total doses of 4.2 and 19.2 Gy. Life shortening was 36 and 274 days; similar effects were obtained by irradiation of female mice.

Tanaka et al.[38] employed 2,000 male and 2,000 female 8-week-old B6C3F1 mice in an investigation of low-dose γ-ray WBI for approximately 400 consecutive days. The dose rates were 0, 0.05, 1, and 20 mGy/d. Even at these very low doses, life span declined consistently with increasing dose.

Caratero et al.[39] delivered duration-of-life WBI to three groups of 300 female C57BL mice (a total of 900 mice). The mean survival times were 550, 673, and 674 days for cumulative total doses of 0, 70, and 140 mGy, a significantly increased life span at both dose levels.

EXTRAPOLATION OF OBSERVED LOW-DOSE RISKS TO LOWER DOSES

At doses below those where significant risks have been demonstrated in human populations (below 50–100 mSv [protracted

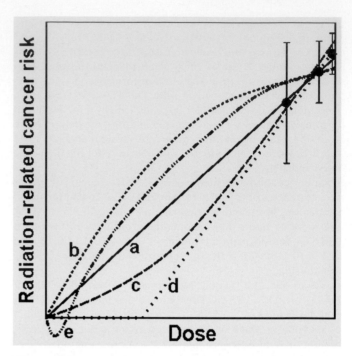

Figure 7.1. Schematic of different possible extrapolations of measured radiation risks down to very low doses, all of which could, in principle, be consistent with higher-dose epidemiological data. *a*: linear extrapolation; *b*: downwardly curving (decreasing slope); *c*: upwardly curving (increasing slope); *d*: threshold; *e*: hormetic.

exposure] or 10–50 mSv [acute exposure]), we cannot use epidemiological data alone to establish the shape of the dose-response relation. All the dose-response relations shown in Figure 7.1 are possible descriptors of low-dose radiation oncogenesis—and different endpoints may well exhibit differently shaped dose-response relations.

LINEAR DOSE-RESPONSE RELATIONS

At the low and intermediate doses that are amenable to statistically meaningful analysis, many data sets are available, both from epidemiological and laboratory studies, that are consistent with a linear dose-response relation. The data have been extensively reviewed in a recent NCRP Report,[40] which concluded "*although other dose-response relationships for the mutagenic and carcinogenic effects of low-level radiation cannot be excluded, no alternate dose-response relationship appears to be more plausible than the linear-nonthreshold model on the basis of present scientific knowledge*," and likewise in the recent BEIR-VII report "*A comprehensive review of available biological and biophysical data supports a 'linear-no-threshold' (LNT) risk model—that the risk of cancer proceeds in a linear fashion at lower doses without a threshold and that the smallest dose has the potential to cause a small increase in risk to humans.*"[41]

At still lower doses, which may not be amenable to direct study, the *biophysical* rationale for linearity (Fig. 7.1 curve *a*) relates to the unique, stochastic, nature of ionizing-radiation energy deposition. The biophysical rationale is essentially:

1. There is direct epidemiological evidence that an organ dose of 10 mGy of diagnostic x-rays is associated with an increase in cancer risk (specifically childhood cancer after in utero exposure[9,10]).

2. At an organ dose of 10 mGy of diagnostic x-rays, most irradiated cell nuclei will be traversed by one or at most a few physically distant electron tracks. Being physically far separated, it is very unlikely that these few electrons tracks could produce DNA damage in some joint, cooperative way; rather these electron tracks will almost certainly act independently to produce stochastic damage and consequent cellular changes.

3. If the dose is decreased, say by a factor of 10, this will simply result in proportionately fewer electron tracks and fewer hit cells. It follows that those fewer cells that are hit at the lower dose (a) will be subject to the same types of electron damage, and (b) will be subject to the same radiobiological processes, as would occur at 10 mGy.

4. Thus, decreasing the number of damaged cells by a factor of 10 would be expected to decrease the biological response by the same factor of 10, that is, the response would decrease linearly with decreasing dose. This argument suggests that the risk of most radiation-induced endpoints will decrease linearly, without a threshold, from approximately 10 mGy down to arbitrarily low doses.

This biophysical argument for linearity considers radiation effects due to autonomous responses of individual cells. Even for clonally cancers, it is likely that oncogenesis involves, in an essential way, interactions among different cells.[42] Cooperative multicellular radiation effects that have been observed to date, such as bystander effects[43] and delayed-instability,[44,45] show saturation at low doses which, in turn, could underlie downwardly curving dose-response relations (Fig. 7.1 curve *b*, see below).

SCENARIOS IN WHICH AN ASSUMPTION OF LINEARITY COULD UNDERESTIMATE LOW-DOSE RISKS

There is evidence for the presence of downwardly curving (decreasing slope) dose-response relations, both from epidemiologic and laboratory studies. The most recent low-dose A-bomb survivor data for both cancer mortality and cancer incidence appear to exhibit this shape. Of course, the shape of the dose-response at these low doses cannot be unequivocally established through epidemiological studies—and this is even less likely to be feasible at still lower doses.

Such downwardly curving dose-response relations for human responses have been interpreted in several ways. The first is the existence of small subpopulations of individuals who are hypersensitive to radiation.[7] Some genetically based radiosensitive subpopulations have been identified, such as *Atm*[46–48] and *Brca1*[49–51] heterozygotes, though the links with radiation-induced cancer sensitivity are still controversial.[52,53]

A second interpretation of downwardly-curving dose-response relations (Fig. 7.1 curve *b*) is in terms of induced radioresistance, sometimes called *adaptive response*, in which a small "priming" radiation dose (typically 5–100 mGy) decreases the radiosensitivity to subsequent larger radiation exposures, perhaps by upregulating some DNA repair mechanisms. The phenomenon has been reported for carcinogenesis,[54] cellular inactivation,[55] mutation induction,[56] chromosome aberration formation,[57] and *in vitro* oncogenic transformation.[58] There is no evidence to suggest that a priming dose can actually eliminate subsequent radioresponsiveness. Available data suggest that the induced radioresistance is transitory, lasting in the range from

4 to 48 hours, which suggests that the phenomenon could be of limited relevance for prolonged low-dose radiation exposures. In experiments in which the effect has been observed in human cells, there is always considerable interindividual variation. It has been reported that the capacity for induced radioresistance decreases significantly with age.[59]

As discussed above, a third interpretation is that downwardly curving dose-response relations (Fig. 7.1 curve *b*) are the result of bystander effects.[43,60] The bystander effect involves radiation-damaged cells sending out signals to adjacent cells that were not directly hit by the radiation; these signals can potentially result in oncogenic damage to the bystander cells.[61] Bystander effects are characterized by a steep response at low doses, reflecting a large number of cells receiving a damage signal from adjacent radiation-damaged cells. At somewhat higher doses, however, the bystander effect saturates (because all relevant cells that can be affected are already affected), which results in a characteristic downwardly curving dose-response relation such as Figure 7.1 curve *b*.[62] Bystander effects have been extensively demonstrated in the laboratory for α radiation and, to a lesser extent, x-rays.[60] While there is evidence that bystander effects may be relevant to low-dose risks from radon (α particle) exposure,[63] their relevance to low-dose x- or γ-ray risks has yet to be established.

SCENARIOS IN WHICH AN ASSUMPTION OF LINEARITY COULD OVERESTIMATE LOW-DOSE RISKS

A threshold in dose (Fig. 7.1 curve *d*) implies that there is some dose below which the risk of a particular endpoint being induced is zero. A possible example is radiation-induced sarcoma (malignancies originating in connective tissue) that is rarely observed at low doses[64]—potentially in part because non-cycling connective-tissue cells need a large dose to stimulate them to cycle.[65] Thus, for example, after radiotherapy there is a significant risk of secondary sarcomas in or near the high-dose (>50 Gy) treatment region, but not in distant organs exposed to low doses.[66,67] The different risk patterns for sarcomas and carcinomas are borne out in the A-bomb survivors,[68] among whom a significant increase in bone-cancer mortality has not been observed (mean dose: 200 mSv, $p = 0.4$), but a significant increase in carcinomas—which originate in cells which are already cycling—is clearly seen ($p < 10^{-4}$).

A hormetic response (Fig. 7.1 curve *e*) would occur if a given dose of radiation reduced the background incidence of some deleterious endpoint. For example, there have been convincing reports that, for some cell lines and for some animal strains, low and intermediate doses of radiation can reduce oncogenic rates, or enhance longevity (review: Ref. 69), so-called hormetic responses. For example, Maisin et al.[70] report that 138 C57BL mice lived an average of 50 days longer than controls after exposure to an acute x-ray dose of 500 mGy; by contrast, in a larger study, Storer et al.[71] report that 1,390 RFM mice lived an average of 75 days less than controls when exposed to the same acute dose of γ rays.

In those animal experiments in which an increase in lifespan has been observed, the gain has generally not reflected a reduction in malignant disease, but rather an early reduction in mortality from infections and other nonmalignant diseases.[69,70] This finding suggests that a lifespan increase, if real, is less likely to be associated with a radiation-related stimulation of DNA repair mechanisms,[72] and more likely to be associated with a radiation-induced enhancement in the immune system.[73]

SUMMARY: LOW RADIATION DOSES

Above doses of 50 to 100 mSv (protracted exposure) or 10 to 50 mSv (acute exposure), there is direct epidemiological evidence from human populations that exposure to ionizing radiation increases the risk of some cancers. The methodological difficulties inherent in low-dose epidemiological studies suggest that it is unlikely that we will be able to directly and precisely quantify cancer risks in human populations at doses much below 10 mSv. Our inability to quantify such risks does not, however, imply that the corresponding societal risks are necessarily negligible—a very small risk, if applied to a large number of individuals, can result in a significant public health problem.

At present, we cannot be sure of the appropriate dose-response relation to use for risk estimation at very low doses. As discussed above, there are mechanistic arguments suggesting that a linear extrapolation of risks to very low doses is appropriate, but testing such arguments at very low doses, particular in human populations, is generally not feasible. However, the alternate models shown in Figure 7.1, while applicable for some endpoints, are less appropriate than the linear model as a generic descriptor of radiation carcinogenesis at low doses and low-dose rates. This is the logic used by the various regulatory agencies in applying the linear model for radiation protection purposes.[40,41,74,75]

HIGH-DOSE RADIATION RISKS ASSOCIATED WITH RADIOTHERAPY

The ability to predict radiation-induced cancer risks associated with modern radiation therapy protocols should allow the risks of second cancers to be included, and potentially reduced, in radiation therapy treatment plan optimization. This consideration is of mounting importance in light of the increasing number of younger patients undergoing radiation therapy and with progressively longer survival times. As screening programs lead to earlier treatment and at younger ages, and as improvements in radiotherapy result in longer survival times, the issue of radiation-induced second cancers is becoming increasingly important.[76,77] The 5-year relative survival rate for prostate cancer in the United States has increased from about 67% in the mid-1970s to about 98% in the 1990s,[78] while the mean age at diagnosis decreased from 72 to 69.[79] The corresponding 10-year relative survival rates are now 76% for both prostate and breast.

Of particular importance in this regard are radiation-induced second cancers in childhood radiation therapy survivors,[80–82] who (a) are probably inherently more sensitive to radiation-induced carcinogenesis than adults, and (b) hopefully have more years of life remaining.

An example of the magnitude of the risks of concern can be seen from the results of a retrospective tumor-registry–based study[66] that compared second cancers in prostate cancer survivors who had radiotherapy, versus those who had surgery: Here, the risks of developing a radiation-associated second malignancy after prostate cancer radiotherapy were estimated as 1 in 290 (all years), 1 in 125 for 5+ year survivors, and 1 in 70 for 10+ year survivors. As expected, second-cancer risks are

much higher in long-term survivors of pediatric radiotherapy, approaching 25% at 30 years.[81] In this context, it is important to note the increased use of chemotherapy in addition to radiation for pediatric cancers,[83] particularly in regard to acute non-lymphocytic leukemic second cancers.[84]

Using retrospective techniques, many such studies of second-cancer risks after radiation therapy have been reported.[66,77,85–95] However, radiotherapy treatment techniques are constantly changing, particularly in terms of escalating treatment dose,[96–98] altered dose fractionation/protraction,[99–102] and differing normal-tissue dose distributions, such as from intensity-modulated radiation therapy[103,104] and particle-beam therapy.[105,106] Consequently, results from second-cancer studies that are the results of treatments that took place several decades ago cannot generally be directly applied to modern-day treatment methods. Before data do become available, this issue can be addressed by developing models that prospectively predict, through use of organ doses or dose distributions, second cancers associated with current radiation therapeutic treatments. Such models also provide insight into the basic mechanisms of radiation carcinogenesis.[107]

MECHANISMS OF RADIATION-INDUCED CANCER AT RADIOTHERAPEUTIC DOSES

The Standard High-Dose Model

For most sites, radiation therapy can deliver very high doses to regions in organs that are in or close to the target volume.[108] In earlier approaches to high-dose risk estimation, radiation-induced carcinogenesis at high doses was assumed to be governed primarily by two competing cellular processes,[109] "initiation" and "inactivation." *Initiation* is the production of changes that make a stem cell premalignant; examples are chromosomal translocations, such as the Philadelphia chromosome,[110] or other cytogenetic abnormalities such as inversions, small-scale mutations, deletions, duplications, or aneuploidy.[111–113] *Inactivation* prevents a stem cell from having viable progeny, examples being mitotic death or apoptosis.

The assumption that radiation carcinogenesis is primarily governed by initiation and inactivation has generally been quantified using the standard linear-quadratic-exponential (LQE) equation[109]; for reviews, see Refs. 107,114, and 115. The LQE equation describes the excess relative cancer risk (ERR) after a single acute dose of radiation (D) as

$$\text{ERR} = (aD + bD^2) \exp(-\alpha D - \beta D^2) \tag{1}$$

where a and b are linear and quadratic coefficients for initiation, and α and β are linear and quadratic coefficients for inactivation. The LQE equation uses the classic linear-quadratic (LQ) form both for radiation-induced initiation ($aD + bD^2$) and for radiation-induced inactivation $\exp(-\alpha D - \beta D^2)$.

For small and intermediate radiation doses, Eq. (1) predicts that ERR is an increasing function of dose, as is seen epidemiologically.[87,88,116,117] At high doses, however, the exponential cellular inactivation term, $\exp(-\alpha D - \beta D^2)$, in this LQE equation leads to very small predicted ERRs; that is, essentially all radiation-initiated premalignant stem cells would be inactivated by the radiation. As shown in Figure 7.2,[107] this prediction of the LQE equation is inconsistent with recent estimates of radiation-induced solid cancer risks, in that a rapid decrease in the ERR at high doses is not observed.

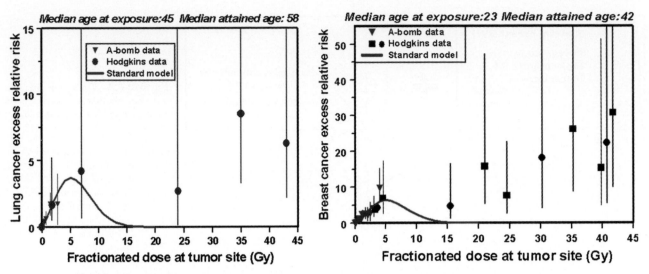

Figure 7.2. ERRs for radiation-induced lung cancer (**left**) and breast cancer (**right**). The lower-dose data points from A-bomb survivors,[118,119] and the data points at high doses are from studies of lung cancer[120] and breast cancer[121,122] after radiotherapy of Hodgkin disease patients. The solid curves in each panel represent fits to the A-bomb data using the standard "initiation + killing" LQE model,[109] which involves a balance solely between induction of premalignant cells and cell killing, without considering cellular repopulation. It is clear that the predictions of this standard LQE model are inconsistent with the high-dose data.

More Realistic High-Dose Models

Consequently, the standard LQE initiation-inactivation model has been extended[107] to include a third mechanism, in addition to initiation and inactivation, of radiation-induced carcinogenesis at high doses. Specifically, symmetric stem-cell proliferation (i.e., a stem cell dividing into two daughter stem cells) occurs in response to radiation-induced cell killing,[123–126] and replenishes the number of stem cells in that organ. Because repopulating cells can only travel very small distances, at least for solid organs, they will have been near the treatment field at the time of irradiation, so will have received significant doses, and so will contain a significant fraction of stem cells with premalignant damage. Symmetric proliferation, which takes place both during and after radiation therapy, will thus increase the high-dose

cancer risk, as any proliferating stem cell that has premalignant damage can pass that damage on to its progeny.

In fact, there is a great deal of quantitative biology in the literature about repopulation kinetics,[123–126] which can be reasonably grafted on to the standard initiation/inactivation model, resulting in a quantitative initiation/inactivation/proliferation model, as discussed in the next section.

PROSPECTIVE ESTIMATION OF RADIOTHERAPY-INDUCED SECOND-CANCER RISKS

The stem cell initiation/inactivation/proliferation model[107,127,128] outlined here provides a practical approach[129] for predicting organ-specific high-dose cancer risks based on (a) cancer risk data from A-bomb survivors (who were exposed to lower doses),

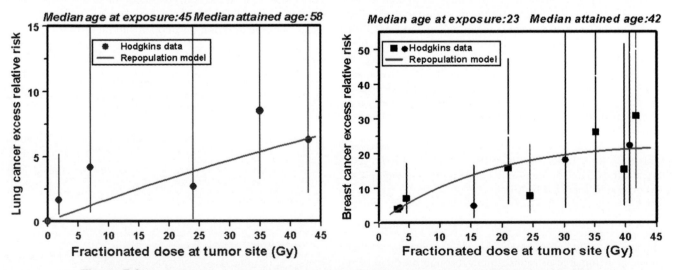

Figure 7.3. Measured and predicted ERRs for lung cancer (**left**) and breast cancer (**right**) induced by high doses of fractionated ionizing radiation. The data points are from studies of second cancers after radiotherapy of Hodgkin disease patients, as in Figure 7.1, and the curves are estimates using the methodology[107] outlined here.

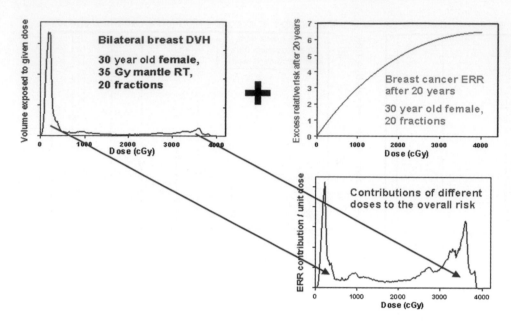

Figure 7.4. Estimation of radiation-induced second-cancer risks based on an appropriate dose-volume histogram (**top left**), in this case for the breasts of a 30-year-old female given 35 Gy of fractionated mantle radiotherapy, and (**top right**) an estimated dose-risk relation (using the approach described in the text) for fractionated radiation-induced breast cancer, 20 years after exposure. For this individual, the result is an estimated[129] ERR for radiation-induced breast cancer, 20 years post exposure, of 2.1 [95% CI: 1.1, 6.1]. The lower graph shows the estimated contribution of different doses within the breasts to the overall ERR.

(b) the demographic variables (age, time since exposure, gender, ethnicity) of the population/individual of interest, and (c) an organ-specific parameter describing radiation-induced cellular repopulation, which has previously been estimated both for breast and lung.[107] First, ERRs are directly estimated for single radiation exposures at moderate doses, based on cancer incidence data among A-bomb survivors.[5,118] Second, a well-established methodology described by Land et al.[130] (and almost identically in the recent BEIR-VII report[131] is used to adjust the dose-dependent ERRs from the A-bomb survivors to apply to the demographics (age, time since exposure, gender, ethnicity) of the individual or group under study. These two steps are implemented through publicly available online software (Interactive RadioEpidemiological Program, IREP[132]). Finally, these moderate-dose ERR estimates for single exposures are adjusted to fractionated high-dose radiation exposure, using the initiation/inactivation/proliferation model[107] outlined above. This augmented cancer risk model is able to well describe demographics-specific epidemiological data for radiotherapy-induced carcinogenesis[107,127]; examples are shown in Figure 7.3.

The approach can, in principle, generate organ-specific ERR estimates for any given radiotherapeutic dose and fractionation scheme, for any given set of demographics (in particular age at exposure, and time post exposure). Essentially all that is needed are dose-volume histogram (DVH) data for the organ or organs of interest. In this "dosimetric + risk-modeling" method, each incremental small volume in the DVH, ΔV_j, is associated with a total dose $D_j = j\Delta D$. Given the associated $\mathrm{ERR}(D_j)$, estimated as described above, the overall predicted ERR is the volume average of these local ERRs, that is, $\mathrm{ERR} = (1/V) \sum_j \mathrm{ERR}(D_j) \Delta V_j$, where V is the organ volume. An example is given in Figure 7.4, based on results reported by Koh et al.[129]

SUMMARY: HIGH RADIATION DOSES

Understanding and quantifying second-cancer risks is the first step toward being able to reduce them through hardware and software optimization—conceptually in the same way as classic early and late sequelae have been reduced by advances in hardware and by increasingly sophisticated treatment planning. This

being said, it is crucial to ensure that any changes in treatment technique designed to decrease second-cancer risks do not impact negatively on primary tumor control.

We are a long way from being able to estimate radiation-induced cancer risks ab initio, that is, solely based on biologically based models. The approach described here, which appears to be reasonably promising, is to use cancer risks originally estimated in A-bomb survivors, modify them for the demographic cohort or individual of interest, and then, guided by available second-cancer risk data, extrapolate these risks to higher doses using the quantitative biological models described here. Finally, combining the results using organ-specific DVHs allows realistic prospective estimates of radiotherapy-related second-cancer risks.

Of course, there remain considerable uncertainties in these modeling approaches. For example, it remains unclear to what extent radiation-induced second-cancer risks depend on the primary cancer, over and above the different dose distributions. A recent study of CNS tumors in survivors of childhood cancers concluded that "after adjustment for radiation dose, neither original cancer diagnosis nor chemotherapy was associated with risk,"[80] but the question is still open and important.

REFERENCES

1. Pochin EE. Problems involved in detecting increased malignancy rates in areas of high natural radiation background. *Health Phys.* 1976;31:148–151.
2. Land CE. Estimating cancer risks from low doses of ionizing radiation. *Science.* 1980;209:1197–1203.
3. Preston DL, Shimizu Y, Pierce DA, et al. Studies of mortality of atomic bomb survivors. Report 13: solid cancer and noncancer disease mortality: 1950–1997. *Radiat Res.* 2003;160:381–407.
4. Pierce DA, Preston DL. Radiation-related cancer risks at low doses among atomic bomb survivors. *Radiat Res.* 2000;154:178–186.
5. Preston DL, Ron E, Tokuoka S, et al. Solid cancer incidence in atomic bomb survivors: 1958–1998. *Radiat Res.* 2007;168:1–64.
6. Pierce DA. Age-time patterns of radiogenic cancer risk: their nature and likely explanations. *J Radiol Prot.* 2002;22:A147–A154.
7. ICRP. Genetic susceptibility to cancer, ICRP Publication 79. *International Commission on Radiological Protection.* Oxford: Pergamon Press; 1999.
8. Herold DM, Hanlon AL, Hanks GE. Diabetes mellitus: a predictor for late radiation morbidity. *Int J Radiat Oncol Biol Phys.* 1999;43:475–479.
9. Doll R, Wakeford R. Risk of childhood cancer from fetal irradiation. *Br J Radiol.* 1997;70:130–139.
10. Mole RH. Childhood cancer after prenatal exposure to diagnostic X-ray examinations in Britain. *Br J Cancer.* 1990;62:152–168.

11. Cardis E, Vrijheid M, Blettner M, et al. The 15-country collaborative study of cancer risk among radiation workers in the nuclear industry: estimates of radiation-related cancer risks. *Radiat Res.* 2007;167:396–416.
12. Wakeford R. More on the risk of cancer among nuclear workers. *J Radiol Prot.* 2009;29:1–4.
13. Muirhead CR, O'Hagan JA, Haylock RG, et al. Mortality and cancer incidence following occupational radiation exposure: third analysis of the National Registry for Radiation Workers. *Br J Cancer.* 2009;100:206–212.
14. Morin Doody M, Lonstein JE, Stovall M, et al. Breast cancer mortality after diagnostic radiography: findings from the U.S. Scoliosis Cohort Study. *Spine.* 2000;25:2052–2063.
15. Ron E, Modan B, Preston D, et al. Thyroid neoplasia following low-dose radiation in childhood. *Radiat Res.* 1989;120:516–531.
16. Ron E, Lubin JH, Shore RE, et al. Thyroid cancer after exposure to external radiation: a pooled analysis of seven studies. *Radiat Res.* 1995;141:259–277.
17. Heyes GJ, Mill AJ, Charles M. Enhanced biological effectiveness of low energy X-rays and implications for the UK breast screening programme (Authors' Reply). *Br J Radiol.* 2006;79:855–857.
18. Borek C, Hall EJ. Transformation of mammalian cells in vitro by low doses of X-rays. *Nature.* 1973;243:450–453.
19. Han A, Elkind MM. Transformation of mouse C3H/10T1/2 cells by single and fractionated doses of X-rays and fission-spectrum neutrons. *Cancer Res.* 1979;39:123–130.
20. Han A, Hill CK, Elkind MM. Repair of cell killing and neoplastic transformation at reduced dose rates of 60Co gamma-rays. *Cancer Res.* 1980;40:3328–3332.
21. Miller RC, Geard CR, Brenner DJ, et al. Neutron-energy-dependent oncogenic transformation of C3H 10T1/2 mouse cells. *Radiat Res.* 1989;117:114–127.
22. Heyes GJ, Mill AJ. The neoplastic transformation potential of mammography X rays and atomic bomb spectrum radiation. *Radiat Res.* 2004;162:120–127.
23. Azzam EI, de Toledo SM, Raaphorst GP, et al. Low-dose ionizing radiation decreases the frequency of neoplastic transformation to a level below the spontaneous rate in C3H 10T1/2 cells. *Radiat Res.* 1996;146:369–373.
24. Elmore E, Lao XY, Ko M, et al. Neoplastic transformation in vitro induced by low doses of 232 MeV protons. *Int J Radiat Biol.* 2005;81:291–297.
25. Redpath JL, Lu Q, Lao X, et al. Low doses of diagnostic energy X-rays protect against neoplastic transformation in vitro. *Int J Radiat Biol.* 2003;79:235–240.
26. Ullrich RL, Jernigan MC, Cosgrove GE, et al. The influence of dose and dose rate on the incidence of neoplastic disease in RFM mice after neutron irradiation. *Radiat Res.* 1976;68:115–131.
27. Ullrich RL, Preston RJ. Myeloid leukemia in male RFM mice following irradiation with fission spectrum neutrons or gamma rays. *Radiat Res.* 1987;109:165–170.
28. Storer JB, Mitchell TJ, Fry RJ. Extrapolation of the relative risk of radiogenic neoplasms across mouse strains and to man. *Radiat Res.* 1988;114:331–353.
29. Thomson JF, Williamson FS, Grahn D. Life shortening in mice exposed to fission neutrons and gamma rays. V. Further studies with single low doses. *Radiat Res.* 1985;104:420–428.
30. Maisin JR, Wambersie A, Gerber GB, et al. Life-shortening and disease incidence in C57Bl mice after single and fractionated gamma and high-energy neutron exposure. *Radiat Res.* 1988;113:300–317.
31. Di Majo V, Rebessi S, Pazzaglia S, et al. Carcinogenesis in laboratory mice after low doses of ionizing radiation. *Radiat Res.* 2003;159:102–108.
32. Covelli V, Di Majo V, Coppola M, et al. The dose-response relationships for myeloid leukemia and malignant lymphoma in BC3F1 mice. *Radiat Res.* 1989;119:553–561.
33. Benjamin SA, Lee AC, Angleton GM, et al. Mortality in beagles irradiated during prenatal and postnatal development. II. Contribution of benign and malignant neoplasia. *Radiat Res.* 1998;150:330–348.
34. Wood DH. Long-term mortality and cancer risk in irradiated rhesus monkeys. *Radiat Res.* 1991;126:132–140.
35. Yochmowitz MG, Wood DH, Salmon YL. Seventeen-year mortality experience of proton radiation in Macaca mulatta. *Radiat Res.* 1985;102:14–34.
36. Upton AC, Randolph ML, Conklin JW, et al. Late effects of fast neutrons and gamma-rays in mice as influenced by the dose rate of irradiation: induction of neoplasia. *Radiat Res.* 1970;41:467–491.
37. Thomson JF, Williamson FS, Grahn D, et al. Life shortening in mice exposed to fission neutrons and gamma rays. II. Duration-of-life and long-term fractionated exposures. *Radiat Res.* 1981;86:573–579.
38. Tanaka S, Tanaka IB III, Sasagawa S, et al. No lengthening of life span in mice continuously exposed to gamma rays at very low dose rates. *Radiat Res.* 2003;160:376–379.
39. Caratero A, Courtade M, Bonnet L, et al. Effect of a continuous gamma irradiation at a very low dose on the life span of mice. *Gerontology.* 1998;44:272–276.
40. NCRP. Evaluation of the linear-nonthreshold dose-response model for ionizing radiation, Report No. 136. *National Council on Radiation Protection and Measurements.* Bethesda, MD: NCRP; 2001.
41. National Research Council of the National Academies. *Health Risks from Exposure to Low Levels of Ionizing Radiation—BEIR VII.* Washington, DC: The National Academies Press; 2006.
42. Barcellos-Hoff MH. It takes a tissue to make a tumor: epigenetics, cancer and the microenvironment. *J Mammary Gland Biol Neoplasia.* 2001;6:213–221.
43. Nagasawa H, Little JB. Unexpected sensitivity to the induction of mutations by very low doses of alpha-particle radiation: evidence for a bystander effect. *Radiat Res.* 1999;152:552–557.
44. Ullrich RL, Davis CM. Radiation-induced cytogenetic instability in vivo. *Radiat Res.* 1999;152:170–173.
45. Little JB. Radiation carcinogenesis. *Carcinogenesis (Oxford).* 2000;21:397–404.
46. Hall EJ, Schiff PB, Hanks GE, et al. A preliminary report: frequency of A-T heterozygotes among prostate cancer patients with severe late responses to radiation therapy. *Cancer J Sci Am.* 1998;4:385–389.
47. Smilenov LB, Brenner DJ, Hall EJ. Modest increased sensitivity to radiation oncogenesis in ATM heterozygous versus wild-type mammalian cells. *Cancer Res.* 2001;61:5710–5713.
48. Swift M, Morrell D, Massey RB, et al. Incidence of cancer in 161 families affected by ataxia-telangiectasia. *N Engl J Med.* 1991;325:1831–1836.
49. Buchholz TA, Wu X, Hussain A, et al. Evidence of haplotype insufficiency in human cells containing a germline mutation in BRCA1 or BRCA2. *Int J Cancer.* 2002;97:557–561.
50. Rothfuss A, Schutz P, Bochum S, et al. Induced micronucleus frequencies in peripheral lymphocytes as a screening test for carriers of a BRCA1 mutation in breast cancer families. *Cancer Res.* 2000;60:390–394.
51. Xia F, Powell SN. The molecular basis of radiosensitivity and chemosensitivity in the treatment of breast cancer. *Semin Radiat Oncol.* 2002;12:296–304.
52. Broeks A, Russell NS, Floore AN, et al. Increased risk of breast cancer following irradiation for Hodgkin's disease is not a result of ATM germline mutations. *Int J Radiat Biol.* 2000;76:693–698.
53. Shafman TD, Levitz S, Nixon AJ, et al. Prevalence of germline truncating mutations in ATM in women with a second breast cancer after radiation therapy for a contralateral tumor. *Genes Chromosomes Cancer.* 2000;27:124–129.
54. Bhattacharjee D, Ito A. Deceleration of carcinogenic potential by adaptation with low dose gamma irradiation. *In Vivo.* 2001;15:87–92.
55. Joiner MC, Marples B, Lambin P, et al. Low-dose hypersensitivity: current status and possible mechanisms. *Int J Radiat Oncol Biol Phys.* 2001;49:379–389.
56. Ueno AM, Vannais DB, Gustafson DL, et al. A low, adaptive dose of gamma-rays reduced the number and altered the spectrum of S1-mutants in human-hamster hybrid AL cells. *Mutat Res.* 1996;358:161–169.
57. Wolff S. The adaptive response in radiobiology: evolving insights and implications. *Environ Health Perspect.* 1998;106(suppl 1):277–283.
58. Azzam EI, Raaphorst GP, Mitchel RE. Radiation-induced adaptive response for protection against micronucleus formation and neoplastic transformation in C3H 10T1/2 mouse embryo cells. *Radiat Res.* 1994;138:S28–S31.
59. Gadhia PK. Possible age-dependent adaptive response to a low dose of X-rays in human lymphocytes. *Mutagenesis.* 1998;13:151–152.
60. Ballarini F, Biaggi M, Ottolenghi A, et al. Cellular communication and bystander effects: a critical review for modelling low-dose radiation action. *Mutat Res.* 2002;501:1–12.
61. Sawant SG, Randers-Pehrson G, Geard CR, et al. The bystander effect in radiation oncogenesis: I. Transformation in C3H 10T1/2 cells in vitro can be initiated in the unirradiated neighbors of irradiated cells. *Radiat Res.* 2001;155:397–401.
62. Brenner DJ, Little JB, Sachs RK. The bystander effect in radiation oncogenesis: II. A quantitative model. *Radiat Res.* 2001;155:402–408.
63. Brenner DJ, Sachs RK. Do low dose-rate bystander effects influence domestic radon risks? *J Radiat Biol.* 2002;78:593–604.
64. White RG, Raabe OG, Culbertson MR, et al. Bone sarcoma characteristics and distribution in beagles fed strontium-90. *Radiat Res.* 1993;136:178–189.
65. Hall EJ. Do no harm—normal tissue effects. *Acta Oncol.* 2001;40:913–916.
66. Brenner DJ, Curtis RE, Hall EJ, et al. Second malignancies in prostate carcinoma patients after radiotherapy compared with surgery. *Cancer.* 2000;88:398–406.
67. Kuttesch JF Jr, Wexler LH, Marcus RB, et al. Second malignancies after Ewing's sarcoma: radiation dose-dependency of secondary sarcomas. *J Clin Oncol.* 1996;14:2818–2825.
68. Pierce DA, Shimizu Y, Preston DL, et al. Studies of the mortality of atomic bomb survivors. Report 12, Part I. Cancer: 1950–1990. *Radiat Res.* 1996;146:1–27.
69. Upton AC. Radiation hormesis: data and interpretations. *Crit Rev Toxicol.* 2001;31:681–695.
70. Maisin JR, Gerber GB, Vankerkom J, et al. Survival and diseases in C57BL mice exposed to X rays or 3.1 MeV neutrons at an age of 7 or 21 days. *Radiat Res.* 1996;146:453–460.
71. Storer JB, Serrano LJ, Darden EB Jr, et al. Life shortening in RFM and BALB/c mice as a function of radiation quality, dose, and dose rate. *Radiat Res.* 1979;78:122–161.
72. Pollycove M, Feinendegen LE. Molecular biology, epidemiology, and the demise of the linear no-threshold (LNT) hypothesis. *CR Acad Sci III.* 1999;322:197–204.
73. Xu Y, Greenstock CL, Trivedi A, et al. Occupational levels of radiation exposure induce surface expression of interleukin-2 receptors in stimulated human peripheral blood lymphocytes. *Radiat Environ Biophys.* 1996;35:89–93.
74. UNSCEAR. *2006 Report. Vol 1: Effects of Ionizing Radiation.* New York, United Nations; 2008.
75. ICRP. The 2007 Recommendations of the International Commission on Radiological Protection. *Ann ICRP.* 2007;37:1–332.
76. Travis LB. Therapy-associated solid tumors. *Acta Oncol.* 2002;41:323–333.
77. Curtis RE, Freedman DM, Ron E, et al. eds. *New Malignancies Among Cancer Survivors: SEER Cancer Registries, 1973–2000.* Bethesda: NIH Publication No. 05-5302; 2006.
78. Jemal A, Tiwari RC, Murray T, et al. Cancer statistics, 2004. *CA Cancer J Clin.* 2004; 54:8–29.
79. Farkas A, Schneider D, Perrotti M, et al. National trends in the epidemiology of prostate cancer, 1973 to 1994: evidence for the effectiveness of prostate-specific antigen screening. *Urology.* 1998;52:444–448.
80. Neglia JP, Robison LL, Stovall M, et al. New primary neoplasms of the central nervous system in survivors of childhood cancer: a report from the Childhood Cancer Survivor Study. *J Natl Cancer Inst.* 2006;98:1528–1537.
81. Bhatia S, Yasui Y, Robison LL, et al. High risk of subsequent neoplasms continues with extended follow-up of childhood Hodgkin's disease: report from the Late Effects Study Group. *J Clin Oncol.* 2003;21:4386–4394.
82. Gold DG, Neglia JP, Dusenbery KE. Second neoplasms after megavoltage radiation for pediatric tumors. *Cancer.* 2003;97:2588–2596.
83. Donaldson SS, Hancock SL, Hoppe RT. The Janeway lecture. Hodgkin's disease—finding the balance between cure and late effects. *Cancer J Sci Am.* 1999;5:325–333.
84. Inskip PD, Curtis RE. New malignancies following childhood cancer in the United States, 1973–2002. *Int J Cancer.* 2007;121:2233–2240.
85. van Leeuwen FE, Travis LB. Second Cancers. In: Devita VT, Hellman S, Rosenberg SA, eds. *Cancer: Principles and Practice of Oncology.* Philadelphia, PA: Lippincott, Williams & Wilkins; 2004.
86. Ron E. Cancer risks from medical radiation. *Health Phys.* 2003;85:47–59.

87. Little MP. Comparison of the risks of cancer incidence and mortality following radiation therapy for benign and malignant disease with the cancer risks observed in the Japanese A-bomb survivors. *Int J Radiat Biol.* 2001;77:431–464.

88. Travis LB, Andersson M, Gospodarowicz M, et al. Treatment-associated leukemia following testicular cancer. *J Natl Cancer Inst.* 2000;92:1165–1171.

89. Weiss HA, Darby SC, Fearn T, et al. Leukemia mortality after X-ray treatment for ankylosing spondylitis. *Radiat Res.* 1995;142:1–11.

90. Curtis RE, Boice JD Jr, Stovall M, et al. Relationship of leukemia risk to radiation dose following cancer of the uterine corpus. *J Natl Cancer Inst.* 1994;86:1315–1324.

91. Boice JD Jr, Engholm G, Kleinerman RA, et al. Radiation dose and second cancer risk in patients treated for cancer of the cervix. *Radiat Res.* 1988;116:3–55.

92. Inskip PD, Kleinerman RA, Stovall M, et al. Leukemia, lymphoma, and multiple myeloma after pelvic radiotherapy for benign disease. *Radiat Res.* 1993;135:108–124.

93. Boice JD Jr, Blettner M, Kleinerman RA, et al. Radiation dose and leukemia risk in patients treated for cancer of the cervix. *J Natl Cancer Inst.* 1987;79:1295–1311.

94. Little MP, Weiss HA, Boice JD Jr, et al. Risks of leukemia in Japanese atomic bomb survivors, in women treated for cervical cancer, and in patients treated for ankylosing spondylitis. *Radiat Res.* 1999;152:280–292.

95. Thomas DC, Blettner M, Day NE. Case-control study of acute and nonlymphocytic leukemia. *J Natl Cancer Inst.* 1992;84:1600–1601.

96. Zelefsky MJ, Fuks Z, Hunt M, et al. High-dose intensity modulated radiation therapy for prostate cancer: early toxicity and biochemical outcome in 772 patients. *Int J Radiat Oncol Biol Phys.* 2002;53:1111–1116.

97. Arriagada R, Komaki R, Cox JD. Radiation dose escalation in non-small cell carcinoma of the lung. *Semin Radiat Oncol.* 2004;14:287–291.

98. Mangar SA, Huddart RA, Parker CC, et al. Technological advances in radiotherapy for the treatment of localised prostate cancer. *Eur J Cancer.* 2005;41:908–921.

99. Stitt JA. High dose rate brachytherapy in the treatment of cervical carcinoma. *Hematol Oncol Clin North Am.* 1999;13:585–593, vii–viii.

100. Nguyen LN, Ang KK. Radiotherapy for cancer of the head and neck: altered fractionation regimens. *Lancet Oncol.* 2002;3:693–701.

101. Vicini FA, Vargas C, Edmundson G, et al. The role of high-dose rate brachytherapy in locally advanced prostate cancer. *Semin Radiat Oncol.* 2003;13:98–108.

102. Pollack A, Hanlon AL, Horwitz EM, et al. Dosimetry and preliminary acute toxicity in the first 100 men treated for prostate cancer on a randomized hypofractionation dose escalation trial. *Int J Radiat Oncol Biol Phys.* 2006;64:518–526.

103. Hall EJ, Wuu CS. Radiation-induced second cancers: the impact of 3D-CRT and IMRT. *Int J Radiat Oncol Biol Phys.* 2003;56:83–88.

104. Bucci MK, Bevan A, Roach M III. Advances in radiation therapy: conventional to 3D, to IMRT, to 4D, and beyond. *CA Cancer J Clin.* 2005;55:117–134.

105. Cox JD. Proton beam radiation therapy in the treatment of cancer. *Clin Adv Hematol Oncol.* 2004;2:355–356.

106. Suit H, Goldberg S, Niemierko A, et al. Proton beams to replace photon beams in radical dose treatments. *Acta Oncol.* 2003;42:800–808.

107. Sachs RK, Brenner DJ. Solid tumor risks after high doses of ionizing radiation. *Proc Natl Acad Sci USA.* 2005;102:13040–13045.

108. Stovall M, Smith SA, Rosenstein M. Tissue doses from radiotherapy of cancer of the uterine cervix. *Med Phys.* 1989;16:726–733.

109. Gray LH. Radiation biology and cancer. In: *Cellular Radiation Biology; A Symposium Considering Radiation Effects in the Cell and Possible Implications for Cancer Therapy, a Collection of Papers.* Baltimore, MD: William and Wilkins Co.; 1965:8–25.

110. Radivoyevitch T, Hoel DG. Modeling the low-LET dose-response of BCR-ABL formation: predicting stem cell numbers from A-bomb data. *Math Biosci.* 1999;162:85–101.

111. Whang-Peng J, Young RC, Lee EC. Cytogenetic studies in patients with secondary leukemia/dysmyelopoietic syndrome after different treatment modalities. *Blood.* 1988;71:403–414.

112. Christiansen DH, Andersen MK, Desta F. Mutations of genes in the receptor tyrosine kinase (RTK)/RAS-BRAF signal transduction pathway in therapy-related myelodysplasia and acute myeloid leukemia. *Leukemia.* 2005;19:2232–2240.

113. Duesberg P, Rasnick D, Li R, et al. How aneuploidy may cause cancer and genetic instability. *Anticancer Res.* 1999;19:4887–4906.

114. Bennett J, Little MP, Richardson S. Flexible dose-response models for Japanese atomic bomb survivor data: Bayesian estimation and prediction of cancer risk. *Radiat Environ Biophys.* 2004;43:233–245.

115. Dasu A, Toma-Dasu I, Olofsson J, et al. The use of risk estimation models for the induction of secondary cancers following radiotherapy. *Acta Oncol.* 2005;44:339–347.

116. Little MP. Risks associated with ionizing radiation. *Br Med Bull.* 2003;68:259–275.

117. Preston DL, Kusumi S, Tomonaga M, et al. Cancer incidence in atomic bomb survivors. Part III. Leukemia, lymphoma and multiple myeloma, 1950–1987. *Radiat Res.* 1994;137:S68–9S7.

118. Thompson DE, Mabuchi K, Ron E, et al. Cancer incidence in atomic bomb survivors. Part II: Solid tumors, 1958–1987. *Radiat Res.* 1994;137:S17–S67.

119. Land CE, Tokunaga M, Koyama K, et al. Incidence of female breast cancer among atomic bomb survivors, Hiroshima and Nagasaki, 1950–1990. *Radiat Res.* 2003;160:707–717.

120. Gilbert ES, Stovall M, Gospodarowicz M, et al. Lung cancer after treatment for Hodgkin's disease: focus on radiation effects. *Radiat Res.* 2003;159:161–173.

121. Travis LB, Hill DA, Dores GM, et al. Breast cancer following radiotherapy and chemotherapy among young women with Hodgkin disease. *JAMA.* 2003;290:465–475.

122. van Leeuwen FE, Klokman WJ, Stovall M, et al. Roles of radiation dose, chemotherapy, and hormonal factors in breast cancer following Hodgkin's disease. *J Natl Cancer Inst.* 2003;95:971–980.

123. Sacher GA, Trucco E. Theory of radiation injury and recovery in self-renewing cell populations. *Radiat Res.* 1966;29:236–256.

124. Brown JM. The effect of acute x-irradiation on the cell proliferation kinetics of induced carcinomas and their normal counterpart. *Radiat Res.* 1970;43:627–653.

125. von Wangenheim KH, Siegers MP, Feinendegen LE. Repopulation ability and proliferation stimulus in the hematopoietic system of mice following gamma-irradiation. *Exp Hematol.* 1980;8:694–701.

126. Cheshier SH, Morrison SJ, Liao X, et al. In vivo proliferation and cell cycle kinetics of long-term self-renewing hematopoietic stem cells. *Proc Natl Acad Sci USA.* 1999;96:3120–3125.

127. Shuryak I, Sachs RK, Hlatky L, et al. Radiation-induced leukemia at doses relevant to radiation therapy: modeling mechanisms and estimating risks. *J Natl Cancer Inst.* 2006;98:1794–1806.

128. Sachs RK, Shuryak I, Brenner D, et al. Second cancers after fractionated radiotherapy: stochastic population dynamics effects. *J Theor Biol.* 2007;249:518–531.

129. Koh ES, Tran TH, Heydarian M, et al. A comparison of mantle versus involved-field radiotherapy for Hodgkin's lymphoma: reduction in normal tissue dose and second cancer risk. *Radiat Oncol.* 2007;2:13.

130. Land C, Gilbert E, Smith JM, et al. *Report of the NCI-CDC Working Group to Revise the 1985 NIH Radioepidemiological Tables.* DHHS Publication No. 03-5387. Bethesda, MD: NIH; 2003.

131. NRC. *Health Risks from Exposure to Low Levels of Ionizing Radiation—BEIR VII.* Washington, DC: The National Academies Press; 2006.

132. Kocher DC, Apostoaei AI, Henshaw RW, et al. Interactive RadioEpidemiological Program (IREP): a web-based tool for estimating probability of causation/assigned share of radiogenic cancers. *Health Phys.* 2008;95:119–147.

Kiyohiko Mabuchi, Saeko Fujiwara
Dale L. Preston, Yukiko Shimizu
Nori Nakamura, Roy E. Shore

Atomic-Bomb Survivors: Long-term Health Effects of Radiation

INTRODUCTION

The atomic bombs exploded about 500 to 600 m above the ground on August 6, 1945 in Hiroshima and 3 days later in Nagasaki, and the people of each city were exposed in a matter of seconds to doses of penetrating ionizing radiation ranging from lethal to almost negligible, depending on their location and shielding. The numbers of deaths before the end of 1945 were estimated to be between 90,000 and 120,000 in Hiroshima (with a population of about 330,000 at that time) and between 60,000 and 80,000 in Nagasaki (with a population of about 250,000). Those acute deaths were attributable to radiation, burns, and other physical injuries.[1] On October 12, 1945 the United States formed a "Joint Commission for the Investigation of the Effects of the Atomic Bomb in Japan" to conduct a coordinated study cooperating with Japanese scientists already on the scene.[2] On November 26, 1946, President Truman approved a directive to the National Academy of Science/National Research Council "to undertake a long range, continuing study of the biological effects and medical effects of the atomic bomb on man." This led to the establishment of the Atomic Bomb Casualty Commission (ABCC) in 1947. In 1975, ABCC became the Radiation Effects Research Foundation (RERF), which has continued research on the health effects of atomic-bomb survivors and their children with financial and scientific support provided from the Japanese and US governments.

At the outset, ABCC studies of radiation effects focused on specific topics of interest, such as hematology, growth and development, and cataracts. Those studies were mostly in the form of case reports or case series without a clearly defined population base. The notable exception was a study by Neel and Schull of genetic effects of the atomic bombs with a clear study design and well-defined objectives.[3] An important turning point in the history of studies of health effects at ABCC, and subsequently at RERF, was the formulation of a Unified Study Program by the Francis Committee in 1955.[4] The unified study program instituted continuing epidemiological follow-up of mortality and cancer incidence, morbidity surveillance based on biennial health examinations (Adult Health Study [AHS]), and postmortem detection in a fixed-sample population of atomic-bomb survivors and control subjects (Life Span Study [LSS]). Later, a second cohort of *in utero* exposed persons and

controls (*In Utero* Cohort), and still another cohort of children of exposed and nonexposed parents were added (F1 Cohort). Follow-up of those cohorts of over 200,000 people in Hiroshima and Nagasaki continues today at RERF (Table 8.1), together with a multitude of special studies ranging from epidemiology, clinical, pathology, and cell and molecular biology.

THE BOMBS AND RADIATION DOSIMETRY

The bomb detonated in Hiroshima was a unique gun-type device ("Little Boy") with a 16-kiloton yield and the height of the burst was 600 m above the ground. The hypocenter was near the city center and the time of detonation was 8:15 AM, August 6, 1945 (Fig. 8.1). The bomb detonated in Nagasaki was a plutonium implosive device ("Fat Man") with a 21-kiloton yield. The height of the burst was 503 m above the ground and the hypocenter was in Urakami valley in a residential/industrial area about 1.5 km north of the city center.[5] While radiation doses were not directly measured soon after the bombings, various special methods have been devised to make retrospective estimates of the radiation doses and fluences that were received at relatively unshielded locations. Additional information useful for retrospective estimation of radiation doses has been obtained from measurements of tested nuclear weapons and simulation using other sources.[5–7]

The availability of reliable and well-characterized radiation dose estimates for individual members of these cohorts is fundamental to the assessment of the health effects of radiation among the survivors and their children. ABCC and later RERF have undertaken continuous and extensive efforts to collect information and establish systems for estimating individual doses from the bombs. Several successively improved dosimetry systems have been developed by extramural working groups and collaboratively implemented by ABCC and RERF investigators. The evolution of the atomic-bomb dosimetry systems, starting from T57D (Tentative 1957 Dosimetry) to the current Dosimetry System 2002 (DS02), is summarized by Cullings et al.[7]

The doses were from penetrating external radiations arising from a large, localized source. This makes it possible to calculate doses systematically because estimated doses are

TABLE 8.1	Radiation Effects Research Foundation (RERF) Cohorts	
Cohort	Subjects	Follow-up (Calendar Years); Major Study Activities
Life Span Study (LSS)	120, 321 persons consisting of proximally and distally exposed atomic-bomb survivors; 26,580 nonexposed city residents not in city at the time of the bombs	Mortality follow-up (1950–) Cancer incidence follow-up (1958–) Autopsy program (1950s–1985) Mail surveys (1965, 1969, 1979, 1991, 2009)
Adult Health Study (AHS)	A subset of 19,961 LSS subjects, including a core of 4,993 proximally exposed survivors and subjects with lesser exposures	Biennial clinical health examination (1958–) *Ad hoc* cancer screening Thyroid examinations Bone density examinations Ophthalmologic examinations
In Utero Study	3,289 persons who were *in utero* at the time of the bomb	Mortality follow-up (1945)
Adult Health Study—*In Utero*	1,568 persons—a subset of the *In Utero* Study Cohort	Biennial clinical health examination (1958–) Mental retardation, IQ, school performance
F1 Study	76,814 persons born to parents, at least one of whom were proximally exposed, born to parents, at least one of whom were distally exposed, or born to nonexposed parents	Mortality follow-up (1946–) Cytogenetic studies Biochemical genetic studies Molecular genetic studies
F1 Clinical Study	11,951 persons—a subset of the F1 Study Cohort	Clinical health examination (2002–2006)
Total	**~212,100 persons**	

essentially the function of the distance from the hypocenter, external shielding (building structure and terrain), and self-shielding (age, orientation, and position for organ doses). In ABCC/RERF dosimetry systems, information on the distance and shielding is obtained from a number of early studies carried out at ABCC starting in 1947 and other official sources. Among the most important is a large-scale field investigation conducted in the 1950s that provides detailed external shielding histories for proximal survivors. Crude shielding category information (e.g., in a house or other wooden structures, or in the open with little or no shielding) is also available from the ABCC/RERF Master File cards and Master Sample Questionnaires administered to persons of interest to ABCC/RERF or members of the major cohort samples. Self-shielding by the human body is estimated using standardized human phantoms that were developed based on anthropometric data for the Japanese population of 1945. Figure 8.2 provides an overview of source terms, transport models, and shielding models used in the latest dosimetry system.[7] Figure 8.3A and B provides a further illustration of how physical fluences are calculated at various levels in finally estimating organ doses. Dose estimates are available for 15 organs (bladder, brain, breast, colon, eye lens, lung, liver, bone marrow, ovary, pancreas, skeleton, stomach, testes, thyroid, and uterus).

The dosimetry systems provide estimates only for direct exposure to the penetrating radiation, that is, neutron and γ rays, emitted by the bombs within a few minutes of detonation

at locations within a few kilometers of the hypocenter. Residual radiation could have occurred from the neutron activation of materials in the soil and structures near the hypocenter, or from local fallout of debris from the bombs. None of the ABCC/RERF dosimetry systems have attempted to estimate individual doses from residual radiation. Doses from residual

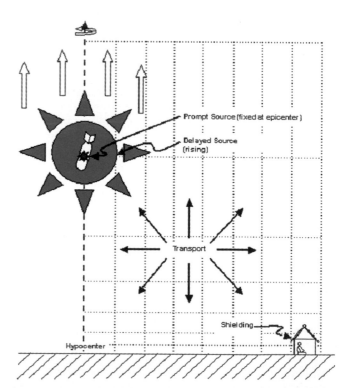

Figure 8.2. Comprehensive atomic-bomb survivor dosimetry providing a source term, a transport model and shielding models. (Reprinted from Cullings HM, et al. Dose estimation for atomic bomb survivor studies: its evolution and present status. *Radiat Res.* 2006;166 (1 pt 2): 219–254, with permission.)

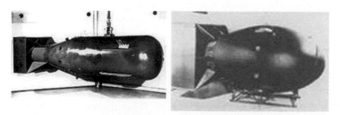

Figure 8.1. Hiroshima and Nagasaki bombs.

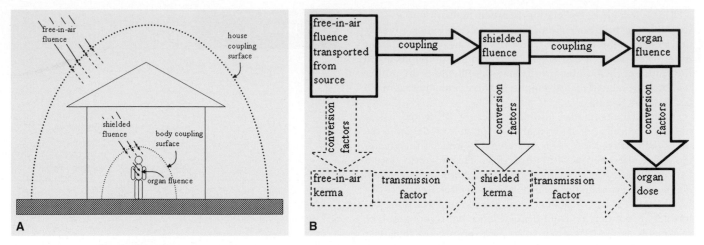

Figure 8.3. **A:** Physical schematic of fluences calculated in DS02 and the surfaces for forward-adjoint Monte Carlo coupling. Fluences for only one of 240 angular directions are depicted. Forward fluences are solid arrows and coupled adjoint fluences are dashed arrows. **B:** Computational schematic of dosimetric quantities calculated by DS02. Calculation of organ doses for survivors with full coded shielding information proceeds by the pathway in bold outline. Conversion factors are also be used to calculate free-in-air and shielded kerma for the same survivors, establishing transmission factors as ratios of shielded to free-in-air kerma and organ dose to shielded kerma. Averages of these transmission factors are used to calculate doses for survivors with less shielding information, via the pathway in dashed outline. (Reprinted from Cullings HM, et al. Dose estimation for atomic bomb survivor studies: its evolution and present status. *Radiat Res.* 2006;166(1 pt 2):219–254, with permission.)

radiation can depend on many identifiable and unidentifiable factors and thus are essentially impossible to estimate but are considered small based on a variety of soil radionuclide measurements.[6]

The current dosimetry system, DS02, originates from the concern that the previous dosimetry (DS86) may have underestimated neutrons at a distance beyond 1.5 km from the Hiroshima hypocenter. This resulted in a comprehensive reevaluation of the survivor dosimetry system, including the bomb source terms, transport models, activation measurement data, and additional sample analyses. As it turned out, an anticipated increase in contributions from neutrons in Hiroshima did not materialize, but the primary change was an increase of 10% in γ rays for both Hiroshima and Nagasaki (Fig. 8.4). This change results in a small (about an 8%) decrease in cancer risk estimates at low doses but virtually no other apparent changes in the shape of the dose response or the temporal patterns of the risk.[8] As of this writing, DS02 doses have been used in analyses of the LSS cancer and leukemia mortality[8] and solid cancer incidence,[9,10] *in utero* solid cancer incidence,[11] and AHS thyroid examination data,[12] as presented in this chapter. Other risk data referred to are based mostly on the previous dose dosimetry system, DS86. However, the major findings on the risk and temporal patterns are only slightly affected by the use of different dosimetry systems.[8]

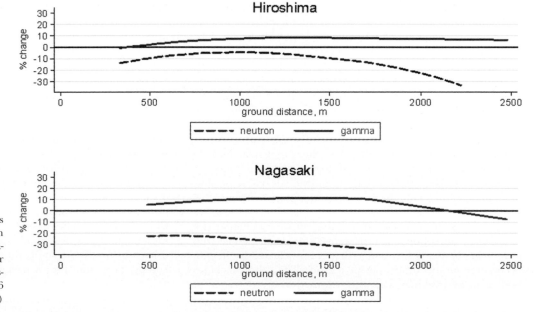

Figure 8.4. DS02/DS86 changes in colon dose. (Reprinted from Cullings HM, et al. Dose estimation for atomic bomb survivor studies: its evolution and present status. *Radiat Res.* 2006;166(1 pt 2):219–254, with permission.)

There is a close correlation between neutron and γ doses such that any inference about a neutron contribution to radiation effects in the RERF data must rely very heavily on intercity differences, which are affected by errors in assumptions about the nature of the bombs. Unfortunately, while there are quite a few neutron-related measurements in Hiroshima, there is much less data for Nagasaki.

Individual organ dose estimates used in RERF risk assessment are typically calculated as the sum of the γ ray dose plus ten times the neutron dose. This weighted dose reflects the greater biological effectiveness of neutron dose. This weighted dose is expressed as Gray (Gy) in this chapter. Since human data do not enable us to estimate the relative biological effectiveness (RBE) of neutrons for carcinogenic effects, the use of a weighting factor of 10 is not derived from firm evidence but is thought to be reasonable as a first approximation for exposure at a total dose of about 1 Gy. The neutron RBE is an important issue, but it is not feasible to estimate the neutron RBE from the RERF data[13] because of the high correlation between γ and neutron doses, the small fraction of the total dose from neutrons, and the potential for bias in intercity comparisons. However, the choice of reasonable weights for neutron doses, for example, in the range 5 to 50, should have a relatively small effect on risk estimates.

Uncertainties about survivor location and shielding are a major source of the random error in individual dose estimates. A statistical method is used to adjust for the impact of those random errors on individual dose estimates. The error-adjusted dose estimates,[14] assuming 35% random errors in individual dose estimates, are typically used in RERF risk analysis.

LIFE SPAN STUDY

The earliest, most authentic enumeration of atomic-bomb survivors, obtained at the time of the 1950 National Census, indicated that there were about 284,000 survivors (159,000 in Hiroshima and 125,000 in Nagasaki). This served as the basis for selecting survivors to be enrolled into the LSS cohort.[15] The LSS cohort consists of about 120,000 people. That number includes about 94,000 atomic-bomb survivors: (a) 54,000 persons who were within 2.5 km of the hypocenter at the time of the bombings (exposed to relatively high doses of radiation) and (b) about 40,000 city-, age- and gender-matched survivors who were between 2.5 and 10 km of the hypocenter (with relatively low or negligible doses of radiation). The cohort also includes about 26,000 unexposed subjects who were residents of Hiroshima or Nagasaki but were not in either city at the time of the bombs. Individual dose estimates are available for 93% of all the survivors in the cohort or for about 80% of those who are within 2.5 km of the hypocenter. About 100,000 survivors are thought to have been exposed to the bombs within 2.5 km of the hypocenter, and thus the LSS cohort appears to include roughly half of these survivors with high radiation exposure.[16]

In order to be in the LSS cohort, individuals had to be alive in 1950, and thus risk assessment for the period during 1945 to 1950 is not possible with the cohort data. Several features of this cohort are considered advantageous for radiation risk estimates. The cohort subjects were a sample of people who were living in a largely urban area and not selected for health, occupation, or any other specific reasons. The cohort includes both men and women who were exposed to a wide range of radiation doses at all different ages in life. As will be presented

TABLE 8.2	LSS Cohort, Vital Status, as of January, 2000	
Age at Exposure (yr)	People	Alive
0–9	17,833	15,988 (90%)
10–19	17,563	13,425 (76%)
20–29	10,891	6,490 (60%)
30–39	12,270	2,762 (23%)
40–49	13,503	254 (2%)
50+	14,551	7 (0%)
Total	86,611	38,926 (45%)

Source: Adapted from Preston, DL, Pierce DA, et al. Effect of recent changes in atomic bomb survivor dosimetry on cancer mortality risk estimates. *Radiat Res.* 2004;162(4):377–389.

later, gender, age at exposure, and attained age (or time since exposure) are significant modifiers of the radiation-related risk for cancer and many other health conditions, and thus have an important implication in estimating radiation risks from medical, occupational, or environmental exposures. The LSS cancer and leukemia data are the most important source of epidemiological information used in lifetime risk estimation by the national and international radiation authorities, such as the National Research Council and the United Nation's Scientific Committee of the Effects of Atomic Radiation (UNSCEAR).

As of the latest mortality follow-up (January 1, 2000),[8] 45% of the survivors (with dose estimates) were alive (Table 8.2). However, a large majority of young survivors are still alive; in particular, most (83%) of over 35,000 people who were exposed under 20 years of age are still alive, and this is the major source of uncertainty in estimating lifetime risk of cancer and other illnesses.

FOLLOW-UP

The LSS cohort has been followed up for vital status and causes of death, beginning in 1950 (Table 8.1). Virtually complete tracing of the cohort members through the Japanese family registry system is unique, but there are limitations in diagnostic accuracy and relevance of diseases reported on death certificates. Starting in 1958, information on incident cancers became available through linkage to tumor/tissue registries in Hiroshima and Nagasaki.[17] The tumor registry data provide more accurate diagnostic information and cover less fatal cancers, such as cancers of the breast, thyroid, and skin, which are radiation sensitive but underrepresented in death certificate information. Diagnosis date reported for incident cancer is a better indicator of disease onset than date of death resulting from cancer. Since cancer incidence data are available only within the scope of the Hiroshima and Nagasaki prefecture-wide registries, LSS cancer incidence analyses include adjustment for people's migratory movements.[18]

A number of mailed questionnaire surveys have been conducted among the members of the LSS (Table 8.1). Information on socioeconomic, lifestyle, and other factors collected from the mail surveys has been used in investigating whether these factors may confound the association of radiation and disease or how they modify the radiation effects. An extensive autopsy program, most actively carried out during the 1950s and 1960s, provided information on the accuracy and type of misclassification of death certificate data.

The AHS is a clinical follow-up of a subset of the LSS. The AHS subjects have been invited to biennial clinical examination at RERF starting in 1958, with a remarkably high participation rate of 70% to 80%. The biennial examination includes general physical examination, history taking, a series of clinical laboratory tests, and *ad hoc* studies on specified conditions (e.g., thyroid disease, ophthalmologic conditions). The follow-up information provides longitudinal morbidity and laboratory data and is an important complement to the assessment of noncancer diseases and conditions.

As with the LSS, the *In Utero* and F1 cohorts are also followed up for mortality and cancer incidence. A subset (about half) of the *In Utero* cohort has also undergone biennial health examination as part of the AHS program. During 2002 to 2006, a subset of about 12,000 of the F1 cohort underwent health examination for the first time (Table 8.1).

DESCRIBING RADIATION RISKS

Two types of risk calculation are used in describing the magnitude of a disease impact of exposure in epidemiological studies. The excess absolute risk (EAR) refers to the difference in the rate of occurrence of disease between an exposed population and a comparable population with no exposure. The relative risk (RR) is the ratio of the occurrence rate in the exposed population to that in the nonexposed population. The excess relative risk (ERR) is the RR − 1, which is essentially identical to the ratio of the EAR to the occurrence rate in the nonexposed comparison population. While the ERR is a measure of the strength of the effect of exposure and may have biological significance, the EAR is a measure of the absolute size of the effect, which may be of public health or clinical significance and is sometimes designated as the "attributable risk."

It is important to note that excess risks, both absolute and relative, can vary not only with radiation dose but also with age at exposure, time after exposure (attained age), gender and other factors, such as smoking. Modification of radiation risk by those factors occurs because baseline disease rates depend on those factors (such as attained age, gender, calendar time) or because differences in sensitivity may vary with these factors (e.g., age at exposure). Risk estimates are usually reported for a specific dose, for example, 1 Gy, for a specified combination of other factors, for example, for a person at attained age of 70 after exposure at age 30. The EAR is used to refer to the estimated number of excess cases per 10,000 persons per year per Gy while the ERR per Gy refers to the estimated ERR for persons exposed at 1 Gy. Risk estimates are typically calculated using regression models that include age at exposure (e), attained age (a), gender (s), city (c, Hiroshima or Nagasaki), and other factors, as needed.

Typically, an ERR model has the form:

$$\lambda_0(c,s,a,b)\,[1 + \text{ERR}(d,e,s,a)],$$

where $\lambda_0(c, s, a, b)$ is the baseline disease rate (i.e., the rate for people with zero dose) and the function ERR (d, e, s, a) describes the relative change in rates associated with dose d allowing for effects of age at exposure, gender, and attained age. The general form of an EAR model is:

$$\lambda_0(c,s,a,b) + \text{EAR}(d,e,s,a).$$

TABLE 8.3	Numbers of Deaths from Leukemia, Solid Cancer, and Noncancer Diseases in the LSS Cohort, 1950 to 2000

	Follow-up from 1950 through 2000	
Causes of Death	*Total Deaths Observed*	*Excess Deaths*
Solid cancers	10,127	479
Leukemia	296	93
Non–cancer diseases[a]	31,881	250

[a]For noncancer diseases, the follow-up period is from 1950 through 1997.

Source: Adapted from Preston DL, et al. Effect of recent changes in atomic bomb survivor dosimetry on cancer mortality risk estimates. *Radiat Res.* 2004;162(4):377–389.

The ERR and EAR functions are described as parametric functions of the form $\rho(d)\varepsilon(e, s, a)$ in which $\rho(d)$ describes the shape of the dose-response function, for example, linear, linear quadratic, threshold, etc., and ε (e, s, a) describes risk variation with gender, time, or other factors.

HEMATOPOIETIC CANCERS

Leukemia

By the late 1940s, there were suggestions of an increased risk of leukemia among the atomic survivors, and hematologists in Hiroshima and Nagasaki formed the Leukemia Registry to monitor cases of leukemia and other hematological malignancies among the survivors.[19] The earliest evidence of an increased risk of leukemia among the survivors was reported in 1952.[20] The latest published LSS mortality data for leukemia are through 2000; there were 296 leukemia deaths in the cohort (Table 8.3), and 93 (46%) of these are estimated to be excess deaths attributable to radiation exposure among the survivors exposed to >0.005 Gy (Table 8.4).[8] This proportion increases with increasing dose and reaches approximately 90% among those exposed to doses >1 Gy.

TABLE 8.4	Observed and Expected Deaths from Leukemia. LSS Mortality, 1950 to 2000

Dose (Gy)	*Subjects*	*Observed*	*Expected*	*Fitted Excess*
0 (<0.005)	37,407	92	84.9	0
0.005–0.1	30,387	69	72.1	4
01–0.2	5,841	14	14.5	5
0.2–0.5	6,304	27	15.6	10
0.5–1.0	3,963	30	9.5	19
1.0–2.0	1,972	39	4.9	28
>2.0	737	25	1.6	28
Total	**86,611**	**296**	**203**	**93**

Source: Adapted from Preston DL, et al. Effect of recent changes in atomic bomb survivor dosimetry on cancer mortality risk estimates. *Radiat Res.* 2004;162(4):377–389.

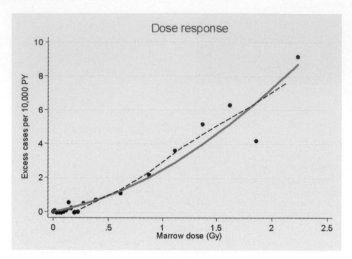

Figure 8.5. Dose response for leukemia, LSS mortality, 1950–2000. (Reprinted from Preston DL, et al. Effect of recent changes in atomic bomb survivor dosimetry on cancer mortality risk estimates. *Radiat Res.* 2004;162(4):377–389, with permission.) Shape of the leukemia dose response shown in terms of dose-category–specific gender-averaged EAR estimates with nonparametric smooth curves. Dose-response functions are standardized to risks in 1970 after exposure to age 20 to 39.

The shape of the dose response for leukemia is nonlinear, with an upward curvature in the bone marrow dose range of 0 to 3 Gy (Fig. 8.5),[8,16] and is best described by a linear-quadratic function. The nonlinear dose-response pattern is different from the linear one seen for solid cancers (as shown later). Leukemia also demonstrates a unique temporal pattern in which the radiation-related risk is strongly modified by age and time after exposure. Figure 8.6 illustrates the remarkably high excess risk in the earlier years among those exposed at a young age, which is followed by a rapid decline with time. Up till now, the majority of the excess leukemia deaths from radiation among those exposed as children occurred during the follow-up period before 1975.[16] For those exposed at older ages, on the other hand, the excess radiation-related risk has declined less sharply

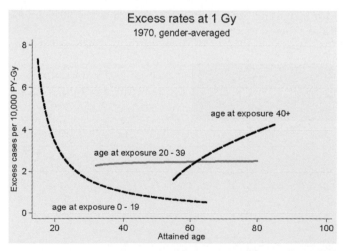

Figure 8.6. Age-time patters for leukemia EAR. LSS mortality 1950 to 2000. (Reprinted from Preston DL, et al. Effect of recent changes in atomic bomb survivor dosimetry on cancer mortality risk estimates. *Radiat Res.* 2004;162(4):377–389, with permission.) Gender-averaged EAR estimates in 1970 after exposure at age 0 to19, 20 to 39, and 40.

and remained through the latest follow-up period. There is still evidence of persistently increased risk of leukemia among the current survivors.[21,22]

Separate analyses of incidence data on specific leukemia subtypes indicate that a strong dose response exists for three types of leukemia, that is, acute lymphocytic, acute myelogenous, and chronic myelocytic leukemia, but not for adult T-cell leukemia, which is endemic in Nagasaki.[23] A radiation effect on chronic lymphocytic leukemia has not been clear with the atomic-bomb survivor data because of the extremely small number of cases of this type of leukemia, which is rare in Japan, unlike western countries. The rapid decline in radiation-related leukemia risk seen in those exposed as a child, as shown in the mortality data above, is evident for all the three types while a slower decline in the risk over time among those exposed at older ages is seen for acute myelocytic leukemia.

Death certificate data on nonneoplastic diseases of the blood and blood-forming organs include a substantial number of misclassified leukemia or other hematopoietic malignancies. A review of medical records available for blood diseases reported on LSS death certificates showed that some of these deaths in fact are from neoplastic conditions, including myelodysplastic syndrome, leukemia, and other cancers. There was a significantly increased ERR of 2.0 for all nonneoplastic blood diseases as a group with an indication of a possible strong radiation effect for myelodysplastic syndrome.[24]

Lymphomas and Multiple Myeloma

Evidence of a radiation effect on lymphoma is inconsistent in general and also with the LSS data. The latest LSS incidence data show suggestive evidence of an increased radiation-related risk for non-Hodgkin lymphoma for males (EAR = 0.6), but not for females.[23] More recently, a parallel analysis of the lymphoma mortality data in the male atomic-bomb survivors and male workers at a US nuclear weapons facility suggested a protracted latency for radiation-related lymphoma that exceeded 35 years after irradiation.[21,22] The LSS data have shown no indication of a radiation effect on Hodgkin lymphoma.

An increased risk of multiple myeloma associated with radiation has been found in the LSS mortality study[16] as well as a previous incidence study.[25] However, this was not confirmed by an in-depth study of hematologically reviewed cases, suggesting the discrepancy may be due to disease misclassification among the small number of cases of multiple myeloma, which is a rare disease in Japan.[23]

Solid Cancers

LSS mortality data continue to be a principal source of information for radiation risk assessment. For cancer, attention increasingly is being given to incidence data that provide better statistical precision, diagnostic validity, and coverage of many radiation-sensitive cancers. The discussion of solid cancers and specific cancer sites in this chapter focuses on findings from the latest LSS solid cancer incidence data for the follow-up period of 1958 to 1998,[9,10] but also refers to relevant findings from mortality and other special cancer studies.

Different from leukemia, temporal patterns of radiation-related risks for solid cancers characteristically show a gradual increase that starts several years after the bombs and that is roughly in proportion to the age-related increase in baseline

TABLE 8.5			Observed and Fitted[a] Solid Cancer Cases by Dose Category and Attributable Fraction, LSS Cancer Incidence, 1958 to 1998				
Dose Category[b]	*Subjects*	*Person (yr)*	*Cases*	*Background*	*Fitted Excess*	*Attributable Fraction*[c] *(%)*	
<0.005	60,792	1,598,944	9,597	9,537	3	0.0	
0.005–0.1	27,789	729,603	4,406	4,374	81	1.8	
0.1–0.2	5,527	145,925	968	910	75	7.6	
0.2–0.5	5,935	153,886	1,144	963	179	15.7	
0.5–1	3,173	81,251	688	493	206	29.5	
1–2	1,647	41,412	460	248	196	44.2	
2+	564	13,711	185	71	111	61.0	
Total	**105,427**	**2,764,732**	**17,448**	**16,595**	**853**	**10.7**	

[a]Estimates of background and fitted excess cases are based on an ERR model with a linear dose response effect, allowing for modification by gender, age at exposure, and attained age.
[b]Weighted colon dose in Gy.
[c]Attributable fraction—percentage of cases attributable to radiation exposure among those exposed to at least 0.005 Gy.
Source: Adapted from Preston DL, et al. Solid cancer incidence in atomic bomb survivors: 1958–1998. *Radiat Res.* 2007;168:1–64.

cancer rates. Although solid cancers include a multitude of disease entities with varying pathogenesis and etiology, there is sufficient rationale for knowing the radiation risk for all solid cancers as a group. The atomic-bomb survivors received whole-body exposure from penetrating radiation, and consequently, significantly increased radiation-related risks have been observed for cancers of a large number of organ sites. Further, there are indications that data for many other cancer sites, for which statistical significance has not been obtained, are generally consistent with radiation-related risk. Pooling of all solid cancers enhances statistical precision, which is especially important in determining the shape of the dose response at low doses—a matter of special concern in radiological protection. Pooled data also help to understand how the radiation risk is modified by age, time, and gender, and, as it turns out, the pattern of radiation-related risk found for solid cancers as a group is observed for most individual cancer sites. This is not to ignore the inherent variability in radiation response expected for different tissues and organs. There are a few significant and noteworthy cancer site–specific differences, as discussed in the subsequent section.

Shape of Dose Response

There are 17,448 solid cancer incident cases in the subcohort of over 100,000 LSS subjects, included in the incidence analyses. Of those cases, 853 were estimated to be attributable to radiation, and this represents 11% (attributable fraction) of all solid cancers among the survivors exposed to >0.005 Gy (mean, 0.23 Gy) (Table 8.5). The attributable proportion increases with increasing dose and reaches 48% among those who received at least 1 Gy. The dose-related increase is well described by a linear dose-response relationship, while a linear-quadratic trend or a dose-threshold model does not fit the data any better than a linear model (Fig. 8.7). The dose response is largely determined from data in the dose range of 0.2 to 2 Gy. However, it is relevant to note that about 75% of the survivors in the cohort were exposed at doses between 0.005 and 0.2 Gy, which is the range of doses of primary interest for low-dose risk estimation. Relevant findings are that a statistically significant dose response is observed even over the lowest dose range of only

0 to 0.15 Gy and that the trend in this range is consistent with that for the full dose range, supporting an approximately linear dose response down to the lowest dose range. The solid cancer risk estimate based on the LSS data has also been found to be statistically consistent with that from a large international pooled analysis of nuclear industry workers who were exposed at low doses (mean, about 0.020 Sv).[25a]

The ERR/Gy for solid cancer incidence is estimated to be 0.47 (or 47%) for a person aged 70 years who was exposed to the bombings at age 30, and this estimate is identical to that for solid cancer mortality.[26] The corresponding estimate of an EAR for solid cancer incidence of 52 per 10,000 person-year-Gy is almost twice as high as that of 30 for solid cancer mortality. This reflects the higher baseline cancer incidence rates compared to cancer mortality rates.

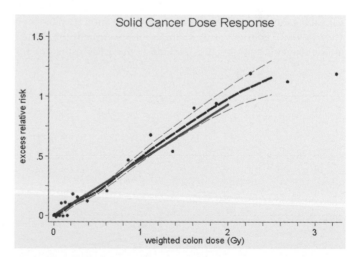

Figure 8.7. Solid cancer dose response, LSS cancer incidence, 1958–1998. (Reprinted from Preston DL, et al. Effect of recent changes in atomic bomb survivor dosimetry on cancer mortality risk estimates. *Radiat Res.* 2004;162(4):377–389, with permission.) The thick solid line is the fitted linear gender-averaged ERR dose response at age 70 following exposure at age 30. The points are nonparametric estimates of the ERR in dose categories. The thick dashed line is a nonparametric smooth of the category-specific estimates and the thin dashed lines are one standard error above and below the smoothed estimate.

TABLE 8.6	Radiation-Risk Parameter Estimates: All Solid Cancers and Non-Gender–Specific Solid Cancers, LSS Cancer Incidence, 1958 to 1998					
	Risk Per Gy[a]				*Age at exposure[b] (% change per decade increase)*	*Attained Age[b] (Power)*
Model	*Male*	*Female*	*Sex-Averaged*	*Sex Ratio (F:M)*		
ALL SOLID CANCERS						
ERR/Gy	0.35	0.58	0.47	1.6	−17%	−1.65
	(0.28; 0.43)[c]	(0.43; 0.69)	(0.40; 0.54)	(1.31; 2.09)	(−25%; −7%)	(−2.1; −1.2)
EAR	43.2[d]	59.8	51.5	1.4	−24%	2.38
	(32.7; 55.1)	(51.0; 69.1)	(43.3; 60.2)	(1.10; 1.79)	(−32%; −16%)	(1.9; 2.8)
NON-GENDER–SPECIFIC SOLID CANCERS[e]						
ERR/Gy	0.34	0.61	0.48	1.8	−10%	−2.09
	(0.27; 0.42)[c]	(0.50; 0.73)	(0.39; 0.56)	(1.31; 2.09)	(−20%; −1%)	(−2.6; −1.5)
EAR	47.9[d]	44.1	46.0	0.9	−19%	2.52
	(36.4; 60.8)	(36.6; 52.0)	(37.9; 54.6)	(0.72; 1.20)	(−29%; −9%)	(2.0; 3.1)

[a]At age 70 following exposure at age 30.
[b]Models include both attained-age and age-at-exposure effects.
[c]90% CI.
[d]Excess cases per 10,000 PY-Gy.
[e]Excludes cancers of the breast, prostate, and genital organs.
Source: Adapted from Preston DL, et al. Solid cancer incidence in atomic bomb survivors: 1958–1998. *Radiat Res.* 2007;168:1–64.

Effects of Gender and Age on Solid Cancer Risk

Some of the most important knowledge gained from the long-term follow-up study is how the radiation-related risk of cancer (and also of most other conditions) varies by age at exposure, time since exposure (or attained age in this cohort), and gender. Differences in the temporal patterns of the risk may be expected from age- or gender-related differences in cell or tissue sensitivity, but observed differences also can be a consequence of how the risk is computed compared to varying baseline disease rates (over time and by age and gender).

As seen in Table 8.6, both the ERR and the EAR estimates for solid cancers are about 50% higher for women than for men (female:male gender ratio of 1.6 and 1.4, respectively). When gender-specific cancers are excluded, the ERR estimates for men and women are essentially unchanged, but the EAR for women decreases so that there is no longer a gender difference in EAR. The reduction in the female EAR is largely due to the removal of a very high radiation-related risk of breast cancer among them. The high gender ratio for the ERR results from the approximately equal EAR being divided by the lower baseline rates of nongenital cancers in women.

Figure 8.8 illustrates that the excess risks are highly dependent on age at exposure and attained age. The ERR for persons exposed to the bombs at a younger age is higher than those exposed at an older age, but it declines over time (with increasing attained age) (left panel). It is important to note, however, that the EAR increases rapidly with age, that is, that the radiation-related excess absolute cancer rate is increasing with age with no apparent indication of abating (right panel). That

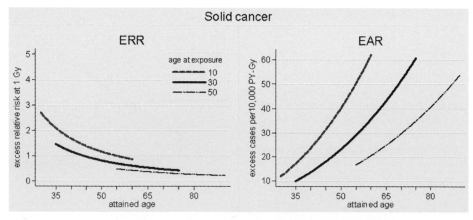

Figure 8.8. Age dependence for the solid cancer ERR (**left panel**) and EAR (**right panel**) for exposure ages of 10, 30, and 50 years. LSS cancer incidence, 1958 to 1998. Variation in solid cancer excess risks at 1 Gy with attained age for persons exposed at age 10, 30, and 50. The left panel presents the fitted ERR estimates; the right panel indicates excess rate (EAR) estimates. The curves are gender-averaged risks following exposure to 1 Gy. (Reprinted from Preston DL, et al. Solid cancer incidence among atomic bomb survivors, 1958–1998. *RERF Update.* 2007;18:9–13, with permission.)

TABLE 8.7	Site-Specific Gender Averaged ERR and EAR, LSS Cancer Incidence, 1958 to 1998				
Site	Total Cases	Excess Cases	Attributable Fraction[a] (%)	ERR/Gy[b] (90% CI)	EAR[b]
All solid	17,448	853	10.7	0.47 (0.04; 0.54)	52 (43; 60)
Oral cavity	277	16	11.4	0.39 (0.11; 0.76)	0.56 (0.20; 1.2)
Esophagus	352	16	10.2	0.52 (0.15; 1.0)	0.58 (0.18; 1.1)
Stomach	4,730	151	7.2	0.34 (0.22; 0.47)	9.1 (6.1; 14)
Colon	1,516	78	11.4	0.54 (0.30; 0.81)	8.0 (4.4; 12)
Rectum	838	14	3.7	0.19 (−0.04; 0.47)	0.56 (−0.13; 1.4)
Liver	1,494	54	8.1	0.30 (0.11; 0.55)	4.3 (0.0; 7.2)
Gall bladder	549	−2	−1.0	−0.05 (<−0.3; 0.3)	−0.01 (<−0.1; 0.51)
Pancreas	512	11	4.8	0.26 (<−0.07; 0.68)	0.46 (−0.13; 1.5)
Lung	1,759	117	14.7	0.81 (0.56;1.1)	7.5 (5.1; 10)
Non–melanoma skin	330	40	23.2	0.17 (0.003; 0.55)	0.35 (0.03; 1.1)
Female breast	1,073	147	27.1	0.87 (0.55; 1.3)	9.2 (6.8; 12)
Uterus	1,162	12	1.9	0.10 (−0.09; 0.33)	0.56 (<0; 1.9)
Ovary	245	11	10.3	0.61 (0.00; 1.5)	0.56 (0.02; 1.3)
Prostate	387	4	2.2	0.11 (−0.10; 0.54)	0.34 (−0.64; 1.6)
Kidney and URT	167	2	2.7	0.13 (−0.25; 0.75)	0.08 (−0.16; 0.44)
Bladder	469	35	16.4	1.23 (0.59; 2.1)	3.2 (1.1; 5.4)
Brain, CNS	281	19	13.0	0.62 (0.21; 1.2)	0.51 (0.17; 0.95)
Thyroid	471	63	24.5	0.57 (0.24; 1.1)	1.2 (0.5; 2.2)
Other	836	65	16.4	0.91 (0.5; 1.4)	5.0 (2.7; 7.7)

[a]Attributable fraction—percentage to cases attributable to radiation exposure among those exposed to at least 0.005 Gy.
[b]ERR at 1 Gy or EAR per 10,000 person-year Gy at age 70 years after exposure at age 30 year.
Adapted from Preston DL, et al. Solid cancer incidence in atomic bomb survivors: 1958–1998. *Radiat Res.* 2007;168:1–64.

pattern suggests that the radiation-related excess risk may persist throughout one's lifetime, and this trend is seen for most of the cancer sites as well.

SITE-SPECIFIC CANCER RISKS

Table 8.7 presents the risk estimates, ERR and EAR, for different cancer sites. Dose responses are significant for cancers of the oral cavity, esophagus, stomach, colon, liver, lung, nonmelanocytic skin, female breast, ovary, urinary bladder, brain/central nervous system (CNS), and thyroid. Radiation-related risks are also increased, though not significantly, for virtually all the remaining cancer sites.

In ranking the ERRs for different cancer sites, the highest ERRs (higher than 0.8, or 80%/Gy) are found for bladder, female breast, and lung cancers and relatively high ERRs (higher than 0.5 or 50%) for cancers of the brain/CNS, ovary, thyroid, colon, and esophagus (Fig. 8.9). For those cancer sites, contributions of radiation exposure to the increased risk are relatively high. A different ranking is seen when one examines EARs, which have clinical or public health implications. High EARs, which reflected high numbers of excess cancers, are seen for cancers of the female breast (9.2), stomach (9.1), colon (8.0), lung (7.5), liver (4.3), bladder (3.2), and thyroid (1.2) in a descending order (Table 8.7). For stomach and liver cancers, the ERR of about 0.3 is modestly high, but the excess in

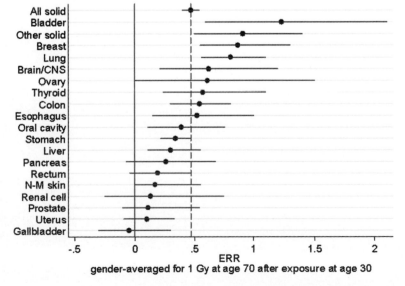

Figure 8.9. Site-specific ERR estimates with 90% confidence intervals. LSS Cancer Incidence, 1958 to 1998. The ERRs are gender averaged and correspond to the fitted risk at age 70 for a person exposed to 1 Gy at age 30. The solid vertical line indicates no excess risk and the dashed vertical line represents the standardized ERR for all solid cancers as a group. N-M skin refers to non-melanoma skin. (Reprinted from Preston DL, et al. Solid cancer incidence among atomic bomb survivors, 1958–1998. *RERF Update.* 2007;18:9–13, with permission.)

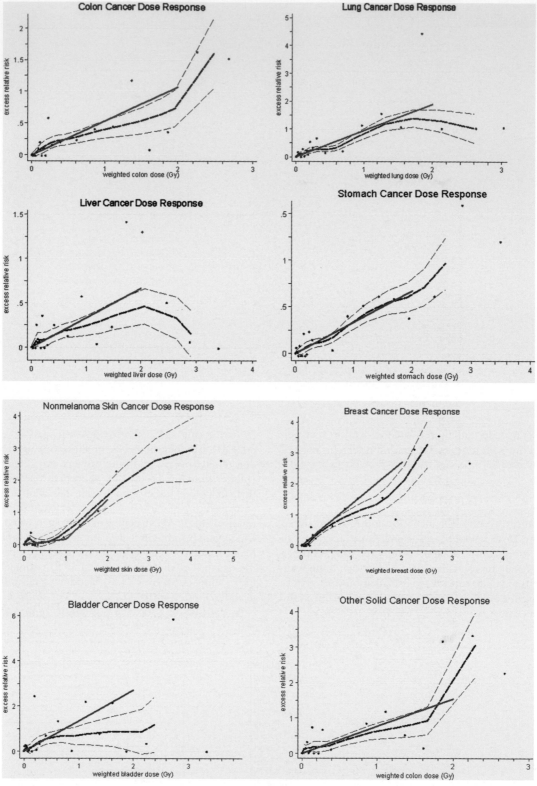

Figure 8.10. Dose response for cancer of the stomach, colon, liver, lung, nonmelanocytic skin, breast, bladder, thyroid, and other sites. LSS cancer incidence, 1958 to 1998. The thick solid line is the fitted linear gender-averaged ERR dose response at age 70 following exposure at age 30. The points are non–parametric estimates of the ERR in dose categories. The thick dashed line is a nonparametric smooth of the category-specific estimates and the thin dashed lines are one standard error above and below the smoothed estimate. (Reprinted from Preston DL, et al. Solid cancer incidence among atomic bomb survivors, 1958–1998. *RERF Update.* 2007;18:9–13, with permission.)

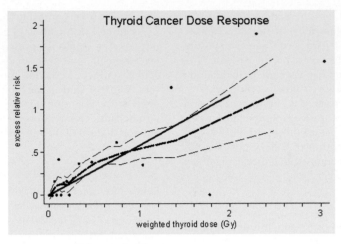

Figure 8.10. (*Continued*)

absolute risks is very high because of the high baseline rates for these cancers in Japan. If one examines excess cancer mortality (not shown) rather than incidence, the ordering of EARs is slightly different yet: stomach, lung, liver, female breast, and colon (largest to smaller), in part reflecting the relatively low fatality of breast and colon cancers.[26]

Oral Cavity and Esophagus

Cancers of the oral cavity are a relatively rare but heterogeneous group of cancers, with some subsites sharing common risk factors, such as smoking and heavy alcohol consumption. The numbers of cases with specific cancer subsite sites are small, but noteworthy is a strong dose response found for the relatively rare tumors of the salivary gland. The estimated ERR of 1.8 for salivary gland cancer (data not shown) is among the highest of all the site-specific estimates. The significant dose response for cancers of the oral cavity and pharynx (ERR = 0.52) as a whole is mostly derived from that for cancer of the salivary glands. Previous pathology studies in the LSS showed that, among various histological subtypes of salivary tumors, a dose response was exceptionally strong for mucoepidermoid carcinoma and Warthin tumor,[27,28] suggesting a remarkable type specificity.

There also is a significant dose response for cancer of the esophagus, with an ERR estimate of 0.52. An increased ERR for esophageal cancer has also been seen in the LSS mortality data.[26]

Stomach

While stomach cancer rates have declined recently in Japan, this cancer is still the most common malignancy in Japan.[29] In the LSS, over 4,700 incident stomach cancer cases make up 27% of all solid cancer cases. For those with stomach doses of >0.005 Gy, 7% of the stomach cancers are related to radiation exposure, and the attributable proportion increases to over 30% among those with doses of ≥1 Gy. The dose response is linear with no indication of nonlinearity (Fig. 8.10).

The gender averaged ERR is 0.34, but the gender-specific ERR is twice as high for females as for males (Fig. 8.11, top panel). The EAR of about 9.5 is similar for males and females. Since the baseline rates for this cancer in the cohort are over twice as high for males as for females, these findings together suggest that the radiation-related risk for stomach cancer adds to, rather than

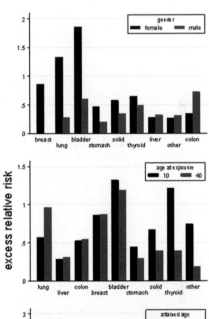

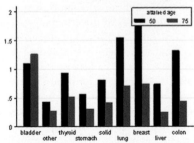

Figure 8.11. Modifying effects of gender, age at exposure, and attained age for major cancer sites. LSS cancer incidence, 1958 to 1998. Comparison of site-specific gender (**top panel**), age at exposure (**middle panel**), and attained age (**bottom panel**) effects on standardized ERR/Gy estimates for selected sites and all solid cancers. The gender-specific estimates correspond to the fitted ERR/Gy at age 70 for a person exposed at age 30. The age-at-exposure–specific estimates are gender-averaged ERR estimates at age 70 following exposure at age 10 (*left bar*) or age 40 (*right bar*). Attained-age-specific estimates are gender averaged ERR estimates at ages 50 (*left bar*) and 75 (*right bar*) following exposure at age 30. Within each panel the sites are ordered based on the magnitude of the ratio of the effect pairs. (Reprinted from Preston DL, et al. Solid cancer incidence among atomic bomb survivors, 1958–1998. *RERF Update.* 2007;18:9–13, with permission.)

multiplies, the baseline rates and that the gender difference in the ERR reflects the lower baseline rates for females. Neither the ERR nor the EAR significantly vary with age at exposure while the ERR decreases and EAR increases as the baseline rates increase with attained age, as would be expected if the radiation effect on stomach cancer were additive to the baseline risk.

Based on clinical and laboratory data using stored sera obtained from the AHS subjects, it appears that radiation risk is seen especially among nonsmokers and those with diffuse-type cancer.[30] Dietary factors (consumption of fruit, vegetables, soy products, or green tea) have no demonstrable modifying effect on the radiation risk of gastric cancer.[31]

Colon and Rectum

Historically, the colon cancer rates were much lower in Japan than in western countries, but they have now risen to about the same level as in the United States.[29] Colon cancer represents the third leading cancer in the cohort. The rectal cancer rates, which have risen less sharply than colon cancer rates in Japan, are roughly equal to those in the west. The LSS dose response for colon cancer incidence is essentially linear, with no indication of nonlinearity (Fig. 8.10). Rectal cancer incidence, however, has not significantly been associated with radiation exposure.

Unlike most solid cancers for which the ERR for females exceeds that for males, both the ERR and the EAR for colon cancer incidence are higher for males than for females. The ERR is not influenced by age at exposure but tends to decline with increasing attained age (Fig. 8.11, two bottom panels). The EAR significantly increases with increasing attained age and, for a given attained age, is higher for those exposed at a younger age (younger birth cohort). Those findings are consistent with the notion that radiation may be acting multiplicatively with factors responsible for the increasing trend for colon cancer over time in Japan.

An earlier site-specific study found no significant difference in the dose response for cancers of the cecum/ascending, transverse/descending, and sigmoid colon.[32]

Liver

Liver cancer is the fourth most common cancer in the cohort, and this reflects high rates of this cancer, especially in males in Japan.[29] The high rates of liver cancer, mostly hepatocellular carcinoma, in Japan have been attributed largely to hepatitis C viral infection (80%) and, to a lesser extent, to hepatitis B viral infection (16%).[33] There is a significant linear dose response for liver cancer with no indication of nonlinearity (Fig. 8.10). About 5% of liver cancers among those exposed at >0.005 Gy are estimated to be due to radiation exposure.

The ERR of 0.3 is nearly identical for males and females (Fig. 8.11, top panel), but the EAR is about three times higher in males than in females. Since the baseline rates are 3 to 4 times higher in males than in females, this pattern of the gender difference suggests that radiation exposure may act multiplicatively with factors responsible for the baseline gender difference. A previous analysis demonstrated an unusual age-at-exposure pattern, that is, very little radiation effects for those exposed under age 10,[34] and this was supported by the latest incidence data. At this point, we do not understand the basis for this anomalous finding. The ERR decreases with increasing attained age as seen for many other solid cancers (Fig. 8.11, bottom panel).

Because it is a common site of metastatic disease, liver cancers reported on death certificates, or even reported to tumor registries, can be unreliable. In a previous study of liver cancers as confirmed by a pathology review,[34,35] a significant linear dose response was found for primary liver cancer. The dose response was essentially due to the radiation effect on hepatocellular carcinomas, which accounted for about 85% of primary liver cancers. A further study using biomarkers for hepatitis viral infection suggested a supermultiplicative interaction of radiation exposure with hepatitis C viral infection for hepatocellular carcinoma risk[36] but no evidence of the interaction with hepatitis B viral infection.

Lung

Lung cancer rates in Japan have been steadily increasing during the past several decades, most likely due to changes in smoking habits. Lung cancer is the second most common cancer in the LSS. There is a significant linear dose response for lung cancer incidence (Fig. 8.10). It is estimated that 15% of lung cancer cases among those exposed at >0.005 Gy are related to radiation exposure (Table 8.7). The radiation effect on lung cancer is among the strongest of all solid cancer risks, as measured in terms of ERR or EAR.

The ERR estimate for males is almost five times lower than that for females—the largest gender difference of all organ-specific ERR estimates (Fig. 8.11, top panel). However, the EAR estimate is not significantly different for males and females, suggesting that the gender difference in ERRs largely reflects lower baseline rates of lung cancer in females. Unlike most other solid cancers, which show a decline in ERR with increasing age at exposure, the lung cancer ERR appears to increase with increasing age at exposure (Fig. 8.11, middle panel). The EAR does not vary by age at exposure but increases with attained age. A plausible explanation for this unique ERR pattern may be that those who were young at exposure have a greater smoking risk (due to higher smoking intensity) than those who were older and that the smoking-radiation effects are more additive than multiplicative. The most recent analysis of the joint effects of smoking and radiation exposure in the LSS based on individual smoking data supported the additive nature of the joint effect, although the pattern of interaction was quite complex.[37] Adjustment for smoking habits reduced the ERR female:male ratio from 4.8 to 1.6, indicating that much of the gender difference in lung cancer radiation risk is due to gender differences in smoking rates.

Skin

Skin cancers, both melanocytic and nonmelanocytic, are rare in Japan. Among nonmelanocytic skin cancer, basal cell carcinoma is much more frequent than squamous cell carcinoma among Caucasians, whereas these two types occur with approximately equal frequency in Japan. The significant dose response found for nonmelanocytic cancer (Table 8.7) is primarily due to the strong dose response for basal cell carcinoma. There is no evidence of radiation effects on squamous cell carcinoma, as previously reported.[38] Basal cell carcinoma is the only cancer for which the data do not support a linear dose response. A model in which there is a spline (i.e., a change in slope) at 1 Gy fits better than a linear model (Fig. 8.10). This model indicates a lower ERR of 1.3 at doses below 1 Gy than that of 2.64 at higher doses. A previous study found the ERR for basal cell carcinoma to decrease markedly with increasing age at exposure.[38] It was not possible to analyze an association between radiation dose and malignant melanoma in the LSS, because only 17 cases occurred in the cohort.

Skin cancer is responsive to both ionizing and ultraviolet irradiation (UV). A separate pathology study[39] reported that the EARs for basal cell carcinoma per unit skin surface area were similar for tumors of UV-exposed and shielded parts of the body. That suggests that radiation-related risk is independent of UV exposure for basal cell carcinoma. A molecular study found that p53 mutations at CpG sites adjacent to pyrimidine dimers were associated with UV exposure, whereas CpG mutations distal from pyrimidine dimers were related to ionizing-radiation dose.[40] Also deletions in the PTCH gene were radiation dose related. Furthermore, 60% of skin cancers in the high-dose group had abnormalities in both the p53 and PTCH genes, compared with 23% of skin cancers in those with low doses.

Breast

Female breast cancer rates have historically been very low in Japan but have increased rapidly in the last several decades, although they are still about 2.5 times lower than in the United States.[41] In the LSS, there are 527 breast cancers among LSS members who received a breast dose of at least 0.005 Gy; of these, about 27% were associated with radiation exposure. The dose response is essentially linear, with no significant nonlinearity (Fig. 8.10). The ERR estimate of 0.87 for this cancer is among the highest of all solid cancer risks (Table 8.7).

Although it has been widely believed that age at exposure is a strong modifier of the breast cancer ERR,[42] the latest LSS data provide no evidence of the modifying effect of age at exposure on the ERR when attained age is included in the model. The ERR decreases significantly with increasing attained age, and age at exposure and attained age seem to have a significant joint effect on the EAR (Fig. 8.12, top panel).

Women who were exposed to the bombs at ages under 20 years have an exceedingly high risk of developing early-onset breast cancer. The risk for breast cancer prior to age 35 is 4.5 times higher in terms of ERR and 3.5 times higher in terms of EAR than expected from the standard models (Fig. 8.12, bottom panel). The higher radiation-related risk of early-onset breast cancer may suggest the presence of a genetically susceptible subgroup or reflect susceptibility of young mammary tissues to carcinogenic initiation.[43]

In an earlier case-control study of breast cancer in the LSS, early age at first full-term pregnancy, multiple births, and lengthy lactation history were protective against breast cancer,[44,45] as expected from numerous other studies. These factors appeared to have a synergistic effect on the radiation-related breast cancer risk.[44,45]

Important information on radiation-related breast cancer risks has also come from studies of women exposed to diagnostic or therapeutic radiation doses, usually delivered at high-dose rates or in fractionation. A pooled analysis has been conducted[46] of several cohorts differing in the nature of exposure and backgrounds, including the LSS[18] and populations

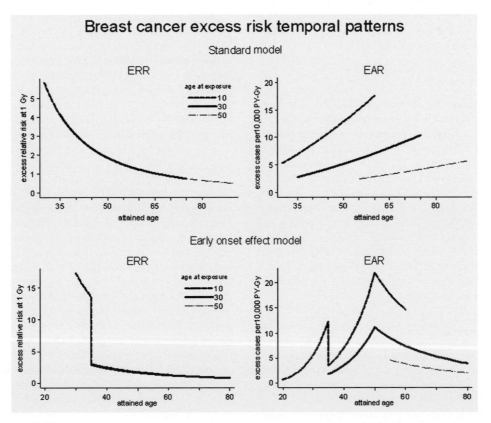

Figure 8.12. Temporal trend for cancer of the breast, LSS cancer incidence, 1958–1998. Temporal patterns and age at exposure variation in the radiation-associated excess breast cancers risks for the standard effect modification model in which excess risks is proportional to a log-linear function of age at exposure and a power of attained age (**top row**) and a model that includes an additional multiplicative effect for early-onset (prior to 35 years of age) cancer (**bottom row**). The panels in the left column compare variation in the ERR/Gy with attained age for ages at exposure of 10, 30, and 50 years. The panels in the right column compare variation in the EAR at 1 Gy with attained age for ages at exposure of 10, 30, and 50 years. (Reprinted from Preston DL, et al. Solid cancer incidence among atomic bomb survivors, 1958–1998. *RERF Update.* 2007;18:9–13, with permission.)

irradiated for tuberculosis fluoroscopic examinations,[47] acute postpartum mastitis,[48] thymic enlargement,[49] benign breast disease,[50] and skin hemangioma.[51,52] No simple unified summary model adequately described the excess breast cancer risk in all groups. The excess breast cancer rates and temporal patterns of the risk were similar for the thymus, tuberculosis and LSS cohorts, suggesting little influence of high-dose rate exposure (thymus patients and atomic-bomb survivors) versus fractionated low-dose rate exposures (tuberculosis patients). The excess rates were higher for the mastitis and benign breast disease patients, possibly reflecting high baseline rates associated with the condition for which they were treated or other factors associated with these benign breast diseases.

As in any other populations, breast cancer in males is rare in Japan. Only nine cases of male breast cancer have been diagnosed in the LSS to date, but a significant dose response was found for this cancer.[53] The ERR of eight is very high but imprecisely estimated because of the small number of cases.

Female Genital Organs

Ovarian cancer is relatively infrequent in Japan, although there has been an increasing trend for this cancer.[41] There is a significant linear dose response for ovarian cancer incidence, with an estimated ERR 0.61 (Table 8.7). Among the various female genital-organ cancers, cancer of the uterine cervix is the most common in this cohort, although cervical cancer rates have declined sharply in recent years in Japan.[54] There are no indications of radiation effects for cancers of the cervix or corpus, or cancers of the uterus as a whole.

Urinary Bladder

The incidence of cancer of the urinary bladder has been increasing but still is relatively infrequent in Japan.[41] There is a significant linear dose response for bladder cancer incidence (Fig. 8.10), with an ERR estimate of 1.23, which is the highest of all solid cancer ERRs (Table 8.7). The ERR is three times as high among females as males (Fig. 8.11, top panel) while the slight gender difference in the EAR is insignificant. Given the higher baseline rate for males, this suggests that the radiation effect is additive with respect to other factors (e.g., smoking and possible occupational exposure) contributing to the gender difference in baseline rates. The bladder cancer ERR is not significantly modified by age at exposure or attained age; in fact, it is the only major radiation-associated tumor site for which the ERR does not vary by attained age.

Brain/Central Nervous System

Brain/CNS tumors are rare in Japan as in other countries. There has been an increasing temporal trend in the incidence rates, probably largely attributable to the increasing use of new imaging diagnostic techniques.[55] An estimated linear ERR of 0.62 is significant (Table 8.7), but it is not possible to evaluate these data for linearity or nonlinearity, or modifying effects of age and gender because of the relatively small numbers. In a previous pathology study of brain/CNS tumors, the most common type in this cohort was meningioma followed by neuroepithelial tumor, schwannoma, and pituitary tumor.[56] Significant radiation effects were seen for schwannomas (ERR = 1.2), and suggestive dose-dependent excesses were seen for pituitary tumors, meningiomas, and gliomas.[38] The ERRs tended to be

higher for men than for women, and higher for younger ages at exposure.

Thyroid

Thyroid cancer rates are relatively high in Japan, and over 90% are papillary thyroid cancers, possibly owing to the high levels of iodine in the diet. Thyroid cancer was one of the first solid cancers associated with ionizing radiation.[57] A landmark in the study of radiation and thyroid cancer was a 1995 pooled analysis of seven of the largest studies, including the LSS, which reported a linear dose-response and a strong age-at-exposure effect such that exposure in childhood confers the largest risk and little risk is seen after adult exposure.[58]

Analysis of updated LSS thyroid cancer incidence data continues to show an essentially linear dose response (Fig. 8.10), although there is a suggestion that risk per unit dose is somewhat larger at lower doses and less at higher doses. The gender-averaged ERR is 0.57, with females having a 30% insignificantly higher risk. However, because females have a higher baseline risk of thyroid cancer, the EAR is 3.6 times as high among females as males. There is also a nearly significant age-at-exposure effect across the age range, such that persons exposed early in life have greater radiation risk in both relative and absolute terms (Fig. 8.11, middle panel). Finally, there is an attained-age effect such that the ERR decreases with increasing age.

Among about 4,100 participants in the AHS who received an ultrasound thyroid screening, 87 thyroid cancers were identified.[12] The thyroid cancer radiation risk tended to vary by age at exposure, with estimates of ERR being 3.5, 1.5, and 0.3 for ages 0 to 9, 10 to 19, and 20+ at the time of radiation exposure. Of those with known histopathology, 92% were papillary cancers. A case-control study of nonradiation risk factors for thyroid cancer did not find that smoking or alcohol consumption modified the radiation risk for thyroid cancer.[59]

Other Sites

Among the various other cancer sites, the gallbladder, pancreas, prostate, and kidney are relatively frequent sites of cancer in the cohort (Table 8.7). For all those sites, with the notable exception of cancer of the gallbladder, there are suggestive, positive dose-response relationships, being consistent with increased risks associated with radiation. ERR estimates are 0.26 for pancreas, 0.11 for prostate, and 0.13 for kidney cancers. An ERR estimate for gallbladder cancer of −0.05 is not significantly lower than zero (no radiation effect), but the upper bound of the confidence interval is lower than the ERR for all solid cancers, suggesting reduced radiation sensitivity of this organ.

There are a substantial number of cancer cases (about 840) at sites other than those discussed above. Those include cancers of ill-defined sites (25%) and numerous subsites. There is a significant linear dose response for this heterogeneous group (Fig. 8.11), with a large ERR estimate of 0.91 (Table 8.7). The largest subgroups of this collection of cancers are cancers of the larynx and the urothelial system. There is no indication of a radiation effect for cancer of the larynx but a significant dose response is seen for cancers of the urothelial system, with an estimated ERR of 2.8. After removing cancers of the larynx and urothelial systems, the dose response still remains significant.

Gender and Age Effects on Site-Specific Cancer Risks

Looking at gender differences in the ERR for various cancer sites (Fig. 8.11, top panel), higher ERRs for women and men are noted for most cancer sites with the largest gender (female:male) ratio for lung and bladder cancers. For both of those cancer sites, baseline cancer rates are much lower in women than in men, possibly reflecting the difference in smoking rates, so the differences in ERR are not reflected in EAR differences. Colon cancer is a notable exception as it is the only major site for which the ERR is higher for men than women.

With regard to the effects of age at exposure, ERRs are generally higher or similar for those exposed at younger (age 10) versus older ages (age 40) (Fig. 8.11, middle panel). The only exception is lung cancer for which the ERR increases with increasing age at exposure. As discussed above, previous analysis showed that this peculiar age-at-exposure trend is diminished when adjusted for smoking rates, which differ greatly by age and birth cohorts.[37] The higher ERR for thyroid cancer among those exposed to the atomic bombs at a young age is evident. The temporal pattern of the breast cancer ERR that has previously been described by the age-at-exposure effect is now captured by the deceasing ERR with attained age (Fig. 8.11, upper panel).

The ERR decreases with increasing attained age for most cancer sites (Fig. 8.11, bottom panel), with the exception of bladder cancer. This decreasing trend is most marked for colon, liver, and breast cancers. There is little evidence of an age-at-exposure effect for these cancer sites, the baseline cancer rates of which have been increasing.

DISEASES OTHER THAN CANCER

The principal source of morbidity information on diseases other than cancer (noncancer diseases) is the AHS. Initial selection of the approximately 20,000 subjects in this subset of the LSS was weighted toward individuals who had received higher doses, so as to be maximally informative regarding radiation effects. AHS subjects have undergone biennial health examinations with remarkably high participation rates since 1958. Morbidity events are reported or detected at the time of health examination, with an additional follow-up for diagnosis. The AHS provides longitudinal data on physiological changes and other subclinical characteristics and is a sampling frame for *ad hoc* studies focusing on special disease endpoints. The AHS is especially valuable for evaluating non-cancer radiation effects because population-based disease incidence registries exist only for cancer. All medical and technical personnel involved with clinical examinations, laboratory tests, and other data gathering are blinded as to the individuals' doses, so as not to introduce biases into the results.

Lens Opacities

Cataracts were first observed in cases who had received very high doses within 3 to 4 years after the bombings.[60] A thorough ophthalmologic examination of AHS subjects in the early 1960s identified posterior subcapsular opacities as the ocular lesion most characteristic of radiation exposure at relatively high doses, that is, >3 Gy.[61] A larger study conducted in 1978 to 1980 confirmed those findings among the subset with high doses who showed an excess of lenticular changes and opacities.[62] There was a suggestion that those younger at exposure may be more radiosensitive to the induction of lenticular changes and opacities. A subsequent reanalysis of those

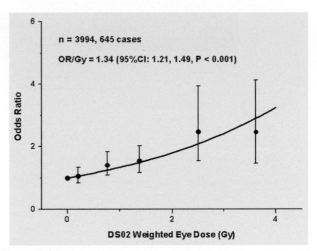

Figure 8.13. Dose response for postoperative cataract. AHS 2000 to 2002. Dose response for 3,761 AHS subjects who underwent medical examinations during 2000 to 2002 for whom radiation dose estimates were available, including 479 postoperative cataract cases. (Reprinted from Nakashima E, et al. A reanalysis of atomic-bomb cataract data, 2000–2002: a threshold analysis. *Health Phys.* 2006;90(2):154–160, with permission.)

data estimated a dose threshold at about 1.5 Gy with an upper confidence limit of 1.8.[63] This was essentially consistent with the judgments made for several decades by radiation protection advisory bodies, such as the International Commission on Radiation Protection[64] and the US National Council on Radiation Protection and Measurements.[65] Those bodies indicated there is a dose threshold such that excess opacities are unlikely to be found below 2 Gy nor cataracts that cause visual impairment below 5 Gy.

Ophthalmologic screening recently conducted (2000–2002) in the AHS subjects found a dose-dependent excess for posterior subcapsular opacities (44% excess at an eye dose of 1 Gy) and a slightly smaller excess for cortical opacities (30% excess at 1 Gy).[66,67] The best estimate of a dose threshold is 0.7 Gy for posterior subcapsular opacities and 0.6 Gy for cortical cataracts. Because of the wide confidence intervals of those estimates, however, the data cannot rule out a lack of a dose threshold and are only marginally consistent with a 2-Gy dose threshold.

However, most of the opacities detected in those ophthalmologic examinations were of relatively low grade and had little or no adverse effect on visual acuity.[66] To assess vision-impairing cataracts, a further study was conducted using history of cataract surgeries as the outcome measure. This study found a 39% excess risk of cataract surgery at 1 Gy (Fig. 8.13). The best estimate for a threshold dose was only 0.1 Gy with an upper confidence bound of 0.8 Gy,[68] so that it is statistically incompatible with a dose threshold of 2 or more Gy, as propounded by the radiation protection bodies. It is the strongest, though not the only, evidence that is prompting those bodies to reconsider what appropriate maximum levels should be set to protect workers (e.g., interventional cardiologists) and others who may receive substantial ocular radiation exposures.

Thyroid Diseases and Hyperparathyroidism

Recently, a thyroid disease screening was conducted in both Hiroshima and Nagasaki survivors some 55 years after the atomic bombs.[12] The investigations involved thyroid ultrasound with a standardized radiological review, clinical laboratory tests, and fine-needle biopsy for nodules >1 cm. A significant linear

TABLE 8.8	Estimated Excess Odds Ratios (EOR) for Thyroid Disease, AHS, 2000 to 2003		
Diagnosis	*No. of Cases*	*EOR/Gy[a] (95% CI)*	*p*
Solid nodule	464	2.01 (1.33–2.94)	<0.001
Malignant tumor	70	1.95 (0.67–4.92)	<0.001
Benign tumor	156	1.53 (0.76–2.67)	<0.001
Other	258	1.67 (0.93–2.83)	<0.001
Cyst	244	0.89 (0.48–1.47)	<0.001
Positive antithyroid antibodies	898	−0.07 (−0.16–0.04)	0.20
Positive TPOAb	427	0.01 (−0.12–0.19)	0.91
Positive TgAb	761	−0.04 (−0.13–0.09)	0.52
Antithyroid antibodies-positive hypothyrodism	102	0.01 (−0.20–0.40)	0.92
Antithyroid antibodies-negative hypothyroidism	81	0.17 (−0.12–0.67)	0.31
Graves disease	38	0.49 (−0.06–1.69)	0.10
Total number examined	**2,637**		

[a]EOR for a person exposed at age 10. This is approximately equivalent to an ERR.
TPOAb, antithyroid peroxidase antibody; TgAb, antithyroglobulin antibody.
Source: Adapted from Imaizumi M, Usa T, et al. Radiation dose-response relationships for thyroid nodules and autoimmune thyroid diseases in Hiroshima and Nagasaki atomic bomb survivors 55–58 years after radiation exposure. *JAMA.* 2006;295(9):1011–1022.

radiation dose response was found for thyroid nodules, with an excess odds ratio (or ERR) per Gy of 2.01 for solid nodule as a group (1.95 for malignant nodule, 1.53 for benign nodule) and that of 0.89 for thyroid cysts (Table 8.8). The radiation-related odds ratios for nodules decreased significantly with increasing age at exposure; this trend existed for both benign and malignant nodules. No significant dose response was found for autoimmune thyroid diseases, that is, positive antithyroid antibodies, antithyroid antibody-positive, or Grave disease.

Hyperparathyroidism is caused most commonly by an adenoma and less frequently by hyperplasia or cancer of the parathyroid gland. The prevalence of hyperparathyroidism has been found to increase with radiation dose, with an estimated relative risk of 4.1 at 1 Gy. Some evidence exists that the effect of radiation on hyperparathyroidism is greater for individuals who were younger at the time of bombing.

Cardiovascular and other late-onset diseases

Indications for radiation effects on cardiovascular disease and other late-onset diseases emerged from a series of analyses of LSS mortality data. Significant radiation dose-related increases were first reported in 1992 for diseases other than cancer (noncancer diseases) as a group and for several disease categories, that is, diseases of the circulatory, digestive, and respiratory systems (Table 8.9).[69] Deaths from heart disease and stroke make up more than half (54%) of noncancer disease deaths, and the radiation dose response is significant for both categories of circulatory disease. Deaths from diseases of the respiratory system and digestive disease are less frequent, 12% and 10% of all noncancer disease deaths, respectively. Subsequently, more detailed analysis of updated mortality data showed that the dose-related increase in the risk of noncancer diseases cannot be

TABLE 8.9	ERRs and Estimated Numbers of Radiation-related Deaths from Noncancer Diseases, LSS mortality, 1968 to 1997		
Cause	*ERR/Sv*	*Deaths[a]*	*Estimated Number of Radiation-Associated Deaths*
All non–cancer diseases	0.14 (0.08; 0.2)[b]	14,459	273 (176; 375)[b]
Heart disease	0.17 (0.08; 0.26)	4,477	101 (47; 161)
Stroke	0.12 (0.02; 0.22)	3,954	64 (14; 118)
Respiratory disease	0.18 (0.06; 0.32)	2,266	57 (19; 98)
Pneumonia	0.16 (0.00;0.32)	1,528	33 (4; 67)
Digestive disease	0.15 (0.00; 0.32)	1,292	27 (0; 58)
Cirrhosis	0.19 (−0.05; 0.5)	567	16 (−2; 37)
Infectious disease	−0.02 (<−0.2; 0.25)	397	−1 (−14; 15)
Tuberculosis	−0.01 (<−0.2; 0.4)	237	−0.5 (−2; 13)
Other diseases	0.08 (−0.04; 0.23)	2,073	24 (−12; 64)
Urinary diseases	0.25 (−0.01; 0.6)	515	17 (−1; 39)

[a]Deaths among proximal survivors between 1968 and 1997.
[b]90% confidence interval.
[c]Excluding diseases of the blood and blood-forming organs.
Source: Adapted from Preston DL, Shimizu Y, et al. Studies of mortality of atomic bomb survivors. Report 13: Solid cancer and noncancer disease mortality: 1950–1997. *Radiat Res.* 2003;160(4):381–407.

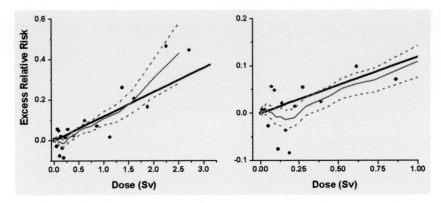

Figure 8.14. Noncancer dose-response function. LSS mortality, 1968 to 1997. The solid straight line indicates the fitted linear ERR model without any effect modification by age at exposure, sex, or attained age. The points are dose category-specific ERR estimates, the solid curve is a smoothed estimate derived from the points, and the dashed lines indicate upper- and lower- one-standard error bounds on the smoothed estimate. The right panel shows the low-dose portion of the dose-response function. (Reprinted from Preston DL, et al. Studies of mortality of atomic bomb survivors. Report 13: Solid cancer and noncancer disease mortality: 1950–1997. *Radiat Res.* 2003;160(4):381–407, with permission.)

explained by smoking or other confounding risk factors examined, possible bias associated with the selection of the survivors, or cancer to noncancer misclassification of causes of death.[24] The RR of noncancer disease is small. An ERR estimate of 0.14 for mortality from all noncancer diseases is about one third of that of 0.47 for all solid cancer mortality. However, because of the relatively high baseline noncancer disease rates, the estimated number of excess noncancer deaths is close to two thirds of that for all solid cancers (Table 8.9; Table 13 from Preston).[26]

There is a significant curvature in the noncancer disease dose response for the follow-up period before 1967,[26] whereas there is no evidence of nonlinearity for noncancer mortality for the later period (1968–1997) (Fig. 8.14). There is a considerable uncertainty regarding the dose response at doses below about 0.5 Gy.[26] Reviewing existing epidemiological data on noncancer diseases following radiation exposure, the UNSCEAR concluded that there is little evidence, outside the atomic-bomb studies, to support an association between fatal cardiovascular disease and radiation exposure in the range of doses <1 to 2 Gy.[70] Similar conclusions have been reached by some[71,72] while others have pointed out that the radiation-related cardiovascular risk in the atomic-bomb survivors is consistent with the high-dose data after adjusting for dose fractionation effects.[73]

Periodic analyses of the AHS biennial examination data have also identified radiation-related increased risks for several major noncancer disease categories[74,75] (Table 8.10). Significant radiation effects were found for chronic liver disease (including fatty liver, alcoholic liver disease, and chronic hepatitis), uterine myoma, cataract, and hypertension.

CARDIOVASCULAR DISEASE AND RELATED CONDITIONS. The latest LSS mortality data (for 1950–2003) on different categories of cardiovascular diseases provided an ERR estimate of 0.09 for stroke based on a linear dose response model, but an indication of upward curvature implied relatively little risk at low doses. For heart disease, an ERR estimate was 0.14 and linear dose response model provided the best fit, suggesting an excess risk at lower doses.[75a] A special study of incident cases of myocardial infarction ascertained from the AHS examination and other medical

sources showed a significant dose response with an estimated relative risk of myocardial infarction at 1 Gy of 1.17, which is similar to the mortality risk estimate.[76] The dose response remained significant after adjusting for blood pressure and serum cholesterol levels.

Subclinical endpoints of cardiovascular and related changes have also been studied in the AHS population. Longitudinal analyses of biennial blood pressure measurements and total serum cholesterol levels since 1958 demonstrated a small but statistically significant radiation effect on temporal or age-related trends for both systolic and diastolic blood pressure[77] as well as cholesterol levels.[78] Therefore, radiation effects on atherosclerotic changes are evident at the preclinical level. Other cardiovascular-related radiation effects seen are dose-related differences in lipid profiles (increased total cholesterol and triglycerides, decreased HDL) that may suggest a mechanism linking radiation exposure to fatty liver as well as aortic arch calcification, hypertension, and ischemic heart diseases.[79]

Some biological insights regarding the radiation effect on atherosclerosis come from study results pointing to radiation effects on long-term inflammatory responses. A significant association between radiation dose and increased inflammatory responses, as measured by leukocytosis, accelerated erythrocyte sedimentation rates or acute phase proteins, has been noted in this population for some time.[80,81] That association has been reexamined using an additional set of inflammatory tests[82]; after allowing for the effect of smoking, radiation dose was found to be associated with increases in levels of α1-globulin, α2-globulin, and sialic acid as well as leukocyte counts and erythrocyte sedimentation rates. In another study,[83] C-reactive protein levels were found to increase significantly with radiation dose (an increase of about 28% at 1 Gy), as did interleukin 6 levels, by 9.3% at 1 Gy.

LIVER DISEASE AND HEPATITIS VIRAL INFECTION. As seen in Table 8.9, over half of radiation-related excess deaths from digestive disease in the LSS are from liver cirrhosis.[26] In Japan, the predominant causes of chronic hepatitis are hepatitis C virus (HCV) and hepatitis B virus (HBV) infection. Among the atomic-bomb survivors, the prevalence of HBV surface antigen positivity has been found to be increased with radiation dose, but not that of

TABLE 8.10	Estimated Relative Risk[a] at 1 Gy for Noncancer Disease Incidence, AHS, 1958 to 1998		
	No. of Cases	*Estimated RR at 1 Sv*	*(95% CI)*
Hypertension	5,035	1.05	(0.99, 1.00)
Hypertension, quadratic model	5,035	1.03	(1.01, 1.06)
Hypertensive heart disease	1,886	0.99	(0.91, 1.09)
Ischemic heart disease	1,546	1.05	(0.95, 1.16)
Myocardial infarction	117	1.12	(0.84, 1.60)
Myocardial infarction, at age <40, quadratic model for 1968–1998	78	1.17	(0.97, 1.56)
Occlusion, stenosis	440	1.06	(0.89, 1.30)
Aortic aneurysm	184	1.02	(0.78, 1.41)
Stroke	184	1.08	(0.90, 1.31)
Stroke, including ill-defined cerebrovascular diseases	729	1.07	(0.92, 1.24)
Thyroid disease	964	1.38	(1.22, 1.57)
Cataract	3,484	1.11	(1.03, 1.19)
Gastric ulcer	930	1.00	(0.88, 1.12)
Chronic liver disease and cirrhosis	1,774	1.12	(1.03, 1.22)
Cholelithiasis	959	1.00	(0.89, 1.12)
Calculus of kidney and ureter	323	1.16	(0.96, 1.43)
Cervical polyp, female	281	1.13	(0.90, 1.45)
Hyperplasia of prostate, male	461	0.90	(0.78, 1.06)
Dementia	316	1.20	(0.92, 1.59)
Parkinson disease	97	0.99	(0.73, 1.58)
Glaucoma	211	0.73	(0.72, 0.89)
Total study subjects	10,339		

[a]Relative risks estimated by a linear model, unless otherwise specified.
Source: Adapted from Yamada M, Wong FL, et al. Noncancer disease incidence in atomic bomb survivors, 1958–1998. *Radiat Res.* 2004;161(6):622–632.

anti-HBV core antibody positivity,[84,85] suggesting that radiation may reduce the ability to clear HBV infection. However, the extent to which that postulated mechanism may contribute to the risk of chronic hepatitis or liver cirrhosis in the survivors remains unclear. With respect to HCV infection, there is no indication for a dose-related increase in the prevalence of anti-HCV antibody positivity.[85] It is possible that the strong synergistic interaction between radiation and HCV infection, as seen for liver cancer (see "Solid Cancer" section), may also be involved in the progression of liver disease associated with HCV infection.[84]

Growth and Development

Following an earlier finding on radiation-related reduction in weight and height at ages <10 years,[86] a further longitudinal analysis has been conducted of measured heights (stature) in the AHS subjects for a 30-year period (1958–1998).[87] A significant reduction in stature associated with radiation exposure was found for persons who were exposed to the bomb at ages <19 years. Estimated effects per Gy were a 1.2 to 2.0 cm reduction for those exposed before 1 year of age.

Radiation effects on the development of female or male reproductive organs among atomic survivors are not clear. Effects on age at menarche and menopause among female survivors also remain unclear. Investigations to measure the level of fertility or prevalence of sterility have been hampered by the difficulty in controlling the influence of social and other factors.[88]

Psychological Effects

The extent of psychological and social effects of the atomic bombing in Hiroshima and Nagasaki was well captured by an in-depth interview study conducted by Lifton in 1962[89] and numerous other anecdotal reports.[90] However, little epidemiological data are available on long-term psychological effects among the survivors. A survey conducted 17 to 20 years after the bombs found that people who were in the city at the time of the bombs reported higher frequencies of anxiety and somatization symptoms than those who were not in the city.[90] Anxiety and somatization disorders have been most frequently found in people with posttraumatic syndrome. In the atomic-bomb survivors, the prevalence of anxiety and somatization symptoms was higher among those who reported acute radiation symptoms. Paradoxically, however, the anxiety and somatization prevalence increased with increasing distance from the hypocenter. The latter trend, which parallels the LSS finding on the decreasing suicide rates with increasing dose,[24,69] remains unexplained.

Aging and Life Shortening

Several clinical endpoints for aging-related conditions have been investigated in the AHS. Thus far, none has been found to be radiation-dose dependent, including osteoporosis as measured by incidence of vertebral fracture and bone mineral density,[91] incidence of Alzheimer dementia or vascular dementia,[92] prostatic hyperplasia, or Parkinson disease.[75]

More broadly, the effects of radiation, especially at low doses, on life expectancy have been the subject of general debate. This has been investigated by analyzing the LSS all-cause mortality data.[93] Relative mortality rates and survival distribution associated with radiation doses were calculated by cohort-based estimation of baseline mortality. Median life expectancy decreased with increasing doses at a rate of about 1.3 years/Gy, but declined more rapidly at high doses. Median loss of life was

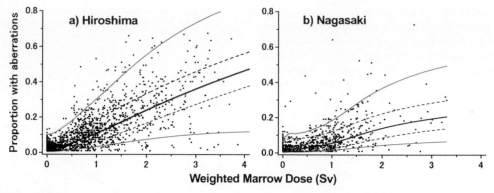

Figure 8.15. Chromosomal aberrations and dose. Proportion of cells with aberration as a function of dose (DS86). The thick curve is a nonparametric estimate of the dose-response function. The dashed lines are 95% prediction limits assuming that cells with aberrations follow a binomial random variation. The outer curves are 95% prediction limits incorporating binomial sampling error and the additional variability from errors in individual dose estimates. (Reprinted from Kodama Y. Stable chromosome aberrations in atomic bomb survivors: results from 25 years of investigation. *Radiat Res.* 2001;156(4):337–346, with permission.)

about 2 months for those with doses below 1 Gy and 2.6 years for those with doses of over 1 Gy. It was estimated that, at 1 Gy, the proportion of total life lost was roughly 60% from solid cancer, 30% from diseases other than cancer, and 10% from leukemia.

Cytogenetic Changes and Somatic Mutations

More than six decades after the atomic bombs, effects of radiation are still observed among the survivors in the frequency of somatic mutations, notably chromosomal aberrations in lymphocytes, and changes in lymphoid cell composition and functions (see next section). Various assays of gene mutations in blood cells in the survivors have been studied, but chromosomal aberrations remain the best indicator of radiation doses that survivors received decades earlier.

Stable chromosomal aberrations were examined in more than 3,000 survivors over a 25-year period starting in the late 1960s to detect cells with a least one translocation or inversion in Giemsa-stained cultures.[94] A highly significant and nonlinear dose response was seen when aberration frequencies were plotted against DS86 doses (Fig. 8.15). As pointed out elsewhere,[95] individual aberration frequencies, when regressed on the physical dose estimates (DS86), exhibited considerably more scatter than predicted for binomial data. This "overdispersion" is due at least in part to imprecision in dose estimates derived from incomplete or approximate information about survivor location and shielding at the time of the bombings. The contribution of a subgroup of people with altered radiosensitivity to the overdispersion is considered small given the small proportion of such subgroups in the general population. The downward curvature in the dose-response relationship at high doses may also be a consequence of random errors in survivor dose estimates. The city difference in the slope of the dose response (lower in Nagasaki) (Fig. 8.15) cannot be explained by differences in the contribution of neutrons but is rather likely due to differences in detection efficiency of translocations by the Giemsa stain methods. Preliminary results from a new study underway using the fluorescence in situ hybridization technique show smaller city differences.

Various assays of somatic mutation have been tested in the survivors, including T-cell hypoxanthine phosphoribosyl-transferase gene, human leukocyte antigen-A gene and T-cell receptor (TCR-α

and TCR-β) genes, and erythrocyte mutation at glycophorin A (GPA) gene. Among these only GPA assay has been found to be capable of detecting long-term radiation effects.[96] However, a major limitation is that this assay is useful for people with M/N heterozygosity, who are 50% of the general population. This and a large individual variability of the mutation frequency make this assay less useful than cytogenetic methods.[97]

Immune Response

Radiation-related changes seen in T-lymphoid cell composition are described by decreased proportions of CD4 helper cells as well as CD4 and CD8 naïve T-cells. Also, radiation-related impairments in T-cell function have been suggested by decreases in T-cell response to mitogens, for example, phytohemagglutinin, alloantigens (mixed lymphocyte reaction) and superantigen, and the ability to produce interleukin 2. On the other hand, dose-dependent increases in proportions of B-cells and inflammatory cytokine levels have been observed.[98,99] Mechanisms by which exposure to radiation from the bombs have led to these long-lasting immunological changes are not well understood. However, it has been suggested that perturbed T-cell homeostasis may accelerate immunological aging and play a role in persistent inflammation involved in the development of atherosclerotic cardiovascular disease. AHS data have not provided evidence of a radiation effect on autoimmune diseases, such as rheumatoid arthritis,[100,101] Sjögren syndrome,[102] or, as indicated above, autoimmune thyroid diseases.[12]

IN UTERO EXPOSURE

The *In Utero* Cohort comprises about 3,300 individuals who were born to mothers pregnant at the time of the bomb[11,103] (Table 8.1). As with the LSS, the *in utero* cohort is followed up for mortality and cancer incidence and a subset is clinically followed as part of the AHS program.

LEUKEMIA AND SOLID CANCERS

During the first 15 years of life in this group of children, there was only one death from leukemia or cancer. A girl who received a relatively high dose (1.43 Gy) died from liver cancer at age 6 years.[103,104] The chance that a cancer unrelated to radiation would occur at such a high dose appears small because only 29 of the 807 person exposed *in utero* (>0.01 Gy) had higher doses, that is, $p = 29/807 = 0.036$.[103,104] This would translate into a large ERR, but with an extremely wide confidence interval. Reviewing the childhood cancer data, ICRP concluded that the dose response from the atomic-bomb study is compatible with the risk estimates seen in the medical irradiation studies but only weakly supportive of them.[105]

The uniqueness of the atomic-bomb *in utero* cohort lies with the follow-up data for adult cancers, about which there are no other informative studies. A recent report of the atomic-bomb study compared the risk estimates for those exposed *in utero* and during childhood as to the incidence of adult solid cancer (at ages 12–55).[11] There was a statistically significant dose dependence for the *in utero* group as well as for the childhood cohort. However, while the EAR increased with time/age for those exposed in childhood, the EAR was relatively flat with increasing age for those exposed *in utero* (Fig. 8.16). At present, it does not appear that *in utero* exposure confers greater adult-cancer risk than childhood exposure, but the difference between the *in utero* and childhood exposure EARs is only suggestive at this point, so further follow-up to older ages is needed.

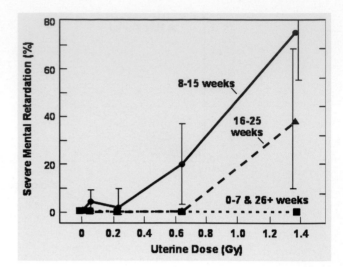

Figure 8.17. Mental retardation by weeks of postconception and dose.

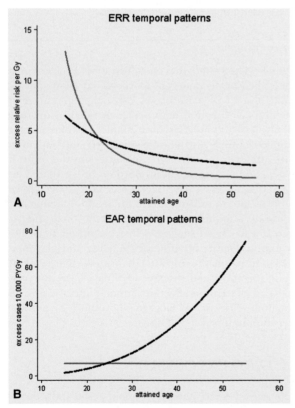

Figure 8.16. Temporal pattern of radiation-associated solid cancer incidence risks among atomic-bomb survivors exposed *in utero* or as young children. The plots describe variation in (**A**) ERRs, and (**B**) EARs following exposure to a radiation dose of 1 Gy. No statistically significant differences between *in utero* (*solid lines*) and early childhood (*dashed lines*) exposure temporal trends were observed for either the ERR or the EARs. (Reprinted from Preston D, et al. Solid cancer incidence in atomic bomb survivors exposed *in utero* or as young children. *J Natl Cancer Inst.* 2008;100(6):428–436, with permission.)

In that regard, it is of interest to note that chromosomal aberration data for the survivors who were exposed *in utero* and had their blood lymphocytes examined at age around 40 years did not indicate any sign of a radiation effect[106] while their mothers did show a clear dose response as seen in other survivors. The finding that chromosome aberrations do not persist after fetal irradiation may be related to the fact that the bone marrow niche for the hematopoietic stem cells is only established sometime after birth in mice[107] and suggests that the aberrant stem cells may perish before they settle in the bone marrow niche. It remains to be known if this characteristic is tissue specific or will have an influence on cancer risk following fetal exposure to radiation.

NEUROLOGICAL EFFECTS

Early studies of neurological effects conducted among children exposed *in utero* are another source of unique information. An increase of frank mental retardation was found among those who were exposed at 16 to 25 weeks and especially at 8 to 15 weeks postconception.[108] But no effects were seen before 8 weeks or after 25 weeks (Fig. 8.17).[109] The prevalence of the effect was estimated to be about 40% at 1 Gy in the 8 to 15 week group, but there appeared to be a dose threshold, which was estimated to be at about 0.6 Gy with a lower confidence limit of 0.3 Gy. Thus, it is unlikely that mental retardation would occur as a result of *in utero* brain doses of <0.3 Gy.[105] The mental retardation was often accompanied by a reduced head size. The most pronounced mental-retardation effects were seen in the period at about 8 to 12 weeks after conception, and MRI examination of several such cases showed an inappropriate migration of neurons to the cerebrum (ectopic gray matter) or faulty brain architecture.[110]

Although the number of cases with frank mental retardation was small, an IQ test administered to about 1,670 school-age children who were *in utero* at the time of the bombs showed a general decrease in IQ amounting to about 25 IQ points at 1 Gy for those who were ages 8 to 15 weeks postconception at exposure.[105] There was other corroborative evidence as well. The records of the highly standardized Japanese primary school grading system showed a dose-dependent decrease in school achievement scores among those who were exposed at 8 to 25 weeks postconception.[105,111] Another study showed a dose-related increase within the 8- to 25-week postconception group in the percentage who had had afebrile seizures of unknown cause.[112]

OTHER DISEASES

Recent AHS data provide some evidence, though limited by the small cohort size, of increased risks of late adult-onset diseases associated with *in utero* radiation exposure. Health examination data of about 1,000 *in utero* AHS subjects showed a radiation-related increase in systolic blood pressure measured during adolescence, with an estimated dose effect of 2.09 mm Hg/Gy.[113] A separate study of examination data during the period 1978 to 2003[114] found a significant association of radiation dose with cardiovascular disease (myocardial infarction or stroke) and hypertension among a group of 1,053 childhood-exposed subjects but not among a smaller group of 506 *in utero* exposed subjects. However, the estimated risks associated with *in utero* exposure, with very wide confidence intervals, were not significantly different from that with childhood exposure.

In a thyroid examination study of about 300 AHS subjects with *in utero* exposure, a dose response for thyroid nodules was not significant, possibly due to the small number of cases but an estimated odds ratio at 1 Gy of 2.78 was similar to that in the postnatally exposed population.[115]

GENETIC EFFECTS: SECOND GENERATION (F1)

Immediately following the atomic bombings, a major public concern arose about the possible genetic effect of radiation in the children of the survivors, and ABCC decided to plan and initiate a large-scale study to assess the frequency of birth defects and other pregnancy outcomes. This monumental work was started in 1948 by Neel and Schull[3] and involved population-based recruitment of 77,000 pregnant women in Hiroshima and Nagasaki, clinical follow-up of these pregnancies starting at the fifth month of gestation through births and questionnaire administration on survivor location and shielding.

The details of the study design, execution and results from early ABCC studies are compiled in "The Children of Atomic Bomb Survivors."[116] Past and present major genetic studies are summarized in Table 8.11.[117]

UNTOWARD PREGNANCY OUTCOMES AND SEX RATIO

The endpoints of untoward pregnancy outcomes included congenital malformations, stillbirth, and prenatal deaths (death within 1 week after birth). During the period of 1948 to 1954, 77,000 newborns were examined and autopsies were also carried out. The results initially were analyzed using crude measures of radiation exposure and later using DS86 dose estimates. No evidence of the effect of parental radiation exposure was found on the frequency of untoward pregnancy outcomes as defined by congenital malformation, stillbirth and perinatal death.[3]

The experimental finding that the proportion of male offspring decreased following maternal irradiation in fruit flies had prompted an investigation to see if the same trend had been observable in the offspring of the survivors. However, no shift in sex ratio was found in the survivor's offspring.[3,118] The discrepancy is explained as follows. In the flies, male offspring are preferentially lost due to an increased frequency of recessive lethal mutations in the maternal X chromosome, but females are protected from this effect because the two X chromosomes are fully active. In mammalian females, by contrast as it was discovered, one of the two X-chromosomes is inactivated (Lyonization) and hence females may not be protected from the detrimental effects of radiation-induced mutations.

CYTOGENETICS

The Giemsa staining method was used to examine blood lymphocytes from 8,322 exposed children and 7,976 unexposed children. Those subjects were selected from members of the F1 cohort for epidemiological follow-up (see below). The frequency of individuals with cytogenetic abnormality (either numerical or structural) was 0.5% to 0.6% in both groups.[119] *De novo* structural rearrangements (both parents normal) were seen in 0.02%, with no indication of a parental radiation exposure effect.

TABLE 8.11	**Major Genetic Studies at ABCC-RERF: Past and Present**		
Study	*No. of Study Subjects*	*Study Period*	*Study Descriptions*
Birth defects and other untoward pregnancy outcomes	77,000	1948–1954	Congenital malformations, stillbirth, perinatal death
Sex ratio	140,000	1948–1966	Search for x-chromosomal recessive lethal mutations
Cytogenetics	16,000	1967–1985	Solid Giemsa method
Biochemical genetic studies	23,000	1975–1984	Electrophoretic variants and erythrocyte enzyme activity
Molecular genetic studies	1,000 child-parent trios	1980s–present	Lymphoblastoid cell lines: two-dimensional DNA electrophoresis, minisatellite mutations, microarray-based comparative genomic hybridization
Epidemiological follow-up	77,000	1946-present	Mortality and cancer incidence follow-up
Clinical health examination	10,000	2002–2006	Prevalence of adult-onset multifactorial diseases

Source: Adapted from Nakamura N. Genetic effects of radiation in atomic-bomb survivors and their children: past, present and future. *J Radiat Res (Tokyo)*. 2006;47(suppl B):B67–B73.

BIOCHEMICAL GENETICS

In a study to detect electrophoretic variants of serum proteins (30 different proteins in 13,000 exposed offspring and 11,000 controls), the number of new mutations found was small (3 in each group) and there was no indication of a radiation effect.[120]

MOLECULAR GENETIC STUDIES

In the mid-1980s, systematic blood collection was initiated to establish immortalized (EBV transformed) lymphoblastoid cell lines from father-mother-child trios. Several studies using these cell lines are ongoing, including mutation frequency at minisatellite loci, deletion mutation using two-dimensional gel electrophoresis technique, or microarray-based comparative genomic hybridization method. Thus far, no discernible effects of parental exposure have been observed.[117]

CANCER AND OTHER MULTIFACTORIAL DISEASES

Following the completion of the early genetic study by Neel and Schull, the need for long-term surveillance of the survivors' offspring was recognized and this led to the formation of the F1 Cohort for epidemiological follow-up. An original cohort of about 59,500 offspring born to parents, one or both of whom were in Hiroshima or Nagasaki at the time of the bomb, were later expanded to include about 77,000 offspring born between 1946 and 1984[121–123] (Table 8.1). As with the LSS, the F1 cohort is followed up for mortality and cancer incidence.

The most recent mortality and cancer incidence data show no evidence of a parental dose-related effect on cancer or noncancer mortality.[124] In the latest mortality study of 40,500 offspring, for whom both paternal and maternal dose estimates are available, hazard ratios for noncancer deaths are 1.01 associated with paternal exposure at 100 mGy and 0.99 associated with maternal exposure at the same dose. Hazard ratios for cancer mortality are 0.95 associated with paternal exposure and 1.00 associated with maternal exposure. For subjects with both parents exposed, the adjusted hazard ratios are 1.16 for

noncancer mortality and 0.96 for cancer mortality. None of those are statistically significant. Analysis of cancer incidence data also provided no evidence of a radiation effect from either paternal or maternal radiation exposure.[123]

The first study to examine whether parental radiation exposure leads to increased heritable risk of common adult-onset multifactorial diseases (i.e., hypertension, diabetes mellitus, hypercholesterolemia, ischemic heart disease, and stroke) was conducted in the clinical examination program involving nearly 12,000 offspring of atomic-bomb survivors who had reached a median age of about 50 years. Data indicated no evidence of association between prevalence of multifactorial diseases in the offspring and parental radiation exposure.[125] Continued follow-up to older ages is clearly needed to investigate the impact of possible genetic effects on disease morbidity and mortality.

SUMMARY AND FUTURE

To date, more than half a century after the bombings, a major overt effect of acute exposure to external radiation is seen in the increased incidence and mortality risks of hematopoietic and solid cancers that adversely affect the longevity and quality of life of the survivors. There is emerging evidence of dose-related increases in risks, also both mortality and incidence, of cardiovascular and several other late-onset noncancer diseases. The persistent nature of the radiation-related risk for solid cancer and noncancer diseases, which may last for one's life time as the current follow-up data suggest, is a matter of concern and scientific importance. New insights into the nature of the radiation-related risk are needed and will undoubtedly come from further follow-up investigations. In the LSS, people exposed to the atomic bombs prior to age 20 comprise the largest proportion (about 70%) of those who are alive (as of 1997, the latest follow-up year) and they generally have larger radiation-related risks than those exposed at older ages. Therefore, the numbers of deaths from all causes and cancer each year will continue to increase through around 2020 (Fig. 8.18).[24] The current risk model predicts that more than about half of the radiation-related excess deaths in the LSS are yet to occur.

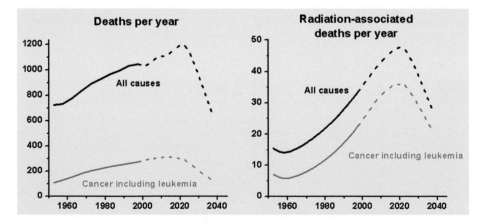

Figure 8.18. Total and radiation-associated deaths per year for all causes and for cancers including leukemia. LSS cohort. The solid lines show the data for the 1950 to 1997 follow-up period while the dashed lines are projections based on the ERR models. The solid cancer model includes both age-at-exposure and attained-age effects while the linear constant relative risk model was used for noncancer. Background rates were projected assuming the birth cohort effects seen in the cohort to date will continue into the future. (Reprinted from Preston D. Studies of mortality of atomic bomb survivors. Report 13: Solid cancer and noncancer disease mortality: 1950–1997. *Radiat Res.* 2003;160(4):381–407, with permission.)

Much has been learned about the dose response for solid cancers and how it is modified by gender, age, and time. Much more, however, needs to be learned about organ-specific cancer risks and their risk modifiers. Our understanding of the radiation-related risk for many cancer sites is still limited, largely because of statistical imprecision due to limited numbers of cases. An attempt has been made and should continue to develop statistical methods to improve organ-specific risk estimates given this limitation.[126] While statistical precision may be improved as numbers of cases will increase in future follow-up, more importantly, further insights are needed about how the radiation-related risk is modified by other risk factors, for example, smoking, female reproductive factors, viral infection, nutrition, etc. Further knowledge in this area will help in extrapolating the risk data from the Japanese population to others with differing disease background. It should be reminded that the patterns of cancer rates are rapidly changing in Japan and becoming similar to the patterns seen in the United States and other western countries. Biological samples for many of the survivors offer opportunities for learning more about radiation carcinogenesis at more fundamental levels and can be capitalized upon.

Some long-term radiation effects on diseases other than cancer are just coming into sight and will become clearer as young survivors become older. Radiation effects on cardiovascular and other late-onset diseases are just being unraveled. The lack of a population-based disease reporting system for noncancer disease incidence hampers a systematic monitoring of disease occurrence. However, the AHS database has effectively identified a number of specific diseases associated with radiation (e.g., thyroid nodule, hyperthyroidism, hypertension, liver disease) and shed light on radiation-related changes that have possible biological implications. More advances can be expected from this approach.

The RERF cohorts of the children exposed to the bomb in *utero* is small but very unique. The RERF data on pediatric cancer risk following *in utero* exposure are largely negative, most likely due to the small cohort size, but a radiation-related increase has been seen for solid cancers occurring in early adult years. The current data suggest the tapering off of the radiation-related cancer risk as the *in utero* survivors age, but this remains to be seen. At the same time, there is an emerging trend of a radiation-related risk of noncancer disease. More follow-up is needed to determine the long-term health consequences of neurological effects and late effects in this population.

The initial study of genetic effects conducted starting soon after the bombs revealed no demonstrable adverse effect on birth defects, other undesirable pregnancy outcomes or other indicators of genetic effects. Given the relatively low parental doses, the negative results do not necessarily indicate that there is no effect. Rather, these and other data from the ongoing RERF studies have been and will continue to be used to estimate the upper bound of the risk. Additional data on adult-onset multifactorial disease (such as diabetes and circulatory disease) are expected to provide additional information unavailable elsewhere, as will data on late-onset Mendelian diseases.

The studies of the atomic-bomb survivors and their children have contributed a large amount of scientific knowledge on the health effects of radiation exposure. The atomic-bomb cohort studies are widely acknowledged as the "gold standard" in studies of radiation health effects and radiological protection. That is a result of the availability of well-characterized

radiation dose estimates and well-defined populations that have been followed up with remarkable efficiency. The atomic-bomb survivor studies do not provide the full answer regarding radiation effects, as they represent responses to single acute external radiation exposure. Nevertheless, these studies provide by far the strongest foundation for human radiation risk assessment.

REFERENCES

1. Shigematsu I, Akiba S. Sampling of atomic bomb survivors and method of cancer detection in Hiroshima and Nagasaki. In: Shigematsu I, Kagan A, eds. *Cancer in Atomic Bomb Survivors*. Tokyo: Japan Scientific Societies Press; 1986.
2. Beebe GW. Reflections on the work of the atomic bomb casualty commission in Japan. *Epidemiol Rev.* 1979;1:184–210.
3. Neel JV, Schull WJ. *The Effect of Exposure to the Atomic Bombs on Pregnancy Termination in Hiroshima and Nagasaki*. National Academy of Sciences—National Research Council; 1956.
4. Francis TJ Jr, Jablon S, Moore FE, et al. *Report of an Ad Hoc Committee for Appraisal of the ABCC Program 1955*. Hiroshima: Radiation Effects Research Foundation; 1959.
5. Radiation Effects Research Foundation. *Reassessment of the Atomic Bomb Radiation Dosimetry for Hiroshima and Nagasaki— Dosimetry System 2002*. Hiroshima Radiation Effects Research Foundation; 2005.
6. Radiation Effects Research Foundation. *US-Japan Joint Reassessment of Atomic Bomb Radiation Dosimetry in Hiroshima and Nagasaki. Dosimetry System 1986. Final Report*. Hiroshima Radiation Effects Research Foundation; 1987.
7. Cullings HM, Fujita S, Funamoto S, et al. Dose estimation for atomic bomb survivor studies: its evolution and present status. *Radiat Res.* 2006;166(1 pt 2):219–254.
8. Preston DL, Pierce DA, Shimizu Y, et al. Effect of recent changes in atomic bomb survivor dosimetry on cancer mortality risk estimates. *Radiat Res.* 2004;162(4):377–389.
9. Preston DL, Ron E, Tokuoka S, et al. Solid cancer incidence among atomic bomb survivors, 1958–1998. *RERF Update.* 2007;18:9–13.
10. Preston DL, Ron E, Tokuoka S, et al. Solid cancer incidence in atomic bomb survivors: 1958–1998. *Radiat Res.* 2007;168:1–64.
11. Preston DL, Cullings HM, Suyama A, et al. Solid cancer incidence in atomic bomb survivors exposed in utero or as young children. *J Natl Cancer Inst.* 2008;100(6):428–436.
12. Imaizumi M, Usa T, Tominaga T, et al. Radiation dose-response relationships for thyroid nodules and autoimmune thyroid diseases in Hiroshima and Nagasaki atomic bomb survivors 55–58 years after radiation exposure. *JAMA.* 2006;295(9):1011–1022.
13. Shimizu Y, Kato H, Schill WJ. Studies of the mortality of A-bomb survivors. 9. Mortality, 1950–1985: Part 2. Cancer mortality based on the recently revised doses (DS86). *Radiat Res.* 1990;121(2):120–141.
14. Pierce DA, Stram DO, Vaeth M. Allowing for random errors in radiation dose estimates for the atomic bomb survivor data. *Radiat Res.* 1990;123(3):275–284.
15. Beebe G, Usagawa M. *The Major ABCC Samples*. Hiroshima: Radiation Effects Research Foundation; 1968.
16. Pierce DA, Shimizu Y, Preston DL, et al. Studies of the mortality of atomic bomb survivors. Report 12, Part I. Cancer: 1950–1990. *Radiat Res.* 1996;146(1):1–27.
17. Mabuchi K, Soda M, Ron E, et al. Cancer incidence in atomic bomb survivors. Part I: Use of the tumor registries in Hiroshima and Nagasaki for incidence studies. *Radiat Res.* 1994;137 (2 Suppl):S1–S16.
18. Thompson DE, Mabuchi K, Ron E, et al. Cancer incidence in atomic bomb survivors. Part II: Solid tumors, 1958–1987. *Radiat Res.* 1994;137(2 suppl):S17–S67.
19. Finch SC, Hrubec Z, Nefzger MD, et al. Detection of leukemia and related disorders. Hiroshima and Nagasaki research plan. *ABCC TR*. Hiroshima: ABCC; 1965.
20. Folley JH, Borges W, Yamawaki T. Incidence of leukemia in survivors of the atomic bomb in Hiroshima and Nagasaki, Japan. *Am J Med.* 1952;311–321.
21 Richardson D, Sugiyama H, Nishi N, et al. Ionizing radiation and leukemia mortality among Japanese atomic bomb survivors, 1950–2000. *Radiat Res.* 2009;172(3):368–382.
22. Richardson D, Sugiyama H, Wing S, et al. Positive associations between ionizing radiation and lymphoma mortality among men. *Am J Epidemiol.* 2009;169(8):969–976.
23. Preston DL, Kusumi S, Tomonaga M, et al. Cancer incidence in atomic bomb survivors. Part III. Leukemia, lymphoma and multiple myeloma, 1950–1987. *Radiat Res.* 1994;137(2 suppl):S68–S97.
24. Shimizu Y, Pierce DA, Preston DL, et al. Studies of the mortality of atomic bomb survivors. Report 12, Part II. Noncancer mortality: 1950–1990. *Radiat Res.* 1999;152(4):374–389.
25. Ichimaru M, Ishimaru T, Mikami M, et al. Multiple myeloma among atomic bomb survivors in Hiroshima and Nagasaki, 1950–76: relationship to radiation dose absorbed by marrow. *J Natl Cancer Inst.* 1982;69(2):323–328.
25a. Cardis E, Vrijheid M, Blettner M, et al. Risk of cancer after low doses of ionising radiation: retrospective cohort study in 15 countries. *Brit Med J.* 2005; 331(7508):77–83.
26. Preston DL, Shimizu Y, Pierce DA, et al. Studies of mortality of atomic bomb survivors. Report 13: Solid cancer and noncancer disease mortality: 1950–1997. *Radiat Res.* 2003;160(4): 381–407.
27. Land CE, Saku T, Hayashi Y, et al. Incidence of salivary gland tumors among atomic bomb survivors, 1950–1987. Evaluation of radiation-related risk. *Radiat Res.* 1996;146(1):28–36.
28. Saku T, Hayashi Y, Takahara O, et al. Salivary gland tumors among atomic bomb survivors, 1950–1987. *Cancer.* 1997;79(8):1465–1475.
29. The Research Group for Population-based Cancer Registration in Japan. 2003 Cancer incidence and incidence rates in Japan in 1998: estimates based on data from 12 population-based cancer registries. *Jpn J Clin Oncol.* 2003;33(5):241–245.

30. Suzuki G, Cullings H, Fujiwara S, et al. Low-positive antibody titer against Helicobacter pylori cytotoxin-associated gene A (CagA) may predict future gastric cancer better than simple seropositivity against *H. pylori* CagA or against *H. pylori*. *Cancer Epidemiol Biomarkers Prev.* 2007;16(6):1224–1228.
31. Sauvaget C, Lagarde F, Nagano J, et al. Lifestyle factors, radiation and gastric cancer in atomic-bomb survivors (Japan). *Cancer Causes Control.* 2005;16(7):773–780.
32. Nakatsuka H, Shimizu Y, Yamamoto T, et al. Colorectal cancer incidence among atomic bomb survivors, 1950–80. *J Radiat Res.* 1992;33:342–361.
33. Yoshizawa H. Hepatocellular carcinoma associated with hepatitis C virus infection in Japan: projection to other countries in the foreseeable future. *Oncology.* 2002;62 (Suppl 1):8–17.
34. Cologne JB, Tokuoka S, Beebe GW, et al. Effects of radiation on incidence of primary liver cancer among atomic bomb survivors. *Radiat Res.* 1999;152(4):364–373.
35. Fukuhara T, Sharp GB, Mizuno T, et al. Liver cancer in atomic-bomb survivors: histological characteristics and relationships to radiation and hepatitis B and C viruses. *J Radiat Res.* 2001;42:117–130.
36. Sharp GB, Mizuno T, Cologne JB, et al. Hepatocellular carcinoma among atomic bomb survivors: significant interaction of radiation with hepatitis C virus infections. *Int J Cancer.* 2003;103(4):531–537.
37. Pierce DA, Sharp GB, Mabuchi K. Joint effects of radiation and smoking on lung cancer risk among atomic bomb survivors. *Radiat Res.* 2003;159(4):511–520.
38. Ron E, Preston DL, Kishikawa M, et al. Skin tumor risk among atomic-bomb survivors in Japan. *Cancer Causes Control.* 1998;9(4):393–401.
39. Kishikawa M, Koyama K, Iseki M, et al. Histologic characteristics of skin cancer in Hiroshima and Nagasaki: background incidence and radiation effects. *Int J Cancer.* 2005;117(3):363–369.
40. Mizuno T, Tokuoka S, Kishikawa M, et al. Molecular basis of basal cell carcinogenesis in the atomic-bombsurvivorpopulation:p53andPTCHgenealterations. *Carcinogenesis.* 2006;27(11):2286–2294.
41. IARC. *Cancer Incidence in Five Continents.* Lyon:International Agency for Research on Cancer; 2002.
42. Ronckers CM, Erdmann CA, Land CE. Radiation and breast cancer: a review of current evidence. *Breast Cancer Res.* 2005;**7**(1):21–32.
43. Land CE, Tokunaga M, Koyama K, et al. Incidence of female breast cancer among atomic bomb survivors, Hiroshima and Nagasaki, 1950–1990. *Radiat Res.* 2003;160(6):707–717.
44. Land CE, Hayakawa N, Machado SG, et al. A case-control interview study of breast cancer among Japanese A-bomb survivors. I. Main effects. *Cancer Causes Control.* 1994;5(2):157–165.
45. Land CE, Hayakawa N, Machado SG, et al. A case-control interview study of breast cancer among Japanese A-bomb survivors. II. Interactions with radiation dose. *Cancer Causes Control.* 1994;5(2):167–176.
46. Preston DL, Mattson A, Holmberg E, et al. Radiation effects on breast cancer risk: a pooled analysis of eight cohorts. *Radiat Res.* 2002;158(2):220–235.
47. Boice JD Jr, Preston DL, Davis FG, et al. Frequent chest X-ray fluoroscopy and breast cancer incidence among tuberculosis patients in Massachusetts. *Radiat Res.* 1991;125(2):214–222.
48. Shore RE, Hildreth N, Woodard E, et al. Breast cancer among women given X-ray therapy for acute postpartum mastitis. *J Natl Cancer Inst.* 1986;77(3):689–696.
49. Hildreth N, Shore RE, Dvoretsky PM. The risk of breast cancer after irradiation of the thymus in infancy. *N Engl J Med.* 1989;321(19):1281–1284.
50. Mattson A, Ruden BI, Hall P, et al. Radiation-induced breast cancer: long-term follow-up of radiation therapy for benign breast disease. *J Natl Cancer Inst.* 1993;85(20):1679–1685.
51. Lindberg S, Karlsson A, Arvidsson B, et al. Cancer incidence after radiotherapy for skin haemangioma during infancy. *Acta Oncologica.* 1995;34(6):735–740.
52. Lundell M, Mattson A, Hakulinen T, et al. Breast cancer after radiotherapy for skin hemangioma in infancy. *Radiat Res.* 1996;145:225–230.
53. Ron E, Ikeda T, Preston DL, et al. Male breast cancer incidence among atomic bomb survivors. *J Natl Cancer Inst.* 2005;97(8):603–605.
54. Ioka A, Tsukuma H, et al. Trends in uterine cancer incidence in Japan 1975–98. *Jpn J Clin Oncol.* 2003;33(12):645–646.
55. Yonehara S, Brenner A, Kishikawa M, et al. Clinical and epidemiologic characteristics of first primary tumors of the central nervous system and related organs among atomic bomb survivors in Hiroshima and Nagasaki, 1958–1995. *Cancer.* 2004;101(7):1644–1654.
56. Preston DL, Ron E, Yonehara S, et al. Tumors of the nervous system and pituitary gland associated with atomic bomb radiation exposure. *J Natl Cancer Inst.* 2002;94(20):1555–1563.
57. Duffy BJ Jr, Fitzgerald PJ. Cancer of the thyroid in children: a report of 28 cases. *J Clin Endocrinol Metab.* 1950;10(10):1296–1308.
58. Ron E, Lubin JH, Shore RE, et al. Thyroid cancer after exposure to external radiation: a pooled analysis of seven studies. *Radiat Res.* 1995;141(3):259–277.
59. Nagano J, Mabuchi K, Yoshimoto Y, et al. A case-control study in Hiroshima and Nagasaki examining non-radiation risk factors for thyroid cancer. *J Epidemiol.* 2007;17(3):76–85.
60. Vogan DG, Martin SF, Kimura S. Atom bomb cataracts. *Science.* 1949;110(2868):654.
61. Miller RJ, Fujino T, Nefzger M. Lens findings in Atomic bomb survivors. A review of major ophthalmic surveys at the atomic Bomb Casualty Commission (1949–1962). *Arch Ophthalmol.* 1967;78(6):697–704.
62. Choshi K, Takaku I, Mishima H, et al. Ophthalmologic changes related to radiation exposure and age in adult health study sample, Hiroshima and Nagasaki. *Radiat Res.* 1983;96(3):560–579.
63. Otake M, Neriishi K, Schull WJ. Cataract in atomic bomb survivors based on a threshold model and the occurrence of severe epilation. *Radiat Res.* 1996;146(3):339–348.
64. ICRP. *1990 Recommendations of the International Commission on Radiological Protection.* Oxford: Pergamon Press; 1990.
65. National Council on Radiation Protection and Measurements. *Limitations of Exposure to Ionizing Radiation. Report 116.* Bethesda, MD: National Council on Radiation Protection and Measurements; 1993.
66. Minamoto A, Taniguchi H, Yoshitani N, et al. Cataract in atomic bomb survivors. *Int J Radiat Biol.* 2004;80(5):339–345.
67. Nakashima E, Neriishi K, Minamoto A. A reanalysis of atomic-bomb cataract data, 2000–2002: a threshold analysis. *Health Phys.* 2006;90(2):154–160.
68. Neriishi K, Nakashima E, Minamoto A, et al. Postoperative cataract cases among atomic bomb survivors: radiation dose response and threshold. *Radiat Res.* 2007;168(4):404–408.
69. Shimizu Y, Kato H. Schull WJ. Studies of the mortality of A-bomb survivors. 9. Mortality, 1950–1985: Part 3. Noncancer mortality based on the revised doses (DS86). *Radiat Res.* 1992;130(2):249–266.
70. United Nations Scientific Committee on the Effects of Atomic Radiation. 2008. *Effects of Ionizing Radiation. Annex b: Epidemiological Evaluation of Cardiovascular Disease and Other Noncancer Diseases Following Radiation Exposure.* New York, NY, 2008.
71. McGale P, Darby SC. Low doses of ionizing radiation and circulatory diseases: a systematic review of the published epidemiological evidence. *Radiat Res.* 2005;163(3):247–257.
72. Little M, Tawn EJ, Tzoulaki I, et al. A systematic review of epidemiological associations between low and moderate doses of ionizing radiation and late cardiovascular effects, and their possible mechanisms. *Radiat Res.* 2008;169(1):99–109.
73. Schultz-Hector S, Trott KR. Radiation-induced cardiovascular diseases: is the epidemiologic evidence compatible with the radiobiologic data? *Int J Radiat Oncol Biol Phys.* 2007;67(1):10–18.
74. Wong FL, Yamada M, Sasaki H, et al. Noncancer disease incidence in the atomic bomb survivors: 1958–1986. *Radiat Res.* 1993;135(3):418–430.
75. Yamada M, Wong FL, et al. Noncancer disease incidence in atomic bomb survivors, 1958–1998. *Radiat Res.* 2004;161(6):622–632.
75a. Shimizu Y, Kodama K, Nishi N, et al. Radiation exposure and circulatory disease risk: Hiroshima and Nagasaki atomic bomb survivor data, 1950–2003. *BMJ.* 2010:340:b5349.
76. Kodama K, Fujiwara S, Yamada M, et al. Profiles of non-cancer diseases in atomic bomb survivors. *World Health Stat Quar—Rapport Trimestriel de Statistiques Sanitaires Mondiales.* 1996;49(1):7–16.
77. Sasaki H, Wong FL, Yamada M, et al. The effects of aging and radiation exposure on blood pressure levels of atomic bomb survivors. *J Clin Epidemiol.* 2002;55(10):974–981.
78. Wong FL, Yamada M, Sasaki H, et al. Effects of radiation on the longitudinal trends of total serum cholesterol levels in the atomic bomb survivors. *Radiat Res.* 1999;151(6):736–746.
79. Akahoshi M, Amasaki Y, Soda M, et al. Effects of radiation on fatty liver and metabolic coronary risk factors among atomic bomb survivors in Nagasaki. *Hypertens Res.* 2003;26(12):965–970.
80. Neriishi K, Matuso N. Relationship between radiation exposure and serum protein alpha and beta globulin fractions. *Nagasaki Med J.* 1986;61:449–454.
81. Sawada H, Kodama K. Adult Health Study Report 6. Results of Six Examination Cycles, 1968–1980. *RERF Technical Report—RERF 86.* Hiroshima and Nagasaki; 1986.
82. Neriishi K, Nakashima E, Delongchamp RR. Persistent subclinical inflammation among A-bomb survivors. *Int J Radiat Biol.* 2001;77(4):475–482.
83. Hayashi T, Kusunoki S. Radiation dose-dependent increases in inflammatory response markers in A-bomb survivors. *Int J Radiat Biol.* 2003;79(2):129–136.
84. Fujiwara S, Kusumi S, Cologne JB, et al. Prevalence of anti-hepatitis C virus antibody and chronic liver disease among atomic bomb survivors. *Radiat Res.* 2000;154(1):12–19.
85. Fujiwara S, Sharp GB, Cologne JB, et al. Prevalence of hepatitis B virus infection among atomic bomb survivors. *Radiat Res.* 2003;159(6):780–786.
86. Otake M, Fujikoshi Y, Funamoto S, et al. Evidence of radiation-induced reduction of height and body weight from repeated measurements of adults exposed in childhood to the atomic bombs *Radiat Res.* 1994;140(1):112–122.
87. Nakashima E, Fujiwara S, Funamoto S. Effect of radiation dose on the height of atomic bomb survivors: a longitudinal study. *Radiat Res.* 2002;158(3):346–351.
88. Blot WJ, Sawada H. Fertility among female survivors of the atomic bombs of Hiroshima and Nagasaki. *Am J Hum Genet.* 1972;24(6 pt 1):613–622.
89. Lifton RJ. *Death in Life—Survivors of Hiroshima.* New York: Random House; 1967.
90. Yamada M, Izumi S. Psychiatric sequelae in atomic bomb survivors in Hiroshima and Nagasaki two decades after the explosions. *Soc Psychiatry Psychiatr Epidemiol.* 2002;37(9):409–415.
91. Fujiwara S, Mizuno S, Ochi S, et al. The incidence of thoracic vertebral fractures in a Japanese population, Hiroshima and Nagasaki, 1958–86. *J Clin Epidemiol.* 1991;44(10):1007–1014.
92. Yamada M, Sasaki H, Mimori Y, et al. Prevalence and risks of dementia in the Japanese population: RERF's adult health study Hiroshima subjects. Radiation Effects Research Foundation. *J Am Geriatr Soc.* 1999;47(2):189–195.
93. Cologne JB, Preston DL. Longevity of atomic-bomb survivors. *Lancet.* 2000;356(9226):303–307.
94. Kodama Y, Pawel D, Nakamura N, et al. Stable chromosome aberrations in atomic bomb survivors: results from 25 years of investigation. *Radiat Res.* 2001;156(4):337–346.
95. Stram DO, Sposto R, Preston DL, et al. Stable chromosome aberrations among A-bomb survivors: an update. *Radiat Res.* 1993;136(1):29–36.
96. Akiyama M, Kyoizumi S, Kusunoki Y, et al. Monitoring exposure to atomic bomb radiation by somatic mutation. *Environ Health Perspect.* 1996;104(suppl 3):493–496.
97. Kleinerman RA, Romanyukha AA, Schauer DA, et al. Retrospective assessment of radiation exposure using biological dosimetry: chromosome painting, electron paramagnetic resonance and the glycophorin a mutation assay. *Radiat Res.* 2006;166(1 pt 2):287–302.
98. Kusunoki Y, Hirai Y, Hakoda M, et al. Uneven distributions of naive and memory T cells in the CD4 and CD8 T-cell populations derived from a single stem cell in an atomic bomb survivor: implications for the origins of the memory T-cell pools in adulthood. *Radiat Res.* 2002;157(5):493–499.
99. Kusunoki Y, Hayashi T. Long-lasting alterations of the immune system by ionizing radiation exposure: implications for disease development among atomic bomb survivors. *Int J Radiat Biol.* 2008;84(1):1–14.

100. Fujiwara S, Carter RI, Akiyama M, et al. Autoantibodies and immunoglobulins among atomic bomb survivors. *Radiat Res.* 1994;137:89–95.

101. Akiyama M. Late effects of radiation on the human immune system: an overview of immune response among the atomic-bomb survivors. *Int J Radiat Biol.* 1995;68(5):497–508.

102. Hida A, Akahoshi M, Takagi Y, et al. Prevalence of Sjogren syndrome among Nagasaki atomic bomb survivors. *Ann Rheum Dis.* 2008;67(5):689–695.

103. Delongchamp RR, Mabuchi K, Yoshimoto Y, et al. Cancer mortality among atomic bomb survivors exposed in utero or as young children, October 1950-May 1992. *Radiat Res.* 1997;147(3):385–395.

104. Jablon S, Kato H. Childhood cancer in relation to prenatal exposure to atomic-bomb radiation. *Lancet.* 1970;2(681):1000–1003.

105. International Commission on Radiological Protection. Biological effects after prenatal irradiation (embryo and fetus). Publication 90. *Ann ICRP.* 2003;33(1–2):1–200.

106. Ohtaki K, Kodama Y, Nakano M, et al. Human fetuses do not register chromosome damage inflicted by radiation exposure in lymphoid precursor cells except for a small but significant effect at low doses. *Radiat Res.* 2004;161(4):373–379.

107. Nakano M, Kodama Y, Ohtaki K, et al. Chromosome aberrations do not persist in the lymphocytes or bone marrow cells of mice irradiated in utero or soon after birth. *Radiat Res.* 2007;167(6):693–702.

108. Otake M, Schull WJ. In utero exposure to A-bomb radiation and mental retardation; a reassessment. *Br J Radiol.* 1984;57(677):409–414.

109. Otake M, Schull WJ, Lee S. Threshold for radiation-related severe mental retardation in prenatally exposed A-bomb survivors: a re-analysis. *Int J Radiat Biol.* 1996;70(6):755–763.

110. Schull WJ, Nishitani H, Hasuo K, et al. Brian abnormalities among the mentally retarded prenatally exposed atomic bomb survivors. *RERF Technical Report 13–91.* 1991.

111. Schull WJ, Norton S, Jensh RP. Ionizing radiation and the developing brain. *Neurotoxicol Teratol.* 1990;12(3):249–260.

112. Dunn K, Yoshimaru H, Otake M, et al. Prenatal exposure to ionizing radiation and subsequent development of seizures. *Am J Epidemiol.* 1990;131(1):114–123.

113. Nakashima E, Akahoshi M, Neriishi K, et al. Systolic blood pressure and systolic hypertension in adolescence of atomic bomb survivors exposed in utero. *Radiat Res.* 2007;168(5):593–599.

114. Tatsukawa Y, Nakashima E, Yamada M, et al. Cardiovascular disease risk among atomic bomb survivors exposed in utero, 1978–2003. *Radiat Res.* 2008;170(3):269–274.

115. Imaizumi M, Ashizawa K, Neriishi K, et al. Thyroid diseases in atomic bomb survivors exposed in utero. *J Clin Endocrinol Metab.* 2008;93(5):1641–1648.

116. National Academy of Sciences. *The Children of Atomic Bomb Survivors. A Genetic Study.* Washington, DC: National Academy Press; 1991.

117. Nakamura N. Genetic effects of radiation in atomic-bomb survivors and their children: past, present and future. *J Radiat Res (Tokyo).* 2006;47(Suppl B):B67–B73.

118. Schull WJ, Neel JV, Hashizume A, et al. Some further observations on the sex ratio among infants born to survivors of the atomic bombings of Hiroshima and Nagasaki. *Am J Hum Genet.* 1966;18(4):328–338.

119. Awa AA, Bloom AD, Yoshida MC, et al. Cytogenetic study of the offspring of atom bomb survivors. *Nature* 1998;218(5139):367–368.

120. Neel JV, Satoh C, Goriki K, et al. Search for mutations altering protein charge and/or function in children of atomic bomb survivors: final report. *Am J Hum Genet.* 1988;42(5):663–676.

121. Kato H, Schull WJ, Neel JV. A cohort-type study of survival in the children of parents exposed to atomic bombings. *Am J Hum Genet.* 1966;18(4):339–373.

122. Yoshimoto Y, Neel JV, Schull WJ, et al. Malignant tumors during the first 2 decades of life in the offspring of atomic bomb survivors. *Am J Hum Genet.* 1990;46:1041–1052.

123. Izumi S, Suyama A, Soda M, et al. Cancer incidence in children and young adults did not increase relative to parental exposure to atomic bombs. *Br J Cancer.* 2003;89(9):1709–1713.

124. Izumi S, Suyama A, Koyama K. Radiation-related mortality among offspring of atomic bomb survivors: a half-century of follow-up. *Int J Cancer.* 2003;107(2):292–297.

125. Fujiwara S, Suyama A, Cologne JB, et al. Prevalence of adult-onset multifactorial disease among offspring of atomic bomb survivors. *Radiat Res.* 2008;170(4):451–457.

126. Pawel D, Preston DL, Pierce D, et al. Improved estimates of cancer site-specific risks for A-bomb survivors. *Radiat Res.* 2008;169(1):87–98.

Harald Paganetti, Torunn Yock
Nancy J. Tarbell, Alexei Trofimov

Optimization of Radiotherapy Treatment Delivery Technology to Minimize Radiation Injury

INTRODUCTION

Eradicating cancerous cells is the main goal in radiation oncology. Ideally, this would be achieved without irradiating any normal tissues. However, because of uncertainties in the target definition as well as in the dose deposited during delivery, healthy tissues are usually included within the outlined target volume. To reach the tumor, the beam of ionizing radiation needs to traverse healthy tissues, sometimes including critical organs, which are often adjacent to, or even overlap with, the target. In line with the general objective in radiation therapy to eradicate tumor cells while minimizing toxicity, the drive behind the development of new technologies and new treatment approaches is to enable one to balance the trade-offs between delivering high volume-conformal dose to the target and limiting the doses to critical structures within tolerance levels, and to provide tools that help advance both goals simultaneously.

Generally, there is assumed to be no advantage from irradiation of any healthy tissues anywhere in the body. A de facto standard for defining normal tissue tolerances was set in 1991[1] as a function of volume of normal tissue irradiated (1/3, 2/3, and 3/3 volume) based on 5% risk of complication within 5 years and 50% risk of complication within 5 years. Recently, these data were updated by using more recent results on normal tissue dose-volume tolerances by analyzing three-dimensional conformal radiation therapy (3DCRT) treatments.[2]

Consequentially, for a delivery technique or modality to achieve reduction in tissue toxicity, it must provide tools to minimize the amount of dose deposited in the beam path proximally (entry dose) and distally (exit dose) to the tumor, as well as laterally (beam penumbra). As an improvement of earlier "2D" treatments, 3DCRT beams are planned based on CT images, and the beams-eye view of the target, with beam modifiers (e.g., wedges) applied to increase dose conformity.

Some of the novel treatment technologies for external beam treatments aim mainly at improved dose conformity in the high-dose region and a reduction of dose to critical structures in the medium-dose region. For example, intensity-modulated x-ray therapy (IMRT) yields highly conformal dose to the target but does not reduce total dose outside the target volume when compared to 3DCRT. IMRT does offer improved dose conformity, compared to 3DCRT, by allowing the delivery of inhomogeneous photon fluence distributions. Currently, most radiation therapy departments are capable of delivering IMRT, most commonly by modulating the beam fluence distributions with a multileaf collimator (MLC).[3] The desired fluence map can be very complex and can only be obtained using inverse planning optimization algorithms. The MLC leaves can be used to allow a step-and-shoot or a dynamic sliding-window delivery.

Similarly, in tomotherapy, the photon fluence map is modulated using a rotating fan beam and a binary collimator in order to create nonuniform photon fluence.[4] The dose can be delivered with helical scans or in a slice-by-slice mode. The CyberKnife system uses a linear accelerator on a robotic arm to deliver uneven fluence maps leading to a conformal dose distribution.[5] Besides these main treatment modalities using photon beams, there are several modalities using other particles, such as electrons, protons, or heavy ions.

Proton therapy receives a growing interest because of the physical characteristics of the depth dose curve of proton and ion beams. The dose peaks at a well-defined depth in tissue allowing highly conformal dose distributions that are comparable or even more conformal than is achievable with IMRT. The depth-dose curve with the Bragg peak can be modulated (into a spread-out Bragg peak [SOBP]) to achieve a homogeneous dose distribution across the target volume. This is done either passively by using a scattering system or actively using magnetically deflected pencil beams.[6] The latter technique also allows the delivery of intensity-modulated fields, that is, intensity-modulated proton therapy (IMPT).[7] Because of the lack of exit dose for proton therapy fields, the total dose (integral dose) absorbed in the patient is typically a factor of two to three lower with protons when compared with 3DCRT or IMRT. It is speculated that particles even heavier than protons are able to improve dose conformity and integral dose ratio even further. Additional advantages of ion therapy may lie in their increased relative biological effectiveness (RBE).

The technical ability to deliver highly target-conformal dose distributions of complex shape, in theory, should allow a reduction in the irradiated volume of normal tissue. However, the complex distributions are also more vulnerable to the uncertainties in localization, set-up, and delivery, both intrafractionally and interfractionally. This fact has triggered the development and clinical introduction of advanced imaging techniques leading to image-guided radiation therapy (IGRT).

As new technologies allowed for increased precision of tumor imaging conformity of delivery of radiation to the volume of interest, the very definition of the radiation target has changed to include various planning volumes. The uncertainty in the definition of the target volume is a limiting factor in itself. Even with the best of imaging, the clinician is left deciding how much to allow for microscopic spread of disease in defining the area that need to be treated. Recently, several targeting and delivery techniques have been proposed, which utilize biological and functional information in order to further optimize radiotherapy treatment.

Thus, the developments in the practice of radiation oncology and the technology of imaging and radiation delivery are inseparable and provide motivation to each other for further refinements and advances. The focus of this chapter is on differences in dose to organs at risk among different treatment modalities and on methods to optimize treatment delivery technologies with respect to integral dose and scattered dose.

RADIATION INJURY IN CANCER THERAPY

RADIATION THERAPY TARGETS

Currently, the common definition of target volumes in treatment planning is that recommended by the International Commission on Radiation Units and Measurements (ICRU).[8–10] Per ICRU recommendation, the target volume should include the visible tumor (i.e., the gross tumor volume, GTV), the volume surrounding the GTV to account for possible microscopic tumor spread (i.e., clinical target volume, CTV), the volume surrounding the CTV to account for motion of the CTV or GTV (i.e., the internal target volume, ITV), and the volume surrounding the CTV or ITV to account for setup uncertainties and other uncertainties (i.e., the planning target volume, PTV). Organs at risk can be defined in a similar way, that is, with the planning organ at risk volume.

The CTV and PTV are frequently defined by expanding the volume using margins. The choice of CTV margins is defined by the clinical experience, and the expansion is often limited to the tissues that are likely to contain the microscopic extensions of the tumor. On the other hand, PTV margins are typically made based on the estimates of the uncertainties of the target position (which includes both the patient immobilization, and the internal motion or intrafractional changes in the anatomy).

Thus, healthy tissues are commonly included in the target volumes in radiation therapy and receive the dose of the same order as the cancerous tissues. Consequently, a delivery technology that allows for reduction in target margins generally yields improved sparing of uninvolved tissues. The introduction of CT-based 3D-conformal treatment planning in the 1970s led to significant reduction in the volume of irradiated tissue, due to better accounting for the shape of the target volume and improved precision of dose calculation.

RADIATION DOSE DISTRIBUTIONS AND ORGANS AT RISK

When describing dose to the patient, we typically distinguish between the treated volume and the irradiated volume. The

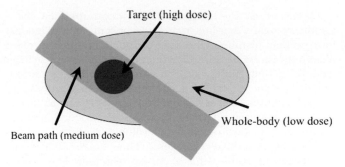

Figure 9.1. Schematics of dose areas in a patient during radiation therapy.

treated volume is defined as the volume enclosed by an isodose surface, selected and specified by the radiation oncologist as being appropriate to achieve the purpose of treatment (e.g., tumor eradication, palliation). The irradiated volume is defined as the volume that receives a dose that is considered significant in relation to normal tissue tolerance. Volumes in the patient receiving dose can thus be separated into three regions (Fig. 9.1): (1) the target (tumor), characterized by the PTV treated with the therapeutic dose; (2) organs at risk typically defined in the tumor vicinity (these may intersect with the beam path and are allowed to receive low-to-intermediate doses); and (3) the rest of the patient body, which may receive low doses. This chapter does focus on radiation injuries in two of these areas. First, we consider the healthy tissue directly irradiated by being in the beam path. The dose level would be typically between 1 and 40 Gy over the course of a treatment. These organs would be part of the volume imaged for treatment planning purposes. Second, we consider the volume not directly irradiated but receiving some dose (typically below 1 Gy over the course of a treatment) due to scattering of primary radiation or due to secondary radiation induced by the primary radiation beam.

Dose delivered to healthy tissues can lead to severe side effects, for example, affecting the functionality of organs or even causing a second cancer. In the tumor and along the path of the therapeutic radiation field, one may have to accept a small risk for developing even significant side effects because of the therapeutic benefit. Such effects are not necessarily proportional to dose. For example, if the dose is prescribed with the aim to kill tumor cells, without leaving behind the cells with the potential for mutation, the risk for radiation-induced cancer within the target area might be smaller than the risk in the surrounding tissues receiving intermediate doses as illustrated in Figure 9.2.

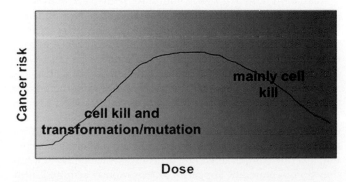

Figure 9.2. Second cancer risk as a function of dose and the main biological effects.

Organs at risk can be divided into two groups. First, there are those organs that are part of the patient volume imaged for treatment planning. Those are considered in the treatment planning process by using dose constraints and are receiving typically medium doses (>1% of the prescribed target dose). The dose is due to scattering of the particle beam and due to the fact that these organs lie within the primary beam path. The total dose delivered is termed integral dose. Second, there are organs further away from the target volume receiving low doses (<1% of the prescribed target dose). These organs are typically not imaged or outlined for treatment planning. This dose is due to large-angle scattering of the beam or due to secondary particles emitted in nuclear or atomic physics interactions of the primary beam with matter.

REDUCING RADIATION INJURIES TO DEFINED "ORGANS AT RISK" RECEIVING HIGH-TO-INTERMEDIATE DOSES

The dose deliverable to the target structure(s) is mostly limited by the dose constraints for organs at risk. New technologies therefore mostly aim at (1) improving dose conformity to the target and (2) reducing the total (integral) dose to the patient.

Because of the long life expectancy post treatment and the potential severity of radiation effects on a growing individual, long-term side effects are of particular concern in the pediatric patient population. Pediatric malignancies are cured now nearly 80% of the time due to dramatic improvements in surgery, chemotherapy, and radiotherapy.[11,12] However, radiotherapy late effects of treatment are well documented in the literature.[13–15] In summary of the growing literature, in addition to the side effects that adults experience,[1] radiotherapy in children impairs growth and development of soft tissue, bone, and nerve. The negative effects are directly correlated with dose and volume of normal tissue irradiated, and inversely correlated with age at irradiation. When certain parts of the body are irradiated and fail to keep pace with the growth of other parts of the body, cosmetic and functional outcomes will result. For example, a limb length discrepancy resulting from ipsilateral radiotherapy for a pelvic Ewing sarcoma can lead to back pain and scoliosis requiring treatment over a lifetime. The late effects depend on the site of the body treated and vary dramatically. It is clear, however, that childhood cancer survivors are more likely to have treatment-related chronic conditions and require more medical care and services, and score lower on measures of quality of life.[16–18]

Radiation dose to growing nontumor pediatric tissues stunts further development and the effects of which are reported most comprehensively in the pediatric population who have received brain radiotherapy. Brain tumors account for over 50% of solid tumors and many will require radiotherapy. Therefore, the effects of radiotherapy on the developing brain warrant special mention. It has been clearly documented that radiotherapy has a profound effect on the developing brain with younger patients faring worse.[19] Deficits in neurocognitive function become more pronounced with time from treatment[20] in part because these children are unable to acquire new skills and information at a rate comparable to their healthy same-age peers, while they do not generally appear to lose previously acquired information and skills.[21] Whole-brain radiotherapy is worse than partial-brain radiotherapy, and the effect is exacerbated with

higher radiation dose and the addition of chemotherapy.[22] Merchant et al.[23,24] demonstrate with mathematical models that the adverse effects of radiotherapy to the brain on neurocognition are directly correlated to dose and volume in a continuous fashion.

Throughout the history of clinical radiation oncology, the introduction of new technologies has been driven by the desire to reduce treatment toxicities, which often required modifications in the treatment planning procedures that offered to achieve better sparing of healthy tissues surrounding the therapy targets. Depth-dose tables and water-equivalent body models have long been replaced with computer-based dose calculation and treatment planning based on 3D imaging.

3D planning became commonplace with the wide clinical introduction of computed tomography (CT) scanning. It allowed better correlation of the dose with the internal anatomy, as the beam directions and contributions from individual fields could be adjusted or optimized to avoid critical organs. The dose had to be calculated directly, based on the selected beam configuration and relative weights, or fluxes of x-rays to be delivered by each beam. These weights were essentially "educated guesses" based on the experience of clinicians and physicists involved in treatment planning.

The ability to further segment individual beams into "beamlets" of varying intensity in IMRT increased the number of variables beyond what could be handled with traditional "forward" (from the incoming beam flux to dose to tissue) planning, and called for introduction of "inverse" planning methods: where the beamlet intensities are determined by computer in optimization process, based on the desired dose distribution.

3D-Conformal and Intensity-Modulated Therapy

The main advantage of intensity-modulated treatments, compared to 3D-conformal therapy, as well as the often-cited motivation behind the introduction into the clinic was the ability of IMRT to conform to concave nonconvex targets, which is especially beneficial when such concavities are found in the close proximity of critical organs. It was estimated that 30% of PTV shapes treated in RT clinics exhibit concavities[25] and thus could significantly benefit from IMRT.

With the wide clinical introduction and availability of linear accelerator-based IMRT, most cases treated presently are not concave targets. Notwithstanding, even in these cases, thanks to distribution optimization using inverse planning methods, IMRT can still provide conformation to the target and sharper lateral penumbra that are advantageous compared to those achieved with forward planning methods.

Of note is that, because large sections of the field are blocked with MLC leaves at most times, IMRT delivery typically requires higher flux of x-rays (greater number of monitor units, MU, of radiation) per field. An increase by a factor of 3 is expected as the rule of thumb. Because the MLC leaves do not attenuate x-rays completely, and roughly 2% to 3% pass through, the out-of-field dose with IMRT due to transmission scales roughly with the ratio of MU, compared to "open field" 3D-conformal treatments.

The use of advanced imaging and immobilization methods led to higher fidelity of target localization for IMRT and allowed for reduction in planning margins in many sites (e.g., to 3 mm or smaller for head and neck treatments set-up with the electronic portal imaging device (EPID), or prostate treatments with cone-beam CT used for set-up). Treatment verification is another important part of treatment delivery. IGRT aims to monitor the tumor position continuously throughout the treatment, either directly or via surrogate markers, to ensure sufficiently precise targeting.

Clinical Experience with IMRT

Since clinical introduction of IMRT began in early 1990s, the safety of the procedure had been quickly established, and the promise of reduced toxicity with more conformal distributions has been confirmed in randomized studies. In head and neck irradiation, significant reduction of dose to the parotid glands was widely documented. Kuppersmith et al.[26] noted that the incidence of acute toxicity was drastically lower than that seen with conventional radiotherapy. Chao et al.[27] concluded that sparing of the parotid glands with IMRT translated into appreciable reduction in xerostomia and improvement in the patients' quality of life. In prostate cancer treatments, Zelefsky et al.[28] reported the combined rates of acute grade 1 and 2 rectal toxicities and the risk of late grade 2 rectal bleeding were significantly lower in the IMRT patients, while urinary toxicities were comparable. Mundt et al.[29] reported that IMRT treatment was well tolerated and associated with less acute gastrointestinal sequelae than conventional 3DCRT of whole pelvis in patients with gynecologic malignancies. Nutting et al.[25] reported significant sparing of the fraction of bowel receiving more than 35 to 50 Gy from pelvic node irradiation (to 50 Gy) of prostate cancer patients with IMRT compared to 3DCRT.

Tomotherapy

Tomotherapy is an example of rotational therapy, in which the target is irradiated with a set of intensity-modulated fan beams, rotated around the patient along a helical path.[4] The MLCs used to modulate the narrow fan beams in tomotherapy have lower transmission,[30] compared to the MLCs used for standard IMRT (in which the leaves often need to travel over 10 cm during field delivery). The use of significantly larger number of independent beam angles in tomotherapy, compared to IMRT (which rarely uses more than seven beams), may provide appreciable advantage in certain anatomical configurations.

Aoyama et al.[31] evaluated the integral dose received by patients during treatments for prostate carcinoma for 3D-conformal, linac-based IMRT and tomotherapy. On average, for five patients, both tomotherapy and IMRT reduced the total integral dose to the whole body by 5% compared to 3D-conformal therapy (leaf transmission was not considered). At the same time, the integral (and mean) dose to surrounding critical organs, including rectal wall and penile bulb, was reduced by over 10% with tomotherapy, compared to standard linac-based IMRT.

Other groups reported significant reduction of acute toxicity with helical tomotherapy, compared to 3D-conformal treatments[32] and reduction in gastrointestinal toxicity compared to IMRT, although possibly at the cost of increased genitourinary toxicity.[33] A similar level of reduction in the incidence of xerostomia in the treatment of nasopharyngeal carcinoma, with both tomotherapy and linac-based IMRT compared to 3DCRT, has been reported.[34]

Particle Therapy

The Bragg peak, characteristic of depth dose curves of proton and other heavy particles, provides possibility to reduce irradiation of the tissue in transit to, and, especially, distally to the tumor. Proton therapy is the most clinically accepted modality of particle therapy. Radiation therapy is also delivered with heavier nuclei (mostly carbon ions, but also helium, beryllium). The radiation from carbon ions is characterized by higher RBE, compared to protons, especially toward the end of range, in the vicinity of Bragg peak. Heavy ions are also less affected by scattering as they pass through the tissue, which makes the lateral penumbra of the dose from a beam of carbon ions rather independent of the depth, while the proton penumbra increases with depth.

In particle physics, protons and neutrons, as well as pi-mesons, are classified collectively as "hadrons," or heavy particles (as opposed to light "leptons"). However, the term "hadron therapy" is frequently used in the literature as a synonym of heavy-ion (e.g., helium, carbon) therapy.

While IMRT has been reputed to be an answer to diminishing neurocognitive deficits in the pediatric population as a result of radiotherapy, there are data suggesting that even low doses of radiotherapy to large volumes are detrimental.[23,24] Such studies help make the argument that particle therapy, which can reduce the total integral approach will be far more successful in reducing the side effects from radiation therapy.[35–40]

Proton radiotherapy has the ability to significantly limit the low-dose radiation beyond the treatment volume. There have been multiple dosimetric studies clearly demonstrating superior normal tissue sparing and decreased integral dose with protons,[36,37,41–46] many of which have already been summarized. However, until recently, there were only two proton centers capable of treating large fields operating in the United States, and only a handful around the world. One of the areas of greatest benefit appears to be in the use of protons for medulloblastoma. Because the treatment volume is so large (craniospinal irradiation), the amount of normal tissue spared is very significant and will be discussed later in the chapter. There are few studies to date reporting the reduced late effects in the pediatric population due to small numbers of patients treated with long-term follow-up. However, the lack of dose delivered to the esophagus, ovaries, and gastrointestinal tract is strikingly different when compared to other techniques. Massachusetts General Hospital has shown that the benefits in the orbital rhabdomyosarcoma (RMS) population are significant[37,38] when compared to the photon late effects of historical controls in the same population. The sparing with protons was primarily seen in dose to the lens and normal brain where low-dose radiotherapy can have important adverse effects. Additional late effect data from prospective clinical trials will be forthcoming for pediatric patients and include parameningeal RMS, low-grade gliomas as well as childhood medulloblastoma, and other pediatric brain tumors.[47]

Particle Range Uncertainties

While it is often advertised that protons deliver essentially no dose beyond the particle's range in tissue, the presence of proton range uncertainty remains a possible limiting factor in the application of fuller clinical engagement of the sharp distal fall-off of the proton Bragg peak. Particle range uncertainty is mainly due to the variations between the planning imaging data, which are usually recorded a few days before the treatment begins, and the actual patient anatomical state, and setup during treatment delivery. Other factors contributing to the range uncertainty include the spread in the energy of the incoming beam, noise and artifacts in imaging data, as well as the uncertainty of estimating the stopping power (amount of interaction and local energy loss by protons) from the images (especially where metal implants and inserts are present). The overall uncertainty for protons is assumed to be of the order of a few percentage of the range (e.g., 3%[48]) or 1 to 3 mm. Moyers et al.[49] have proposed a formalism to calculate the distal and proximal margins to account for range variations. From our current clinical experience, this appears to be to be a minor factor in the majority of patients treated as demonstrated radiographically in craniospinal irradiation.[35]

The use of in vivo range verification during treatment delivery is one possibility to ensure safe and precise localization of the distal gradient of Bragg peak, to achieve better sparing of critical structures. Several techniques for range verification and range visualization have been developed, including PET scanning[50] and T1-weighted magnetic resonance images post treatment.[35]

Another way to make use of the distal gradient for organ sparing is by modeling the range uncertainty probabilistically, and accounting for this uncertainty in treatment plan optimization,[51] or considering the "worst case" outcomes: this approach results in plans that are less sensitive affected by range variations, compared to standard optimization techniques.

Intensity-Modulated Therapy with Protons and Other Particles

Proton beam therapy is delivered by two treatment techniques. The majority of patients are currently treated with passive scattering technique, but some institutions are moving toward the beam scanning technique. Passive scattering needs various scatterers, beam-flattening devices, collimators, and energy modulation devices. Additionally, for each patient, individual apertures and compensators have to be designed and built. In proton beam scanning, the prescribed dose is delivered by scanning narrow proton pencil beams across the targeted volume, while modulating the intensity of the beam, the dwell time per position, or both. With the narrow scanned beams and no scattering devices necessary, the interaction of protons with the gantry material is minimized, as is the number of externally created secondary particles, such as neutrons.

Proton beam scanning can be used to deliver any proton treatment plan deliverable with passive scattering. However, it offers the additional advantage of delivering IMPT. Unlike SOBP proton field treatments, in which each field delivers a uniform (within a few percentage) dose to the whole target volume, individual IMPT fields typically deliver nonuniform dose distributions, which combine to produce the desired therapeutic dose distribution. As with the x-rays, IMPT offers improved conformity of dose distributions to the target volume and increased sparing of healthy tissue compared to both 3D-conformal particle therapy and photon IMRT.

Proton IMPT treatments are routinely delivered at the Paul Scherer Institute (PSI) in Switzerland.[52] The experience at PSI demonstrated improved tissue sparing in a number of sites, including intracranial, nasopharyngeal, and paraspinal lesions.[53–55] Therapy with scanned carbon ion beams was, until recently, routinely performed at the German Society for Heavy Ion Research (GSI, Darmstadt)[56] and is to be resumed at the new heavy-ion therapy center in Heidelberg (HIT).

Comparative Treatment Plans

The proton dose localization in Bragg peak provides an obvious advantage compared to the depth dose curve of megavoltage x-rays, in regard to target conformation and reduction in the integral dose to nontarget tissues. While the clinical significance of this reduction in the dose bath is often not clear or certain, a wide spectrum of diseases and sites are presently treated at proton centers. Over four decades of experience with proton therapy confirmed that, while it may not be universally superior to other radiotherapy modalities, it is indeed a safe and efficient treatment. Various opinions have been voiced on whether or not randomized clinical trials are needed before any further expansion of the proton therapy application although most do not believe randomized trials are needed in pediatrics.[57–59]

Prostate carcinoma is the only disease for which randomized phase III trials comparing proton and x-ray therapy have been conducted and documented. Massachusetts General Hospital (MGH) reported on high-dose irradiation boosting with protons in 202 patients with stage T3-4 disease. All patients received 50.4 Gy with photons, and were then randomized either to receive a conformal proton boost to a total dose of 75.6 Gy-equivalent, or to proceed with the photon-only treatment to 67.2 Gy. A significant gain in local disease control was observed in the proton-boost arm at 5 to 8 years, for the subset of patients.[60]

Treatment planning studies investigated relative dosimetric advantages of proton-only therapy, compared to both 3D-conformal and IMRT therapy with x-rays.[61–64] Protons were shown to substantially reduce the integral dose to the patient, the mean doses to rectum and bladder, and, in general, the volumes of tissue irradiated to below 50% of the prescription dose (Fig. 9.3). Depending on specifics of planning and treatment techniques, improved sparing was observed in the whole rectum, and rectal wall V50, V70, V78,[64] or bladder V60 and V70,[63] for target doses of 78 and 79.2 Gy, respectively. The increased risk of late and acute rectal toxicity has been previously correlated with larger rectal V60, V75[65,66] and other dose-volume metrics in the high-dose range. Further improvements in rectal sparing are expected with intensity-modulated proton therapy.

Of all tumor sites, the protons' ability to significantly reduce the mean dose delivered to critical organs, or, in some cases, to spare them completely, is perhaps the most valuable in craniospinal irradiation[36] and in head and neck treatments[67] (Fig. 9.4). Common complications with photons include

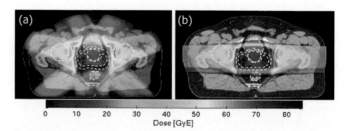

Figure 9.3. Dose distributions from (a) IMRT and (b) 3D-conformal proton therapy treatment plans for a case of prostate carcinoma. Dashed white lines designate the outlines of the prostate gland, seminal vesicles, PTV, and the organs at risk: rectum, bladder, and femoral heads (for more details, see Ref. 63).

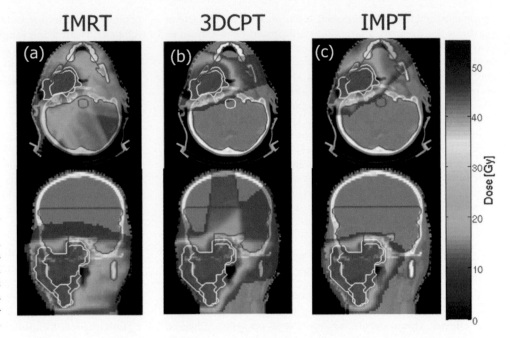

Figure 9.4. Dose distributions from RMS treatment plans: (**A**) IMRT, (**B**) 3D-conformal proton therapy, and (**C**) IMPT. The target volumes (gross tumor volume, lymph nodes, clinical target volume) are outlined in white and other structures in purple. Patient data were provided by Dr. N. Liebsch (Massachusetts General Hospital, Boston, MA).

dysphagia, neurocognitive decline, endocrine dysfunction as well as hearing loss and the risk of second malignancy.[15,47] Kozak et al.,[68] reported significantly superior sparing of optic nerves, retina, parotid glands, temporal brain lobes, cochlea, with protons, compared to IMRT, for ten parameningeal RMS patients. In a comparison of IMRT and protons plans (both 3D-conformal and IMPT) for childhood ependymoma by MacDonald et al.,[69] the latter achieved a significantly improved

sparing of a number of critical organs, which included cochlea, pituitary gland, hypothalamus, and temporal brain lobe. IMPT was shown to have potential to further the clinical advantage of proton therapy[69,70] and to reduce the estimated risk of second cancers.[70]

In the treatment of paraspinal sarcomas and retroperitoneal sarcomas (Fig. 9.5), the limited dose tolerance of the many surrounding radiosensitive structures (e.g., spinal cord, cauda equina,

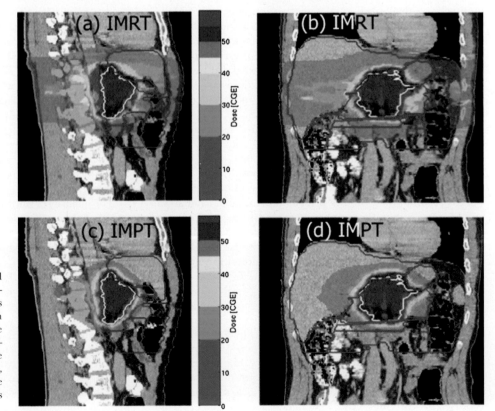

Figure 9.5. A case of retroperitoneal sarcoma. Dose distributions from intensity-modulated therapy with (**A, B**) x-rays (IMRT), and (**C, D**) protons (IMPT) in sagittal and coronal sections through the isocenter. The clinical target volume is outlined in white. Purple lines designate the outlines of critical structures: liver, stomach, small bowel, duodenum. Patient data were provided by Dr. T. DeLaney (Massachusetts General Hospital, Boston, MA).

esophagus, small and large bowel) often presents an obstacle in reaching the prescribed target dose. Improved dose conformation with IMRT of retroperitoneal malignancies was shown to lead to the reduced small bowel dose with IMRT,[71] with expected reduction in gastrointestinal toxicity. The analysis of clinical outcomes for patients treated with high-dose fractionated radiation therapy using 3D treatment planning and combined proton and photon beams to portions of the cauda equina by Pieters et al.[72] suggests that the probability of neurotoxicity is a relatively steep function of dose. Thus, in many cases, even a modest reduction in the mean and maximum dose to organs is reasonably expected to lead to reduced toxicity rates in these patients. IMPT has been shown to have a strong potential to reduce the irradiation of critical structures, especially with increased distance from the target, and allow for dose escalation.[52,53,73]

REDUCING RADIATION INJURIES DUE TO LOW (SCATTERED AND SECONDARY) DOSES

The radiation injuries described above are of concern in the intermediate-dose regions and can be divided into early and late effects. These should be avoided if possible. However, within the field of irradiation, one may have to accept a significant risk for normal tissue toxicity, which is outweighed by the therapeutic benefit.

Besides dose deposited in tissues in the vicinity of the target, there can be dose more distant to the target. This is caused by radiation being scattered at large angles in the treatment head, radiation leakage through the treatment head, and by secondary radiation, that is, radiation generated by interactions of the primary radiation with material in the treatment head or the patient. Some treatment techniques, while aiming at highly conformal dose to the target, do not necessarily deliver lower dose to areas distant to the target. It has been cautioned that compared with conventional radiotherapy, the use of IMRT could result in a higher incidence of radiation-induced second cancers. This risk has been argued in proton therapy as well but it is more likely that protons will decrease the risk of second malignancies because of the decrease in integral dose to normal tissue as discussed earlier.[74–77] Because doses are very low (typically <1% of the prescribed dose), the main concerns are late effects and, in particular, second cancers.

Criteria for a malignancy to be classified as a radiation-induced second tumor are as follows[78]: (1) the tumor occurs within "nonirradiated" tissue, (2) the histology of the second tumor is different from that of the original disease, (3) the existence of a latency period for a radiation-associated tumor, (4) the second tumor was not present at the time of irradiation, and (5) the patient does not have a cancer-prone syndrome.

Treatment-related cancers are a well-recognized side effect in radiation oncology.[79,80] The cumulative risk for the development of second cancers over a 25-year follow-up interval has been estimated as ranging from 5% to 12%[81–84] with radiation therapy as a predisposing factor.[81,85–87] Radiation can cause intracranial tumors after therapeutic cranial irradiation for leukemia,[88] tinea capitis,[89,90] and intracranial tumors.[91–93] The median latency of second cancers has been reported as 7.6 years in one group of patients.[94] In patients with pituitary adenoma, a cumulative risk of secondary brain tumors of 1.9% to 2.4% at approximately 20 years after radiotherapy and a latency period for tumor occurrence of 6 to 21 years were reported.[95,96] Brenner et al.[97] examined second cancers from

prostate radiotherapy and found that the absolute risk was 1.4% for patients surviving longer than 10 years. Data on radiation-induced cancer and mortality after exposure to low-doses data have been summarized in the BEIR VII (Biological Effects of Ionizing Radiation) report for various organs.[98]

3DCRT and IMRT

In IMRT, the photon fluence is modulated using an MLC. This allows higher dose conformity than with 3DCRT. However, the increased ability of shaping the prescribed dose distribution comes with a price. Parts of the radiation field generated in the treatment head are blocked at any given time during IMRT delivery. This has two consequences. First, there will be dose outside a treated volume caused by leakage radiation through the MLC. The spatial distribution of the resulting dose and its magnitude depends on the design and operation of the MLC and the patterns of modulation specified by the treatment planning algorithm, that is, the sequencing algorithm. Second, because less dose is delivered per unit time, an IMRT treatment plan results in an increase in MU by a factor of around 3.[99] As a consequence, treatment will be prolonged, which increases radiation scattered from collimators and beam modifiers.

The magnitude of such doses is well understood and there are numerous publications on scattered doses in photon therapy.[100–107] The AAPM Radiation Therapy Task Group analyzed the scattered dose in photon beams.[108] Further, the majority of published studies on scattered and secondary doses in radiation therapy beams have been summarized in a review.[109]

The difference between 3DCRT and IMRT in terms of scattered or leakage radiation can be significant.[99,110] Typically, the dose decreases exponentially with distance from the field edge.[100,103,106] Dose equivalent values of approximately 0.1 to 5 mSv per treatment Gy at 1 m from the isocenter were reported.[111–119] Verellen and Vanhavere[120] determined whole-body equivalent doses of $1.6 \times 10{-}2$ mSv per MU with IMRT delivery. Since late effects are of particular concern for pediatric patients, scattered doses in pediatric IMRT were studied by Klein et al.[121] They showed that the scattered dose increase with increasing beam energy distant to the field but decreases with increasing beam energy closer to the field edge. This demonstrates that treatment head leakage dominates distant to the field, while close to the field scattering is the main contributor.

Studies on scattered doses have also been conducted for serial tomotherapy[120,122] and helical tomotherapy.[123] Further, significantly higher scattered doses than with IMRT were reported for CyberKnife treatments.[124]

The majority of photon treatments are done with 6-MV beam energy. For treating deep-seated tumors in the pelvic region, higher photon energies are frequently being used. Photons with energies above approximately 8 MV can cause nuclear interactions in the beam path, which leads to neutron radiation. Neutrons originate from the flattening filter, the bremsstrahlung target, shielding material, and from scattering in the treatment room. The average energy of these neutrons is about 1 MeV,[125] which is in the range where the quality factor for neutrons is the greatest. Because neutrons have a higher RBE compared to photons, a weighting factor needs to be applied (see Section 3.3). The absorbed dose due to neutrons produced in soft tissue irradiated by a 25-MV beam was found to be <40 mGy per treatment Gy.[126] Mainly due to secondary neutrons, a dose of several mSv per treatment Gy was reported for 18-MV IMRT delivery.[127–130]

Obviously, significance has to be measured not in dose but in risk for radiation injury, such as the development of a second cancer. It has been estimated that we might see an elevated risk for developing a second malignancy when using IMRT instead of 3DCRT.[75,97,99] Specifically, the impact of secondary neutrons in IMRT on cancer risk has been assessed.[131,132] The comparison of the relative risk for late effects between IMRT and 3DCRT is not straightforward. As discussed in the previous section, we also have to consider the intermediate-dose levels. IMRT might be able to reduce the volume of healthy tissue receiving intermediate doses, which in turn may lead to a decrease in secondary sarcomas and carcinomas.[75] Kry et al.[76,133] reported scattered photon and neutron doses using photon energies from 6- to 15-MV showing significant differences between IMRT and 3DCRT for the risk of second malignancies. The maximum risk for a fatal second malignancy was 2.1% for 10-MV IMRT.

Radiation-induced sarcomas occur mainly in tissues that receive higher doses of radiation.[134] One might thus argue that it is unlikely that a difference exists between 3DCRT and IMRT, since the high-dose volume is similar. Concerning radiation-induced carcinomas, there is likely to be an increased incidence after IMRT treatments compared to 3DCRT because of a larger volume irradiated to lower doses. Hall and Wuu[75] estimated that an additional 0.5% of surviving patients will develop a second malignancy as a result of this factor and that an additional 0.25% of surviving patients will develop a radiation-induced malignancy because of increased MU in IMRT.

IMRT and Protons

When moving from IMRT to proton therapy, dose conformity may or may not increase significantly. However, there will be less integral dose when using protons instead of IMRT. The main consequence is that, on average, organs at risk will receive lower dose in the intermediate-dose regions, as discussed in the section "Radiation Injury in Cancer Therapy." Nevertheless, protons show a similar disadvantage as IMRT in the existence of a low secondary dose bath to the whole body of the patient. While in IMRT this dose is caused by the "exit" irradiation distal to the target, scattered photons or secondary neutrons, the low-dose bath in proton therapy is caused mainly by secondary neutrons.[135] Neutrons as a by-product of proton radiation are produced in the treatment head and the patient. The contribution from the treatment head typically dominates.[136,137] The neutron yield depends on the material in the beam path and, hence, on the design of the beam line and treatment head. Since the treatment head geometry is field dependent, there can be quite a variation when comparing secondary radiation for different patient fields. It has been shown that for most treatment heads, the neutron dose will increase with decreasing aperture opening, that is, with decreasing field size. This is because small field sizes impinging on the patient require a big part of the primary beam to be blocked. This is associated with neutron production in the blocking material.

Scattered radiation from therapeutic proton beams has been studied extensively.[136,138–148] Choosing a worst-case scenario for their delivery system, Yan et al.[142] measured neutron doses of 1 to 15 mSv per treatment Gy in a 160-MeV passively scattered proton beam. Similar neutron doses were reported by others,[147] decreasing from 6.3 to 0.6 mSv/Gy with increasing distance to isocenter and increased as the range modulation increased. For

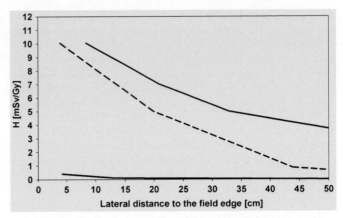

Figure 9.6. Neutron equivalent dose per treatment dose as a function of distance to the field edge as measured for two proton beam fields (*solid lines*). The two results refer to the highest[142] and the lowest[146] measured doses for passive scattered proton beams reported in the literature, thus illustrating the dependency on field characteristics. The dashed line shows one example for the scattered photon dose as measured for a 6-MV IMRT treatment.[121]

a small aperture opening, equivalent doses up to 20 mSv/Gy were reported.[148] The results from various studies vary significantly because neutron doses decrease rapidly with lateral distance from the proton field making it heavily dependent on the point of interest. Other parameters influencing neutron doses are aperture, air gap, beam energy, and treatment head design.[146] Because of the significant influence of the patient's aperture, neutron doses would typically increase with decreasing field size. For the much smaller neutron component generated in the patient, this effect would be reversed.

Experimental data on scattered or secondary doses are typically obtained in well-defined phantom geometries, that is, the results show the dose as a function of distance relative to the treated volume. Figure 9.6 shows measured and calculated doses as a function of lateral distance to the field edge for two proton beams and one IMRT beam. The neutron dose to proton patients was also compared with the x-ray dose from CT imaging.[137] It turned out that, as an example, for young patients the secondary dose to the thyroid received in the course of proton therapy for a brain lesion can be in the order of more than 20 times the dose from a chest CT exam.

The magnitude of second cancer risk in patients treated with proton radiation has been estimated utilizing computer simulations of organ doses.[149,150] One study considered organ specific neutron equivalent doses for proton therapy brain fields and applied organ specific risk models[98] to assess the risk for developing solid cancers and leukemia.[150] It was found that young patients are subject to significantly higher risks than adult patients due to geometric differences and age dependency of risk models. Specifically, a comparison of the lifetime risks showed that breast cancer should be the main concern for females, whereas for males, risks for lung cancer were more significant. Other than for pediatric patients, leukemia was the leading risk for an adult. It was also found, however, that most of the calculated lifetime risks were below 1% for a considered 70-Gy treatment and that most of the risks were significantly below the (natural) baseline risk.

Second malignancies are a major source of morbidity and mortality in pediatric cancer survivors and protons decrease the volume and dose to normal tissues compared with photon techniques. Although IMRT affords great conformality to the target volume at high doses, due to the increased volume of tissue receiving lower doses it may nearly double the risk of second malignancy compared with 3D conformal techniques.[75] The second malignancy rates in children from incidental normal tissue dose are on the order of 2% to 10% by 15 to 20 years after radiotherapy.[94,151,152] Miralbell et al.[153] demonstrated expected second malignancy risks in a modeling study comparing proton and photon techniques and found the expected risks for second malignancy using protons to be significantly less dependent on the case and the treatment technique.

There is little published literature on the second malignancy rates in the children treated with proton radiotherapy. Recently, the comparative risk for developing second malignancies from scattered photon dose in IMRT and secondary neutron dose in proton therapy has been assessed by analyzing clinical data.[154] The study matched patients treated with proton radiation therapy from 1974 to 2001 at the Harvard Cyclotron Laboratory and photon patients from the Surveillance, Epidemiology, and End Results cancer registry.[155] Patients were matched patients by age at radiation treatment, year of treatment, cancer histology, and site of treatment. After adjusting for gender and the age at treatment, the results indicated that the use of proton radiation therapy may be associated with a lower risk of a second malignancy compared to photon radiation therapy.

Protons and Scanned Protons

There are two different beam delivery methods in proton therapy, the passive scattering technique and the scanning technique.[156] The first method needs various scatterers, beam-flattening devices, collimators, and energy modulation devices. Additionally, for each patient, individual apertures and compensators are required. In proton beam scanning, a proton pencil beam is magnetically scanned over the target volume without the need for beam shaping scattering devices. Because of fewer scattering devices, the scanning method produces a lower neutron background than passive scattering.[141]

Since computer simulations have shown that in today's treatment head designs, roughly 60% to 95% of the neutrons in the patient are generated in the treatment head (i.e., only 5% to 40% in the patient), we can assume that proton beam scanning reduces the neutron dose exposure significantly, in particular for small treatment fields (i.e., small aperture openings in scattering systems). For a the proton beam scanning system at the PSI, neutron equivalent doses between 2 and 5 mSv/Gy were measured for target volumes of 211 (sacral chordoma) and 1,253 cm³ RMS, respectively, and 0.002 to 8 mSv/Gy for lateral distances of 100 to 7 cm from isocenter.[141]

Scanned proton beams are believed to result in a lower second cancer risk than passive scattered protons or photons.[141,153] Miralbell et al.[153] assessed the potential influence of improved dose distribution with proton beams compared to photon beams on the incidence of treatment-induced second cancers in pediatric oncology. The study involved two children, one with a parameningeal RMS and one with a medulloblastoma. It was shown that scanned proton beams reduce the incidence of

radiation-induced second cancers for the RMS patient by a factor of >2 and for the medulloblastoma case by a factor of 15 when compared with IMRT. Because the contribution from secondary neutrons can be neglected for scanned beams, the improvement is simply due to a smaller irradiated high-dose volume.

Biological Effectiveness of Low Doses

The RBE is being used in proton therapy to relate proton doses to photon dose. Typically, a generic RBE of 1.1 is applied because the variations in proton RBE are judged to be smaller than the uncertainties in RBE values as a function of dose, dose rate, fractionation, endpoint, and beam characteristics. For high doses, where only deterministic effects play a role, the RBE is a valid concept. The RBE is only defined in combination with a reference radiation for a given biological effect.

In the low-dose region, that is, for secondary radiation, the term "radiation weighting factor" instead of RBE emphasizes the fact that the quality or weighting factor is typically not endpoint or dose dependent. Weighting factors are a set of values (as a function of radiation and energy) agreed upon for radiation protection estimations. The radiation weighting factor scales the absorbed dose and results in the organ equivalent dose. It is defined as a function of the type, and sometimes the energy, of the radiation and converts the absorbed dose in Gy to Sievert (Sv).[157]

For risk estimations, a linear dose-response relationship is typically assumed for most endpoints (exceptions include e.g., leukemia). However, the dose needs to be converted into an equivalent dose in order to reflect the relative effectiveness of different radiation modalities.

The dose deposited by neutron radiation is typically quite low in photon (high energy) as well as proton beams. However, due to their physical interaction mechanisms, as for example characterized by their track structure, their effectiveness is much higher than that of photon beams. Furthermore, the biological effectiveness increases with decreasing dose. The big uncertainties in neutron RBE data have led to the adoption of pragmatic judgments and recommendation by international committees for practical purposes. To estimate the biological effectiveness of neutrons as a function of neutron energy, the International Commission of Radiation Protection (ICRP) recommends the use of a bell-shaped curve with a maximum of 20 at neutron energies around 1 MeV (thus these neutrons would be 20 times more effective than photons at the same dose). Luckily, although most of the neutrons in the patient will be around 1 to 2 MeV where the weighting factor is highest, most of the dose deposited by neutrons comes from higher energy neutrons, resulting in a much lower weighting factor. Nevertheless, uncertainties and even ambiguities exist about how these weighting factors are used. In particular, the calculation of neutron equivalent dose for an organ requires the knowledge about the underlying neutron energy distribution, information obtainable only from dedicated experiments or Monte Carlo calculations.

Neutron quality factors are subject to significant uncertainties, which could affect risk estimations, in particular at low doses. There are not sufficient amount of data to define the radiation effectiveness of neutrons for epidemiological endpoints. The quality factor recommendation by the ICRP may not reflect reality at the very low doses as it does focus on radiation protection rather than radiation epidemiology. The ICRP explicitly states that the term effective dose is a quantity for use in radiation protection and not in epidemiology. These limitations have to be considered when analyzing secondary doses.

REFERENCES

1. Emami B, Lyman J, Brown A, et al. Tolerance of normal tissue to therapeutic irradiation. *Int J Radiat Oncol Biol Phys.* 1991;21:109–122.
2. Milano MT, Constine LS, Okunieff P. Normal tissue tolerance dose metrics for radiation therapy of major organs. *Semin Radiat Oncol.* 2007;17:131–140.
3. Bortfeld, T. Optimized planning using physical objectives and constraints. *Semin Radiat Oncol.* 1999;9:20–34.
4. Mackie TR, Holmes T, Swerdloff S, et al. Tomotherapy: a new concept for the delivery of dynamic conformal radiotherapy. *Med Phys.* 1993;20:1709–1719.
5. Adler JR Jr, Chang SD, Murphy MJ, et al. The Cyberknife: a frameless robotic system for radiosurgery. *Stereotact Funct Neurosurg.* 1997;69:124–128.
6. Paganetti H, Bortfeld T. Proton therapy. In: Schlegel W, Bortfeld T, Grosu AL, eds. *New Technologies in Radiation Oncology.* Heidelberg: Springer. ISBN 3-540-00321-5 2005.
7. Lomax A. Intensity modulation methods for proton radiotherapy. *Phys Med Biol.* 1999;44:185–205.
8. ICRU. *Prescribing, Recording, and Reporting Photon Beam Therapy.* Bethesda, MD: International Commission on Radiation Units and Measurements, 1993; Report No. 50.
9. ICRU. *Prescribing, Recording and Reporting Photon Beam Therapy (Supplement to ICRU Report 50).* Bethesda, MD: International Commission on Radiation Units and Measurements, 1999; Report No. 62.
10. ICRU. *Prescribing, Recording, and Reporting Proton-Beam Therapy.* Bethesda, MD: International Commission on Radiation Units and Measurements, 2007; Report No. 78.
11. NCI. Fact Sheet 04/22/2005. Available at: http://www.cancer.gov/cancertopics/factsheet/Sites-Types/childhood 2005
12. Ries LAG, Harkins D, Krapcho M, et al. SEER cancer statistics review, 1975–2003. Available at: http://seer.cancer.gov/csr/1975_2003/2006
13. Bhat SR, Goodwin TL, Burwinkle TM, et al. Profile of daily life in children with brain tumors: an assessment of health-related quality of life. *J Clin Oncol.* 2005;23:5493–5500.
14. Geenen MM, Cardous-Ubbink MC, Kremer LC, et al. Medical assessment of adverse health outcomes in long-term survivors of childhood cancer. *JAMA.* 2007;297:2705–2715.
15. Shih HA, Loeffler JS, Tarbell NJ. Late effects of CNS radiation therapy. *Cancer Treat Res.* 2009;150:23–41.
16. Hjern A, Lindblad F, Boman KK. Disability in adult survivors of childhood cancer: a Swedish national cohort study. *J Clin Oncol.* 2007;25:5262–5266.
17. Oeffinger KC, Mertens AC, Sklar CA, et al. Chronic health conditions in adult survivors of childhood cancer. *N Engl J Med.* 2006;355:1572–1582.
18. Speechley KN, Barrera M, Shaw AK, et al. Health-related quality of life among child and adolescent survivors of childhood cancer. *J Clin Oncol.* 2006;24:2536–2543.
19. Mulhern RK, Palmer SL, Merchant TE, et al. Neurocognitive consequences of risk-adapted therapy for childhood medulloblastoma. *J Clin Oncol.* 2005;23:5511–5519.
20. Mulhern RK, Merchant TE, Gajjar A, et al. Late neurocognitive sequelae in survivors of brain tumours in childhood. *Lancet Oncol.* 2004;5:399–408.
21. Palmer SL, Goloubeva O, Reddick WE, et al. Patterns of intellectual development among survivors of pediatric medulloblastoma: a longitudinal analysis. *J Clin Oncol.* 2001;19:2302–2308.
22. Bull KS, Spoudeas HA, Yadegarfar G, et al. Reduction of health status 7 years after addition of chemotherapy to craniospinal irradiation for medulloblastoma: a follow-up study in PNET 3 trial survivors on behalf of the CCLG (formerly UKCCSG). *J Clin Oncol.* 2007;25:4239–4245.
23. Merchant TE, Kiehna EN, Li C, et al. Modeling radiation dosimetry to predict cognitive outcomes in pediatric patients with CNS embryonal tumors including medulloblastoma. *Int J Radiat Oncol Biol Phys.* 2006;65:210–221.
24. Merchant TE, Kiehna EN, Li C, et al. Radiation dosimetry predicts IQ after conformal radiation therapy in pediatric patients with localized ependymoma. *Int J Radiat Oncol Biol Phys.* 2005;63:1546–1554.
25. Nutting C, Dearnaley DP, Webb S. Intensity modulated radiation therapy: a clinical review. *Br J Radiol.* 2000;73:459–469.
26. Kuppersmith RB, Greco SC, Teh BS, et al. Intensity-modulated radiotherapy: first results with this new technology on neoplasms of the head and neck. *Ear Nose Throat J.* 1999;78:238, 241–236, 248 passim.
27. Chao KSC, Deasy JO, Markman J, et al. A prospective study of salivary function sparing in patients with head and neck cancers receiving intensity modulated or three-dimensional radiation therapy: initial results. *Int J Radiat Oncol Biol Phys.* 2001;49:907–916.
28. Zelefsky MJ, Fuks Z, Happersett L, et al. Clinical experience with intensity modulated radiation therapy (IMRT) in prostate cancer. *Radiother Oncol.* 2000;55:241–249.
29. Mundt AJ, Lujan AE, Rotmensch J, et al. Intensity-modulated whole pelvic radiotherapy in women with gynecologic malignancies. *Int J Radiat Oncol Biol Phys.* 2002;52:1330–1337.
30. Balog JP, Mackie TR, Wenman DL, et al. Multileaf collimator interleaf transmission. *Med Phys.* 1999;26:176–186.
31. Aoyama H, Westerly DC, Mackie TR, et al. Integral radiation dose to normal structures with conformal external beam radiation. *Int J Radiat Oncol Biol Phys.* 2006;64:962–967.
32. Cozzarini C, Fiorino C, Di Muzio N, et al. Significant reduction of acute toxicity following pelvic irradiation with helical tomotherapy in patients with localized prostate cancer. *Radiother Oncol.* 2007;84:164–170.
33. Keiler L, Dobbins D, Kulasekere R, et al. Tomotherapy for prostate adenocarcinoma: a report on acute toxicity. *Radiother Oncol.* 2007;84:171–176.
34. Lee N, Xia P, Quivey JM, et al. Intensity-modulated radiotherapy in the treatment of nasopharyngeal carcinoma: an update of the UCSF experience. *Int J Radiat Oncol Biol Phys.* 2002;53:12–22.
35. Krejcarek SC, Grant PE, Henson JW, et al. Physiologic and radiographic evidence of the distal edge of the proton beam in craniospinal irradiation. *Int J Radiat Oncol Biol Phys.* 2007;68:646–649.
36. St. Clair WH, Adams JA, Bues M, et al. Advantage of protons compared to conventional X-ray or IMRT in the treatment of a pediatric patient with medulloblastoma. *Int J Radiat Oncol Biol Phys.* 2004;58:727–734.
37. Yock T, Schneider R, Friedmann A, et al. Proton radiotherapy for orbital rhabdomyosarcoma: clinical outcome and a dosimetric comparison with photons. *Int J Radiat Oncol Biol Phys.* 2005;63:1161–1168.
38. Friedmann AM, Tarbell NJ, Schaefer PW, et al. Case records of the Massachusetts General Hospital. Weekly clinicopathological exercises. Case 4: 2004. A nine-month-old boy with an orbital rhabdomyosarcoma. *N Engl J Med.* 2004;350:494–502.
39. Kirsch DG, Tarbell NJ. New technologies in radiation therapy for pediatric brain tumors: the rationale for proton radiation therapy. *Pediatr Blood Cancer.* 2004;42:461–464.
40. Kirsch DG, Tarbell NJ. Conformal radiation therapy for childhood CNS tumors. *Oncologist.* 2004;9:442–450.
41. Archambeau JO, Slater JD, Slater JM, et al. Role for proton beam irradiation in treatment of pediatric CNS malignancies. *Int J Radiat Oncol Biol Phys.* 1992;22:287–294.
42. Fuss M, Hug EB, Schaefer RA, et al. Proton radiation therapy (PRT) for pediatric optic pathway gliomas: comparison with 3D planned conventional photons and a standard photon technique. *Int J Radiat Oncol Biol Phys.* 1999;45:1117–1126.
43. Fuss M, Poljanc K, Miller DW, et al. Normal tissue complication probability (NTCP) calculations as a means to compare proton and photon plans and evaluation of clinical appropriateness of calculated values. *Int J Cancer (Radiat Oncol Invest).* 2000;90:351–358.
44. Lin R, Hug EB, Schaefer RA, et al. Conformal proton radiation therapy of the posterior fossa: a study comparing protons with three-dimensional planned photons in limiting dose to auditory structures. *Int J Radiat Oncol Biol Phys.* 2000;48:1219–1226.
45. Lomax AJ, Bortfeld T, Goitein G, et al. A treatment planning inter-comparison of proton and intensity modulated photon radiotherapy. *Radiother Oncol.* 1999;51:257–271.
46. Suit HD, Goldberg S, Niemierko A, et al. Proton beams to replace photon beams in radical dose treatments. *Acta Oncol.* 2003;42:800–808.
47. Yock TI, Tarbell NJ. Technology insight: proton beam radiotherapy for treatment in pediatric brain tumors. *Nat Clin Pract Oncol.* 2004;1:97–103.
48. Bussiere MR, Adams JA. Treatment planning for conformal proton radiation therapy. *Technol Cancer Res Treat.* 2003;2:389–399.
49. Moyers MF, Miller DW, Bush DA, et al. Methodologies and tools for proton beam design for lung tumors. *Int J Radiat Oncol Biol Phys.* 2001;49:1429–1438.
50. Parodi K, Paganetti H, Shih HA, et al. Patient study of in vivo verification of beam delivery and range, using positron emission tomography and computed tomography imaging after proton therapy. *Int J Radiat Oncol Biol Phys.* 2007;68:920–934.
51. Unkelbach J, Chan TC, Bortfeld T. Accounting for range uncertainties in the optimization of intensity modulated proton therapy. *Phys Med Biol.* 2007;52:2755–2773.
52. Lomax AJ, Boehringer, T, Coray A, et al. Intensity modulated proton therapy: a clinical example. *Med Phys.* 2001;28:317–324.
53. Lomax AJ, Pedroni E, Rutz H, et al. The clinical potential of intensity modulated proton therapy. *Z Med Phys.* 2004;14:147–152.
54. Weber DC, Lomax AJ, Rutz HP, et al. Spot-scanning proton radiation therapy for recurrent, residual or untreated intracranial meningiomas. *Radiother Oncol.* 2004;71:251–258.
55. Weber DC, Rutz HP, Pedroni ES, et al. Results of spot-scanning proton radiation therapy for chordoma and chondrosarcoma of the skull base: the Paul Scherrer Institute experience. *Int J Radiat Oncol Biol Phys.* 2005;63:401–409.
56. Schulz-Ertner D, Nikoghosyan A, Thilmann C, et al. Results of carbon ion radiotherapy in 152 patients. *Int J Radiat Oncol Biol Phys.* 2004;58:631–640.
57. Glimelius B, Montelius A. Proton beam therapy—do we need the randomised trials and can we do them? *Radiother Oncol.* 2007;83:105–109.
58. Suit H, Kooy H, Trofimov A, et al. Should positive phase III clinical trial data be required before proton beam therapy is more widely adopted? No. *Radiother Oncol.* 2008;86:148–153.
59. Goitein M, Cox JD. Should randomized clinical trials be required for proton radiotherapy? *J Clin Oncol.* 2008;26:175–176.
60. Shipley WU, Verhey LJ, Munzenrider JE, et al. Advanced prostate cancer: the results of a randomized comparative trial of high dose irradiation boosting with conformal protons compared with conventional dose irradiation using photons alone. *Int J Radiat Oncol Biol Phys.* 1995;32:3–12.
61. Mock U, Bogner J, Georg D, et al. Comparative treatment planning on localized prostate carcinoma conformal photon versus proton-based radiotherapy. *Strahlenther Onkol.* 2005;181:448–455.
62. Zhang X, Dong L, Lee AK, et al. Effect of anatomic motion on proton therapy dose distributions in prostate cancer treatment. *Int J Radiat Oncol Biol Phys.* 2007;67:620–629.
63. Trofimov A, Nguyen PL, Coen JJ, et al. Radiotherapy treatment of early-stage prostate cancer with IMRT and protons: a treatment planning comparison. *Int J Radiat Oncol Biol Phys.* 2007;69:444–453.
64. Vargas C, Fryer A, Mahajan C, et al. Dose-volume comparison of proton therapy and intensity-modulated radiotherapy for prostate cancer. *Int J Radiat Oncol Biol Phys.* 2008;70:744–751.
65. Benk VA, Adams JA, Shipley WU, et al. Late rectal bleeding following combined X-ray and proton high dose irradiation for patients with stages T3–T4 prostate carcinoma. *Int J Radiat Oncol Biol Phys.* 1993;26:551–557.
66. Hartford AC, Niemierko A, Adams JA, et al. Conformal irradiation of the prostate: Estimating long-term rectal bleeding risk using dose-volume histograms. *Int J Radiat Oncol Biol Phys.* 1996;36:721–730.
67. Chan AW, Liebsch NJ. Proton radiation therapy for head and neck cancer. *J Surg Oncol.* 2008;97:697–700.
68. Kozak KR, Adams J, Krejcarek SJ, et al. A dosimetric comparison of proton and intensity-modulated photon radiotherapy for pediatric parameningeal rhabdomyosarcomas. *Int J Radiat Oncol Biol Phys.* 2008;74:197–186.

69. MacDonald SM, Safai S, Trofimov A, et al. Proton radiotherapy for childhood ependymoma: initial clinical outcomes and dose comparisons. *Int J Radiat Oncol Biol Phys.* 2008;71:979–986.

70. Steneker M, Lomax A, Schneider U. Intensity modulated photon and proton therapy for the treatment of head and neck tumors. *Radiother Oncol.* 2006;80:263–267.

71. Koshy M, Landry JC, Lawson JD, et al. Intensity modulated radiation therapy for retroperitoneal sarcoma: a case for dose escalation and organ at risk toxicity reduction. *Sarcoma.* 2003;7:137–148.

72. Pieters RS, Niemierko A, Fullerton BC, et al. Cauda equina tolerance to high-dose fractionated irradiation. *Int J Radiat Oncol Biol Phys.* 2006;64:251–257.

73. Weber DC, Trofimov AV, Delaney TF, et al. A treatment plan comparison of intensity modulated photon and proton therapy for paraspinal sarcomas. *Int J Radiat Oncol Biol Phys.* 2004;58:1596–1606.

74. Hall EJ. Intensity-modulated radiation therapy, protons, and the risk of second cancers. *Int J Radiat Oncol Biol Phys.* 2006;65:1–7.

75. Hall EJ, Wuu C-S. Radiation-induced second cancers: the impact of 3D-CRT and IMRT. *Int J Radiat Oncol Biol Phys.* 2003;56:83–88.

76. Kry SF, Salehpour M, Followill DS, et al. The calculated risk of fatal secondary malignancies from intensity-modulated radiation therapy. *Int J Radiat Oncol Biol Phys.* 2005;62: 1195–1203.

77. Paganetti H, Bortfeld T, Delaney TF. Neutron dose in proton radiation therapy: in regard to Eric J. Hall (*Int J Radiat Oncol Biol Phys.* 2006;65:1–7). *Int J Radiat Oncol Biol Phys.* 2006;66:1594–1595; author reply 1595.

78. Cahan WG, Woodard HQ, Higonbotham NL, et al. Sarcoma arising in irradiated bone: report of eleven cases. *Cancer.* 1948;1:3–29.

79. Schottenfeld D, Beebe-Dimmer JL. Multiple cancers. In: Schottenfeld D, Fraumeni JF Jr, eds. *Cancer Epidemiology and Prevention.* Oxford Press, USA; 2006:1269–1280.

80. van Leeuwen FE, Travis LB. Second cancers. In: Devita VT, et al., eds. *Cancer: Principles and Practice of Oncology.* 7th ed. Lippincott, Philadelphia; 2005:2575–2602.

81. de Vathaire F, Francois P, Hill C, et al. Role of radiotherapy and chemotherapy in the risk of second malignant neoplasms after cancer in childhood. *Br J Cancer.* 1989;59:792–796.

82. Hawkins MM, Draper GJ, Kingston JE. Incidence of second primary tumours among childhood cancer survivors. *Br J Cancer.* 1987;56:339–347.

83. Olsen JH, Garwicz S, Hertz H, et al. Nordic Society of Paediatric Haematology and Oncology Association of the Nordic Cancer Registries. Second malignant neoplasms after cancer in childhood or adolescence. *Br Med J.* 1993;307:1030–1036.

84. Tucker MA, Meadows AT, Boice JD Jr, et al. Cancer risk following treatment of childhood cancer. In: Boice JD Jr, Fraumeni JF Jr, eds. *Radiation Carcinogenesis: Epidemiology and Biological Significance.* Raven Press, NY; 1984:211–224.

85. Potish RA, Dehner LP, Haselow RE, et al. The incidence of second neoplasms following megavoltage radiation for pediatric tumors. *Cancer.* 1985;56:1534–1537.

86. Strong LC, Herson J, Osborne BM, et al. Risk of radiation-related subsequent malignant tumors in survivors of Ewing's sarcoma. *J Natl Cancer Inst.* 1979;62:1401–1406.

87. Tucker MA, D'Angio GJ, Boice JD Jr, et al. Bone sarcomas linked to radiotherapy and chemotherapy in children. *N Engl J Med.* 1987;317:588–593.

88. Neglia JP, Meadows AT, Robison LL, et al. Second neoplasms after acute lymphoblastic leukemia in childhood. *N Engl J Med.* 1991;325:1330–1336.

89. Ron E, Modan B, Boice JD, et al. Tumors of the brain and nervous system after radiotherapy in childhood. *N Engl J Med.* 1988;319:1033–1039.

90. Sadetzki S, Flint-Richter P, Ben-Tal T, et al. Radiation-induced meningioma: a descriptive study of 253 cases. *J Neurosurg.* 2002;97:1078–1082.

91. Kaschten B, Flandroy P, Reznik M, et al. Radiation-induced gliosarcoma: case report and review of the literature. *J Neurosurg.* 1995;83:154–162.

92. Liwnicz BH, Berger TS, Liwnicz RG, et al. Radiation-associated gliomas: a report of four cases and analysis of postradiation tumors of the central nervous system. *Neurosurgery.* 1985;17:436–445.

93. Simmons NE, Laws ER Jr. Glioma occurrence after sellar irradiation: case report and review. *Neurosurgery.* 1998;42:172–178.

94. Kuttesch JF Jr, Wexler LH, Marcus RB, et al. Second malignancies after Ewing's sarcoma: radiation dose-dependency of secondary sarcomas. *J Clin Oncol.* 1996;14:2818–2825.

95. Brada M, Ford D, Ashley S, et al. Risk of second brain tumour after conservative surgery and radiotherapy for pituitary adenoma. *Br Med J.* 1992;304:1343–1346.

96. Minniti G, Traish D, Ashley S, et al. Risk of second brain tumor after conservative surgery and radiotherapy for pituitary adenoma: update after an additional 10 years. *J Clin Endocrinol Metab.* 2005;90:800–804.

97. Brenner DJ, Curtis RE, Hall EJ, et al. Second malignancies in prostate carcinoma patients after radiotherapy compared with surgery. *Cancer.* 2000;88:398–406.

98. BEIR. Health risks from exposure to low levels of ionizing radiation, *BEIR VII, Phase 2.* National Research Council. National Academy of Science, Washington, DC; 2006.

99. Followill D, Geis P, Boyer A. Estimates of whole-body dose equivalent produced by beam intensity modulated conformal therapy. *Int J Radiat Oncol Biol Phys.* 1997;38:667–672.

100. Fraass BA, van de Geijn J. Peripheral dose from megavolt beams. *Med Phys.* 1983;10: 809–818.

101. Greene D, Chu GL, Thomas DW. Dose levels outside radiotherapy beams. *Br J Radiol.* 1983;56:543–550.

102. Greene D, Karup PG, Sims C, et al. Dose levels outside radiotherapy beams. *Br J Radiol.* 1985;58:453–456.

103. Kase KR, Svensson GK, Wolbarst AB, et al. Measurements of dose from secondary radiation outside a treatment field. *Int J Radiat Oncol Biol Phys.* 1983;9:1177–1183.

104. Keller B, Mathewson C, Rubin P. Scattered radiation dosage as a function of x-ray energy. *Radiology.* 1974;111:447–449.

105. Lillicrap SC, Morgan HM, Shakeshaft JT. X-ray leakage during radiotherapy. *Br J Radiol.* 2000;73:793–794.

106. McParland BJ. Peripheral doses of two linear accelerators employing universal wedges. *Br J Radiol.* 1990;63:295–298.

107. Sherazi S, Kase KR. Measurements of dose from secondary radiation outside a treatment field: effects of wedges and blocks. *Int J Radiat Oncol Biol Phys.* 1985;11:2171–2176.

108. Stovall M, Blackwell CR, Cundiff J, et al. Fetal dose from radiotherapy with photon beams: report of AAPM radiation therapy committee task group no. 36. [Erratum in *Med Phys.* 1995;22:353–1354.] *Med Phys.* 1995;22:63–82.

109. Xu XG, Bednarz B, Paganetti H. A review of dosimetry studies on external-beam radiation treatment with respect to second cancer induction. *Phys Med Biol.* 2008;53:R193–R241.

110. Williams PO, Hounsell AR. X-ray leakage considerations for IMRT. *Br J Radiol.* 2001;74: 98–100.

111. Agosteo S, Foglio Para A, Maggioni B, et al. Radiation transport in a radiotherapy room. *Health Phys.* 1995;68:27–34.

112. Gudowska I. Measurements of neutron radiation around medical electron accelerators by means of 235U fission chamber and indium foil activation. *Radiat Prot Dosimetry.* 1988;23:345–348.

113. McCall RC, Jenkins TM, Shore RA. Transport of accelerator produced neutrons in a concrete room. *IEEE Trans Nucl Sci.* 1979;26:1593–1597.

114. McGinley PH. Photoneutron fields in medical accelerator rooms with primary barriers constructed of concrete and metals. *Health Phys.* 1992;63:698–701.

115. Palta JR, Hogstrom KR, Tannanonta C. Neutron leakage measurements from a medical linear accelerator. *Med Phys.* 1984;11:498–501.

116. Sanchez F, Madurga G, Arrans R. Neutron measurements around an 18 MV linac. *Radiother Oncol.* 1989;15:259–265.

117. Sherwin AG, Pearson AJ, Richards DJ, et al. Measurements of neutrons from high energy electron linear accelerators. *Radiat Prot Dosimetry.* 1988;23:337–340.

118. Tosi G, Torresin A, Agosteo S, et al. Neutron measurements around medical electron accelerators by active and passive detection techniques. *Med Phys.* 1991;18:54–60.

119. Uwamino Y, Nakamura T, Ohkubo T, et al. Measurement and calculation of neutron leakage from a medical electron accelerator. *Med Phys.* 1986;13:374–384.

120. Verellen D, Vanhavere F. Risk assessment of radiation-induced malignancies based on whole-body equivalent dose estimates for IMRT treatment in the head and neck region. *Radiother Oncol.* 1999;53:199–203.

121. Klein EE, Maserang B, Wood R, et al. Peripheral doses from pediatric IMRT. *Med Phys.* 2006;33:2525–2531.

122. Mutic S, Low DA. Whole-body dose from tomotherapy delivery. *Int J Radiat Oncol Biol Phys.* 1998;42:229–232.

123. Ramsey C, Seibert R, Mahan SL, et al. Out-of-field dosimetry measurements for a helical tomotherapy system. *J Appl Clin Med Phys.* 2006;7:1–11.

124. Petti PL, Chuang CF, Smith V, et al. Peripheral doses in CyberKnife radiosurgery. *Med Phys.* 2006;33:1770–1779.

125. Zanini A, Durisi E, Fasolo F, et al. Monte Carlo simulation of the photoneutron field in linac radiotherapy treatments with different collimation systems. *Phys Med Biol.* 2004;49:571–582.

126. Ing H, Nelson WR, Shore RA. Unwanted photon and neutron radiation resulting from collimated photon beams interacting with the body of radiotherapy patients. *Med Phys.* 1982;9:27–33.

127. Reft CS, Runkel-Muller R, Myrianthopoulos L. In vivo and phantom measurements of the secondary photon and neutron doses for prostate patients undergoing 18 MV IMRT. *Med Phys.* 2006;33:3734–3742.

128. Barquero R, Mendez R, Vega-Carrillo HR, et al. Neutron spectra and dosimetric features around an 18 MV linac accelerator. *Health Phys.* 2005;88:48–58.

129. Chibani O, Ma C-MC. Photonuclear dose calculations for high-energy photon beams from Siemens and varian linacs. *Med Phys.* 2003;30:1990–2000.

130. Lin JP, Chu TC, Lin SY, et al. The measurement of photoneutrons in the vicinity of a Siemens Primus linear accelerator. *Appl Radiat Isot.* 2001;55:315–321.

131. Nath R, Epp ER, Laughlin JS, et al. Neutrons from high-energy x-ray medical accelerators: an estimate of risk to the radiotherapy patient. *Med Phys.* 1984;11:231–241.

132. Hall EJ, Martin SG, Amols H, et al. Photoneutrons from medical linear accelerators - radiobiological measurements and risk estimates. *Int J Radiat Oncol Biol Phys.* 1995;33: 225–230.

133. Kry SF, Salehpour M, Followill DS, et al. Out-of-field photon and neutron dose equivalents from step-and-shoot intensity-modulated radiation therapy. *Int J Radiat Oncol Biol Phys.* 2005;62:1204–1216.

134. Kalra S, Grimer RJ, Spooner D, et al. Radiation-induced sarcomas of bone: factors that affect outcome. *J Bone Joint Surg Br.* 2007;89:808–813.

135. Paganetti H. Nuclear interactions in proton therapy: dose and relative biological effect distributions originating from primary and secondary particles. *Phys Med Biol.* 2002;47: 747–764.

136. Jiang H, Wang B, Xu XG, et al. Simulation of organ specific patient effective dose due to secondary neutrons in proton radiation treatment. *Phys Med Biol.* 2005;50:4337–4353.

137. Zacharatou-Jarlskog C, Lee C, Bolch W, et al. Assessment of organ specific neutron doses in proton therapy using whole-body age-dependent voxel phantoms. *Phys Med Biol.* 2008;53:693–714.

138. Agosteo S, Birattari C, Caravaggio M, et al. Secondary neutron and photon dose in proton therapy. *Radiother Oncol.* 1998;48:293–305.

139. Binns PJ, Hough JH. Secondary dose exposures during 200 MeV proton therapy. *Radiat Prot Dosimetry.* 1997;70:441–444.

140. Roy SC, Sandison GA. Scattered neutron dose equivalent to a fetus from proton therapy of the mother. *Radiat Phys Chem.* 2004;71:997–998.

141. Schneider U, Agosteo S, Pedroni E, et al. Secondary neutron dose during proton therapy using spot scanning. *Int J Radiat Oncol Biol Phys.* 2002;53:244–251.

142. Yan X, Titt U, Koehler AM, et al. Measurement of neutron dose equivalent to proton therapy patients outside of the proton radiation field. *Nucl Instrum Methods Phys Res A.* 2002;476:429–434.

143. Tayama R, Fujita Y, Tadokoro M, et al. Measurement of neutron dose distribution for a passive scattering nozzle at the Proton Medical Research Center (PMRC). *Nucl Instrum Methods Phys Res A.* 2006;564:532–536.

144. Wroe A, Rosenfeld A, Schulte R. Out-of-field dose equivalents delivered by proton therapy of prostate cancer. *Med Phys.* 2007;34:3449–3456.

145. Zacharatou-Jarlskog C, Paganetti H. Sensitivity of different dose scoring methods on organ specific neutron doses calculations in proton therapy. *Phys Med Biol.* 2008;53:4523–4532.

146. Mesoloras G, Sandison GA, Stewart RD, et al. Neutron scattered dose equivalent to a fetus from proton radiotherapy of the mother. *Med Phys.* 2006;33:2479–2490.

147. Polf JC, Newhauser WD. Calculations of neutron dose equivalent exposures from range-modulated proton therapy beams. *Phys Med Biol.* 2005;50:3859–3873.

148. Zheng Y, Newhauser W, Fontenot J, et al. Monte Carlo study of neutron dose equivalent during passive scattering proton therapy. *Phys Med Biol.* 2007;52:4481–4496.

149. Brenner DJ, Hall EJ. Secondary neutrons in clinical proton radiotherapy: a charged issue. *Radiother Oncol.* 2008;86:165–170.

150. Zacharatou-Jarlskog C, Paganetti H. The risk of developing second cancer due to neutron dose in proton therapy as a function of field characteristics, organ, and patient age. *Int J Radiat Oncol Biol Phys.* 2008;69:228–235.

151. Broniscer A, Ke W, Fuller CE, et al. Second neoplasms in pediatric patients with primary central nervous system tumors: the St. Jude Children's Research Hospital experience. *Cancer.* 2004;100:2246–2252.

152. Jenkinson HC, Hawkins MM, Stiller CA, et al. Long-term population-based risks of second malignant neoplasms after childhood cancer in Britain. *Br J Cancer.* 2004;91:1905–1910.

153. Miralbell R, Lomax A, Cella L, et al. Potential reduction of the incidence of radiation-induced second cancers by using proton beams in the treatment of pediatric tumors. *Int J Radiat Oncol Biol Phys.* 2002;54:824–829.

154. Chung CS, Keating N, Yock T, et al. comparative analysis of second malignancy risk in patients treated with proton therapy versus conventional photon therapy. *Int J Radiat Oncol Biol Phys.* 2008;72:S8.

155. SEER. Cancer Statistics Review 1975–2000. Available at: http://seer.cancer.gov/csr/197-2000.

156. Blattmann H. Beam delivery systems for charged particles. *Radiat Environ Biophys.* 1992;31:219–231.

157. ICRP. *Relative Biological Effectiveness (RBE), Quality Factor (Q), and Radiation Weighting Factor (wR).* International Commission on Radiological Protection. Oxford: Pergamon Press; 2003:92.

Toxicity Due to Systemic Radiotherapy

NORMAL TISSUE TOXICITY FROM RADIONUCLIDE THERAPY: DETERMINANTS AND MODULATORS

There is an increasing body of information on normal tissue toxicities associated with systemic radionuclide exposure from therapy, diagnostic procedures, and environmental sources (including accidents and acts of war). The lack of standard toxicity scoring criteria that can be uniformly applied to multiple therapeutic modalities hampers comparisons and establishment of reliable organ tolerance limits from radionuclide exposure. The International Atomic Energy Agency (IAEA) has sponsored conferences to address this issue.[1] Among their findings is the important observation that late toxicity is underreported. The IAEA conference report includes several recommendations for improving the capture of adverse events from radionuclide therapy.[1]

Reports of normal tissue toxicity from radionuclide exposure are more limited than toxicity data for external beam radiation. In general, normal organs appear to tolerate higher doses of radiation from radionuclides than from high dose rate conventional external beam radiation therapy, but with a larger degree of variability. There are a number of well-established factors that influence radionuclide toxicity and may, in part, contribute to the variability of effects reported in the literature. These include age, gender, genetic makeup, immune factors, physiologic conditions, radionuclide characteristics, dose rate, heterogeneous dose distribution, and radioprotector/sensitizer use.

Even with systemic administration, the distribution of radionuclides in the targeted tumor or organ, as well as normal tissues, is usually very heterogeneous. This complicates accurate dose quantitation and greatly affects organ toxicity. For example, the liver tolerance for arterially targeted ^{90}Y-microspheres is more than twice that for intravenously administered ^{90}Y-antibody conjugates, which are much more homogeneously distributed.[2,3] Dose/volume histogram analysis may better predict toxicity.[3–5] For a complete assessment of toxicity, the heterogeneity of dose deposition from radionuclides must be considered at both the cellular and the subcellular level.[6]

RADIONUCLIDE CHARACTERISTICS

Different forms of radionuclide therapy can produce variable effects as shown by the comparison of gene expression after

α and γ radiation.[7] A recent study directly comparing the therapeutic efficacy of α versus β radioimmunoconjugates with rituximab showed superior efficacy of the α emitter.[8] However, radioprotectors were less effective with α emitters than when used with β and γ emitters.[9] Even among the β emitters, there can be differences in toxicity and efficacy, perhaps secondary to low dose rate and radiation-induced bystander effects, both of which are areas of active investigation.[10–14]

DOSE RATE

Differential dose rates and cumulative doses to subregions of normal organs, such as the kidney, can significantly affect toxicity and will be discussed later in this chapter. For example, the effects of model assumptions using kidney subregions as described in the MIRD no. 19 pamphlet for dosimetry calculations are consistent with clinical outcome when the biological equivalent dose is computed.[15,16] This model uses linear quadratic equations (α/β ratios) that have been extensively applied for external beam radiation.[17,18] In the linear quadratic model, the linear (α component) corresponds to a single lethal ionization event. Two closely spaced ionizations are required for the β component, which is influenced by such factors as the rate of repair.

PHYSIOLOGIC CONDITIONS

Conditions such as nutritional status, anemia, disease spread in organs, hypoxia, exposure to carcinogens, status of recovery from prior therapy, and other physiologic stressors can influence radiation tolerance.[19] For example, hypertension and diabetes are associated with poorer renal tolerance to pretargeted radioimmunotherapy (RIT).[20] On the other hand, physiologic changes associated with modifiers of radiation, such as use of the radioprotectant amifostine, improved renal tolerance among patients receiving this therapy. Combining "protective measures" of fractionation of radionuclide administration, the radioprotector amifostine and infusion of dextran + lysine have allowed for a 35% to 50% increase in cumulative administered activity within renal tolerance.[20] Animal studies indicate that posttreatment renal-active medications, in addition to those during radiation, can decrease the risk of renal toxicity. In these studies of an ^{225}Ac-conjugate, furosemide increased excretion of ^{221}Fr and its daughter ^{213}Bi. A protective effect was also associated with prolonged spironolactone (a renin-angiotensin-aldosterone system antagonist) treatment.[21]

It may be impossible to totally separate "physiology" from radiobiologic and genetic factors influencing radiosensitivity, as these are likely to be confounding variables. For example, a physiologically stressed system may have suboptimal sublethal repair capacity. Genetic factors leading to hypertension, diabetes, and anemia, in addition to the genetic background of the patient, influence the inherent sensitivity to γ radiation[22,23] and can contribute to and modify the toxic manifestations of radionuclide exposure.

As above, there are multiple radiobiologic factors that influence toxicity and must be taken into consideration for individualized toxicity predictions. Adjustment for a few factors has been reported to improve dose/response relationships. Much work is still needed to more fully elucidate modifying factors for the mitigation of radiation toxicity.[24,25] An updated compendium of normal organ toxicity dose/response relationships and more detailed discussion of modifying factors was recently published.[26]

RADIOIMMUNOTHERAPY AND SYSTEMICALLY TARGETED RADIATION THERAPY

RADIOIMMUNOTHERAPY

Systemically targeted radiation therapy can be delivered using a carrier or targeting moiety, such as an antibody or peptide, to which is linked a radionuclide. Unconjugated radionuclides can be used for purposes of thyroid ablation, treatment of diffuse intraperitoneal disease (e.g., ovarian cancer), or the treatment of diffuse bone metastases. The unconjugated radionuclides in clinical use may be selectively taken up by the targeted tissue (e.g., ^{131}I for the treatment of thyroid cancer) or may provide for irradiation of serosal surfaces (e.g., ^{32}P for intraperitoneal treatment of ovarian cancer). The toxicity of systemic or intracavitary (with a component of systemic distribution) radiotherapy is determined by a number of factors including properties of the targeting agent and radionuclide, dose, disease distribution and tumor burden, bone marrow reserve, and prior cytotoxic therapies. The remainder of this chapter will discuss dose-limiting toxicities (DLTs), toxicity profiles, and potential late effects of these therapies.

RIT and other forms of systemically targeted radiation therapy use antibodies, antibody fragments, constructs, fusion peptides or peptides to target radiation-emitting radionuclides to tumors.[27] In most cases, the radionuclide is chemically linked to the carrier or targeting agent. Alternatively, a pretargeting approach can be used, in which the targeting agent is administered first, followed in some cases by a clearing agent to remove the antibody or targeting moiety that has not bound to tumor and is still in the circulation. Lastly, in the pretargeting regimen, a therapeutic radionuclide-hapten complex is administered, which then binds to the antibody or targeting agent that has localized in tumor, with unbound radionuclide being rapidly excreted in the urine. Pretargeting has the potential advantage of increasing the relative uptake of the radionuclide in tumor compared with normal tissues, with enhanced tumor:whole body and tumor:normal organ ratios compared with those generally obtained with directly radiolabeled antibodies.[27]

At present, there are only two radiolabeled monoclonal antibodies approved by the FDA. Both of these are anti-CD 20 antibodies, labeled with either ^{131}I (tositumomab) or ^{90}Y (ibritumomab tiuxetan), and are approved for the treatment of low-grade or transformed B cell non-Hodgkin lymphoma (NHL) in patients who have failed at least one course of chemotherapy[28,29] with/without rituximab.[30,31] The discussion of toxicity associated with RIT will be focused on these two antibodies, since they have been extensively studied, and their toxicity profile is similar to that of other directly labeled monoclonal antibodies.

At nonmyeloablative doses, the DLT of RIT is myelosuppression, using a variety of antibodies and radionuclides.[27] In the pivotal trials[28,29] that led to FDA approval of the two radiolabeled anti-CD20 monoclonal antibodies above, the recommended dose for therapy in patients with platelet counts greater than 150,000 was the activity of ^{131}I-tositumomab estimated to deliver a whole-body dose of 75 cGy or 0.4 mCi/kg of ^{90}Y-ibritumomab tiuxetan. These doses were found to result in transient and reversible myelosuppression and an overall toxicity profile that was acceptable and well tolerated by most patients.[28,29]

Hematologic toxicity from a large number of patients in multiple trials with both ^{131}I-tositumomab[32] and ^{90}Y-ibritumomab tiuxetan (0.4 mCi/kg ^{90}Y dose for patients with platelet counts 150,000/mm^3 and above; 0.3 mCi/kg ^{90}Y for patients with platelet counts 100,000–149,000/mm^3)[33] is summarized in Table 10.1 in terms of median nadir counts and time to recovery for thrombocytopenia, neutropenia, and anemia. As can be seen, grade 3 and 4 hematologic toxicity was common. The time to nadir was approximately 4 to 7 weeks for ^{131}I-tositumomab, with the median time to nadir for ^{90}Y-ibritumomab tiuxetan of 7 to 9 weeks, which is much later than the myelosuppression that is usually observed with chemotherapy. Persistent myelosuppression was present in a small percentage of treated patients. Five to seven percent of patients treated with ^{131}I-tositumomab with grade 3/4 toxicity did not recover to grade 2 or better, with slightly less than 5% of patients treated with ^{90}Y-ibritumomab tiuxetan having severe cytopenias lasting more than 12 weeks. The extent and duration of myelosuppression correlated with the extent of bone marrow involvement with lymphoma (increased involvement results in more targeting of the marrow by the anti-CD20 antibodies) and the number of prior chemotherapy regimens/purine analogues. Up to 22% of patients required hematologic support with growth factors and/or transfusion (Table 10.2).[28–33]

The mean dose to red marrow was 0.65 mGy/mBq (range 0.5–1.1 mGy/mBq) for ^{131}I-tositumomab[32] and 71 cGy (range: 18–221 cGy) for ^{90}Y-ibritumomab tiuxetan, respectively.[34] Studies with both of these radiolabeled antibodies included an unlabeled antibody arm. As expected, the hematologic toxicity was significantly greater in the arms with the radiolabeled antibody,[28,35] demonstrating the important contribution of the radiation associated with RIT to toxicity. With both radiolabeled antibodies, nonhematologic toxicity was mild, usually grade 1 and 2, and reversible. The most common nonhematologic side effects of the treatment were asthenia, nausea, chills, and fever, some of which were attributable to mild infusion reactions or the antibody itself.[28,29,34]

The treatment regimen for ^{131}I-tosimumomab utilizes medication to block the uptake of the radiolabeled I by the thyroid. Nevertheless, the blockade is not complete, and hypothyroidism has been observed. Depending upon the patient population, the incidence of hypothyroidism based on elevated thyroid stimulating hormone (TSH) or initiation of thyroid replacement therapy was 13% to 18%, with a median time to development of

TABLE 10.1	Integrated Safety Analysis of Hematologic Toxicity		
	¹³¹I-Tositumomab (n = 230)	*⁹⁰Y-Ibritumomab Tiuxetan (n = 349)*	
		0.4 mCi/kg ⁹⁰Y Dose	*0.3 mCi/kg ⁹⁰Y Dose*
ENDPOINT			
Platelets			
Median nadir (cells/mm³)	43,000	41,000	24,000
% of patients <50,000/mm³	53%	61%	78%
Median duration of platelets <50.000/mm³ (days)	32[a]	24[b]	35
% of patients with platelets <25,000/mm³	21%	—	—
% of patients with platelets <10,000/mm³		10%	14%
ABSOLUTE NEUTROPHIL COUNT (ANC)			
Median nadir (cells/mm³)	690	800	600
% of patients with ANC <1,000 cells/mm³	63%	57%	74%
Median duration of ANC <1,000 cells/mm³ (days)	31[a]	22[b]	29
% of patients with ANC <500 cells/mm³	25%	30%	35%
HEMOGLOBIN			
Median nadir (gm/dL)	10	10.5 (pivotal study)	
% of patients with hemoglobin <8 g/dL	29%	17%	20%
Median duration of hemoglobin <8.0 g/dL (days)	23[a]	14[b]	14[a]
% of patients with hemoglobin <6.5 g/dL	5%	3%	8%

[a]Time to recovery to baseline grade.
[b]Duration measured from date of last laboratory test before the development of grade 3 or 4 toxicity to the date of the first value of grade 2 toxicity.

hypothyroidism of 15 to 16 months, and cumulative incidences of hypothyroidism at 2 and 5 years of 9% to 11% and 17% to 19%, respectively.[32] Cases of myelodysplasia syndrome (MDS) and acute leukemia have also been reported following treatment with both of these radiolabeled antibodies. Specifically, MDS or acute myeloid leukemia (AML) has occurred in 2% of patients treated with ⁹⁰Y-ibritumomab tiuxetan 8 to 34 months after treatment.[36] With median follow up of 29 months, 44 cases of MDS and/or secondary leukemia have been reported in 995 patients treated with ¹³¹I-tositumomab.[32] In order to put this in perspective, it is important to note that the incidence of MDS is 4% to 8% in patients with NHL without prior high dose-dose therapy or RIT.[37,38] These patients are commonly treated with alkylating agents, which are known risk factors for both MDS and leukemia, resulting in an incidence of MDS of 1% to 1.5% per year, 2 to 9 years following chemotherapy.[37]

RIT has also been administered into cavities, such as the peritoneal cavity for the treatment of ovarian cancer. With these approaches, there is a component of systemic distribution, and hematologic toxicity has been dose limiting.[27] There can also be toxicities unique to the route of administration (e.g., bowel adhesions/obstruction associated with intraperitoneal therapy). Again, myelosuppression has been the DLT with pretargeting

TABLE 10.2	Type of Supportive Care	
	¹³¹I-Tositumomab (n = 230)	*⁹⁰Y-Ibritumomab Tiuxetan (n = 349)*
G-CSF	12%	13%
Erythropoietin	7%	8%
Platelet transfusions	15%	22%
Packed RBCs	16%	20%

strategies.[27] Properties of the antibody can also contribute to the toxicity profile. An example of this occurred in phase I/II trials that used an antibody that crossreacted with gastrointestinal epithelium and renal tubules, in which grade 4 diarrhea and renal toxicity were observed.[39] Interestingly, these toxicities were observed only at estimated doses far in excess of normal organ tolerance to conventional high dose radiation therapy, demonstrating the importance of dose rate as a determinant of toxicity with RIT.[39]

As can be seen above, myelosuppression is the primary DLT in most RIT studies using nonmyeloablative doses. The use of RIT as a component of preparatory regimens for bone marrow or stem cell transplants has provided information on second organ toxicity at these higher doses of RIT. In a protocol combining RIT with chemotherapy prior to transplant, the MTD was defined as the dose of ¹³¹I-tositumomab that gave no more than 25 Gy to any normal organ, when combined with VP-16 (60 mg/kg) and cyclophosphamide (100 mg/kg).[40] In these studies, the second organ DLT was cardiopulmonary toxicity. It is expected that with ⁹⁰Y-labeled antibodies in this setting, that hepatic toxicity will be dose limiting.

RADIONUCLIDE THERAPY FOR PALLIATION OF SYMPTOMATIC BONE METASTASES

Radionuclides can be used to palliate painful bone metastases in patients with involvement of multiple skeletal sites with associated osteoblastic responses.[41–43] Efficacious radionuclides have an affinity for bone and behave like calcium analogues, with preferential uptake in sites of osteogenesis. There are currently three radionuclides (³²P, ⁸⁹Sr, ¹⁵³Sm) approved for this indication in the United States. The emission properties and dose to bone surface and red marrow are summarized in Table 10.3. The DLT of all of these radionuclides is myelosuppression, specifically

TABLE 10.3	Properties of Radionuclides Approved for Use in the United States for Palliative Treatment of Bone Metastases		
	^{32}P	^{89}Sr	^{153}Sm
$t_{1/2}$ (days)	14.3	53	1.95
β emission	E_{max} 1.71 MeV	E_{max} 1.46 MeV	640–810 KeV
γ emission	—	—	103 KeV
cGy/mCi bone surface	37.0	63.0	25.0
cGy/mCi red bone marrow	28.0	40.7	5.7

thrombocytopenia. ^{32}P will be discussed later for use in other indications, and is rarely used any more for the treatment of bone metastases because of its relatively undesirable biodistribution, with a low bone surface:red marrow ratio and relatively more uptake in soft tissues that other radionuclides now available.[41]

The recommended dose of ^{89}Sr is 4 mCi or 40 to 60 uCi/kg. Platelet counts typically drop approximately 30% compared with baseline, with a nadir 12 to 16 weeks following treatment. There is also a corresponding decrease in white blood cells (WBC) that is somewhat variable, with recovery over approximately 6 months following treatment, provided there is no progressive disease and/or the patient does not receive additional cytotoxic therapies in the interim.[41–44] The recommended dose of ^{153}Sm is 1.0 mCi/kg. WBC and platelets nadir at 40% to 50% of baseline counts within 3 to 5 weeks of treatment and tend to return to pretreatment levels by 8 weeks.[41,42,45] Grade 4 hematologic toxicity is rare with this administered dose. As with all therapies that affect the bone marrow, there is cumulative damage and decreased bone marrow reserve, which can decrease tolerance for subsequent cytotoxic therapy.[41,42,45]

Rhenium-186 HEDP (^{186}Re) is approved for use in Europe and is in clinical trials in the United States.[41] It is of interest because of its relatively short half-life of 89.3 hours, relatively high energy β emission of 1.07 MeV, and γ emission at 137 KeV, which is easily imaged with a γ camera. It is hoped that these properties will enable multiple dosing.[41] As with the other radionuclides above, thrombocytopenia is the DLT, with a nadir at approximately 4 weeks to approximately 47% of baseline.[46] The MTD seems to be determined in part by the extent of prior cytotoxic therapy, with a lower MTD in breast cancer patients than patients with prostate cancer.[47] Another interesting radionuclide in clinical development is ^{117m}Sn-DTPA,[41] which is not a β emitter, but rather decays with the emission of monoenergetic conversion electrons, that should result in a relatively lower bone marrow dose and improved bone surface: red bone marrow ratio. Also promising and in early clinical trials are the α-emitting bone-seeking agents such as ^{223}Ra,[48] which have a theoretical advantage over other radionuclides studied to date because of the short path length and high LET of α particles produced, which should result in further improvement in bone surface:marrow dose ratios.

^{131}I, ^{32}P, AND ^{166}HO THERAPY FOR THE TREATMENT OF SOLID TUMORS, POLYCYTHEMIA VERA, AND MULTIPLE MYELOMA

^{131}I has been used therapeutically for decades to treat hyperthyroidism as well as some forms of thyroid cancer.[41] It is very rapidly and efficiently taken up by the thyroid, with 95% of the dose delivered to follicular epithelium within the thyroid gland. ^{131}I has a $t_{1/2}$ of 8.1 days and β emission of 364 keV, which are desirable properties for therapy. When used to treat residual/recurrent disease following surgery for well-differentiated papillary or follicular thyroid cancer, ablative doses of ^{131}I are commonly given 3 to 6 weeks following surgery and are generally well tolerated. Side effects can include nausea, vomiting, sialoadenitis, transient swelling, and pain at sites of metastasis, and bone marrow suppression. Radiation sickness has been reported with doses in excess of 300 mCi.[41]

The properties of ^{32}P have been summarized in Table 10.3. In addition to use for the treatment of painful bone metastases, ^{32}P has also been used in several other clinical settings,[41] including the treatment of patients with polycythemia vera (PCV), malignant pleural effusions, and peritoneal carcinomatosis secondary to ovarian cancer.

For patients with PCV, intravenous administration of 3 to 5 mCi ^{32}P can provide effective cytoreductive and antithrombotic therapy, with decreased red blood cell (RBC) and platelet counts within 10 to 12 weeks of therapy.[49] Because of the delay in response, ^{32}P is used in combination with phlebotomy. A single treatment with 2.8 to 3.5 mCi/m^2 has been reported to result in a complete remission rate of 98% of patients. This treatment was well tolerated and allowed for retreatment at 3 to 6 month intervals. Unfortunately, ^{32}P was found to be associated with an increased incidence of malignancy, especially MDS and acute leukemia, in which there is dose-response relationship between dose and incidence of disease. For this reason, ^{32}P therapy has been largely replaced by newer therapies such as α-interferon and anagrelide, which do not have a significant mutagenic risk. Currently, use of ^{32}P is largely restricted to patients with PCV over the age of 70 years, especially in those elderly patients with poor venous access and/or poor compliance.[41,49]

^{32}P has also been used to treat the serosal lining of cavities and associated malignant effusions. For example, pleural effusions have been treated with some success using 10 mCi ^{32}P that is injected into the pleural space following drainage of the pleural effusion.[41] ^{32}P found greater use when administered intraperitoneally (ip) (10–20 mCi) for the treatment of micrometastatic ovarian cancer. As with any intracavitary treatment, there is a component of systemic distribution that contributes to the toxicity profile.[41] In a GOG-OCSG trial no. 7602, that compared melphalan to 15 uCi ^{32}P ip, nearly 75% of the patients had no side effects. Other patients did have mild to moderate gastrointestinal symptoms, with four cases of bowel obstruction and one of bacterial peritonitis.[50] A follow-up GOG study compared high dose cyclophosphamide/cisplatin to ^{32}P in resectable Stage II and poor prognosis Stage I patients. There was a trend

($p = 0.075$) toward improved progression-free survival with the chemotherapy regimen, but no difference in overall survival. More patients treated with ^{32}P had bowel problems, and some had suboptimal distribution of the radionuclide within the peritoneal cavity due to prior adhesions and areas of loculation. Based on these results, cisplatin-based chemotherapy became the standard of care and largely replaced the use of ^{32}P in this setting.[51]

^{166}Ho-1,4,7,10-tetraazacyclododecane-1,4,7,10-tetramethylene-phosphonic acid (^{166}Ho-DOTMP) has been studied in combination with melphalan as a preparatory regimen for autologous peripheral blood stem cell transplantation (ASCT) for the treatment of multiple myeloma. ^{166}Ho was selected for this indication because of its high energy β (1.85 MeV), which delivers high dose radiation to both bone and bone marrow, and relatively short $t_{1/2}$ of 26.8 hours, which allows for infusion of stem cells within 6 to 8 days.[52] Initially, in a single agent dose-escalation phase 1 trial, doses up to 2,100 mCi were administered, with a resulting red marrow dose of up to 41 Gy. At these doses, there was no extramedullary toxicity.[52] This trial provided a basis for two subsequent phase 1/2 studies to determine the MTD of ^{166}Ho in combination with melphalan when used as a conditioning regimen prior to ASCT. Median skeletal uptake was 24% and the median total therapy activity injected was 2,113 mCi (range: 460–4,476 mCi). Median doses to the bladder wall, bone marrow, bone surfaces, and kidney were 4,250, 3,120, 5,640, and 430 cGy, respectively. Importantly, there were no significant differences in the time to engraftment for any of the ^{166}Ho dose levels studied, and no differences in the level of transfusion support for any of the treatment groups.

There were, however, some important late toxicities, consisting of 27 of 83 patients who experienced grade 2 and 3 hemorrhagic cystitis (only 1 of whom received continuous bladder irrigation), 7 patients with severe thrombotic microangiopathy (TMA) and 30% of patients with grade 2 to 4 renal toxicity. Of note, there were no severe cases of TMA in patients receiving ^{166}Ho doses lower than 30 Gy, and most of the renal toxicity was observed with doses that delivered in excess of 40 Gy to the bone marrow. The median dose to the kidney of patients with severe TMA nephropathy was 710 cGy, which demonstrates the probable contribution of the initial high dose rate irradiation of the kidney, secondary to rapid urinary excretion of the untargeted ^{166}Ho. These data suggest that an administered dose that delivers 30 cGy to the bone marrow could be a well-tolerated dose for subsequent studies of this conditioning regime.[52] In a retrospective analysis, ^{166}Ho combined with melphalan demonstrated a trend toward a higher complete remission rate than melphalan alone in patients undergoing ASCT.[53]

Lastly, ^{166}Ho has demonstrated efficacy when administered intra-arterially (20 mCi/cm tumor diameter, not to exceed 200mCi) in patients with large single hepatocellular carcinoma tumors, with a response rate of 78%. Thirty-one patients out of 54 had a complete response, with a median duration of 27 months. The most common grade 3 and 4 toxicities were cytopenias, transaminase elevation, and hyperbilirubinemia.[54]

PEPTIDE RECEPTOR RADIONUCLIDE THERAPY

Peptide receptor radionuclide therapy is another form of systemically targeted radiotherapy in which the peptide/ligand for a receptor overexpressed on tumor is linked to a radionuclide for therapy. Examples of this approach include the use of

^{131}I-mIBG for the treatment of neuroblastoma (in combination with ASCT)[55] and ^{177}Lu-DOTA-Try3-octreotate[56,57] or ^{90}Y-DOTA-Tyr3-octreotate[56,57] for the treatment of neuroendocrine tumors. This therapy has been reported to be of clinical benefit in a subset of patients. Common toxicities consist of nausea, vomiting, grade 2 and 3 cytopenias, and occasionally renal toxicity in patients with preexisting renal insufficiency.

RISK OF MALIGNANCY INDUCTION FROM RADIONUCLIDE EXPOSURE

As with all sources of radiation, radionuclide exposure can be associated with the induction of secondary malignancies. This is assessed as an increased stochastic risk, and not as a graded toxicity. Although most data have been reported for adults, there is an age influence for low dose malignancy induction that is important for children.[58,59] For example, there is a continuously decreasing risk of thyroid cancer for each decade of age at low-level radiation exposure, whereas for breast cancer the sex-averaged risk is greatest in the second decade and then declines with advancing age.[60] This has held true for the data from the Chernobyl accident, where children had an inverse risk with age, from age 0 to 17.[61] Extensive data are provided in BEIR (biologic effects of ionizing radiation) reports that provide information on malignancy risk estimates from populations of atomic bomb survivors, and those exposed for medical and occupational purposes.[62] The linear relationship between exposure level and malignancy, plus failure to find a threshold, has increased concerns for excess medical exposure, whether for diagnostic or therapeutic purposes.

On the other end of the age spectrum, second malignancy is more likely as age advances in lymphoma patients treated with multimodality therapy. The risk of MDS and acute leukemia was discussed earlier in this chapter. Importantly, in some NHL patients, treated with RIT who subsequently developed MDS, dysplasia was present prior to the radionuclide therapy.[29] Due to decades of experience, there are more data on carcinogenic effects for 131I exposure than other entities. In addition to MDS, there is increased risk of thyroid cancer and colon cancer.[63] Some of the risk of a second malignancy among thyroid cancer patients, attributed to 131I therapy, may be due to a genetic predisposition or other factors, since the risk in this 131I-treated population actually decreases for lung and cervix cancer.[64] Hematologic and bone malignancies have a stronger association with bone-seeking radionuclides than 131I. Tools such as The Radiation Dose Assessment Resource, RADAR,[65] provide aid in predicting risks of malignancy induction. Some of the informational sources also take into account some of the known determinants (e.g., age and sex) of risk for the induction of second malignancies. There is also concern for non–malignant health hazards from radionuclides that require further study, such as cataract development and earlier death.[66]

CONCLUSION

While less is known about normal tissue toxicity from radionuclide therapy than from external beam radiation therapy, there is an increasing body of information suggesting that normal organs can tolerate higher doses of relatively low dose rate radiation associated with radionuclide therapy compared to high dose rate conventional radiation therapy. Important determinants of radionuclide toxicity include the heterogeneous distribution of radionuclides in targeted tumors as well as normal organs, patient characteristics, radionuclide emission properties, dose rate factors, and concomitant use of radioprotectors or radiosensitizers. Future studies should help to more fully elucidate determinants of toxicity as well as modifying factors for the mitigation of radionuclide toxicity, to facilitate the development of strategies to further improve the therapeutic index of these therapies.

REFERENCES

1. Davidson SE, Trotti A, Ataman OU, et al. Improving the capture of adverse event data in clinical trials: the role of the International Atomic Energy Agency. *Int J Radiat Oncol Biol Phys.* 2007;69:1218–1221.
2. Tempero M, Leichner P, Baranowska-Kortylewicz J, et al. High-dose therapy with ⁹⁰Yttrium-labeled monoclonal antibody CC49: a phase I trial. *Clin Cancer Res.* 2000;6:3095–3102.
3. Yorke ED, Jackson A, Fox RA, et al. Can current models explain the lack of liver complications in Y-90 microsphere therapy? *Clin Cancer Res.* 1999;5:3024s–3030s.
4. Kennedy AS, Nutting C, Coldwell D, et al. Pathologic response and microdosimetry of (90) Y microspheres in man: review of four explanted whole livers. *Int J Radiat Oncol Biol Phys.* 2004;60:1552–1563.
5. Sarfaraz M, Kennedy AS, Lodge MA, et al. Radiation absorbed dose distribution in a patient treated with yttrium-90 microspheres for hepatocellular carcinoma. *Med Phys.* 2004;31:2449–2453.
6. Neti PV, Howell RW. Log normal distribution of cellular uptake of radioactivity: implications for biologic responses to radiopharmaceuticals. *J Nucl Med.* 2006;47:1049–1058.
7. Martin S, Kronenwett R, Vandenbulcke K, et al. Targeted alpha radiation and gamma rays induce significantly different molecular responses in human leukemic lymphocytes as revealed by gene expression profiling. *J Nucl Med.* 2005;46(suppl 2):192.
8. Dahle J, Bruland OS, Larsen RH. Relative biologic effects of low-dose–rate alpha-emitting ²²⁷Th-rituximab and beta-emitting ⁹⁰Y-tiuxetan-ibritumomab versus external beam x-radiation. *Int J Radiat Onc Biol Phys.* 2008;72:186–192.
9. Narra VR, Harapanhalli RS, Howell RW, et al. Vitamins as radioprotectors in vivo. I. Protection by vitamin C against internal radionuclides in mouse testes: implications to the mechanism of damage caused by the Auger effect. *Rad Res.* 1994;137:394–399.
10. Mothersill C, Seymour C. Low-dose radiation effects: experimental hematology and the changing paradigm. *Exp Hematol.* 2003;31:437–445.
11. Mothersill C, Seymour C. Radiation-induced bystander effects, carcinogenesis and models. *Oncogene.* 2003;22:7028–7033.
12. Albanese J, Dainiak N. Modulation of intercellular communication mediated at the cell surface and on extracellular, plasma membrane-derived vesicles by ionizing radiation. *Exp Hematol.* 2003;31:455–464.
13. Boyd M, Ross SC, Dorrens J, et al. Radiation-induced biologic bystander effect elicited in vitro by targeted radiopharmaceuticals labeled with alpha-, beta-, and auger electron-emitting radionuclides. *J Nucl Med.* 2006;47:1007–1015.
14. Kassis AI. Therapeutic radionuclides: biophysical and radiobiologic principles. *Sem Nucl Med.* 2008;38:358–366.
15. Bouchet LG, Bolch WE, Blanco HP, et al. MIRD pamphlet No. 19: absorbed fractions and radionuclide S values for six age-dependent multiregion models of the kidney. *J Nucl Med.* 2003;44:1113–1147.
16. Wessels BW, Konijnenberg MW, Dale RG, et al. MIRD pamphlet No. 20: the effect of model assumptions on kidney dosimetry and response: implications for radionuclide therapy. *J Nucl Med.* 2008;49:1884–1899.
17. Barendsen GW. Dose fractionation, dose-rate and iso-effect relationships for normal tissue responses. *Int J Radiat Oncol Biol Phys.* 1982;8:1981–1997.
18. Thames HD, Hendry JH. *Fractionation in Radiotherapy.* Philadelphia, PA: Taylor and Francis; 1987.
19. Brill AB, Stabin M, Bouville A, et al. Normal organ radiation dosimetry and associated uncertainties in nuclear medicine, with emphasis on iodine-131. *Radiat Res.* 2006;166 (1 pt 2):128–140.
20. Valkema R, Pauwels SA, Kvols LK, et al. Long-term follow-up of renal function after peptide receptor radiation therapy with (90)Y-DOTA(0),Tyr(3)-octreotide and (177)Lu-DOTA(0), Tyr(3)-octreotate. *J Nucl Med.* 2005;46(suppl 1):83S–91S.
21. Jaggi JS, Seshan SV, McDevitt MR, et al. Mitigation of radiation nephropathy after internal alpha-particle irradiation of kidneys. *Int J Radiat Oncol Biol Phys.* 2006;64(5):1503–1512.
22. Ho AY, Fan G, Atencio DP, et al. Possession of ATM sequence variants as predictor for late normal tissue responses in breast cancer patients treated with radiotherapy. *Int J Radiat Oncol Biol Phys.* 2007;69:677–684.
23. Williams JR, Zhang Y, Zhou H, et al. Overview of radiosensitivity of human tumor cells to low-dose-rate irradiation. *Int J Radiat Oncol Biol Phys.* 2008;72(3):909–917. Review.
24. Siegel JA, Yeldell D, Goldenberg DM, et al. Red marrow radiation dose adjustment using plasma FLT3-L cytokine levels: improved correlations between hematologic toxicity and bone marrow dose for radioimmunotherapy patients. *J Nucl Med.* 2003;44(1):67–76.
25. Juweid ME, Zhang CH, Blumenthal RD, et al. Prediction of hematologic toxicity after radioimmunotherapy with (131)I-labeled anticarcinoembryonic antigen monoclonal antibodies. *J Nucl Med.* 1999;40(10):1609–1616.
26. Meredith R, Wessels B, Knox S. Risks to normal tissues from radionuclide therapy. *Semin Nucl Med.* 2008;38(5):347–357.
27. Meredith RF, Wong JYC, Knox SJ. Targeted radionuclide therapy. In: Gunderson LL, Tepper JE, eds. *Clinical Radiation Oncology.* 2nd ed. London, Elsevier Church Livingstone; 2007: chap 21, 407–435.
28. Witzig TE, Gordon LI, Cabanillas F, et al. Randomized controlled trial of yttrium-90-labeled ibritumomab tiuxetan radioimmunotherapy versus rituximab immunotherapy for patients with relapsed or refractory low-grade, follicular, or transformed B-cell non-Hodgkin's lymphoma. *J Clin Oncol.* 2002;20(10):2453–2463.
29. Kaminski MS, Zelenetz AD, Press OW, et al. Pivotal study of iodine I 131 tositumomab for chemotherapy-refractory low-grade or transformed low-grade B-cell non-Hodgkin's lymphomas. *J Clin Oncol.* 2001;19:3918–3928.
30. Horning SJ, Younes JB, Lucas, et al. Rituximab treatment failures: tositumomab and iodine ¹³¹I tositumomab (Bexxar) can produce meaningful durable responses. *Blood.* 2002;100:1385.
31. Witzig TE, Flinn IW, Gordon LI, et al. Treatment with ibritumomab tiuxetan radioimmunotherapy in patients with rituximab-refractory follicular non-Hodgkin's lymphoma. *J Clin Oncol.* 2002;20:3262–3269.
32. Bexxar package insert—complete citation to follow Bexxar Therapeutic Regimen Product Information. Corixa, Seattle Wash, 2003.
33. Witzig TE, White CA. Safety of yttrium-90 ibritumomab tiuxetan radioimmunotherapy for relapsed low-grade, follicular, or transformed non-Hodgkin's lymphoma. *J Clin Oncol.* 2003;21(7):1263–1270.
34. Wiseman GA, White CA, Sparks RB, et al. Biodistribution and dosimetry results from a phase III prospectively randomized controlled trial of Zevalin radioimmunotherapy for low-grade, follicular, or transformed B-cell non-Hodgkin's lymphoma. *Crit Rev Oncol Hematol.* 2001;39(1–2):181–194.
35. Davis TA, Kaminski MS, Leonard JP, et al. The radioisotope contributes significantly to the activity of radioimmunotherapy. *Clin Cancer Res.* 2004;10(23):7792–7798.
36. Zevalin package insert—IDEC Pharmaceuticals Corp., San Diego, CA, 2001.
37. Pedersen-Bjergaard J, Ersbøll J, Sørensen HM, et al. Risk of acute nonlymphocytic leukemia and preleukemia in patients treated with cyclophosphamide for non-Hodgkin's lymphomas. Comparison with results obtained in patients treated for Hodgkin's disease and ovarian carcinoma with other alkylating agents. *Ann Intern Med.* 1985;103(2):195–200.
38. Greene MH, Young RC, Merrill JM, et al. Evidence of a treatment dose response in acute nonlymphocytic leukemias which occur after therapy of non-Hodgkin's lymphoma. *Cancer Res.* 1983;43(4):1891–1898.
39. Knox SJ, Goris ML, Tempero M, et al. Phase II Trial of Yttrium-⁹⁰-DOTA-Biotin pretargeted by NR-LU-10 antibody/streptavidin in patients with metastatic colon cancer. *Clin Cancer Res.* 2000;6:406–414.
40. Press OW, Eary JF, Gooley T, et al. A phase I/II trial of iodine-131-tositumomab (anti-CD20), etoposide, cyclophosphamide, and autologous stem cell transplantation for relapsed B-cell lymphomas. *Blood.* 2001;98(4):2535–2543.
41. Massey R. Current use of therapeutic radiopharmaceuticals for patient care, American Pharmaceutical Association Annual Meeting, March 2000, Washington, DC.
42. Siberstein EB, Buscombe JR, McEwan A, et al. Society of Nuclear Medicine Procedure Guideline for Palliative Treatment of Bone Metastases, Society of Nuclear Medicine Procedure Guidelines Manual; 2003:147–153.
43. Bouchet LG, Bolch WE, Goddu SM, et al. Considerations in the selection of radiopharmaceuticals for palliation of bone pain from metastatic osseous lesions. *J Nucl Med.* 2000;41(4):682–687.
44. Metastron (strontium-89 chloride injection) Package insert, Arlington Heights, IL: Medi-Physics Inc.; 1993.
45. Quadramet Package insert (Samarium SM 158 Lexidronam Injection), Richmond, CA: Berlex Laboratories; 1999.
46. de Klerk JMH, van het Schip AD, Zonnenberg BA, et al. Evaluation of thrombocytopenia in patients treated with rhenium-186-HEDP: guidelines for individual dosage recommendations. *J Nucl Med.* 1994;35(9):1423–1428.
47. de Klerk JMH, van het Schip AD, Zonnenberg BA, et al. Phase 1 study of rhenium-186 -HEDP in patients with bone metastases originating from breast cancer. *J Nucl Med.* 1996;37(2):244–249.
48. Nilsson S, Franzén L, Parker C, et al. Bone-targeted radium-223 in symptomatic, hormone-refractory prostate cancer: a randomised, multicentre, placebo-controlled phase II study. *Lancet Oncol.* 2007;8(7):587–594.
49. Barbui T, Finazzi G. Treatment of polycythemia vera. *Haematologica.* 1998;83(2):143–149.
50. Young RC. Initial therapy for early ovarian carcinoma. *Cancer.* 1987;60(8 suppl): 2042–2049.
51. Young RC, Brady MF, Nieberg RK, et al. Adjuvant treatment for early ovarian cancer: a randomized phase III trial of intraperitoneal ³²P or intravenous cyclophosphamide and cisplatin—a gynecologic oncology group study. *J Clin Oncol.* 2003;21(23):4350–4355.
52. Giralt S, Bensinger W, Goodman M, et al. ¹⁶⁶Ho-DOTMP plus melphalan followed by peripheral blood stem cell transplantation in patients with multiple myeloma: results of two phase 1/2 trials. *Blood.* 2003;102(7):2684–2691. Epub 2003 May 1.
53. Christoforidou AV, Saliba RM, Williams P, et al. Results of a retrospective single institution analysis of targeted skeletal radiotherapy with ¹⁶⁶holmium-DOTMP as conditioning regimen for autologous stem cell transplant for patients with multiple myeloma. Impact on transplant outcomes. *Biol Blood Marrow Transplant.* 2007;13:543–549.
54. Sohn JH, Choi HJ, Lee JT, et al. Phase II study of transarterial holmium-166-chitosan complex treatment in patients with a single, large hepatocellular carcinoma. *Oncology.* 2009;76(1):1–9. Epub 2008 Nov 17.
55. Ladenstein R, Pötschger U, Hartman O, et al. 28 years of high-dose therapy and SCT for neuroblastoma in Europe: lessons from more than 4000 procedures. *Bone Marrow Transplant.* 2008;41(suppl 2):S118–S127.
56. Kwekkeboom DJ, Mueller-Brand J, Paganelli G, et al. Overview of results of peptide receptor radionuclide therapy with 3 radiolabeled somatostatin analogs. *J Nucl Med.* 2005;46: 62–66.
57. Hörsch D, Prasad V, Baum RP. Longterm outcome of peptide receptor radionuclide therapy (PRRT) in 454 patients with progressive neuroendocrine tumors using yttrium-90

and lutetium-177 labelled somatostatin receptor targeting peptides. *J Clin Oncol.* 26:2008 (May 20 suppl; abstr 4517).

58. Royal HD. Effects of low level radiation-what's new? *Semin Nucl Med.* 2008;38(5):392–402.

59. Tronko MD, Howe GR, Bogdanova TI, et al. A cohort study of thyroid cancer and other thyroid diseases after the Chernobyl accident: thyroid cancer in Ukraine detected during first screening. *J Natl Cancer Inst.* 2006;98:897–903.

60. Preston DL, Ron E, Tokuoka S, et al. Solid cancer incidence in atomic bomb survivors: 1958–1998. *Radiat Res.* 2007;168(1):1–64.

61. NCRP (National Council on Radiation Protection and Measurement): Report No. 136 Evaluation of the Linear-Nonthreshold Dose-Response Model for Ionizing Radiation. Bethesda, MD, National Council on Radiation Protection and Measurement, 2001.

62. BEIRVII: Health Risks from Exposure to Low Levels of Ionizing Radiation is available from the National Academies Press, 500 Fifth Street, NW, Washington, DC, 20001.

63. Rubino C, Adjadj E, Doyon F, et al. Radiation exposure and familial aggregation of cancers as risk factors for colorectal cancer after radioiodine treatment for thyroid carcinoma. *Int J Radiat Oncol Biol Phys.* 2005;62:1084–1089.

64. Subramanian S, Goldstein DP, Parlea L, et al. Second primary malignancy risk in thyroid cancer survivors: a systematic review and meta-analysis. *Thyroid.* 2007;17:1277–1288.

65. www.doseinfo-radar.com

66. Vrijheid M, Cardis E, Ashmore P, et al. Mortality from diseases other than cancer following low doses of ionizing radiation: results from the 15-Country Study of nuclear industry workers. *Int J Epidemiol.* 2007;36(5):1126–1135.

CHAPTER

11

Brenda Shank

Toxicity Due to Total Body Irradiation

INTRODUCTION

The effects of irradiation to the entire human body have been studied in uncontrolled situations, for example in warfare (Hiroshima, Nagasaki) and in radiation accidents, including external exposure to high activity radiation sources, as well as in well-publicized incidents, such as that at Chernobyl, in which both external exposure and internal ingested and inhaled exposure were issues. Meaningful analyses of specific organ toxicities are difficult to assess in such situations, in which exact dose, dose rate, and dose distribution information are unavailable. The data from Chernobyl dramatize the high incidence of thyroid papillary cancer in children concentrated in the city of Gomel in Belarus, apparently caused by exposure to radioactive iodine-131, the fallout of which was concentrated throughout the northern part of Chernobyl and southern part of Gomel Province.[1]

Radiation effects have also been studied in considerable detail in the controlled situations of total body irradiation (TBI) for hematopoietic cell transplantation (HCT), an all-encompassing term for *bone marrow transplantation* (BMT) or *stem-cell transplantation*, in which we have accurate knowledge of total dose, dose rate, dose fractionation, type of irradiation, dose distribution in the body, and other parameters that ultimately govern the effects of irradiation.

In addition to the above studies in humans, *in vitro* cellular studies and *in vivo* animal studies have also contributed to our understanding of the effects of whole-body irradiation (WBE). In this chapter, the emphasis will be on controlled studies of TBI in humans, but laboratory studies will be cited when their conclusions can contribute significantly to our understanding. Our knowledge of radiation syndromes comes primarily from animal studies and radiation accidents in humans.

RADIATION PARAMETERS INFLUENCING WHOLE-BODY EFFECTS

DOSE HOMOGENEITY

In radiation accidents, delivered dose may differ greatly for different organs, depending on distance from the source, partial shielding of some areas of the body by interposed objects, or even by the body itself for deeper organs. When TBI is delivered, homogeneity may be well controlled, that is, within 5% or, at

most, 10% of a given prescribed dose. This is achieved by using a large source-to-isocenter distance, with the body perpendicular to the source as much as possible, and extended, that is, standing on a special support stand, or lying down, with at least a 10-cm margin of the beam edge around the head and extremities.

Additionally, for energies higher than that of cobalt-60 (1.25 MV), a tissue-equivalent screen is needed between the patient and the beam, to allow adequate buildup of the dose upon entry into the skin to prevent underdosage for a distance beneath the skin. Half of a given TBI treatment is generally given from one direction and the other half from the opposite direction (e.g., anterior-posterior/posterior-anterior), so that the final dose to the skin surface depends on exit dose from the opposing beam as well.

Tissue compensators have also been used at thinner areas of the body (neck, feet, etc.) to increase homogeneity, especially when beam energies of 10 MV or greater have been used.

DOSE RATE AND TOTAL DOSE

Organ effects are highly dependent upon total dose, dose rate, and fractionation (number of fractions, or treatments, given and time interval between fractions). When TBI is delivered in a single dose, dose rate must be kept low to minimize organ toxicity, especially interstitial pneumonitis (IP) in lung, but also cataracts of the lens, and veno-occlusive disease (VOD) of the liver. For example, with a single total dose of 10 Gy, it is necessary to use a dose rate of ≤0.05 Gy/min to decrease the probability of IP. For fractionated TBI schedules, dose rate is less important, although for fraction sizes of 2 Gy or more, a dose-rate effect was still observed, in a mouse study.[2]

At the large source-to-isocenter distances used for TBI at most medical centers to ensure that the entire unflexed body is in the beam with sufficient margin around a patient, the dose rate is usually in the desired range. For infants, who may be treated horizontally on a mat on the floor (with a shorter source-to-isocenter distance), it may be necessary to reduce the dose rate by means of Pb (lead) attenuators.

ORGAN PROTECTION

For high dose TBI, lung shielding has been frequently used. Most commonly, partially attenuating shields (one-half-value layer) have been used throughout a treatment course.[3] Partial shielding of liver and kidneys has also been used to decrease the incidence of VOD and renal dysfunction.[4]

RADIATION SYNDROMES

The *prodromal syndrome (or stage)* is a complex of early symptoms that may occur 5 to 10 minutes after WBE, characterized primarily by anorexia, nausea and vomiting, and easy fatiguability. The time of onset, maximum severity, and duration of symptoms are a function of total dose. Without marrow or stem-cell support, the $LD_{50/60}$ (dose at which there is 50% lethality by 60 days) is about 3 to 4 Gy. At higher (supralethal) doses, other early symptoms and signs may also be observed, such as diarrhea, intestinal cramps, fever, headache, and, ultimately, fluid loss, dehydration, weight loss, and hypotension. A severe prodromal response portends a poor prognosis. The symptoms may last for a few minutes to a few days. A *latent period* of up to 1 week duration may then follow, during which time the patient may appear and feel relatively well. Ultimately, however, at supralethal doses, death will ensue from one or more of three distinct syndromes: hematopoietic syndrome, gastrointestinal syndrome, and cerebrovascular syndrome (Table 11.1).

The *hematopoietic syndrome* results from the death of mitotically active blood precursor cells in the bone marrow, which would normally replace white and red blood cells and platelets at the end of their normal life spans. Doses between 3 and 8 Gy are likely to cause death by this mechanism, if no stem cell support is given. Circulating lymphocyte counts decrease first, within 24 hours; the lymphocyte count nadir has been considered one of the best clinical dosimeters. For a nadir no less than $1,200/mm^3$, clinical support has not been needed.[5] Neutrophil counts increase initially, with increased maturation in the marrow and mobilization, followed by a rapid decline by the second day, which continues more slowly over the next 1 to 3 weeks. With the loss of these two cell types, the individual is susceptible to life-threatening infection. This risk is exacerbated by the loss of intestinal mucosa (see below and Chapter 38), providing an entryway for organisms, especially bacteria, leading to potential septicemia and death.

Additionally, platelet levels fall in parallel with neutrophil counts, increasing the risk of death from hemorrhage. The incidence of hematopoietic death peaks at around day 30, and recovery of hematopoiesis, when radiation doses are low enough, usually occurs at about 60 days. The changes in white blood count and platelets in two patients who received a single fraction of TBI (1.25 Gy) of a planned fractionated course are illustrated in Figure 11.1.[6] Anemia is not a problem in otherwise healthy humans after an acute exposure, due to the long half-life of erythrocytes (~120 days), and their recovery of production over 1 to 2 months.

The *gastrointestinal syndrome* occurs at doses of the order of 10 Gy or greater, leading initially to anorexia and intractable diarrhea. The small bowel, in this situation, becomes denuded of mucosal endothelium as a result of stem cell loss; dehydration, weight loss, and exhaustion ensue, with death in 5 to 10 days. Death cannot be ascribed totally to a pure gastrointestinal syndrome, since bacteria colonize the surfaces and walls of the intestine as well, and the immune system is compromised from hematopoietic failure. Several firefighters involved in the Chernobyl incident, including some who received marrow transplantation, suffered from symptoms of the gastrointestinal syndrome. With

TABLE 11.1	Radiation Syndromes Resulting from Whole-Body Exposure				
Syndrome	*Dose (Gy)[a]*	*Prodromal Symptoms*	*Prodromal Timing (Dose-dependent)*	*Syndrome Symptoms/Signs*	*Death/Time Frame*
Hematopoietic	~1–10	Anorexia, nausea, vomiting, fatiguability	5–10 minutes to 1–2 days for onset; duration of minutes to a few days.	Anorexia, fever associated with infection, hemorrhage. Decreased lymphocyte, neutrophil, and platelet counts. May be a latent period of 1 or more weeks prior to symptoms.	$LD_{50/60}$ = 3–4 Gy (without stem cell support). Full recovery possible at higher doses with stem cell support. Death peaks at ~30 days. Hematopoietic recovery at ~60 days.
Gastrointestinal	>10	Anorexia, severe nausea and vomiting; intractable diarrhea and intestinal cramping.	Increased severity in a few minutes to hours. Duration ~2 days.	Dehydration, weight loss, electrolyte imbalance, diarrhea. Latent period <1 week. Denudation of small bowel endothelium and hematopoietic failure also causing infection.	Death in 5–10 days.
Cerebrovascular	≥100	Severe nausea and vomiting; watery diarrhea; disorientation, headache, loss of consciousness.	Severe symptoms within minutes. Duration ~2 days.	Watery diarrhea; hypotension, respiratory distress; impaired vision, coma.	Death in 1–2 days in 100%. Possibly related to intracranial pressure, due to small blood vessel leakage and anoxia.

[a]Absorbed dose in Gy refers to photon irradiation equivalency.

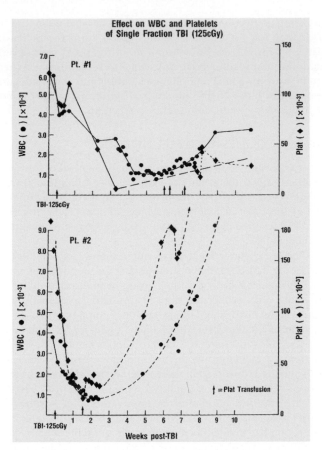

Figure 11.1. Changes with time (weeks post-TBI) in peripheral blood white cells (WBC) and platelets (Plat) after a single fraction of TBI (125 cGy) in two patients (Pt. no. 1 and Pt. no. 2.). (Reprinted from Shank B, O'Reilly RJ, Cunningham I, et al. Total body irradiation for bone marrow transplantation: the Memorial Sloan-Kettering Cancer Center experience. *Radiother Oncol.* 1990;1(suppl 1):58–81 with permission.)

planned TBI for HCT, many components of the hematopoietic and gastrointestinal syndromes are mitigated by supportive care, including transfusions, growth factors, antibiotics, and, of course, by the regrowth of the transplanted stem cells. In mouse studies, significant survival benefit has been seen by the addition of pleiotropic cytokines to antimicrobial supportive care.[7]

The *cerebrovascular syndrome* occurs at doses of 100 Gy or greater. Central nervous system death is secondary to damage to the vascular endothelium, leading to increased intracranial pressure as leakage from blood vessels occurs, and anoxia. Direct neuronal damage occurs only following extremely high doses (1,000 Gy) and, fortunately, has been seen only in animal studies. Death occurs rapidly with this syndrome (1–2 days), as hypotension, mental incapacitation, and coma develop quickly.

ACUTE TOXICITIES OF TBI FOR HCT

Acute toxicities may develop within hours or a few days after TBI. These are usually the result of edema, parenchymal cell loss, and/or inflammation. The most common acute side effects after TBI for HCT are nausea and vomiting, which are less intense with fractionated regimens compared to single-dose regimens.[6] The most effective agents for treatment of this complication have been the 5-hydroxytryptamine subtype 3 antagonists,

ondansetron and granisetron.[8–10] Dexamethasone added to granisetron resulted in better emetic control than granisetron alone in a study of 50 patients conditioned for HCT with chemotherapy with or without TBI; nonserious side effects were more frequent, however, such as insomnia, headache, flushing, and hyperglycemia.[11]

Nausea and vomiting, along with other acute side effects of oral mucositis, diarrhea, and parotiditis were all less with twice-daily hyperfractionated irradiation compared with single-dose irradiation in a study that randomized dose rate but not fractionation.[12,13] Dose rate per se had no effect on these toxicities. No parotiditis occurred with fractionated TBI (12 Gy in six fractions) in another study, compared with a 40% incidence with single-dose TBI.[14] Acute parotiditis during or after TBI was a predictor of IP in one small study.[15] Fatigue occurs over the course of TBI. Some patients may develop erythema of the skin and, later, even hyperpigmentation.

LATE TOXICITIES OF TBI FOR HCT

LUNG: INTERSTITIAL PNEUMONITIS

After HCT, one of the major contributors to mortality has been IP, with a minimum incidence of about 20%, even in patients who have not received TBI as a part of their preparative regimen. Many factors play a role in IP development, including infectious agents (e.g., cytomegalovirus or *Pneumocystis carinii*), graft-versus-host disease (GVHD), and innate patient characteristics (older age, greater body weight, or greater body surface area).[16]

The importance of TBI as a risk factor may be altered by changes in fractionation, dose rate, and total lung dose, as seen in many reported studies. There is a lower incidence of IP and fewer fatalities from IP when fractionated TBI is used than when single-dose TBI is used as part of the preparative regimen for transplantation, even though a higher total dose has been used with the fractionated regimens. This has been found in a large number of nonrandomized studies (17–26) and in a randomized study.[27]

Dose rate is important primarily with single-dose TBI. Very low dose rates (0.025 Gy/min) result in a low incidence of IP (10%) and fatal IP (5%), but these necessitate a very lengthy treatment time, as long as 7 hours.[28] An unacceptably high IP incidence (8 of 11 patients), with 50% mortality, was found in a study with a high instantaneous dose rate (0.21–0.235 Gy/min).[25] Two studies suggest that with sufficiently fractionated TBI, dose rate loses its importance, which is understandable if the dose per fraction is within the shoulder of the cell survival curve for the tissue of interest (e.g., lung), and the time between fractions is long enough for repair to take place between fractions.[12,29] Two reports suggest that with a regimen of 12 Gy in six fractions, dose rate may still have an influence, with higher dose rates increasing the risk of IP.[30,31] On the other hand, in the low-dose-rate arm of one of the above studies, no significant difference in IP was found between single-dose and hyperfractionated TBI.[12]

The influence of total dose on the incidence of IP may be seen in studies where lung blocks have been used in some of the patients. In one study, IP was reduced to 8% when lung shields were used, compared to 27% incidence without such shields.[32] In another study with static intensity-modulating compensators constraining the lung dose to 11 Gy, the IP rate was lowered to

8.5%, compared with 22.2% when lung dose was 12 Gy.[33] The benefit was even greater in the pediatric patients, 4.2% at 11 Gy versus 25% at 12 Gy. In a multivariate logistic regression analysis of published IP data, it was reported that a conditioning regimen of 12 Gy in six daily fractions induced an IP incidence of 11% without lung shielding, but with shielding of the lung to 50% of this dose, the incidence was lowered to 2.3%.[34] However, when lung dose reduction by shielding was attempted in a randomized study with a single-dose 10-Gy regimen, IP was essentially the same for 6-Gy lung dose (23%) versus 8-Gy (28%), and, unfortunately, relapse was found to be higher in the 6-Gy group.[35]

LIVER: VENO-OCCLUSIVE DISEASE

Hepatic VOD, also known as *sinusoidal obstruction syndrome*, is a relatively common complication occurring within the first month following HCT. Endothelial cell damage results in sinusoidal obstruction, with or without venular occlusion. This potentially fatal syndrome includes symptoms of jaundice, painful hepatomegaly, fluid retention, and weight gain. TBI and chemotherapy are the principal causes of VOD although its etiology is multifactorial. A higher total dose was implicated in one study (>12 Gy compared with 12 Gy).[36] Fractionated TBI (12–14 Gy) has usually resulted in a lower incidence of VOD when compared with single-dose (10 Gy) TBI,[12,22,37–40] although there have been a few exceptions.[12,14,41]

In single-dose regimens, dose rate plays a role, with minimal VOD observed at dose rates of 0.07 Gy/min or less, compared with an incidence of as high as 50% with dose rates of 0.18 to 1.20 Gy/min.[42]

Strategies to reduce the incidence of VOD include using a lower total dose of TBI, increased fractionation including hyperfractionation (multiple small fractions per day separated by at least 5 hours to allow for normal tissue repair), and nonmyeloablative regimens (very low dose TBI and less intense chemotherapy).

KIDNEY: NEPHRITIS AND CHRONIC RENAL FAILURE

Effects of TBI on kidney have been very difficult to distinguish from the effects of systemic agents used prior to or during the course of transplantation and recovery, such as antibiotics, cyclosporin for GVHD prophylaxis, cytosine arabinoside (AraC), etc. Renal dysfunction was strongly correlated with total TBI dose in two studies.[43,44] In one study in which renal dose was limited to 12 Gy by CT planning, with a TBI fractionation of 12 Gy in six fractions, 2 Gy/fraction twice daily, there was only one case of radiation nephritis, 24 months after marrow transplantation, in the 59 patients who had no pretreatment creatinine elevation.[45] In another study, there was no relationship of renal dysfunction to TBI dose (>12 Gy vs. ≤12 Gy), but there was a possible compensatory effect of a decreased fraction size (1.75 Gy) in the >12 Gy group compared to a fraction size of 2 Gy in the ≤12 Gy group.[46]

Single-dose TBI to only 7.5 Gy was shown to be significantly associated with severe chronic renal failure after allogeneic transplantation (6.3%), compared with only 0.8% with fractionated TBI (either 12 Gy in six fractions or 14.4 Gy in eight fractions).[47]

An interesting retrospective review and analysis of the literature regarding late renal toxicity found that in the reports involving adults only, the only significant variable related to its incidence was total dose.[48] In the reports involving pediatric patients only, the use of cyclosporine or teniposide was significant, but no radiation-related variables were significant. When studies involving mixed populations (adults and children) were grouped with the adults-only studies, significant variables were total dose, dose rate, and number of fractions.

BRAIN: COGNITIVE DYSFUNCTION

Few studies have looked at cognitive function after TBI for transplantation. A study in children who received low-dose cranial irradiation for marrow transplantation showed no significant changes in IQ or in an adaptive behavior scale.[49] Hyperfractionated TBI resulted in no alterations in cognitive testing in a study of 58 patients.[50]

One study has related increasing cognitive dysfunction to increasing TBI dose, by both univariate and multivariate analyses.[51] Another study by the same group demonstrated that 75% of adults with malignant disease (primarily leukemia), who were candidates for BMT had cognitive impairment prior to the transplantation procedure, when tested for 11 functional indices.[52] Most common was memory impairment. Prior history of cranial irradiation was the variable most strongly associated with impaired function, but there were also trends possibly implicating high-dose AraC, as well as treatment of central nervous system disease with intrathecal chemotherapy. Children with acute lymphocytic leukemia who had more than one course of cranial irradiation had greater decrements in IQ and achievement.[53]

TBI was one risk factor, among many others, for higher delirium severity, but not for the incidence of delirium in adults who underwent HCT.[54] In children who had undergone HCT, TBI was one of the risk factors for severe neurologic events; other factors were transplant from an allogeneic donor, especially if unrelated, and development of severe acute GVHD.[55]

EYE: CATARACTS

With single-dose TBI, it has been found that the incidence of cataract development is very high, 80% to 100%, when patients are followed 8 to 10 years.[56–62] As many as 59% of these patients required cataract surgery.[57]

The incidence of cataract development is considerably less (5%–30%) when TBI is fractionated,[22,56–58,60,62–67] with only about 20% requiring surgery.[56,57,61] One exception is a study with rapid fractionation (10.5–12 Gy in only 1.5–3 days), in which 63% of patients developed cataracts.[68] TBI given at a high dose rate increases the development and severity of cataracts,[63,69] as does prior cranial irradiation.[70,71] Factors unrelated to irradiation that increase the risk of cataracts include steroid use,[56,64,72] the use of non–T-cell-depleted grafts,[61,67] GVHD development,[56] and the use of busulfan.[73]

Total dose to the eyes plays a significant role in cataract development and severity as shown in studies with eye shielding. In a study of children with hematologic disorders who underwent TBI in only one or two fractions prior to BMT, cataract incidence was 31% in 139 children with eye shielding compared to 90% in 49 children without shielding.[74] Severe cataracts were only 3% with shielding compared to 38% without shielding. This same group has studied the parameters for the linear quadratic formula for the lens based on results in patients treated with single-dose TBI and BMT,[75] excluding those patients who received heparin or posttransplant steroids. The values of the parameters for lens were characteristic of late-responding tissues and allowed prediction of cataract formation, based on TBI dose and dose rate.

ENDOCRINE SYSTEM: THYROID AND GONADAL DYSFUNCTION

Many abnormalities in endocrine function have been described after HCT and reviewed extensively in the literature[76,77]; these include hypothyroidism, growth deficits, impaired sexual development, and infertility. Fractionated TBI has resulted in decreased morbidity when compared with single-dose TBI.

Thyroid function has been shown to be impaired more frequently when transplant regimen include TBI.[78,79] In several studies, a much higher incidence of compensated hypothyroidism and overt hypothyroidism was found in children who had received single-dose TBI (10 Gy) compared with those who had received fractionated TBI (12–15.75 Gy over 4–7 days).[60,76,80–82]

Gonadal function was depressed in the majority of patients who received single-dose TBI in one study, but was less frequently altered in patients who received fractionated TBI, as measured by basal and stimulated luteinizing hormone levels and follicle-stimulating hormone levels.[78] With single-dose TBI (10 Gy), the development of secondary sexual characteristics was significantly delayed in 71% of girls and 83% of boys, but with fractionated TBI (12–15.75 Gy), about 49% of girls and 58% of boys experienced delayed development.[83] Although most women develop primary gonadal failure, a few have recovered, and pregnancies have occurred.[76,80,84,85,86] In a single-center study, women who had undergone HCT, especially if they had received TBI, were at a high risk for spontaneous abortion, preterm labor, and delivery of low–birth-weight babies.[86]

GROWTH: RETARDATION FROM BONE AND HORMONAL EFFECTS

There are two causes of growth retardation in children who have received TBI: depressed growth hormone and a direct radiation effect on bone growth. Growth hormone deficiency is found in about 30% to 70% of children who have received TBI, but if they have had prior cranial irradiation, this incidence climbs to as high as 82%.[83] Less growth retardation occurs with fractionated TBI compared with single-dose TBI.[87–89]

SECONDARY MALIGNANCIES

An association between irradiation for transplantation and the development of secondary malignancies (SM) has been controversial. An analysis from Seattle with 2,246 patients (320 with aplastic anemia and 1,926 with hematologic malignancies) yielded a 1.4% incidence of SM and implicated TBI as well as the use of antithymocyte globulin for GVHD as risk factors.[90] An analysis of European BMT data that compared immunosuppression versus BMT for patients with severe aplastic anemia showed that patients who were immunosuppressed had a greater cumulative incidence of cancer at 10 years (18.8%) compared with those who had a transplant (3.1%).[91] In the patients in the BMT group who developed solid tumors, there was a relative risk of 9.6 for the use of irradiation in the conditioning regimen. Inexplicably, all the patients who developed solid tumors were male.

An analysis of 493 non–Hodgkin lymphoma patients who had undergone autologous HCT found 22 patients who had developed persistent cytopenia in at least one cell line and with morphologic or cytogenetic evidence of therapy-related myelodysplastic syndrome or acute myelogenous leukemia (AML).[92] TBI was independently associated with an increased risk of developing myelodysplastic syndrome or AML.

A high incidence of thyroid cancer (14% at 8–17.3 years post-TBI) was found in a study of late effects in 42 children who were treated with TBI prior to HCT.[93] The authors indicated that this rate was similar to the 12% incidence of thyroid cancer for the 56 children in another study who were followed for more than 10 years after allogeneic BMT.[94] In a comparison of matched populations of children treated with autologous BMT prepared with regimens either with or without TBI, 9% (3/32) developed a papillary thyroid carcinoma at a mean of 6 years after treatment in the TBI group.[79] None developed thyroid carcinoma in the chemotherapy-only group. Other investigators have suggested no association with irradiation.[95,96] A more extensive discussion of irradiation related to BMT as a major risk factor for solid tumor development, and as a contributing factor for leukemia development, is summarized in a review.[97]

CONCLUSIONS

The effects of WBE, as described in this chapter, involve multiple organ systems. With high doses in radiation accidents or in warfare, these effects can be devastating, leading to death, through protean changes in the hematopoietic, gastrointestinal, and cerebrovascular systems. In a controlled manner, however, TBI may be utilized productively to aid in decreasing tumor burden and helping to immunosuppress diseased patients who need HCT. By increasing dose fractionation, and/or decreasing dose rate, and by shielding sensitive organs, tissue damage may be minimized to a great degree; however, we must be aware of, and treat to the best of our knowledge and abilities, the wide-ranging multiorgan effects of this useful treatment tool.

REFERENCES

1. Satow Y. General review of the late effects of the Chernobyl accident: comparison between Chernobyl and Hiroshima. In: Takeichi N, Satow Y, Masterson RH, eds. *The Chernobyl Accident: Thyroid Abnormalities in Children, Congenital Abnormalities and Other Radiation Related Information—The First Ten Years*. 1st ed. Hiroshima: Hiroshima-Nagasaki Peace Foundation; 1996.
2. Tarbell NJ, Amato DA, Down JD, et al. Fractionation and dose rate effects in mice: a model for bone marrow transplantation in man. *Int J Radiat Oncol Biol Phys*. 1987;13:1065–1069.
3. Shank B, Hopfan S, Kim JH, et al. Hyperfractionated total body irradiation for bone marrow transplantation: I. Early results in leukemia patients. *Int J Radiat Oncol Biol Phys*. 1981;7:1109–1115.
4. Lawton CA, Barber-Derus S, Murray KJ, et al. Technical modification in transplant. *Int J Radiat Oncol Biol Phys*. 1992;17:319–322.
5. Thoma GE Jr, Wald N. The diagnosis and management of accidental radiation injury. *J Occup Med*. 1959;1:421–447.
6. Shank B, O'Reilly RJ, Cunningham I, et al. Total body irradiation for bone marrow transplantation: the Memorial Sloan-Kettering Cancer Center experience. *Radiother Oncol*. 1990;1(suppl):68–81.
7. Hérodin F, Grenier N, Drouet M. Revisiting therapeutic strategies in radiation casualties. *Exp Hematol*. 2007;35(4 suppl 1):28–33.
8. Spitzer TR, Friedman CJ, Bushnell W, et al. Double-blind, randomized, parallel-group study on the efficacy and safety of oral granisetron and oral ondansetron in the prophylaxis of nausea and vomiting in patients receiving hyperfractionated total body irradiation. *Bone Marrow Transplant*. 2000;26:203–210.
9. Spitzer TR, Bryson JC, Cirenza E, et al. Randomized double-blind, placebo-controlled evaluation of oral ondansetron in the prevention of nausea and vomiting associated with fractionated total body irradiation. *J Clin Oncol*. 1994;12:2432–2438.
10. Tiley C, Powles R, Catalano J, et al. Results of a double blind placebo controlled study of ondansetron as an antiemetic during total body irradiation in patients undergoing bone marrow transplantation. *Leuk Lymphoma*. 1992;7:317–321.

11. Matsuoka S, Okamoto S, Watanabe R, et al. Granisetron plus dexamethasone versus granisetron alone in the prevention of vomiting induced by conditioning for stem cell transplantation: a prospective randomized study. *Int J Hematol.* 2003;77:86–90.
12. Ozsahin M, Pene F, Touboul E, et al. Total body irradiation before bone marrow transplantation; results of two randomized instantaneous dose rates in 157 patients. *Cancer.* 1992;69:2853–2865.
13. Belkacemi Y, Pene F, Touboul E, et al. Total body irradiation before bone marrow transplantation for acute leukemia in first or second complete remission. Results and prognostic factors in 326 consecutive patients. *Strahlenther Onkol.* 1998;174:92–104.
14. Valls A, Granena A, Carreras E, et al. Total body irradiation in bone marrow transplantation: fractionated versus single dose. Acute toxicity and preliminary results. *Bull Cancer.* 1989;76:797–804.
15. Oya N, Sasai K, Tachiiri S, et al. Influence of radiation dose rate and lung dose on interstitial pneumonitis after fractionated total body irradiation: acute parotitis may predict interstitial pneumonitis. *Int J Hematol.* 2006;83:86–91.
16. Shank B. Total body irradiation. In: Gunderson LL, Tepper JE. *Clinical Radiation Oncology.* 2nd ed. New York, NY: Churchill Livingstone; 2006.
17. Pino y Torres JL, Bross DS, Lam W-C, et al. Risk factors in interstitial pneumonitis following allogeneic bone marrow transplantation in adult patients. *Int J Radiat Oncol Biol Phys.* 1982;8:1301–1307.
18. Cosset JM, Baume D, Pico JL, et al. Single dose versus hyperefractionated total body irradiation before allogeneic bone marrow transplantation: a non-randomized comparative study of 54 patients at the Institut Gustave-Roussy. *Radiother Oncol.* 1989;15:151–160.
19. Shank B, Chu FCH, Dinsmore R, et al. Hyperfractionated total body irradiation for bone marrow transplantation. Results in seventy leukemia patients with allogeneic transplants. *Int J Radiat Oncol Biol Phys.* 1983;9:1607–1611.
20. Sutton L, Kuentz M, Cordonnier C, et al. Allogeneic bone marrow transplantation for adult acute lymphoblastic leukemia in first complete remission: factors predictive of transplant-related mortality and influence of total body irradiation modalities. *Bone Marrow Transplant.* 1993;12:583–589.
21. Socie G, Devergie A, Girinsky T, et al. Influence of the fractionation of total body irradiation on complications and relapse rate for chronic myelogenous leukemia. *Int J Radiat Oncol Biol Phys.* 1991;20:397–404.
22. Kim TH, McGlave PB, Ramsay N, et al. Comparison of two total body irradiation regimens in allogeneic bone marrow transplantation for acute non-lymphoblastic leukemia in first remission. *Int J Radiat Oncol Biol Phys.* 1990;19:889–897.
23. Blume KG, Forman SJ, Snyder DS, et al. Allogeneic bone marrow transplantation for acute lymphoblastic leukemia during first complete remission. *Transplant.* 1987;43:389–392.
24. Devergie A, Reiffers J, Vernant JP, et al. Long-term follow-up after bone marrow transplantation for chronic myelogenous leukemia: factors associated with relapse. *Bone Marrow Transplant.* 1990;5:379–386.
25. Kim TH, Rybka WB, Lehnert S, et al. Interstitial pneumonitis following total body irradiation for bone marrow transplantation using two different dose rates. *Int J Radiat Oncol Biol Phys.* 1985;11:1285–1291.
26. Bacigalupo A, van Lint MT, Frassoni F, et al. Late complications of allogeneic bone marrow transplantation. *Med Oncol Tumor Pharmacother.* 1991;8:261–263.
27. Thomas ED, Clift RA, Hersman J, et al. Marrow transplantation for acute nonlymphoblastic leukemia in first remission using fractionated or single-dose irradiation. *Int J Radiat Oncol Biol Phys.* 1982;8:817–821.
28. Barrett A, Depledge MH, Powles RL. Interstitial pneumonitis following bone marrow transplantation after low dose rate total body irradiation. *Int J Radiat Oncol Biol Phys.* 1983;9:1029–1033.
29. Gogna NK, Morgan G, Downs K, et al. Lung dose rate and interstitial pneumonitis in total body irradiation for bone marrow transplantation. *Australas Radiol.* 1992;36:317–320.
30. Beyzadeoglu M, Oysul K, Dirican B, et al. Effect of dose-rate and lung dose in total body irradiation on interstitial pneumonitis after bone marrow transplantation. *Tohoku J Exp Med.* 2004;202:255–263.
31. Carruthers SA, Wallington MM. Total body irradiation and pneumonitis risk: a review of outcomes. *Br J Cancer.* 2004;90:2080–2084.
32. Labar B, Bognanic V, Nemet D, et al. Total body irradiation with or without lung shielding for allogeneic bone marrow transplantation. *Bone Marrow Transplant.* 1992;9:343–347.
33. Schneider RA, schultze J, Jensen JM, et al. Long-term outcome after static intensity-modulated total body radiotherapy using compensators stratified by pediatric and adult cohorts. *Int J Radiat Oncol Biol Phys.* 2008;70:194–202.
34. Sampath S, Schultheiss TE, Wong J. Dose response and factors related to interstitial pneumonitis after bone marrow transplant. *Int J Radiat Oncol Biol Phys.* 2005;63:876–884.
35. Girinsky T, Socie G, Ammarguellat H, et al. Consequences of two different doses to the lungs during a single dose of total body irradiation: results of a randomized study on 85 patients. *Int J Radiat Oncol Biol Phys.* 1994;30:821–824.
36. McDonald GB, Hinds MS, Fisher LD, et al. Veno-occlusive disease of the liver and multiorgan failure after bone marrow transplantation: a cohort study of 355 patients. *Ann Intern Med.* 1993;118:255–267.
37. Deeg HJ, Sullivan KM, Buckner CD, et al. Marrow transplantation for acute non lymphoblastic leukemia in first remission: toxicity and long-term follow-up of patients conditioned with single dose or fractionated total body irradiation. *Bone Marrow Transplant.* 1986;1:151–157.
38. McDonald GB, Sharma P, Matthews DE, et al. Veno-occlusive disease of the liver after bone marrow transplantation: diagnosis, incidence, and predisposing factors. *Hepatology.* 1984;4:116–122.
39. Resbeut M, Cowen D, Blaise D, et al. Fractionated or single-dose total body irradiation in 171 acute myeloblastic leukemias in first complete remission: is there a best choice? *Int J Radiat Oncol Biol Phys.* 1995;31:509–517.
40. Girinsky T, Benhamou E, Bourhis J-H, et al. Prospective randomized comparison of single-dose versus hyperfractionated total body irradiation in patients with hematologic malignancies. *J Clin Oncol.* 2000;18:981–986.
41. Belkacemi Y, Ozsahin M, Rio B, et al. Is veno-occlusive disease incidence influenced by the total body irradiation technique? *Semin Oncol.* 1995;171:694–697.
42. Shulman HM, Hinterberger W. Hepatic veno-occlusive disease-liver toxicity syndrome after bone marrow transplantation. *Bone Marrow Transplant.* 1992;10:197–214.
43. Rhoades JL, Lawson CA, Cohen EP, et al. Incidence of bone marrow transplant nephropathy (BMT-Np) after twice-daily hyperfractionated total body irradiation [abstract]. *Cancer J Sci Am.* 1997;3:116.
44. Miralbell R, Bieri S, Mermillod B, et al. Renal toxicity after allogeneic bone marrow transplantation: the combined effects of total body irradiation and graft-versus-host disease. *J Clin Oncol.* 1996;14:579–585.
45. Borg M, Hughes T, Horvath N, et al. Renal toxicity after total body irradiation. *Int J Radiat Oncol Biol Phys.* 2002;54:1165–1173.
46. Esiashvili N, Chiang K-Y, Hasselle MD, et al. Renal toxicity in children undergoing total body irradiation for bone marrow transplant. *Radiother Oncol.* 2009;90:242–246.
47. Delgado J, Cooper N, Thomson K, et al. The importance of age, fludarabine and total body irradiation in the incidence and severity of chronic renal failure after allogeneic hematopoietic cell transplantation. *Biol Blood Marrow Transplant.* 2006;12:75–83.
48. Cheng JC, Schultheiss TE, Wong YC. Impact of drug therapy, radiation dose, and dose rate on renal toxicity following bone marrow transplantation. *Int J Radiat Oncol Biol Phys.* 2008;71:1436–1443.
49. Kramer JH, Crittenden MR, Halberg FE, et al. A prospective study of cognitive functioning following low-dose cranial radiation for bone marrow transplantation. *Pediatrics.* 1992;90:447–450.
50. Wenz F, Steinvorth S, Lohr F, et al. Prospective evaluation of delayed central nervous system (CNS) toxicity of hyperfractionated total body irradiation (TBI). *Int J Radiat Oncol Biol Phys.* 2000;48:1497–1501.
51. Andrykowski MA, Altmaier EM, Barnett RL, et al. Cognitive dysfunction in adult survivors of allogeneic marrow transplantation: relationship to dose of total body irradiation. *Bone Marrow Transplant.* 1990;6:269–276.
52. Andrykowski MA, Schmitt FA, Gregg ME, et al. Neuropsychologic impairment in adult bone marrow transplant candidates. *Cancer.* 1992;70:2288–2297.
53. Mulhern RK, Ochs J, Fairclough D, et al. Intellectual and academic achievement status after CNS relapse: a retrospective analysis of 40 children treated for acute lymphoblastic leukemia. *J Clin Oncol.* 1987;5:933–940.
54. Fann JR, Roth-Roemer S, Burington BE, et al. Delirium in patients undergoing hematopoietic stem cell transplantation. *Cancer.* 2002;95:1971–1981.
55. Faraci M, Lanino E, Dini G, et al. Severe neurologic complications after hematopoietic stem cell transplantation in children. *Neurology.* 2002;59:1895–1904.
56. Deeg HJ, Flournoy N, Sullivan KM, et al. Cataracts after total body irradiation and marrow transplantation: a sparing effect of dose fractionation. *Int J Radiat Oncol Biol Phys.* 1984;10:957–964.
57. Benyunes MC, Sullivan KM, Deeg HJ, et al. Cataracts after bone marrow transplantation: long-term follow-up of adults treated with fractionated total body irradiation. *Int J Radiat Oncol Biol Phys.* 1995;32:661–670.
58. Livesey SJ, Holmes JA, Whittaker JA. Ocular complications of bone marrow transplantation. *Eye.* 1989;3:271–276.
59. Calissendorff B, Bolme P, el Azazi M. The development of cataract in children as a late side-effect of bone marrow transplantation. *Bone Marrow Transplant.* 1991;7:427–429.
60. Sanders JE. Late effects in children receiving total body irradiation for bone marrow transplantation. *Radiother Oncol.* 1990;1(suppl):82–87.
61. Hamon MD, Gale RP, MacDonald ID, et al. Incidence of cataracts after single fraction total body irradiation: the role of steroids and graft versus host disease. *Bone Marrow Transplant.* 1993;12:233–236.
62. Flowers MED, Deeg HJ. Delayed complications after hematopoietic transplantation. In: Blume HG, Forman SJ, Appelbaum FR, eds. *Hematopoietic Cell Transplantation.* 3rd ed. Malden, MA: Blackwell Publishing, Inc.; 2004.
63. Ozsahin M, Belkacemi Y, Pene F, et al. Total body irradiation and cataract incidence: a randomized comparison of two instantaneous dose rates. *Int J Radiat Oncol Biol Phys.* 1994;28:343–347.
64. Dunn JP, Jabs DA, Wingard J, et al. Bone marrow transplantation and cataract development. *Arch Ophthalmol* 1993;111:1367–1373.
65. Lappi M, Rajantie J, Uusitalo RJ. Irradiation cataract in children after bone marrow transplantation. *Graefes Arch Clin Exp Ophthalmol.* 1990;228:218–221.
66. Belkacemi Y, Labopin M, Vernant JP, et al. Cataracts after total body irradiation and bone marrow transplantation in patients with acute leukemia in complete remission: a study of the European Group for Blood and Bone Marrow Transplantation. *Int J Radiat Oncol Biol Phys.* 1998;41:659–668.
67. Aristei C, Alessandro M, Santucci A, et al. Cataracts in patients receiving stem cell transplantation after conditioning with total body irradiation. *Bone Marrow Transplant.* 2002;29:503–507.
68. Bray LC, Carey PJ, Proctor SJ, et al. Ocular complications of bone marrow transplantation. *Br J Ophthalmol.* 1991;75:611–614.
69. Beyzadeoglu M, Dirican B, Oysul K, et al. Evaluation of fractionated total body irradiation and dose rate on cataractogenesis in bone marrow transplantation. *Haematologia (Budap).* 2002;32:25–30.
70. Fife K, Milan S, Westbrook K, et al. Risk factors for requiring cataract surgery following total body irradiation. *Radiother Oncol.* 1994;33:93–98.
71. Zierhut D, Lohr F, Schraube P, et al. Cataract incidence after total body irradiation. *Int J Radiat Oncol Biol Phys.* 2000;46:131–135.
72. Van Kempen-Harteveld ML, Struikmans H, Kal HB, et al. Cataract after total body irradiation and bone marrow transplantation: degree of visual impairment. *Int J Radiat Oncol Biol Phys.* 2002;52:1375–1380.
73. Holmstrom G, Borgstrom B, Calissendorff B. Cataract in children after bone marrow transplantation: relation to conditioning regimen. *Acta Ophthalmol Scand.* 2002;80:211–215.

74. Van Kempen-Harteveld ML, van Weel-Sipman MH, Emmens C, et al. Eye shielding during total body irradiation for bone marrow transplantation in children transplanted for a hematological disorder: risks and benefits. *Bone Marrow Transplant.* 2003;31:1151–1156.

75. Van Kempen-Harteveld ML, Belkacemi Y, Kal HB, et al. Dose-effect relationship for cataract induction after single-dose total body irradiation and bone marrow transplantation for acute leukemia. *Int J Radiat Oncol Biol Phys.* 2002;52:1367–1374.

76. Sanders JE, Long-term Follow-up Team. Endocrine problems in children after bone marrow transplant for hematologic malignancies. *Bone Marrow Transplant.* 1991;8(suppl1):2–4.

77. Sanders JE. Endocrine complications of high-dose therapy with stem cell transplantation. *Pediatr Transplant.* 2004;8(suppl 5):39–50.

78. Carlson K, Lönnerholm G, Smedmyr B, et al. Thyroid function after autologous bone marrow transplantation. *Bone Marrow Transplant.* 1992;10:123–127.

79. Flandin I, Hartmann O, Michon J, et al. Impact of TBI on late effects in children treated by megatherapy for Stage IV neuroblastoma. A study of the French Society of Pediatric Oncology. *Int J Radiat Oncol Biol Phys.* 2006;64:1424–1431.

80. Söönders JE, Seattle Marrow Transplant Team. The impact of marrow transplant preparative regimens on subsequent growth and development. *Semin Hematol.* 1991;28:244–249.

81. Thomas BC, Stanhope R, Plowman PN, et al. Endocrine function following single fraction and fractionated total body irradiation for bone marrow transplantation in childhood. *Acta Endocrinol.* 1993;128:508–512.

82. Berger C, Le-Gallo B, Donadieu J, et al. Late thyroid toxicity in 153 long-term survivors of allogeneic bone marrow transplantation for acute lymphoblastic leukemia. *Bone Marrow Transplant.* 2005;35:991–995.

83. Sanders JE. Growth and development after hematopoietic cell transplantation. In: Blume HG, Forman SJ, Appelbaum FR, eds. *Hematopoietic Cell Transplantation.* 3rd ed. Malden, MA: Blackwell Publishing, Inc.; 2004.

84. Samuelsson A, Fuchs T, Simonsson B, et al. Successful pregnancy in a 28-year-old patient autografted for acute lymphoblastic leukemia following myeloablative treatment including total body irradiation. *Bone Marrow Transplant.* 1993;12:659–660.

85. Giri N, Vowels MR, Barr AL, et al. Successful pregnancy after total body irradiation and bone marrow transplantation for acute leukaemia. *Bone Marrow Transplant.* 1992;10:93–95.

86. Sanders JE, Hawley J, Levy W, et al. Pregnancies following high-dose cyclophosphamide with or without high-dose busulfan or total-body irradiation and bone marrow transplantation. *Blood.* 1996; 87:3045–3052.

87. Hovi L, Saarinen UM, Siimes MA. Growth failure in children after total body irradiation preparative for bone marrow transplantation. *Bone Marrow Transplant.* 1991; 8(suppl1):10–13.

88. Brauner R, Fontoura M, Zucker JM, et al. Growth and growth hormone secretion after bone marrow transplantation. *Arch Dis Child.* 1993;68:458–463.

89. Cohen A, Rovelli A, Bakker B, et al. Final height of patients who underwent bone marrow transplantation for hematologic disorders during childhood: a study by the Working Party for Late Effects-EBMT. *Blood.* 1999;93:4109–4115.

90. Sullivan KM, Mori M, Sanders J, et al. Late complications of allogeneic and autologous marrow transplantation. *Bone Marrow Transplant.* 1992;10(suppl 1):127–134.

91. Socie G, Henry-Amar M, Bacigalupo A, et al. Malignant tumors occurring after treatment of aplastic anemia: the European Bone Marrow Transplantation—Severe Aplastic Anemia Working Party. *N Engl J Med.* 1993;329:1152–1157.

92. Hosing C, Munsell M, Yazji S, et al. Risk of therapy-related myelodysplastic syndrome/acute leukemia following high-dose therapy and autologous bone marrow transplantation for non-Hodgkin's lymphoma. *Ann Oncol.* 2002;13:450–459.

93. Faraci M, Barra S, Cohen A, et al. Very late nonfatal consequences of fractionated TBI in children undergoing bone marrow transplant. *Int J Radiat Oncol Biol Phys.* 2005;63:1568–1575.

94. Cogen A, Rovelli A, van Lint MT, et al. Secondary thyroid carcinoma after allogeneic bone marrow transplantation during childhood. *Bone Marrow Transplant.* 2001;28:1125–1128.

95. Kolb HJ, Guenther W, Duell T, et al. Cancer after bone marrow transplantation. *Bone Marrow Transplant.* 1992;10:135–138.

96. Neglia J, Shapiro R, Haake R, et al. Second neoplasms following bone marrow transplantation (BMT) [abstract]. *Blood.* 1992;80:169a.

97. Shank B. Chemo-radiation induced carcinogenesis: the bone marrow transplant model. In: Rosenthal CJ, Rotman M, eds. *Infusion Chemotherapy—Irradiation Interactions.* Amsterdam: Elsevier Science; 1998.

12

C. Norman Coleman
Judith L. Bader

Response to Radiological and Nuclear Terrorism

INTRODUCTION

Following the end of the Cold War and prior to September 11, 2001, the possibility of a nuclear attack on the United States received rare public discussion. Privately, governmental nuclear weapons policies were still in evolution and focused on disarmament and the prevention of nuclear proliferation. Few countries had nuclear weapons. In this environment, investment in the radiation medical sciences and physical weapons-related technology had stabilized or decreased, and new nuclear power plants were not a key part of US energy policy. The 9/11 attacks on the United States have resulted in dramatic changes, with a major new public and governmental focus on nuclear weapon detection, antiproliferation, antiterrorism, and comprehensive preparedness planning, along with the acknowledged need for nuclear power and other technologies to play a role in energy independence for the country.[1,2]

This chapter emphasizes key Department of Health and Human Services (HHS) activities and programs relating to the medical planning for radiological and nuclear terrorism, which is, for convenience, called collectively *radiation events*. The context for HHS activities in the complex, newly designed larger national planning efforts is described briefly. In greater detail, this chapter focuses especially on medical consequence management for radiation mass casualty events, including development of response plans, acquisition of physical and personnel assets, and the development of a framework to deliver resources and medical countermeasures to affected populations. Consequence management includes many activities other than medical activities, including issues related to the military, transportation, communication, critical infrastructure, law enforcement, and security, but these issues are beyond the scope of this chapter. Obviously, counterproliferation and nonproliferation are preferred strategies, with detection and interdiction being crucial to avoiding a radiation event. Nonetheless, detailed consequence management strategies and activities must also be designed and exercised in advance, with all relevant partners nationally and internationally.

Many US government agencies have some or major focus on radiological and nuclear issues. The key agencies include the Departments of Energy, Defense, Homeland Security, the Environmental Protection Agency, various intelligence agencies, the Justice Department, and Nuclear Regulatory Commission (NRC), and the Department of HHS. Integration of these functions for planning and response is the focus of the new National Response Framework (NRF)[3] and within that document the Nuclear/Radiological Incident Annex (list of acronyms at end of chapter). The organizational chart of comprehensive responses for the federal government is detailed in a subdocument of the NRF that includes the 15 emergency support functions (ESFs).[4] ESF no. 8 is Public Health and Medical Services for which HHS is the lead federal agency. HHS also participates in a supportive role in several of the other ESFs. The operational framework for personnel, equipment, and venues for responses to major events is presented in the National Incident Management System (NIMS),[5] the details of which are currently under revision, and a parallel document is the Hospital Incident Command System.

In addition, the Department of Homeland Security has published 15 detailed prototypes of mass casualty events[6]; no. 1 is a mass casualty improvised nuclear device (IND) event, and no. 11 is a radiological dispersal device (RDD) event. These detailed scenarios are intended to assist federal, state, tribal, and local government planning and coordination efforts by providing very specific conditions against which to activate planning, logistic, operational, and administration functions. Although any terrorist event is unlikely to mirror these events exactly, planning required to respond to these events would likely touch on most of the issues involved in that type of scenario.

Each US government agency is required to respond directly to the overarching and critically important Executive Branch's National Security Presidential Directive-17/Homeland Security Presidential Directive 4, [6,7] which provides three pillars of our "National Strategy to Combat Weapons of Mass Destruction." As stated in a document entitled the pillars are as follows:

1. **Counterproliferation to Combat WMD Use**

   The possession and increased likelihood of use of WMD by hostile states and terrorists are realities of the contemporary security environment. It is therefore critical that the US military and appropriate civilian agencies be prepared to deter and defend against the full range of possible

WMD employment scenarios. We will ensure that all needed capabilities to combat WMD are fully integrated into the emerging defense transformation plan and into our homeland security posture. Counterproliferation will also be fully integrated into the basic doctrine, training, and equipping of all forces, in order to ensure that they can sustain operations to decisively defeat WMD-armed adversaries.

2. **Strengthened Nonproliferation to Combat WMD Proliferation**
   The United States, our friends and allies, and the broader international community must undertake every effort to prevent states and terrorists from acquiring WMD and missiles. We must enhance traditional measures—diplomacy, arms control, multilateral agreements, threat reduction assistance, and export controls—that seek to dissuade or impede proliferant states and terrorist networks, as well as to slow and make more costly their access to sensitive technologies, material, and expertise. We must ensure compliance with relevant international agreements, including the Nuclear Nonproliferation Treaty, the Chemical Weapons Convention, and the Biological Weapons Convention. The United States will continue to work with other states to improve their capability to prevent unauthorized transfers of WMD and missile technology, expertise, and material. We will identify and pursue new methods of prevention, such as national criminalization of proliferation activities and expanded safety and security measures.

3. **Consequence Management to Respond to WMD Use**
   Finally, the United States must be prepared to respond to the use of WMD against our citizens, our military forces, and those of friends and allies. We will develop and maintain the capability to reduce to the extent possible the potentially horrific consequences of WMD attacks at home and abroad.

The US government has also engaged with international partners[8] in radiation response and planning efforts as well as with state, local, and tribal governments; hospitals; and professional societies.

BACKGROUND AND DESCRIPTION OF POTENTIAL MASS CASUALTY RADIATION EVENTS

Radiation events have the potential to cause unintended exposure and/or contamination, with or without physical damage to the environment. The extent of infrastructure damage, casualties, and fatalities from a radiation event will obviously be event specific.

A radiation event may be obvious as with IND or explosive RDD (Fig. 12-1). It may be more subtle with a nonexplosive RDD or radiological exposure device (RED). These may be discovered by a monitoring device such as an environmental device in a public facility or a portal monitor at a medical facility. An event may be announced by a terrorist group to create chaos and terror and, conceivably, it may be a false alarm to cause disruption. Or, an event may not be recognized for some time until some astute clinician recognizes potential radiation-induced symptoms or syndromes or public health surveillance detects the event. Clearly, the suspicion of a radiation event by knowing the symptoms and signs of irradiated victims will help in the speed of detection of a surreptitious event.

Figure 12-1 highlights features of the spectrum radiation events. The general response philosophy has been to prepare for the worst possible event, the IND realizing that solutions for that will subsume many, but not all, of the issues of a RDD.

For an IND, national planning activities have focused on a 10-kiloton (kT) event, as that is specified for planning purposes

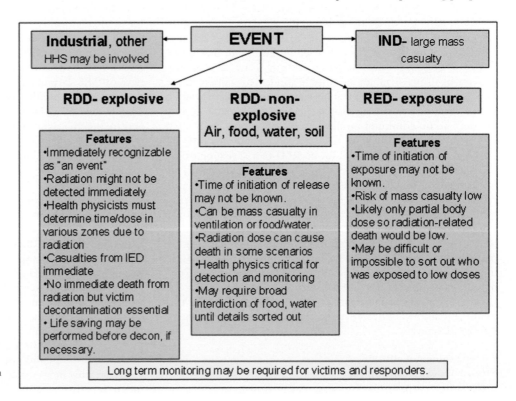

Figure 12.1. Spectrum of radiation events.

in the National Planning Scenarios.[6] Many factors will impact the initial damage from an IND, including location (which city/place, where in that city, size of the population, time of day, height of the detonation (air vs. ground blast), size of device, completeness of detonation, weather conditions, building construction, electromagnetic pulse, and others). Any IND detonation will produce terrible devastation with many thousands of people killed from the blast and with a spectrum of injuries including one or more of blast injury, crush injury, skin burns from radiation, burn from fire, radiation injury, glass injury, retinal burns, and injury resulting from the flash blindness with secondary vehicle accidents.

Victims with major radiation plus other injury or burn (combined injury) are unlikely to survive very long after the initial event, and it may be difficult for responders to reach such victims, particularly those close to the epicenter, within the first hours to days. There will be tens of thousands needing immediate medical care, tens of thousands who will need medical care in the subsequent few weeks, many thousands seeking immediate medical attention from fear of injury, and hundreds of thousands who will need an estimate of their risk from the radiation along with advice and assurance. There are a number of reports in the unclassified, unofficial literature that provide potential details. Bell and Dallas[1] modeled both a 20-kT and a 550-kT IND detonation well as the 10-kT detonation from the National Planning Scenario no. 1.[6] Newer models include potentially more accurate estimates of what will happen within an urban setting including impact of sheltering in place, urban canyon effects (particularly important for an RDD), rapid changes in fall out dose, and estimates of damage to physical infrastructure.

For an RDD, the consequence depends on the radionuclide, its size, and mode of dispersal. For an explosive RDD, medical and physical effects start at an actual "time zero." Radiation exposure that can be measured or estimated would be a result of the time within the contaminated zone. A key feature of an explosive RDD or "dirty bomb" is that the airborne radioactivity settles to the ground within about 20 to 30 minutes, so that it is a radioactive footprint rather than plume in the air that is the source of ongoing radiation. RDD airborne dispersal is almost entirely by unpredictable low altitude winds, particularly those in urban canyons. Expert RDD modelers have indicated that it will be necessary to measure the dispersion of radioactivity and not depend on computer models.[9]

For a nonexplosive RDD (e.g., spreading radionuclides in the food or water supply) and for an RED (e.g., creating exposure by hiding a source in a public place), there probably will be no "time-zero" or known time the event began. Detection will require alert clinicians to identify symptom clusters in patients or detection by routine environmental surveillance. It may not be possible to time and quantify the exposure or contamination or even identify the true denominator of those affected. As with past events, there will likely be many hundreds to thousands times more who worry about having received radiation compared to the number who actually did.

After exposure to radiation, the population is at risk for the Acute Radiation Syndrome (ARS), which classically includes 4 subsyndromes:

• Hematologic syndrome
• Gastrointestinal syndrome
• Central nervous system (neurovascular) syndrome
• Cutaneous syndrome

Newer research has suggested that ARS can also be considered a multiorgan dysfunction system, rather than four discrete subsyndromes. Delayed effects of radiation are also of concern, including those related to carcinogenesis and normal tissue damage.

Contamination after radiation events may be internal via inhalation, ingestion, or absorption through the skin or open wounds. Radionuclides of concern may emit α, β, or γ radiation that result in exposure. Radionuclide internal contamination can also affect normal tissues via chemical damage to tissues.

ENGAGING THE US MEDICAL ESTABLISHMENT AFTER 9/11

The events of September 11 promptly initiated the engagement and collaboration of the radiation oncology and biology communities to discuss what knowledge and capabilities existed that could contribute to radiological and nuclear terrorism preparedness and response and what gaps required attention.[10]

Much of the initial focus was on understanding normal radiation tissue injury, and the assessment of existing and potential new radiation protectors/mitigators, biodosimetry, and training and education.[11,12]

The generic concept of radiation protectors was subclassified into its key components[12]:

• Pre-exposure protectors
• Postexposure mitigators
• Treatment

Mitigators would reduce the medical consequences in order to save lives and reduce the need for in-patient medical care after radiation exposure and the development of the ARS.

Radiation-specific mitigators after exposure are effective only during a limited time window, and this must be accounted for in the medical response planning. Drugs that require delivery in less than a few hours or agents that require complex handling might be unsuitable in a mass casualty event. Treatment would be planned for potentially salvageable patients who develop ARS symptoms as well as those who are highly likely to do so. Some currently available drugs such as the granulocyte colony-stimulating factor (G-CSF) function as both mitigators and treatments, as seen in animal models.[10,13] Nonspecific radiation exposure symptom mitigators (as for nausea and vomiting) would also be required in a mass casualty event, and their stockpiling, storage, and prompt delivery would also require advanced planning.

Because there was no coordinated research and development strategy before September 11, a science-based comprehensive planning structure had to be created. Through excellent collaboration and coordination among experts throughout government and academia, including advisory working groups through the White House Office of Science and Technology Policy, a radiation research and development plan was created[10,14,15] and implemented led by National Institutes of Allergy and Infectious Diseases[16] on behalf of all NIH bioterrorism programs. Investment in these new programs was funded by funds that supplemented the existing NIH research budget, so that terrorism response did not replace other research.

Before this new civilian R and D structure was established, initial medical response recommendations came from the Armed Forces Radiobiology Research Institute (AFRRI).[17] Their plans were specifically designed for military use but had much in common with the civilian response.

After 9/11, several papers were key to informing the civilian sector and were critical to the development of early planning concepts. The medical response paper by Mettler and Voelz in 2002[18] discussed the radiation event issue in general terms, and the now classic report by Waselenko et al. addressed the issue of the ARS and its medical management.[13] Other expert recommendations from earlier research were also consulted,[19] indicating a resurgence in interest in radiation injury.

ENGAGING THE DEPARTMENT OF HHS AND ITS PARTNERS

HHS's approach developed through Assistant Secretary for Preparedness and Response (ASPR)[20] to planning for radiation event responses had several objectives:

- Develop a general response algorithm with standardized concepts and terminology for planners and responders. For response planners, HHS has developed systems that take into account the presence of radiation.[21]
- Develop a just-in-time information system for medical management that would be up-to-date and easily accessible and useable. To that end, the Radiation Event Medical Management (REMM) web portal has been created by HHS and the National Library of Medicine.[22,23]
- Exercise the response capability through simulations and exercises and through ongoing improvement in models and capabilities.
- Develop a robust enterprise to tackle the development of countermeasures.
- Develop a robust geographic information system linking operational information with infrastructure assets.
- Develop a robust responder corps to assist state and local responders.

A good deal of the HHS radiation response planning work has been recently published in the medical literature.[21,22,24,25] Updates and revision of planning and response are constantly ongoing, reflected in both public and classified documents. Some key planning documents are available in redacted form on the ASPR website.[20]

Two very recent publications from the HHS Office of the ASPR provide an in-depth discussion of the organization of the federal response[24] and the model for the organization of the medical response that takes into account the radiation effect on victims and the radiation limits of responders.[21] These publications include detailed referencing of the statutes, directives, and websites of the various agencies involved. REMM[23] is another source of updated information in this rapidly emerging field. This chapter provides an overview and does not repeat these details.

The overall initial approach to organize the response uses a time-oriented algorithm called the *Chain of Medical Response.*[24] This was derived from the various documents that assign responsibility to Agencies and Departments. Steps are not entirely linear, and there are branching points at which multiple next-steps occur. This Chain of Response has 17 steps from event to event detection to initial response to coordinated communications to comprehensive response once in-field data became available to engagement of federal response to expert centers for definitive

care to long-term follow-up for those at risk of long-term consequences, primarily radiation-inducible cancer. In addition to the initial structuring of the HHS response, it was critical to define how HHS would interact with the many external Agencies and Departments that participate in the response. Federal agency responsibility is based on authorizing legislation and presidential directives. To practice the response and define gaps, there are mandated, periodic exercises including major national level exercises involving federal, state, local, and tribal planners and responders. Lessons learned from exercises and real-life events are captured, evaluated, and implemented to help refine and improve the planning and response processes. In addition, new resources constantly need to be evaluated and integrated in the plans, with a balance on present needs, future products and evolving science, cost, and technology.

Before the federal response can be mounted, the local incident commander (IC) will assume responsibility using a standard organizational structure based on National Incident Management Structure or NIMS.[5] Federal agencies will be contacted and will have immediate involvement for an IND but much less of an initial role with smaller radiation events. Health, medical, and environmental physicists will be essential to define the scope of the event, first locally and then at higher levels. For an IND, federal response will rely on environmental monitoring by Interagency Modeling and Atmospheric Assessment Center.[26] On scene measurement of dose rate will include information from first responders and also from federal teams (Department of Energy [DOE], Environmental Protection Agency [EPA], Department of Defense [DOD], and others) that will provide expertise. For an RDD, analysis of the radionuclide may be done on the scene with gamma spectrometer and also might require analysis by the Center for Disease Control and Prevention (CDC) radiobioassay laboratory. The interagency physicists will coordinate their response through the Advisory Team and provide information regarding exposure and risk to the IC.

Providing up-to-date and credible information is essential. Federal agencies will coordinate their response through the NICCL (National Incident Communication Conference Line) and will work with the local IC. Key decisions will be recommendations as to who needs to shelter-in-place, who needs to be evacuated, and who is not at risk for exposure and can remain home. An initial response to shelter-in-place requires being in a facility or building that offers reasonable protection so that knowledge of the city and its construction will be important in decision making. Newer nuclear detonation response computer models that estimate damage to infrastructure and effects on people now include "protection factors" based on the materials used to construct buildings. The complex models are available to help guide responders plan for casualties as well as to recommend to incident managers in real time whether and when to recommend sheltering in place versus evacuation. These will be forthcoming in the Draft Protective Action Recommendations (PARs).[27]

Medical care will be initiated by the first responders and local medical facilities. For small events, the local and regional facilities possibly with some federal resources should be sufficient. For a moderate-to-large radiation event, regional and national resources will be required. This includes the National Disaster Medical System (NDMS)[28] and the Radiation Injury Treatment Network (RITN),[29,30] as well as individual expert volunteers.[24] There is a need for radiation oncologists and physicists to be on the volunteer rosters.

Medical resources will come from local, state, and regional facilities and stockpiles.[31] States will support one another's medical response through Emergency Management Assistance Compacts (EMACs).[32] The CDC manages the Strategic National Stockpile (SNS)[31] that includes medicines and supplies for a range of threats. The SNS can have resources on the scene by 24 hours. The SNS has "push-packs" ready for transport and also has contracts for surge capacity with vendors, referred to as *Vendor-Managed Inventory* (VMI). This obviates the need to buy and then dispose of large quantities of unused drugs, particularly drugs that have routine clinical use. The VMI is essentially a bubble in the routine supply line such that the surge in drugs comes from a stock that will otherwise be used in clinical care, for example, to prevent neutropenia from cancer treatment.

Present data suggest that the use of G-CSF will be useful as a radiation mitigator for the acute radiation hematological syndrome. Current animal data indicate that this cytokine is most effective if started as soon as possible, and it may have only limited efficacy as a mitigator after the first 24 hours. To meet the 24-hour window requirement, HHS is working with event mod-

elers, SNS, RITN, and the Veteran's Administration to explore the possibility of having multiple facilities, each with a modest bubble in their supply on hand so that there is a reasonable and geographically dispersed supply locally in the aggregate. This approach, still in the planning stage, is referred to as *User-Managed Inventory* (UMI) or virtual SNS. It not only allows each city and region to have additional "first doses" available but also distributes the supply among a number of facilities.

Putting all of the response together is referred to as the *Concept of Operations* or CONOPS. In developing the HHS and Federal CONOPS, there was not a standardized system of how to organize the medical response accounting for the presence of radiation. Figure 12-2 illustrates the RTR system, which stands for Radiation TRiage, TReatment, and Transport.[21] It is *not a traditional mass casualty triage system*, such as START of JumpSTART[33,34] (see Ref. 21 for detailed discussion). The RTR1 to RST3 sites will form spontaneously after an event with RTR1 being closest to the epicenter, RTR2 near the plume/footprint, and RTR3 being outside the radiation zone. Medical Care sites will be preidentified as will major anticipated Assembly Centers. HHS is working on a computerized geographical information system mapping

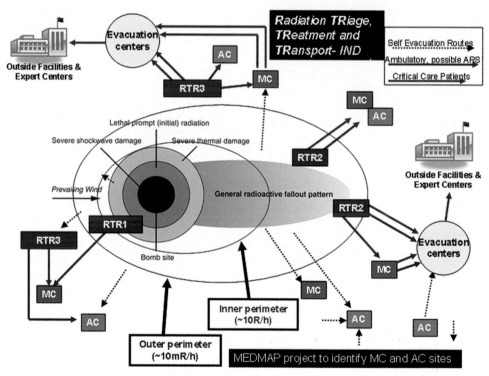

Figure 12.2. Diagram of the RTR medical response system for an IND incident (21). The epicenter, initial destruction pattern, and plume direction will determine where medical triage will occur. RTR sites will typically form spontaneously and will be of three general types: RTR1, near the blast where casualties will have primarily physical trauma from blast and thermal effects and potentially prompt or fall-out related radiation injury; RTR2, near the plume where casualties will have primarily radiation injury with varying to no physical trauma; and RTR3, not limited by radiation, where casualties may have physical trauma from blast or thermal, but will likely be unexposed to radiation due to their location primarily outside the blast and fall out zones. Definitive medical care will be provided at MC sites to which medical supplies and personnel will be sent. These may involve expert care centers, alternate care centers, definitive care centers, etc. throughout the region or nation. AC (assembly sites) will be collection points for displaced persons and for victims not requiring immediate medical attention who need guidance, possible triage, and disposition. Major transportation hubs will include airports, seaports, railroad stations, and designated highway or other road routes. Victim flow will be mainly away from the incident although many people not too far from the incident will be able to safely stay in their homes. At all RTR sites and AC sites, efforts will be made to track all victims and evacuees as they are moved to MC sites nearby or by transport to the region or nationally. An ongoing HHS project called *MEDMAP project* will preidentify the MC and AC sites and have an immediately available up-to-date interactive map to use during a response. This will allow the immediate identification of what facilities are available, which are off line and how far into regional and national resources the response will go. Reprinted from Hrdina CM, Coleman CN, Bogucki S, et al. The "RTR" medical response system for nuclear and radiological mass casualty events: a functional TRiage-TRansport-TReatment medical response model. *J Prehospital Disaster Med.* 2008. In press.

project for MC and AC sites throughout the United States. These data will be meshed graphically with real-time radiation location estimates. The project is called the *MEDMAP project.*

Fear of radiation and antiradiation sentiment make it necessary that responses involve credible experts, both government and nongovernment, to educate and inform the public and guide public policy. Developing effective public messaging has been a major focus of HHS planning at HHS, CDC, and among grantees. It is recognized that many people without physical trauma or radiation exposure will require psychological counseling.

ENGAGING THE NONFEDERAL GOVERNMENT AND THE PRIVATE SECTOR

While the federal role in radiation events will be essential, basic planning and responding must also be done at the state, local, and tribal levels, as federal response assets will not be available for some time after the event. Thus, there are wide-ranging needs and opportunities for radiation experts to train and help.[25] Indeed, as described in detail in the recent publication from ASPR,[24] the HHS planning and response program integrates many factors:

- basic understanding of radiation physics and biology
- biology of tissue injury and the stress response
- regenerative medicine
- health physics
- computer modeling
- medical response operations and logistics
- medical treatment algorithms and guidelines for the wide spectrum of civilian population
- systems approaches to event management including triage, treatment, and transport
- training, equipping, and transporting caregivers for medical and psychological problems and fatality management
- sophisticated risk assessment, management algorithms, and surveillance plans for potential long-term effects of radiation injury

We envision this multiexpert response to be bidirectional, iterative, comprehensive, and creative. Additional participants are welcome including the ongoing efforts from American Society of Therapeutic Radiology and Oncology, American Society of Hematology, National Marrow Donor Program, American Society of Bone Marrow Transplantation, Health Physics Society, American Society of Clinical Oncology, and others. Volunteering with one's state and with the federally coordinated programs such as Emergency System for Advance Registration of Volunteer Health Professionals (ESARVP) are good options.

Should a radiation event occur, radiation oncologists and physicists may well get a call from the local responders.[35] Even those who may have minimal interest and/or time should be familiar with the resources available. The HHS-sponsored REMM[23] website (http://remm.nlm.gov) provides key background information for those without formal Radiation Medicine training, and other training assets are available on the CDC Radiation Emergency website (http://www.bt.cdc.gov/radiation/).[36]

There is a long history of Protective Action Guidelines (PAGs) addressing acceptable thresholds and responses for occupational radiation exposure and exposure during small radiation accidents, including those at Nuclear Power Plants from agencies such as OSHA, EPA, NRC, Radiation Emergency Assistance Center/Training Site (REAC/TS) of the DOE. After 9/11, additional attention had to be directed to developing PAGs[37] for the general public and responders during radiation exposures associated with terrorist events event. An important document from Federal Emergency Management Agency was published in the Federal Register in August 2008,[37] which addresses PAGs during INDs and RDDs. An additional document is currently being prepared by an interagency group[27] that will supersede this document and update older documents that do not address mass casualty terrorist events.

BIODOSIMETRY AND MEDICAL COUNTERMEASURES

Individual victim dose assessment is an important factor for determining who will:

- need immediate medical care
- likely need care in the next 1 to 3 weeks,
- need some evaluation for radiation-induced cancer risk weeks, months, or years later
- not require further medical management for radiation effect

The present approach is to "bin" people initially into three major groups for those who have had a whole or major partial body exposure of

- <2 Gy who need no intervention for ARS;
- 2 to 4 Gy, who need evaluation by RITN or similar expert for potential ARS and who should receive a radiation mitigator for ARS; and
- 4 Gy, who need immediate medical mitigation and treatment.

Figure 12-3 indicates how biodosimetry (biomarker of dose received) and radiobioassay (analysis of internal contamination by radionuclide) might be used to assess victims. Lymphocytes are especially sensitive to radiation-induced intermitotic death, and the rate of decline (depletion kinetics) is used to estimate dose. The calculation of the neutrophil/lymphocyte ratio over time may be a better measure and that is being explored.[38] Cytogenetic analysis of radiation-induced aberrations, primarily dicentrics, in lymphocytes is especially useful for risk assessment, but due to the time required to create the metaphase spread, it is limited in the very acute phase (first 72 hours). It can be useful for the secondary triage. The goal of new rapid techniques is to have a reliable single point assay to help triage victims into risk groups. These include invasive (e.g., molecular, cellular) and noninvasive (e.g., electron paramagnetic resonance or EPR) techniques.[39]

The conceptual model for a new radiation laboratory network (Rad-LN) is in Figure 12-4 and described in the legend. This is an evolving setting with improvement in the current technologies including automation and artificial intelligence for cytogenetics, novel molecular diagnostics, and new methodologies for radiobioassay. Hematology surge capacity will require regional resources including the RITN centers.

Medical countermeasures will be used to reduce the medical consequences of radiation terrorist events. Radiation is unlike infectious agents for which there may be pre-exposure

ASPR **Assessing exposure and contamination conceptual approach** In addition to medical history

Event	Radio-bioassay (analyze the radionuclide)	Triage by hematology	"Rapid" biodosimetry (molecular) in development	Cytogenetics (dicentrics)
RDD, explosive	+ + + +	+	+ +	+ + +
RDD, non-explosive	+ + + +	+	+ +	+ + +
RED	+	+ +	+ + +	+ +
IND	+ + +	+ + + +	+ + + +	+ + + +
Concerned citizens or uncertain history	+ + + +	+	+ + +	+ + + +

Figure 12.3. Biodosimetry for triage and treatment. In addition to medical history and an estimate of possible physical dose from models and actual measurements, laboratory assessment is critical in triage and management. This table indicates what assays would be used. The column in gray is how new rapid dosimetric techniques under development might be used to enhance or replace current methodologies. These include noninvasive technologies.

prophylaxis. Since the time of a radiation event will not be known, the focus of the radiation medical countermeasures program has been postexposure mitigation and treatment. While radioprotectors such as amifostine have use in clinical oncology, there is no indication for this in emergency response as the radiation dose that first responders would be permitted or willing to receive with their consent would likely be 1 Gy or lower. Should there be an agent that is demonstrated to reduce radiation-induced cancer and be sufficiently nontoxic and easy to administer, this would certainly be a consideration for use by responders entering a radiation zone as well as potential victims.

The requirement for postexposure use has opened up new areas of research in radiation biology. A phrase we have used *Late effects occur late* emphasizes that there are ongoing processes following the initial dose of radiation that take time to produce clinical manifestations. Indeed, the term DEARE—*Delayed Effects of Acute Radiation Exposure*—was coined to emphasize that even early organ injury can take months to develop as with lung and renal injury; that is, there is an "incubation period" from radiation to manifest organ system dysfunction.

The medical countermeasures are now developed under the guidance of the HHS Public Health Emergency Medical

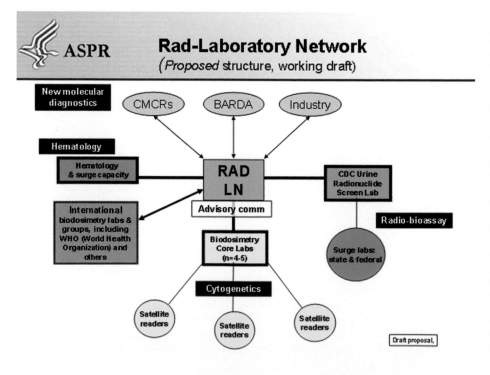

Figure 12.4. Proposed configuration of a Rad-LN. A Rad-LN is under development. The figure illustrates how such a network might look. There would be ongoing development to improve current techniques, such as automation and use of artificial intelligence for the dicentric chromosome assay, and to create new methods using molecular, cellular, and tissue techniques. The latter might even be noninvasive such as electron spin resonance. Cytogenetics would be done by having core laboratories prepare samples, and if their capacity were exceeded for reading samples, a network of experts would be available, including international partners (World Health Organization and the International Atomic Energy Agency). For an RDD, bioassay is necessary, particularly urine analysis for screening. CDC has a radiobioassay laboratory to identify and quantify a range of radionuclides. They collaborate with state laboratories. Radiation safety and nuclear medicine laboratories can assist in mass screening as well.

Countermeasures Enterprise (PHEMCE), which serves to coordinate communication and programs among entities involved in medical countermeasure development, acquisition, and deployment.[40,41] PHEMCE is coordinated by the HHS ASPR and includes three other HHS agencies—CDC, FDA, and NIH—and collaborates with the Departments of Defense, Homeland Security, Veterans Affairs, and Agriculture, and also other interagency stakeholders. PHEMCE has taken an end-to-end approach including research, development, acquisition, storage, maintenance, deployment, and policy for utilization. The 2007 *HHS PHEMCE Implementation Plan for CBRN Threats*[42] identified the top-priority targets for medical countermeasure research, product development, and acquisition.

The spectrum of injuries for which development of radiation medical countermeasures are desirable includes:

- ARS—hematological, gastrointestinal, central nervous system, cutaneous, and the delayed toxicity for pulmonary and renal;
- Combined injury—radiation plus other injury;
- Radionuclide internal contamination (for a select group of radionuclides); and
- Carcinogenesis and cataractogenesis and other late effects.[16,42]

Coordination among those developing medical products and those planning the response is critical so that the drugs deployed are compatible with the CONOPS and that the CONOPS be adapted to the extent possible so that an effective medical countermeasure can be deployed. For example, a drug that must be administered within a few hours of an IND would not be feasible. For agents that require administration within 24 hours of the exposure to be effective, ASPR is developing new models such as the UMI, described above. Updates on the opportunities and progress in medical countermeasure development can found on the websites from National Institute of Allergy and Infectious Diseases[16] and Biomedical Advanced Research and Development Authority.[43]

MEDICAL MANAGEMENT

A general outline of the sequence of events for medical management of a radiation event is:

- Ensuring safety of the operational field for responders and establishing security
- Initiating primary mass casualty triage
- Performing life-saving interventions on site
- Initiating secondary triage of victims to the appropriate venues
- Performing decontamination that does not interfere with life-saving treatment
- Estimating victim radiation dose via multiple means
- Initiation of potential medical countermeasures for those who need prompt attention
- Counseling those who need to return for additional evaluation for long-term effects

An RED or a nonexplosive RDD (Fig. 12-1) will not likely have a time-zero so that victims will present with symptoms of radiation injury and, as for an RDD of any type, concern of internal contamination. The initial injuries for an explosive RDD will be from the explosive device. For an IND, many people will be killed by the explosion and fireball, and many will have severe physical trauma and burns along with radiation from the initial

detonation and fallout. Of those who have only radiation exposure, most will be from the fallout where the time within the fallout and footprint zones will determine the total dose.

Contamination can be external from material on the victim or internal from inhalation, ingestion, or wound contamination. Radiation exposure comes from the initial flash of an IND and from the radiation emitted by radioactive material that comprises the fallout and footprint even though it may not actually come in contact with victims. The radiation dose received by a victim may be inhomogeneous with partial body shielding (e.g., by buildings) from the initial flash and by heterogeneous contamination. Exposure from the fallout and footprint may be heterogeneous and dose rate effects may reduce the medical consequences. Thus, history of victim location, victim symptoms and signs, and laboratory studies will be used to try to estimate the likelihood of a victim having received a sufficiently high enough dose of radiation so that the ARS may be possible.

The ARSs are organ-system based although it must be remembered that in significant whole body exposure, the physiological response results from the response of all the organs to radiation,[44] and medical management will require a suite of medical countermeasures along with excellent supportive care. Following exposure to radiation, there may be initial symptoms followed by a latency period in which the victim feels well followed by manifestation of organ injury. At higher exposure doses, there will be more initial symptoms, with a shorter the latency period (or none at all) and more severe organ dysfunction. The rapidly proliferating organ systems demonstrate the earliest effects with the hematological system being the most sensitive. There is dose-related lymphopenia shortly after exposure due to intermitotic apoptosis followed in a few days to weeks by neutropenia and thrombocytopenia. At a whole body or substantial body dose of 2 Gy, consideration is given to utilizing mitigators (bone marrow cytokines), and with a dose around 3.5 to 4 Gy, it is very likely that hospitalization will be needed. The LD_{50}, the dose at which half the people will die, is approximately 3.5 Gy; however, it may be 1 to 2 Gy higher with aggressive supportive care. Thus, while the use of mitigators may reduce the likelihood of developing cytopenia such that hospitalization may not be required, and may reduce risk of mortality, aggressive supportive care is *the most important* intervention for hematological ARS.

The next most sensitive organ but with shorter latency is the gastrointestinal tract. Rapid cell turnover of the gastrointestinal mucosa will lead to manifestation of the syndrome within a week when the dose is >6 Gy. At a very high dose, >10 Gy, there is the cerebrovascular syndrome characterized by major cardiovascular collapse by 24 to 48 hours. The cutaneous syndrome will occur at approximately 4 to 6 Gy with skin erythema and potentially skin denudation.

Clinicians should be aware that most of the information on ARS comes from Hiroshima and Nagasaki as well as more recent accidental and industrial exposures from events with a limited number of victims. A major mass casualty event will have more unknowns regarding dose rate, concomitant physical injury, comorbid conditions of victims, and mass panic so that the symptoms of radiation injury such as nausea and vomiting may not be reliable. There are few individuals worldwide with expertise and experience in treating radiation victims. As medical responders have access to expert advice, the approach taken by HHS was to work with the National Library of Medicine[22] to develop a just-in-time, web-based algorithm based response system, the REMM, targeted to medical responders.[23]

After 9/11, HHS OASPR recognized that as important as a radiation terrorist event would be (with an IND being a very high consequence but very low probability event), most medical responders would be unlikely to want to spend their limited professional education time and efforts in this area, given the pressing other priorities in their daily lives and the greater likelihood of other mass casualty scenarios. HHS sponsored the development of the REMM website with input from national and world-renowned experts. The system has undergone usability testing and is continuously updated. REMM is available on the web, as a down load to a laptop or home computer and as a PDA. There are management algorithms for exposure, contamination, both or neither. The numerous features include a dose calculator, a review of radionuclides of interest, a list of countermeasures with doses, decontamination information and videos, a dictionary and large bibliography, a large library of multimedia assets to teach complex radiation issues to clinicians without expertise Radiation Medicine, and a simple explanation of potential radiation mass casualty events, among other topics.

A key concept behind REMM is the importance of dose in medical management. For an IND, the initial triage is to place radiation victims into three broad categories based on their need for immediate treatment, treatment within the next few weeks, and no treatment for ARS:

- 4 Gy
- 2 to 4 Gy
- <2 Gy

Victims with combined injury with an estimated whole body radiation dose of >2 Gy will need ARS management[13] as combined injury lowers the threshold for illness and mortality compared to radiation exposure alone. It is acknowledged that there will be uncertainty in deciding into which category any patient belongs so that these dose groups are conservatively low. Following this initial field triage, secondary venue triage will also occur, based on symptoms, additional biodosimetry, and clinical evolution, including consideration of the European system.[45] The importance of RITN and the RTR/MEDMAP programs is that victims can be distributed throughout the state, region, or country so that expert care can be administered. For the ARS hematological syndrome, there will be a latency period of up to 3 to 4 weeks so that many patients can be managed as outpatients as is done in oncology care. Thus, the HHS CONOPS is being built around the use of REMM, RITN, NDMS, voluntary assistance, and a national response.[24]

This chapter does not cover the details of medical management that are available in REMM. Additional management guidelines are available from the CDC,[36] AFRRI,[17] REAC/TS,[46] and other sites, accessible from their own sites and/or with links to REMM.[23]

SUMMARY

Preparedness for response to a mass casualty radiation event requires a broad range of expertise. The medical planning is being done with consideration of key issues from basic science through to the delivery of care to many thousands of victims.

It is hoped, of course, that an actual response for a mass casualty event will never be needed. Nonetheless, radiation preparation efforts are likely to have benefits to nonterrorism applications, including cancer care.

The highlights of the HHS preparedness activities include:

- Radiological/nuclear preparation is part of All Hazards approach, so that models and plans can be used for other natural and man-made disasters.
- Medical response to the spectrum of potential radiation events is planned, including response for smaller industrial accidents.
- Radiation external exposure effects are dose-related
  - ARS and its subsyndromes—hematological, gastrointestinal, cutaneous, central nervous system
  - DEARE result from initial exposure but can have longer latency period. Thus, there is an "incubation period" during which intervention may mitigate clinical manifestations.
- Countermeasures for internal radiation contamination require mitigating the chemical effects of the radionuclide as well as its radiation effects, and each nuclide is different.
- Algorithm-based approach (like Advanced Cardiac Life Support) has been used to develop the CONOPS. This includes
  - The overall response using the Chain of Medical Response (from event to long-term follow-up)
  - Medical management for exposure, contamination and both (REMM)
- Emergency response will depend on physical infrastructure and the presence of radiation. A response system has been developed for radiation events:
  - **RTR** response model
  - PAGs are available and PARs are in preparation (may be available by publication time). These can be used to plan the activities of first responders.
- Victim dose is estimated by both physical dosimetry and biodosimetry (biomarkers)
  - The potential future development of a national Rad-LN must balance investment in current technique and developing technology and have a flexible model for surge capacity.
- Medical countermeasures may contain drugs that are used for other medical treatments (oncology/hematology). Dual-use agents are a key to the PHEMCE strategy.
  - Response will require a suite of medical countermeasures as radiation injury, and mass casualty events will produce multiorgan injury.
  - A major program is supported through the National Institutes of Allergy and Infectious Diseases.
  - The medical countermeasures have time-critical windows of efficacy so that the CONOPS and medical drug delivery must be closely linked.
  - The SNS will provide countermeasures and resources in support of the local/regional responders.
  - Novel models to facilitate countermeasure delivery are being developed such as the "UMI" in addition to the SNS and VMI.
- REMM provides just-in-time information and can be readily updated. This is the essential source of information (www.remm.nlm.gov). Readers are encouraged to download REMM and join the Listserv.
- Close collaboration within HHS and with interagency partners is essential part of our planning

- PHEMCE is coordinating HHS efforts of ASPR, CDC, FDA, and NIH.
- Other agencies closely involved are DHS, DOD, VA, DOE (REAC/TS), and USDA.

There are unique opportunities for scientists, physicists, and clinicians to participate in the range of activities at the federal, state, and local level (24,25) to enhance the science, preparedness, and confidence of the public and to provide active participants with a sense of contribution to society and the common good.

REFERENCES

1. Bell WC, Dallas C. Vulnerability of populations and the urban health care systems to nuclear weapon attack—examples from four American cities. *Int J Health Geogr.* 2007;6:5.
2. Carter AB, May MM, Perry WJ. Center for Strategic and International Studies, and the Massachusetts Institute of Technology. The day after: action following a nuclear blast in a U.S. City. *Washington Quart.* 2007;30:19–22.
3. National Response Framework. Available at: http://www.fema.gov/emergency/nrf/. Accessed November 24, 2008.
4. Emergency support functions. Available at: http://www.fema.gov/pdf/emergency/nrf/nrf-esf-intro.pdf. Accessed November 14, 2008.
5. National Incident Management System description. Available at: http://www.nrt.org/Production/NRT/NRTWeb.nsf/AllAttachmentsByTitle/SA-385aNIMS-90-web/$File/NIMS-90-web.pdf?OpenElement. Accessed November 14, 2008.
6. National Planning Scenarios. Available at: http://media.washingtonpost.com/wp-srv/nation/nationalsecurity/earlywarning/NationalPlanningScenariosApril2005.pdf. Accessed November 24, 2008.
7. National Security Presidential Directive 17, combat weapons of mass destruction. Available at: http://www.fas.org/irp/offdocs/nspd/nspd-17.html. Accessed November 3, 2008.
8. Global Initiative to combat nuclear terrorism, Department of State. Available at: http://www.state.gov/t/isn/c18406.htm. Accessed November 3, 2008.
9. Harper FT, Musolino SV, Wente WB. Realistic radiological dispersal device hazard boundaries and ramifications for early consequence management decisions. *Health Phys.* 2007;93(1):1–16.
10. Coleman CN, Blakely WF, Fike JR, et al. Molecular and cellular biology of moderate-dose (1–10 Gy) radiation and potential mechanisms of radiation protection: report of a workshop at Bethesda, Maryland, December 17–18, 2001. *Radiat Res.* 2003;159:812–834. Review.
11. Coleman CN, Stone HB, Alexander GA, et al. Education and training for radiation scientists: radiation research program and American Society of Therapeutic Radiology and Oncology Workshop, Bethesda, Maryland, May 12–14, 2003. *Radiat Res.* 2003;160:729–737.
12. Stone HB, Moulder JE, Coleman CN, et al. Models for evaluating agents intended for the prophylaxis, mitigation and treatment of radiation injuries. Report of an NCI Workshop, December 3–4, 2003. *Radiat Res.* 2004;162:711–728.
13. Waselenko JK, MacVittie TJ, Blakely WF, et al. Medical management of the acute radiation syndrome: recommendations of the Strategic National Stockpile Radiation Working Group. *Ann Intern Med.* 2004;140:1037–1051.
14. Coleman CN, Stone HB, Moulder JE, et al. Medicine. Modulation of radiation injury. *Science.* 2004;304:693–694.
15. Pellmar TC, Rockwell S; Radiological/Nuclear Threat Countermeasures Working Group. Priority list of research areas for radiological nuclear threat countermeasures. *Radiat Res.* 2005;163:115–123. Review.
16. NIAID Medical countermeasures against radiation and nuclear threats. Program of the National Institutes of Allergy and Infectious Diseases. Available at: http://www3.niaid.nih.gov/topics/radnuc/. Accessed November 14, 2008.
17. Armed Forces Radiobiology Research Institute. Available at: http://www.afrri.usuhs.mil/. Accessed November 14, 2008.
18. Mettler FA Jr, Voelz GL. Major radiation exposure—what to expect and how to respond. *N Engl J Med.* 2002;346:1554–1561.
19. Goans RE, Waselenko JK. Medical management of radiological casualties. *Health Phys.* 2005;89:505–512.
20. Office of the Assistant Secretary for Preparedness and Response. Available at: http://www.hhs.gov/aspr/. Accessed November 14, 2008.
21. Hrdina CM, Coleman CN, Bogucki S, et al. The "RTR" medical response system for nuclear and radiological mass casualty events: a functional TRiage-TRansport-TReatment medical response model. *J Prehospital Disaster Med.* 2009;24:167–78.
22. Bader JL, Nemhauser J, Chang F, et al. Radiation Event Medical Management (REMM): web site guidance for health care providers. *Prehosp Emerg Care.* 2008;12:1–11.
23. Radiation Event Medical Management, REMM. Available at: www.remm.nlm.gov. Accessed November 15, 2008.
24. Coleman CN, Hrdina C, Bader J, et al. Medical response to a radiological/nuclear event: Integrated Plan from the Office of the Assistant Secretary for Preparedness and Response, Department of Health and Human Services. *Ann Emerg Med.* 2009;53:213–222.
25. Coleman CN, Parker GW. Radiation terrorism: WHAT society needs from the radiobiology-radiation protection and radiation oncology communities. *J Radiol Prot.* 2009;29:159–69.
26. Interagency Monitoring and Assessment Center. Available at: https://eed.llnl.gov/sub-page.php?cat_id=4. Accessed November 14, 2008.
27. Protective Action Recommendations: Planning Guidance for Response to a Nuclear Detonation. Under review.
28. National Disaster Medical System. Available at: http://www.hhs.gov/aspr/opeo/ndms/index.html. Accessed November 24, 2008.
29. Radiation Injury Treatment Network. http://bloodcell.transplant.hrsa.gov/ABOUT/RITN/index.html. Accessed November 14, 2008.
30. Weinstock DM, Case C Jr, Bader JL, et al. Radiologic and nuclear events: contingency planning for hematologists/oncologists. *Blood.* 2008;111:540–545.
31. Center for Disease Control and Prevention: Strategic National Stockpile. Available at: http://www.bt.cdc.gov/Stockpile/. Accessed November 14, 2008.
32. Emergency Medical Assistance Compact. Available at: http://www.emacweb.org/. Accessed November 14, 2008.
33. START triage system. Available at: http://www.start-triage.com/. Accessed November 24, 2008.
34. JumpSTART triage system. Available at: http://www.jumpstarttriage.com/. Accessed November 24, 2008.
35. Emergency System for Advanced Registration of Volunteer Health Professionals (ESAR-VHP). Available at: http://www.medicalreservecorps.gov/File/2008_NLC/DayThree/JenniferHannah.pdf. Accessed November 24, 2008.
36. Center for Disease Control and Prevention—Radiation Studies Branch. Available at *http://www.cdc.gov/nceh/radiation/.* Accessed November 24, 2008.
37. Planning Guidance for Protection and Recovery Following Radiological Dispersal Device (RDD) and Improvised Nuclear Device (IND) Incidents. Available at: http://www.fema.gov/good_guidance/download/10260. Accessed November 14, 2008.
38. Fliedner TM, Chao NJ, Bader JL, et al. Approaches to radiation emergency medical preparedness and assistance: A US/European Consultation Workshop. *Stem Cells.* 2009;27:1205–11.
39. Grace MB, Moyer BR, Ramakrishan N, et al. Rapid radiation dose assessment for radiological public health emergencies: roles of NIAID, BARDA and the FDA. BioDose 2008 meeting Health Physics (submitted), 2010;98:172–78.
40. Grace MB, Moyer BR, Prasher JM, et al. The U.S. Government's medical countermeasure portfolio for nuclear and radiological emergencies: synergy from interagency cooperation. *Health Phys.* (submitted).
41. Public Health Emergency Medical Countermeasures Enterprise. Available at: http://www.hhs.gov/aspr/barda/phemce/index.html. Accessed November 15, 2008.
42. The 2007 HHS PHEMCE Implementation Plan for CBRN Threats. Available at: http://www.hhs.gov/aspr/barda/phemce/strategy. Accessed November 15, 2008.
43. Biomedical Advanced Research and Development Authority. Available at: http://www.hhs.gov/aspr/barda/index.html. Accessed November 15, 2008.
44. Bertho JM, Roy L, Souidi M, et al. New biological indicators to evaluate and monitor radiation-induced damage. *Radiat Res.* 2008;169:543–550.
45. Fliedner TM, Friesecke I, Beyer K, eds. *Medical Management of Radiation Accidents: Manual on the Acute Radiation Syndrome.* Oxford: British Institute of Radiology; 2001.
46. Radiation Emergency Assistance Center/Training Site at Oak Ridge Institute for Science and Education. Available at: http://orise.orau.gov/reacts/. Accessed November 24, 2008.

Francis A. Cucinotta

Radiation Effects of Space Travel

INTRODUCTION

Space radiation is a major limitation for long-term space travel.[1-4] There are two sources of radiation in space: the galactic cosmic rays (GCR) and solar particle events (SPEs). The GCR comprise protons, helium, and high energy and charge (HZE) nuclei along with secondary radiation, including neutrons and recoil nuclei, produced by nuclear reactions in spacecraft or tissue.[2] The product of the particle fluence (F) by the linear energy transfer (LET) is the absorbed dose ($D = F \times \text{LET}$ in units of Gray [Gy]), and when weighted by a relative biological effectiveness (RBE) factor or quality factor (QF), a biological dose equivalent is defined ($H = D \times \text{QF}$ in units of Sievert [Sv]). HZE nuclei are characterized as high LET radiation, which have a large RBE to γ rays. There are important questions about the validity of a scaling approach based on RBEs for GCR because of possible unique biological damage from HZE nuclei. SPEs consist of low-to-high energy protons (up to several hundred MeV) that are effectively absorbed by shielding; however, the time of onset of SPEs is difficult to predict. Radiation protection for space travel has several unique considerations compared to Earth-based radiation protection.[5] The types of radiation and lack of human epidemiology data thereof, which leads to large uncertainties in risk projection models, are the most critical differences, especially for longer space missions. The goals of space travel and the small population of individuals selected to participate in space missions are also important considerations.

Effective doses from GCR of up to 2 mSv/day accumulate in interplanetary space, and approximately half this value on planetary surfaces or in low Earth orbit (LEO).[2,3] Figure 13.1 shows the badge dosimetry values from all past NASA missions along with tissue-weighted effective doses for astronauts.[7] Also shown are biodosimetry results from astronauts returning from the International Space Station (ISS) or Russian Mir space station and projections for a 1,000-day Mars mission. Spaceflight in LEO, such as 6-month ISS missions, is partially protected by the Earth's magnetic field and the solid shielding of the planet. GCR and SPE interact with the Earth's atmosphere and magnetospheres to produce the trapped radiation often called the Van Allen belts[5,6] as discovered by James Van Allen in 1958. Astronauts on ISS missions have average effective doses of 80 mSv,[7] much higher exposures than Earth-based radiation workers (nuclear power plants, hospitals, accelerators, etc.) and the uncertainties due to the type of radiation in space are a large safety concern. In future, missions away from the Earth's protection of duration from 2 to 3 years

for Mars exploration would result in cumulative GCR exposures of >1 Sv and upper 95% confidence intervals for fatal cancer of >10% are estimated.[3,8] At this time, it is not clear if such exposures would prevent long-term space travel due to both safety and costs. Many scientific gaps related to risk estimation and mitigation approaches must be addressed through research to support a mission decision. Space radiation risks include cancer, acute radiation sickness (ARS), and degenerative risks to the central nervous system (CNS) and heart, and cataracts. NASA has set radiation limits for each of these risks and supports radiobiology research to understand and mitigate risks for future space missions.

RADIATION PROTECTION AT NASA

Because of the types of radiation in space and the possibility of prolonged (chronic) irradiation over many months, the concepts used for risk projection on Earth must be modified. In 1989, the NCRP Report No. 98[6] recommended that NASA use age- and gender-dependent career dose limits based on a common excess risk limit of 3% risk of fatal cancer. The limiting level of 3% risk was based on several criteria including comparison to dose

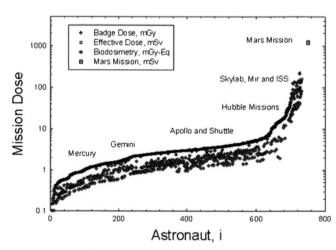

Figure 13.1. Summary of mission badge dose, effective dose, and population average biological dose equivalent for astronauts on all NASA space missions, including Mercury, Gemini, Apollo, Skylab, Apollo-Soyuz, Space Shuttle, NASA-Mir space station, and ISS missions. Also shown is estimate for Mars mission. (Redrawn from Cucinotta FA, Kim MH, Willingham V, et al. Physical and biological organ dosimetry analysis for International Space Station astronauts. *Radiat Res.* 2008;170:127–138.)

TABLE 13.1	Career Effective Dose Limits for 1-year Missions	
	E(mSv) for a 3% REID (Average Life-loss per Death, yr)	
Age at Exposure, yr	*Males*	*Females*
30	620 (15.7)	470 (15.7)
35	720 (15.4)	550 (15.3)
40	800 (15.0)	620 (14.7)
45	950 (14.2)	750 (14.0)
50	1150 (12.5)	920 (13.2)
55	1470 (11.5)	1120 (12.2)

limits for ground radiation workers and to rates of occupational death in the so-called less-safe industries such as deep sea fishing and mining. It was noted[6] that astronauts face many other risks, and adding a large radiation risk was not justified. The average years of life loss from low LET radiation–induced cancer death is about 15 years for workers of age 40 years.[5] Studies for tumor induction in small animals suggest an earlier appearance of cancer for high LET radiation compared to low LET radiation.[2,5] A comparison of radiation-induced cancer deaths to cancer fatalities in the US population is also complex because of the smaller years of life loss from cancers in the general population where most cancer deaths occur above age 70 years.

Age- and gender-dependent dose to fatal cancer risk conversions are updated by NASA as new information is obtained.[8,9] Table 13.1 shows the current age at exposure and gender-dependent limits. Lifetime cancer risks limits are calculated in terms of the quantity Risk of Exposure-Induced Death (REID) with the acceptable risk limit up to a 3% REID. The REID differs from increased cancer risk by counting radiation deaths that would occur anyway in a population but occurring at an earlier age due to radiation exposure. New risk estimates based on the BEIRV VII[10] and UNSCEAR[11] reports are being evaluated at this time, which is compared in Table 13.2 for the case of 6-month stays on the Earth's moon. Uncertainties at the 95% confidence level would exceed the 3% risk limit level in several cases for such lunar missions. Age is the most critical factor in the current model based on the NCRP Report No. 132[5] and the UNSCEAR model.[11]

However, the BEIR VII model[10] ignores any dependence of age at exposure dependence for exposures over age 30 years, with the exception for the reduction in radiation risks that occurs late in life due to nonradiation causes of death as described by a life table. In design studies at NASA, selecting astronauts for older age at exposure (50 years or more) is cost effective to reduce mission risks compared to adding radiation shielding or shortening mission length. Therefore, understanding the biology of the age dependence of cancer risk is a vital concern.

Additional radiation limits for clinically significant noncancer effects are also followed by NASA as described by Table 13.3. The method used for evaluating the equivalent dose for noncancer effects[5] is similar to cancer; however, it uses the unit of "Gy-equivalent" to distinguish effective doses based on RBE for noncancer effects from those based on Q-values to be used for estimating cancer risks. Because RBEs for noncancer effects may depend on dose, the RBE used for specifying the Gy-equivalent are the values determined at the threshold dose for the noncancer effect being evaluated. Noncancer risks considered are cataracts, skin damage, and CNS and heart disease risks. A limit to the exposure to the blood forming organs (BFO) ensures that severe harm to the blood system does not occur and also is protective against the prodromal risks. Information on noncancer late effects is very immature and it is difficult to project how such risks depend on radiation quality and dose rate, or if dose thresholds occur. The severity of the risks is also an important consideration when compared to the risk of cancer death.

TABLE 13.2	Estimates of the % of REID for Cancer and 95% Confidence Intervals for a 180-day Mission to the Earth's Moon		
Age, yr	*Current NASA Model*	*UNSCEAR*	*BEIR-VII*
MALES			
35	0.71 [0.21, 2.6]	0.86 [0.25, 3.2]	0.68 [0.28, 2.5]
45	0.53 [0.16, 2.0]	0.66 [0.19, 2.5]	0.65 [0.27, 2.4]
55	0.36 [0.11, 1.35]	0.48 [0.14, 1.8]	0.60 [0.25, 2.2]
FEMALES			
35	0.86 [0.25, 3.2]	1.19 [0.35, 4.4]	0.96 [0.4, 3.5]
45	0.64 [0.19, 2.4]	0.86 [0.25, 3.2]	0.92 [0.38, 3.4]
55	0.43 [0.13, 1.6]	0.57 [0.17, 2.1]	0.83 [0.35, 3.1]

Results are for solar minimum for males and females of different ages behind 20 g/cm² aluminum shields. Comparisons are made of the current model of radiation mortality rates used at NASA as recommended by the NCRP,[5] and recommendations from the BEIRVII[10] and UNSCEAR reports.[11] Confidence intervals are calculated as described in Ref. 8.

TABLE 13.3	Dose Limits for Short-term or Career Noncancer Effects (in mGy-Eq or mGy)		
Organ	*30-day Limit*	*1-Yr Limit*	*Career Limit*
Lens[a]	1,000 mGy-Eq	2,000 mGy-Eq	4,000 mGy-Eq
Skin	1,500	3,000	6,000
BFO	250	500	Not applicable
Heart[b]	250	500	1,000
CNS[c]	500	1,000	1,500
CNS[c] ($Z \geq 10$)	—	100 mGy	250 mGy

[a]Lens limits are intended to prevent early (<5 year) severe cataracts (e.g., from a SPE). An additional cataract risk exists at lower doses from cosmic rays for subclinical cataracts, which may progress to severe types after long latency (>5 year) and are not preventable by existing mitigation measures; however, they are deemed an acceptable risk to the program.
[b]Heart doses calculated as average over heart muscle and adjacent arteries.
[c]CNS limits should be calculated at the hippocampus.

Only a few persons are selected for space travel and they will incur many occupational risks due to possible failure of rocket launch, life support, and Earth atmosphere re-entry systems. Other health risks of concern are bone loss due to microgravity and psychological effects. Astronauts undergo a rigorous selection process to ensure their competence for a wide range of mission performance capabilities. Astronaut selection for radiation resistance has not been considered in the past or current space programs; however, if the ability to make such determinations becomes possible, it would be debated as a method to lower mission costs and risks. It is unlikely that mechanisms that confer radiation sensitivity for high doses (>1 Gy) of low LET radiation will carry over unamended for considering risks for high LET radiation or low dose-rate exposures because distinct biological response mechanisms occur.

UNCERTAINTIES

NASA has recognized the importance of the uncertainties in risk projection models for radiation exposure, and uncertainty assessment is a requirement for mission design optimization and radiation protection. Mission safety can only be predicted within a defined confidence level, corresponding to the statistical nature of such a calculation. Large uncertainties limit the value of a median projection or so-called point estimate of risk. Radiation limits have been implemented at NASA based on the NCRP recommendations[5] for organ dose methodologies and point estimates for cancer risks; however, NASA applies these with an ancillary requirement to protect against the upper bound of the 95% confidence level of the risk projection calculated by propagation of the errors in factors that enter the projection models. In support of the principle of As Low As Reasonably Achievable, mission design and operations must include cost versus benefit analyses of approaches to improve crew safety with higher confidence. Such analyses are often limited by the uncertainties in risk projections because the benefit of mitigation measures cannot be adequately stated if uncertainties are large.

Figure 13.2 illustrates the current estimates of uncertainty factors that enter risk projection models and the wide range uncertainty bands for different types of radiation exposure. Estimates of the uncertainties for cancer risk from low LET

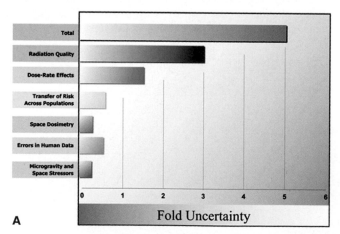

A

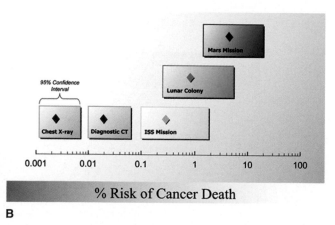

B

Figure 13.2. Uncertainties in space and terrestrial radiation exposures.[3] Panel (**A**) presents estimates of uncertainties in projecting cancer risks for space and terrestrial exposures. Several factors such as radiation quality effects, space physics, and microgravity do not contribute on Earth and lead to large increases in risk projections. Predicting risks to individuals is difficult as there are very few quantitative measures of individual sensitivity. Only a select few individuals enjoy space travel and projecting risks for individuals rather than populations will be of utmost importance for space missions to Mars. The extrapolation from experimental models to humans is perhaps the greatest challenge to cancer risk assessments. The uncertainties are larger for astronauts in space compared to typical exposures on Earth as illustrated in panel (**B**), which shows the current estimates of cancer risks and 95% confidence bands for adults of age 40 years, the typical age of astronauts on space missions for several terrestrial exposures and missions on the ISS, a lunar colony, and the projections for a Mars mission.

radiation, such as x-rays and γ-rays, have been reviewed several times in recent years and indicate that the major uncertainty is the extrapolation of cancer effects data from high to low dose rates.[10,12] Other projection model uncertainties include the transfer of risk across populations and sources of error in epidemiology data including dosimetry, bias, and statistical ones. Major uncertainties are predicting the cancer risks from the protons and heavy ions and secondary radiation in space, and in space dosimetry.[2,3] The limited understanding of the radiobiology of HZE nuclei has been estimated to be the largest contributor to the uncertainty for space radiation effects.[1,3] SPEs present distinct challenges since their time of onset, size, and spectral characteristics cannot be predicted reliably.[13] SPE challenges include specifying mission design criteria based on a well-defined worse case[14] and the development of real-time response models.

SPACE RADIATION ENVIRONMENTS

The GCR comprise protons, helium, and HZE nuclei along with secondary radiation including neutrons and high LET recoil nuclei, produced by nuclear reactions in spacecraft or tissue. Most cosmic rays probably originate in our galaxy, especially in supernova explosions,[2] although the highest energy components ($\geq 10^{17}$ eV amu^{-1}) are of extragalactic origin. The particle composition of the GCR is about 88% protons, 9% helium ions, and 3% heavy ions.[2] The energy spectrum of the GCR has a median value near 1,000 MeV/nucleon, and consequently these particles are so penetrating that shielding can only partially reduce the doses absorbed by the crew. Therefore, current shielding approaches cannot be considered a solution for the space radiation problem with the exception of SPEs, which are effectively absorbed by shielding.

The sun's 11-year solar cycle modulates GCR doses by about twofold over the course of a solar cycle[15] with the lowest doses occurring at solar maximum when the solar wind is strongest. The solar wind is a plasma of both positive and negative particles trapped in a magnetic field emanating from the Sun. The solar wind is really an extension of the solar corona to at least several astronomical units from the Sun (1 AU ≈ 1.5×10^8 km). It is composed mostly of protons and persists through variable parts of the quiet Sun's output. A solar flare is an intense local brightening on the face of the Sun close to a sunspot. The solar abnormality results in an alteration of the general outflow of solar plasma at moderate energies and local solar magnetic fields carried by that plasma. As the solar plasma envelops the Earth, the magnetic screening effects inherent in plasmas act to shield the Earth from GCR (this is known as a Forbush decrease), while contributing far more radiation of their own. When the solar plasma interacts with the geomagnetic field, a disturbance or storm occurs. During an intense magnetic disturbance, the Earth's magnetic fields, that is, the Van Allen radiation belts, are compressed into the Earth's atmosphere in polar regions, and trapped electrons in the belt are lost.

In association with many of the optical flares occurring from time to time on the solar surface, large fluxes of solar energetic particles are sometimes accelerated and emitted, and these emissions of solar cosmic radiation are designated SPEs. SPEs with periods of several hours to days represent one of several short-lived manifestations of the active Sun. At solar maximum, the probability of SPEs increases with five to ten proton events

per year occurring with little warning. The solar wind and SPEs are composed of the same types of particles, mostly protons with the next significant component being helium nuclei. These two groups of particles are distinguished by their numbers and their speed or energy. Heavier nuclei, mostly in the carbon, nitrogen, and oxygen group, have also been observed from major SPEs. Kim et al.[14] have considered the nearly 400 SPEs observed in the space age and data on large SPEs inferred from ice-core samples since 1450. Figure 13.3 shows results where the BFO dose is plotted versus the integral fluence of protons with energies about 100 MeV from the largest historical events. Tolerance levels are also shown based on the variability of the energy spectra of protons from event to event. Lethal doses are not plausible when adequate shielding of 5 cm or more are provided for protection.

SPACE RADIOBIOLOGY

The initial biophysical events caused by HZE tracks in cells and tissue differ from other types of radiation such as γ-rays or α particles leading to different biological risks. For the particles composing space radiation, energy deposition is highly localized along the trajectory of each particle with lateral diffusion of energetic electrons (δ-rays) away from the nuclei's path. In deep space, δ-rays from HZE nuclei and protons traverse each cell in space about once per day.[16] The rate of energy deposition per unit length of a particle trajectory is described by the LET. The unit generally used in radiobiology for LET is the kiloelectron volt per micrometer, or keV/μm. The LET of charged particles changes as a function of the particle velocity, β or kinetic energy, and its charge, Z approximately in proportion to Z^2/β^2. As the velocity (or the energy) of a particle increases, the LET decreases to a minimum near a velocity of approximately 90% of the speed of light; at higher energies, the LET increases very slowly due to relativistic effects. High-energy charged particles lose energy when they traverse any material. As they slow

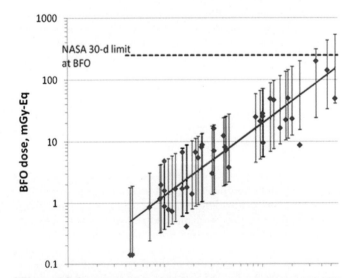

Figure 13.3. BFO dose versus integral fluence of solar protons with energy more than 100 MeV, Φ_{100} for the historically largest SPEs. Calculations assume shielding by a 15 g/cm^2 sphere polyethylene in interplanetary space. The best linear fit regression line is shown, along with 90% tolerance limits. The current NASA 30-day limit at BFO is shown as the horizontal dashed line.

down, the LET increases to a maximum and then very rapidly decreases to zero. The low-energy maximum in LET occurs very close to the point where the charged particle loses its remaining energy and stops. Nuclear fragmentation and other nuclear interactions, including projectile fragmentation of the primary ion and target fragmentation of tissue constituents, occur as ions traverse tissue. For proton and HZE nuclei irradiation, target fragmentation, including secondary neutron production, introduces an additional high LET component into the radiation field.[17]

Oxidative damage to DNA and non-DNA targets in the cell nucleus, cytoplasm, or extracellular matrix varies with LET. For example, yields of OH$^-$ and aqueous electrons, e$^-_{aq}$ decrease with increasing LET, while yields of H_2O_2 and H_2 increase with increasing LET.[18] These differences in the types and spatial distribution of oxidative species that change with radiation quality are expressed in distinctions in the types and complexity of DNA damage that occurs and in signaling cascades that respond to oxidative damage such as TGFβ and the ERK signal transduction pathways. The effectiveness of radioprotectors or pharmaceutical countermeasures that act as antioxidants could also be impacted by such differences in the types and spatial dependence of oxidative species for different radiation qualities.

Biophysical models have shown that the energy deposition events by high LET radiation produce differential DNA lesions, including complex DNA breaks, and that there are qualitative differences between high- and low-LET radiation both in the induction and repair of DNA damage. The number of DNA single-strand breaks (SSB) and double-strand breaks (DSB) produced by radiation varies little with radiation type; however, for high-LET radiation, a higher fraction of DNA damages are complex, that is, clusters containing mixtures of two or more of the various types of damages (SSB, DSB, etc.) within a localized region of DNA.[19] Complex damage is uncommon for endogenous damage or low-LET radiation and has been associated with the increased RBE of densely ionizing radiation. The repair of DSB is known to occur through direct end-joining and homologous recombination processes. For high-LET radiation, where complex DSB occur with high frequency, repair is often incomplete leading to cell death and the misrejoining of unrepairable ends with other radiation-induced DSB leads to large DNA deletions and simple and complex chromosome aberrations.[2,3]

ACUTE RISKS

For SPEs, dose rates are in the low-to-intermediate range (<0.5 Gy/h) and large variations of organ doses at different tissue sites occur, even for the largest SPEs. These factors significantly reduce the probability of severe damage to the BFO system or acute death. Therefore, the major acute risks of concern for SPE are the prodromal effects also called ARS with components including nausea, vomiting, fatigue, and reduced performance.[20] SPE doses of >0.1 Gy are extremely improbable in LEO due to the protection of the Earth's magnetic field and are not a concern for ISS missions. The highest ARS concern is for lunar missions[20] where extensive time outside of a habitat is likely or in transit to or from Mars. The Mars atmosphere is equivalent to about 20 cm of CO_2 shielding providing protection from ARS on the Mars surface. SPEs attenuate quickly in

tissue; however, very high skin doses are possible from a large SPE that could compromise immune defense mechanisms. Other space factors including microgravity, sleep deprivation, altered circadian rhythms, and reduced access to medical care are a concern in estimating ARS risks.

The ratio of skin to deep-seated organ doses for solar protons may vary up to 10-fold with average values of about twofold behind shielding. This variation is more extreme than for γ-rays and introduces uncertainties in the risks of ARS from available human data or experimental studies in animals. Reduced dose rates are known to be sparring for blood system damage; however, it is not clear how the different specific components of ARS are modulated at lower dose rates or if cumulative dose is the determinant on outcome for SPE exposures that most likely occur with 1 to 2 days.[20]

CANCER RISKS

Animal studies generally demonstrate that HZE nuclei have a higher carcinogenic effectiveness than low-LET radiation. RBEs have been measured for a small number of HZE nuclei types or LETs in mice or rats for tumors of the skin, liver, and of Harderian or mammary gland, and with values as high as 25 to 40 observed for iron nuclei.[21–23] The risk and detriment of cancer is not fully characterized until the relationship between radiation quality and latency, where tumors appear earlier after high-LET irradiation, is adequately described. Recent studies have debated the relative importance of DNA damage and mutation or extracellular matrix remodeling and other so-called nontargeted effects (NTE) as initiators of carcinogenesis. Tissue effects independent of DNA damage that have been associated with cancer initiation or progression include genomic instability,[24] extracellular matrix remodeling,[25] persistent inflammation, and oxidative damage.

NTE including bystander effects and genomic instability in the progeny of irradiated cells are a major interest in radiation protection challenging the traditional paradigm of dose responses that increase linearly with dose with no threshold as motivated by a DNA mutation mechanism or other targeted DNA effects (TE). Evidence for NTE is more extensive for high LET radiation than for low LET; however, it has largely been observed in cell culture models.[24] Studies of genomic instability in mice support NTE models[25]; however, it has proven difficult to directly observe NTE on tumor induction in mice or other species. Bystander experiments *in vitro* suggest that NTE may occur with a shallow or nearly constant dose response above a very low dose threshold (<0.01 Gy).

Tumor response data in mice irradiated with HZE nuclei are best described by an NTE model at low dose.[26] Figure 13.4 shows comparison of the NTE model to the data of Alpen et al.[21] plotted as tumor prevalence versus the number of ions per cell nucleus. The dose-response for iron nuclei is similar to found for other tissues and rodents, and shows that at a fluence of less than one iron nuclei per 100 cells can more than double the tumor incidence. The RBE in the NTE model for an ion of dose D_I continues to increase with decreasing dose and can be represented by the equation:

$$RBE_{NTE} = RBE_{NTE}\left(1 + \frac{D_{cr}}{D_I}\right)$$

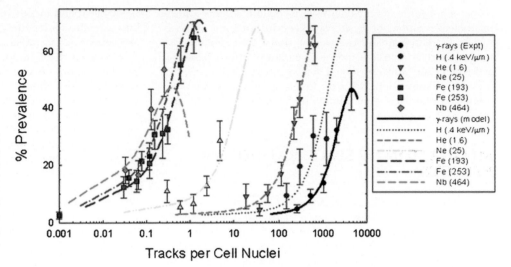

Figure 13.4. Comparison of NTE model to experiments for prevalence of Harderian gland tumors[21] versus the number of radiation tracks (ions) per cell nuclei (cell diameter of 5.5 μm) from Cucinotta and Chappell.[26] Error bars represent standard errors. For γ-rays, a mean LET of 0.23 keV/μm is used to convert dose to number of radiation tracks.

where D_{cr} is the dose where the TE and NTE are equal and estimated to be in the range from 0.05 to 0.2 Gy for heavy ions.[26] RBEs in the NTE model increase as the dose is decreased and become much higher than the TE model at the dose of interest for space travel. The shape of the tumor response curve and RBE values found in the NTE model have important implications for space travel because the shallow nonlinear dose responses predicted at GCR heavy ion dose rates (<0.2 Gy/yr) would alter how mission design factors such as duration and radiation shielding are analyzed for radiation protection purposes.

CNS RISKS

Acute and late CNS risks from space radiation are of concern for space exploration missions to the moon or Mars. Acute CNS risks include altered cognitive function, reduced motor function, and behavioral changes, all of which may affect performance and human health. Late CNS risks are possible neurological disorders such as Alzheimer disease, dementia, or premature aging. The possibility of HZE nuclei causing CNS damage at low dose was noted after the Apollo astronauts observed light flashes during dark adaptation.[27] These visual sensations are related to the passage of HZE particles through the retina, or proton-induced nuclear interactions in the eye. The microlesion concept considers stochastic tissue events that occur to columns of damaged cells along the path of HZE nuclei and the possibility of unique types of tissue damage occurring even at low doses. Microlesion formation is of special concern for damage to the CNS, where fully differentiated structures are present.[6] However, it could also play a role in increased effectiveness for HZE nuclei in highly structured tissues.

CNS effects[1,2] that have been observed in animal models include altered motor function or performance,[28] accelerated striatal aging,[29] late degradation of DNA,[30] altered dopamine function,[28] and neurodegeneration.[2,31] The Casarett model[32] predicts that the appearance of late degenerative effects to the CNS and other tissues could be advanced by many years after radiation exposure in what has been called "radiation accelerated aging." This effect would have an increasing severity with increasing HZE fluence or dose, and appears to be relevant

in describing the increased incidence of cataracts observed in astronauts exposed to moderate doses of space radiation.[33]

Accumulating data indicate that radiation not only affects differentiated neural cells, but also the proliferation and differentiation of neuronal precursor cells and adult neuronal stem cells. Recent evidence points out that neuronal progenitor cells are sensitive to radiation with LET and dose-dependent responses (reviewed in Ref. 2). Studies on low-LET radiation show that radiation stops not only the generation of neuronal progenitor cells, but also their differentiation into neurons and other neural cells. Studies with HZE nuclei of activated microglia indicate that changes in neurogenesis are associated with a significant dose-dependent inflammatory response even 2 months after irradiation.[2] Such studies suggest that the pathogenesis of radiation-induced cognitive injury may involve loss of neural precursor cells from the subgranular zone (SGZ) of the hippocampal dentate gyrus and alterations in neurogenesis.[2] Further research is necessary to quantify the significance of such studies to humans and to further define radiation quality, dose, and dose-rate dependencies.

DEGENERATIVE TISSUE RISKS

An increased occurrence of cataracts has been documented in astronauts returning from past space missions including Apollo, Skylab, and space shuttle missions.[33,34] The increased risks were observed at much lower doses than would be expected from low LET studies with significant relative risk factors of >2 at space lens dose equivalents as low as 8 mSv. Posterior subcapsular and cortical cataracts are most often associated with radiation exposure. The formation of these two types of cataracts appears to be associated with space irradiation according to NASA study.[34] The low dose with no or very low dose threshold estimated for space radiation cataract risks suggests a stochastic effect originating from a small number of damaged cells or small region of tissue. However, the clinical significance of cataracts requires further study to understand their importance in radiation protection.[35]

More recently, results from human epidemiology studies of several cohorts have raised a concern for increased risks of heart disease at low dose.[11] Little et al.[36] provide a comprehensive review of the data and perform a meta-analysis to estimate the excess relative risk for coronary heart disease and stroke among the atomic-bomb survivors, and several cohorts of nuclear weapons or reactor workers. Information on dose-rate and radiation quality is extremely sparse for estimating risk to the heart. A plausible model of radiation effects based on arthrosclerosis[37] suggests several mechanisms including cell killing and inflammation. RBEs or dose-rate modifiers in experimental systems are largely undefined for heart disease risks from space radiation.[2]

MITIGATION OF SPACE RADIATION EFFECTS

The understanding of countermeasures (including shielding) to space radiation risks is hindered at this time because the large uncertainties in risk projection models indicate a lack of mechanistic understanding and data for assessing the possible need or effectiveness of countermeasures for specific space missions. GCR nuclei of average energy can penetrate a substantial thickness of materials, on the order of 10s to 100s of centimeters of water or aluminum. If they suffer nuclear interactions, the lighter secondary products will lose energy at a lower rate and therefore will be able to penetrate even further. For this reason, it is not possible to provide sufficient material to fully absorb all types of radiation in space. In addition, the relative effectiveness of nuclei will change as a function of depth of penetration, because the composition of the nuclei changes and because the LET of each nuclei changes as it loses energy and slows down inside the material. Hydrogen-rich materials are the most efficient for both GCR and SPE because they are more efficient per unit mass in slowing down ions and producing little secondary radiation. Inaccuracies in risk assessment models prevent the proper evaluation of shielding amounts and types, thus reducing the ability of NASA to apply cost-benefit analysis to shielding evaluations.

Biological countermeasures will be difficult to assess for space radiation effects because more than one risk occurs and there are potential interactions between acute and late effect protection mechanisms. Dietary antioxidants and anti-inflammatory drugs are expected to provide risk reduction for low LET radiation delivered at high dose and dose rate; however, their effectiveness at low dose rates and for high LET radiation is less clear. Phosphorothioates and other aminothiols, which are usually administered shortly before irradiation, are effective in tissue protection against ionizing radiation, with the compound ethyol (also known as amifostine or WR-2721) approved in many countries for clinical use during chemotherapy and radiotherapy cancer treatments.[38,39] Unfortunately, amifostine and other thiols have significant side effects, including nausea, vomiting, vasodilatation, and hypotension. The use of these compounds in space flights for protection against chronic exposure to cosmic radiation is not likely. Dietary supplements maybe ineffective or cause harm,[40] while naturally occurring antioxidants are less effective than phosphorothioate agents in protection against high-dose acute radiation burden. Nutritional antioxidants have a low toxicity, can be used for prolonged time, and they seem to play a key role in the prevention of cancer. However, the storage of such foods for long-term space flights is an unsolved technology problem. Retinoids and vitamins (A, C, and E) are well known and studied natural radioprotectors.[4] Hormones (e.g., melatonin), glutathione, superoxide dismutase, phytochemicals from plant extracts (including green tea and cruciferous

vegetables), and metals (especially selenium, zinc, and copper salts) are also under study as dietary supplements for individuals overexposed to radiation.[4]

Effectiveness of antioxidants in space is further complicated by the presence of HZE nuclei. In principle, antioxidants should provide reduced or no protection against densely ionizing radiation, because direct effect is more important than free radicals–mediated indirect radiation damage at high LET. However, some recent experiments suggest that an efficient radioprotection by dietary supplements can be achieved even in case of exposure to high-LET radiation. Ascorbate reduces the frequency of mutations in human-hamster hybrid cells exposed to high-LET C-ions.[41] Vitamin A strongly reduces the induction of fibroma in rats exposed to swift Fe ions.[42] Dietary supplementation with Bowan-Birk protease inhibitors, L-selenomethionine, or a combination of selected antioxidant agents[2] is also of potential benefit.

REFERENCES

1. National Academy of Sciences (NAS). National Academy of Sciences Space Science Board, Report of the Task Group on the Biological Effects of Space Radiation. *Radiation Hazards to Crews on Interplanetary Missions.* Washington, DC: National Academy of Sciences; 1996.
2. National Council on Radiation Protection and Measurements, Information needed to make radiation protection recommendations for space missions beyond Low-Earth Orbit. *NCRP Report No. 153,* Bethesda MD: NCRP; 2006.
3. Cucinotta FA, Durante M. Cancer risk from exposure to galactic cosmic rays: implications for space exploration by human beings. *Lancet Oncol.* 2006;7:431–435.
4. Durante M, Cucinotta FA. Heavy ion carcinogenesis and human space exploration. *Nature Rev Cancer.* 2008;8:465–472.
5. National Council on Radiation Protection and Measurements, Recommendations of Dose Limits for Low Earth Orbit. *NCRP Report 132.* Bethesda MD: NCRP; 2000.
6. National Council on Radiation Protection and Measurements (NCRP). Guidance on radiation received in space activities. *NCRP Report 98.* Bethesda MD: NCRP; 1989.
7. Cucinotta FA, Kim MH, Willingham V, et al. Physical and biological organ dosimetry analysis for International Space Station astronauts. *Radiat Res.* 2008;170:127–138.
8. Cucinotta FA, Kim MY, Ren L. Evaluating shielding effectiveness for reducing space radiation cancer risks. *Radiat Meas.* 2006;41:1173–1185.
9. Preston DL, Shimizu Y, Pierce DA, et al. Studies of mortality of atomic bomb survivors. report 13: solid cancer and non-cancer disease mortality: 1950–1997. *Radiat Res.* 2003;160:381–407.
10. National Academy of Sciences Committee on the Biological Effects of Radiation, BEIR-VII. *Health Risks from Exposure to Low Levels of Ionizing Radiation.* Washington, DC: National Academy of Sciences Press; 2006.
11. United Nations Scientific Committee on the Effects of Atomic Radiation, Sources and Effects of Ionizing Radiation. *UNSCEAR 2006 Report to the General Assembly, with Scientific Annexes.* New York: United Nations; 2006.
12. National Council on Radiation Protection and Measurements (NCRP). Uncertainties in fatal cancer risk estimates used in radiation protection. *NCRP Report 126.* Bethesda MD: NCRP; 1997.
13. National Research Council (NRC) Aeronautics and Engineering Board. *Managing Space Radiation Risk in the New Era of Space Exploration.* Washington, DC: National Academies Press; 2008.
14. Kim MY, Hayat MJ, Feiveson AH, et al. Prediction of frequency and exposure level of solar particle events. *Health Phys.* 2009;97:68–81.
15. Badhwar GD, Cucinotta FA, O'Neill PM. An analysis of interplanetary space radiation exposure for various solar cycles. *Radiat Res.* 1994;138:201–208.
16. Cucinotta FA, Nikjoo H, Goodhead DT. The effects of delta rays on the number of particle-track traversals per cell in laboratory and space exposures. *Radiat Res.* 1998;150:115–119.
17. Wilson JW, Townsend LT, Shinn JL, et al. Galactic cosmic ray transport methods, past, present, and future. *Adv Space Res.* 1994;10:841–852.
18. Meesungoen J, Jay-Gerin JP. High-LET radiolysis of liquid water with $1H^+$, $4He^{2+}$, $12C^{6+}$, and $20Ne^{9+}$ ions: effects of multiple ionization. *J Phys Chem A.* 2005;109:6406–6419.
19. Goodhead DT. Initial events in the cellular effects of ionizing radiations: clustered damage in DNA. *Int J Radiat Biol.* 1994;65:7–17.
20. Hu S, Kim MY, McClellan G, et al. Modeling the acute health effects to astronauts from exposure to solar particle events. *Health Phys.* 2009;96:465–476.
21. Alpen EL, Powers-Risius P, Curtis SB, et al. Tumorigenic potential of high-Z, high-LET charged particle radiations. *Radiat Res.* 1993;88:132–143.
22. Dicello JF, Cucinotta FA, Gridley D, et al. In vivo mammary tumorigenesis in the Sprague–Dawley rat and microdosimetric correlates. *Phys Med Biol.* 2004;49:3817–3830.
23. Weil MM, Bedford JS, Bielefeldt-Ohmann H, et al. Incidence of acute myeloid leukemia and hepatocellular carcinoma in mice irradiated with 1 GeV/nucleon ^{56}Fe ions. *Radiat Res.* 2009;172:213–219.
24. Kadhim MA, Macdonald DA, Goodhead DT, et al. Transmission of chromosomal instability after plutonium α-particle irradiation. *Nature.* 1992;355:738–740.
25. Barcellos-Hoff MH, Park C, Wright EG. Radiation and the microenvironment—tumorigenesis and therapy. *Nature Rev Cancer.* 2005;5:867–875.

26. Cucinotta FA, Chappell LJ. Non-targeted effects and the dose response for heavy ion tumors. *Mutat Res.* 2010;687:49–53.
27. Charman WN, Dennis JA, Fazio GG, et al. Visual sensations produced by single fast particles. *Nature.* 1971;230:522–524.
28. Rabin BM, Joseph JA, Shukitt-Hale B, et al. Effects of exposure to heavy particles on a behavior medicated by the dopaminergic system. *Adv Space Res.* 2000;25:2065–2074.
29. Joseph JA, Hunt WA, Rabin BM, et al. Possible "accelerated striatal aging" induced by ^{56}Fe heavy particle irradiation: implications for manned space flights. *Radiat Res.* 1992;130:88–95.
30. Lett JT, Williams GR. Effects of LET on the formation and fate of radiation damage to photoreceptor cell component of the rabbit retina: implications for the projected manned mission to Mars. In: Swenberg CE, Horneck G, Stassinopoulos EG, eds. *Biological effects of Solar and Galactic Cosmic Radiation.* Part A. NY: Plenum Press; 1993:185–201.
31. Rola R, Sarrkissan V, Obenaus A, et al. High-LET radiation induced inflammation and persistent changes in markers of hippocampal neurogenesis. *Radiat Res.* 2005;165:556–560.
32. Rubin P, Casarett GW. *Clinical Radiation Pathology.* Philadelphia, PA: Saunders; 1968.
33. Cucinotta FA, Manuel F, Jones J, et al. Space radiation and cataracts in astronauts. *Radiat Res.* 2001;156:460–466.
34. Chylack LT, Peterson LE, Feiveson A, et al. NASCA Report 1: cross-sectional study of relationship of exposure to space radiation and risk of lens opacity. *Radiat Res.* 2009;172:10–20.
35. Blakely EA, Kleiman NJ, Neriishi K, et al. Radiation cataractogenesis: epidemiology and biology. *Radiat Res.* 2010;173:709–717.
36. Little MP, Tawn EJ, Tzoulaki I, et al. Review and meta-analysis of epidemiological associations between low/moderate doses of ionizing radiation and circulatory disease risks, and their possible mechanisms. *Radiat Environ Biophys.* 2010; Doi: 10.1007/s00411-009-0250.
37. Little MP, Gola A, Tzoulaki I. A model of cardiovascular disease giving a plausible mechanism for the effect of fractionated low-dose ionizing radiation exposure. *PLOS Comput Biol.* 2009;5:1–11.
38. Sauvaget C, Kasagi F, Waldren CA. Dietary factors and cancer mortality among atomic-bomb survivors. *Mutat Res.* 2004;551:145–152.
39. Weiss JF, Landauer MN. Radioprotection by antioxidants. *Ann NY Acad Sci.* 2000;99:44–60.
40. Waldren CA, Vannais DB, Ueno AM. A role for long-lived radicals (LLR) in radiation-induced mutation and persistent chromosomal instability: counteraction by ascorbate and RibCys but not DMSO. *Mutat Res.* 2004;551:255–265.
41. Burns FJ, Tang M, Frenkel K, et al. Induction and prevention of carcinogenesis in rat skin exposed to space radiation. *Radiat Environ Biophys.* 2007;46:195–199.
42. Bjelakovic G, Nikolova D, Gluud LL, et al. Mortality in randomized trials of antioxidant supplements for primary and secondary prevention: systematic review and meta-analysis. *JAMA.* 2007;297:842–857.

14

Roger M. Macklis

Radiation Injuries in Nuclear Power Plant Operation

INTRODUCTION

As world energy needs become prominent topics in international economic and civic agendas, traditional energy sources such as coal and hydroelectric power are being challenged by other more carbon-efficient approaches to energy production and transmission. Although nuclear power plants fell into disfavor in the second half of the 20th century due to safety and environmental concerns, many analysts are now rethinking the role of nuclear power as a sustainable energy source capable of large-scale production and minimal long-term carbon emission and greenhouse gas production.[1]

As interest in nuclear technology rebounds, newer approaches to safer nuclear power plant operation are once again beginning to attract commercial and academic attention. In the 2008 US presidential election, both candidates affirmed their support for further exploration of safe nuclear energy alternatives. Indeed, though nuclear energy was not a core part of his preelection agenda, an election website for President Barack Obama noted that "nuclear power represents more than 70% of our noncarbon generated electricity. It is unlikely that we can meet our aggressive climate goals if we eliminate nuclear power as an option."[2] In the United States as well as other countries, ongoing concerns about safe operation, waste storage, and protection against terrorist targeting remain substantial impediments to popular acceptance of nuclear power as major energy alternatives.[3] It is apparent that we will need to develop new types of risk mitigation strategies for the new millennium.[4]

EARLY HISTORY

Historical discussions of nuclear accidents and radiation injuries generally begin with an acknowledgement of the many poorly publicized injuries that took place in the early decades after the discovery of radioactivity and radiation therapy.[5,6]

After the Curies discovered radium and radioactivity in 1898 (a discovery thread for which multiple Nobel Prizes were subsequently awarded including two to Marie Curie herself), many early investigators were exposed to injury through excessively prolonged and poorly protected radiation activities.[7] Indeed, Marie Curie herself died at age 64 of preleukemia, and by the 1920s, the risk of work-related radiogenic cancers was well recognized. Radiation protection strategies were widely discussed for the laboratory and the industrial sectors, though critics remained concerned that long-term, low-level radiation-related risks were still not fully appreciated or regulated. It was not until the devastating atomic bomb explosions of Hiroshima and Nagasaki that the world fully appreciated that radioactive materials could be toxic not only to the immediately exposed cohort but also to individuals who never had direct contact exposure to dangerous radioactive compounds except as indirect regional "fallout." Detailed accounts of early experimental medical and military injuries have been summarized recently[7,8] and will not be further explored in this chapter. Instead, the chapter focuses on recent-era injuries and accidental deaths from acute and chronic radiation exposure experiences taking place in nuclear power plants in the United States and abroad, and some recent approaches to mitigating these risks.

Several serious accidents involving nuclear power plants occurred in the 1950s.[8] Some of these events are already well documented in the literature and reportedly involved serious or even fatal injuries in small cohorts of immediately exposed industrial personnel. Similarly, industrial nuclear accidents reported in the 1960s and 1970s occurred in multiple workplace locations but generally involved only limited numbers of serious injuries or deaths. The two well-known exceptions to this generally safe industrial disaster record involve the previously secret Russian Mayak reprocessing plant disaster of 1957[10] and the now infamous Chernobyl disaster of 1986.[11] Both of these incidents involved significant acute and chronic contamination events and loss of life, and it is from these two major nuclear plant disasters that much of the available emergency response information and predictions have been formulated.

MAYAK 1957 INCIDENT

The *Mayak* installation (Russian for *beacon*) was located approximately 72 km northwest of Chelyabinsk in Russia. It was built in total secrecy as part of the cold war Soviet nuclear weapons program. The plant was designed to reprocess plutonium from decommissioned bombs and nuclear reactors, and was subsequently used as a source of commercial tritium and other isotopes. A number of poorly documented injuries and deaths reportedly occurred involving plant workers injured in chronic radiation exposures and nearby lake contamination episodes. On September 29, 1957, the cooling system for a tank storing thousands of tons of dissolved nuclear waste leaked at the site, releasing approximately 20 MCi (7.4×10^{17} Bq) of radioactivity. At least 200 people died of the ensuing radiation exposure and more than 10,000 people were ultimately evacuated. Almost 500,000 people may have been exposed to some significant radiation levels related to the accident. The episode was not publicly revealed until after the fall of the Soviet Union though knowledgeable people in both military and industrial enclaves in the East and West had long heard rumors of the Mayak affair. On the International Nuclear Events Scale of 0 to 7, the Mayak event was rated as "level 6," the most serious nuclear industrial disaster before Chernobyl.

1986 CHERNOBYL DISASTER

On April 26, 1986, reactor number 4 at the Chernobyl nuclear power plant in the Ukraine exploded, resulting in the near-term death or serious injury of several hundred people in the area.[11] Of the 237 workers thought to be at greatest risk of exposure during the incident, approximately 140 later showed clinical evidence suggestive of acute radiation syndrome (ARS). Of these, approximately 60 showed evidence of cutaneous radiation syndrome and 28 died of the immediate consequences of this syndrome. Only a handful of patients died of radiation-related hematopoietic syndrome and marrow failure, though thousands more were exposed to a significant radiation level and thus must be considered at permanent risk for hematopoietic malignancies and chronic diseases. To date, only a few cases of leukemia or myelodysplastic syndrome have been documented in the exposed cohort, and solid tumor rates have been surprisingly low.[9] Less severe diseases attributed to chronic Chernobyl radiation exposures including benign cutaneous sequela, cataracts, fertility problems, and Hashimoto thyroiditis have been well documented in survivors. Though an international attempt at allogeneic bone marrow transplant was made in several dozen severely exposed cases in the months immediately following, there is ongoing controversy as to whether this heroic rescue attempt using poorly HLA-matched unrelated donors resulted in more or fewer postmanagement complications and deaths. As a result, other more recent nuclear power plant disasters have been approached somewhat more conservatively and deliberately, with human leukocyte antigen (HLA)-matched or partially matched allogeneic marrow transplant treated as a last resort for those thought to have no chance of autologous recovery.

Based on this limited historical experience set, appropriate management guidelines for victims of a nuclear power plant disaster are currently works in progress. In general, the management approaches can be divided into four different strategic components[12]:

A. Classical response and prevention strategies such as protective barriers and radioactive source-subject proximity limits
B. Identification of suspected radiation exposure patients via dosimetry and clinical syndromes
C. Accepted radioprotectors and pharmacologic mitigation strategies
D. New classes of proposed radiation antidotes and pharmacologic countermeasures

PREVENTION, EVALUATION AND MITIGATION OF EXPOSURE

CLASSICAL PROTECTION MEASURES, SITE SECURITY, AND RECOGNITION OF EXPOSURE SYNDROMES

The oldest and most obvious protective measures used to minimize radiation injury risks involve effective physical shielding and increasing source to subject distance, and these strategies still play major roles in formulating frontline responses to any nuclear incident. As soon as a suspected or confirmed accidental exposure event takes place, trained teams with appropriate equipment should be deployed to estimate the type and degree of radiation exposure or byproducts released. Active sources or areas at risk of further contamination must be identified, secured, shielded, and (where feasible) removed. Access to at-risk sites must be controlled and all potentially exposed personnel identified and triaged for possible medical evaluation and treatment. These general disaster response strategies are dealt with in greater detail in recently updated emergency services handbooks.[13] For decontamination and radiation exposure level estimation, several new triage exposure estimates and biodosimetry approaches are being evaluated.[14] Clearly, decontamination should be done in such a way that time intervals spent by responding personnel near radiation sources and contaminated areas are minimized and accurately recorded. Because radioactivity exposure falls off according to the inverse square law, simply doubling the observer's distance from a source will reduce exposure by a factor of 4. Similarly, minimizing time spent in proximity to a radioactive source will greatly decrease the likelihood of hazardous exposures. High-density shielding materials (e.g., lead barriers or other dense metal container devices) play major roles in "first responder" attempts to decontaminate and safeguard exposed areas while minimizing risk to emergency response decontamination personnel. Experts recommend establishing a secure decontamination center with showers, replacement clothing, and radiologic detectors to identify and remove radioactive sources and any contaminated clothing. Geiger-Müller survey meters and ion chambers are generally considered the most useful on-site instruments. For most minimal exposure situations, universal precautions with immediate removal of contaminated clothing and replacement with protective gear and good hand washing hygiene are usually considered adequate to minimum risk of long-term radiation damage. Minimally exposed psychological casualties ("the worried well") must also be anticipated and referred for evaluation after any public radiation contamination incident. Rapid patient triage by teams trained to identify both medical injuries and radiation exposure histories are critical in a confirmed or suspected nuclear contamination event. Priority is usually given to medical triage and urgent care of medical injuries with occult contamination and fleeting or low-level exposures regarded as secondary concerns. These issues are addressed in greater detail in available emergency care manuals.[15,16]

IDENTIFICATION AND DOSIMETRIC EVALUATION OF EXPOSED VICTIMS

Acute Radiation Syndrome (ARS) as a Clinical Entity

Classic ARS involves a constellation of findings in virtually all organ systems.[12] The most significant and characteristic findings for ARS are generally observed in irradiated hematopoietic, GI, neurologic, and renal systems. The full-blown description of ARS is thus divided into the bone marrow or hematopoietic syndrome (usually described for dose ranges of 0.7 to 10 Gy of total body irradiation [TBI]), the gastrointestinal syndrome (typical seen at doses >6 Gy and prominent after 10 Gy), and the disastrous cardiovascular and CNS syndromes (seen with flash exposure doses in the range of 50 Gy or more).[17] For each of these syndromes, the time course may be divided into a prodromal stage, a latent stage, and a stage of frank radiation exposure illness prior to eventual recovery or death. In general, the sooner the exposed casualty shows the onset of symptoms after exposure, the higher the probable absorbed radiation levels and the more dangerous the exposure. For primates, body doses greater than about 6 to 10 Gy, survival is deemed unlikely without urgent hospitalization and full access to supportive therapies such as blood products, antibiotics, and aggressive skin care. For doses >20 Gy of total body exposure, survival is considered unlikely using any currently known technologies. Note that these dose ranges apply to total body exposures; accidental or therapeutic radiation delivered to limited body regions may exceed these levels by a factor of 10 or more without permanent or serious physiologic damage. Details of the classic ARS findings, dose ranges, and time course projections are described in more detail in Chapter 11 on whole body effects of radiation.

Estimation of Acute Exposure and Expected Toxicity

Radiation exposure estimates after a nuclear power plant incident may be performed using methods quite similar to strategies developed for other total or partial body radiotherapy exposures.[16] Initial estimates typically involve a dosimetric approximation based on the known or estimated distance from the exposure source, the degree of interposed shielding, and the duration of exposure. For many situations, however, these details may not be known with any precision. While knowledge about the position of the involved individual, the degree of shielding, and the exact type of emission and exposure events may be available for a situation in which an individual is exposed to a well-controlled commercial radioactive source, exposures such as those likely to be seen in a disaster scene like Chernobyl will probably involve much higher levels of dosimetric uncertainty. For this reason, recent interest has developed around attempts to formulate and validate methodologies to provide valid and reproducible biomarkers to estimate cumulative radiation exposure and to make that estimate in time to enact protective or mitigating medical strategies.

The circulating blood lymphocyte count has been shown to represent a convenient minimally invasive biomarker for acute total body radiation exposures.[12] As soon as practical after the exposure has occurred (or is suspected), a complete blood count (CBC) with differential white blood cell count should be drawn and analyzed. Serial CBC analyses usually show a marked lymphocyte depression over the first 2 to 3 days after an acute exposure. The degree and velocity of the decline in absolute lymphocyte count have been validated as useful biomarkers and are now part of the first-responder strategy. Serial CBC and differential evaluations should be obtained and analyzed every 4 to 6 hours for the next few days. The shape of the graph tracing will often correlate with the timing for expected onset of clinical symptoms such as nausea, vomiting, itching, cutaneous changes, and diarrhea. If applicable, serial photos should be taken and time-stamped to show changes over time. Individuals exposed to the same radiation dose over a more protracted period of time will show very different effects as physiologic recovery measures begin to come into play. Note that these biomarkers relate only to the radiation-related aspects of an exposure. In cases of a physical explosion or a conventional detonation blast, explosion injuries may occur concurrently with radiation injuries and may produce a much more complicated and life-threatening situation.

Other biomarkers being developed include cytogenetic evaluation with analysis of dicentric chromosomal changes, and analysis of other types of chromosomal aberrations. Various automated and high-throughput models of potential chromosome screening systems are under development for potential use in estimating approximate absorbed doses after accidental or deliberate radiation exposures.[17]

The Spectrum of Clinical Symptoms Seen in Acute Radiation Syndrome

Exposure of most or all of the body to acute radiation doses of 1 Gy or more can be expected to initiate the classic symptoms associated with ARS.[17] The duration of each phase of ARS and the time interval between exposure and symptoms will often show tight correlation with the severity of the exposure. For a total body exposure of >10 Gy, nausea and vomiting as well as neurocognitive problems such as dizziness or loss of consciousness have been observed within minutes. Fever and bloody diarrhea may be observed within hours. Cardiovascular instability, erythema, and disorientation may persist over the first 24 to 48 hours. As WBC and platelets fall, serious problems related to bleeding and infection become part of the radiation exposure picture. The risk of sepsis has been reported to be highest in week 4 to 6 after high-level abdominal radiation exposure. Malaise, nausea, and apathy may become chronic findings and may be difficult to differentiate from other syndromes related to extreme stress. Characteristic skin reactions may help differentiate various contributing or overlapping factors. In general, any patient suspected of high-level radiation exposure should be admitted to a hospital for complete workup and expert management.

ACCEPTED RADIOPROTECTORS AND PHARMACOLOGIC MITIGATION STRATEGIES

Potassium Iodide (KI) Supplements and Similar Chemical Blockers of Radioiodine Incorporation

Situations such as the Chernobyl disaster in which volatile radioactive gasses are discharged into the environment may warrant treatment of small or large populations with potassium preparations (KI or KIO_3) in order to block uptake by the thyroid gland of iodine-131 produced as a consequence of nuclear accidents.[18-21] Rates of thyroid cancer were reported to increase by a factor of up to 100 beginning about 4 years after the Chernobyl disaster. Some regional facilities stockpile emergency stores of KI or KIO_3 in either liquid or solid form with instructions to distribute the stock to individuals in regions at risk. This is especially important for children whose thyroids are quite active and thus may be particularly prone to exposure-related leukemia and solid tumors. The use of KI is dealt with in greater detail in Chapter 27, Head and Neck. It must be noted that this sort of radioprotector will only be effective against radioactive iodine exposures and similar classes of radioactive material exposures. The use of KI offers essentially no protection against other types of radiation injuries or cancers, and some states have deliberately refused the Nuclear Regulatory Commission (NRC) offer of KI stockpile due to concern that the public may incorrectly assume that all types of radiogenic cancers are prevented by the medication. The American Thyroid Association recommends the distribution of these agents to people living within 50 miles of an operating nuclear reactor. In addition to general medical management with fluid support, wound care, and blood products, some types of pharmaceutical protective measures should be considered for patients with potential high-level industrial radiation.

Amifostine (Ethyol)

Amifostine[22] is a member of a well-known class of free radical scavengers with a chemistry related to their sulftydryl compound chemistry. This class of protectors has been under evaluation since the 1940s when cysteine ($SH-CH_2-CH-NH_2/COOH$) was identified as a compound capable of increasing the tolerance of mice to TBI of injected shortly before radiation exposures. These compounds have a free SH group at one end of the molecule and a basic moiety such as an amoire or quanidine group at the other end. The best evaluated of this class of protectors is amifostine (Ethyol) previously identified as WR-2721 and said to be the secret compound carried by astronauts to be used in the event of a major solar flare. Amifostine is FDA approved for protection of both chemotherapy and radiotherapy toxicities, and a recent American Society of Clinical Oncology (ASCO) update supported its use as a xerostomia prevention agent in patients undergoing radiotherapy to the head and neck. Its potential as an emergency radioprotector is currently unknown and under evaluation. More information on Amifostine can be found in Chapter 5.

Cytokines, Growth Factor, and Stem Cell Transplant Technologies

The area of cytokine investigation has been aided substantially by pharmacologic interest in hematopoietic system repair and recovery after exposure to cytotoxic cancer therapeutics.[23] The use of granulocyte colony-stimulating factor (G-CSF), granulocyte macrophage colony-stimulating factor (GM-CSF), and related hematopoietic growth factors now represents a multibillion dollar component of the pharmaceutical industry, and the reader is referred to recent reviews of this field reported in Chapter 5 or a full description of the utility and toxicities of these agents in various clinical contexts. Recent areas of cytokine repair process investigations have focused on signal transduction networks involving multiple partially related families of

molecular signals in the TGF, epidermal growth factor (EGF), and tumor necrosis factor (TNF) families and the coordinated stress responses observed at the interface of cellular repair, repopulation, and inflammation. Many types of normal tissues have been shown to display radiation-induced acute-phase inflammatory responses that may be observed within hours of radiation exposure and may recur weeks or months later. These networks are presumed to represent evidence of evolutionarily conserved tissue repair enhancement circuitry seen in higher organisms. Some tissues appear to show higher levels of radioresistance after initial "priming" of the proinflammatory pathways by low dose radiation. Signal transduction coordinators such as transforming growth factor (TGF)-β and related molecules may be involved in several components of healthy tissue repair and potentially may accelerate healing when used as emergency intervention agents. It appears that TGF-β may play a key role in the stimulation of matrix protein synthesis, inhibition of matrix degeneration, and control of integrin expression. The fact that this pathway has been implicated in both radiation repair and radiation damage and that conflicting dose response data have been produced using different experimental systems underlines the fact that these powerful tissue remodeling signals will require extensive preclinical and clinical evaluation prior to being recommended for emergency use after a nuclear power plant incident or a similar emergency event. In a similar fashion, mucosal repair enhancement molecules such as compounds related to keratinocyte growth factor (KGF) are now entering large-scale clinical trials as mucosal protectors in oncology.

One important new product in this category, palifermin, is a recombinant form of KGF, and was recently approved for prophylaxis against severe mucositis associated with hematopoietic stem cell transplant.[24] In recent guidelines issued by the ASCO, palifermin is recommended in case of stem cell transplant undergoing TBI. This was the first new issuance of radiation protection guidelines since 2002 and will presumably find utility in the radioprotection of patients with disaster-precipitated high dose TBI or accidental oropharyngeal exposures similar to the therapeutic indications in oncology guidelines. The stockpiling and use of palifermin and other cytokines as emergency protectors is entirely hypothetical and logistically problematic.

NEWER EXPERIMENTAL APPROACHES TO RADIOPROTECTION AND PHARMACOLOGIC RADIATION EXPOSURE MITIGATION

A number of different new lines of investigation are being undertaken at different centers, many centering on the activation of signaling pathways capable of regulating critical elements of the cellular apoptotic pathways.[25] In some cases, investigators are attempting to interrupt major normal tissue cell suicide induction pathways such as those under the control of the proapoptotic master regulator p53.[26] These investigations attempt to understand how normal tissue suicide circuits, sometimes apparently activated by stress responses to genotoxic signals such as ionizing radiation, can be controlled.

In other cases, the research centers on the activation of major antiapoptotic signaling circuits such as nuclear factor-kappa beta (NF-kB); a transcription factor thought to utilize the IKB-kinase B-network to reduce cell suicide as an acute toxicity of ionizing radiation.[26,27] Of note, these apoptosis-control therapeutics are still in very early phases of testing and due to the subject nature of the condition being discussed, ethical principle prevents true normal subject efficacy testing since this would require potentially hazardous experimental radiation exposures for the subjects. However, preclinical testing is allowed by the FDA using a combination of safety testing in patient groups exposed to the genetic radiation together with analogous animal studies in primates and other mammals. This sort of preclinical testing is currently in progress for one candidate molecule, CBLB502. This compound was purified from flagellin protein from salmonella typhimurium and appears to exert potent activation and radioprotection of gut and other critical tissues.[26] Other related bacterial-derived molecules are being evaluated for hematopoietic protection and mucosal rehealing after radiation. Preclinical studies involving mice with syngeneic tumors indicate substantial protection against the harmful effects of both radiation and certain chemotherapeutic compounds without compromising cytotoxicity against target tumor cells.

In addition to the compounds mentioned above, several newer families of potential future medications are currently in early or intermediate stages of development. Some of these compounds fall into well-known families of active agents (e.g., a member of the steroid family named 5-androstenedial with putative activity in strengthening cellular elements of the immune system), and others fall into entirely new categories of potentially active agents (e.g., large and small molecules being developed to target the cell-adhesion mediators such as members of the integrin family). In both cases, molecules with known activity in networks active in inflammation and cell communication control are now being re-evaluated with an eye to potential roles in emergency measures for radioprotection and tissue damage control. In the fall of 2008, the US National Institute of Allergy and Infectious Disease (NIAID, the branch of the Departments of Health and Human Services charged with antiterrorist countermeasure progress) announced 25 new awards for expanding the research capacity in the area of radiation countermeasures. Although aimed primarily at radioprotectants capable of rapid deployment in case of radioterrorism and military exposures, the resulting knowledge base should have clear-cut applicability to industrial disasters such as power plant malfunction and accidental contamination events.

At present, we must regard all of the partially validated potential emergency response radioprotectors as works in progress and it remains to be seen whether some or all of these candidate radioprotectors will ever prove clinically useful. Nevertheless, the potential for accidental or deliberate radiation overdoses as part of an industrial accident or deliberate radioterrorist events (e.g., the feared "dirty bomb" scenario) suggests that efforts to develop new types of acute exposure radioprotectors and radiation countermeasures are an urgent healthcare priority in the modern era. As nuclear power continues to regain a dominant role in plans for cost-effective world energy production with low carbon emission, new classes of radiation antidotes will be required for stockpiling and emergency response treatments. Until acknowledged medical radioprotectors, countermeasures, and antidotes are developed and deployed and until the public feels comfortable with their availability as emergency safety responses, it is unlikely that nuclear power plants will be generally accepted as a viable source of future energy. There is some urgency attached to these developments since nuclear energy appears to be one of the most promising approaches for meeting the world's energy needs for the 21st century.

REFERENCES

1. Ansolabehere S, Deutch J, Driscoll E, et al. The future of nuclear power: an interdisciplinary MIT Study. 2003;1–16. Available at: http://we.mit-edu/nuclearpower/. Accessed October 13, 2008.
2. Briscoe D. Obama's Nuclear Reservations Political squabbling over how to store waste could hold back the industry. Newsweek Project Green. 2008. Available at: http://newsweek.com/id/170348. Accessed 02/06/2009.
3. Wikipedia. Nuclear power debate. Available at: http://en.wikipedia.org/wiki/Nuclear_debate. Accessed October 13, 2008.
4. Dunn P. Safe Nuclear Power and Green Hydrogen Fuel. PHYSorg.com. 2005. Available at: http://www.physorg.com/news8956.html. Accessed February 6, 2009.
5. Macklis RM. Radithor and the era of mild radium therapy. *JAMA*. 1990;264:614–618.
6. Macklis RM. The great radium scandal. *Sci Am*. 1993;269(2):94–99.
7. Weart SR. *Nuclear Fear a History of Images*. Massachusetts: President and Fellows of Harvard College; 1988.
8. List of civilian nuclear accidents, Available at: http://en.wikipedia.org/wiki/List_of_civilian_nuclear_accidents. Accessed October 13, 2008.
9. Gottlober P, Steinert M, Weiss M, et al. The outcome of local radiation injuries: 14 years of follow-up after the Chernobyl accident. *Radiat Res*. 2001. Available at: http://www/ncbi.nlm.nih.gov/pubmed/11182791. Accessed October 13, 2008.
10. Mayak. Available at: http://en.wikipedia.org/wiki/Mayak. Accessed November 9, 2008.
11. Gottlober P, Steinert M, Weiss M, et al. The outcome of local radiation injuries: 14 years of follow-up after the Chernobyl accident. *Radiat Res*. 2001;155:409–416.
12. Turai I, Veress K, Gunalp B, et al. Medical response to radiation incidents and radionuclear threats. *Br Med J*. 2004;328(7439):568–572.
13. "Emergency Department Management of Radiation Casualties": a public service by the Health Physics Society for hospital staff training. Jerrold T. Bushberg, PhD, UC Davis Health System, 2007.
14. Prasanna P, Krasnopolsky K, Livingston G, et al. Laboratory automation for Cytogenetic Biodosimetry and Laboratory Comparison of the Dicentric Assay. Radioprotection 2008, Vol. 43, no. 5, DOI: 10.1051/radiopro:2008518.
15. Keys DG. *Medical Response to Terrorism*. Philadelphia, PA: Lippincott Williams & Wilkins; 2004
16. Acute Radiation Syndrome: A Fact Sheet for Physicians: a report by the Centers for Disease Control and Prevention. Washington, DC: CDC, 03/18/2005.
17. Hall EJ, Giaccia AJ. *Radiobiology for the Radiologist*. Philadelphia, PA: Lippincott Williams & Wilkins; 2006.
18. Moulder JE. Post-irradiation approaches to treatment of radiation injuries in the context of radiological terrorism and radiation accidents: a review. *Int J Radiat Biol*. 2004;80:3–10.
19. Meincke V, van Beuningen D, Sohns T, et al. Medical management principles for radiation accidents. *Mil Med*. 2003;168:219–222.
20. Turai I, Veress K, Gunalp B, et al. Medical response to radiation incidents and radionuclear threats. *Br Med J*. 2004;328:568–572.
21. Product Review: Potassium Iodide (KI) and Potassium Iodate (KIO$_3$): Radioprotective Agents: a report by ConsumerLab.com. 06/12/2007.
22. Yu Z, Eaton JW, Persson HL. The radioprotective agent, amifostine, suppresses the reactivity of intralysosomal iron. *Redox Rep*. 2003;8:347–355.
23. Neta R, Oppenheim JJ, Douches SD. Interdependence of the radioprotective effects of human recombinant interleukin 1∝, tumor necrosis factor ∝, granulocyte colony-stimulating factor, and murine recombinant granulocyte-macrophage colony-stimulating factor. *J Immunol*. 1988;140:108–111.
24. Hensley M, Hagerty K, Kewalramani T, et al. The American Society of Clinical Oncology 2008 Clinical Practice Guideline Update: Use of Chemotherapy and Radiation Therapy Protectants. Expert Panel on the Use of Chemotherapy and Radiation Therapy Protectants. *J Oncol Pract*. 2008;4(6 November):277–279.
25. NIAID Announces 25 New Awards to Develop Radiation Countermeasures: a report of the U.S. Department of Health and Human Services: National Institute of Allergy and Infectious Diseases. 10/07/2008.
26. Burdelya LG, Krivokrysentko VI, Tallant TC, et al. An Agonist of Toll-Like Receptor 5 Has Radioprotective Activity in Mouse and Primate Models. 03/2008,10.1126/science.1155193.
27. Strom E, Sathe S, Komarov PG, et al. Small-molecule inhibitor of p53 binding to mitochondria protects mice from gamma radiation. *Nat Chem Biol*. (published on-line 23 Jul 2006).

Marco De Santis
Gianluca Straface

Effect of Radiation on the Embryo and Fetus

INTRODUCTION

Ionizing radiation is produced by high-energy electromagnetic waves such as x-rays and gamma rays. X-rays and gamma rays differ only in the origin of radiation; x-rays are produced by transitions in electron energy states, whereas gamma rays are emitted by atomic nuclei involved in radioactive decay. Charged particles such as α and β particles emitted by radionuclides can also produce ionization.

The amount of radiation can be measured in two different ways: Exposure to ionizing radiation, produced by x-rays or gamma rays from any source, is measured in roentgens (R), while the radiation dose absorbed in tissue is measured in Gray (Gy) or rad (1 Gy = 100 rad, 1 cGy = 1 rad, 1 mGy = 0.1 rad). The exposure of a human tissue to 1 R yields approximately 1 rad (1 cGy) of absorbed dose, depending on the energy of the radiation and the tissue under consideration. However, different kinds of ionizing radiation can deposit the same total energy but produce different degrees of biological damage. A biologically equivalent dose, expressed in Seivert (Sv) or rem (1 Sv = 100 rem, 1 mSv = 0.1 rem), reflects the differing biological effects of specific types of radiation. For the types of radiation typically used for diagnostic or therapeutic purposes, rem, rad, cGy, and cSv are interchangeable[1,2] (Table 15.1).

The risk of exposure to ionizing radiation is increasing in the general population. A recent review pointed out a 121% increase in diagnostic testing involving ionizing radiation for pregnant women during the last decade, with a 25% increase in the use of computerized tomography (CT) scanning scan each year.[3] At the same time, there has been growing concern, both in public opinion and among health care workers, regarding the possible risks related to ionizing radiation in pregnancy. Some studies have shown that a significant percentage of Canadian family doctors (6%) and gynecologists (5%) suggest the termination of a pregnancy in women having undergone abdominal CT scan.[4] Pregnant women exposed to low-dose ionizing radiation have also been shown to greatly overestimate the radiation-related risk to the unborn fetus.[5]

From the available studies, it is clear that gestational age and radiation dose are the most important determinants of potential noncancer health effects. Our current knowledge about the effects of ionizing radiation led to the elaboration of some basic tenets:

- During the first 2 weeks after conception, exposure to a dose of radiation >0.1 Gy can cause the death of the embryo.[6] Embryos surviving such a dose will not be at a risk significantly higher than baseline for developing a malformation.

- In all stages of gestation radiation-induced, noncancer health effects are undetectable for fetal doses below 0.05 Gy. Most authors agree that a dose of 0.05 Gy represents the limit below which no noncancer effects are produced at any stage of gestation. In rodents, a small risk may exist for malformations, as well as effects on the central nervous system (CNS) in the 0.05 to 0.10 Gy range for some stages of gestation. However, the threshold dose for congenital birth defects in the human embryo or fetus is most likely between 0.10 and 0.20 Gy.

- From the 16th week of gestation to birth, radiation-induced, noncancer health effects are unlikely for exposures below about 0.50 Gy. Although some authors suggest that a small

TABLE 15.1		Main Radiation Measures	
Measure	*SI*	*Use*	*Equivalence*
Roentgen (R)	C/kg	Exposure	1 R = 2.58 × 10⁻⁴ C/kg
Rad (rad)	Gray (Gy)	Absorbed dose	1 rad = 0.01 Gy
Rem (rem)	Sievert (Sv)	Biologically equivalent dose	1 rem = 0.01 Sv

Source: Modified from De Santis M, Di Gianantonio E, Straface G, et al. Ionizing radiations in pregnancy and teratogenesis. A review of literature. *Reprod Toxicol*. 2005;20:323–329.

TABLE 15.2		Stochastic Versus Deterministic Effects of Radiation		
	Threshold Dose	*Dose-related Probability*	*Dose-related Severity*	*Examples*
Deterministic	Yes	Yes	Yes	Most adult normal tissue toxicities (e.g., cataract formation) Fetal malformation Mental retardation from *in utero* radiation exposure
Stochastic	No	Yes	No	Carcinogenesis Mutagenesis

risk exists for impaired brain function above 0.10 Gy in the 16- to 25-week stage of gestation, most researchers agree that after about 16 weeks' gestation, the threshold for congenital effects is approximately 0.50 to 0.70 Gy.[7]

STOCHASTIC VERSUS DETERMINISTIC EFFECTS

Radiation-induced health effects in humans can be divided into two main categories (Table 15.2). Stochastic effects (phenomena involving probability) refer to induction of diseases such as cancer or genetic disease that can result from a point mutation. A risk for induction of stochastic effects is presumed to exist even at low doses; and while the risk increases with increasing dose, the severity of the resulting effect is not dose dependent. Deterministic effects require multicellular injury and appear to have a threshold dose below which deleterious effects do not occur.[2] For deterministic effects, below a certain threshold dose, radiation-related risks are equivalent in exposed populations and control populations who have received only background radiation.[8] Radiation carcinogenesis is considered a stochastic effect, while the induction of birth defects by radiation (teratogenesis) is considered a deterministic effect.

RADIATION TERATOGENESIS

IRRADIATION OF GERM CELLS PRIOR TO CONCEPTION

The radiation-induced health effects on the germ cells, expressed by a reduced fertility, are well known (see Chapters 34 and 35). Since it is known that the most critical target for ionizing radiation is DNA, parental germ cells are clearly at risk for radiation-induced mutations. From this point of view, the most radiosensitive period is during rapid cell division in the testis. This occurs during spermatogenesis and may involve a period of up to 6 months prior to ejaculation. On the other hand, the oocytes, resting in suspended meiosis I, are relatively resistant to radiation-induced mutations. However, during the 6 or 7 weeks prior to ovulation, when the first meiotic division starts, oocytes become sensitive to radiation-induced damage as well. But even during this period of increased radiosensitivity, the magnitude of the genetic risk due to any kind of preconception radiation exposure appears to be negligible.[2,9]

EXPOSURE POST CONCEPTION

In order to assess the teratogenic risk of radiation exposure after conception, the stage of embryogenesis at the time of the exposure must be considered. During the first 2 weeks after conception, a blastocyst implantation failure may occur if the radiation dose is above 0.1 Gy. During the preimplantation period (approximately the first 14 days after conception or 3–4 weeks after last menstruation), the risk of lethal effects to the embryo is greatest and consequently the risk of teratogenic effects is extremely low. Therefore, it is well known that, during this period, radiation exposure will either be lethal or have no effect ("all or none"). Since at this stage the embryo is composed of only a few cells, the loss of a single progenitor cell can cause death and failure of the blastocyst to implant in the uterus.[1]

The period of organogenesis (from the third to the eighth week after conception) is the period of highest risk for radiation-induced malformations. The developing CNS is exquisitely sensitive to radiation-induced malformations during this period.[10] Other organs systems display sensitivity depending on the precise timing of irradiation in relationship to their period of development.

The fetal period (from 8 weeks until the end of gestation) is generally a time of decreasing sensitivity to radiation teratogenesis for the fetus; nevertheless, the CNS, which continues to develop throughout gestation, retains sensitivity to radiation.[11]

Brent summarized the stochastic and deterministic effects of ionizing radiation on the embryo and fetus. The results are based on thousands of experimental studies on animals as well as human epidemiologic studies. Estimates of the threshold doses for congenital malformations, growth retardation, pregnancy loss, and neurological effects all exceed 0.20 Gy. Growth retardation and fetal death exhibit even higher thresholds, depending on the stage of gestation.[12,13] The major congenital anomalies caused by in utero irradiation are microcephaly, mental retardation and other CNS defects, and growth retardation[12–14] (Table 15.3).

Microcephaly is the most common malformation reported after exposure to high doses of in utero irradiation.

Much information on the effects of acute exposure to ionizing radiation comes from epidemiological studies of children born to atomic bomb survivors. One limitation of these studies is that they examined the effects of a single, high-dose exposure and not of intermittent low-dose exposures typically experienced in medical, occupational, or environmental situations.[14] Other sources of information are animal studies and studies of patients treated with a radiotherapeutic procedure before or during pregnancy.

In a study of women treated with radiotherapy for uterine cancer during pregnancy, Goldstein and Murphy reported that within a sample of 74 newborns, 34%, exposed to doses >1 Gy (>100 rads), showed congenital malformations. Specifically, most of them (23%) showed microcephaly, but genital hypoplasia,

TABLE 15.3	Ionizing Radiation and Congenital Malformations	
Malformations	*Estimated Threshold Dose*	*Gestational Age at Greatest Risk*
Microcephaly	≥20 Gy	8–15
Mental retardation	0.06–0.31 Gy between 8 and 15 weeks	
	0.25–0.28 Gy between 16 and 25 weeks	
	>50 Gy after 25 weeks	
Reduction in IQ	0.1 Gy	8–15
Other malformations (skeleton, genitals, eyes)	≥0.20 Gy	3–11

Sources: De Santis M, Di Gianantonio E, Straface G, et al. Ionizing radiations in pregnancy and teratogenesis. A review of literature. *Reprod Toxicol.* 2005;20:323–329; Schull WJ, Neel JV. Atomic bomb exposure and the pregnancies of biologically related parents. A prospective study of the genetic effects of ionizing radiation in man. *Am J Public Health Nations Health.* 1959;49(12):1621–1629.

cleft palate, hypospadias, microphthalmia, cataracts, strabismus, retinal degeneration, and optic athropy were also reported. Almost all microcephalic children in this report were mentally retarded and had short stature as well.[15,16] Furthermore, the incidence of microcephaly rose with increasing exposure.[2]

Another important deduction of the researchers was that 70% of children with malformations were exposed to radiation during the first 5 months of gestation. Using these data, other authors observed that *in utero* exposure to ionizing radiation was associated with congenital malformations only for exposures between approximately the 3rd and the 19th weeks of gestation and that microcephaly occurred only for exposure prior to the 17th week.[12]

Debakan came to a similar conclusion gathering all the case studies existing in literature up to that time (26 case studies) of women receiving pelvic radiation during pregnancy for various indications. He observed that all the women were exposed to very high radiation doses (>2.5 Gy) and that the majority of cases of mental retardation and other major malformations occurred for exposures between the 3rd and the 11th week of gestation. Furthermore, growth retardation, microcephaly, and mental retardation were the only congenital anomalies observed in the interval between 10 and 20 weeks. No malformations were observed for exposure beyond the 20th week of gestation.[17]

Microcephaly also developed in many children of atomic bomb survivors, exposed *in utero* to doses between 0.1 and 1.5 Gy.[18,19] Otake and Schull found a 4.2% incidence of microcephaly (62/1,473) and 1.7% of mental retardation (26/1,473) among Hiroshima and Nagasaki survivors irradiated *in utero*. Mental retardation was not always associated with microcephaly, and many children born with cranial malformations who were not mentally retarded were exposed before 7 weeks following conception.[20]

Whether radiation-induced mental retardation is truly a deterministic effect has been most controversial. In 1984, Otake and Schull put forth a no-threshold model for mental retardation, proposing simply a dose-dependent effect for severe mental retardation with a risk doubled with exposures of 0.02 Gy. Furthermore, they suggested that the likelihood of developing severe mental retardation in the first 8 weeks was near or equal to zero, that the maximum risk for irradiation occurred between the 8th and the 15th week, decreasing between the

16th and the 25th week. After the 25th week of gestation and for exposures of <100 rads, no case of severe mental retardation was reported.[21]

On reanalysis of their data, they later supported a threshold dose between 0.12 and 0.23 Gy for exposures in the 8th and the 15th week period and about 0.21 Gy between the 16th and the 25th week. In 1999, they concluded that the threshold dose for mental retardation was approximately 0.18 Gy (0.06–0.31 Gy) for exposures between the 8th and the 15th week of gestation and that, in later stages of gestation, this threshold dose could increase up to 0.25 to 0.28 Gy.[22–24] Also in 1999, Miller proposed a threshold dose of 0.5 Gy, which is much higher than exposures received during most common diagnostic radiology procedures.[25]

Otake and Schull demonstrated that *in utero* exposure to ionizing radiation was not only associated with severe mental retardation but also that a direct, deleterious effect on IQ existed with a maximum linear dose effect between the 8th and the 15th week and a reduction of 21 to 29 IQ points per Gy. In the period between the 16th and the 25th week, the reduction was approximately 13 to 21 points per Gy. No effect on IQ reduction was observed for exposure doses of <0.1 Gy.[22–24,26] Others have also observed a reduction of about 30 IQ points per Sievert between the 8th and the 15th week, whereas a lesser effect is observed between the 16th and the 25th week.[27] The search for a threshold dose related to the effect of radiation on IQ did not lead to a clear conclusion even if, according to some authors, this dose could be approximately 10 cGy.[28]

CARCINOGENESIS

The association between *in utero* exposure to radiation and development of leukemia and other childhood cancers has been recognized for over 30 years.[10] Whether the carcinogenic effects for a given dose of radiation vary on the basis of gestation period has not been determined. At this time, the carcinogenic risk is assumed to be constant throughout pregnancy. However, analysis of experimental studies carried out on animals suggests that the carcinogenic effects of radiation are greatest in late fetal development, and are much less in the stages of blastogenesis and organogenesis. Einhorn suggested that the period of organogenesis could be more resistant to the carcinogenic

TABLE 15.4	Estimated Risk for Cancer from Prenatal Radiation Exposure	
Radiation Dose	*Estimate Childhood Cancer Incidence*[a,b]	*Estimated Lifetime[c] Cancer Incidence*[d] *(Exposure at Age 10)*
No radiation exposure above background	0.3%	38%
0.00–0.05 Gy	0.3%–1%	38%–40%
0.05–0.50 Gy	1%–6%	40%–55%
>0.50 Gy	>6%	>55%

[a]Data published by the International Commission on Radiation Protection.
[b]Childhood cancer mortality is roughly half of childhood cancer incidence.
[c]The lifetime cancer risks from prenatal radiation exposure are not yet known. The lifetime risk estimates given are for Japanese males exposed at age 10 years from models published by the United Nations Scientific Committee on the Effects of Atomic Radiation.
[d]Lifetime cancer mortality is roughly one third of lifetime cancer incidence.
Source: Prenatal Radiation Exposure: A Fact Sheet for Physicians. Department of Health and human Services. Center for Disease Control and Prevention. Available at: www.bt.cdc.gov/radiation

effect of radiation, possibly due to regulatory factors that are highly active against the carcinogenic effects of radiation.[29] Some experimental studies have indicated that juvenile mice are more sensitive to the oncogenic effects of radiation than the embryo.[30–32]

Many studies have tried to determine the magnitude of cancer risk in childhood after prenatal exposure to ionizing radiation, but this estimate proved to be very difficult due to the conflicting data available to date. Evidence for a causal association derives almost entirely from case-control studies, whereas practically all cohort studies find no association, most notably in the atomic bomb survivors. Although it is likely that in utero radiation exposure represents a leukemogenic risk to the fetus, the magnitude of the risk remains uncertain.[33–35]

Currently, it is believed that *in utero* exposure to a radiation dose of 1 to 2 cGy may increase the risk of leukemia by a factor of 1.5 to 2 above natural incidence.[36] The British Oxford Survey of Childhood Cancer estimated the cancer risk following in utero exposure to ionizing radiation to be 0.022/Gy.[37] A study carried out in the United Kingdom on women who underwent diagnostic radiology examinations in the late pregnancy in the period 1958 to 1961 estimated the risk to be 0.04 to 0.05/Gy.[38]

The causal nature of the risk of cancers other than leukemia is less convincing, and the similar RR (relative risk) determined from different studies for virtually all forms of childhood cancer suggests an underlying bias. Few studies have supported a potential risk of adult cancer after in utero exposure to radiation.

Among atomic bomb survivors exposed *in utero*, there were only 18 cases of cancer in the years 1950 to 1984, 5 of them in the "zero-dose" group. Two of these subjects had childhood cancer (both were exposed to 0.30 Gy). All the others developed cancer in adulthood. The estimated relative risk for cancer for exposure to 1 Gy was 3.77.[39]

Therefore, at the moment, it is not clear if in utero exposure to ionizing radiation is a causal or a concausal factor for leukemia incidence in childhood. Surely, genetic and environmental factors contribute to a larger extent than radiation. The fact that atomic bomb survivors exposed in utero to radiation doses up to 500 rads did not show a significant increase in childhood cancers makes clear the complexity of this phenomenon. However, a low carcinogenic risk cannot be completely excluded.[36,40]

How should we interpret the cancer risk for an in utero exposure of 10 cGy or less? The pregnant woman should be counseled that the radiation-related risk is insignificant compared with the risk of spontaneous incidence of cancer and reproductive effects in general (Table 15.4).

EXPOSURE TO DIAGNOSTIC RADIATION

There is general agreement that fetal exposure of <5 cGy is not considered teratogenic.[2,5,11–14] It is important to stress that the risks are determined by the dose to the fetus, which is likely to be much less than the maternal exposure. The vast majority of diagnostic radiology procedures result in a fetal dose <5 cGy, even those procedures that may expose the fetus to higher levels of risk such as barium enema (0.07 Gy), abdominal and pelvic CT (0.0088 and 0.025 Gy), and nuclear medicine procedures.[41–43]

Several studies carried out on women who had received diagnostic x-ray procedures at different stages of gestation showed no evidence of an increased risk of malformation.[42,44,45] Even the incidence of mental retardation did not show an increased frequency in a study by Mole (4–10/1,000/cGy).[46] The highest fetal dose (117 mGy) administered in the period of greater sensitivity (8–15 week) was much lower than the threshold dose for severe mental retardation of 390 to 460 mGy (39–46 cGy) reported by Otake et al.[47] On the basis of these considerations it is evident that, for diagnostic doses, the risk of severe mental retardation is negligible.[11] With regard to the risk of IQ reduction, considering the 25 to 29 points reduction per Gy reported by Otake et al., the majority of diagnostic procedures should lead to reductions in IQ of about 0.2 points.[42,47,48]

The National Council on Radiation Protection and Measurements report 54 states that: "The risk of abnormality is considered negligible at 5 rads (0.05 Gy) or less when compared to the other risks of pregnancy, and the risk of malformations is significantly increased above control levels only at doses above 15 rads (0.15 Gy). Therefore, exposure of the fetus to radiation arising from diagnostic procedures would rarely be a cause, by itself, for terminating a pregnancy."[49]

PROFESSIONAL EXPOSURE

The International Commission on Radiological Protection (ICRP) states that the level of protection for the embryo of a pregnant woman exposed to radiation at work should be similar to that provided for the general population. Furthermore, the ICRP states that the fetus should be protected by the application of an additional equivalent dose limit of 2 mSv to the maternal abdominal surface from the diagnosis of pregnancy to the end of gestation, being understood that the dose limit for the fetus is 1 mSv.[50]

The NCRP recommends a total equivalent dose limit of 500 mrem for the embryo or the fetus. Moreover, once the diagnosis of pregnancy has been made, the dose should not be >50 mrem for each month. These recommendations were elaborated in order to limit the dose to the fetus in case of professional exposure.[51] In recent years, protection measures for professional exposure have been revised according to the principle of keeping radiation "as low as reasonably achievable." Radiation exposure should be as low as possible, even if the health worker is not pregnant. Every measure taken in order to reduce radiation dose to the mother will also reduce the dose to the fetus.[51]

No evidence of an increased risk of malformations compared to the general population was found in 9,208 pregnancies of radiographers (both men and women). This study showed only a borderline risk of chromosome anomalies and childhood cancer.[52] A study carried out on 27,181 pregnancies of 13,600 nuclear industries workers (men and women) found no increased risk of malformation, but an increased risk of early miscarriage or stillbirth was detected. This increased risk for fetal death was not confirmed by other studies that analyzed populations who lived near nuclear plants.[53,54]

Analysis of the effect on the Chernobyl population after the disaster, showed an increased incidence of malformations, abortion and preterm labour.[55] Similarly, an observational study carried out in Germany on the prevalence of children with Down syndrome between 1980 and 1989 showed an increase in the number of cases in only 1 month, right after the Chernobyl disaster.[56]

PATERNAL EXPOSURE

Some studies investigated the percentage of malformations among newborns whose fathers were previously exposed to radiotherapy for testicular cancer, but no significant differences were found compared to the general population.[57] Even in the offspring of male survivors of the atomic blasts in Hiroshima and Nagasaki survivors, no increase in the percentage of malformations, fetal death, or low birthweight was found.[58,60]

The available studies have found no association between paternal irradiation and childhood cancer risk.[58,59,60]

CONCLUSION

Every living being is exposed to in utero radiation (background radiation). Background radiation includes cosmic rays from outer space, terrestrial radiation from the earth and building materials, and naturally occurring radioisotopes (ingested or inhaled). It has been estimated that background radiation contributes an exposure of approximately 0.075 to 0.1 rem (0.75–1.0 mSv) during the period of gestation.[1] Estimates of the spontaneous risks are 15% to 20% for abortion, 3% for major malformations, 4% for intrauterine growth retardation, and 8% to 10% for late-onset genetic diseases. These risks are considerably greater than the risk attributed to an exposure of 1 rem (10 mSv) during gestation. Brent calculated the risk of 1 rad (1 cGy) to be approximately 0.003%. Thus, the risks associated with low-dose radiation exposures such as those used during medical procedures are many thousands of times smaller than the spontaneous risks.[61,62]

RECOMMENDATIONS

Unnecessary radiation exposure should always be avoided. If an exposure is unavoidable, the following criteria should be applied:

1. Total exposure can be limited by minimizing the time of exposure;
2. The distance from the radiation source should be maximized;
3. Shielding should be used whenever possible.

Finally, patients should be counseled that the risk is extremely small for a fetal dose below 5 cGy but that there is a significant possibility of damage for fetal doses >50 cGy.

REFERENCES

1. Jankowski CB. Radiation and pregnancy. Putting the risks in proportion. *Am J Nurs.* 1986; 86:260–265.
2. Brent R, Meistrich M, Paul M. Ionizing and nonionizing radiations. In: Paul M, ed. *Occupational and Environmental Reproductive Hazards: A Guide for Clinicians.* Baltimore, MD: Williams & Wilkins; 1993:165–200.
3. Lazarus E, De Benedictis C, Mayo-Smith WW, et al. Use of radiological examinations in pregnant women: a ten year review-1997–2006. Radiological Society of North America Scientific Assembly and Annual Meeting 2007, Chicago, 436.
4. Ratnapalan S, Bona N, Chandra K, et al. Physicians' perceptions of teratogenic risk associated with radiography and CT during early pregnancy. *Am J Roentgenol.* 2004;182(5): 1107–1109
5. Bentur Y, Horlatsch N, Koren G. Exposure to ionizing radiation during pregnancy: perception of teratogenic risk and outcome. *Teratology.* 1991;43(2):109–112.
6. International Commission on Radiological Protection, eds. *Annals of the ICRP, Publication 84: Pregnancy and Medical Radiation 30 (1).* Tarrytown, NY: Pergamon, Elsevier Science, Inc.; 2000.
7. Prenatal Radiation Exposure: A Fact Sheet for Physicians. Department of Health and human Services. Center for Disease Control and Prevention. Available at: www.bt.cdc.gov/radiation
8. Bentur Y. Ionizing and nonionizing radiation in pregnancy. In: Koren G, ed. *Maternal-Fetal Toxicology. A Clinician's Guide.* 3rd ed. New York, NY: Marcel Dekker Inc; 2001.
9. Russell LB. Information from specific-locus mutants on the nature of induced and spontaneous mutations in the mouse. In: Ramel C, Lambert B, Magnusson J, eds. *Genetic Toxicology of Environmental Chemicals. Part B: Genetic Effects and Applied Mutagenesis.* New York, NY: A. R. Liss, Inc., 1986:37–447.
10. Mole RH. Detriment in human after irradiation in utero. *Int J Radiat Biol.* 1991;60: 561–564.
11. De Santis M, Di Gianantonio E, Straface G, et al. Ionizing radiations in pregnancy and teratogenesis. A review of literature. *Reprod Toxicol.* 2005;20:323–329.
12. Brent RL. Utilization of developmental basic science principles in the evaluation of reproductive risks from pre- and postconception environmental radiation exposures. *Teratology.* 1999;59:182–204.
13. Boice JD Jr. Studies of atomic bomb survivors. Understanding radiation effects. *JAMA.* 1990;264 (5):622–623.
14. Brent RL. Saving lives and changing family histories: appropriate counseling of pregnant women and men and women of reproductive age, concerning the risk of diagnostic radiation exposures during and before pregnancy. *Am J Obstet Gynecol.* 2009;200(1):4–24.
15. Goldstein L, Murphy DP. Microcephalic idiocy following radium therapy for uterine cancer during pregnancy. *Am J Obstet Gynecol.* 1929;18:189–195, 289–293.
16. Goldstein L, Murphy DP. Etiology of ill health in children born after maternal pelvic irradiation. Part II. Defective children born after postconceptional maternal irradiation. *Am J Roentgenol.* 1929;22:322–331.
17. Debakan AS. Abnormalities in children exposed to X-radiation during various stages of gestation: tentative timetable of radiation injury to the human fetus I. *J Nucl Med.* 1968;9(9):471–477.

18. Plummer G. Anomalies occurring in children exposed in utero to the atomic bomb in Hiroshima. *Pediatrics.* 1952;10(6):687–693.

19. Blot WJ, Miller RW. Mental retardation following in utero exposure to the atomic bomb of Nagasaki and Hiroshima. *Radiology.* 1973;106:617–619.

20. Otake M, Schull WJ. Radiation-related small head sizes among prenatally exposed atomic bomb survivors. Technical Report Series, RERF 6-92, 1992.

21. Otake M, Schull WJ. In utero exposure to A-bomb radiation and mental retardation: a reassessment. *Br J Radiol.* 1984;57:409–414.

22. Schull WJ, Otake M. Effects on intelligence of prenatal exposure to ionizing radiation. Hiroshima, Japan: Radiation Effects Research Foundation; 1986.

23. Schull WJ, Otake M. Cognitive function and prenatal exposure to ionizing radiation. *Teratology.* 1999;59:222–226.

24. Otake M, Schull WJ, Lee S. Threshold for radiation-related severe mental retardation in prenatally exposed A-bomb survivors: a reanalysis. *Int J Radiat Biol.* 1996;70:755–763.

25. Miller RW. Severe mental retardation and cancer among atomic bomb survivors exposed in utero. *Teratology.* 1999;59:234–235.

26. Schull WJ. *Effects of Atomic Radiation: A Half-Century of Studies from Hiroshima and Nagasaki.* New York, NY: Wiley-Liss & Sons, Inc.; 1995.

27. Smith H. The detrimental health effects of ionizing radiation. *Nucl Med Commun.* 1992;13(1):4–10.

28. Streffer C, Shore R, Konermann G, et al. Biological effects after prenatal irradiation (embryo and fetus). A report of the International Commission on Radiological Protection. *Ann ICRP.* 2003;33(1–2):5–206.

29. Einhorn L. Can prenatal irradiation protect the embryo from tumor-development. *Acta Oncologica* 1991;30(3):291–299.

30. Brent RL. Radiation-induced embryonic and fetal loss from conception to birth. In: Porter IH, Hook EB, eds. *Human Embryonic and Fetal Death.* New York, NY: Academic Press; 1980:177–181

31. Rugh R, Duhamel L, Skareoff L. Relation of embryonic and fetal X-irradiation to life time average weights and tumor incidence in mice. *Proc Soc Exp Biol Med.* 1966;121:714–718.

32. Reincke U, Stutz E, Wegner G. Tumoren nach einmaliger Roentgenbestrahlen weisser Ratten in verscheidenem Lebensalter. *Z Krebsforsch.* 1964;66:165–186.

33. Boice JD, Miller RW. Childhood and adult cancer after intrauterine exposure to ionizing radiation. *Teratology.* 1999;59:227–233.

34. Wakeford R, Little MP. Risk coefficients for childhood cancer after intrauterine irradiation: a review. *Int J Radiat Biol.* 2003;79:203–209.

35. Doll R, Wakeford R. Risk of childhood cancer from fetal irradiation. *Br J Radiol.* 1997;70:130–139.

36. Brent, RL. The effects of embryonic and fetal exposure to x-ray, microwaves, and ultrasound. *Clin Perinatol.* 1986;13(3):615–648.

37. Bithell JF, Stiller CA. A new calculation of the carcinogenic risk of obstetric X-raying. *Stat Med.* 1988;7:857–864.

38. Mole RH. Childhood cancer after prenatal exposure to diagnostic X-ray examinations in Britain. *Br J Cancer.* 1990;62(1):152–168.

39. Yoshimoto Y, Mabuchi K. Mortality and cancer risk among offspring (F₁) of atomic bomb survivors. *J Radiat Res (Tokyo).* 1991;32(suppl):294–300.

40. Miller RW. Epidemiological conclusions from radiation toxicity studies. In: Fry RJ, Grahn D, Griem ML, Rust JH, eds. *Late Effects of Radiation.* London: Taylor & Francis; 1970.

41. Wagner LK, Lester RG, Saldana LR. *Exposure of the Pregnant Patient to Diagnostic Radiations: A Guide to Medical Management.* 2nd ed. Madison, WI: Medical Physics Publishing; 1997.

42. Osei EK 1999, Faulkner K. Fetal position and size data for dose estimation. *Br J Radiol.* 1999;72:363–370.

43. Sharp C, Shrimpton JA, Bury RF. *Diagnostic Medical Exposures: Advice in Exposure to Ionising Radiation during Pregnancy.* National Radiological Protection Board; Chilton, Didcot, Oxon, UK; 1998.

44. Kinlen LJ. Diagnostic irradiation, congenital malformations and spontaneous abortion. *Br J Radiol.* 1968;41:648–654.

45. Bohnen N, Ragozzino MW, Kurland LT. Effect of diagnostic radiation during pregnancy on head circumference at birth. *Int J Neurosci.* 1996;87:175–180.

46. Mole RH. Radiation effects on pre-natal development and their radiological significance. *Br J Radiol.* 1979;614(52):89–101.

47. Otake M, Schull WJ, Yoshimaru, H. Brain damage among the prenatally exposed. *J Radiat Res.* 1991;32.

48. Hu Y, Yao J. Long-term effects of prenatal diagnostic X-rays on childhood physical and intellectual development. *J Radiol Prot.* 1994;14:251–255.

49. NRCP. Medical radiation exposure of pregnant and potentially pregnant women. Report No. 54. Washington, USA: NRCP; 1977.

50. International Commission on Radiological Protection, eds. *Annals of the ICRP, Publication 90: Biological Effects After Prenatal Irradiation (Embryo and Fetus) 33 (1–2).* Tarrytown, NY: Pergamon, Elsevier Science, Inc.; 2003.

51. National Council on Radiation Protection and Measurements, *Limitation of Exposure to Ionizing Radiation,* NCRP Report No. 116, Bethesda, MD, 1993.

52. Roman E, Watson A, Beral V, et al. Case-control study of leukaemia and non-Hodgkin's lymphoma among children aged 0–4 years living in west Berkshire and north Hampshire health districts. *Br Med J.* 1993;306:615–621.

53. Doyle P, Maconochie N, Roman E, et al. Fetal death and congenital malformation in babies born to nuclear industry employees: report from the nuclear industry family study. *Lancet.* 2000;356:1293–1299.

54. Dummer TJB, Dickinson HO, Pearce MS, et al. Stillbirth rates around the nuclear installation at Sellafield, North West England: 1950–1989. *Int J Epidemiol.* 1998;27:74–82.

55. Castronovo FP Jr. Teratogen update: radiation and Chernobyl. *Teratology.* 1999;60(2):100–106.

56. Sperling K, Pelz J, Wegner RD, et al. Frequency of trisomy 21 in Germany before and after the Chernobyl accident. *Biomed Pharmacother.* 1991;45(6):255–262.

57. Senturia YD, Peckham CS, Peckham MJ. Children fathered by men treated for testicular cancer. *Lancet.* 1985;2(8458):766–769.

58. Schull WJ, Neel JV. Atomic bomb exposure and the pregnancies of biologically related parents. A prospective study of the genetic effects of ionizing radiation in man. *Am J Public Health Nations Health.* 1959;49(12):1621–1629.

59. Miller RW. Relation between cancer and congenital defects: an epidemiologic evaluation. *J Natl Cancer Inst.* 1968;40(5):1079–1085.

60. Koren G, ed. *Maternal-Fetal Toxicology. A Clinician's Guide.* 3rd ed. New York, NY: Marcel Dekker Inc.; 2001.

61. Brent RL. The effect of embryonic and fetal exposure to X-ray, microwaves, and ultrasound: counseling the pregnant and nonpregnant patient about these risks. *Semin Oncol.* 1989;16(5):347–368.

62. De Santis M, Cesari E, Nobili E, et al. Radiation effects on development. *Birth Defects Res C.* 2007;81:177–182.

Nadia N. Issa Laack
Paul D. Brown

Cognitive Sequelae of Brain Radiation

INTRODUCTION

Radiotherapy (RT) is a proven curative and palliative therapeutic tool in the treatment of a wide variety of primary and metastatic brain tumors. Recent advances in multimodality therapy have led to improvement in survival for many cancer patients. As survival has improved, more attention has been directed toward long-term treatment-related morbidity. Specifically, the effect of RT on the long-term cognitive performance has become a major concern. Analyses of neurocognitive function are confounded by numerous other factors such as the tumor itself, surgery, chemotherapy, concurrent medical illnesses, neurologic comorbidity, and medications. These competing risks make determination of the contribution of RT to the patient's total impairment difficult. This chapter attempts to review the pathophysiologic mechanisms of RT-induced central nervous system (CNS) injury, discusses the incidence and factors determining risk of cognitive dysfunction in adults and children, summarizes the data on prevention of and treatment of injury, and presents areas for future research and intervention based on our current pathophysiologic understanding.

PATHOPHYSIOLOGY OF CNS INJURY

Because the morbidity caused by cranial irradiation can be devastating, the radioresponse of normal CNS tissues has been extensively studied and reviewed.[1–7] More recently, molecular and cellular biologic research have begun to shed light on the biochemical processes that may be responsible for RT-induced CNS injury.[8–10] The typical response after radiation to the whole-brain or large-volume brain irradiation has classically been divided into three categories, acute, subacute, and late, based on the timing of onset of symptoms.[6,11] Acute effects

are reversible and occur during the first weeks of fractionated radiation. Acute effects are characterized by drowsiness, headache, nausea, emesis, and worsening of preexisting focal symptoms. Increased cerebral edema is believed to be the cause of the symptoms, and treatment with dexamethasone usually results in symptomatic improvement.[6] A prospective study using positron emission tomography (PET) to document CNS metabolism and blood flow supports this hypothesis. CNS blood flow measured by ^{15}O–H_2O PET increased at 3 weeks and decreased at 6 months after RT. Compared to baseline, metabolism measured by FDG-PET decreased in association with increasing dose at 3 weeks (during RT) and 6 months after RT.[12] Early delayed or subacute encephalopathy typically presents at 1 to 6 months after completion of RT and is also reversible. Typical symptoms include headache, somnolence, fatigability, and deterioration in preexisting deficits.[13] Subacute encephalopathy is believed to be secondary to diffuse demyelination.[7,14] Although corticosteroids are useful in ameliorating symptoms, the syndrome typically resolves spontaneously within several months after presentation.[13]

Late delayed effects generally appear >6 months after irradiation and are often irreversible and progressive.[4] Late delayed injury is generally localized to the white matter and is thought to be secondary to vascular injury, demyelination, and ultimately necrosis. Therapeutic radiation trials suggest the risk of necrosis is low, generally between 2% and 7% at 5 years, even with the relatively high doses used to treat primary brain tumors.[15] Long-term follow-up of children receiving therapeutic cranial radiation demonstrates a higher risk of cerebral vascular disease including small vessel disease and atrophy as well as stroke and moyamoya syndrome, supporting a vascular mechanism of injury. Rates of significant vascular events have been reported to be as high as 4% at 5 years after moderate to high-dose RT, which, although is overall quite low, is higher than expected in an age-matched healthy population and would be expected to increase over time in long-term survivors.[16–18] Diffusion tensor imaging studies show progressive, dose-dependent demyelination that begins focally in high-dose regions during radiation and becomes diffuse independent of dose beyond 7 months after RT.[14] Radiation necrosis is the culmination of both parenchymal injury and loss of normal vascularity and generally is seen 18 to 24 months after the completion of RT.[1]

Late effects can be further characterized as focal radiation necrosis, diffuse white matter injury, and combined therapy leukoencephalopathy.[1] Symptoms vary depending on type and location of injury. In focal radiation necrosis, symptoms include seizures, symptoms of increased intracranial pressure, and neuroanatomic-specific symptoms. MRI reveals an area of irregular enhancement often with surrounding edema.

Focal radiation necrosis is often difficult to distinguish from recurrent or progressive tumor (Fig. 16.1), and although PET and magnetic resonance spectroscopy (MRS) may help differentiate the two, tissue biopsy is currently required to make a definitive diagnosis.[19,20] Symptoms of diffuse white matter injury range from mild lassitude to significant memory loss and severe dementia.[1] Combined therapy leukoencephalopathy can be similar to diffuse white matter injury but can also include ataxia, confusion, dysarthria, seizures, and ultimately incapacitating dementia or death.[21,22] Imaging findings are similar to that of diffuse white matter injury but also may include dystrophic calcification of the basal ganglia and gray-white matter interface.[1]

The tolerance of the normal CNS to RT refers to the incidence of severe morbidity (usually necrosis) and mortality after cranial RT. Based on both mathematical models and results of

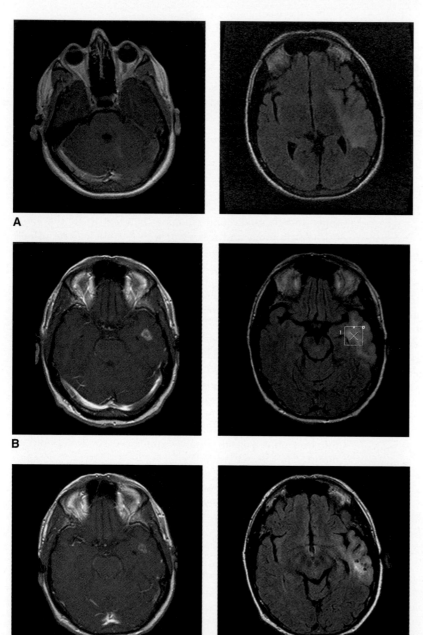

Figure 16.1. **A:** MR imaging of 62-year-old male with grade 2 oligodendroglioma showing no contrast enhancement on T1 (*left*) with gadolinium and hyperintense T2 signal as well as fullness of sulci on FLAIR axial images (*right*). **B:** 6 months after completion of 54-Gy conformal RT, the patient developed contrast-enhancing lesion in left temporal lobe (*left*). Decrease mass effect noted on T2 FLAIR image (*right*). MRS showed elevated lactate peak consistent with radionecrosis. **C:** 3 years after RT. Slow involution of area of radionecrosis. Note generalized mild cerebral atrophy, worse in left temporal lobe in region of RT.

treatment of primary CNS tumors, the TD 5/5 or 5% probability of necrosis at 5 years after RT is approximately 50 Gray (Gy) for whole-brain radiation and 60 Gy for partial brain irradiation.[6,23] These estimates are very crude and do not take into account factors known to influence CNS tolerance such as different fractionation schedules, concurrent medical illnesses (diabetes, hypertension), and adjunctive therapy.[11,24] Because survival after treatment of cranial neoplasms is improving, evaluation of treatment outcome has moved toward the detection of more subtle evidence of radiation toxicity (i.e., neurocognitive deterioration) that may occur independent of overt necrosis.

Cognitive dysfunction is often seen in the absence of radionecrosis or other imaging abnormality suggesting a cellular or molecular mechanism of radiation injury. Two primary mechanisms of radiation injury have been proposed, the vascular injury hypothesis and the neuroglial hypothesis. The vascular hypothesis is based primarily on data that are convergent with the mechanisms of injury leading to radionecrosis but on a microscopic scale. Death of endothelial cells in the microvasculature has been shown to begin during RT.[8] This is the mechanism partially responsible for the acute edema that develops during therapy and is often treated with corticosteroids. Over the following weeks to months, there continues to be progressive loss of endothelia. Similar to atherosclerotic vessel disease, the abnormal endothelial surface is "sticky" and platelets then adhere to the exposed matrix. These fine capillaries are then partially or fully occluded by thrombi. This is followed by abnormal endothelial proliferation.[1,8] Some of the abnormalities noted include thickening of the basement membranes and replacement of the lumen by collagen, fibrinoid necrosis of small arterial vessels, accelerated atherosclerosis, vascular insufficiency, and infarction.[8] Autopsy studies confirm that the microscopic vascular changes are similar to the small vessel disease seen in vascular dementia.[25–27] Over time, loss of capillary vasculature results in brain atrophy, specifically loss of white matter, which can eventually be seen on radiographic imaging.[28–31]

Although radiographically, loss of white matter or disruption of the structure of normal appearing white matter is prominent after cranial RT, physiologically, the hippocampal-dependent functions of learning, memory, and spatial information processing seem to be preferentially affected by RT.[27,32–37] In addition, cognitive effects associated with radiographic changes are associated with high dose cranial RT. Recent data suggest a cellular and molecular response occurs in the CNS in response to even very low doses of radiation. Neural stem cells, present in the hippocampus, continue to generate progenitor cells that can differentiate into neurons, even into adulthood and are suspected to be a target of low-dose radiation injury.[38–40] Neurogenesis in adults is associated with learning and new memory.[41] Evidence is accumulating that radiation reduces neurogenesis in the hippocampus and causes an inflammatory response that alters the neural microenvironment and may mediate the radiation injury. Monje et al. elegantly demonstrate *in vitro* and in an *in vivo* rat model that low doses of radiation (2 Gy) reduce the number of newborn neurons in the hippocampus as well as induce a microglial inflammatory response. The activation and proliferation of microglia in hippocampus were found to be responsible for the effects on neurogenesis and neurodifferentiation. Interestingly, the authors also noted loss of normal association between neuron progenitors and microvasculature, an association that is necessary for neuron differentiation.[39]

A recent study using boron-neutron capture technique, which allows selective irradiation of either the microvasculature or neural parenchyma, suggests the neural parenchyma is responsible for the majority of the decline in neurogenesis in response to ionizing radiation.[42] Other researchers have confirmed the role of the hippocampal neurogenesis in the response to radiation injury[33,43–46] including a study using heavy charged particles and similar doses (0.5–4.0 Gy) in a mouse model of brain radiation exposure.[47]

Recently, clinical support for this hypothesis has been presented in the form of a case-control autopsy series. In a report of four patients of varying ages and receiving various radiation doses, a 10- to 100-fold reduction in neuron granule cells in hippocampus was documented in the patients who had received radiation. In one particularly interesting case, a patient who had previously received whole-brain RT (WBRT) received focal radiation to the left hippocampus and temporal lobe 1 month prior to her death. Comparison of the left and right hippocampus in the same patient revealed 79% fewer newborn cells, 59% fewer dividing cells, as well as a twofold increase in activated microglia on the side irradiated twice, which the authors conclude provide clinical support to their *in vitro* and *in vivo* data.[40,48]

It is becoming increasingly clear that the pathophysiology of late RT injury is dynamic, complex, and a result of inter- and intracellular interactions between the vasculature and many of the parenchymal cell lines.[39] Recent cellular studies have also implicated astrocytes, microglia, neurons, and neuronal stem cells as modulators of the CNS response to radiation and shown that there are different responses to low- and high-dose radiation.[3,39] Based on these data, interest has developed in understanding the neural microenvironment that may be responsible for the propagation of radiation injury with hopes of developing a more targeted approach to treating or preventing radiation injury. Because radiation injury is associated with an inflammatory response, including the formation of radical oxygen species and release of inflammatory cytokines, which appear to contribute to impaired neurogenesis, blocking the inflammatory cascade would be expected to reduce the radiation effect on impaired neurogenesis.[38,49] Indomethacin, a nonsteroidal anti-inflammatory, was effective in reducing the number of activated microglia and increased the rate of neurogenesis twofold when given before and after RT in a mouse model of radiation injury.[38] Glutamate via NMDA-receptor pathway is also hypothesized to be a potential mediator of radiation injury.[50] Glutamate is the primary neurotransmitter involved in the excitotoxicity mechanism of neuron degeneration and death seen in similar forms of neurodegenerative dementia, specifically vascular dementia.[51] WBRT results in impairment of spatial learning and memory in rats that correlates with alterations of the NMDA receptor in the hippocampus.[33] Other proposed molecules or pathways for possible mediation of inflammatory injury are the superoxide dismutase pathway, which may mediate free-radical formation after radiation[52]; renin-angiotensin pathway and angiotensin II, an inflammatory cytokine associated with radiation injury and inflammation[53]; and the VEGF pathway, which is associated with radiation necrosis.[49]

In summary, the latent period after RT is believed to an active phase where cytokines and growth factors play an important role in cellular communication. Apoptosis, or programmed cell death, may be the mechanism of glial and endothelial destruction. Injury to astrocytes and microglia may disrupt the balance

TABLE 16.1	Factors Associated with Increased Risk of Brain Injury After RT
Risk Factor	*Increased Risk of Radiation Injury*
Dose	Higher total dose
Volume	Larger brain volume
Age	Infants, young children
Host factors	Vascular comorbidities (diabetes, atherosclerosis, hypertension), tumor type (PCNSL)
Concurrent medical therapy	Concurrent use of chemotherapy (e.g., methotrexate)

of growth factors necessary for glial growth and endothelial stability.[9] The pathophysiology of radiation injury suggests a complex association of vascular and neuroglial injury as well as changes in the neural microenvironment and microglia that result in both cellular and eventually anatomic changes in the brain.[11]

COGNITIVE EFFECTS IN ADULTS

The majority of data suggesting cognitive toxicity after RT are from patients receiving therapeutic radiation.[4] The next section of this chapter reviews the quantitative data available to describe the scope and severity of radiation injury as well as clinical risk factors for the development of cognitive injury (Table 16.1).

BRAIN METASTASES

The treatment of brain metastasis is controversial in the neuro-oncology community. This is largely because of the concerns of cognitive sequelae of whole-brain radiation in populations of patients who are experiencing improvements in survival due to advances in chemotherapy to control systemic disease.[54,55] Because of these cognitive concerns, more focal RT, such as stereotactic radiosurgery (SRS) for individual metastases, is being studied as a method to reduce the potential cognitive effects of therapy.

WBRT is the primary treatment for metastatic disease to brain. Most patients are treated with a short course of large-fraction radiation (e.g., 30 Gy in ten fractions). In one of the earliest reports detailing cognitive decline after RT, DeAngelis et al. identified 12 patients with brain metastases who developed delayed complications of WBRT with an incidence of dementia of 1.9% to 5.1% in the two populations reviewed. Although the total dose of WBRT was only 2,500 to 3,900 cGy, daily fractions of 300 to 600 cGy were employed in these patients. The authors noted large daily fraction sizes predispose patients to delayed neurologic toxicity, and they recommended more protracted schedules (smaller fraction sizes) to improve the safety and efficacy of WBRT for "good-risk" patients with brain metastases.[56]

Retrospective studies such as this are limited by the lack of baseline testing. Tumor characteristics and progression have a significant role in cognitive dysfunction that confounds neurocognitive data for patients who have received RT, especially in retrospective studies.[11] In the largest prospective

neurocognitive study of patients receiving WBRT, 90% of patients were cognitively impaired in one or more domain at baseline, *prior* to radiation. The authors also noted that 60% of patients experienced neurocognitive decline in one or more domain at 6 months after WBRT but that neurocognitive decline correlated closely with progressive disease. Although tumor progression had the strongest impact on neurocognitive outcome, statistically significant declines at 6 months were seen in some domains, particularly early and delayed memory, even in patients without progressive disease.[57]

Exposure to neurotoxic chemotherapy and high total radiation dose are also associated with an increased risk of radiation injury to the brain. Progressive multifocal leukoencephalopathy is a rare but devastating toxicity that has been reported to occur in patients after exposure to certain neurotoxic chemotherapy agents such as methotrexate or rituximab alone,[58,59] and has also been documented with combined-modality (radiation and chemotherapy) therapy. Five patients in one report of long-term survivors after 40 to 50 Gy WBRT with concurrent cis-platinum based chemotherapy for metastatic germ cell tumors developed progressive multifocal leukoencephalopathy. The initial study included 60 patients with CNS metastatic disease, 30 of whom succumbed to their disease, leaving 30 patients who survived for assessment of long-term toxicity. MRI revealed gliosis and diffuse atrophy. All five patients had significant neurologic disability and three eventually died. This report confirms the importance of total dose and volume as well as concurrent use of potentially additive neurotoxic agents in the risk of CNS injury.[60]

The importance of volume of radiated brain is also associated with risk of cognitive injury. SRS for brain metastasis is highly focused RT to small volumes (usually tumors <3 cm) but very large fraction sizes (12–25 Gy) given generally in a single treatment. In a recent study comparing SRS to WBRT for patients with up to up to three brain metastasis, 49% of patients in the WBRT group experienced declines in learning and memory at 4 months compared to only 23% in the SRS group. The study is small, and critics note a substantial difference in survival in the two groups, strongly suggesting the patients may not have been well matched for prognostic factors.[61,62] Additionally, at 4 months, cognitive function after RT is at a nadir due to subacute or early delayed effects of RT that gradually resolve over time (Fig. 16.2).[63] In a recent report of long-term survivors

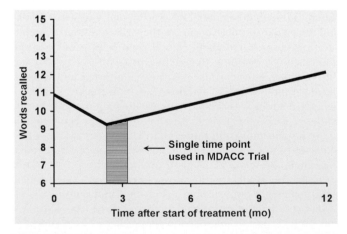

Figure 16.2. Hopkins verbal learning test words recalled by time after start of RT in brain tumor patients. (From Armstrong CL, et al. Radiotherapeutic effects on brain function: double dissociation of memory systems. *Neuropsychiatry Neuropsychol Behav Neurol.* 2000;13(2):101–111.)

TABLE 16.2	Cognitive Outcomes after Whole-Brain RT for Brain Metastases in Prospective Trials with Baseline Testing				
Author	Number Receiving RT	Radiation Total Dose/Fraction Size (Gy)	Timing of Neurocognitive Assessment	Type of Neurocognitive Assessment	Neurotoxicity After RT
Regine et al.[134]	445 patients on study; 359 with neurocognitive assessment	30/10 or 54.4/ 1.6 bid	2- and 3-mo post-RT outcomes reported	MMSE	MMSE decreased 0.5–0.6 for patients with tumor control MMSE decreased 1.9–6.3 for patients with progressive disease
Penitzka et al.[135]	64 total WBRT; 36 for brain metastasis	40/20	3-,6- and 9-mo outcomes reported	90-min battery (intelligence, attention, memory)	No declines noted
Meyers et al.[57]	401 total	30/10	Q1 mo × 6 mo then Q3 mo until death	45-minute battery (memory, motor speed/dexterity, executive function)	90% of patients impaired at baseline (before RT); NCF measured at 2 mo post-RT correlated with tumor progression
Li et al.[64]	208 (135 assessable with MRI data)	30/10	Q1 mo × 6 mo then Q3 mo until death	45-minute battery (memory, motor speed/dexterity, executive function)	Control group of Meyers'[57] study. Tumor regression at 2 mo correlated with delay in NCF decline. 15-mo survivors had stable or improving NCF
Aoyama et al.[65]	132 total; 65 received WBRT	30/10 with SRS boost vs. SRS alone (18–25 Gy)	Median 5.3 mo (range 0.7–58.7)	MMSE	Addition of WBRT improved average time until MMSE decline over SRS alone (7.6 mo vs. 16.5 mo, $p = 0.05$)
Corn et al.[136]	156	37.5/15 ± thalidomide	Q2 mo	MMSE	Neurocognitive failure defined as MMSE <23; 35% failed at 12 mo post-RT
Chang et al.[62]	58 total; 28 received WBRT	30/12 with SRS boost vs. SRS alone (15–24 Gy)	4 mo	HVLT (learning and memory)	HVLT decline at 4 mo more frequent after WBRT + SRS than SRS alone (49% vs. 23%)

MMSE, Folstein Mini-Mental State Examination; RT, radiotherapy; WBRT, whole-brain radiotherapy; MRI, magnetic resonance imaging; NCF, neurocognitive function; SRS, stereotactic radiosurgery; HVLT, Hopkins verbal learning test.

(15 months) after WBRT, neurocognitive function correlated most strongly with tumor progression such that patients with sustained reduction of tumor burden actually had improved neurocognitive function.[64] The effect of tumor control on neurocognitive function was also seen in a similar study of SRS with or without WBRT. Patients neurocognitive function again correlated with tumor progression, and because SRS alone patients experienced earlier brain relapse, time to neurocognitive decline as measured by Mini-Mental Status Exam (MMSE) was shorter in the SRS alone group.[65] Although it is generally accepted that there is a volume effect of RT such that larger volumes of irradiated brain may result in a higher risk of cognitive injury, these studies illustrate the complex association between effects of tumor control, dose per fraction, and volume of radiation with radiation injury.

Overall, it is difficult to determine the effects of RT from the other confounding variables in patients with brain metastasis. Large fraction sizes are associated with dementia and cognitive decline after WBRT as are high total dose and concurrent use of chemotherapy. Large-volume RT is more likely to have a higher risk of cognitive injury in comparison to partial brain volumes although it seems progression of brain metastasis is the dominant cause of cognitive deterioration in this population (Table 16.2).

LOW-GRADE GLIOMAS

The role of cranial RT in the management of low-grade gliomas has also generated much controversy in the neuro-oncology community. Because of their longer progression-free survival, patients with low-grade glioma have sufficient time to "develop" late radiation neurotoxicity,[36] which has been documented in a number of retrospective studies.[66–70]

Prospective studies have found an increased risk of cognitive injury with higher total dose.[71] In a prospective North Central Clinical Trial Cooperative Group (NCCTG)-led intergroup trial, 203 eligible/analyzable adult patients with supratentorial low-grade gliomas were randomized to a lower dose (50.4 Gy per 28 fractions) or a higher dose (64.8 Gy per 36 fractions) of

TABLE 16.3	Cognitive Outcomes after RT for Low-Grade Gliomas in Prospective Trials with Baseline Testing				
Author	Histology (Number Receiving RT)	Radiation Total Dose/ Fraction Size (Gy)	Mean Follow-up (yr)	Type of Neurocognitive Assessment	Neurotoxicity After RT
Glosser et al.[137]	Chordoma, chondrosarcoma (17)	Proton RT median 68.4 CGE/1.8 CGE	4	Intelligence/conceptual reasoning, language and visuospatial processing, memory, attention, motor function	No; mild decline in psychomotor speed with high doses
Vigliani et al.[74]	LGG, AA (17)	54/1.8	4	2.5-hour battery (intelligence, attention, memory)	No; transient decline in reaction time
Armstrong et al.[73]	LGG, pituitary, pineal, meningioma (26)	Mean 54.6/1.8–2.0	3	4-hour battery (intelligence, attention, memory, verbal learning, cognitive flexibility, psychomotor skills, language)	No; mild decline in visual memory after 5 yr
Brown et al.[72]	LGG (203)	50.4/1.8 or 64.8/1.8	7.4 (median)	MMSE and NFS	5.3% with MMSE decline at 5 yr
Torres et al.[75]	Meningioma, LGG, GBM, ependymoma, adenoma (15)	Mean 54/1.8	2	Memory, attention, and processing speed	No decline up to 2 yr after RT; decline in memory and attention only if tumor progression
Laack et al.[36]	LGG (20)	50.4/28 or 64.8/33	3	4-hour battery (intelligence, attention, memory, verbal learning, cognitive flexibility, psychomotor skills, language)	No decline up to 5 yr after RT; mild decline in 64.8 Gy arm in immediate verbal memory, learning, and spatial problem solving

AA, anaplastic astrocytoma; GBM, glioblastoma multiforme; LGG, low-grade glioma; MMSE, Folstein Mini-Mental State Examination; NFS, neurologic function scores; RT, radiotherapy.

localized radiation therapy. Grade 3 to 5 radiation neurotoxicity (necrosis, encephalitis, death) developed in six patients in the high-dose arm (2-yr actuarial rate of 5%) and in one patient in the low-dose arm (2-year actuarial rate of 2.5%).[15] Brown et al. reviewed the cognitive performance data collected prospectively in these patients. MMSEs and neurologic function scores (NFS) recorded at baseline and at each study evaluation were analyzed to assess cognitive and physical function over time. Median follow-up was 7.4 years in the 101 patients alive at the time of analysis.[72] The percentages of patients without tumor progression who experienced significant deterioration of their MMSE scores from baseline at years 1, 2, and 5 were 8.2%, 4.6%, and 5.3% respectively. In contrast, the majority of patients with an abnormal baseline MMSE score (<27) experienced significant gains (59%, 50%, and 67% at years 1, 2, and 5, respectively). Although these results are encouraging, one of the major limitations in this study is the insensitivity of the measurement tool, the MMSE, relative to sophisticated neuropsychometric tests. The first 20 patients (10 in each dose arm) treated on this protocol (who agreed to further assessment) did undergo an extensive battery of neuropsychometric tests at baseline (before RT) and at 18-month intervals for up to 5 years after completing RT. No significant decline of new learning, intellectual, or memory function for the two dose groups over the period of follow-up in these patients was found.[36] Other centers have conducted prospective neuropsychometric testing before and after RT and found similar results with little

evidence of widespread neurocognitive deficits due to radiation therapy.[63,73–75] The results from these trials are similar to the data observed in brain metastasis patients in that higher total dose, larger fraction sizes, and larger brain volumes are associated with increased risk of cognitive decline after RT; however, the preponderance of prospective data shows the risk of significant cognitive decline after focal, moderate-dose RT to be very low (Table 16.3).

PRIMARY CENTRAL NERVOUS SYSTEM LYMPHOMA (PCNSL)

Primary central nervous system lymphoma (PCNSL) is a malignant brain tumor sensitive to both chemotherapy and radiation. Historically patients were treated with WBRT alone. Median survival after WBRT alone is approximately 12 to 18 months[76] with a high incidence of neurotoxicity in the long-term survivors. Recently, combined modality treatment has been shown to improve survival. Although survival has increased in some reports to over 40 months, the incidence of neurotoxicity is still high.[77–80] Combined therapy may cause severe leukoencephalopathy and brain atrophy. Symptoms of dementia-ataxia syndrome typically occur 4 months to several years after treatment.[81] Elderly patients appear to be particularly at risk. Reports of 8% to 50% incidence of severe dementia after WBRT with or without chemotherapy are found in the literature with the incidence rising to 62% to 82% for patients older than 60 years.[82,83] CNS lymphoma has a predisposition for perivascular infiltration, which may play a role in the breakdown of the blood-brain barrier (BBB).[80] Disruption of the BBB may place the CNS at higher risk of late toxicity after cranial irradiation.[84] Attempts to improve toxicity with hyperfractionation (a smaller fraction of radiation given more than once a day) have been unsuccessful.[79] The severity of neurotoxicity after RT for PCNSL testifies to the variety of confounding variables that influence neurocognitive effects of radiation. In PCNSL, older age, the infiltrative nature of the tumor itself,[83] and adjuvant use of neurotoxic chemotherapeutic agents[85] result in high rates of neurocognitive dysfunction after radiation.

COGNITIVE EFFECTS IN CHILDREN

Since the time of the atomic bomb exposures of Hiroshima and Nagasaki, studies of radiation exposure, primarily prenatally, have been associated with increased risk of mental retardation and cognitive deficits.[86] The window of greatest sensitivity was found to be between 8 and 25 weeks of gestation. MRI studies revealed abnormally situated gray matter suggesting altered neuronal migration. Microcephaly was also noted in this cohort and associated with overall growth retardation as well as mental retardation. After birth, radiation effects on the brain are less pronounced and gross structural abnormalities are generally not seen.[87] However, the developing brain continues to exhibit increased sensitivity to ionizing radiation in comparison with adults. Although the exquisite sensitivity of the developing brain declines gradually over time, the exact age the brain takes on a more adult susceptibility pattern is unknown. Data in pediatric LGG suggest minimal IQ falloff after age 12.[88]

Similar to adults, most data describing the cognitive effects of radiation exposure come from therapeutic radiation studies. Leukemia is the most common childhood malignancy. The BBB reduces penetration of chemotherapy agents and the CNS is considered to be a "sanctuary site" for harboring residual tumor cells that eventually result in relapse. Early in the treatment of pediatric leukemia, cranial or craniospinal RT was used in combination with chemotherapy to consolidate CNS therapy of leukemia patients. Because these patients were being treated prophylactically, the potential cognitive effects of tumor and surgery are removed, and this should be an informative group to evaluate the effects of RT. Results have been mixed with some studies showing neurocognitive decline after 18 Gy when compared to children who did not receive RT,[89] while other studies have not documented a detectable decline after similar doses. A prospective trial evaluating neurocognitive outcome in children with childhood acute lymphoblastic leukemia (ALL) treated with 18, 24 Gy, or no cranial RT showed no difference between the groups.[90] However, 22% to 30% experienced significant cognitive decline over time with females and young age being associated most closely with risk of cognitive injury. Unfortunately, even in this more ideal cohort, the effect of RT alone is difficult to distinguish, and the CNS toxic chemotherapy agent, methotrexate, used in this trial was suspected to have a role in the cognitive decline found in the nonirradiated group. Methotrexate has been associated with cognitive decline in subsequent ALL studies as well.[91] Although disruption of the integrity of normal appearing white matter and white matter volume loss, specifically in the temporal lobes, hippocampi,

and thalami, is documented by diffusion-tensor imaging and MRI in long-term survivors of ALL, it is difficult to determine the contribution of cranial RT to this finding.[92,93] Smaller white matter volumes are associated with larger deficits in attention, intelligence, and academic achievement[94] in this population as well.

The most complete data on long-term cognitive effects after brain radiation are from St. Jude Children's Research Hospital. Merchant et al.[88,95-97] have reported on 5-year neuropsychiatric data after radiation for a variety of tumor types including ependymoma, LGG, medulloblastoma, and craniopharyngioma. IQ losses after RT ranged from 2 to 4 points per year. Age and volume of brain, especially supratentorial brain, receiving different doses of RT were associated with cognitive injury such that the youngest patients and those receiving the highest dose to the largest brain volume were most affected. Interestingly, even infants (>12 months) receiving very high dose of highly focal or conformal RT to the posterior fossa for ependymoma showed minimal cognitive decline. A modest but significant decline in reading scores was seen over time, but math and spelling performance remained stable. This was felt to be due to the minimal supratentorial radiation exposure and more minor contribution of the cerebellum to cognitive function, confirming the importance of volume and location of radiation to risk of cognitive injury.[98]

Therapeutic doses of RT are clearly associated with cognitive impairment in young children, with the risk increasing both with decreasing age and increasing radiation dose and volume. Although higher dose RT is associated with increased risk of radiation injury, recent data suggest that even very low doses of RT, such as those administered during diagnostic imaging studies such as computed tomography (CT), may also result in late cognitive impairment. In a population-based cohort study from Sweden, over 3,000 male infants (<18 months) who were treated with cutaneous RT for hemangiomas were found to have a lower rates of high-school graduation and lower scores on standardized tests of learning ability and logical reasoning than the unirradiated cohort. The calculated dose to the cortical brain was estimated to be 10 cGy, similar to the radiation exposure from a head CT. A dose-response relationship was also observed such that infants receiving >25 cGy were more likely to experience declines in learning and logical reasoning. Although an epidemiologic study, Sweden has a nationalized health system and requires cognitive testing for all males prior to the required military service at age 18 resulting in a reliable and complete data set for this report. The study is limited by the inability to compare irradiated infants with a similar cohort of patients with hemangiomas who did not receive radiation. However, the dose-response effects on neurocognitive function support the role for radiation exposure as at least a contributor to cognitive outcomes in this cohort.[99] Previous epidemiologic data for children receiving CT in early childhood or cranial radiation exposure for ringworm treatment revealed similar findings. Children receiving low doses (1–1.5 Gy) of cranial radiation in those reports had lower school examination scores, IQ scores, and psychological test scores.[87] These data support the increased radiosensitivity of the developing brain to even very low doses of radiation.

The exquisite sensitivity of neural stem cells in the hippocampus to ionizing radiation may explain recent accumulating data that even low radiation doses may contribute to changes in cognitive function. Mouse models of radiation injury support a role for even very low doses of radiation on the neural microenvironment. Gene expression profiles in mice radiated with 10 cGy showed high degree of concordance with the unirradiated aging human brain and brain tissue from Alzheimer patients. This transcriptional response was not seen after higher doses (2 Gy) of radiation.[100]

Taken together, the available evidence suggests an increased risk of neurocognitive toxicity in children with even moderate dose radiation. Risk of cognitive injury is most strongly associated with age, with the youngest patients being the most vulnerable to radiation injury. It is possible that even diagnostic doses of radiation may affect cognitive development in infants. Volume and brain location are also critical with supratentorial brain being more commonly associated with increased risk of late cognitive injury. Current therapeutic trials in the pediatric population aim to minimize total radiation dose, delay RT when safe for as long as possible, and minimize volume of brain irradiated to minimize the risk of cognitive injury.

RADIATION EXPOSURE

Although the vast majority of cognitive outcome data have been derived from radiation therapy patients, longitudinal data on populations exposed to ionizing radiation after nuclear incidents or other incidental exposures also provide insight into the cognitive effects of radiation.

The Chernobyl nuclear reactor accident exposed hundreds of thousands of people in the Ukraine, including infants and children, to a range of radiation doses. The WHO as well as American and Israeli researchers have found no significant association of radiation exposure with cognitive impairment in the prenatally exposed, infants, and young children. Cognitive impairment was documented by Ukrainian researchers, but these results have not been independently verified.[101] In a 4-year longitudinal study, researchers performed neuropsychiatric testing on healthy Ukrainian volunteers living >200 km away from the accident site to populations with varying degrees of radiation exposure. Testing began 8 years after radiation exposure and was repeated annually for 4 years. Significant cognitive declines were seen in all exposed groups and correlated with degree of radiation exposure. Memory, learning, and visual-motor slowing were preferentially affected. The estimated brain radiation dose to the different groups was not reported. The study did not control for other general health effects of acute and chronic radiation exposure, such as endocrine or metabolic deficiencies. Nevertheless, these data may suggest a risk of long-term neurocognitive effects after radiation exposure.[102]

PREVENTION AND TREATMENT OF COGNITIVE SEQUELAE

It is becoming increasingly clear that the pathophysiology of late RT injury is dynamic, complex, and a result of intercellular and intracellular interactions between the vasculature and many of the parenchymal cell lines.[38] Recent cellular studies have also implicated astrocytes, microglia, neurons, and neuron stem cells as modulators of the CNS response to radiation.[3,38] Hippocampal-dependent functions of learning, memory, and spatial information processing seem to be preferentially affected by RT. Rational design of preventive strategies requires a pathophysiologic understanding of the intracellular mechanisms.

Hippocampal-sparing RT is currently being evaluated as a potential mechanism to reduce radiation morbidity (Fig. 16.3). Advances in RT treatment delivery and target localization allow delineation of hippocampus and avoidance of high doses of RT to that region.[103–105] The threshold dose for radiation injury to the hippocampus is unknown, so it is unclear whether the doses achievable will result in clinically significant improvements in cognitive function.

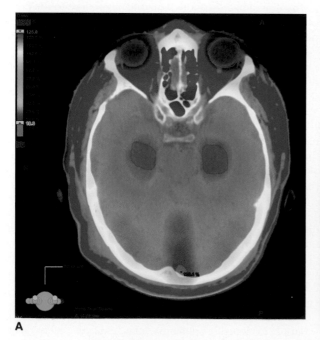
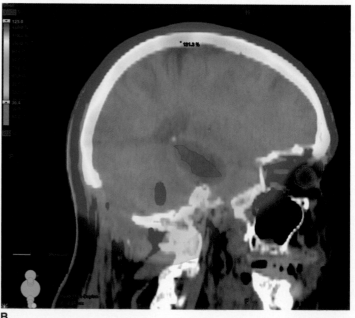

A   **B**

Figure 16.3. Radiation isodose curves depicting hippocampus-sparing WBRT. Hippocampus receives <20% of the radiation prescription dose.

Fike et al.[106] showed that a-difluoromethylornithine (DFMO, a polyamine synthesis inhibitor), reduced the volume of radionecrosis and contrast-enhancement in dog brain. Kondziolka et al. used U-74389G, a 21-aminosteroid that is selective to the endothelium, administered intravenously approximately 1 hour prior to gamma-knife treatment for rat C6-glioma. The drug prevented the development of perifocal edema and radiation-induced vascular damage in the surrounding healthy rat brain.[107]

Based on the neuroglial hypothesis, mediators of neurogenesis have also been proposed for prevention of radiation injury. Lithium prevents apoptosis of neural stem cells in the hippocampus after radiation and has been used in a phase I trial in humans.[108] Tianeptine, a clinically effective antidepressant, has been shown to stimulate neurogenesis and prevent apoptosis in the hippocampus in mouse models.[109] Pretreatment with melatonin has been shown to reduce the decline in neurogenesis seen after brain radiation *in vivo*. Melatonin was noted to be a free-radical scavenger that may mediate the protective effect in the hippocampus.[110] A recent prospective trial in humans, however, did not support a role for melatonin in preserving neurologic function although cognitive function was not the primary outcome of the trial.[111] Pioglitazone, an anti-inflammatory agent, has also been shown to prevent cognitive dysfunction in rats when administered prior to RT.[112]

Erythropoietin (EPO) has shown promise in preventing and reversing radiation-induced cognitive injury in animals. EPO in cell media is able to prevent neuronal death secondary to radicals generated by sodium nitroprusside that have similar activity to the hydroxyl radical (an agent with a prominent role in mediating radiation-related injury).[113,114] Studies in rats have shown that EPO is produced by astrocytes[115] and neurons[116] and prevents glutamate-induced neuronal death *in vitro*.[115] EPO has been shown to improve cognitive performance in mice[117] and ischemia-induced cognitive impairment in gerbils.[118]

The Radiation Therapy Oncology Group (RTOG) is currently conducting a prospective randomized trial evaluating memantine for the prevention of cognitive dysfunction after WBRT. Memantine, an NMDA-receptor channel blocker,[119] has been shown to prevent propagation of vascular injury in mouse stroke models[120] and has been shown to improve cognitive function in vascular dementia patients.[121,122] Further elucidation of the cellular interactions between the different CNS cell types will lead to a better understanding of the radiation response of the brain as well as targets for therapeutic intervention.

Treatment of cognitive sequelae of cranial radiation is limited at this time.[123] Methylphenidate has been used in a few small series of patients exhibiting neurobehavioral slowing with good response.[124–126] Patients who develop psychomotor slowing, decline in executive functioning, or general apathy may particularly benefit.[125] Unfortunately, a phase III, placebo-controlled trial did not confirm a benefit in cognitive function of quality of life in patients receiving RT for brain tumors.[127,128]

Histologic evidence supports a role for vascular injury as a cause of late radiation injury. Hyperbaric oxygen (HBO) has been reported to improve radiation fibrosis and vascular injury at other anatomic sites.[129] Unfortunately, a phase I/II trial of HBO for seven patients with cognitive deficits after cranial radiation did not support a benefit for these patients.[130] Because demyelination has also been implicated in late radiation injury, oligodendroglial cells have been studied as potential therapeutic target. A study by Groves et al.[131] showed that transplantation of purified O-2A (oligodendrocyte type 2 astrocyte) cells

into demyelinated lesions caused by radiation and ethidium bromide resulted in remyelinization of the lesions by the O-2A cells. O-2A and other cells capable of myelinating lesions in the brain can be derived from totipotent embryonal stem cells.[132]

Donepezil has been used as in the treatment of Alzheimer dementia and showed promise in the treatment of radiation induced cognitive injury in a phase II trial.[133] A phase III, placebo-controlled trial has been performed to confirm this finding, the results of which are still pending. Therapy trials such as this one are similarly confounded by the same factors that prohibit study of radiation effects on cognition in adults (the tumor itself, surgery, other medications), and it may be difficult to detect improvements in cognition if the overwhelming etiology for cognitive dysfunction is due to irreversible tumor or other causes.

CONCLUSIONS

Cognitive impairment after CNS radiation can range from mild apathy to incapacitating dementia. Cognitive deterioration may occur in patients undergoing WBRT, hypofractionated RT, and concurrent neurotoxic chemotherapy and is likely due to late delayed effects of RT. Certain tumor types such as primary CNS non-Hodgkin lymphoma[134–139] place patients at particular risk for cognitive injury after radiation. Young children and elderly patients are also more susceptible to radiation injury. In infants and very young children, even diagnostic doses of RT may result in detrimental cognitive effects. The hippocampus may mediate the effects of RT on cognition.

Recent cellular, molecular, and biochemical work has been instrumental in elucidating the mechanism of the CNS response to radiation. In the future, we can expect the rational development of selective radiosensitizers and radioprotective agents to reduce the morbidity of cranial RT, especially in children. Development of targeted therapeutic agents is also needed for patients in whom RT cannot be avoided.

REFERENCES

1. Schultheiss TE, Kun LE, Ang KK, et al. Radiation response of the central nervous system. *Int J Radiat Oncol Biol Phys.* 1995;31(5):1093–1112.
2. Dropcho EJ. Central nervous system injury by therapeutic irradiation. *Neurol Clin.* 1991;9(4):969–988.
3. Tofilon PJ, Fike JR. The radioresponse of the central nervous system: a dynamic process. *Radiat Res.* 2000;153(4):357–370.
4. Kramer S. The hazards of therapeutic irradiation of the central nervous system. *Clin Neurosurg.* 1968;15:301–318.
5. Hopewell JW, Wright EA. The nature of latent cerebral irradiation damage and its modification by hypertension. *Br J Radiol.* 1970;43(507):161–167.
6. Sheline GE, Wara WM, Smith V. Therapeutic irradiation and brain injury. *Int J Radiat Oncol Biol Phys.* 1980;6(9):1215–1228.
7. van der Kogel AJ. Radiation-induced damage in the central nervous system: an interpretation of target cell responses. *Br J Cancer Suppl.* 1986;7:207–217.
8. Belka C, Budach W, Kortmann RD, et al. Radiation induced CNS toxicity—molecular and cellular mechanisms. *Br J Cancer.* 2001;85(9):1233–1239.
9. Nieder C, Andratschke N, Price RE, et al. Innovative prevention strategies for radiation necrosis of the central nervous system. *Anticancer Res.* 2002;22(2A):1017–1023.
10. Monje ML, Mizumatsu S, Fike JR, et al. Irradiation induces neural precursor-cell dysfunction. *Nat Med.* 2002;8(9):955–962.
11. Laack NN, Brown PD. Cognitive sequelae of brain radiation in adults. *Semin Oncol.* 2004;31(5):702–713.
12. Hahn CA, Zhou SM, Raynor R, et al. Dose-dependent effects of radiation therapy on cerebral blood flow, metabolism, and neurocognitive dysfunction. *Int J Radiat Oncol Biol Phys.* 2009;73(4):1082–1087.
13. Boldrey ES, Sheline G. Delayed transitory clinical manifestation after radiation treatment of intracranial tumors. *Acta Radiol.* 1967;5:5–10.
14. Nagesh V, Tsien CI, Chenevert TL, et al. Radiation-induced changes in normal-appearing white matter in patients with cerebral tumors: a diffusion tensor imaging study. *Int J Radiat Oncol Biol Phys.* 2008;70(4):1002–1010.

15. Shaw E, Arusell R, Scheithauer B, et al. Prospective randomized trial of low- versus high-dose radiation therapy in adults with supratentorial low-grade glioma: initial report of a North Central Cancer Treatment Group/Radiation Therapy Oncology Group/Eastern Cooperative Oncology Group study [see comments]. *J Clin Oncol.* 2002;20(9):2267–2276.

16. Keene DL, Johnston DL, Grimard L, et al. Vascular complications of cranial radiation. *Childs Nerv Syst.* 2006;22(6):547–555.

17. Kikuchi A, Maeda M, Hanada R, et al. Moyamoya syndrome following childhood acute lymphoblastic leukemia. *Pediatr Blood Cancer.* 2007;48(3):268–272.

18. Ishikawa N, Tajima G, Yofune N, et al. Moyamoya syndrome after cranial irradiation for bone marrow transplantation in a patient with acute leukemia. *Neuropediatrics.* 2006;37(6):364–366.

19. Di Chiro G, Oldfield E, Wright DC, et al. Cerebral necrosis after radiotherapy and/or intraarterial chemotherapy for brain tumors: PET and neuropathologic studies. *AJR Am J Roentgenol.* 1988;150(1):189–197.

20. Schlemmer HP, Bachert P, Henze M, et al. Differentiation of radiation necrosis from tumor progression using proton magnetic resonance spectroscopy. *Neuroradiology.* 2002;44(3):216–222.

21. Price RA, Jamieson PA. The central nervous system in childhood leukemia. II. Subacute leukoencephalopathy. *Cancer.* 1975;35(2):306–318.

22. Doyle DM, Einhorn LH. Delayed effects of whole brain radiotherapy in germ cell tumor patients with central nervous system metastases. *Int J Radiat Oncol Biol Phys.* 2008;70(5):1361–1364.

23. Emami B, Lyman J, Brown A, et al. Tolerance of normal tissue to therapeutic irradiation. *Int J Radiat Oncol Biol Phys.* 1991;21(1):109–122.

24. Shaw E. Central nervous system tumors: overview. In: Gunderson LL, Tepper JE, eds. *Clinical Radiation Oncology.* Philadelphia, PA: Churchill Livingstone; 2000:314–335.

25. Brown WR, Moody DM, Thore CR, et al. Vascular dementia in leukoaraiosis may be a consequence of capillary loss not only in the lesions, but in normal-appearing white matter and cortex as well. *J Neurol Sci.* 2007;257(1–2):62–66.

26. Brown WR, Blair RM, Moody DM, et al. Capillary loss precedes the cognitive impairment induced by fractionated whole-brain irradiation: a potential rat model of vascular dementia. *J Neurol Sci.* 2007;257(1–2):67–71.

27. Moretti R, Torre P, Antonello RM, et al. Neuropsychological evaluation of late-onset post-radiotherapy encephalopathy: a comparison with vascular dementia. *J Neurol Sci.* 2005;229-230:195–200.

28. Fujii O, Tsujino K, Soejima T, et al. White matter changes on magnetic resonance imaging following whole-brain radiotherapy for brain metastases. *Radiat Med.* 2006;24(5):345–350.

29. Reddick WE, Glass JO, Palmer SL, et al. Atypical white matter volume development in children following craniospinal irradiation. *Neuro-Oncol.* 2005;7(1):12–19.

30. Reddick WE, Glass JO, Helton KJ, et al. A quantitative MR imaging assessment of leukoencephalopathy in children treated for acute lymphoblastic leukemia without irradiation. *Am J Neuroradiol.* 2005;26(9):2371–2377.

31. Shibamoto Y, Baba F, Oda K, et al. Incidence of brain atrophy and decline in mini-mental state examination score after whole-brain radiotherapy in patients with brain metastases: a prospective study. *Int J Radiat Oncol Biol Phys.* 2008;72(4):1168–1173.

32. Raber J, Rola R, LeFevour A, et al. Radiation-induced cognitive impairments are associated with changes in indicators of hippocampal neurogenesis. *Radiat Res.* 2004;162(1):39–47.

33. Shi L, Adams MM, Long A, et al. Spatial learning and memory deficits after whole-brain irradiation are associated with changes in NMDA receptor subunits in the hippocampus. *Radiat Res.* 2006;166(6):892–899.

34. Nagel BJ, Delis DC, Palmer SL, et al. Early patterns of verbal memory impairment in children treated for medulloblastoma. *Neuropsychology.* 2006;20(1):105–112.

35. Nagel BJ, Palmer SL, Reddick WE, et al. Abnormal hippocampal development in children with medulloblastoma treated with risk-adapted irradiation. *Am J Neuroradiol.* 2004;25(9):1575–1582.

36. Laack NN, Brown PD, Ivnik RJ, et al. Cognitive function after radiotherapy for supratentorial low-grade glioma: a North Central Cancer Treatment Group prospective study. *Int J Radiat Oncol Biol Phys.* 2005;63(4):1175–1183.

37. Armstrong CL, Hunter JV, Ledakis GE, et al. Late cognitive and radiographic changes related to radiotherapy: initial prospective findings. *Neurology.* 2002;59(1):40–48.

38. Monje ML, Palmer T. Radiation injury and neurogenesis. *Curr Opin Neurol.* 2003;16(2):129–134.

39. Monje ML, Mizumatsu S, Fike JR, et al. Irradiation induces neural precursor-cell dysfunction. *Nat Med.* 2002;8(9):955–962.

40. Monje ML, Vogel H, Masek M, et al. Impaired human hippocampal neurogenesis after treatment for central nervous system malignancies. *Ann Neurol.* 2007;62(5):515–520.

41. Barani IJ, Benedict SH, Lin PS. Neural stem cells: implications for the conventional radiotherapy of central nervous system malignancies. *Int J Radiat Oncol Biol Phys.* 2007;68(2):324–333.

42. Otsuka S, Coderre JA, Micca PL, et al. Depletion of neural precursor cells after local brain irradiation is due to radiation dose to the parenchyma, not the vasculature. *Radiat Res.* 2006;165(5):582–591.

43. Andres-Mach M, Rola R, Fike JR. Radiation effects on neural precursor cells in the dentate gyrus. *Cell Tissue Res.* 2008;331(1):251–262.

44. Andres-Mach M, Rosi S, Rola R, et al. Radiation effects on neurogenic regions in the mammalian forebrain. *Future Neurol.* 2007;2(6):647–659.

45. Limoli CL, Giedzinski E, Rola R, et al. Radiation response of neural precursor cells: linking cellular sensitivity to cell cycle checkpoints, apoptosis and oxidative stress. *Radiat Res.* 2004;161(1):17–27.

46. Mizumatsu S, Monje ML, Morhardt DR, et al. Extreme sensitivity of adult neurogenesis to low doses of X-irradiation. *Cancer Res.* 2003;63(14):4021–4027.

47. Rola R, Fishman K, Baure J, et al. Hippocampal neurogenesis and neuroinflammation after cranial irradiation with 56Fe particles. *Radiat Res.* 2008;169(6):626–632.

48. Monje M. Cranial radiation therapy and damage to hippocampal neurogenesis. *Dev Disabil Res Rev.* 2008;14(3):238–242.

49. Kim JH, Brown SL, Jenrow KA, et al. Mechanisms of radiation-induced brain toxicity and implications for future clinical trials. *J Neuro-Oncol.* 2008;87(3):279–286.

50. Orrego F, Villanueva S. The chemical nature of the main central excitatory transmitter: a critical appraisal based upon release studies and synaptic vesicle localization. *Neuroscience.* 1993;56(3):539–555.

51. Danysz W, Parsons CG, Karcz-Kubicha M, et al. GlycineB antagonists as potential therapeutic agents. Previous hopes and present reality. *Amino Acids.* 1998;14(1–3):235–239.

52. Rola R, Zou Y, Huang TT, et al. Lack of extracellular superoxide dismutase (EC-SOD) in the microenvironment impacts radiation-induced changes in neurogenesis. *Free Radic Biol Med.* 2007;42(8):1133–1145.

53. Robbins ME, Diz DI. Pathogenic role of the renin-angiotensin system in modulating radiation-induced late effects. *Int J Radiat Oncol Biol Phys.* 2006;64(1):6–12.

54. Smalley SR, Laws ER Jr, O'Fallon JR, et al. Resection for solitary brain metastasis. Role of adjuvant radiation and prognostic variables in 229 patients. *J Neurosurg.* 1992;77(4):531–540.

55. Kelly K, Bunn PA Jr. Is it time to reevaluate our approach to the treatment of brain metastases in patients with non-small cell lung cancer? *Lung Cancer.* 1998;20(2):85–91.

56. DeAngelis LM, Delattre JY, Posner JB. Radiation-induced dementia in patients cured of brain metastases. *Neurology.* 1989;39(6):789–796.

57. Meyers CA, Smith JA, Bezjak A, et al. Neurocognitive function and progression in patients with brain metastases treated with whole-brain radiation and motexafin gadolinium: results of a randomized phase III trial. *J Clin Oncol.* 2004;22(1):157–165.

58. Ram R, Ben-Bassat I, Shpilberg O, et al. The late adverse events of rituximab therapy—rare but there! *Leuk Lymphoma.* 2009;50:1083–1095.

59. Matsubayashi J, Tsuchiya K, Matsunaga T, et al. Methotrexate-related leukoencephalopathy without radiation therapy: distribution of brain lesions and pathological heterogeneity on two autopsy cases. *Neuropathology.* 2009;29(2):105–115.

60. Doyle DM, Einhorn LH. Delayed effects of whole brain radiotherapy in germ cell tumor patients with central nervous system metastases [see comment]. *Int J Radiat Oncol Biol Phys.* 2008;70(5):1361–1364.

61. Chang EL, Wefel JS, Maor MH, et al. A pilot study of neurocognitive function in patients with one to three new brain metastases initially treated with stereotactic radiosurgery alone. *Neurosurgery.* 2007;60(2):277–283; discussion 283–284.

62. Chang EL, Wefel JS, Hess KR, et al. Neurocognition in patients with brain metastases treated with radiosurgery or radiosurgery plus whole-brain irradiation: a randomized controlled study. *Lancet Oncol.* 2009;10:1037–1044.

63. Armstrong CL, Corn BW, Ruffer JE, et al. Radiotherapeutic effects on brain function: double dissociation of memory systems. *Neuropsychiatry Neuropsychol Behav Neurol.* 2000;13(2):101–111.

64. Li J, Bentzen SM, Renschler M, et al. Regression after whole-brain radiation therapy for brain metastases correlates with survival and improved neurocognitive function. *J Clin Oncol.* 2007;25(10):1260–1266.

65. Aoyama H, Tago M, Kato N, et al. Neurocognitive function of patients with brain metastasis who received either whole brain radiotherapy plus stereotactic radiosurgery or radiosurgery alone. *Int J Radiat Oncol Biol Phys.* 2007;68(5):1388–1395.

66. Gregor A, Cull A, Traynor E, et al. Neuropsychometric evaluation of long-term survivors of adult brain tumours: relationship with tumour and treatment parameters. *Radiother Oncol.* 1996;41(1):55–59.

67. Surma-aho O, Niemela M, Vilkki J, et al. Adverse long-term effects of brain radiotherapy in adult low-grade glioma patients. *Neurology.* 2001;56(10):1285–1290.

68. Asai A, Matsutani M, Kohno T, et al. Subacute brain atrophy after radiation therapy for malignant brain tumor. *Cancer.* 1989;63(10):1962–1974.

69. Taphoorn MJ, Schiphorst AK, Snoek FJ, et al. Cognitive functions and quality of life in patients with low-grade gliomas: the impact of radiotherapy. *Ann Neurol.* 1994;36(1):48–54.

70. Klein M, Heimans JJ, Aaronson NK, et al. Effect of radiotherapy and other treatment-related factors on mid-term to long-term cognitive sequelae in low-grade gliomas: a comparative study. *Lancet.* 2002;360(2):1361–1368.

71. Kiebert GM, Curran D, Aaronson NK, et al. EORTC Radiotherapy Co-operative Group. Quality of life after radiation therapy of cerebral low-grade gliomas of the adult: results of a randomised phase III trial on dose response (EORTC trial 22844). *Eur J Cancer.* 1998;34(12):1902–1909.

72. Brown P, Buckner J, O'Fallon J, et al. Effects of radiotherapy on cognitive function in patients with low-grade glioma measured by the Folstein Mini-Mental State Examination. *J Clin Oncol.* 2003;21(13):2519–2524.

73. Armstrong CL, Hunter JV, Ledakis GE, et al. Late cognitive and radiographic changes related to radiotherapy: initial prospective findings [see comments]. *Neurology.* 2002;59(1):40–48.

74. Vigliani MC, Sichez N, Poisson M, et al. A prospective study of cognitive functions following conventional radiotherapy for supratentorial gliomas in young adults: 4-year results. *Int J Radiat Oncol Biol Phys.* 1996;35(3):527–533.

75. Torres IJ, Mundt AJ, Sweeney PJ, et al. A longitudinal neuropsychological study of partial brain radiation in adults with brain tumors. *Neurology.* 2003;60(7):1113–1118.

76. Nelson DF, Martz KL, Bonner H, et al. Non-Hodgkin's lymphoma of the brain: can high dose, large volume radiation therapy improve survival? Report on a prospective trial by the Radiation Therapy Oncology Group (RTOG): RTOG 8315. *Int J Radiat Oncol Biol Phys.* 1992;23(1):9–17.

77. Herrlinger U, Schabet M, Brugger W, et al. Primary central nervous system lymphoma 1991–1997: outcome and late adverse effects after combined modality treatment. *Cancer.* 2001;91(1):130–135.

78. Bessell EM, Graus F, Lopez-Guillermo A, et al. CHOD/BVAM regimen plus radiotherapy in patients with primary CNS non-Hodgkin's lymphoma. *Int J Radiat Oncol Biol Phys.* 2001;50(2):457–464.

79. DeAngelis LM, Seiferheld W, Schold SC, et al. Combination chemotherapy and radiotherapy for primary central nervous system lymphoma: Radiation Therapy Oncology Group Study 93-10. *J Clin Oncol.* 2002;20(24):4643–4648.

80. O'Brien P, Roos D, Pratt G, et al. Phase II multicenter study of brief single-agent methotrexate followed by irradiation in primary CNS lymphoma. *J Clin Oncol.* 2000;18(3):519–526.

81. Keime-Guibert F, Napolitano M, Delattre JY. Neurological complications of radiotherapy and chemotherapy. *J Neurol.* 1998;245(11):695–708.

82. Basso U, Brandes AA. Diagnostic advances and new trends for the treatment of primary central nervous system lymphoma. *Eur J Cancer.* 2002;38(10):1298–1312.

83. Laack N, Ballman K, Brown PD, et al. Whole-brain radiotherapy (WBRT) and high-dose methylprednisolone (HDMP) for elderly patients with primary central nervous system lymphoma (PCNSL): results of North Central Cancer Treatment Group (NCCTG) 96–72–51. *Int J Radiat Oncol Biol Phys.* 2004;60(1 Suppl):S260.

84. Rubin P, Gash DM, Hansen JT, et al. Disruption of the blood-brain barrier as the primary effect of CNS irradiation. *Radiother Oncol.* 1994;31(1):51–60.

85. Blay JY, Conroy T, Chevreau C, et al. High-dose methotrexate for the treatment of primary cerebral lymphomas: analysis of survival and late neurologic toxicity in a retrospective series. *J Clin Oncol.* 1998;16(3):864–871.

86. Otake M, Schull WJ. Review: radiation-related brain damage and growth retardation among the prenatally exposed atomic bomb survivors. *Int J Radiat Biol.* 1998;74(2):159–171.

87. Verheyde J, Benotmane MA. Unraveling the fundamental molecular mechanisms of morphological and cognitive defects in the irradiated brain. *Brain Res Rev.* 2007;53(2):312–320.

88. Merchant TE, Kun L, Wu S, et al. A phase II trial of conformal radiotherapy for pediatric low grade glioma. *J Clin Oncol.* 2009.

89. Spiegler BJ, Kennedy K, Maze R, et al. Comparison of long-term neurocognitive outcomes in young children with acute lymphoblastic leukemia treated with cranial radiation or high-dose or very high-dose intravenous methotrexate [see comment] [erratum appears in *J Clin Oncol.* 2006;24(32):5181]. *J Clin Oncol.* 2006;24(24):3858–3864.

90. Mulhern RK, Fairclough D, Ochs J. A prospective comparison of neuropsychologic performance of children surviving leukemia who received 18-Gy, 24-Gy, or no cranial irradiation. *J Clin Oncol.* 1991;9(8):1348–1356.

91. Waber DP, Turek J, Catania L, et al. Neuropsychological outcomes from a randomized trial of triple intrathecal chemotherapy compared with 18 Gy cranial radiation as CNS treatment in acute lymphoblastic leukemia: findings from Dana-Farber Cancer Institute ALL Consortium Protocol 95-01. *J Clin Oncol.* 2007;25(31):4914–4921.

92. Dellani PR, Eder S, Gawehn J, et al. Late structural alterations of cerebral white matter in long-term survivors of childhood leukemia. *J Magn Reson Imaging.* 2008;27(6):1250–1255.

93. Mabbott DJ, Noseworthy MD, Bouffet E, et al. Diffusion tensor imaging of white matter after cranial radiation in children for medulloblastoma: correlation with IQ. *Neuro-Oncology.* 2006;8(3):244–252.

94. Reddick WE, Shan ZY, Glass JO, et al. Smaller white-matter volumes are associated with larger deficits in attention and learning among long-term survivors of acute lymphoblastic leukemia. *Cancer.* 2006;106(4):941–949.

95. Merchant TE, Kiehna EN, Li C, et al. Modeling radiation dosimetry to predict cognitive outcomes in pediatric patients with CNS embryonal tumors including medulloblastoma. *Int J Radiat Oncol Biol Phys.* 2006;65(1):210–221.

96. Merchant TE, Kiehna EN, Kun LE, et al. Phase II trial of conformal radiation therapy for pediatric patients with craniopharyngioma and correlation of surgical factors and radiation dosimetry with change in cognitive function. *J Neurosurg.* 2006;104(Suppl 2):94–102.

97. Merchant TE. Craniopharyngioma radiotherapy: endocrine and cognitive effects. *J Pediatr Endocrinol.* 2006;19(Suppl 1):439–446.

98. Conklin HM, Li C, Xiong X, et al. Predicting change in academic abilities after conformal radiation therapy for localized ependymoma. *J Clin Oncol.* 2008;26(24):3965–3970.

99. Hall P, Adami HO, Trichopoulos D, et al. Effect of low doses of ionising radiation in infancy on cognitive function in adulthood: Swedish population based cohort study. *Br Med J.* 2004;328(7430):19–21.

100. Lowe XR, Havenaar JM. Early brain response to low-dose radiation exposure involves molecular networks and pathways associated with cognitive functions, advanced aging and Alzheimer's disease. *Radiat Res.* 2009;171(1):53–65.

101. Bromet EJ, Havenaar JM. Psychological and perceived health effects of the Chernobyl disaster: a 20-year review. *Health Phys.* 2007;93(5):516–521.

102. Gamache GL, Levinson DM, Reeves DL, et al. Longitudinal neurocognitive assessments of Ukrainians exposed to ionizing radiation after the Chernobyl nuclear accident. *Arch Clin Neuropsychol.* 2005;20(1):81–93.

103. Barani IJ, Cuttino LW, Benedict SH, et al. Neural stem cell-preserving external-beam radiotherapy of central nervous system malignancies. *Int J Radiat Oncol Biol Phys.* 2007;68(4):978–985.

104. Ghia A, Tome WA, Thomas S, et al. Distribution of brain metastases in relation to the hippocampus: implications for neurocognitive functional preservation. *Int J Radiat Oncol Biol Phys.* 2007;68(4):971–977.

105. Gutierrez AN, Westerly DC, Tome WA, et al. Whole brain radiotherapy with hippocampal avoidance and simultaneously integrated brain metastases boost: a planning study. *Int J Radiat Oncol Biol Phys.* 2007;69(2):589–597.

106. Fike JR, Gobbel GT, Marton LJ, et al. Radiation brain injury is reduced by the polyamine inhibitor alpha- difluoromethylornithine. *Radiat Res.* 1994;138(1):99–106.

107. Kondziolka D, Mori Y, Martinez AJ, et al. Beneficial effects of the radioprotectant 21-aminosteroid U-74389G in a radiosurgery rat malignant glioma model. *Int J Radiat Oncol Biol Phys.* 1999;44(1):179–184.

108. Yang, ES, Li BSY, Hallahan DE. Lithium-mediated neuroprotection during cranial irradiation: a phase I trial. *Int J Radiat Oncol Biol Phys.* 2007:S586–687.

109. Akyurek S, Senturk V, Oncu B, et al. The effect of tianeptine in the prevention of radiation-induced neurocognitive impairment. *Med Hypotheses.* 2008;71(6):930–932.

110. Manda K, Ueno M, Anzai K. Cranial irradiation-induced inhibition of neurogenesis in hippocampal dentate gyrus of adult mice: attenuation by melatonin pretreatment. *J Pineal Res.* 2009;46(1):71–78.

111. Berk L, Berkey B, Rich T, et al. Randomized phase II trial of high-dose melatonin and radiation therapy for rpa class 2 patients with brain metastases (RTOG 0119). *Int J Radiat Oncol Biol Phys.* 2007;68(3):852–857.

112. Zhao W, Payne V, Tommasi E, et al. Administration of the peroxisomal proliferator-activated receptor gamma agonist pioglitazone during fractionated brain irradiation prevents radiation-induced cognitive impairment. *Int J Radiat Oncol Biol Phys.* 2007;67(1):6–9.

113. Senzer N. Rationale for a phase III study of erythropoietin as a neurocognitive protectant in patients with lung cancer receiving prophylactic cranial irradiation. *Semin Oncol.* 2002;29(6 Suppl 19):47–52.

114. Sakanaka M, Wen TC, Matsuda S, et al. In vivo evidence that erythropoietin protects neurons from ischemic damage. *Proc Natl Acad Sci USA.* 1998;95(8):4635–4640.

115. Morishita E, Masuda S, Nagao M, et al. Erythropoietin receptor is expressed in rat hippocampal and cerebral cortical neurons, and erythropoietin prevents in vitro glutamate-induced neuronal death. *Neuroscience.* 1997;76(1):105–116.

116. Bernaudin M, Bellail A, Marti HH, et al. Neurons and astrocytes express EPO mRNA: oxygen-sensing mechanisms that involve the redox-state of the brain. *Glia.* 2000;30(3): 271–278.

117. Hengemihle JM, Abugo O, Rifkind J, et al. Chronic treatment with human recombinant erythropoietin increases hematocrit and improves water maze performance in mice. *Physiol Behav.* 1996;59(1):153–156.

118. Catania MA, Marciano MC, Parisi A, et al. Erythropoietin prevents cognition impairment induced by transient brain ischemia in gerbils. *Eur J Pharmacol.* 2002;437(3): 147–150.

119. Chen HS, Pellegrini JW, Aggarwal SK, et al. Open-channel block of N-methyl-D-aspartate (NMDA) responses by memantine: therapeutic advantage against NMDA receptor-mediated neurotoxicity. *J Neurosci.* 1992;12(11):4427–4436.

120. Chen HS, Wang YF, Rayudu PV, et al. Neuroprotective concentrations of the N-methyl-D-aspartate open-channel blocker memantine are effective without cytoplasmic vacuolation following post-ischemic administration and do not block maze learning or long-term potentiation. *Neuroscience.* 1998;86(4):1121–1132.

121. Wilcock G, Mobius HJ, Stoffler A, et al. A double-blind, placebo-controlled multicentre study of memantine in mild to moderate vascular dementia (MMM500). *Int Clin Psychopharmacol.* 2002;17(6):297–305.

122. Orgogozo JM, Rigaud AS, Stoffler A, et al. Efficacy and safety of memantine in patients with mild to moderate vascular dementia: a randomized, placebo-controlled trial (MMM 300). *Stroke.* 2002;33(7):1834–1839.

123. Butler JM, Rapp SR, Shaw EG. Managing the cognitive effects of brain tumor radiation therapy. *Curr Treat Options Oncol.* 2006;7(6):517–523.

124. Meyers CA, Weitzner MA, Valentine AD, et al. Methylphenidate therapy improves cognition, mood, and function of brain tumor patients. *J Clin Oncol.* 1998;16(7):2522–2527.

125. Weitzner MA, Meyers CA, Valentine AD. Methylphenidate in the treatment of neurobehavioral slowing associated with cancer and cancer treatment. *J Neuropsychiatry Clin Neurosci.* 1995;7(3):347–350.

126. DeLong R, Friedman H, Friedman N, et al. Methylphenidate in neuropsychological sequelae of radiotherapy and chemotherapy of childhood brain tumors and leukemia. *J Child Neurol.* 1992;7(4):462–463.

127. Gleason Jr JF, Case D, Rapp SR, et al. Symptom clusters in patients with newly-diagnosed brain tumors. *J Support Oncol.* 2007;5(9):427–433, 436.

128. Butler JM Jr, Case LD, Atkins J, et al. A phase III, double-blind, placebo-controlled prospective randomized clinical trial of d-threo-methylphenidate HCl in brain tumor patients receiving radiation therapy. *Int J Radiat Oncol Biol Phys.,* 2007;69(5):1496–1501.

129. Plafki C, Carl UM, Glag M, et al. The treatment of late radiation effects with hyperbaric oxygenation (HBO). *Strahlenther Onkol.* 1998;174(Suppl 3):66–68.

130. Hulshof MC, Stark NM, van der Kleij A, et al. Hyperbaric oxygen therapy for cognitive disorders after irradiation of the brain. *Strahlenther Onkol.* 2002;178(4):192–198.

131. Groves AK, Barnett SC, Franklin RJ, et al. Repair of demyelinated lesions by transplantation of purified O-2A progenitor cells. *Nature.* 1993;362(6419):453–455.

132. Brustle O, Jones KN, Learish RD, et al. Embryonic stem cell-derived glial precursors: a source of myelinating transplants. *Science.* 1999;285(5428):754–756.

133. Shaw EG, Rosdhal R, D'Agostino RB, Jr, et al. Phase II study of donepezil in irradiated brain tumor patients: effect on cognitive function, mood, and quality of life. *J Clin Oncol.* 2006;24(9):1415–1420.

134. Regine WF, Scott C, Murray K, et al. Neurocognitive outcome in brain metastases patients treated with accelerated-fractionation vs. accelerated-hyperfractionated radiotherapy: an analysis from Radiation Therapy Oncology Group Study 91-04. *Int J Radiat Oncol Biol Phys.* 2001;51(3):711–717.

135. Penitzka S, Steinvorth S, Sehlleier S, et al. Assessment of cognitive function after preventive and therapeutic whole brain irradiation using neuropsychological testing]. *Strahlenther Onkol.* 2002;178(5):252–258.

136. Corn BW, Moughan J, Knisely JP, et al. Prospective evaluation of quality of life and neurocognitive effects in patients with multiple brain metastases receiving whole-brain radiotherapy with or without thalidomide on Radiation Therapy Oncology Group (RTOG) trial 0118. *Int J Radiat Oncol Biol Phys.* 2008;71(1):71–78.

137. Glosser G, McManus P, Munzenrider J, et al. Neuropsychological function in adults after high dose fractionated radiation therapy of skull base tumors. *Int J Radiat Oncol Biol Phys.* 1997;38(2):231–239.

138. Buckner JC, Gesme D, O'Fallon JR, et al. Phase II trial of procarbazine, lomustine, and vincristine as initial therapy for patients with low-grade oligodendroglioma or oligoastrocytoma: efficacy and associations with chromosomal abnormalities. *J Clin Oncol.* 2003;21(2):251–255.

139. Meyers CA, Hess KR, Yung WK, et al. Cognitive function as a predictor of survival in patients with recurrent malignant glioma. *J Clin Oncol.* 2000;18(3):646–650.

Helen A. Shih
Jay S. Loeffler

Hypothalamic-Pituitary Axis

GROSS ANATOMY, LOCATION, IMAGING OF NORMAL STRUCTURE

The hypothalamic-pituitary axis (HPA) comprises the hypothalamus, pituitary, and neuronal tracks bridging these two structures. Functionally, it includes endocrine organs of the thyroid, adrenal glands, and gonads. The hypothalamus lies in the deep anterior midline brain, inferior to the thalamus as its name suggests. The pituitary stalk connects the hypothalamus to the pituitary gland. The optic chiasm sits anterior to the pituitary stalk, otherwise known as the *infundibulum*. A normal pituitary gland is 7 to 10 mm in diameter but many normal variations exist. The gland itself is housed within the sella turcica, a bony out pouching of the posterior sphenoid bones. The pituitary gland is flanked by the cavernous sinuses on both sides. The sphenoid sinus lies immediately inferior and anterior to the sella.

The pituitary gland is a complex organ. It comprises three lobes: the adenohypophysis anteriorly, the neurohypophysis posteriorly, and the pars intermedia or intermediate lobe. The adenohypophysis, or anterior lobe, is the largest of the three lobes and produces multiple hormones that act upon downstream endocrine glands. The neurohypophysis, or posterior lobe, is contiguous with the hypothalamus via the median eminence and does not produce hormones but rather retains and releases hormones that are produced by the hypothalamus. The intermediate lobe is the smallest of the pituitary lobes, comprising a thin layer of cells separating the anterior and posterior lobes.

The bony landmarks of the sella and sphenoid sinuses are easily seen on plain film and computed tomography. The wall of the sella includes the tuberculum sellae anteriorly and the dorsum sella posteriorly. The sella abuts the anterior clinoids on both sides superioanteriorly and similarly the posterior clinoids superioposteriorly. Both the hypothalamus and the pituitary gland are best imaged by magnetic resonance imaging (MRI). The pituitary is best viewed on coronal or sagittal planes and can be followed in its attachment via the pituitary stalk to the hypothalamus. The pituitary has a homogeneous appearance on T1 weighting and enhances with gadolinium. The pattern of enhancement varies with time of imaging with sequential enhancement from the neurohypophysis, followed by the infundibulum, then the adenohypophysis lastly.

HISTOLOGICAL ANATOMY OF STRUCTURE—FUNCTIONAL UNITS IMPORTANT IN RADIATION DAMAGE

The hypothalamus produces a number of hormones that regulate pituitary function. These include growth hormone–releasing hormone (GHRH), corticotrophin-releasing hormone (CRH), thyroid-releasing hormone (TRH), and gonadotropin-releasing hormone (GnRH).

Hormonal production in the pituitary is divided by the individual cells that are differentiated by the lobes of the gland. The adenohypophysis produces a number of hormones, namely adrenocorticotropic hormone (ACTH), growth hormone (GH), thyroid-stimulating hormone (TSH), luteinizing hormone (LH), and follicular-stimulating hormone (FSH). The posterior lobe does not produce hormones but stores and releases the hypothalamic hormones antidiuretic hormone (ADH, also known as *vasopressin*) and oxytocin. The intermediate lobe of the pituitary produces melanocyte-stimulating hormone.

The perfusion of the pituitary gland may be a factor in determining the late effects of ionizing irradiation. The posterior lobe is supplied by the inferior hypophyseal artery. The anterior lobe, infundibulum, and median eminence are all supplied by the superior hypophyseal artery. The capillaries that feed the anterior pituitary lobe do not have the typical blood-brain barrier and thus provide vascular access for the pituitary hormones. Both hypophyseal arteries ultimately arise from the internal carotid arteries.

The specific cells that produce each of these hormones vary in their radiation sensitivity and are discussed in this chapter based upon both animal data and clinical experiences.

DATA FOR FRACTIONATED AND SINGLE-DOSE EFFECTS ON STRUCTURE

Sensitivity of the HPA to ionizing radiation is well documented, but the degree of tolerance and functional compromise of the HPA varies among the specific hormonal axes and details of radiation exposure. Single high-dose radiation exposure by stereotactic radiosurgery (SRS) is commonly used with treatment of hypersecreting pituitary adenomas. It is associated with a more rapid normalization of hypersecretion than fractionated radiation therapy. Both forms of radiotherapy harbor the risk of functional compromise to the remaining normal HPA axes and even to the originally hypersecretory axis. Fortunately, deficiencies within the HPA can generally be physiologically corrected with modern medical therapies.

ANIMAL DATA

Experimental data evaluating the radiation effects on the HPA are sparse due to the difficulty of developing useful systems to study. Because much of the concerning radiation effects are delayed by years, preclinical studies require ample time, expense, and an infrastructure to maintain and support such investigations. Most animal data utilize systems in which the bulk of the cranium of the animal is irradiated. Results are often hypothesized as an effect of HPA irradiation, but whether effects may be dependent entirely on the result of some other cranial structure cannot be entirely discounted.

Available biological studies document a variety of cellular and physiologic responses to radiation exposure, many with uncertain significance. A single fraction of 10 Gy is frequently chosen in animal studies because of its estimated effect to be equivalent to 24 Gy in 2-Gy fractions, a common cranial dose used in treating pediatric leukemia.[1] Multiple studies have documented that a single fraction of 10 Gy to the cranium of rats results in an acute increase in corticosterone and ACTH levels within 4 to 6 hours.[2,3] This is followed by a rise in corticotropin-releasing factor (CRF) mRNA 3 days later, possibly indicating a continued stimulatory effect on this axis and ultimately an acute and sustained response to stress. There appears to be a dose sensitivity threshold with GH-secreting cells being more sensitive to doses of larger than 3 Gy per fraction based upon a study of rat pituitary cells irradiated with a single dose between 1 and 15 Gy.[4] This was in contrast to other pituitary cell types such as basophilic cells that secrete gonadotropins or TSH that showed far greater radiation tolerance to single fraction doses with a threshold exceeding 10 Gy. High-dose cranial irradiation at 40 Gy in a single fraction is associated with increased apoptosis in the pituitary, but the significance of this in the setting of supratherapeutic dose to the pituitary is unclear.[5] Developmental effects of cranial irradiation indicate a dichotomy in which lower doses of 5 to 6 Gy in a single fraction given to immature female rats lead to an accelerated onset of puberty, whereas higher doses (≥9 Gy) lead to delayed sexual development.[6]

Another animal model used has been partial cranial irradiation of 8-week-old male rats in which the entire HPA was included.[7] Using this technique, investigators delivered 20 to 24 Gy in a single fraction and rats were assessed for their pituitary hormonal content as a surrogate of hormonal function at 8, 14, and 20 weeks. Compared to control rats, irradiated animals demonstrated a significant decrease in both body weight and pituitary gland size and showed a time- and dose-dependent pituitary insufficiency. Control rats demonstrated an increase in both body size and pituitary gland weight over this time period. Aside from these differences, the treated rats seemed grossly normal in appearance and behavior. However, hormonal content within the pituitary glands decreased with both increased time from irradiation and increased dose

administered. GH and prolactin (PRL) showed the greatest sensitivity followed by TSH, and lastly by LH and ACTH. Twenty weeks following 24 Gy, there was approximately 90% reduction in GH and PRL content in the pituitaries of the irradiated animals compared to controls. Similarly, TSH, LH, and ACTH demonstrated a maximum decrease of pituitary content of approximately 20%, 30%, and 40%, respectively, at 20 weeks' follow-up after 24 Gy. These data demonstrate the dose- and time-dependent increase of pituitary dysfunction. In another report, stunting of growth and weight gain in rats receiving 10-Gy cranial irradiation appeared to continue on a progressively worsening trajectory likely well beyond the last captured measurement at 150 days.[1]

HUMAN DATA

The degree and time to which functional damage to the HPA is manifested by ionizing radiation depends upon dose, fractionation, and volume of HPA exposed to radiation. Low doses of 20 Gy can cause GH deficiency, whereas higher doses of 30 to 50 Gy will almost certainly cause deficiency of one or more other hormones with onset of signs or symptoms occurring more rapidly with higher doses or larger radiation fraction size. The differential effect of HPA sensitivity to radiation exposure suggests effects are a result of direct radiation sensitivity rather than a secondary effect such as vascular insufficiency. It is worth remembering that the HPA is more sensitive to irradiation during childhood and becomes slightly more resilient with age.[8,9]

TOTAL BODY IRRADIATION

Radiation exposure in the setting of total body irradiation (TBI) is associated with multiple endocrinological changes. These represent a unique setting in which both the central structures, namely HPA, and the peripheral organs, namely the thyroid, adrenals, and gonads, are all irradiated. In one report, 20 patients underwent bone marrow transplantation involving TBI and had late endocrine function assessment at a median of 3.3 years.[10] Nineteen patients received TBI with 12 Gy in five fractions and one patient receiving total nodal irradiation to 8 Gy in five fractions. Five patients had a decreased GH response to GHRH challenge. The direct effect of end endocrine organ irradiation was found to be the largest determinant of net endocrine dysfunction with direct thyroid, ovarian, and testicular irradiation being the primary contributing factors. Similar findings of GH deficiency and decreased height were found with TBI of 18 children treated with 12 Gy in 6 fractions.[11] Such blunting effect on the GH axis as a result of low-dose fractionated TBI is not uniformly found. One report of ten patients treated with TBI of 12 Gy in five fractions did not find any primary HPA deficits when tested at a range of 2 to 11 years after irradiation.[12] There are few data on single fraction TBI, but one report of 10 Gy TBI delivered in one fraction found these children experienced a more severe GH deficiency with stunted height than those treated with fractionated TBI of 12 Gy.[11] The damage appeared to arise secondary to effects on the HPA since normal growth rates were achieved in such patients treated with exogenous GH supplementation.

TABLE 17.1	Radiation Delivered in these Three Plans to the Hypothalamus, Pituitary Stalk, and Pituitary Gland as Compared to the Tumor											

Percentage of Structure Volume Receiving Percentage Dose

Structure	Tumor			Pituitary			Stalk			Hypothalamus		
% Dose	3D CRT	IMRT	SRT	3D CRT	IMRT	SRT	3D CRT	IMRT	SRT	3D CRT	IMRT	SRT
102	36.47	33.2	98.8	32.8	55.4	99.7	0.0	0.0	0.0	0.0	0.0	0.0
100	94.9	89.4	99.8	98.8	91.2	100	12.5	0.0	0.0	0.0	0.0	0.0
95	100	100	100	100	100	100	45.8	61.8	15.8	0.0	0.0	0.0
90	100	100	100	100	100	100	58.3	80.9	35.1	0.0	0.0	0.0
80	100	100	100	100	100	100	100	100	70.2	0.0	2.4	0.0
60	100	100	100	100	100	100	100	100	100	7.7	10.2	8.7
40	100	100	100	100	100	100	100	100	100	26.3	23.4	37.9
20	100	100	100	100	100	100	100	100	100	63.8	52.9	88.5

3D CRT, 3D conformal radiation therapy; IMRT, intensity-modulated radiation therapy; SRT, stereotactic radiotherapy.

INTENTIONAL FRACTIONATED RADIATION THERAPY TO THE HPA

The overall incidence of hypopituitarism after fractionated radiotherapy to the HPA is approximately 20% at 5 years. Rates increase 50% to 80% by 20 years based upon data from patients with acromegaly who received pituitary irradiation. Data are limited but this rate will likely continue to trend upward with longer follow-up. A recent retrospective series of fractionated radiation therapy that includes a mix of conventional—two-to three-field treatments and five-field stereotactic delivery found new hypopituitarism in 37 of 100 patients at a median follow-up of 6.7 years.[12] Mean dose was 45 Gy with a range of 43 to 50.3 Gy delivered. This is consistent with majority of other reported experiences and has held with time. Littley et al.[13] reported on 251 patients treated for a variety of cranial irradiation indications, the majority, that is, 227 cases, being for pituitary adenomas. Doses of 12 Gy fractionated did not result in detectable HPA deficiency but beginning at doses of 20 Gy, there were detectable deficits in all of thyroid, cortisol, and gonadotropin levels and an elevation in PRL levels. The degree of HPA dysfunction increased with radiation dose most notably with thyroid function in which 52% of patients treated with 42 to 45 Gy developed hormonal deficiency. Time to onset of the hormonal effect was shorter with higher doses, particularly between fractionated doses of 35 to 45 Gy as compared to 20 Gy. Risk of HPA deficits after irradiation appears to be influenced by surgical manipulation prior to irradiation.[14] Sensitivity of individual hormonal axes was variable among patients with the exception of GH, which was consistently the most sensitive with regard to time to deficit.[14]

Listed in Table 17.1 are the published series of pituitary adenoma irradiation with mean or median follow-up data of at least 5 years that include reported rates of new or progressive hypopituitarism. Overall, about half of patients experienced at least one dysfunctional axis at 10 years' follow-up after irradiation for a pituitary adenoma. Risk factors for causing pituitary dysfunction include concomitant irradiation of the hypothalamus,[15] higher dose,[15] and larger baseline tumor volume in the case of nonfunctioning adenomas.[16] Patients with preexisting pituitary deficiency, typically as a result of disease or surgical intervention, were more susceptible to further pituitary hormonal deficits following conventional radiation therapy.[17,18]

FRACTIONATED RADIATION THERAPY: INCIDENTAL HPA IRRADIATION

The robustness of the HPA is demonstrated by patients who received incidental HPA irradiation on a background of typically normal HPA function. These retrospective studies constitute an array of patients exposed to radiation for purposes of treatment of a variety of CNS conditions and head and neck malignancies. Even with technical advancements allowing for increasing radiation sparing of surrounding normal tissues, radiation targets abutting the HPA result in unavoidable irradiation (Figs. 17.1–17.3).

Patients with craniopharyngiomas represent one cohort who receive incidental HPA radiation due to the proximity

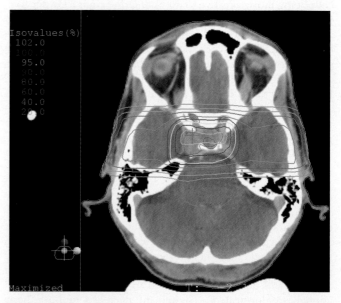

Figure 17.1. Comparison of radiation therapy delivery techniques. Sample radiation plans using modern techniques of 3D conformal radiation therapy (Fig. 17.1), intensity-modulated radiation therapy (Fig. 17.2), and stereotactic radiotherapy (Fig. 17.3) demonstrate that increasing conformality decreases dose to large regional structures such as the brain. Those normal structures most intricately involved with targets such as the HPA complex with a cavernous sinus–based meningioma as depicted here continue to receive unavoidable radiation.

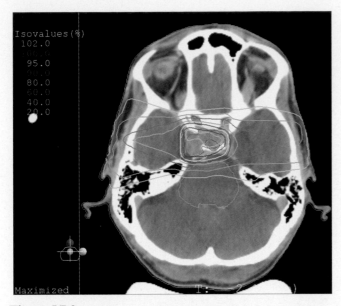

Figure 17.2. 3D Conformal radiation therapy.

to the intended tumor target. In a study of 40 patients with craniopharyngioma treated with surgery and stereotactic radiotherapy to 52.2 Gy in 1.8 Gy fractions, 50% of patients developed new pituitary deficiency after surgery and only two patients developed further new deficits at a median follow-up of 98 months.[19] In contrast, a similar study of 39 patients with craniopharyngioma treated with surgery and fractionated radiation to 50 Gy documented pituitary hormonal deficits postoperatively and postradiation therapy at 74% and 82%, respectively. New pituitary deficits after irradiation occurred in 42% of patients at a median follow-up of 40 months.[20] Such discrepancies in data may be due to the inherent limitations of retrospective studies, differences in the definitions of hypopituitarism that vary widely by each axis, and differences of presentation of data

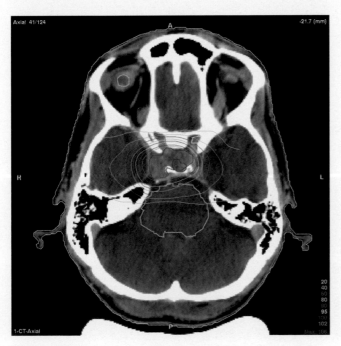

Figure 17.3 Stereotactic radiotherapy.

by each investigator (e.g., new versus progressive hormonal deficiencies). Data with high-dose proton radiation therapy for craniopharyngiomas show a high incidence of hypopituitarism although largely present after surgical intervention prior to radiotherapy.[21] Thirteen of 15 patients, including all five pediatric cases, harbored some postoperative but preradiation therapy hypopituitarism. The remaining two patients developed some pituitary deficiency following irradiation. This would be expected where the target for craniopharyngiomas is juxtaposed to the HPA, making collateral irradiation to this normal structure unavoidable even with the greater conformality of proton radiotherapy.

Similar reports of late effects in patients treated with radiation for other intracranial but non-HPA indications also give insight into the radiosensitivity of the HPA. One such study evaluated 32 patients, ages 6 to 65, who received cranial irradiation for non–HP related indications but who received incidental HPA doses of 39.6 to 70.3 Gy.[22] Baseline levels were available and response to stimulation of hormonal axes was assessed at 2 to 13 years after irradiation. Among the 23 patients who did not receive direct thyroid irradiation, 65% had a hypothalamic or pituitary-related hypothyroid deficiency with the dose of radiation correlating with the severity of dysfunction. Oligomenorrhea was present in 70% of premenopausal women, and a low testosterone level was present in 30% of men. Normal response to GnRH stimulation in both genders was consistent with a hypothalamic deficiency as opposed to pituitary dysfunction. An elevated PRL was detected in half of patients and was more common after cranial irradiation in adults as compared to children. Only 9% of patients had entirely normal neuroendocrine function. Despite the limitations of being retrospective and possibly confounded by disease extending to and perhaps involving the HPA, these data reflect the large impact of cranial irradiation on the HPA.

Long-term follow-up for patients irradiated for head and neck malignancies provides yet another source of understanding radiation late effects. This patient population is particularly attractive because often there is no intracranial extension and thus no mass effect on the HPA that may contribute to HPA dysfunction. Bhandare et al.[23] recently reported on 312 patients irradiated for head and neck malignancies all without intracranial extension of disease and thus with presumptive baseline normal HPA function. At a median clinical follow-up of 5.6 years, 44 (14.1%) of patients experienced some clinical hypopituitarism. Of these, 14 patients were found to have hypothalamic dysfunction and 30 patients had pituitary deficiency. Among 68 patients who were clinically asymptomatic and tested, 33.8% were found to harbor subclinical hypopituitarism. Between 5- and 10-year follow-ups, there was an increase in both clinical hypopituitarism (7%–28%) and subclinical hypopituitarism (15%–35%). A similar study evaluating 166 head and neck malignancy patients who received a median of 50 Gy and 57 Gy to the hypothalamus and pituitary, respectively, found 81% of patients developed an HPA deficiency.[8] Overall, 67% of patients harbored a hypothalamic deficiency and 40% had a primary pituitary deficiency. With the exception of cortisol, all other HPA deficiencies had a median time of detection between 2 and 4 years following the completion of radiotherapy. Median time to cortisol deficiency was 6 years. Snyers et al.[24] evaluated 76 patients with sinonasal cancers treated predominantly with surgery and radiation. An initial biochemical deficit in insulin-like growth factor-1 (IGF-1) was detected in 57% of patients

TABLE 17.2   HPA After Fractionated Radiation Therapy for Pituitary Adenomas

Study	RT	No. of Patients and Type	Median Follow-up	Dose (Gy)	LC	Normalized Function	Total Hypopituitarism	RT Hypopituitarism
Brada et al.[33]	Conv	411 mix	10.5 y	45 (45–50)	88%/20 y	na	30%/10 y (sup)	na
Tsang et al.[34]	Conv	128 NFA	8.3 y	45	91%/10 y	50%/19 y	68%*/10 y	23%*[a]
Zierhut et al.[35]	Conv	70 mix / 68 funct	6.5 y (avg)	45.5 (40–60)	95% all	na	na	27%F, 19%G, 19%ACTH, 13%TSH, 12%PRL[a]
McCord et al.[36]	Conv	141 mix	9.2 y	47.2 (42–55)	93%/15 y	90%c/p	49%[a]	24%
Rush and Cooper[37]	Conv	70 mix	8 y	45 (43.2–50.4)	97%	78%–100%	42% sup	
Landolt et al.[38]	Conv	50 acro	7.5 y (avg)	40 (40–56)	100%	?	na	16%nl ⇒sup
Powell et al.[39]	Conv	32 acro	5.2 y (avg)	47.4 (45–54)		50%/7.1 y	30% pre	32%/10 y new
Barrande et al.[18]	Conv	128 acro	11.5 y	52 (43.5–60.5)		44%	82%/10 y[a]	34%
Biermasz et al.[17]	Conv	36 acro	10 y	40 (25–50)		53%/10 y	58%/15 y (sup)	47%
Epaminonda et al.[40]	Conv	67 acro / 26 acro	10 y / min15 y	54 (40–75)	na	71%/15 y / 58%/8 y / 65%/15y	na	60%/med4–7 y
Cozzi et al.[41]	Conv	49 acro	14 y	46	96%	16%/10y	35%pre	10%/10y
Colin et al.[42]	SRT	110 mix	6.8 y	50.4	99%	42%cr / 100%cr+pr	24% F/L, 12% ACTH, 14% T	36.7%
Minniti et al.[43]	Conv	47 acro	12 y	45–50	95%/15 y	77%/15 y	85%/15 y	52%
Jenkins et al.[44]	Conv	884 acro	7 y	45	na	60%/10 y / 77%/20y	44%–58%/ax10 y	15%–27%/axis[a]
Jallad et al.[45]	Conv	95 acro	5.9 y (avg)	50 (32.4–60)	100%	54%	11%baseline	44%/5.9 y
Langsenlehner et al.[46]	Conv	87 mix	15 y	50.4 (46–54)	95%/15 y	92%	97%/10 y	88%
Minniti et al.[47]	Conv	40 ACTH	9 y	45–50	93%/10 y	84%/10 y	76%/10 y	51%
Van den Bergh et al.[48]	Mix	76 NFA	7.7 y	45–55.8	95%/10 y	na	79%/10 y[a]	61% nl ⇒sup[a]
Snead et al.[12]	Mix	100 mix	6.7 y	45 (43–50.4)	88%/10 y	na	na	35%

[a]Minimum hypopituitarism rate, report by separate axes.

was found to be largely subclinical. Among the 24% true HPA deficits detected, defined as persistent deficit with provocative testing, the mean doses to the hypothalamus and pituitary were 51.6 and 56 Gy, respectively. Among patients without detectable HPA deficits at last follow-up, the mean doses to the hypothalamus and pituitary were 44.3 and 51 Gy, respectively. Lam et al.[25] report a 62% rate of neuroendocrine dysfunction at 5 years among 31 adult nasopharyngeal carcinoma patients who received a mean of 40 Gy to the hypothalamus and 62 Gy to the pituitary. GH deficiency was both the most common and earliest of deficits to occur, affecting 63.5% of the patients. Deficiencies in gonadotropins, ACTH, and TSH occurred at 5-year rates of 31%, 27%, and 15%, respectively. Hyperprolactinemia was detected in 13% of patients at 2 years after irradiation and rose to 23% at 5 years. The cumulative incidence of any hypopituitarism was 0%, 3.5%, 11.5%, 20%, and 30% at 1, 2, 3, 4, and 5 years. Another study of 107 patients with skull base tumors that were predominantly chordomas or chondrosarcomas found 5-year effects on the HPA of 72% hyperprolactinemia, 30% hypothyroidism, 29% hypogonadism, and 19% hypoadrenalism.[15] Minimum doses of ≥50 Gy to the pituitary were associated with HPA dysfunction. Similarly, maximum dose of ≥70 Gy to the pituitary or ≥50 Gy to the hypothalamus was associated with an increased rate of neuroendocrine dysfunction.

Other retrospective data have shown the responsiveness of the HPA is altered after cranial radiotherapy. Depressed GH response to GHRH stimulation has been documented following childhood cranial irradiation. Achermann et al.[26] studied five male adult long-term survivors of cranial irradiation who were irradiated at a median time of 13.7 years prior to study for pediatric brain tumors and received >30 Gy. Whether this dose was delivered to the HPA in addition to the primary intended target is unclear, but all individuals demonstrated an attenuated response to GHRH. Similar findings of attenuated GH response to stimulation in adults following childhood cranial irradiation are reported at both lower radiation doses of 18 to 25 Gy[27,28] and at higher doses as used with treating primary CNS solid tumors.[29] Relatively normal pulsatile response was preserved but was blunted and less predictive as compared to controls. These data suggest the anatomic pathways in the HPA remain intact postirradiation.

A unique occurrence in children treated with low-dose cranial irradiation is the development of precocious puberty. The extent to which early-onset puberty is a result of HPA irradiation is unclear since reported series typically involve complex and multiple inciting factors. Quigley et al.[30] describe a group of 45 children with acute lymphoblastic leukemia who survived following treatment that included both cranial irradiation of 24 Gy and a combination of ten drugs including cyclophosphamide and cytarabine, drugs known to cause direct gonadal injury. Despite confirmed biochemical evidence of hypogonadism, puberty occurred in these children approximately a year in advance to the population norm. The mechanism for this effect is not well understood.

STEREOTACTIC RADIOSURGERY

The degree of late adverse effects to high-dose single fraction irradiation to the HPA is only recently becoming fully recognized as longer follow-up date is becoming available. The use of SRS in the management in pituitary adenomas is typically a secondary or tertiary role to medical management and surgery.

Nonetheless, SRS has become increasingly applied within the last decade for refractory disease. Recent studies of acromegaly suggest excellent efficacy of SRS in normalizing overproduction of GH. The risk of hypopituitarism ranges from 6% to 52% by 5 years (Table 17.2). Longer follow-up data of SRS for secreting adenomas suggest rates of hypopituitarism continue to increase with time, up to 69% of patients for a given HPA.[31] The average time to develop hypopituitarism was reported at 48 months in one study that stipulated an inclusion criteria of minimum 5 year follow-up and with a third of patients followed for over 10 years.[32] Larger size of adenomas (>4 cc) has been found in at least one study to be a risk factor for SRS-related HPA dysfunction.[16] Thus, while initial experiences with radiosurgery suggested a much lower rate of HPA injury compared to larger field fractionated techniques, as the radiosurgery results mature it is clear that HPA dysfunction cannot be avoided in some patients.

The only reported SRS experience using proton radiation with at least 5-year follow-up data was two limited series that document similar findings of pituitary deficiency of 52% and 38% at median follow-up time of 62 and 76 months, respectively.[49,50] This is in keeping with the expectation that proton radiation will have the same biological efficacy as photons for a given dose deposition and in the setting of treating pituitary adenomas where there is no sparing of the pituitary. However, there remains a dosimetric benefit of protons in the reduced or eliminated dose to surrounding normal tissues in the cranium, which may have a clinical benefit. Avoidance of dose to the hypothalamus may translate to a long-term lower incidence of multiple axes or complete hypopituitarism (Table 17.3).

BRACHYTHERAPY

A less common form of radiation exposure to the HPA is by brachytherapy, using a β emitter such as phosphorus-32 in liquid form that is injected within sellar cysts such as with recurrent craniopharyngiomas. Whereas this is also a potential source for radiation-related hypopituitarism, most series find that hypopituitarism in this setting is a result of surgical manipulation and/or direct tumor effects.[58,59]

TESTING OF FUNCTION FOLLOWING IRRADIATION, DEFINITION OF TOXICITY

Testing of hypothalamic and pituitary function is sufficiently complex that it ideally should be directed by an endocrinologist. Patients should be screened for medications that may influence endocrine function such as corticosteroids, anti-convulsants, and hormone replacements. Comprehensive blood tests such as blood counts and metabolic panel are important to suggesting potential abnormalities. Because the central neuroendocrine function of the hypothalamus and pituitary is tied intricately with that of the regulated end organ function, both central and peripheral endocrine functions require testing to determine the source of potential dysfunction. Basic definition and screening of each of the hormonal axes are discussed with brief inclusion of secondary studies. These are not comprehensive description of the endocrine physiology. Definitions of hypopituitarism for each axis are variable but common ranges or more widely accepted definitions are provided. For all patients, evaluation should include MRI of the HPA region.

TABLE 17.3		SRS Experiences with Median Follow-up ≥5 years						
Study	RT	Follow-up (mo)	No. of Patients	Median Dose (Gy)	LC	Normalized Function	Total Hypopituitarism	RT Hypopituitarism
Thorén et al.[51]	GK	64	21 GH	40–70 (1–3fx)	na	81% pr+	29% pre	24%
Höybye et al.[31]	GK	17 y	18 ACTH	30–120 (est)[a] 70 med[b]	100%	83%	8/17go pre 0/14ACpre 0/16tsh pre	3/17go 7/14ACTH 11/16tsh 69% min
Iwai et al.[52]		60	34 NFA	14	93%/5 y	na	na	6.5%
Voges et al.[53]	linac	82	142 mix (8–20)	15.3 (mean)	96.5%	51%/5 y	47.4% pre	12.3%
Liscák et al.[54]	GK	60	140 NFA	20	100%	na	90% pre	1.4%
Petit et al.[50]	pr	76	22 GH	20	100%	95%c/p	na	38%
Pollock et al.[55]	GK	63	46 GH	20	100%	60%/5 y	35% pre	33%/5 y
Vik-Mo et al.[56]	GK	67	53 GH	26.5	100%	86%/10 y	30% pre	13%sup
Losa et al.[57]	GK	69	83 GH	21.5	97.6%	60.2%	21%go pre 5%thy pre 2.4%adr pre	8.5%
Petit et al.[49]	pr	62	33 Cush	20	100%	79%c/p	na	52%
Pollock et al.[16]	GK	64	62 NFA	16 (11–20)	95%/7 y	na	na	32%/5 y
Castinetti et al.[32]	GK	97 avg	76 mix	28 (mean)	100%	44.7%	na	21%

[a]Treatments range one to four sessions of SRS, each to unique sites.
[b]Median dose in two fractions, dose to target periphery per gamma knife convention.

SOMATOTROPIC AXIS

This axis is driven by the production of GHRH that is released by the hypothalamus. GHRH stimulates GH secretion by the pituitary. GH level of <2 mg/mL is a relatively new definition of GH deficiency. Many studies have previously used a definition of <5 mg/mL. GH level itself is not a reliable measure of overall GH production because of normal fluctuation of levels throughout the day. IGF-1 is a more reliable indicator of overall activity of this axis. It stimulates GH production. Exogenous challenge by GHRH and/or arginine can be done to assess the response of the pituitary. Alternatively, an insulin tolerance test can be performed. These provocative assays should be performed by an experienced endocrinologist. Clinical GH deficiency is frequently asymptomatic and does not need supplementation in the postpubertal state. Less commonly, there may be symptoms of fatigue or sense of less general well-being that may be causes to provide supplementation. Again, an endocrinologist is the appropriate specialist to both make this decision and provide pharmacotherapy.

CORTICOSTEROID AXIS

CRH is released by the hypothalamus and stimulates ACTH release by the pituitary. ACTH stimulates adrenal gland production of cortisol. Direct measure of cortisol is one method of testing adrenal gland function. Deficiency of this axis is typically first assessed by documenting low cortisol levels at multiple time points since normal diurnal fluctuations exist. Serum and salivary levels are common assays. Low/normal levels of ACTH may indicate HPA deficiency. CRH stimulation test differentiates between hypothalamic versus pituitary deficiency. Inferior petrosal sinus sampling can confirm pituitary origin of overstimulation in this axis and determine potential laterality

of a pituitary adenoma. Clinical hypocortisolemia is commonly characterized by fatigue, light headedness, weakness, weight loss, joint or muscle aches, and depressive affect.

GONADAL AXIS

GnRH is released by the hypothalamus and stimulates LH and FSH release from the pituitary. These pituitary hormones go on to stimulate gonads with differential effect by gender. Estradiol is predominantly released by the ovaries in women with variable levels depending upon premenopausal/postmenopausal status. There is also a minor component of production by adipose tissue. Testosterone measurements should include both the total and free components. Testosterone is predominantly released by the testes in men. Low LH and low testosterone in men indicate central hypogonadism with deficiency in HPA.

Low/normal LH and low estradiol in premenopausal women indicate low GnRH production. GnRH challenge can differentiate hypothalamic versus pituitary deficiency but should be administered by a trained endocrinologist. Clinical hypogonadism in premenopausal women may manifest as loss of menses, decreased libido, hot flashes, and sleep disturbances. In men, decreased libido, muscle mass, fatigue, and impotence may occur.

THYROID AXIS

TRH is released by the hypothalamus and stimulates TSH from the pituitary. TSH stimulates thyroid hormone production by the thyroid gland. Deficiencies in this axis are often differentiated between primary and secondary hypothyroidism. Elevated TSH levels suggest either decrease production of thyroid hormones by the thyroid, or less commonly is a result of increase production of TRH. Low TSH levels suggest hypothalamic deficiency. Serum free T4 is a direct measure of active hormone and thyroid gland function. Serum total T4 includes free and bound forms of T4 and is interpreted in context of other related thyroid assays.

Serum total T3 is often normal except when severe hypothyroidism occurs and also requires context of other related thyroid assays for appropriate interpretation. In hypothalamic hypothyroidism, there is low serum free T4 and low TSH, yet normal basal and peak response to TRH. Clinical hypothyroidism is classically characterized by increased fatigue, lethargy, cold intolerance, dry skin and hair, weight gain, and constipation.

LACTOTROPH AXIS

PRL is produced by the hypothalamus and released by the posterior lobe of the pituitary. Hyperprolactinemia may result as a decline in production or disruption in flow of dopamine from the hypothalamus to the pituitary. Dopamine has an inhibitory effect on pituitary release of PRL. Clinical hyperprolactinemia for men and postmenopausal women may present with galactorrhea. For premenopausal women, lactation and loss of menses may occur. For all people, loss of libido and headaches are common symptoms.

ANTIDIURETIC HORMONE AXIS

ADH (vasopressin) is released by the pituitary and increases fluid resorption in the kidneys, thereby maintains physiologic fluid homeostasis. ADH levels increase when there is decreased fluid consumption or when greater losses of fluid occur (e.g., increased sweat production or gastrointestinal loss). Sodium is a key serum electrolyte affected by ADH and may be high with ADH deficiency. A decrease of ADH production can occur as a result of primary disease involvement (e.g., tumor) or as a result of surgical manipulation, resulting in diabetes insipidus. It is consistently never seen as a result of radiation exposure. Patients receiving cranial irradiation are often subjected to risk factors or direct disease involvement of the HPA, and in these cases screening this axis for deficiency should be considered.

TIME, DOSE, VOLUME RECOMMENDATIONS

The lack of appreciation of the HPA function and sensitivity to radiation has led to inadvertently greater irradiation and injury. With greater awareness, a conscious avoidance or minimization of irradiation of the HPA can have a significant quality-of-life (QOL) impact on these patients. Collectively, avoiding doses >30 Gy delivered at no >2 Gy fractions in adults will markedly decrease risk of radiation-induced HPA dysfunction but rates will still increase with time. Thus, there is never a period of observation when patients are risk free from developing HPA dysfunction, and these patients need to be followed by neuroendocrine studies over their entire lives. Doses above 50 Gy in standard fractionation to the HPA will likely demonstrate a much faster onset of HPA dysfunction with higher risk of affecting multiple axes with higher doses. SRS does seem to induce a faster onset of HPA dysfunction. Most therapeutic SRS doses to the pituitary for treatment of adenomas will pose a high risk of causing other hormonal deficiencies.

Perhaps the fortunate aspect of HPA irradiation is that supplementation of all vital hormonal functions is available such that with appropriate surveillance and treatment, there is no absolute dose to the HPA at which irradiation would be profoundly debilitating or fatal so long as appropriate medical intervention is available. However, there is a variable decrement to QOL in patients with hypopituitarism such that irradiation of the HPA should still be avoided when possible. In a case control study, 99 patients with nonfunctioning pituitary adenomas treated with surgery of which 37% also received radiation therapy were found to have a significantly worse QOL after either treatment, particularly in regard to effect of fatigue.[60] Controls were 125 unaffected individuals and the assay used was a battery of 4 well-established QOL questionnaires. Specific problems included socialization, emotional well-being, physical problems, and general self-health perception. Data were not stratified by those who receive radiation specifically, but if HPA deficits have a QOL impact then radiation exposure is almost certainly a contributing factor. Similarly, a more recent and larger series from the same investigators reported on 403 patients with mixed pituitary adenomas who achieved hormonal or tumor growth control yet self-reported an overall low QOL.[60] These patients were compared to 440 controls. The depressed QOL was uniformly found across the same four QOL questionnaires. Patients affected with acromegaly or Cushing disease reported the worse QOL. These investigators provide additional possible causes for these findings stating current methods of hormonal correction are imperfect to simulating normal physiology.[61] Serum level of hormones is an imperfect surrogate of hormonal presence and activity in tissue, particularly when these are exogenous supplements. Many hormones are secreted in pulsatile fashion or have fluctuating levels in response to stresses, time of day, health, and other activities. The pharmacokinetics of supplements is typically not the same as endogenous hormones, often with very disparate half-lives. Together, the inability to restore physiologic hormonal physiology by current supplementation emphasizes the importance of avoiding irradiation and its associated hypopituitarism when possible.

There are multiple factors that contribute to radiation tolerance of tissues. In normal healthy tissues, the intrinsic radiation tolerances are estimated from data of prior experiences with irradiation. While there are general tissue tolerances that have become accepted in clinical practice, the exact tolerance of many tissues for a given individual is unknown. Sporadically, unusual sensitivity to an extremely low dose of radiation occurs. Thus, when possible, the smallest volume and dose of radiation should be used to minimize risk of radiation-related adverse events. Because the effects in organs such as the HPA are delayed by many years, the full long term consequences are often difficult to appreciate. In addition, the cause for radiation exposure may impact on radiation tolerance. That is, tissues that are potentially compromised prior to irradiation such as from disease or tumor involvement may have a lower radiation dose tolerance. In the case of the HPA, baseline disease states may actually affect the function of the HPA such that hormonal dysfunction exists at baseline. These factors should be weighed by the treating physician during radiation planning and patients should be appropriately counseled regarding the additional risk of radiation-related HPA adverse effects.

STRATEGIES FOR AVOIDING TOXICITY

Avoidance of hypopituitarism is best achieved by avoidance of irradiation of the hypothalamus and pituitary gland. Whereas avoidance of unnecessary pituitary irradiation has been generally intuitive, the importance of also avoiding unnecessary hypothalamic irradiation should also be recognized.[8,15,22,23,25] Increasingly conformal methods of radiotherapy delivery and improved imaging have enabled progressively smaller volumes to be targeted and treated with accuracy. For cranial radiation therapy in which the HPA is not the target, the HPA should be defined and consciously avoided such that beam arrangements can be chosen to eliminate unnecessary exit dose into it. For radiation treatment planning by intensity-modulated radiation therapy, the HPA can be labeled as a *radiation-sensitive structure*, thereby minimizing dose to it.

For treatments in which the HPA structures are inclusive within the radiation targets such as for pituitary adenomas, fractionated radiation therapy may help preserve existing HPA function or at least delay time to loss of function. This adverse effect must be weighed with the purpose of radiotherapy since radiosurgical treatment may offer faster normalization of a hypersecretory adenoma. The impact of hypopituitarism may be a lesser concern in such patients who are typically monitored closely for their neuroendocrine function and often harbor other neuroendocrine deficits for which they are already receiving replacement. For radiation therapy treatments such as whole-brain radiation therapy in which the entire HPA is included with fractionated radiation, smaller fraction size may have a decreased risk of neuroendocrine deficiency but again this unclear benefit should be balanced with the primary intention for radiation therapy.

Lastly, the risk of HPA dysfunction after irradiation is partly a function of the baseline health of the patient and HPA. Those people with central causes of hormonal deficiencies will be at inherently higher risk for further deficits following irradiation.

TREATMENT OF INJURY

Despite its complexity and importance in homeostasis, the HPA can be functionally compensated by pharmacologic supplementation and affected persons can lead largely normal lives. Perhaps the most salient point is that patients treated with cranial irradiation whether for a pituitary etiology meriting therapeutic irradiation or incidental irradiation for another indication for cranial irradiation all require surveillance for HPA dysfunction. Because decrement in the HPA function occurs gradually over months to years and can be clinical insidious, annual HPA functional screening is recommended. Patients to be treated with radiation with expected HPA exposure should be cautioned on the importance of neuroendocrine screening and specifically the possibility of late radiation effects years following the time of radiation therapy. Because neuroendocrine screening and evaluation of abnormalities can be fairly complex, patients should be ideally followed by an endocrinologist. Most deficiencies of the HPA can be adequately supplemented. Even fertility can sometimes be regained with appropriate hormonal therapy. Ovulation was reestablished in four of six women with suspected hypothalamic hypogonadism as a result of pituitary irradiation, with or without surgery by replacement with exogenous GnRH.[62]

REFERENCES

1. Schunior A, Zengel AE, Mullenix PJ, et al. An animal model to study toxicity of central nervous system therapy for childhood acute lymphoblastic leukemia: effects on growth and craniofacial proportion. *Cancer Res.* 1990;50:6455
2. Lebaron-Jacobs L, Wysocki J, Griffiths NM. Differential qualitative and temporal changes in the response of the hypothalamus-pituitary-adrenal axis in rats after localized or total-body irradiation. *Radiat Res.* 2004;161:712–722.
3. Velickovic N, Djordjevic A, Matic G, et al. Radiation-induced hyposuppression of the hypothalamic-pituitary adrenal axis is associated with alterations of hippocampal corticosteroid receptor expression. *Radiat Res.* 2008;169:397–407.
4. Hochberg Z, Kuten A, Hertz P, et al. The effect of single-dose radiation on cell survival and growth hormone secretion by rat anterior pituitary cells. *Radiat Res.* 1983;94:508–512.
5. Nakasu S, Nakasu Y, Fukami T, et al. Immunohistochemical proliferation markers may overestimate the growth potential afterionizing radiation: in vivo study in the rat anterior pituitary gland. *Neurol Med Chir (Tokyo).* 2003;43:521–526.
6. Roth C, Schmidberger H, Schaper O, et al. Cranial irradiation of female rats causes dose-dependent and age-dependent activation or inhibition of pubertal development. *Pediatr Res.* 2000;47:586–591.
7. Robinson ICAF, Fairhall KM, Hendry JH, et al. Differential radiosensitivity of hypothalamo-pituitary function in the young adult rat. *J Endocrinol.* 2001;169:519–526.
8. Samaan NA, Schultz PN, Yang KP, et al. Endocrine complications after radiotherapy for tumors of the head and neck. *J Lab Clin Med.* 1987;109:364–372.
9. Brauner R, Czernichow P, Rappaport R. Greater susceptibility to hypothalamopituitary irradiation in younger children with acute lymphoblastic leukemia. *J Pediatr.* 1986;108:332.
10. Kauppila M, Koskinen P, Irjala K, et al. Long-term effects of allogeneic bone marrow transplantation (BMT) on pituitary, gonad, thyroid and adrenal function in adults. *Bone Marrow Transplant.*1998;22:331–337.
11. Brauner R, Adan L, Souberbielle JC, et al. Contribution of growth hormone deficiency to the growth failure that follows bone marrow transplantation. *J Pediatr.* 1997;130:785–792.
12. Snead FE, Amdur RJ, Morris CG, et al. Long-term outcomes of radiotherapy for pituitary adenomas. *Int J Radiat Oncl Biol Phys.* 2008;71:994–998.
13. Littley MD, Shalet SM, Beardwell CG, et al. Radiation-induced hypopituitarism is dose-dependent. *Clin Endocrinol (Oxf).* 1989;31:363–373.
14. Littley MD, Shalet SM, Beardwell, et al. Hypopituitarism following external radiotherapy for pituitary tumours in adults. *Q J Med.* 1989;70:145–160.
15. Pai HH, Thornton A, Katznelson L, et al. Hypothalamic/pituitary function following high-dose conformal radiotherapy to the base of skull: demonstration of a dose-effect relationship using dose-volume histogram analysis. *Int J Radiat Oncol Biol Phys.* 2001;49:1079–1092.
16. Pollock BE, Cochran J, Natt N, et al. Gamma knife radiosurgery for patients with nonfunctioning pituitary adenomas: results from a 15-year experience. *Int J Radiat Oncl Biol Phys.* 2008;70:1325–1329.
17. Biermasz NR, van Dulken H, Roelfsema F. Long-term follow-up results of postoperative radiotherapy in 36 patients with acromegaly. *J Clin Endocrinol Metab.* 2000;85:2476–2482.
18. Barrande G, Pittino-Lungo M, Coste J, et al. Hormonal and metabolic effects of radiotherapy in acromegaly: long-term results in 128 patients followed in a single center. *J Clin Endocrinol Metab.* 2000;85:3779–3785.
19. Combs SE, Thilmann C, Huber PE, et al. Achievement of long-term local control in patients with craniopharyngiomas using high precision stereotactic radiotherapy. *Cancer.* 2007;109:2308–2314.
20. Minniti G, Saran F, Traish D, et al. Fractionated stereotactic conformal radiotherapy following conservative surgery in the control of craniopharyngiomas. *Radiother Oncol.* 2007;82:90–95.
21. Fitzek MM, Linggood RM, Adams J, et al. Combined proton and photon irradiation for craniopharyngioma: long-term results of the early cohort of patients treated at Harvard Cyclotron Laboratory and Massachusetts General Hospital. *Int J Radiat Oncol Biol Phys.* 2006;64:1348–1345.
22. Constine LS, Woolf PD, Cann D, et al. Hypothalamic-pituitary dysfunction after radiation for brain tumors. *N Engl J Med.* 1993;328:87–94.
23. Bhandare N, Kennedy L, Malyapa RS, et al. Hypopituitarism after radiotherapy for extracranial head and neck cancers. *Head Neck.* 2008;30:1182–1192.
24. Snyers A, Janssens GORJ, Twickler MB, et al. Malignant tumors of the nasal cavity and paranasal sinuses: long-term outcome and morbidity with emphasis on hypothalamic-pituitary deficiency. *Int J Radiat Oncol Biol Phys.* 2009;73:1343–1351.
25. Lam KS, Tse VK, Wang C, et al. Effects of cranial irradiation on hypothalamic-pituitary function—a 5-year longitudinal study in patients with nasopharyngeal carcinoma. *Q J Med.* 1991;78:165–176.
26. Achermann JC, Brook CGD, Hindmarsh PC. The GH response to low-dose bolus growth hormone-releasing hormone ($GHRH(1-29)NH_2$) is attenuated in patients with longstanding post-irradiation GH insufficiency. *Eur J Endocrinol.* 2000;142:359–364.
27. Lannering B, Rosberg S, Marky I, et al. Reduced growth hormone secretion with maintained periodicity following cranial irradiation in children with acute lymphoblastic leukaemia. *Clin Endocrinol (Oxf).* 1995;42:153–159.
28. Brennan BMD, Rahim A, Mackie EM, et al. Growth hormone status in adults treated for acute lymphoblastic leukaemia in childhood. *Clin Endocrinol (Oxf).* 1998;48:777–783.
29. Darzy KH, Pezzoli SS, Thorner MO, et al. The dynamics of growth hormone (GH) secretion in adult cancer survivors with severe GH deficiency acquired after brain irradiation in childhood for nonpituitary brain tumors: evidence for preserved pulsatility and diurnal variation with increased secretory disorderliness. *J Clin Endocrinol Metab.* 2005;90:2794–2803.
30. Quigley C, Cowell C, Jimenez M, et al. Normal or early development of puberty despite gonadal damage in children treated for acute lymphocytic leukemia. *N Engl J Med.* 1989;321:143–151.

31. Höybye C, Grenbäck E, Rähn T, et al. Adrenocorticotropic hormone-producing pituitary tumors: 12- to 22-year follow-up after treatment with stereotactic radiosurgery. *Neurosurgery*. 2001;49:284–292.

32. Castinetti F, Nagai M, Morange I, et al. Long-term results of stereotactic radiosurgery in secretory pituitary adenomas. *J Clin Endocrinol Metab*. 2009;94: [epub ahead of print].

33. Brada M, Rajan B, Traish D, et al. The long-term efficacy of conservative surgery and radiotherapy in the control of pituitary adenomas. *Clin Endocrinol (Oxf)*. 1993;38:571–578.

34. Tsang RW, Brierley JD, Panzarella T, et al. Radiation therapy for pituitary adenoma: treatment outcome and prognostic factors. *Int J Radiat Oncol Biol Phys*. 1994;30:557–565.

35. Zierhut D, Flentje M, Adolph J, et al. External radiotherapy of pituitary adenomas. *Int J Radiat Oncol Biol Phys*. 1995;33:307–314.

36. McCord MW, Buatti JM, Fennell EM, et al. Radiotherapy for pituitary adenoma: long-term outcome and sequelae. *Int J Radiat Oncol Biol Phys*. 1997;39:437–433.

37. Rush S, Cooper PR. Symptom resolution, tumor control, and side effects following postoperative radiotherapy for pituitary macroadenomas. *Int J Radiat Oncol Biol Phys*. 1997;37:1031–1034.

38. Landolt AM, Haller D, Lomax N, et al. Stereotactic radiosurgery for recurrent surgically treated acromegaly: comparison with fractionated radiotherapy. *J Neurosurg*. 1998;88:1002–1008.

39. Powell JS, Wardlaw SL, Post KD, Freda PU. Outcome of radiotherapy for acromegaly using normalization of insulin-like growth factor I to define cure. *J Clin Endocrinol Metab*. 2000;85:2068–2071.

40. Epaminonda P, Porretti S, Cappiello V, et al. Efficacy of radiotherapy in normalizing serum IGF-I, acid-labile subunit (ALS) and IGFBP-3 levels in acromegaly. *Clin Endocrinol (Oxf)*. 2001;55:183–189.

41. Cozzi R, Barausse M, Asnaghi D, et al. Failure of radiotherapy in acromegaly. *Eur J Endocrinol*. 2001;145:717–726.

42. Colin P, Jovenin N, Delemer B, et al. Treatment of pituitary adenomas by fractionated stereotactic radiotherapy: a prospective study of 110 patients. *Int J Radiat Oncol Biol Phys*. 2005;62:333–341.

43. Minniti G, Jaffrain-Rea M-L, Osti M, et al. The long-term efficacy of conventional radiotherapy in patients with GH-secreting pituitary adenomas. *Clin Endocrinol (Oxf)*. 2005;62:210–216.

44. Jenkins PJ, Bates P, Carson MN, et al. Conventional pituitary irradiation is effective in lowering serum growth hormone and insulin-like growth factor-I in patients with acromegaly. *J Clin Endocrinol Metab*. 2006;91:1239–1245.

45. Jallad RS, Musolino NR, Salgado LR, et al. Treatment of acromegaly: is there still a place for radiotherapy? *Pituitary*. 2007;10:53–59.

46. Langsenlehner T, Stiegler C, Quehenberger F, et al. Long-term follow-up of patients with pituitary macroadenomas after postoperative radiation therapy: analysis of tumor control and functional outcome. *Strahlenther Onkol*. 2007;183:241–247.

47. Minniti G, Osti M, Jaffrain-Rea ML, et al. Long-term follow-up results of postoperative radiation therapy for Cushing's disease. *J Neurooncol*. 2007;84:79–84.

48. Van den Bergh ACM, van den Berg G, Schoorl MA, et al. Immediate postoperative radiotherapy in residual nonfunctioning pituitary adenoma: beneficial effect on local control without additional negative impact on pituitary function and life expectancy. *Int J Radiat Oncol Biol Phys*. 2007;67:863–869.

49. Petit JH, Biller BM, Yock TI, et al. Proton stereotactic radiotherapy for persistent ACTH-producing adenomas. *J Clin Endocrinol Metab*. 2008;93:393–399.

50. Petit JH, Biller BM, Coen JJ, et al. Proton stereotactic radiotherapy for persistent GH-producing adenomas. *Endocr Pract*. 2007;13:726–734.

51. Thorén M, Rähn T, Guo WY, et al. Stereotactic radiosurgery with the cobalt-60 gamma unit in the treatment of growth hormone-producing pituitary tumors. *Neurosurgery*. 1991;29:663–668.

52. Iwai Y, Yamanaka K, Yoshioka K, et al. Radiosurgery for nonfunctioning pituitary adenomas. *Neurosurgery*. 2005;56:699–705.

53. Voges J, Kocher M, Runge M, et al. Linear accelerator radiosurgery for pituitary macroadenomas: a 7-year follow-up study. *Cancer*. 2006;107:1355–1364.

54. Liscák R, Vladyka V, Marek J, et al. Gamma knife radiosurgery for endocrine-inactive pituitary adenomas. *Acta Neurochir (Wien)*. 2007;149:999–1006.

55. Pollock BE, Jacob JT, Brown PD, et al. Radiosurgery of growth hormone-producing pituitary adenomas: factors associated with biochemical remission. *J Neurosurg*. 2007;106:833–838.

56. Vik-Mo EO, Øksnes M, Pedersen P-H, et al. Gamma knife stereotactic radiosurgery for acromegaly. *Eur J Endocrinol*. 2007;157:255–263.

57. Losa M, Gioia L, Picozzi P, et al. The role of stereotactic radiotherapy in patients with growth hormone-secreting pituitary adenoma. *J Clin Endocrinol Metab*. 2008;93:2546–2552.

58. Pollock BE, Lunsford LD, Kondziolka D, et al. Phosphorus-32 intracavitary irradiation of cystic craniopharyngiomas: current technique and long-term results. *Int J Radiat Oncol Biol Phys*. 1995;33:437–446.

59. Hasegawa T, Kondzilka D, Hadjipanayis CG, et al. Management of cystic craniopharyngiomas with phosphorus-32 intracavitary irradiation. *Neurosurgery*. 2004;54:813–822.

60. Van der Klaauw AA, Kars M, Biermasz NR, et al. Disease-specific impairments in quality of life during long-term follow-up of patients with different pituitary adenomas. *Clin Endocrinol (Oxf)*. 2008;69:775–784.

61. Romijn JA, Smit JWA, Lamberts SWJ. Intrinsic imperfections of endocrine replacement therapy. *Eur J Endocrinol* 2003;149:91–97.

62. Hall JE, Martin KA, Whitney HA, et al. Potential for fertility with replacement of hypothalamic gonadotropin-releasing hormone in long term female survivors of cranial tumors. *J Clin Endocrinol Metab*. 1994;79:1166–1172.

18

Niranjan Bhandare, James T. Parsons
M. Tariq Bhatti, William M. Mendenhall

Optic Nerve, Eye, and Ocular Adnexa

INTRODUCTION

Intra- and extracranial tumors involving structures adjacent to the optic apparatus are common. These include tumors arising in the nasal cavity, paranasal sinuses, nasopharynx, and central nervous system (CNS), such as meningiomas, pituitary adenomas, craniopharyngiomas, and schwannomas. The preferred treatment for many of these tumors is radical or adjuvant high-dose radiation therapy (RT). Occasionally, the anatomical configuration of the intracranial vault and paranasal sinuses and the possibility of subclinical disease extension through the thin bony walls that separate the paranasal sinuses from the orbits necessitate that the contiguous orbit and medial portions of the eye be included in the planning treatment volume for external-beam RT. RT, in the form of ophthalmic (episcleral) plaque brachytherapy or charged-particle external-beam therapy (protons, heavy ions),[1,2] offers patients with anterior (iris, ciliary body) and posterior (choroidal) uveal melanomas and retinoblastomas a vision-sparing alternative to enucleation.[3,4] Stereotactic radiosurgery (SRS) is also used for the treatment of ocular melanomas, pituitary tumors, and meningiomas that are anatomically close to the visual apparatus.

The proximity of the planning target volume to the visual apparatus poses a challenge in RT treatment planning and delivery since radiation may cause damage to the eye and its surrounding structures. Although the eye and adnexae are vulnerable to radiation, individual parts of the visual system show significant variation in their sensitivity to radiation.[5] Radiation-induced damage to components of the visual pathways leads to morbidities varying in severity and latency. Acute ocular complications to the adnexae and anterior segment include dermatitis, eyelid edema, blepharitis, keratitis, conjunctivitis, and iridiocytis.[2,6] Late ocular adnexal and anterior-segment radiation-induced ocular complications include eyelash loss, cataracts, lacrimal duct atrophy, dry eye (also known as "keratoconjunctivitis sicca" or "xerophthalmia"), corneal ulceration, opacification, iris neovascularization, and secondary glaucoma.[2,6] Acute posterior-segment complications include secondary retinal detachment and vitreous, retinal, or choroidal hemorrhage.[2,6] Radiation-induced retinopathy (RIRN), radiation-induced maculopathy, and radiation-induced optic neuropathy (RION) are the most common late posterior-segment complications. Based on the location of the lesion along

the optic nerve and its clinical manifestations, RION has been divided into two separate entities: anterior radiation-induced optic neuropathy (ARION) and posterior radiation-induced optic neuropathy (PRION).[7,8] Strabismus, scleral atrophy, scleral necrosis, choroidal neovascularization (CNV), and globe perforation though less common, also occur.[2,9] Other complications include orbital hypoplasia, enophthalmos, phthisis bulbi, and in pediatric patients bone maldevelopment and risk of developing a secondary tumor.

DESCRIPTION OF GROSS ANATOMY AND IMAGING OF THE NORMAL STRUCTURE

GROSS ANATOMY

The eye is an externalized portion of the brain. The neural retina is a derivative and extension of the diencephalon, and the optic nerve is structurally and functionally a tract of the CNS rather than a peripheral nerve. The blood vessels of the retina are similar to those of the brain.[10,11] The eye is a slightly asymmetrical sphere with an approximate anteroposterior diameter or length of 24 to 25 mm. It has a volume of about 6.5 cm³. In cross section (Fig. 18.1), the eye is divided into three layers: the external layer, formed by the sclera and cornea; the intermediate layer, divided into two parts, the anterior (iris and ciliary body) and posterior (choroid); and the internal layer, the retina. The conjunctiva is a clear mucous membrane that covers the sclera and lines the inside of the eyelids. Within the eye, there are three chambers: the anterior chamber (between the cornea and the iris), the posterior chamber (between the iris and the crystalline lens), and the vitreous chamber (between the lens and the retina). The first two chambers are filled with aqueous humor, whereas the vitreous chamber is filled with a more viscous fluid, the vitreous humor.

The cornea, a transparent dome-shaped window, covers the front of the eye. It is normally transparent, clear, and devoid of blood vessels. Due to its high concentration of nerve endings (first division of the trigeminal nerve), the cornea is extremely sensitive. The adult cornea comprises five layers: the epithelium, the Bowman membrane, the stroma, Descemet membrane, and the endothelium. The lens is located 1 to 2 mm anterior to the ora serrata retinae and 5 mm below the surface of the cornea.

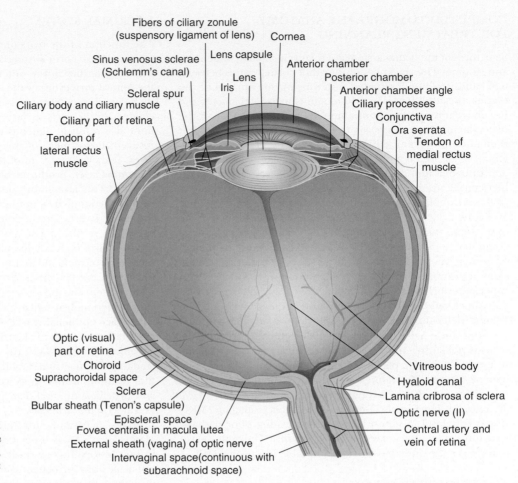

Fibers of ciliary zonule
(suspensory ligament of lens)   Cornea
Sinus venosus sclerae   Lens capsule
(Schlemm's canal)   Anterior chamber
Lens   Posterior chamber
Iris   Anterior chamber angle
Scleral spur   Ciliary processes
Ciliary body and ciliary muscle   Conjunctiva
Ciliary part of retina   Ora serrata
Tendon of   Tendon of
lateral rectus   medial rectus
muscle   muscle

Optic (visual)
part of retina   Vitreous body
Choroid   Hyaloid canal
Suprachoroidal space   Lamina cribrosa of sclera
Sclera   Optic nerve (II)
Bulbar sheath (Tenon's capsule)
Episcleral space   Central artery and
Fovea centralis in macula lutea   vein of retina
External sheath (vagina) of optic nerve
Intervaginal space(continuous with
subarachnoid space)

Figure 18.1. Anatomy of the eye. (From Netter FH. *Atlas of Human Anatomy.* Colacino, S, ed. Summit, NJ: Ciba-Geigy Corporation; 1994: Plate 85.)

Though a multilayer structure, an adult lens mainly contains two easily discernable, morphologically distinct compartments, the fiber cell mass and the epithelium. Whereas the functional phenotype and transparency of the ocular lens is provided by the fiber cell mass, the epithelium is the more active metabolic compartment.

The lacrimal system involves the lacrimal secretory system, lacrimal ducts, ocular surface (cornea and conjunctiva), eyelids, and associated sensory nerves.[12] The lacrimal secretory system[13] is broadly divided into (1) the basic secretors and (2) the reflex secretors. The basic secretors include three sets of glands. First, the mucin secretors consisting of (a) the conjunctival mucin-secreting goblet cells, (b) the crypt of Henle and (c) the glands of Manz. Second, the lacrimal secretors consisting of (a) the accessory lacrimal glands of Kraus and (b) the accessory lacrimal glands of Wolfring, Third, the oil secretors include (a) the tarsal (meibomian) glands and (b) the glands of Zeis. The reflex secretors consist of the main lacrimal gland and accessory palpalbral gland. Two to six excretory ducts along with their blood vessels, lymphatics, and nerves extend from the hilus of the main gland downward through the lacrimal foramen. The ducts continue downward a short distance in the postaponeurotic space and then pierce the posterior lamella of the lavatory and conjunctiva to empty into the conjunctival sac, just above the convex lateral margin of the upper tarsus.

The retina is a multilayered structure. The retina covers about three quarter of the eyeball. Two important areas of the retina are the optic disc and the macula lutea. The optic disc lacks photoreceptors and its center is referred to as the "blind spot." On the temporal side of the disc is the macula. At the center of macula is the fovea. The edge of the retina is defined by the ora serrata.

The optic nerve is formed of axons of ganglion cells and contains the retinal artery and central retinal vein that emerge from a central depression known as the "physiologic cup." The optic nerve is divided into four parts: First, the intraocular optic nerve, which is further divided into (a) the optic-nerve head or optic disc, (b) the prelaminar part located anterior to the lamina cribrosa, (c) the laminar part located within the lamina cribrosa, and (d) the postlaminar part located posterior to the lamina cribrosa. Second, the orbital portion extends from the globe to the apex of the orbit. Third, the intracanalicular part is located within the optic canal. Fourth, the intracranial portion merges into the optic chiasm and then optic tract. The blood supply to the optic nerve is derived from the central retinal artery, posterior ciliary arteries, pial branches of the ophthalmic artery, and branches of the internal carotid artery.[14]

The optic chiasm is located approximately 1 cm above the pituitary, anterior to the infundibulum. The chiasm forms the anterior border of the third ventricle with direct contact with cerebrospinal fluid. It projects into the third ventricle creating superior-inferior fluid recesses, the optic and infundibular recess.

COMPUTED TOMOGRAPHY ANATOMY FOR TREATMENT PLANNING

Structures of the ocular system are relatively small in dimension and volume. The thickness of the adult cornea varies between 0.52- and 0.67-mm;[15] situated 5 mm below the surface of the cornea, the adult lens is 9 to 10 mm in equatorial diameter and has an axial length of about 4 mm.[16] The mean volume of the major lacrimal gland is 0.17 to 0.19 cc in adults.[17] The adult retina occupies about 66% to 75% of the inner surface of the globe. The retina is a disc of approximately 20 to 40-mm diameter with <0.5 mm thickness.[18] The optic nerves vary in length between 35 to 55 mm with an average of 45 mm.[19] Diameters of the retrobulbar optic nerve range between 2.2 and 3.9 mm averaging 2.86[20] to 3.5 mm.[21] The estimated total volume of the optic nerve varies between 0.2 and 0.6 cc. Depending on the computed tomography (CT)-slice thickness, from 10 mm to 1.0 mm, it will appear on one to five slices. The average dimensions of the optic chiasm are 8 mm anterior-posteriorly by 4 mm superoinferiorly and 13 mm laterally.[22,23] The optic nerve maintains an elevation of 45 degrees relative to the orbital roof. The volume determination involves the delineated area and the slice thickness; a 10- or 5- or 3 mm slice thickness for the CT scans is not sufficient to accurately delineate and evaluate the volume of the optic pathway structures with an average diameter of 3.5 mm. To delineate the optic structures accurately, thin slices of 1.0 mm through parts housing the optic nerve are optimal. The use of CT-magnetic resonance imaging (MRI) fusion is helpful in identifying and delineating optic pathway structures (the optic nerve and optic chiasm). The optic nerves and chiasm are often most readily locatable on coronal MRI.

HISTOPATHOLOGY AND PATHOGENESIS

CRYSTALLINE LENS

A radiation-induced cataract is commonly seen as posterior subcapsular cataract (PSC) due to the initial location of its appearance within the lens after radiation exposure. Cataract formation results from irradiation of the germinative zone that consists of mitotically active cells within a ring at the periphery of the lens about 1 mm in front of the lens equator and 3 to 4 mm from the center of the lens.[24,25] The underlying mechanism for the development of radiation-induced cataracts is thought to involve direct DNA damage to germinal epithelial cells at the equator, which is later expressed as opacification when the epithelial cells differentiate into fiber cells and migrate to the PSC location.[26] The resulting defective-lens-fiber formation leads to the accumulation of debris in the posterior subcapsular region. It has been reported that a molecular basis for the origin and development of cataracts involves an altered gene-expression pattern of cyclin-dependent kinase-inhibitor CDKN1A (a human-lens epithelial-cell gene), which misregulates the signal transduction pathways linked to the differentiation and role of linear energy transfer.[27] Changes have also been noted in the subcapsular region[28] with thinning of the anterior subcapsular clear zone. With time, the subcapsular clear zone reforms both anteriorly and posteriorly and the cataract is seen to become separated from the capsule, with depth increasing with time.[29,30] In eyes that have been subjected to high radiation doses, the cataracts progress rapidly to maturity without recovery.[28]

LACRIMAL SYSTEM

The function of the tears under normal conditions is to lubricate, and flush corneal and conjunctival surfaces. By smoothing the irregularities in the outer surface, the tear layer improves the optical properties of the cornea. The term "dry eye" refers to a complex of chronic symptoms that occur secondary to changes in the eye's surface, cornea, and conjunctival epithelium as a result of aqueous insufficiency. Dry eye occurs as a result of impairment of the dynamic stability of the tear-film layer. Tears are made up of three layers. The innermost is the mucinous layer, produced by goblet cells located in the conjunctiva. This layer lubricates the relatively hydrophobic corneal and conjunctival epithelium and provides an anchor for the other layers. The middle is the lacrimal (aqueous) layer produced by the major and accessory lacrimal glands. The topmost layer is the meibomian (lipid) layer derived from the secretions of meibomian and Zeis glands that retard the evaporation of the tear film. The stability of the normal tear film is dependent on the presence of normal epithelial microvilli with adherent brush-like glycol proteins that originate from subsurface epithelial vesicles. Insufficiency of any of the three components, as well as blockage of the lipid component due to chronic inflammation of the meibomian glands after RT, may lead to loss of tear-film stability and rapid breakdown of the tear film resulting in dry spots, corneal ulceration, vascularization and opacification, and damage to the conjunctival epithelium (keratoconjunctivitis sicca).

Acute persistent, involutional atrophy of the meibomian glands after RT was observed in some exenteration specimens in one histopathology study, although the role of this involutional atrophy in ocular symptoms is unclear.[31] The atrophy probably affects the precorneal tear film and may ultimately contribute to corneal and conjunctival irritation. Other eyelid changes include epilation, acute and chronic dermatitis, depigmentation, atrophy, telangiectasia of skin, ectropion, entropion, and second cancers.[5] In some specimens, total loss of the meibomian glands and ducts, remnants of meibomian glands and ducts, or metaplasia of meibomian glands with cystically dilated meibomian ducts containing keratin in their lumina were observed. Other observation included (a) alterations in the palpabral conjunctiva ranging from focal loss of cells to squamous metaplasia; (b) a variable degree of chronic nongranulomatous conjunctivitis of paplabral conjunctiva; (c) focal chalaziain in recently irradiated specimens; (d) absence of the sebaceous gland of Zeis; and (e) modifications of the apocrine gland of Moll including atypicality with dilated lumina and variation in the individual's morphological features. Histopathologic findings indicated that the meibomian glands, which are sebaceous, are more sensitive to radiation and more permanently altered than the sebaceous glands of Zeis. The apocrine glands of Moll appear relatively radioresistant but can also be altered by radiation.[5,31]

Information on effects of radiation on nasolacrimal ducts remains limited as they have not been routinely evaluated for ductal patency after high-dose RT. Development of epiphora secondary to obstruction of previously normal nasolacrimal ducts after radiation in the presence of normal puncta and canaliculi has been reported,[32] although nasolacrimal duct obstruction by tumor invasion in such cases needs to be ruled out. Stenosis of lacrimal canaliculi and puncta after high doses of radiation is more common.[32]

RETINA

The effects of RT on the retina can be acute or chronic.[33] Based on histologic studies in monkeys, Cibis and Brown[34] suggested that acute changes within 6 hours of radiation include nuclear pyknosis, predominantly among rods, and edema restricted to the outer retinal layer. Acute (within hours) destruction of retinal rod cells in the retinas of monkeys was reported after a single exposure of 2,000 R.[34,35]

Nonproliferative radiation retinopathy (NPRR) is an early stage of retinopathy and involves capillary and arteriolar weakening as well as damage that has been noted in histopathologic studies.[36,37] In severely affected capillaries, both pericytes and capillary endothelial cells showed pyknosis, striking vacuolization, and loss of organelles as demonstrated by electron microscopy.[38,39] Endothelial cell injury and loss, primarily in the capillaries, is considered to be a fundamental abnormality of chronic radiation damage.[36,38–41] This leads to capillary closure (observable with fluorescin angiography),[40,42,43] and subsequently retinal ischemia, necrosis of nerve tissue, and fibrovascular proliferation.[38,39,44–46]

While small retinal vessels are commonly involved,[37] larger retinal and choroidal vessels may also be affected later in the course of the disease.[47] As a result of this involvement pattern, the inner retinal layers are preferentially damaged; however, the retinal pigment epithelium (RPE) may also be destroyed.[48] In advanced retinopathy, the choriocapillaris lamina degenerates.[38] Capillary closure compromises retinal circulation resulting in severe capillary nonperfusion. Subsequent retinal ischemia is presumed to release growth factors that lead to neovascularization in the retina, which is referred to as "proliferative retinopathy" (PRR).[39,47] A significantly higher concentration of vascular endothelial growth factor-A (VEGF-A) was found in eyes with neovascularization that were treated with radiation. PRR is a more advanced form of the disease. PRR, central retinal vein occlusion or ischemia of ciliary body may lead to neovascular glaucoma (NVG). The abnormal vessels often grow on the surface of the retina, the optic nerve, the iris.

TRABECULLAR MESHWORK

Neovascularization of the anterior chamber angle, along with its fibrovascular supportive membrane, acts to block the normal structures of the angle and pull the peripheral iris and cornea into apposition, thus blocking the trabecular meshwork. Peripheral anterior synechiae form and may rapidly lead to permanent angle closure. The result is a secondary angle closure without pupil block. An unusual pattern of vascular growth of the neovascular complex and polypoidal lesions around the borders of the subfoveal CNV with pronounced exudation and hemorrhage have been reported and named "radiation-associated choroidal neovasculopathy."[49] In some patients, it can lead to a subtotal or total retinal detachment with further evolution to NVG.

OPTIC NERVE

RION may be a part of a more extensive problem associated with delayed radionecrosis observed in parts of the CNS.[50,51] Pathology of enucleated eye,[52] autopsy findings,[50,53] biopsy results[54] of patients diagnosed with RION have been reported in literature. The features that were consistent in these reports included striking vascular changes, pronounced reactive gliosis, fibrosis, fibrinoid necrosis, hyalinosis, endothelial hyperplasia, narrowing of small vessels supplying the optic nerve and optic chiasm, and occasional occlusion of vessels that may have been secondary to these vascular changes. Demyelination, axonal loss, areas of fibronoid necrosis, regions of fibrous astrocyte proliferation, reactive astrocytosis, and obliterative endatertitis indicated damage to the neural tissue. Limited but significant apoptotic depletion of the oligodendroglial population has been reported after chiasmal irradiation in animal models and was suggested to be related to the development of RION.[55] Decreased numbers of endothelial cells and endothelial cell-lined vessels in human optic nerves that had received high-dose irradiation were observed in enucleated eyes.[56] Despite a number of reports on the pathophysiologic observations of delayed radiation damage to neural tissue,[53,57–61] the role of vascular damage in neural atrophy is still debated. Though there is no consensus on the exact mechanism of radiation injury to the visual pathway or CNS, vascular, cytopathic, chromosomal, and autoallergic factors have been considered to play a part.[50,51,57–60,62,63]

INCIDENCE AND LATENCY

INCIDENCE

Cataract Formation

Information on the incidence of cataract formation after RT remains sparse. Because of the effectiveness and ease of modern surgical techniques for lens replacement after cataract genesis, the development of cataracts is not considered a major complication of RT. The most common complication of plaque therapy for ciliary body melanoma is radiation-induced cataracts (48% for ciliary body melanoma vs. 14% for posterior uveal melanoma).[64,65] Deeg et al.[66] estimated an actuarial incidence of cataracts for patients undergoing total body irradiation (TBI) who were given fractionated (2–2.5 Gy/fraction, total dose of 12–15.75 Gy) and single fraction (10 Gy) RT to be 18% and 80%, respectively. The authors concluded that patients given single-fraction TBI had a 4.7-fold higher relative risk of developing cataracts than those given fractionated doses. Henk et al.[67] reported a 74% incidence of lens opacities in patients who received lens doses in the range of 4.5 to 30 Gy in 10 to 20 fractions.

Dry Eye

Letschert et al.[68] reported an incidence of keratitis in 58% of patients subjected to treatment doses of ≤40 Gy. Dry-eye syndrome was reported in 30% of patients receiving >40 Gy for the treatment of orbital non-Hodgkins lymphoma with fractionated RT. In this study, the doses received by the lacrimal glands may have been higher than the treatment dose but were not estimated. In two studies, the incidence of dry eye was not observed at doses <30 Gy when delivered with standard fractionation (1.8–2.0 Gy).[9,69] Parsons et al.[9] reported that 3 of 16 (19%) patients developed dry eye for doses ≤45 Gy and 100% of patients who received doses >57 Gy developed dry eye. Bassell et al.[69] noted a 4.5% incidence for doses between 30 and 39 Gy, increasing to 23% for doses between 40 and 49 Gy. The incidence of corneal ulceration has been observed for doses over 40 Gy.[68,70]

Radiation-induced Retinopathy

The reports on the incidence of RIRN in patients treated with fractionated RT are variable. Letschert et al.[68] reported a 9% incidence of RIRN in the dose range of 44 to 49 Gy delivered by standard fractionation. Chan and Shukovsky[71] reported a 95% incidence in patients who received >55 Gy treated with 2 Gy/fraction. Parsons et al.[72] reported on 27 eyes in 26 patients who received external-beam RT ranging in doses from 40 Gy to >75 Gy to half or more of the retina developing RIRN. For all patients in the dose range of 45 to 55 Gy, the incidence of RIRN was 53% (8/15), and when excluding the patients with diabetes mellitus, chemotherapy, and high doses per fraction (>3 Gy), the incidence was 22%. Monroe et al.[73] reported a 20% actuarial incidence of retinopathy at both 5 and 10 years and 5- and 10-year incidence of ipsilateral blindness of 16% and 17%, respectively, in patients treated with both once-daily and twice-daily fractionation. The median retinal dose for all patients was 56.85 Gy (range, 5–86 Gy), and in patients with RIRN it was 64.8 Gy (range, 40–86 Gy) delivered to one third of the retina.

Radiation-induced Optic Neuropathy

The reported incidence of RION in all patients after fractionated RT was 10.6% (14/131) by Parsons et al.[8] and 8.8% (24/273) by Bhandare et al.[7] Jiang et al.[74] separated the incidence of RION (8 of 98 patients; 10.2%) from optic-chiasm damage (11 of 208 patients; 5.2%) after fractionated RT for paranasal sinuses. Parsons et al.[8] reported that the 5- and 10-year actuarial incidences of RION above doses of 60 Gy to the optic nerve were 13% and 16%, and Bhandare et al. (2009, unpublished data) observed an overall incidence of 15% and 17%, among all patients. Jiang et al.[74] reported a 5- and 10-year incidence of 34% for a median dose per fraction of 2.2 Gy (range, 1.61–2.76) in the treatment of craniopharyngiomas treated to doses between 51.3 and 70.0 Gy. Flickinger[75] estimated a 5-year cumulative actuarial risk of RION of 30% after fractionated RT for craniopharyngiomas treated to a median total dose of 60 Gy (range, 51.3–70 Gy) at a median dose per fraction of 1.83 Gy, although the doses received by the optic nerve were not reported.

Bilateral Radiation-induced Optic Neuropathy

A number of cases of bilateral RION have been reported in the literature.[7,8,61,74,76] Although bilateral RION has often been considered an optic-chiasm injury,[74] reports of cases of bilateral ARION[7] have indicated the possibility of independent damage in both anterior optic nerves or independent lesions in both posterior optic nerves. The time course of bilateral vision loss varies significantly, from simultaneous vision loss[7] to a difference of 104 months between the eyes.[74] The time variation further adds to the question of whether bilateral vision loss is due to independent bilateral PRION or optic-chiasm damage, as the latter should cause bilateral vision loss nearly simultaneously. In one study, 9 of 11 patients who developed bilateral vision loss received doses ≥60 Gy to the chiasm, 1 patient received 50 Gy, and another 55 Gy.[74] At present, there are insufficient data to compare optic-nerve damage and chiasmal damage independently, but there is no reason to believe that chiasmal tolerance should differ from the optic nerve.

LATENCY

Cataracts

A delay of 3 to 8 years between RT and observed cataract formation has been reported.[67] Patients receiving single-fraction TBI are more likely to develop cataracts within 3 years after RT with the likelihood decreasing thereafter.[66]

Dry Eye

The visual impairment due to dry eye may often be less significant during the first few months after radiation, but corneal stromal edema, clouding, and corneal scarring and vascularization eventually lead to vision loss within 1 year.[32] Parsons et al.[9] reported that most patients who received >45 Gy and developed dry eye were symptomatic within 1 month after radiation, and corneal opacification and vascularization were pronounced within 9 to 10 months after radiation. Patients who received doses >57 Gy developed severe keratoconjunctivitis sicca within 1 to 2 months after RT, frequently followed by corneal opacification within 1 year. Three cases of dry eye with low doses to the lacrimal gland (32 Gy in 16 fractions over 22 days, 35.5 Gy in 20 fractions over 32 days, or 45 Gy in 21 fractions in 29 days) showed slow development of corneal vascularization and opacification within 4 to 10 years. Jiang et al.[74] observed the median time to manifestation of corneal injury to be 9 months (range, 1–31 months) for doses between 41.8 and 74.7 Gy to the lacrimal gland delivered at 1.02 to 3.72 Gy/fraction. Another study suggested the latency of corneal ulceration to be a function of the total radiation dose received by the cornea, with doses over 60 Gy causing a latency of <1 year.[70]

Radiation-induced Retinopathy

The onset of RIRN may be biphasic, presenting some relatively minor changes, like retinal blot hemorrhages or small, isolated cotton wool spots without any vision problems that resolve over time. The latency between RT and clinical manifestations of vascular changes varies, ranging from 7 months to 8.5 years with a median of 1.5 to 2.0 years after external-beam RT[71,77] and between 4 to 32 months after radioactive plaque therapy.[78] RIRN is often clinically manifested 1.5 to 3.0 years after fractionated external-beam treatment.[79] A short latency (<24 months) between RT and the occurrence of RIRN is thought to be a risk factor in the development of proliferative radiation retinopathy (PRR). In contrast, the risk of PRR in patients with NPRR for up to 4 years may be small.[47] A decreased initial visual acuity, which is believed to reflect more severe ischemia, was associated with new-vessel development.[47] Eyes with PRR have a worse prognosis of retaining useful vision than eyes with NPRR.[47] Rubiosis iridis and/or NVG have been observed 17 months to 5.5 years (median, 28 months) after fractionated RT.[47,72]

Radiation-induced Optic Neuropathy

The latency of RION has been reported to vary from 7 months[74] to 14 years.[8] The reported median latency was 28 months according to Parsons et al.,[8] 27 months by Jiang et al.,[74] and 30 months by Bhandare et al.[7] Jiang et al.[74] suggested that the dose per fraction and the total dose were related to the differences in the time of onset, but the latency for RION was not associated with a doses greater than or less than 60 Gy in another study.[7]

FACTORS ASSOCIATED WITH OPHTHALMIC TOXICITY

TREATMENT-RELATED FACTORS

Total Dose, Dose Per Fraction, Fractionation, and Treatment Modality

LENS. A threshold for detectable lens opacity has been reported to be 0.5 to 2.0 Gy in a single exposure,[80] although in some studies only 12% of patients exceeding a dose of 2 Gy have progressive opacities.[81,82] In an earlier study,[83] the lowest total dose that produced lens opacities after a fractionated course of treatment was 400 R and a total dose of 1,150 R (approximately 10 Gy) always led to cataract formation with a mean time of 4 years. While subsequent studies questioned these results and claimed that the tolerance of the lens was higher, their data were admittedly obtained from low-dose seed implants.[84] When delivered as a single fraction, the incidence of cataracts increases over a dose range of 4 to 15 Gy.[66,83] A significant sparing effect of radiation dose fractionation on cataract genesis was observed in one study.[66] The information on the cataract formation as a result of fractionated RT remains sparse. Henk et al.[67] observed that the adult lens can tolerate a total dose of 5 Gy after fractionated RT. At 15 Gy, with a fraction size of 1 Gy to the lens, the probability of visual impairment was 50% over 8 years; doses above 16.5 Gy almost invariably led to visual impairment. Some studies suggested tolerance dose for conventionally fractionated RT to be 12 Gy.[85,86] For eye-plaque brachytherapy for superonasal and inferior tumors of the meridian and apex, dose rates >57 cGy/h are suggested to be predictive factors for radiation-induced cataracts.[64] Radiation-induced cataracts are considered to be a deterministic (nonstochastic) late effect, so that below the threshold the cataracts are not produced and, above the threshold the severity of the biological response is dose related.[87]

LACRIMAL SYSTEM. The incidence of dry eye increases with the total dose received by the respective organs as well as the dose per fraction.[9] In cases of external-beam RT high doses (as with carcinoma), dry eye results in vision loss within 6 to 10 months after treatment. Low doses (as with lymphoma) usually lead to mild symptoms of correctible dry eye and cataract formation.[9] Because the cornea is a superficial structure, the surface dose to the cornea from a single portal would be low compared to the prescription dose, although in a multiportal treatment the contributions to the corneal dose from multiple portals may add up. The dose distribution from lateral portals may vary along the corneal surface. The dose-effect relationship for direct injury to the cornea is difficult to obtain, and changes to the cornea have been associated with irradiation of lacrimal tissue with the corneal complications arising secondary to dryeye syndrome.[9] Starting at 30 Gy, the occurrence of dry eye has been observed to increase steadily with the total dose received by the major lacrimal gland.[9,69] A dose incidence of dry-eye syndrome from Parsons et al.[9] is presented in Figure 18.2.

RADIATION-INDUCED RETINOPATHY. One earlier study[88] suggested 35 Gy as the upper limit of a safe dose, but cases of RIRN have been reported at lower doses such as 11,[89] 12,[90] and 20 Gy.[91,92] A number of factors have been suggested[9] to play a role in the development of RIRN at these low-dose levels, including dosimetry errors,[46] large doses per fraction,[46,92] an associated incidence with the prescription dose rather than

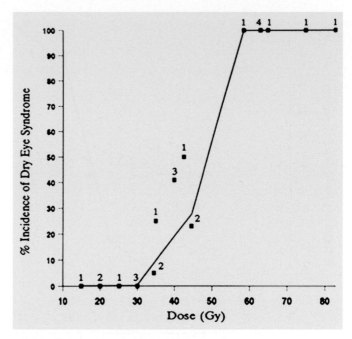

Figure 18.2. The sigmoid dose response curve for dry eye. (Data presented by Parsons JT, Bova FJ, Fitzgerald CR, et al. Severe dry-eye syndrome following external beam irradiation. *Int J Radiat Oncol Biol Phys.* 1994;15;30(4):775–780.)

the retinal dose,[46,89] difficulty with accurately estimating the retinal dose,[89,93] intensive chemotherapy in conjunction with RT,[39] diabetes mellitus,[94] and minor retinal changes that did not lead to vision loss.[40] Despite these contributing factors, there are number of undisputed cases of RIRN documented after a treatment dose of 20 Gy in patients with Grave disease.[95–97] A prospective study documented microvascular abnormalities in some patients before RT that increased after 20 Gy, suggesting that Grave disease may cause or predispose patients to retinopathy.[98] No case of RIRN was observed in 311 patients treated with radiation for Grave ophthalmopathy to total treatment doses of 20 or 30 Gy with 2 Gy/fraction at a follow-up of 1 to 21 years,[79] nor in 59 patients treated to retinal doses of 25 to 40 Gy in 2-Gy fractions.[69]

Mewis[99] reported RIRN in patients given 25 to 30 Gy for choroidal metastases. A number of other studies have reported an increasing incidence of RIRN at doses between 40 and 50 Gy delivered in 1.8 to 2 Gy/fraction.[68,69] Parsons et al. reported incidences of RIRN from doses above 45 Gy to the retina (50% of patients treated to between 45 and 55 Gy), with the percentage incidence increasing consistently with an increase in the total dose received by the retina. A dose incidence of RIRN from Parsons et al.[72] is presented in Figure 18.3.

Monroe et al.[77] also reported steady increases in the incidence of RIRN with increases in the dose to retina over 50 Gy. An increase in dose, whether given by brachytherapy or with external-beam RT, does not necessarily cause radiation retinopathy to develop earlier.[44,100–102]

Increasing fraction sizes have been associated with increases in the incidence of retinal complications.[45,77,88,92,93,100] Excluding the patients for whom factors other than radiation may have contributed to the development of retinopathy (e.g., diabetes, adjuvant chemotherapy), an analysis of patients

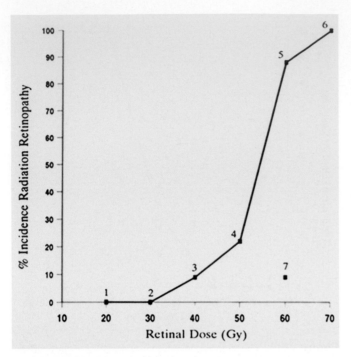

Figure 18.3. The sigmoid dose response curve for RIRN. (Data presented by Parsons JT, Bova FJ, Fitzgerald CR, et al. Radiation retinopathy after external-beam irradiation: Analysis of timedose factors. *Int J Radiat Oncol Biol Phys.* 1994;30:765–773.)

with RIRN showed an increase in incidence with fraction sizes >1.9 Gy, and concluded that in the dose range of 45 to 55 Gy, the risk of RIRN would increase with an increase in fraction size above the standard fraction size of 1.8 to 2.0 Gy.[72] In another study, a fraction size >2 Gy was also associated with increased incidence of RIRN and RION.[103] The literature on the relationship between fractionation (once a day or twice a day) and the incidence of RIRN remains limited. Monroe et al.[77] concluded that hyperfractionation was associated with a lower incidence of RIRN. The benefit of hyperfractionation was most apparent at higher doses (>50 Gy). Of the patients receiving doses >50 Gy to the retina, the incidence of RIRN was significantly lower for patients treated with twice-daily fractionation compared with once-daily fractionation (13% vs. 37%; $p = 0.0037$).

RADIATION-INDUCED OPTIC NEUROPATHY. Irrespective of the treatment modality, whether stereotactic radiotherapy, brachytherapy, or fractionated RT, the total dose received by the optic nerve remains the most important treatment-related risk factor in the incidence of RION. Several studies[7,8,74] agree that the incidences of RION and optic-chiasm injury increase significantly with an increase in the total dose to the optic nerve or optic chiasm when the total dose received by these structures exceeds 55 to 60 Gy using conventional fractionation. A comparison of studies is difficult, however, due to variations in dose-specification criteria; therefore, a specific threshold dose cannot be suggested from these studies. In patients treated with fractionated RT, no case of RION was observed by Parsons et al.[8] at doses <59 Gy. Although Jiang et al.[74] did not observe RION at a total dose <56 Gy, in that dataset the incidence of optic-chiasm injury was observed at 50 Gy. While the incidence

of RION and RIRN at treatment doses of 41 to 43 Gy and 40 Gy, respectively, has been reported,[68] the actual doses received by the optic nerve and the retina have not been estimated and can possibly be higher than the prescription dose. Brown et al.[100] reported severe vision loss due to RION in one diabetic patient treated with 35 Gy.

Among the studies that evaluated the effect of fraction size on the incidence of RION, an actuarial analysis by Bhandare et al.[7] revealed a decrease in the 5-year freedom from RION rate of 93% for a dose per fraction of ≤1.8 Gy to 78% for a dose per fraction of >1.8 Gy ($p = 0.0005$). Parson et al.[8] reported an increase in the percentage incidence from 8% to 40% when patients received >1.9 Gy/fraction. Jiang et al.[74] found that the total dose, *D*, multiplied by the fractional dose, *d*, *Dd*, was significant in vision loss due to RION. Van den Bergh et al.,[104] in a review of several studies of RION in acromegalic patients and in another review of post-RT RION in patients treated for nonfunctioning pituitary adenomas,[105] observed that more than 75% of these patients received doses ≥2.0 Gy/fraction. Though it may not be feasible to determine an optimal treatment threshold or limiting fraction size from these datasets, it would be safe and practical to infer from the present datasets that a fraction size greater than the standard 1.8 to 2.0 Gy/fraction will enhance the incidence of RION or optic-chiasm damage. Harris and Levine[106] reported that a dose per fraction in excess of 2.5 Gy significantly increased the risk of RION. Information on the effect of hyperfractionation on the incidence of RION remains limited. One study[7] reported a possible benefit by using hyperfractionation. A decrease in incidence of RION from 19 of 172 patients (11.0%) to 5 of 101 patients (4.95%) treated with standard and hyperfractionated regimens, respectively. Five- and ten-year actuarial incidences of RION for patients receiving >60 Gy to any segment of the optic nerve decreased from 21% and 23% to 8% and 8% ($p = 0.0024$), respectively. The univariate ($p = 0.0963$) and multivariate ($p = 0.0684$) analysis, however, indicated marginal significance.

The total dose received by the ocular organs depends on the treatment regimen (whether delivered by fractionated RT, SRS, plaque brachytherapy, or charged-particle therapy). Typically, proton irradiation delivers doses in the range of 70% of the prescription dose to the anterior segment, thereby increasing the incidence of adnexal and anterior-segment complications.[2,107] The incidence of cataracts and NVG is heavily dependent on the percentage of the anterior segment in the beam.[108] Higher incidences of anterior-segment complications (dry eye, epiphora, NVG) were observed with charged-particle irradiation (He-ions) than with iodine-125 (^{125}I) radioactive plaques.[64,108–110] The enucleation rate was mainly associated with post-RT treatment complications and was reported to be higher for He-ion irradiation than ^{125}I plaque treatment.[108]

STEREOTACTIC RADIOSURGERY. The information on fractionated RT may contribute to our understanding of RION, but it cannot be generalized into single-fraction high-dose SRS since treatment parameters such as fraction size and overall treatment time play a role in the incidence of the morbidity. Several reports have presented the tolerance of the optic nerve to single-fraction SRS.[53,111–113] Some studies concluded that the tolerance of the anterior optic apparatus is approximately 8 Gy when delivered by a single fraction. Girkin et al.[53] suggested a limiting dose of 8 Gy in patients without prior RT to reduce the incidence of RION. Tishler et al.[111]

found optic-nerve injury in 24% of patients treated with doses >8 Gy, but no such injury for doses <8 Gy delivered by gamma knife or linear accelerator. Stafford et al.[114] observed RION in <2% of patients despite the majority (73%) having received doses >8 Gy to a short segment of the optic apparatus. Duma et al.[113] found no complications of visual pathways when the dose of radiation did not exceed 9 Gy. Other studies concluded that doses up to 10 Gy are well tolerated by most patients.[112,114,115] Leber et al.[112] reported no RION after SRS doses <10 Gy, 26.7% for doses between 10 to 15 Gy, and 77.8% for doses >15 Gy to the optic apparatus. Stafford et al.[114] reported a 1.7% incidence of RION for doses <8 Gy, 1.7% for doses of 8 to 10 Gy, and 6.9% for doses >12 Gy. They concluded that the risk of RION remains low for patients receiving doses up to 12 Gy to the anterior optic pathway (either the optic nerve or chiasm). These studies suggest that with single-fraction RT, the dose to the optic nerve or chiasm should be limited to the range of 8 to 10 Gy with a reported incidence of RION increasing significantly at higher doses.[112,114]

Girkin et al.[53] have summarized the risk factors for RION after radiosurgery.

1. Dose >8 Gy to any part of the optic nerve.[111,116,117]
2. Prior external-beam RT.[53]
3. Prior anterior visual pathway dysfunction secondary to a previous surgery or tumor compression.[112]
4. A treatment plan based on CT rather than MR images.[112,118,119]
5. Large tumor volume (a pituitary tumor larger than 5 mm in diameter).[120,121]
6. A treatment isocenter within 5 mm of the anterior visual pathway.[120]

Chemoradiation

Chemotherapy is commonly used along with RT in the treatment of head-and-neck cancers. Systemic chemotherapy, when delivered with RT, has been implicated in the development of delayed radiation injuries. Cerebral necrosis has been associated with RT combined with intra-arterial, intrathecal, or intravenous chemotherapy,[122,123] but the data on the synergistic effects of chemotherapy delivered along with RT in the development of ocular complications remain sparse. A number of anecdotal reports have suggested an increase in the risk of vision complications with concomitant chemotherapy. Jiang et al.[74] reported that chemoradiation significantly impacted the likelihood of corneal injury and related chemoradiation to differences in latency. Chemoradiation may potentiate the development of RIRN at lower total doses[39] and may shorten the latency between exposure and retinal changes.[100] Monroe et al.[73] found that chemotherapy did not significantly impact RIRN on univariate ($p = 0.358$) and multivariate ($p = 0.87$) analyses.

In a study by Kinyoun et al.,[47] chemotherapy did not increase the risk of developing of PRR. They noted that chemotherapy may decrease the risk of proliferation, speculating that chemotherapy may reduce the release of vasoproliferative factors or the capacity of endothelial cells to proliferate.

There are anecdotal data on the incidence of RION after RT combined with chemotherapy.[124] RION was reported in two patients who received low-dose prophylactic cranial radiation (24 Gy) in conjunction with intrathecal chemotherapy, suggesting that the concomitant chemotherapy predisposes patients to optic neuropathy at a lower dose.[123]

Vincristine,[125–127] nitrosoureas,[128,129] and cisplatin[130] have been associated with cranial-nerve injuries, including injury to the optic nerve. After reviewing the literature pertaining to visual toxicity after chemotherapy, Griffin and Garnick[130a] suggested that 5-fluorouracil and intrathecal methotrxate[54] may contribute to optic-nerve atrophy after cranial RT. Several studies have presented case studies reporting incidences of RION after combined RT and chemotherapy.[54,123,124,131] Adjuvant chemotherapy was not significant on univariate ($p = 0.47$) and multivariate ($p = 0.81$) analysis in a study comparing patients treated with RT alone versus those treated with combined chemotherapy and RT; however, the sample size in that study was small.[7]

There is no other 2-arm study with a statistically significant patient sample in the present literature. The question of whether chemotherapy plus RT will enhance the incidence of RION, RIRN, and other ocular complications through its synergistic effects, and whether these are sequence dependent (i.e., delivered neoadjuvantly, concomitantly, or adjuvantly) and dose dependent requires further studied.

PATIENT-RELATED FACTORS

Age, Race, and Sex

The incidence of RION increases in patients over the age of 50 years treated with doses >60 Gy to the optic nerve.[7,8] Parsons et al.[8] observed that no patient in their dataset below the age of 50 years developed RION. A correlation between advanced age (>50 years) and an increase in the incidence of RIRN has also been reported, yet RION can still occur below the age of 50 years.[7,77] Monroe et al.[73] reported an association between advanced age and RIRN on both univariate ($p = 0.01$) and multivariate ($p = 0.03$) analyses. The investigators of an eye-plaque study also suggested that the age of the patients (>61 years) predicted vision decrease.[64] One study suggested a preponderance of RION in female acromegaly patients versus males with acromegaly.[104] At present, there is no study that has statistically evaluated the influence of race or sex on the incidence of vision loss after RT, particularly RIRN or RION.

Location and Extension of Tumor

The location of the tumor relative to the ocular organs is a determining factor for the dose received by the vision apparatus. The proximity of the treatment site to the eye has been correlated with the incidence of ocular complications, with the rate of occurrence being highest when irradiating the entire eye or orbit (87%), paranasal sinuses (45%), or nasopharynx (36.4%).[132] For plaque applications, the dose to the surrounding structures or the adnexa increases with increasing tumor sizes. The maximum apical tumor height and the basal dimension have been associated with vision loss.[4] The location of the tumor, whether anterior or posterior to the equator, has also been associated with visual outcome.[133] Plaque applications for the of lesions located in the anterior segment show a reduced incidence of posterior-segment complications, while those for the tumors located in the posterior nasal quadrant reduce the dose to the macula, decreasing the incidence of vision loss.[133] The proximity of the posterior tumor margin to the fovea has been associated with the development of maculopathy[3] and suggested to be most significant predictor of nonproliferative RIRN.[134] While some studies observed higher rates of macular and optic-disc complications when treating posterior lesions,[82,135] others did not observe dependence of visual outcome on tumor location.[136,137] The shape of the tumor (mushroom shaped) has also been suggested to predict vision decrease.[64] Tumor thickness and location have been implicated as predictors in charged-particle therapy.[1] Other factors that have been associated with RIRN after plaque therapy include tumor margin of <4 mm to the foveola, tumor limited to the choroid without a ciliary body, and iris involvement.[134] When treating uveal melanoma with both plaque and charged-particle therapy, an involved ciliary body was a risk factor for developing NVG, indicating that the anterior tumor margin is an important determinant.[64] In the treatment of orbital lesions, keratitis was found to be more common in patients with conjunctival lesions (82%) than in patients with intraorbital lesions (45%).[68] More anterior-segment complications (dry eye, epiphora, NVG) were observed with He-ions than with iodine-125 radioactive plaques.[108,109]

Volume Irradiated

The irradiated volume of the ocular organs may be a determining factor in the rate of complications. The irradiated volume of the eye was statistically significant for ocular inflammation in patients with ocular melanoma treated with protons.[137] The volume of retina irradiated is associated with incidence of RIRN. Takeda et al.[138] observed that eyes receiving more than 50 Gy to >60% of the retina were more likely to develop RIRN. A dose-volume analysis using CT in a carbon ion RT study indicated that the volume irradiated to ≥50 GyE ($V_{50\ IC}$) to the iris-ciliary body and irradiation of the optic disc were risk factors for NVG.[139] It has been suggested that a large irradiated volume ($V_{50\ IC}$) of the anterior segment of the eye may result in local ischemic changes or severe complications.[139] The incidence of cataracts and NVG is heavily dependent on the percentage of the anterior segment in the charged-particle beam.[108] Typically, proton irradiation delivers doses in the range of 70% of the prescription dose to the anterior segment, increasing the incidence of adnexal and anterior-segment complications.[2,107]

Pre-existing Conditions

Pre-existing vascular disorders like arteriosclerosis may contribute to the incidence of radiation-induced ocular complications.[40,107] Systemic conditions such as hypertension, diabetes mellitus, and autoimmune disorders have been suggested to make patients more susceptible to RIRN.[44,45,88,94,140] RIRN has been reported in patients with diabetes mellitus after receiving relatively low doses of 30 Gy in 15 fractions.[94] Pre-existing diabetes Mellitus has been suggested to lower the threshold for RIRN in some reports.[100,141] Since both the conditions are microangiopathies, the possibility of a synergistic effect has been anticipated. Although there are many anecdotal reports[40,72,94,97,100,140,142] that have suggested implicating diabetes mellitus in the incidence of RIRN, the data from these reports remain insufficient for conclusion. The incidence of RIRN after relatively low-dose RT (20 Gy delivered in ten fractions) for Grave ophthalmopathy has been reported and attributed to disease conditions and pre-existing retinal microvascular abnormalities.[92,98,140,143] Kinyoun et al.[47] did not observe the suggested risk factors associated with RIRN (i.e., diabetes mellitus, systemic hypertension) to increase the risk of developing PRR.

Diabetes was not observed to be a factor in patients with RION in one study.[8] In another study, the incidence of RION was comparable in patients with diabetes mellitus (1 out of 12 patients; 8%) compared to patients who did not have diabetes (23 out of 261 patients; 9%).[7] A limited dataset in that study of only 8 patients with hypertension who underwent RT found that 25% (2 of 8) of hypertensive patients compared to 8% (22 of 265) of nonhypertensive patients had RION.[7] Whether diabetes and hypertension constitute risk factors of RION and RIRN needs further investigation.

Pituitary Conditions, Acromegaly

The incidence of RION or optic-chiasm damage at doses as low as 40 Gy,[144,145] 40 to 45 Gy,[51,146,147] and 45 to 50 Gy[104,125,128,148] treated with fraction sizes varying between 2.0 and 2.8 Gy has been reported in the literature after treatment for patients with pituitary adenomas or acromegaly. The optic system in patients with pituitary adenomas and acromegaly has been suggested to be more sensitive to radiation damage than patients irradiated for nonfunctioning pituitary adenomas.[51,103,146,149] This may be due to vascular and hormonal changes secondary to acromegaly.[103] The mass effect or surgery in cases of pituitary adenomas may also sensitize the optic system.[51,103,104,146,149] This opinion is not universally accepted.[150,151] Van den Bergh et al.[105] reported a low risk of RION following RT (45–50.4 Gy) for nonfunctioning pituitary adenomas; however, they also reported that even 45 Gy in 25 fractions has been responsible for injury in a few patients, probably due to pre-existing opticochiasmal compression. The optic apparatus in patients with nonfunctioning pituitary adenomas may also be somewhat more susceptible to injury after RT than the optic nerves in patients without pre-existing compression.

OCULAR COMPLICATIONS: DEFINITIONS, CLINICAL MANIFESTATIONS, AND DIAGNOSIS

CATARACTS

A radiation-induced cataract is defined by lens opacity that is not present before radiation treatment. The Lens Opacity Classification System II offers criteria for diagnosing cataracts that consists of sets of standardized color photographs for grading the different forms of cataract using the slit-lamp test. The classification system consists of four classes: nuclear color, nuclear opalescence, cortical grading, and PSC.

DRY-EYE SYNDROME

Dry-eye syndrome, marked by a deficiency in the quantity and quality of tears, is defined by alterations in the production, the ingredients, and the stability of tears as well as changes in the epithelial structure of the conjunctiva and cornea. Pain from dry eye can be significant due to marked innervations of corneal epithelium with numerous nerves. Symptoms and ocular reaction involved in dry eye are presented in Figure 18.4 and Tables 18.1 and 18.2.

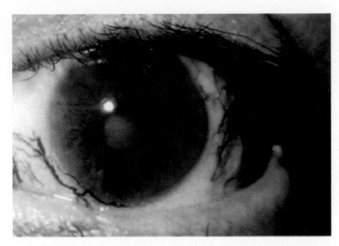

Figure 18.4. Radiation-associated anterior-segment complications: eyelash loss, dry eye, keratitis, and cataract. (From Finger PT. Radiation therapy for choroidal melanoma. *Surv Ophthalmol.* 1997;42(3):215–232. Review.)

TABLE 18.2	Dry-Eye Reactions

Corneal reactions in dry eye
Edema
Opacification
Mucous discharge
Symblepheron

Corneal reactions in severe cases of dry eye
Vascularization
Ulceration
Bacterial infection (streptococcal endophthalmitis)
Thinning of cornea
Perforation of cornea

After any acute reactions subside, the patients who are persistently symptomatic, with punctate epithelial staining of the cornea, normal lid-globe apposition, and reduced marginal tear meniscus, may be diagnosed to have dry eye. Although dry eyes can be diagnosed by symptoms alone, tests can determine both the quality and the quantity of tears. A symptoms-based assessment and diagnosis can be carried out using McMonnies and Ho's dry-eye questionnaires. A slit-lamp test can be performed to document any damage to the eye. The diagnostic criteria for determining dry eye are not well standardized. The diagnosis in severe cases is easy, but mild cases are more difficult to diagnose. The underlying cause is determined by measuring the production, evaporation rate, and quality of the tear film. There are several methods used to evaluate tear production, but, among them, the most widely used are Schirmer test and the tear-break-up-time test because they are easily administered, quick, and inexpensive. An objective diagnostic technique that quantifies the concentration of Ap4A, a molecule that naturally occurs in tears, has been recently described.[32] Corneal epithelial defects, such as abrasions and ulcerations, may be readily visualized by staining with fluorescein.

TABLE 18.1	Dry-Eye Symptoms

Common symptoms of dry eye
Tearing (varying degree)
Increased blinking
Dry, scratchy, gritty, or sandy feeling
Foreign-body sensation
Pain or soreness (varying degree)
Stinging or burning, itching
Redness
Eye fatigue
Contact-lens intolerance
Photophobia
Blurry vision (may be related to tear-film irregularity and may clear temporarily by blinking)

RETINOPATHY

Initial complaints of RIRN often include blurred, diminished vision, floaters, or both.[47] Commonly observed fundoscopic observations of NPRR and PRR are presented in Figure 18.5 and Table 18.3. Macular edema (ME) is the leading cause of vision loss in patients with RIRN.[47] Post RT clinically significant ME is manifested by central macular thickening, hard exudates threatening the macular center or one disc area of thickening in the macula, cystoids or noncystoid ME and serous detachment.[42,44,46,48,152] Intravenous fluorescin angiography (IVFA) of the eyes with RIRN often affirms the pathologies observed on fundoscopic exams. Observations specific to IVFA in RIRN are presented in Figure 18.6 and Table 18.4.

In cases of PRR, the patients may or may not have any symptoms during the growth of neovascularization; however, these blood vessels may lead to vitreous hemorrhage that may result in changes in vision ranging from a few floaters, to cobwebs, to cloudy vision, or to complete, rapid and sudden vision loss. Other observations include rubiosis iridis

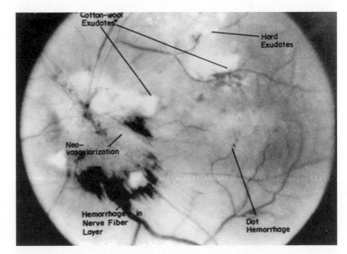

Figure 18.5. Fundoscopic examination of a patient after radiotherapy for fibrosarcoma of the left nasal cavity with a total dose to the retina 60 Gy, delivered in 32 fractions. The patient exhibits edematous with fuzzy margins. Other observations included cotton wool spots, hard exudates, intraretinal and preretinal hemorrhages, and irregular tortuous branch retinal arterioles. (From Parsons JT, Fitzgerald CR, Hood CI, et al. The effects of irradiation on the eye and optic nerve. *Int J Radiat Oncol Biol Phys.* 1983;9(5):609–622.)

TABLE 18.3	Radiation-induced Retinopathy

Fundoscopic observations with NPRR
   Retinal edema associated with infarction ischemia of the area of
      the retina involved in vascular occlusion
   Cotton wool spots
   Telangiectasia
   Capillary obstruction
   Fine and coarse pigmentation mottling with microaneurysms
   Intraretinal microvascular abnormalities including fusiform,
      tortuous, and saccular dilations
Fundoscopic observations with PRR
   Disc and/or retinal neovascularization
   Vitreous, preretinal, disc hemorrhages
   Retinal pigment atrophy
   Retinal (macular) detachment

TABLE 18.4	Radiation-induced Retinopathy

Findings on fluorescin fundus angiography
   Capillary nonperfusion
   Obliteration of retinal vessels (capillaries more susceptible than
      small and main arterioles), capillary closure
   Leakage from intraretinal microvascular abnormalities as well
      as from disc and retinal neovascularization in PRR, at times
      severe enough to cause clinically detectable retinal thickening
   Retinal edema, associated with infarction or ischemia of the area
      of the retina involved in vascular occlusion
   Microaneurysms in areas of capillary occlusion
   Retinal telangiectases and in cases of PRR neovascularization
   Cotton wool spots due to focal occlusion of small retinal
      arterioles, producing infarcts in the retina
   Hard exudates in the macular region indicative of interference
      with the oxidation mechanism in the retina and representing
      lipid material (common in PRR)
   Vascular sheathing

(iris neovascularization), hyphema, and/or NVG (Fig. 18.7). Patients with rubeosis may show a deficit in choriocapillaris circulation on fluorescein fundus angiography. A marked increase in intraocular pressure may occur with the development of severe rubeosis iridis and/or chamber-angle neovascularization. A rise in the intraocular pressure above 23-mm Hg with iris neovascularization, after previously normal pressure, is diagnosed as NVG. NVG has been observed in the weeks to months after the onset of vision deterioration due to RIRN in some patients.[72] Atrophy of the RPE occasionally observed in patients with RIRN is a feature that distinguishes RIRN from diabetic retinopathy.[33] Radiation-induced scleral necrosis is diagnosed when there is sufficient sceral erosion to allow direct visualization of uveal tissue. Radiation vitreous hemorrhage is diagnosed when there is vitreous blood detectable with slitlamp biomicroscopy, indirect ophthalmoscopy, or an A-scan and B-scan ultrasonography.

The pathologic changes in the retina in cases of RIRN are more severe in the posterior than the anterior retina, possibly due to an increased number of capillaries and a higher blood flow in the macular region.[44,102] The peripheral retina may be less susceptible to developing RIRN.[134] In some patients, both visual acuity and the ophthalmoscopic appearance of the fundus may remain normal before vision deteriorates.[152] In others, the pathologic changes precede the onset of visual deterioration by 1 to 2 years.[72]

OPTIC NEUROPATHY

For the proper diagnosis of RION, both pre- and post-RT ophthalmologic evaluations are necessary, along with the long-term ophthalmology follow-up. Clinical manifestations of ARION (Fig. 18.8) differ significantly from PRION. A comparison of the clinical manifestations, fundoscopic and IVFA observations of ARION and PRION is presented in Table 18.5. The lack of an initial fundoscopic and IVFA observation is a common feature of PRION, rendering the diagnosis more difficult, and the diagnosis is often made through the process

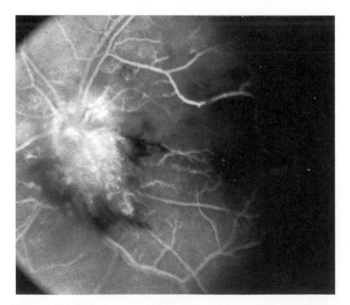

Figure 18.6. Fluorescein angiography observations showed irregular fluorescence of large vessel walls superiorly, extensive fluorescein leaks from neovascular tissue over the disc, and an area of retinal capillary nonperfusion superior to the fovea. (From Parsons JT, Fitzgerald CR, Hood CI, et al. The effects of irradiation on the eye and optic nerve. *Int J Radiat Oncol Biol Phys.* 1983;9(5):609–622.)

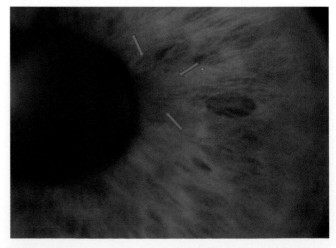

Figure 18.7. Radiation-induced rubiosis iridis.

of elimination of other conditions that may lead to vision loss among post-RT patients who have received high doses of radiation to the optic nerve. The diagnosis of RION is often presumptive, based on the exclusion of other causes leading to vision loss including optic neuritis or other ischemic optic neuropathies such as arteritic and nonarteritic ischemic optic neuropathies.

RADIOGRAPHY IN DIAGNOSIS OF RADIATION-INDUCED OPTIC NEUROPATHY

CT is useful for eliminating compression due to recurrence or progression of tumor in the optic pathway or other intracranial pathologies such as a regrowth of primary tumor, radiation-induced secondary neoplasms, or arachnoidal adhesions around the chiasm leading to vision loss; however, CT is unremarkable for detecting both ARION and PRION, other than the occasional edema, with some level of nonspecific and questionable optic-nerve prominence.[7,8,153] CT abnormalities reported in cases of RION, with or without contrast, pertain to brain tissue in the peritotemporal and frontal regions, as an area of decreased attenuation within white matter, with or without a mass defect, but not specific to the visual pathway.[153,154] Cerebral angiography is not useful for detecting RION as these studies are either normal or demonstrate areas of radionecrosis as a vascular mass.[154,155]

MRI with T1- and T2-weighted images done without administering the contrast medium are usually normal,[148] but occasionally may show swelling of the affected segment of the optic nerve.[156,157] MRI with gadolinium diethylenetriamine pentaacetic acid (Gd-DTPA) exhibits focal contrast enhancement due to leakage attributed to a disruption of the blood-brain barrier in the region of the optic-nerve infarction. Thus, a typical discrete focal contrast enhancement in the posterior optic nerve on MRI with Gd-DTPA has been suggested for the diagnosis of PRION (Fig. 18.9).[54,148,156,157] The enhancement fades within 12 weeks of the onset of PRION symptoms as atrophy supervenes.[158] A lack of specificity remains the limitation of MRI with Gd-DTPA as it does not distinguish PRION from

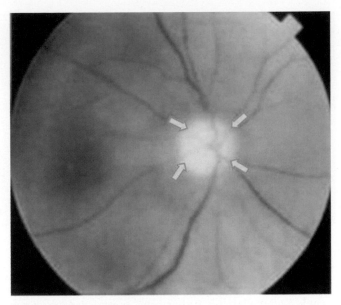

Figure 18.8. Fundus photograph of the right eye. There is pallor of the optic-nerve head (*arrows*) due to radiation injury (radiation induced optic neuropathy).

other pathologies such as optic neuritis. MRI with Gd-DTPA may not be necessary for the diagnosis of ARION since it can be diagnosed by fundoscopic and IVFA examinations. However, the use of MRI in patients who are at high risk of RION during the high-risk period has been recommended in the literature.[158] The visual evoked potential (VEP) is caused by sensory stimulation of a subject's visual field and is observed using electroencephalography. VEP has been reported to be abnormal during the months before vision loss.[159] Abnormal VEP has also been detected when visual function and fundus examination were still normal in patients treated with RT.[160] Besides the routine examination, evaluating the VEP prior to loss of vision in high-risk patients is also suggested by some investigators.[161]

TABLE 18.5	Symptoms of RION	
ARION	*PRION*
Clinical manifestations	
Profound, rapid painless visual loss is commonly observed, along with compromise in visual fields	Though profound, rapid, painless visual loss is commonly observed and gradual vision loss also observed; compromise in visual fields
Marcus Gunn pupil is common	Marcus Gunn pupil is common
Amaurosis fugax (sudden transient blindness lasting a short duration) and transient diplopia may be observed	Amaurosis fugax is commonly observed
Ophthalmoscopic observations	
Pallid optic-nerve edema in the early phase	No optic-nerve edema or swelling observed in early stage
Hyperemic areas with microaneurysms may be observed on the sectors of the optic disc	Hyperemic areas with microaneurysms are not commonly observed on the optic disc
Early phase followed by varying degrees of optic disc pallor and atrophy, with sectoral/segmental or entire disc involvement, leading to a chalky white appearance in the late phase (6–8 weeks after onset)	Disc pallor (sectoral or entire disc) observed only in the late phase (4–6 weeks from onset of visual loss); Optic atrophy with disc pallor leading to a chalky white appearance in the late phase (8–12 weeks after onset).
IVFA	
Filling defects and perfusion delays in the optic disc and peripapillary choroid in arterial, arteriovenous, and venous phases at presentation in early phase	No filling defects and perfusion delays observed at presentation in the early phase.

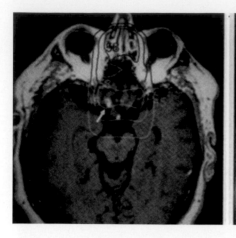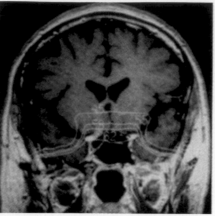

Figure 18.9. A magnetic resonance image (T1 weighted with Gd-DTPA) of typical discrete, focal contrast enhancement in the posterior optic nerve (*arrow*). (From Young WC, Thornton AF, Gebarski SS, et al. Radiation induced optic neuropathy: correlation of MR imaging and radiation dosimetry. *Radiology.* 1992;185:904–907, with permission)

BONE EFFECTS

Other morbidities associated with irradiation of the orbit include alterations in bone growth and second malignancies. In children treated for retinoblastoma, the effect of high-dose RT on the condrocytes of the orbital bones and alterations in the orbit growth owing to enucleation without proper prosthesis is shown to lead to facial asymmetry and deformities (e.g., hypotelorism, endophthalmos, depressed temporal bones, atrophy of the temporalis muscle, and a narrow and deep orbit).[162,163] The increased risk of a second malignancy (infield sarcoma induction) has also been suggested.[164] Follow-up evaluations should include considerations for these complications.

MATHEMATICAL/BIOLOGICAL MODELS

The doses received by the organs of the ocular system depend on the anatomic location of the treatment site (intra- or extraocular tumors), the treatment modality (megavoltage x-ray, plaque brachytherapy, particle therapy), and the patient-specific treatment plan. Organs associated with the ocular system (the lens, the components of the lacrimal system, the retina, the optic nerve, and the chiasm) are small in volume. The small volumes of these organs introduce the uncertainty delineating these organs on CT for the treatment planning, further confounding the uncertainty in the dose-volume histograms and their interpretation. A further lack of understanding of the physiologic phenomena involved in the initiation and progression of some of these complications poses a serious limitation when interpreting dose-volume information. There can be a significant gradient in the doses received by parts of the optic nerve extending from the optic chiasm to the optic disc and retina from the posterior pole to the nasal or temporal ora serrata, as well as those received by the ipsi- and contralateral eyes. The correspondence between the location of the lesion that initiates the infarction and the dose deposited at the location is difficult to establish in cases of RIRN and RION. Although an increase in the irradiated volume of the retina or optic nerve is expected to increase the incidence of RIRN and RION, a dose-volume effect on the incidence of these complications is difficult to establish. The information on dose-volume effects and relevant biological parameters remains limited.

Using a linear quadratic model, van Kempen-Harteveld et al.[137a] obtained a tissue-specific parameter, $\alpha/\beta = 0.75$, and

the rate of repair of sublethal damage, $\mu = 0.65/\text{h}$ (where $\mu = \ln 2/T_{1/2}$), for cataract induction after single-fraction radiation. A sigmoidal dose-response curve for lacrimal gland dysfunction and dry-eye syndrome reported by Parsons et al.[9] showed no incidence of dry eye for total doses <30 Gy, an increase in the incidence to 5% to 25% at doses of 30 to 40 Gy, and 100% incidence at doses >57Gy.

A few studies have attempted the use of Neuret and NTCP modeling for RION. Emami et al.[165] presented information on the tolerance dose for irradiation of the whole optic nerve. Burman et al.[166] applied the empirical Lyman model[167] to the Emami data to represent normal-tissue response under conditions of uniform irradiation to whole and/or partial volumes as a function of dose and volume irradiated. A TD 5/5 of 50 Gy, TD 50/5 of 65 Gy for RION/optic-chiasmal damage, TD 5/5 of 45 Gy, and TD 50/5 of 65 Gy for RIRN were estimated. The Berman–Emami analysis is based on two-dimensional dosimetry generated prior to 1991 at multiple institutions with significant variability in dose specification and the data collection.

Flickinger et al.[168] used the Neuret formulation and estimated 30% actuarial risk of RION for patients receiving a Neuret equivalent of >60 Gy at 1.8 Gy/fraction. Goldsmith et al.[169] constructed two approaches to predict optic-nerve radiation tolerance, limiting the analysis to the lowest reported doses associated with RION in the literature. The first approach uses a model based on optic ret, a unit derived from the nominal standard dose that incorporates total dose and number of fractions into a single quantitative term. A least-square linear regression was calculated for threshold doses on a log-log plot. The proposed model suggested the dose regimens for a low risk of RION in terms of optic ret (890 optic ret = DX $N^{-0.53}$), Optic ret may enable better differentiation of toxic and nontoxic regimens than the ret,[170] and has compared favorably with the Neuret formula.[63] The second approach calculated the RION threshold isotoxicity using the linear quadratic model for a given dose per fraction, and the least square linear regression was calculated for threshold doses on a reciprocal total dose plot yielding an α/β of 3.06. Significance levels of the regression coefficients for both models were determined.[171] The regression coefficient for the optic ret model (0.53) was statistically significant ($p < 0.001$) whereas that for the linear-quadratic model ($p > 0.10$) was not. Shrieve et al.[172] used the opticret model to predict the optic-nerve tolerance following various numbers of fractions. The model predicts a dose of 8.9 Gy to be associated with a low risk of optic neuropathy after a single fraction, and 54 Gy delivered with at least 30 fractions. Although the use of ret was suggested as a predictor of RION toxicity in some studies,[102,103] a subsequent study suggested that ret may not enable good prediction of RION.[106]

Jiang et al.[74] fitted a linear-quadratic model to the RION data, but they did not present a rigorous analysis of the modeling nor did they derive parameters of clinical significance, such as tissue doses for 5%, 10%, and 50% complication (TD 5, TD 10, and TD 50, respectively) or the slope at 50% complication, γ 50, from the data modeling. Estimated α/β and the corresponding 95% confidence intervals from the linear-quadratic fit were as follows: (a) for the data without correction for chemotherapy it was 1.18 Gy (range, –3.2 to 5.5 Gy); (b) including chemotherapy it was 3.04 Gy (range, –3.95 to 10.02 Gy); and (c) after stratifying for chemotherapy it was 2.93 Gy (range, –4.24 to 10.1 Gy). Martel et al.[173] attempted NTCP modeling for six presumed cases of RION in a dataset of 20. Only three patients had typical manifestations of RION resulting in vision loss. The other three were described as "mild optic neuropathy," which included one case of retinopathy and two other cases of transient atypical symptoms. This study used the maximum dose received by the optic nerve for analysis. The maximum dose in any structure could be a dose to a single voxel and cannot be effectively utilized for dose-volume analysis. Although the study presents NTCP modeling for RION using the Lyman model, there are insufficient data for a dose-volume analysis. In this study, NTCP was not estimated by fitting a model to the dataset; instead, NTCP was calculated using model parameter values presented in the Burman-Emami analysis[165,166] for each patient. They concluded that the Lyman model for NTCP overpredicted the incidence of RION for values of *n* = 0.25, *m* = 0.14, TD 50 = 65 Gy, and the agreement was improved for TD 50 = 72 Gy. Unfortunately, insufficient data as well as lack of precision in the study design and data make the results of this study unreliable.

There remain several limitations in the studies in the current literature, such as a relatively small number of patients, variation in the dose specification to optic nerve, thereby making the choice of any specific model for routine clinical utilization difficult. An NTCP modeling of the datasets from literature[7,8,74,165,166] is presented in Figure 18.10 (Bhandare et al., unpublished data, 2009).

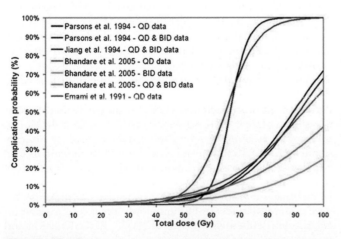

Figure 18.10. NTCP analysis for RION. Logistic regression model fitting to datasets in the literature (From Bhandare et al., unpublished data.)

STRATEGIES FOR AVOIDING TOXICITY

The strategy for dose reduction to the ocular organs depends on the modality of RT used (i.e., megavoltage x-ray, eye plaque, charged-particle therapy). The most potential ocular complications can be anticipated during the course of treatment planning at which time attempts can be made to reduce the dose to ocular structures. Patients should be informed of, and understand, the potential risks. A pre-RT ophthalmology evaluation of patients at high risk for RION is strongly suggested. Continued follow-up in the post-RT period should be carried out on a regular interval, not if or when dictated by the specific vision-related problems. A number of problems, such as dry eye, cataracts, RIRN and/or glaucoma, may occur simultaneously, thereby making the assessment and management difficult. The radiation oncologist and the ophthalmologist must coordinate before, during, and after the course of RT to avoid any pitfalls. Accurate target and critical-organ delineation, three-dimensional conformal and intensity-modulated techniques, and stereotactically aided treatment setups should be helpful in limiting the doses to critical structures.[174] These treatment techniques allow optimal patient positioning, reproducibility of portals and segments, unconventional beam angles, geometric shaping of the radiation beam so that it corresponds to the "beam's eye" view of the target, and geometric shaping of the isodose distribution by altering the beam intensity (fluence). A deliberate inhomogeneity of the dose across the target volume and a minimal or acceptable dose to vital organs can be achieved. IMRT can be viable and valuable in treatments of intra- and extracranial tumors to limit the doses to the optic apparatus and reduce the possibility of orbital hypoplasia, dry-eye syndrome, keratoconjunctivitis sicca, retinopathy, and optic neuropathy. An advantage of IMRT is the sparing of the optic apparatus in the treatment retinoblastoma.[86] Inverse treatment planning with IMRT using multiple segments applied in a conformal fashion to deliver modulated treatment has been shown to reduce the dose significantly to the lacrimal glands.[175] Reductions in the incidences of corneal injury and the grade and progression of conjunctivitis and dry-eye syndrome were observed in a clinical study of patients treated with IMRT for sinonasal cancer.[176] In addition to paying careful attention to the treatment planning, the radiation oncologist must pay careful attention to time-dose parameters (fractionation) and calculate the total dose and fraction size to each of the critical structures in an attempt to limit the volume of tissue receiving that dose.[177] Other suggested measures include using local anesthesia and a lid retractor to retract the upper lateral eyelid from the treatment field, maintaining an open-eye position during the treatment to prevent the bolus effect of the lids on the cornea and conjunctiva, and using a lead shield to protect the lens. Irradiated volume of orbit has been associated with an increase in the ocular toxicity after single-port charged-particle therapy. Lead shielding of the lens was reported to reduce the dose to the germinative zone of the lens to between 36% and 50% of the tumor dose with a Co-60 beam and to 11% to 18% with 5-Mev x-rays in treatment of orbital tumors.[67] Reducing the orbital volume with multiportal irradiation and lowering the dose to the orbital content is suggested to reduce the risk of NVG after charged-particle therapy.[178]

In brachytherapy applications, high-energy Co-60 ophthalmic plaques have been replaced by lower energy ruthenium-106 (^{106}Ru), ^{125}I, and later by palladium-103 (^{103}Pd). Compared to ^{60}Co, both ^{125}I (28 KeV) and ^{106}Ru (primarily a β emitter with a max energy of 3.5 Mev resulting in a typical penetration of 10% of the surface dose to 5–6 mm through water or tissue) were found to deliver significantly less radiation to normal ocular structures. The lower energy ^{103}Pd (21 KeV) has resulted in increased dose to the tumor and decreased radiation to normal ocular tissues compared to ^{125}I.[179] One millimeter of gold shielding will block more than 99.95% of low-energy radiation emitted from either ^{125}I or ^{103}Pd seeds. Used in the low-energy eye plaques, gold shielding blocks the radiation to the sides and posterior of the plaque and protects adnexal structures. It is also associated with a lower incidence of dry eye and NVG.[2]

Morphologic and functional observations in animal experiments have described a prevailing protection profile of amifostine and lidocaine on lacrimal glands, suggesting a prophylactic approach in the radioprotection of lacrimal glands during radiotherapy of the orbital region.[180] Radioprotective agents, including barbiturates and lidocaines, have been promising in animal models.[181] Lidocaine may depress the activity of excitable tissues by blocking voltage-gated sodium channels. Barbiturates may offer a protective effect on neuronal inhibition and blockage of serotonin-induced vasoconstriction by blocking γ- amino-butyric acid receptors. Amifostine (WR-2721), a phosphorothioate, is suggested to modulate the vascular response to radiation in animals.[182] Perhaps the most promising data come from the use of inhibitors of angiotensin-converting enzyme (ACE) to reduce radiation injury. The ACE inhibitor ramipril in animal models showed a threefold increase in the mean peak latency in the VEP of the placebo, whereas 75% of the ramipril group had normal VEP.[183]

TREATMENT OF INJURY

Suspected cases of ocular complications due to RT should be immediately referred to an ophthalmologist for diagnosis and management. The most important aspect of improving or stabilizing the vision is seeing the patient as quickly as possible from the onset of visual loss. The best treatment outcomes were in those patients who were seen and treated by ophthalmologists within 48 to 72 hours of visual loss.

CATARACTS

Not all cataracts require surgical treatment. In most cases, an ophthalmologist can closely monitor the patient's vision over a period of time and recommend treatment if or when there is a sufficient level of visual loss affecting quality of life. Significant improvements in intraocular surgical technique and technology now allow small-incision cataract surgery (e.g., phacoemulsification). Post-RT cataract formation is a completely manageable minor complication. In case of suspicion of an underlying RIRN, retinal function can be evaluated with bright flash electroretinography and transscleral visual evoked response; or in the case of suspicion of RION, a VEP can be performed before cataract extraction since there will be little or no improvement after extraction if RIRN or RION exists.

DRY EYE (XEROPHTHALMIA)

Anterior-segment disease should be managed early and aggressively to avoid corneal complications. Dry-eye syndrome after

RT is usually a chronic problem that varies in severity. The approaches for management and treatment of dry eye include tear stimulation and supplementation, increased tear retention, eyelid cleansing, and suppression of eye inflammation.[184] For cases with mild-to-moderate dry eye, adequate and regular use of artificial tears may be sufficient to prevent corneal complications. Autologous serum eye drops have been suggested to be more effective than artificial tears as they include essential tear components such as epidermal growth factor, hepatocyte growth factor, fibronectin, neurotrophic growth factor, and vitamin A, all of which have been shown to play important roles in the maintenance of a healthy ocular surface epithelial milieu.[185] In addition to lubricating tear ointments, myolytic agents can be used. Consistent with indicated biological mechanisms, sufferers should consume dietary omega-3 fatty acids or its topical application can be helpful in improving the quality of the tear film.[186] Inflammation occurring in response to tear-film hypertonicity can be suppressed by mild topical steroids or with topical immunosuppressants such as cyclosporine.[187] Patients with severe dry eye may benefit from a customized contact lens (Boston scleral lens). The lens rests on the sclera and provides a protective bandage for corneal epithelial defects, creating a fluid-filled layer over the cornea and preventing it from drying. It may not be well tolerated by some patients with severe dry-eye syndrome.[11] For patients with severe dry eye, the lacrimal drainage system can be occluded by the insertion of punctal plugs or cauterization of lacrimal puncta.

In cases of inflammation of the cornea (also known as "keratitis"), the frequent use of artificial tears or ointments to moisten the surface of the eye is recommended. Patching the affected eye during sleep may also promote healing if there is an epithelial defect. Relentless keratitis resulting in irreversible corneal opacification is an indication for corneal transplantation. Ocular inflammation from mild uveitis is usually treated by corticosteroids and cycloplegics. A blind painful, visionless eye may require evisceration or enucleation.

RADIATION-INDUCED RETINOPATHY

Since RIRN and diabetic retinopathy are clinically and histopathologically similar, treatment for RIRN is based on diabetic retinopathy.[77] Visual loss with NPRR is primarily due to the development of ME. Generally, mild and moderate NPRR does not require treatment, unless accompanied by ME. Argon-laser focal photocoagulation to seal the specific leaky blood vessels in a small area of the retina usually near the macula is the treatment of choice for ME. Unfortunately, there is no effective treatment of macular ischemia.

The risk of rapid progression from NPRR to PRR is often determined by fundoscopic and/or angiographic findings. Panretinal photocoagulation (PRP) treatment is used to slow the growth of new abnormal blood vessels that have developed over a wide area of the retina and reduce the risk of progression to high-risk PRR. Kinyoun et al.[43] used PRP in patients with a high risk of neovascularization and reported a regression of new vessels in half of the eyes as well as no recurrent vitreous hemorrhages at 19 to 66 months. In patients at high risk for developing PRR, elective PRP may lower the risk of iris neovascularization (rubeosis) rubeosis or NVG.[72] Early detection and treatment are associated with better visual outcome.[188] Pharmacologic therapy for NPRR without ME is in its early investigational stages. Protein kinase C inhibitors (e.g., ruboxistaurin) and aldose reductase inhibitors have been evaluated in clinical trials for nonproliferative diabetic retinopathy with no evidence of a benefit,[142,189] but their use in NPRR has not yet been studied. Pentoxifylline is known to improve blood flow in ocular diseases associated with capillary nonperfusion, such as central retinal vein occlusion and diabetic retinopathy.[190] Treatment with oral pentoxifylline has been reported to reverse the effects of RIRN in a single case report. However, the authors conceded that the visual improvement seen with pentoxifylline may have been coincidental with the natural history of the disease and may not be a direct effect of pentoxifiline.[191] Hyperbaric oxygen (HBO) treatments and systemic corticosteroids have not shown consistent efficacy in treatment of RIRN.[77,139]

Indications for proliferative retinopathy (PRR) treatment include high-risk proliferative characteristics, rubeosis with or without NVG, moderate-to-severe neovascularization not involving the optic disc, and widespread retinal ischemia and capillary nonperfusion.

A vitreous hemorrhage will usually be absorbed over the course of several weeks to months, resulting in some improvement in vision. Unclearing vitreous hemorrhage can be effectively managed with a pars plana vitrectomy.[43,192]

The action of VEGF is implied in more advanced retinal disease, including proliferative vascular changes and neovascularization secondary to retinal ischemia. VEGF is known to increase retinal vascular permeability and in part, its effects are mediated by protein kinase C.[193] Therefore, inhibition of VEGF or protein kinase C may improve vascular dysfunction. Antiangiogenic VEGF inhibitors such as bevacizumab (Avastin), ranibizumab, and pegaptanib are considered to be most promising pharmacologic treatments for PRR. Progressive reduction in retinal hemorrhages, exudates, cotton wool spots, microangiopathy, decreased ME along with improvement or stabilization of visual acuity was reported in six cases of RIRN after plaque RT by Finger and Chin[194] after use of VEGF inhibitor (bevacizumab). Rapid improvement of radiation-induced NVG and exudative retinal detachment after intravitreal application of ranibizumab in a case was reported Dunavoelgyi et al.[195] Rapid resolution of neovascularization and control of intraocular pressure after treatment with bevacizumab in three cases of NVG were reported by Chilov et al.[196] Pharmacologic therapy for the treatment of PRR is still investigational. Pharmacologic agents such as intravitreal glucocorticoids (e.g., triamcinolone acetonide) may reduce neovascularization. Other treatment options for treatment of NVG after radiation include PRP, peripheral retina cryotherapy, and photodynamic therapy with verteporfin.

RADIATION-INDUCED OPTIC NEUROPATHY

Most of the treatment options for the treatment of RION have emerged from the experience based upon treatment of arteritic and nonarteritic ischemic optic neuropathies.[197,198] A number of management options for RION have been considered, with some options being tried and reported.[51,63,199,200] These include: (1) systemic corticosteroids; (2) HBO; (3) anticoagulants; (4) combination treatment regimens; (5) optic-nerve sheath fenestration; and (6) angiogenesis inhibitors.

1. *Systemic corticosteroids*: Use of systemic corticosteroid in the treatment of RION is based on the hypothesis that radiation injury may be initiated by free radicals. Despite reports of occasional vision improvement in some cases, the use

of systemic corticosteroids (prednisone, dexamethasone, methyl-prednisolone) has not been consistently effective in the treatment of RION.[157,161,201]

2. *HBO:* HBO induces high oxygen partial pressure in tissues, reduces edema, initiates activation of fibroblasts and macrophages, stimulates angioneogenesis and collagen synthesis. HBO also has bacteriostatic and bacteriocidal effects.[202] In circumstances of radionecrosis, it is believed that the oxygen levels are too low to support angiogenesis, and that artificially produced higher oxygen levels thus break the cycle of ischemia and necrosis,[203] but the events involved in the mechanism are not clearly understood. Though the utilization of HBO in treatment of radiation-induced necrosis of non-neural tissue,[203] particularly bone,[202] has shown promise, in RION the efficacy of HBO remains questionable. Though vision improvement, partial visual recovery, or arrest of further vision decline has been reported after treatment with HBO,[161,204,205] in other cases the results have been unsatisfactory.[61,153] Anecdotal evidence suggested that HBO may be more beneficial if delivered as early as possible after the onset of vision loss, compared to days or weeks after the onset of RION.[158,204,205] In comparison of three groups of patients, (a) those receiving no treatment, (b) those receiving HBO at 2.0 atm, and (c) those receiving HBO at 2.4 atm, HBO was associated with better outcomes at higher pressures.[206] Furthermore, it has been suggested that patients at high risk for RION (e.g., high dose to the optic nerve, close proximity of lesion to the optic nerve, RION in one eye) should be considered for frequent imaging with MRI during the period of high risk (0–20 months) and if the signs of RION are detected on MRI, patients could be subjected to prophylactic HBO.[158,205]

3. *Anticoagulation*: Anticoagulants inhibit serum protein-mediated coagulation and secondarily reduce platelet aggregation and release.[207,208] It has been postulated that anticoagulation with heparin and warfarin promotes blood flow to irradiated tissue.[60] Though anticoagulation appears to offer some benefits in delayed cerebral radionecrosis, use of anticoagulants (heparin or warfarin) has not shown promise in the treatment of RION.[209] Moreover, stronger circumstantial evidence for lack of benefit from anticoagulation comes from several case reports in which RION has been documented to develop in patients while receiving anticoagulant (warfarin) therapy for other conditions such as cardiac disease.[203,210]

4. *Combination treatment regimens:* A combination of corticosteroid and HBO has been tried with unsatisfactory results. Though stabilization and improvement in vision in some cases have been reported after treatment with combination of corticosteroid and HBO[7,61], this approach has not shown consistency in results. In one series, none of the 11 patients were treated with combination of HBO and corticosteroid had an improvement in vision.[61] Further evidence of the ineffectiveness of combination therapy was described in a case of progressive vision deterioration resulting in bilateral optic atrophy despite treatment with oral anticoagulation and high doses of intravenous methylprednisolone.[211]

5. *Optic-nerve sheet fenestration (ONSF):* ONSF, primarily used in cases of visual loss associated with papilledema (raised intracranial pressure), was postulated to enhance the flow of interstitial fluid across the optic-nerve sheath, although the precise mechanism was not well understood. However, the role of ONSF in treating nonarteritic ischemic optic

neuropathy has been refuted and was determined to be harmful.[212] However, use of ONSF and restoration of vision in three cases of ARION have been reported in one study.[213]

6. *Angiogenesis inhibitors*: Bevacizumab is humanized monoclonal antibody that binds VEGF, inhibiting its binding to the receptors that promote angiogenesis. Selective antibody blocking (anti-VEGF therapy) inhibits the formation of abnormal blood vessels and decreases vascular permeability.[214] Finger[215] presented a case report of treatment of RION after with intravitreal injections of bevasuzimab where the patient showed decreased optic disc microangiopathy and hemorrhage and a well-perfused optic disc appearance with sharp margins and improved vision from 20/32 to 20/20 in several months. Though application of bevasizumab appears promising, the efficacy of bevacizumab needs to be further investigated in patients treated with external-beam RT at high doses who exhibit drastic and delayed vision loss often varying between 20/100 and no light perception.

In summary, despite the many therapeutic options available for treatment of RION to date, none of them has been proven to consistently restore or preserve visual function. A few scattered cases of spontaneous improvement following the onset of RION have been reported, most of which occurred in patients receiving radiation to the anterior optic nerve from plaque therapy for choroidal tumors. The pathologic changes in these patients are characterized by disc swelling, sometimes hemorrhages with retinal exudates, and cotton wool spots,[216] and may represent a special subset of patients with initial and possibly reversible inflammatory component or a phase.[217]

ORBITAL HYPOPLACIA

Another rare but significant morbidity of orbital radiation is orbital hypoplasia, which usually needs no treatment. In severe cases, rebuilding of the bones around the eye may be possible. In extreme cases of enophthalmos, plastic surgery can be done to build up the orbit.

ACKNOWLEDGMENTS. We would like to thank the editorial staff, Jessica Kirwan, Rachelle Dazile, and Cristian Barquero, in the Research Office at the Department of Radiation Oncology at the University of Florida.

REFERENCES

1. Char DH, Castro JR, Kroll SM, et al. Five-year follow-up of helium ion therapy for uveal melanoma. Arch Ophthalmol. 1990;108:209–214.
2. Finger PT. Radiation therapy for choroidal melanoma. Surv Ophthalmol. 1997;42:215–232.
3. Shields CL, Shields JA, De Potter P, et al. Plaque radiotherapy in the management of retinoblastoma. Use as a primary and secondary treatment. Ophthalmology. 1993;100:216–224.
4. Puusaari I, Heikkonen J, Summanen P, et al. Iodine brachytherapy as an alternative to enucleation for large uveal melanomas. Ophthalmology. 2003;110:2223–2234.
5. MacFaul PA, Bedford MA. Ocular complications after therapeutic irradiation. Br J Ophthalmol. 1970;54:237–247.
6. Shields JA, Shields CL. Non-neoplastic conditions that can simulate posterior uveal melanoma and other intraocular neoplasms. In: Intraocular Tumors: An Atlas and Text. 2nd ed. Philadelphia, PA: Lippincott Williams & Wilkins; 2007:171–205.
7. Bhandare N, Monroe AT, Morris CG, et al. Does altered fractionation influence the risk of radiation-induced optic neuropathy? Int J Radiat Oncol Biol Phys. 2005;62:1070–1077.
8. Parsons JT, Bova FJ, Fitzgerald CR, et al. Radiation optic neuropathy after megavoltage external-beam irradiation: analysis of time-dose factors. Int J Radiat Oncol Biol Phys. 1994;30:755–763.
9. Parsons JT, Bova FJ, Fitzgerald CR, et al. Severe dry-eye syndrome following external beam irradiation. Int J Radiat Oncol Biol Phys. 1994;30:775–780.
10. Cohen AL. The retina and optic nerve. In: Moses RA, ed. Adler's Physiology of the Eye: Clinical Application. 7th ed. St. Louis, MO: CV Mosby; 1980:370–410.
11. Parsons JT, Bova FJ, Fitzgerald CR, et al. Tolerance of the visual apparatus to conventional therapeutic irradiation. In: Gutin PH, Leibel SA, Sheline GE, eds. Radiation Injury to the Nervous System. New York, NY: Raven Press, Ltd; 1991:283–302.
12. The definition and classification of dry eye disease: report of the Definition and Classification Subcommittee of the International Dry Eye WorkShop (2007). Ocul Surf. 2007;5:75–92.
13. Jones LT. The lacrimal secretory system and its treatment. Am J Ophthalmol. 1966;62:47–60.
14. Hayreh SS. The 1994 Von Sallman Lecture. The optic nerve head circulation in health and disease. Exp Eye Res. 1995;61:259–272. Review.
15. Hogan JM, Alvaro JA, Weddell J. Cornea. In: Histology of the human eye: An atlas and Textbook. 2nd ed. Philadelphia, PA: Saunders; 1971:55–100.
16. Forrester J, Dick A, McMenamin P, Lee W. The Eye: Basic Sciences in Practice. 3rd Ed. London: Saunders Ltd; 2008.
17. Koutrouza-Tavlaridis N, Elzarka A. Lacrimal gland ultrasound. ASUM Ultrasound Bull. November 6, 2003(4):13–14.
18. Alamouti B, Funk J. Retinal thickness decreases with age: an OCT study. Br J Ophthalmol. 2003;87:899–901.
19. Glasgow, B. Optic nerve—cranial nerve II. http://www.medrounds.org/ocular-pathology-study-guide/2005/10/optic-nerve-cranial-nerve-ii.html. Updated October 22, 2005. Accessed September 25, 2009.
20. Beatty S, Good PA, McLaughlin J, et al. Echographic measurements of the retrobulbar optic nerve in normal and glaucomatous eyes. Br J Ophthalmol. 1998;82:43–47.
21. Karim S, Clark RA, Poukens V, et al. Demonstration of systematic variation in human intraorbital optic nerve size by quantitative magnetic resonance imaging and histology. Invest Ophthalmol Vis Sci. 2004;45:1047–1051.
22. Riodan-Eva P, Hoyt WF. Neuro-ophthalmology. In: Riodan-Eva P, Vaughn D, Asbury T, eds. General Ophthalmology. 15th ed. Stamford, CT: Appleton & Lange; 1998:244.
23. Slamovits TL. Anatomy and physiology of optic chiasm. In: Miller NR, Newman NJ, eds. Clinical Neuro-Ophthalmology. 5th ed. Baltimore, MD: Lippincott Williams & Wilkins; 1998:85–100.
24. Pirie A. Recovery from and protection against radiation damage to the lens. In: Smelser GK, ed. Structure of Eye. New York, NY: Academic Press Inc.; 1961:259–272.
25. Merriam GR Jr, Worgul BV. Experimental radiation cataract—its clinical relevance. Bull N Y Acad Med. 1983;59:372–392.
26. Cogan DG, Donaldson DD, Reese AB. Clinical and pathological characteristics of radiation cataract. AMA Arch Ophthalmol. 1952;47:55–70.
27. Chang PY, Bjornstad KA, Rosen CJ, et al. Effects of iron ions, protons and X rays on human lens cell differentiation. Radiat Res. 2005;164:531–539.
28. Roth J, Brown N, Catterall M, et al. Effects of fast neutrons on the eye. Br J Ophthalmol. 1976;60:236–244.
29. Brown N. Dating the onset of cataract. Trans Ophthalmol Soc U K. 1976;96:18–23.
30. Brown NP, Bron A. Lens Disorders: A Clinical Manual of Cataract Diagnosis. 3rd ed. Oxford: Butterworth-Heinemann; 1996;203.
31. Karp LA, Streeten BW, Cogan DG. Radiation-induced atrophy of the meibomian gland. Arch Ophthalmol. 1979;97:303–305.
32. Peral A, Carracedo G, Acosta MC, et al. Increased levels of diadenosine polyphosphates in dry eye. Invest Ophthalmol Vis Sci. 2006;47:4053–4058.
33. Zamber RW, Kinyoun JL. Radiation retinopathy. West J Med. 1992;157:530–533.
34. Cibis PA, Brown DV. Retinal changes following ionizing radiation. Am J Ophthalmol. 1955;40:84–88.
35. Cibis PA, Noell WK, Eichel B. Ocular effects produced by high-intensity x-radiation. AMA Arch Ophthalmol. 1955;53:651–663.
36. Egbert PR, Fajardo LF, Donaldson SS, et al. Posterior ocular abnormalities after irradiation for retinoblastoma: a histopathological study. Br J Ophthalmol. 1980;64:660–665.
37. Archer DB. Doyne Lecture. Responses of retinal and choroidal vessels to ionising radiation. Eye (Lond). 1993;7(pt 1):1–13.
38. Irvine AR, Alvarado JA, Wara WM, et al. Radiation retinopathy: an experimental model for the ischemic–proliferative retinopathies. Trans Am Ophthalmol Soc. 1981;79:103–122.
39. Irvine AR, Wood IS. Radiation retinopathy as an experimental model for ischemic proliferative retinopathy and rubeosis iridis. Am J Ophthalmol. 1987;103:790–797.
40. Amoaku WM, Archer DB. Cephalic radiation and retinal vasculopathy. Eye (Lond). 1990; 4(pt 1):195–203.
41. Archer DB, Amoaku WM, Gardiner TA. Radiation retinopathy–clinical, histopathological, ultrastructural and experimental correlations. Eye (Lond). 1991;5(pt 2):239–251.
42. Hayreh SS. Post-radiation retinopathy. A fluorescence fundus angiographic study. Br J Ophthalmol. 1970;54:705–714.
43. Kinyoun JL, Chittum ME, Wells CG. Photocoagulation treatment of radiation retinopathy. Am J Ophthalmol. 1988;105:470–478.
44. Bagan SM, Hollenhorst RW. Radiation retinopathy after irradiation of intracranial lesions. Am J Ophthalmol. 1979;88:694–697.
45. Wara WM, Irvine AR, Neger RE, et al. Radiation retinopathy. Int J Radiat Oncol Biol Phys. 1979;5:81–83.
46. Kinyoun JL, Kalina RE, Brower SA, et al. Radiation retinopathy after orbital irradiation for Grave's ophthalmopathy. Arch Ophthalmol. 1984;102:1473–1476.
47. Kinyoun JL, Lawrence BS, Barlow WE. Proliferative radiation retinopathy. Arch Ophthalmol. 1996;114:1097–1100.
48. Kinyoun JL, Zamber RW, Lawrence BS, et al. Photocoagulation treatment for clinically significant radiation macular oedema. Br J Ophthalmol. 1995;79:144–149.
49. Maertens I, van Limbergen E, Leys A. Radiation-associated choroidal neovasculopathy, exudative detachment and neovascular glaucoma. A case report. Bull Soc Belge Ophtalmol. 1999;274:51–56.
50. Crompton MR, Layton DD. Delayed radionecrosis of the brain following therapeutic x-radiation of the pituitary. Brain. 1961;84:85–101.
51. Atkinson AB, Allen IV, Gordon DS, et al. Progressive visual failure in acromegaly following external pituitary irradiation. Clin Endocrinol (Oxf). 1979;10:469–479.

52. Ross HS, Rosenberg S, Friedman AH. Delayed radiation necrosis of the optic nerve. *Am J Ophthalmol.* 1973;76:683–686.
53. Girkin CA, Comey CH, Lunsford LD, et al. Radiation optic neuropathy after stereotactic radiosurgery. *Ophthalmology.* 1997;104:1634–1643.
54. Hudgins PA, Newman NJ, Dillon WP, et al. Radiation-induced optic neuropathy: characteristic appearances on gadolinium-enhanced MR. *Am J Neuroradiol.* 1992;13:235–238.
55. Nagayama K, Kurita H, Nakamura M, et al. Radiation-induced apoptosis of oligodendrocytes in the adult rat optic chiasm. *Neurol Res.* 2005;27:346–350.
56. Levin LA, Gragoudas ES, Lessell S. Endothelial cell loss in irradiated optic nerves. *Ophthalmology.* 2000;107:370–374.
57. O'Connell J, Brunschwig A. Observations on the roentgen treatment of intracranial gliomata with especial reference to the effects of irradiation upon the surrounding brain. *Brain.* 1937;60:230–257.
58. Davidoff LM, Dyke CG, Elsberg CA. The effect of radiation applied directly to the brain and spinal cord. I. Experimental investigations on *Macacus rhesus* monkeys. *Radiology.* 1938;31:451–463.
59. Arnold A, Bailey P, Harvey RA, et al. intolerance of the primate brainstem and hypothalamus to conventional and high energy radiations. *Neurology.* 1954;4:575.
60. Glantz MJ, Burger PC, Friedman AH, et al. Treatment of radiation-induced nervous system injury with heparin and warfarin. *Neurology.* 1994;44:2020–2027.
61. Roden D, Bosley TM, Fowble B, et al. Delayed radiation injury to the retrobulbar optic nerves and chiasm. Clinical syndrome and treatment with hyperbaric oxygen and corticosteroids. *Ophthalmology.* 1990;97:346–351.
62. Raskind R. Central nervous system damage after radiation therapy. *Int Surg.* 1967;48:430–441.
63. Sheline GE, Wara WM, Smith V. Therapeutic irradiation and brain injury. *Int J Radiat Oncol Biol Phys.* 1980;6:1215–1228.
64. Gunduz K, Shields CL, Shields JA, et al. Plaque radiotherapy of uveal melanoma with predominant ciliary body involvement. *Arch Ophthalmol.* 1999;117:170–177.
65. Quivey JM, Char DH, Phillips TL, et al. High intensity 125-iodine (125I) plaque treatment of uveal melanoma. *Int J Radiat Oncol Biol Phys.* 1993;26:613–618.
66. Deeg HJ, Flournoy N, Sullivan KM, et al. Cataracts after total body irradiation and marrow transplantation: a sparing effect of dose fractionation. *Int J Radiat Oncol Biol Phys.* 1984;10:957–964.
67. Henk JM, Whitelocke RA, Warrington AP, et al. Radiation dose to the lens and cataract formation. *Int J Radiat Oncol Biol Phys.* 1993;25:815–820.
68. Letschert JG, Gonzalez GD, Oskam J, et al. Results of radiotherapy in patients with stage I orbital non-Hodgkin's lymphoma. *Radiother Oncol.* 1991;22:36–44.
69. Bessell EM, Henk JM, Whitelocke RA, et al. Ocular morbidity after radiotherapy of orbital and conjunctival lymphoma. *Eye.* 1987;1:90–96.
70. Morita K, Kawabe Y. Late effects on the eye of conformation radiotherapy for carcinoma of the paranasal sinuses and nasal cavity. *Radiology.* 1979;130:227–232.
71. Chan RC, Shukovsky LJ. Effects of irradiation on the eye. *Radiology.* 1976;120:673–675.
72. Parsons JT, Bova FJ, Fitzgerald CR, et al. Radiation retinopathy after external-beam irradiation: analysis of time-dose factors. *Int J Radiat Oncol Biol Phys.* 1994;30:765–773.
73. Monroe AT, Bhandare N, Morris CG, et al. Preventing radiation retinopathy with hyperfractionation. *Int J Radiat Oncol Biol Phys.* 2005;61:856–864.
74. Jiang GL, Tucker SL, Guttenberger R, et al. Radiation-induced injury to the visual pathway. *Radiother Oncol.* 1994;30:17–25.
75. Flickinger JC. Radiation-induced optic neuropathy. *J Neurosurg.* 1991;75:496–497.
76. Wijers OB, Levendag PC, Luyten GP, et al. Radiation-induced bilateral optic neuropathy in cancer of the nasopharynx. Case failure analysis and a review of the literature. *Strahlenther Onkol.* 1999;175:21–27.
77. Monroe AT, Bhandare N, Morris CG, et al. Preventing radiation retinopathy with hyperfractionation [abstract]. *Int J Radiat Oncol Biol Phys.* 2004;60:S188.
78. Gunduz K, Shields CL, Shields JA, et al. Radiation retinopathy following plaque radiotherapy for posterior uveal melanoma. *Arch Ophthalmol.* 1999;117:609–614.
79. Petersen IA, Kriss JP, McDougall IR, et al. Prognostic factors in the radiotherapy of Graves' ophthalmopathy. *Int J Radiat Oncol Biol Phys.* 1990;19:259–264.
80. International Commission on Radiological Protection. Recommendations. Annals of the ICRP. Oxford: Pergamon Press; 1990.
81. Hall EJ. *Radiobiology for the Radiologist.* 3rd ed. Philadelphia, PA: J.B. Lippincott Company; 1988.
82. Mettler FA, Upton AC. *Medical Effects of Ionizing Radiation.* 3rd ed. Orlando, FL: Saunders; 2008;350–356.
83. Merriam GR Jr, Focht EF. A clinical study of radiation cataracts and the relationship to dose. *Am J Roentgenol Radium Ther Nucl Med.* 1957;77:759–785.
84. Britten MJ, Halnan KE, Meredith WJ. Radiation cataract—new evidence on radiation dosage to the lens. *Br J Radiol.* 1966;39:612–617.
85. Rubin P. Law and order of radiation sensitivity. Absolute versus relative. *Front Radiat Ther Oncol.* 1989;23:7–40.
86. Reisner ML, Viegas CM, Grazziotin RZ, et al. Retinoblastoma—comparative analysis of external radiotherapy techniques, including an IMRT technique. *Int J Radiat Oncol Biol Phys.* 2007;67:933–941.
87. Hall EJ. *Radiobiology for the Radiologist.* 4th ed. Philadelphia, PA: J.B. Lippincott Company; 1994.
88. Chacko DC. Considerations in the diagnosis of radiation injury. *JAMA.* 1981;245:1255–1258.
89. Elsas T, Thorud E, Jetne V, et al. Retinopathy after low dose irradiation for an intracranial tumor of the frontal lobe. A case report. *Acta Ophthalmol (Copenh).* 1988;66:65–68.
90. Ingraham HJ, Perry HD, Donnenfeld ED, et al. Glued-on, rigid gas-permeable contact lens for severe radiation-induced keratitis. *Am J Ophthalmol.* 1992;113:538–540.
91. Kim MK, Char DH, Castro JL, et al. Neovascular glaucoma after helium ion irradiation for uveal melanoma. *Ophthalmology.* 1986;93:189–193.
92. Nikoskelainen E, Joensuu M. Retinopathy after irradiation for Graves' ophthalmopathy. *Lancet.* 1989;2:690–691.
93. Perrers-Taylor M, Brinklety D, Reynolds T. Choroidoretinal damage as a complication of radiotherapy. *Acta Radiol.* 1965;431–440.
94. Viebahn M, Barricks ME, Osterloh MD. Synergism between diabetic and radiation retinopathy: Case report and review. *Br J Ophthalmol.* 1991;75:629–632.
95. Gorman CA, Garrity JA, Fatourechi V, et al. The aftermath of orbital radiotherapy for Graves' ophthalmopathy. *Ophthalmology.* 2002;109:2100–2107.
96. Kinyoun JL, Orcutt JC. Radiation retinopathy. *JAMA.* 1987;258:610–611.
97. Marcocci C, Bartalena L, Rocchi R, et al. Long-term safety of orbital radiotherapy for Graves' ophthalmopathy. *J Clin Endocrinol Metab.* 2003;88:3561–3566.
98. Robertson DM, Buettner H, Gorman CA, et al. Retinal microvascular abnormalities in patients treated with external radiation for Graves ophthalmopathy. *Arch Ophthalmol.* 2003;121:652–657.
99. Mewis L, Tang RS, Salmonsen PC. Radiation retinopathy after "safe" levels of irradiation. *Invest Ophthalmol Vis Sci.* 1982;22:222.
100. Brown GC, Shields JA, Sanborn G, et al. Radiation retinopathy. *Ophthalmology.* 1982;89:1494–1501.
101. Lloyd MA, Heuer DK, Baerveldt G, et al. Combined Molteno implantation and pars plana vitrectomy for neovascular glaucomas. *Ophthalmology.* 1991;98:1401–1405.
102. Shukovsky LJ, Fletcher GH. Retinal and optic nerve complications in a high dose irradiation technique of ethmoid sinus and nasal cavity. *Radiology.* 1972;104:629–634.
103. Aristizabal S, Caldwell WL, Avila J. The relationship of time-dose fractionation factors to complications in the treatment of pituitary tumors by irradiation. *Int J Radiat Oncol Biol Phys.* 1977;2:667–673.
104. Van den Bergh AC, Dullaart RP, Hoving MA, et al. Radiation optic neuropathy after external beam radiation therapy for acromegaly. *Radiother Oncol.* 2003;68:95–100.
105. Van den Bergh AC, Schoorl MA, Dullaart RP, et al. Lack of radiation optic neuropathy in 72 patients treated for pituitary adenoma. *J Neuroophthalmol.* 2004;24:200–205.
106. Harris JR, Levene MB. Visual complications following irradiation for pituitary adenomas and craniopharyngiomas. *Radiology.* 1976;120:167–171.
107. Wilson MW, Hungerford JL. Comparison of episcleral plaque and proton beam radiation therapy for the treatment of choroidal melanoma. *Ophthalmology.* 1999;106:1579–1587.
108. Char DH, Quivey JM, Castro JR, et al. Helium ions versus iodine 125 brachytherapy in the management of uveal melanoma. A prospective, randomized, dynamically balanced trial. *Ophthalmology.* 1993;100:1547–1554.
109. Char DH, Castro JR, Quivey JM, et al. Uveal melanoma radiation. 125I brachytherapy versus helium ion irradiation. *Ophthalmology.* 1989;96:1708–1715.
110. Decker M, Castro JR, Linstadt DE, et al. Ciliary body melanoma treated with helium particle irradiation. *Int J Radiat Oncol Biol Phys.* 1990;19:243–247.
111. Tishler RB, Loeffler JS, Lunsford LD, et al. Tolerance of cranial nerves of the cavernous sinus to radiosurgery. *Int J Radiat Oncol Biol Phys.* 1993;27:215–221.
112. Leber KA, Bergloff J, Langmann G, et al. Radiation sensitivity of visual and oculomotor pathways. *Stereotact Funct Neurosurg.* 1995;64(suppl 1):233–238.
113. Duma CM, Lunsford LD, Kondziolka D, et al. Stereotactic radiosurgery of cavernous sinus meningiomas as an addition or alternative to microsurgery. *Neurosurgery.* 1993;32:699–705.
114. Stafford SL, Pollock BE, Leavitt JA, et al. A study on the radiation tolerance of the optic nerves and chiasm after stereotactic radiosurgery. *Int J Radiat Oncol Biol Phys.* 2003;55:1177–1181.
115. Ove R, Kelman S, Amin PP, et al. Preservation of visual fields after peri-sellar gamma-knife radiosurgery. *Int J Cancer.* 2000;90:343–350.
116. Urie MM, Fullerton B, Tatsuzaki H, et al. A dose response analysis of injury to cranial nerves and/or nuclei following proton beam radiation therapy. *Int J Radiat Oncol Biol Phys.* 1992;23:27–39.
117. Mehta MP, Kinsella TJ. Cavernous sinus cranial neuropathies: is there a dose-response relationship following radiosurgery? *Int J Radiat Oncol Biol Phys.* 1993;27:477–480.
118. Carbini CH, Goodman ML, Jones NE. The use of magnetic resonance imaging in performing stereotactic surgery. In: Lunsford LD, ed. *Stereotactic radiosurgery update: Proceedings of Int'l. Stereotactic radiosurgery Symposium.* New York, NY: Elsevier; 1992;67–72.
119. Gerdes JS, Hitchon PW, Neerangun W, et al. Computed tomography versus magnetic resonance imaging in stereotactic localization. *Stereotact Funct Neurosurg.* 1994;63:124–129.
120. Stephanian E, Lunsford LD, Coffey RJ, et al. Gamma knife surgery for sellar and suprasellar tumors. *Neurosurg Clin N Am.* 1992;3:207–218.
121. Flickinger JC, Lunsford LD, Wu A, et al. Treatment planning for gamma knife radiosurgery with multiple isocenters. *Int J Radiat Oncol Biol Phys.* 1990;18:1495–1501.
122. Di Chiro G, Oldfield E, Wright DC, et al. Cerebral necrosis after radiotherapy and/or intraarterial chemotherapy for brain tumors: PET and neuropathologic studies. *Am J Roentgenol.* 1988;150:189–197.
123. Fishman ML, Bean SC, Cogan DG. Optic atrophy following prophylactic chemotherapy and cranial radiation for acute lymphocytic leukemia. *Am J Ophthalmol.* 1976;82:571–576.
124. Guy J, Mancuso A, Quisling RG, et al. Gadolinium-DTPA-enhanced magnetic resonance imaging in optic neuropathies. *Ophthalmology.* 1990;97:592–600.
125. Schatz NJ, Litchenstein S, Corbett JJ. Delayed radiation necrosis of the optic nerves and chiasm. In: Glaser JS, Smith JL, eds. *NeuroOphthalmology: Symposium of the University of Miami and Bascom Palmer Eye Institute.* St. Louis, MO: CV Mosby; 1975:131–139.
126. Norton SW, Stockman JA. Unilateral optic neuropathy following vincristine chemotherapy. *J Pediatr Ophthalmol Strabismus.* 1979;16:190–193.
127. Sanderson PA, Kuwabara T, Cogan DG. Optic neuropathy presumably caused by vincristine therapy. *Am J Ophthalmol.* 1976;81:146–150.
128. Landolt AM. Hazards of radiotherapy in patients with pituitary adenomas. In: Derome PJ, Jedyak CP, Peillon F, eds. *Pituitary Adenomas.* Paris: Asclepios Publishers; 1980:227–231.
129. Lokich JJ, Skarin AT, Frei E III. 1-(2-chloroethyl)-3-cyclohexyhl-1-nitrosourea (methyl CCNU) and adriamycin combination therapy. *Cancer.* 1974;34:1593–1597.

130. Ostrow S, Hahn D, Wiernik PH, et al. Ophthalmologic toxicity after cisdichlorodiammineplatinum (II) therapy. *Cancer Treat Rep.* 1978;62:1591–1594.

130a. Grifffin JD, Garnick MB. Eye toxicity of cancer chemotherapy: a review of the literature. *Cancer.* 1981;48(7):1539–1549.

131. Phillips TL, Fu KK. Quantification of combined radiation therapy and chemotherapy effects on critical normal tissues. *Cancer.* 1976;37:1186–1200. Review.

132. Amoaku WM, Archer DB. Cephalic radiation and retinal vasculopathy. *Eye.* 1990;4:195–203.

133. Finger PT. Tumour location affects the incidence of cataract and retinopathy after ophthalmic plaque radiation therapy. *Br J Ophthalmol.* 2000;84:1068–1070.

134. Gass JDM. *Stereoscopic Atlas of Macular Diseases.* 2 ed. St. Louis, MO: CV Mosby; 1977.

135. Packer S. Iodine-125 radiation of posterior uveal melanoma. *Ophthalmology.* 1987;94:1621–1626.

136. Lumbroso-Le Rouic L, Charif CM, Levy C, et al. 125I plaque brachytherapy for anterior uveal melanomas. *Eye (Lond).* 2004;18:911–916.

137. Lumbroso L, Desjardins L, Levy C, et al. Intraocular inflammation after proton beam irradiation for uveal melanoma. *Br J Ophthalmol.* 2001;85:1305–1308.

137a. van Kempen-Harteveld ML, Belkacémi Y, Kal HB, et al. Dose-effect relationship for cataract induction after single-dose total body irradiation and bone marrow transplantation for acute leukemia. *Int J Radiat Oncol Biol Phys.* 2002;52(5):1367–1374.

138. Takeda A, Shigematsu N, Suzuki S, et al. Late retinal complications of radiation therapy for nasal and paranasal malignancies: relationship between irradiated-dose area and severity. *Int J Radiat Oncol Biol Phys.* 1999;44:599–605.

139. Tasman W, Jaeger EA. *Wills Eye Hospital Atlas of Clinical Ophthalmology.* 2 ed. Philadelphia, PA: Lippincott Williams & Wilkins; 2001.

140. Wakelkamp IM, Tan H, Saeed P, et al. Orbital irradiation for Graves' ophthalmopathy: Is it safe? A long-term follow-up study. *Ophthalmology.* 2004;111:1557–1562.

141. Dhir SP, Joshi AV, Banerjee AK. Radiation retinopathy in diabetes mellitus: Report of a case. *Acta Radiol Oncol.* 1982;21:111–113.

142. The effect of ruboxistaurin on visual loss in patients with moderately severe to very severe nonproliferative diabetic retinopathy: initial results of the Protein Kinase C beta Inhibitor Diabetic Retinopathy Study (PKC-DRS) multicenter randomized clinical trial. *Diabetes.* 2005;54:2188–2197.

143. Miller ML, Goldberg SH, Bullock JD. Radiation retinopathy after standard radiotherapy for thyroid-related ophthalmopathy. *Am J Ophthalmol.* 1991;112:600–601.

144. Al Mefty O, Kersh JE, Routh A, et al. The long-term side effects of radiation therapy for benign brain tumors in adults. *J Neurosurg.* 1990;73:502–512.

145. Macleod AF, Clarke DG, Pambakian H, et al. Treatment of acromegaly by external irradiation. *Clin Endocrinol (Oxf).* 1989;30:303–314.

146. Hammer HM. Optic chiasmal radionecrosis. *Trans Ophthalmol Soc UK.* 1983;103(pt 2):208–211.

147. Tsang RW, Brierley JD, Panzarella T, et al. Role of radiation therapy in clinical hormonally-active pituitary adenomas. *Radiother Oncol.* 1996;41:45–53.

148. Guy J, Mancuso A, Beck R, et al. Radiation-induced optic neuropathy: a magnetic resonance imaging study. *J Neurosurg.* 1991;74:426–432.

149. Bloom B, Kramer S. Secretory tumors of the pituitary gland: conventional radiation therapy in the management of acromegaly. In: Black PM, Zervas NT, Ridgway EC, eds. *Secretory Tumors of Pituitary (Progress in endocrine research and therapy).* 1 ed. New York, NY: Lippincott Williams & Wilkins; 1984:179–190.

150. Eastman RC, Gorden P, Roth J. Conventional supervoltage irradiation is an effective treatment for acromegaly. *J Clin Endocrinol Metab.* 1979;48:931–940.

151. Dowsett RJ, Fowble B, Sergott RC, et al. Results of radiotherapy in the treatment of acromegaly: lack of ophthalmologic complications. *Int J Radiat Oncol Biol Phys.* 1990;19:453–459.

152. Chee PH. Radiation retinopathy. *Am J Ophthalmol.* 1968;66:860–865.

153. Kline LB, Kim JY, Ceballos R. Radiation optic neuropathy. *Ophthalmology.* 1985;92:1118–1126.

154. Martins AN, Johnston JS, Henry JM, et al. Delayed radiation necrosis of the brain. *J Neurosurg.* 1977;47:336–345.

155. Kramer S, Lee KF. Complications of radiation therapy: the central nervous system. *Semin Roentgenol.* 1974;9:75–83.

156. Young WC, Thornton AF, Gebarski SS, et al. Radiation-induced optic neuropathy: correlation of MR imaging and radiation dosimetry. *Radiology.* 1992;185:904–907.

157. Zimmerman CF, Schatz NJ, Glaser JS. Magnetic resonance imaging of radiation optic neuropathy. *Am J Ophthalmol.* 1990;110:389–394.

158. Lessell S. Friendly fire: neurogenic visual loss from radiation therapy. *J Neuroophthalmol.* 2004;24:243–250.

159. Leber KA, Bergloff J, Pendl G. Dose-response tolerance of the visual pathways and cranial nerves of the cavernous sinus to stereotactic radiosurgery. *J Neurosurg.* 1998;88:43–50.

160. Kirkham TH. Neuro-ophthalmic presentations of sarcoidosis. *Proc R Soc Med.* 1973;66:167–169.

161. Boschetti M, De Lucchi M, Giusti M, et al. Partial visual recovery from radiation-induced optic neuropathy after hyperbaric oxygen therapy in a patient with Cushing disease. *Eur J Endocrinol* 2006;154:813–818.

162. Kaste SC, Chen G, Fontanesi J, et al. Orbital development in long-term survivors of retinoblastoma. *J Clin Oncol* 1997;15:1183–1189.

163. Imhof SM, Mourits MP, Hofman P, et al. Quantification of orbital and mid-facial growth retardation after megavoltage external beam irradiation in children with retinoblastoma. *Ophthalmology.* 1996;103:263–268.

164. Wong FL, Boice JD Jr, Abramson DH, et al. Cancer incidence after retinoblastoma. Radiation dose and sarcoma risk. *JAMA.* 1997;278:1262–1267.

165. Emami B, Lyman J, Brown A, et al. Tolerance of normal tissue to therapeutic irradiation. *Int J Radiat Oncol Biol Phys.* 1991;21:109–122.

166. Burman C, Kutcher GJ, Emami B, et al. Fitting of normal tissue tolerance data to an analytic function. *Int J Radiat Oncol Biol Phys.* 1991;21.

167. Lyman JT. Complication probability as assessed from dose-volume histograms. *Radiat Res.* 1985;8(suppl 1):S13–S19.

168. Flickinger JC, Lunsford LD, Singer J, et al. Megavoltage external beam irradiation of craniopharyngiomas: analysis of tumor control and morbidity. *Int J Radiat Oncol Biol Phys.* 1990;19:117–122.

169. Goldsmith BJ, Rosenthal SA, Wara WM, et al. Optic neuropathy after irradiation of meningioma. *Radiology.* 1992;185:71–76.

170. Ellis F. Dose, time and fractionation: a clinical hypothesis. *Clin Radiol.* 1969;20:1–7.

171. Matthews D, Farewell V. Linear regression models for medical data. In: Karger, ed. *Using and Understanding Medical Statistics.* 2nd ed. Basal;1988:124–130.

172. Shrieve DC, Hazard L, Boucher K, et al. Dose fractionation in stereotactic radiotherapy for parasellar meningiomas: radiobiological considerations of efficacy and optic nerve tolerance. *J Neurosurg.* 2004;101(suppl 3):390–395.

173. Martel MK, Sandler HM, Cornblath WT, et al. Dose-volume complication analysis for visual pathway structures of patients with advanced paranasal sinus tumors. *Int J Radiat Oncol Biol Phys.* 1997;38:273–284.

174. Pan CC, Hayman JA. Recent advances in radiation oncology. *J Neuroophthalmol.* 2004;24:251–257.

175. Metcalfe P, Chapman A, Arnold A, et al. Intensity-modulated radiation therapy: not a dry eye in the house. *Australas Radiol.* 2004;48:35–44.

176. Claus F, Boterberg T, Ost P, et al. Short term toxicity profile for 32 sinonasal cancer patients treated with IMRT. Can we avoid dry eye syndrome? *Radiother Oncol.* 2002;64:205–208.

177. Parsons JT. Radiation toxicity to the visual system. *J Neuroophthalmol.* 2004;24:193–194.

178. Rajendran R, Weinberg V, Daftari I. Decreased incidence of neovascular glaucoma by sparing anterior structures of the eye for proton beam therapy of ocular melanoma. [abstract]. *Int J Radiat Oncol Biol Phys.* 2004;60:311–312.

179. Finger PT, Moshfeghi DM, Ho TK. Palladium 103 ophthalmic plaque radiotherapy. *Arch Ophthalmol.* 1991;109:1610–1613.

180. Beutel J, Schroder C, von Hof K, et al. Pharmacological prevention of radiation-induced dry eye-an experimental study in a rabbit model. *Graefes Arch Clin Exp Ophthalmol.* 2007;245:1347–1355.

181. Oldfield EH, Friedman R, Kinsella T, et al. Reduction in radiation-induced brain injury by use of pentobarbital or lidocaine protection. *J Neurosurg.* 1990;72:737–744.

182. Plotnikova ED, Levitman MK, Shaposhnikova VV, et al. Protection of microcirculation in rat brain against late radiation injury by gammaphos. *Int J Radiat Oncol Biol Phys.* 1984;10:365–368.

183. Kim JH, Brown SL, Kolozsvary A, et al. Modification of radiation injury by ramipril, inhibitor of angiotensin-converting enzyme, on optic neuropathy in the rat. *Radiat Res.* 2004;161:137–142.

184. Lemp MA. Management of dry eye disease. *Am J Manag Care.* 2008;14:S88–S101.

185. Kojima T, Higuchi A, Goto E, et al. Autologous serum eye drops for the treatment of dry eye diseases. *Cornea.* 2008;27(suppl 1):S25–S30.

186. Miljanovic B, Trivedi KA, Dana MR, et al. Relation between dietary n-3 and n-6 fatty acids and clinically diagnosed dry eye syndrome in women. *Am J Clin Nutr.* 2005;82:887–893.

187. Lopez FH. Keratoconjunctivitis sicca. Hampton R, ed. http://emedicine.medscape.com/article/1196733-overview. Updated April 21, 2006. Accessed November 19, 2009.

188. Thorne JE, Maguire AM. Good visual outcome following laser therapy for proliferative radiation retinopathy. *Arch Ophthalmol.* 1999;117:125–126.

189. Aiello LP, Davis MD, Girach A, et al. Effect of ruboxistaurin on visual loss in patients with diabetic retinopathy. *Ophthalmology.* 2006;113:2221–2230.

190. Jay WM, Aziz MZ, Chapman JM, et al. Effect of oral or intravenous pentoxifylline on ocular and optic nerve blood flow. *Ophthalmic Res.* 1987;19:318–321.

191. Gupta P, Meisenberg B, Amin P, et al. Radiation retinopathy: the role of pentoxifylline. *Retina.* 2001;21:545–547.

192. Murray TG, Christmas N. 53 year old female complaining of "seeing blood" OU for 4 weeks. http://www.djo.harvard.edu/site.php?url=/physicians/gr/330. Updated 1996. Accessed November 20, 2009.

193. Harhaj NS, Felinski EA, Wolpert EB, et al. VEGF activation of protein kinase C stimulates occludin phosphorylation and contributes to endothelial permeability. *Invest Ophthalmol Vis Sci.* 2006;47:5106–5115.

194. Finger PT, Chin K. Anti-vascular endothelial growth factor bevacizumab (avastin) for radiation retinopathy. *Arch Ophthalmol.* 2007;125:751–756.

195. Dunavoelgyi R, Zehetmayer M, Simader C, et al. Rapid improvement of radiation-induced neovascular glaucoma and exudative retinal detachment after a single intravitreal ranibizumab injection. *Clin Experiment Ophthalmol.* 2007;35:878–880.

196. Chilov MN, Grigg JR, Playfair TJ. Bevacizumab (Avastin) for the treatment of neovascular glaucoma. *Clin Experiment Ophthalmol.* 2007;35:494–496.

197. Hayreh SS, Zimmerman MB, Podhajsky P, et al. Nonarteritic anterior ischemic optic neuropathy: role of nocturnal arterial hypotension. *Arch Ophthalmol.* 1997;115:942–945.

198. Burde RM. Optic disk risk factors for nonarteritic anterior ischemic optic neuropathy. *Am J Ophthalmol.* 1993;116:759–764.

199. Hayreh SS, Podhajsky P, Zimmerman MB. Role of nocturnal arterial hypotension in optic nerve head ischemic disorders. *Ophthalmologica.* 1999;213:76–96.

200. Hayreh SS. Anterior ischemic optic neuropathy. Role of nocturnal arterial hypotension. *Klin Monatsbl Augenheilkd.* 1996;208:aA12-aA17.

201. Piquemal R, Cotter JP, Arsene S, et al. Radiation-induced optic neuropathy 4 years after radiation: report of a case followed up with MRI. *Neuroradiology.* 1998;40:439–441.

202. Al Waili NS, Butler GJ, Beale J, et al. Hyperbaric oxygen and malignancies: a potential role in radiotherapy, chemotherapy, tumor surgery and phototherapy. *Med Sci Monit.* 2005;11:RA279-RA289.

203. Marx RE, Ehler WJ, Tayapongsak P, et al. Relationship of oxygen dose to angiogenesis induction in irradiated tissue. *Am J Surg.* 1990;160:519–524.

204. Guy J, Schatz NJ. Hyperbaric oxygen in treatment of radiation-induced optic neuropathy. *Ophthalmology.* 1986;93:1083–1088.

205. Borruat FX, Schatz NJ, Glaser JS, et al. Visual recovery from radiation-induced optic neuropathy. The role of hyperbaric oxygen therapy. *J Clin Neuroophthalmol.* 1993;13:98–101.

206. Borruat FX, Schatz NJ, Glaser JS, et al. Radiation optic neuropathy: report of cases, role of hyperbaric oxygen therapy, and literature review. *Neuro-ophthalmology.* 1996;16:255–266.

207. Wessler S, Gitel SN. Pharmacology of heparin and warfarin. *J Am Coll Cardiol.* 1986;8: 10B–20B.

208. Choay J. Structure and activity of heparin and its fragments: an overview. *Semin Thromb Hemost.* 1989;15:359–364.

209. Barbosa AP, Carvalho D, Marques L, et al. Inefficiency of the anticoagulant therapy in the regression of the radiation-induced optic neuropathy in Cushing's disease. *J Endocrinol Invest.* 1999;22:301–305.

210. Danesh-Meyer HV, Savino PJ, Sergott RC. Visual loss despite anticoagulation in radiation-induced optic neuropathy. *Clin Experiment Ophthalmol.* 2004;32:333–335.

211. Garrott H, O'Day J. Optic neuropathy secondary to radiotherapy for nasal melanoma. *Clin Experiment Ophthalmol.* 2004;32:330–333.

212. The Ischemic Optic Neuropathy Decompression Trial Research Group. Optic nerve decompression surgery for nonarteritic anterior ischemic optic neuropathy (NAION) is not effective and may be harmful. *JAMA.* 1995;273:625–632.

213. Mohamed IG, Roa W, Fulton D, et al. Optic nerve sheath fenestration for a reversible optic neuropathy in radiation oncology. *Am J Clin Oncol.* 2000;23:401–405.

214. Rosenfeld PJ, Schwartz SD, Blumenkranz MS, et al. Maximum tolerated dose of a humanized anti-vascular endothelial growth factor antibody fragment for treating neovascular age-related macular degeneration. *Ophthalmology.* 2005;112:1048–1053.

215. Finger PT. Anti-VEGF bevacizumab (Avastin) for radiation optic neuropathy. *Am J Ophthalmol.* 2007;143:335–338.

216. Brown GC, Shields JA, Sanborn G, et al. Radiation optic neuropathy. *Ophthalmology.* 1982;89:1489–1493.

217. Levy RL, Miller NR. Hyperbaric oxygen therapy for radiation-induced optic neuropathy. *Ann Acad Med Singapore.* 2006;35:151–157.

Cranial Nerves

Cranial nerve injury is a feared complication of any course of high-dose radiotherapy to the brain or the head and neck region. There are a number of different ways in which cranial nerve dysfunction may occur after radiation injury. Before the cranial nerves exit the brainstem, the rots of the cranial nerves, the nuclei, may be injured by high-dose radiation limited to the brainstem. Emami et al.[1] calculated TD 5/5 values (tolerance dose limits for 5% risks of brainstem injury developing 5 years after radiation) to be 60, 53, and 50 Gy at 2 Gy/fraction for irradiating 1/3, 2/3, and 3/3 of the brainstem, respectively. Urie's[2] estimates of the 1% and 5% radiation tolerance of cranial nerves and their nuclei within the brainstem from a limited group of 27 proton beam patients were 60 and 70 cobalt-Gy-equivalent, respectively.

Radiation injury anywhere along the pathway of cranial nerves may be either direct or indirect. Tumors causing cranial neuropathies from nerve compression or invasion are often the reason that cranial nerves are irradiated in the first place. As some tumors, and especially their neovasculature, react to therapeutic irradiation (intended to eventually relieve tumor nerve compression), interstitial pressure may acutely increase causing indirect injury to the cranial nerve. This can happen within the nerve root in the brainstem during a course of fractionated radiotherapy to a brainstem glioma in a patient not on corticosteroids. I have also seen it happen immediately after finishing conventional fractionated radiotherapy of meningiomas compressing the optic nerve. Acute hearing loss that occurs within 1 week of radiosurgery (RS) to acoustic schwannomas seems to be from this cause. It usually can be reversed by steroids and seems to occur more often in people with histories of sudden drops in their hearing prior to RS who have responded to steroids.

The most direct radiation injury to cranial nerves is the acute axonal degeneration that develops after trigeminal neuralgia RS. A typical gamma knife RS treatment plan for trigeminal neuralgia is shown in Figure 19.1. A maximum dose of 80 Gy is commonly prescribed using 4-mm diameter collimators that usually encompass a 5 to 6 mm segment of the proximal trigeminal nerve within the 50% isodose surface receiving 40 Gy. Pain relief develops in 80% to 90% of patients from 1 day to 3 months following the procedure, with most responses developing between 1 week and 1 month.[3,4] Kondziolka et al.[5] investigated gamma knife trigeminal neuralgia RS in a baboon model, irradiating their trigeminal nerves to 80 and 100 Gy. Pathological examination at 6 months showed axonal degeneration in the center of the two 80-Gy nerves (Fig. 19.2).

Examination of two nerves irradiated to 100 Gy showed axonal degeneration, with myelin vacuolation and expansion of the intercellular matrix (consistent with edema). In one of the two 100-Gy nerves, the entire width was almost completely necrotic, yet the nerve ganglia remained normal including the nerve nuclei and the rest of the brainstem (that received only low-dose irradiation). There did not seem to be any selective sparing of touch over pain fibers. It appears that because touch fibers outnumber pain fibers that touch sensation is more likely to remain intact and is preserved in 90% of trigeminal neuralgia patients after RS.[3]

FACTORS AFFECTING RADIATION SENSITIVITY OF NERVES

A number of factors affect the risk of radiation injury to cranial nerves. The chief factors include the type of nerve being irradiated, total radiation dose, dose per fraction, the length of the nerve irradiated, and individual differences in radiation sensitivity. Aside from known conditions such as ataxia telangectasia resulting in extreme radiation sensitivity (equally affecting resulting tumors and normal tissue), slight variations in radiation sensitivity seem to be present in otherwise normal individuals. If the vascular supply of a cranial nerve has been compromised by surgery or tumor invasion, it may be more difficult for it to withstand the effects of radiotherapy on the vasculature of that nerve. This may be why hearing loss seems to occur at a greater rate in acoustic schwannoma patients irradiated to 45 to 55 Gy than when the same region is irradiated for meningiomas not invading the canal. Similarly, hypertension, diabetes, and peripheral vascular disease could potentially cause subtle increases in radiation sensitivity. Nonrheumatoid collagen vascular diseases, specifically scleroderma, have been associated with late radiation complications, chiefly late fibrosis.[6] This is unlikely to be a problem with intracranial radiotherapy or particularly RS. High-dose radiotherapy of the skull base or head and neck in these individuals could lead to fibrosis that could compromise portions of cranial nerve at or outside of the skull base.

There seems to be a difference in radiation sensitivity between different types of cranial nerves. Special sensory nerves, which include the olfactory, optic, and acoustic/vestibular nerves, seem the most sensitive.[7] Somatic sensory nerves seem to be the next most sensitive nerves followed by the motor nerves as the least

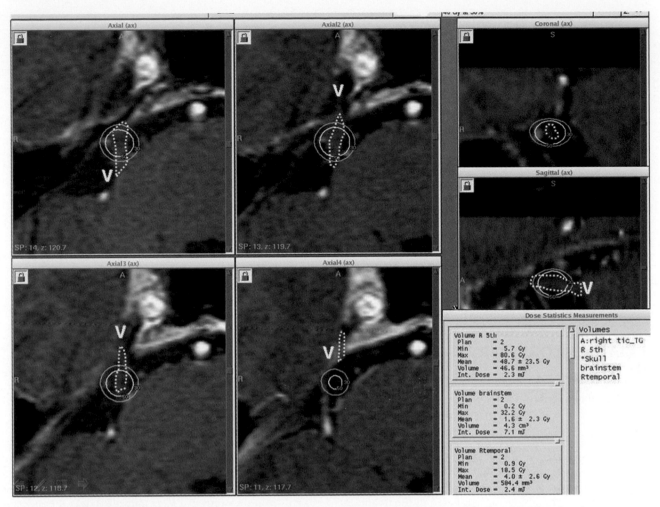

Figure 19.1. A typical gamma knife plan for treatment of trigeminal neuralgia affecting the right trigeminal nerve with 4-mm diameter collimators to a maximum dose of 80 Gy with 40 Gy to the 50% isodose surface (shown) and 24 Gy to 30% isodose surface (outer line shown).

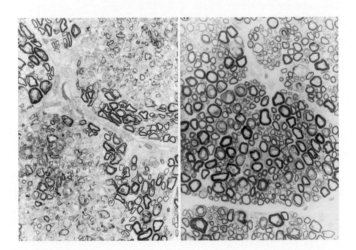

Figure 19.2. Toluidine blue-stained, 1-μm-thick sections of a baboon trigeminal nerve. Left: after 80-Gy RS, axonal degeneration and focal necrosis is identified (original magnification, ×100). Right: adjacent to the radiosurgical target, the appearance of the nerve is normal (original magnification, ×100). (Used from Kondziolka D, et al. Histological effects of trigeminal nerve radiosurgery in a primate model: implications for trigeminal neuralgia radiosurgery. *Neurosurgery.* 2000;46(4):971–976; discussion 976–977, with permission.)

sensitive. This is well illustrated in the diameter/dose-response analysis for acoustic schwannoma RS for 238 patients treated in Pittsburgh from 1987 to 1994 shown in Figures 19.3 to 19.5.[7] Transverse tumor diameter measurements were used to approximate the length of nerve being irradiated. Treatment planning techniques have improved since then, leading to lower risks of

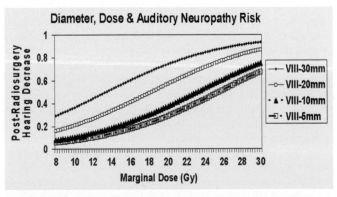

Figure 19.3. Dose-response according to transverse tumor diameter (intracanalicular and extracanalicular) for change in Gardner-Robertson Hearing Grade.

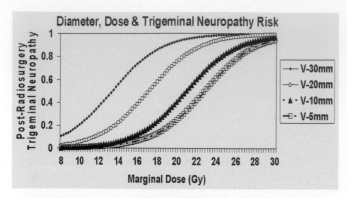

Figure 19.4. Dose-response according to transverse tumor diameter (extracanalicular only) for the development of any new or increased trigeminal neuropathy.

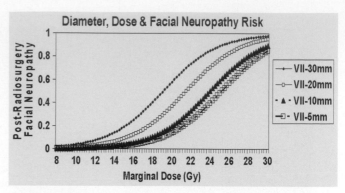

Figure 19.5. Dose-response according to transverse tumor diameter (intracanalicular and extracanalicular) for any new or increased facial weakness developing post-RS.

facial and trigeminal neuropathy than predicted by these curves for doses of 12 to 13 Gy in recent series (0% facial nerve injury and 2% to 3% trigeminal neuropathy for the entire series).[8–10]

SPECIAL SENSORY NERVES: I, II, AND VIII

Most of the time that high-dose radiotherapy is administered to the olfactory region, the sense of smell and a good deal of the sense of taste have already been lost from damage caused by the tumor or surgery. This occurs in the treatment of paranasal sinus carcinomas, olfactory neuroblastomas, and olfactory groove meningiomas. Temporary changes in taste are commonly reported during radiotherapy when the skull base (but not the tongue) is irradiated in the treatment of primary brain tumors. In these cases, the often modest radiation doses administered to the olfactory region seem responsible.

Because of the importance of vision and the wealth of literature on optic neuropathy, radiation injury to the optic nerve was covered in Chapter 19 of this book. The auditory branch of the eighth nerve causes greater concerns for radiation injury than the vestibular branch. Vestibular problems can occur from radiation but are usually transient. Because the brain integrates vestibular input from both cochleas along with touch sensation and visual input to control balance, vestibular symptoms tend to last only until the brain adapts to changes. Acoustic schwannoma patients present more commonly with hearing problems than balance problems despite the fact that these tumors are thought to more commonly arise on the vestibular branch. Patients who present with vestibular problems often see improvement over time with tumor growth during observation or following treatment (surgery or radiation) that results in diminished vestibular function/input from that side. Hearing is best assessed formally with an audiogram. The most important parameters followed on audiograms are the speech discrimination (SD) score and the pure tone average (PTA). The average of the three pure tone levels heard at 500; 1,000; and 2,000 Hz has been exclusively used in the past. Recently, many audiologists and neuro-otologists began to report four-frequency PTAs with results at 3,000 Hz added into the average to better reflect the frequencies of speech. SD scores can vary with amplification and are therefore reported with the decibel level used for

testing. The speech reception threshold provides additional feedback as to how much amplification is needed. Table 19.1 shows the Gardner-Robertson hearing classification system that is widely used to report results after managing acoustic schwannomas with surgery or radiation.[11] The terms "serviceable" or "useful hearing preservation" are used to describe preserved hearing of at least Gardner-Robertson Grade II. Hearing preservation is also often reported as preservation of the same Gardner-Robertson Hearing Grade (excluding those with Grade V hearing without testable SD). Long-term hearing follow-up is essential even after surgery, where delayed hearing loss may develop presumably from vascular compromise. While most other post-RS injuries develop within 2 years, hearing deterioration may develop 3 to 5 years or even longer after RS.[8] Radiation injuries after conventional fractionated radiotherapy (XRT) typically occur at a later time after radiotherapy (rarely before 6 months, as opposed to 6 months being the median time for post-RS injuries).

Figure 19.6 shows the relationship of the cranial nerves in the internal auditory canal and the proximity of the cochlea to most acoustic tumors. The rapid fall-off of radiation dose and the inhomogeneous dose distributions used may account for some differences in hearing and facial nerve preservation

TABLE 19.1	Gardner-Robertson Hearing Classification	
Gardner-Robertson Grade	*PTA*	*% SDᵃ*
I (good-excellent)	0–30 dB	70–100
II (serviceable)	31–50 dB	50–69
III (nonserviceable)	51–90 dB	5–49
IV (poor)	91 dB-max	1–4
V (no hearing)	Not testable	None

PTA is the three-frequency pure tone average from 500, 1,000, and 2,000 Hz.
ᵃ% SD is the speech discrimination score. If the grade assignments differ between the PTA and the % SD values, then the lower grade is to be used.
Source: Gardner G, Robertson JH. Hearing preservation in unilateral acoustic neuroma surgery. *Ann Otol Rhinol Laryngol.* 1988;97(1):55–66.

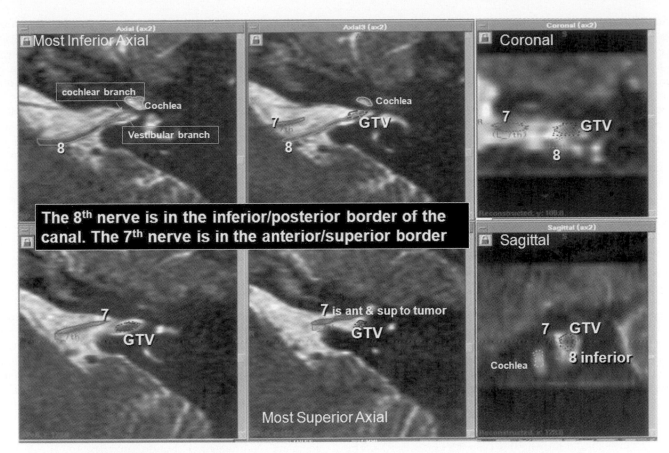

Figure 19.6. Small intracanalicular acoustic neuroma with the cochlea, facial (VII), and auditory/vestibular nerves identified.

between institutions using similar as well as different techniques for RS. In addition to the radiation sensitivity of the auditory nerve itself, the cochlea is a radiosensitive structure that may be damaged by radiation. One of the first demonstrations of the power of intensity-modulated radiotherapy techniques (IMRT) to improve radiotherapy was the ability to reduce the cochlear dose from 54.2 without IMRT to 36.7 Gy with IMRT to preserve hearing in children undergoing posterior fossa irradiation of medulloblastoma.[12] Thirteen percent of the IMRT group developed Grade III or IV hearing loss after chemotherapy and radiotherapy, compared to 64% of the Conventional-RT group ($p <$ 0.014).[12] There are some reports correlating hearing preservation after acoustic schwannoma RS with cochlear dose. While higher doses of radiation were undoubtedly delivered to the cochlea in early RS series and may have been responsible for hearing loss in some cases, modern treatment planning techniques for RS allow greater sparing of the cochlea. A recent study by Kano correlated hearing preservation with mean cochlear dose < 4.2 Gy.[9] This dose cut-off of 4.2 Gy (equivalent at most to 9 Gy at 2 Gy/fraction) seems too low to be a reasonable guideline. It probably reflects the correlation between dose to the cochlea and tumor volume, especially the amount of tumor irradiated within the internal auditory canal. As would be expected from the position of the auditory nerve, the radiation dose absorbed by the auditory nerve will increase as the length and width of the acoustic tumor that must be irradiated within the canal and to a lesser extent outside the canal increase. A mean dose of 8 Gy should be less than or equal to the equivalent dose for the standard recommend fractionated radiotherapy cochlear limit

of 35 Gy (with or without chemotherapy). The dose-response curves for hearing preservation are significantly less steep in Figure 19.3 than the dose-response curves for cranial nerves V and VII. This could be from varying maximum doses received by the vestibular nerve in different treatment plans, different cochlear doses, and varied ability of the acoustic nerve to tolerate radiation because of different degrees of tumor injury prior to RS.

SINGLE INSTITUTION COMPARISONS OF RS AND FRACTIONATED RADIOTHERAPY

Single institution comparisons of RS and stereotactic fractionated radiotherapy were published by groups at Jefferson University in Philadelphia, VU University Medical Center in the Netherlands and Heidelberg.[13–15] Andrews reported Jefferson's comparison of RS in 69 patients to fractionated radiotherapy (50 Gy per 25 fractions) in 56 patients.[13] The first 5 RS patients were treated at Jefferson with a linear accelerator, the rest with gamma knife. Fourteen patients without hearing underwent LINAC RS and 11 with hearing received fractionated radiotherapy with nine 4-Gy fractions. The authors stated that the patients receiving nine 4-Gy fractions would be the subject of a separate report, but it is not clear whether the LINAC RS patients were included in the total of 69 RS patients. The RS patients were treated with a gamma unit *almost* invariably" with a marginal dose of 12 Gy to the 50% isodose volume. Some of the RS patients received higher prescription doses than 12 Gy, but there are no details provided in the chapter. The authors found similar facial and trigeminal neuropathy rates in both the RS and fractionated radiotherapy groups, but hearing loss was significantly higher in the RS group. Because there were only a limited number of patients with serviceable hearing in each group (12 RS and 21 radiotherapy patients) and follow-up was limited, it is unclear that the long-term hearing preservation will be significantly different between the groups. The possibility that hearing loss could occur more slowly after radiotherapy than RS was not considered. Andrews et al. recently reported further improvements in hearing preservation in a more recent group of 46 acoustic schwannoma patients irradiated to 46.8 Gy compared to 43 treated to 50.4 Gy with median audiogram follow-ups of 65 and 53 weeks.[16] The median actuarial hearing preservation time was significantly longer with 46.8 Gy than with 50.4 Gy (165 weeks vs. 79 weeks, $p = 0.0318$). One transient facial neuropathy and no trigeminal neuropathy developed.

Meijer et al.,[14] from Amsterdam, recently reported another single institution comparison of RS and fractionated stereotactic radiotherapy (SRT) for acoustic neuroma. Forty-nine edentulous patients (mean age = 63 years), unable to reliably use a bite block in a relocate-able/noninvasive stereotactic frame, were selected for linear accelerator RS to either 10 or 12.5 Gy marginal dose prescribed to the 80% isodose. Eighty patients with intact dentition (mean age = 43 years) underwent stereotactic fractionated radiotherapy to 20 Gy in four to five fractions prescribed to the 80% isodose volume. They found a higher 5-year rate of trigeminal neuropathy with RS versus radiotherapy (8% vs. 2%, $p = 0.048$). Five-year actuarial tumor control was similar (100% RS vs. 94% SRT), as was facial neuropathy (7% RS vs. 3% SRT) and hearing loss (25% RS vs. 39% SRT). The higher than expected rates of facial and trigeminal neuropathy for the 13-0-12.5 Gy RS group compared to published low-dose RS results with gamma knife may reflect less than fully conformal treatment plans.

Combs et al.[15] reported Heidelberg's comparison of 30 acoustic schwannoma patients undergoing a median LINAC RS dose of 13 Gy to 176 patients receiving a median dose of 57.6 Gy of fractionated SRT after 76 months of median follow-up. Overall, hearing control was comparable between the groups. However, within the RS cohort, patients irradiated to ≤13 Gy had better hearing preservation than those receiving >13 Gy.

SOMATIC SENSORY-TRIGEMINAL NERVE INJURY

Trigeminal nerve injury can manifest with different types and degrees of symptoms. Decreased facial sensation is the most obvious, most expected, and most common type of trigeminal nerve injury. A mild decrease in facial sensation causes little hardship to patients. Complete facial numbness makes it difficult to know where food is in the patient's mouth. Patients need to be careful not to bite their tongue or cheek, and not to drool. Facial numbness also increases the risk of cranial abrasion. Paresthesias and different pain syndromes may develop. Facial sensation may be fully or partly intact but typical trigeminal neuralgia may develop with touch fibers transmitting paroxysms of severe pain. This has been reported to develop in up to 1% of acoustic scwhannoma patients undergoing RS for tumors extending near the trigeminal nerve. When complete facial numbness develops following RS or ablative surgical procedures on the trigeminal nerve like radiofrequency

rhizotomy, deafferentation pain or anesthesia dolorosa may develop. Deafferentation pain is constant pains and less likely to be helped by medications like carbamazepine used for typical trigeminal neuralgia. Patients may have the sensation of facial swelling with either deafferentation pain or trigeminal neuralgia with little or no discernable swelling.

The effects of volume or length of nerve irradiated and dose are evident in both acoustic neuroma RS and trigeminal neuralgia RS. There is no risk of trigeminal neuropathy after RS of intracanalicular acoustic schwannomas because of the much lower doses the trigeminal nerve receives compared to tumors extending into the cerebellar-pontine angle that often push up against the trigeminal nerve. The risk of trigeminal neuropathy in acoustic neuroma RS series treating to 12 to 13 Gy is 2% to 3% with approximately two third of those cases experiencing numbness alone and one third developing paresthesias or typical trigeminal neuropathy.[8] Chan reported the Harvard series of 70 acoustic neuroma patients treated to a median dose of 54 Gy in 30 fractions with a 4% rate of trigeminal neuropathy.[17,18] Trigeminal neuropathy develops in approximately 10% of trigeminal neuralgia patients after irradiation of the trigeminal nerve root with 40 Gy to the 50% isodose volume of a single isocenter with 4-mm diameter collimators (maximum dose: 80 Gy). A blinded randomized trial of RS to two isocenters versus one failed to show that irradiating a longer segment of the trigeminal nerve significantly improved pain control. Only an increase in facial numbness was identified in the two isocenter groups.[18]

Trigeminal neuropathy may develop after RS of cavernous sinus tumors, most commonly meningioma, but also pituitary adenomas, chordomas, or chondrosarcomas. An early study by Tishler et al.[19] correlated RS dose with the risk of injury to nerves in the cavernous sinus. Morita correlated the risk of trigeminal neuropathy to a dose of 19 Gy or greater administered to Meckel's cave (cranial nerve V ganglion).[20] In the Marseille series of 92 cavernous sinus tumors undergoing a median RS dose of 14 Gy, 7/14 cases with pretreatment trigeminal neuropathy improved (3 completely), 1 worsened from tumor recurrence, but no new cases of trigeminal neuropathy developed.[21] Litre reported no case of trigeminal neuropathy after stereotactic irradiation of 100 cavernous sinus meningiomas to 45 Gy in 25 fractions.[22]

Kano reported the Pittsburgh experience in 33 trigeminal schwannoma patients with RS to a median dose of 15 Gy.[23] Neurological symptoms improved in 33% and worsened in 8% with tumor recurrence. No cases of radiation-related trigeminal neuropathy developed. Hamm reported 95% control and no new neuropathy developing out of 19 nonacoustic schwannomas (13 trigeminal) treated to 54 to 59.4 Gy with 1.8 to 2 Gy fractions.[24] Showalter found no difference in tumor control or cranial nerve tolerance in a comparison of 24 nonacoustic schwannomas undergoing radiotherapy to a median dose of 50.4 Gy compared to 15 undergoing RS to a mean dose of 12 Gy.[25] Nineteen of the 39 tumors in that series were trigeminal schwannomas.

MOTOR CRANIAL NERVES

While facial neuropathy is a feared complication of acoustic neuroma RS that helped develop interest in radiation alternatives, it has failed to be much of a problem in recent RS series using modern techniques with 12 to 13 Gy.[8] Initial RS series of patients treated during the 1980s with less sophisticated treatment plans and doses of 15 to 18 Gy reported trigeminal neuropathy rates (temporary plus permanent) in the range of 10% to 30%.[26] None of the 216 acoustic schwannoma patients who underwent primary management with RS to 12 to 13 Gy at the University of Pittsburgh developed either temporary or permanent facial neuropathy. None of the six patients who underwent repeat RS for acoustic schwannoma recurrences have developed facial neuropathy.[27] Cases of facial neuropathy have been reported with these RS doses at other centers, and one temporary case occurred in Pittsburgh in a postoperatively treated case. Facial neuropathy has also been reported in some series of acoustic tumors treated with fractionated radiotherapy.[15,17] Chan reported a 1% rate of facial neuropathy in the Harvard series of acoustic schwannoma patients treated to median dose of 54 Gy in 30 fractions.[17] Out of six facial schwannomas undergoing RS to 12 to 13 Gy, all were controlled and no new facial weakness developed.[28] Similar results were reported in four facial schwannoma patients undergoing SRT in Sapporo.[29,30] Out of 18 patients undergoing RS for nonacoustic schwannonmas at the University of Florida to a mean dose of 13.1 Gy, five developed neurological improvement, one of the two facial schwannoma patients developed a worsened facial weakness, and two cases of hearing deterioration developed.[30]

In the Marseille series of 92 cavernous sinus tumors undergoing a median RS dose of 14 Gy, 23/54 cases with pretreatment oculomotor problems improved (8 completely) and 1 worsened, but no new cases of oculomotor neuropathy developed.[21]

No new neuropathies developed in 33 patients with 34 jugular foramen schwannomas managed by RS (median dose: 14 Gy) at the University of Pittsburgh.[31] Tumor control was 94% at 10 years. Similarly, Genc reported a series of 18 glomus jugulare tumors that underwent RS to a median dose of 15 Gy with 56% reporting improvement, tumor control in 17/18, and no radiation-related neuropathies developing.[32]

Cranial nerve palsies are rare complications of high-dose radiotherapy in nasopharyngeal carcinoma patients (NPC) receiving conventional radiotherapy at 1.8 to 2 Gy/d. Lin et al.[33] reported 19 patients with radiation-related cranial neuropathies who received total dose of 70 to 130 Gy to the nasopharynx and 50 to 90 Gy to the neck. No denominator was provided but the expected incidence is in the range of 1% of patients undergoing this type of treatment. Unilateral vocal cord paralysis alone and hearing loss were excluded. The latency before palsy was 12 to 240 months. Single nerve palsy developed in four patients, including two patients with hypoglossal palsy and two patients with recurrent laryngeal palsy. Two patients had three nerve palsies and 13 patients had 2 nerve palsies each. Vagus and hypoglossal palsy occurred in combination in 11 patients. Overall, 17 patients developed hypoglossal palsies, 11 patients vagus palsies, 6 patients had recurrent laryngeal nerve palsies, and 2 developed accessory palsies (all bilateral). Marked neck fibrosis was documented in 12/19 patients. Vocal cord paralysis caused easy choking and hoarseness with severe respiratory difficulty in two patients who had bilateral vocal cord palsy.

TREATMENT OF RADIATION-RELATED CRANIAL NEUROPATHIES

Patients presenting with acute radiation induced cranial neuropathies usually present without recent imaging to distinguish tumor recurrence from radiation complications. In either case, initial management with corticosteroids seems warranted. If symptoms resolve with steroids and the medication can be tapered and withdrawn without symptomatic recurrence, then no further intervention is required. Because long-term high-dose steroids can cause a host of problems including hyperglycemia, muscle weakness, cushingoid facies, insomnia, irritability and tiredness, other alternatives need to be investigated if steroids cannot be promptly tapered. The combination of pentoxifylline 400 mg BID and vitamin E 400 to 500 IU BID for 6 months or longer was shown in a randomized trial to alleviate late radiation fibrosis from breast cancer radiotherapy.[34] Limited experience in treating post-RS brain injuries appears favorable.[35] Because radiation injury reactions are inflammatory-type reactions that can reach a peak and then subside at least in the brain parenchyma, the effectiveness of interventions like hyperbaric oxygen has been rightly doubted. Anticoagulation is another intervention that has been used with questionable effectiveness.[36] Recently, bevacizumab has shown effectiveness in treating biopsy-proven radiation necrosis.[37]

REFERENCES

1. Emami B, Lyman J, Brown A, et al. Tolerance of normal tissue to therapeutic irradiation. *Int J Radiat Oncol Biol Phys.* 1991;21(1):109–122.
2. Urie MM, Fullerton B, Tatsuzaki H, et al. A dose response analysis of injury to cranial nerves and/or nuclei following proton beam radiation therapy. *Int J Radiat Oncol Biol Phys.* 1992;23(1):27–39.
3. Kondziolka D, Zorro O, Lobato-Polo J, et al. Gamma knife stereotactic radiosurgery for idiopathic trigeminal neuralgia. *J Neurosurg.* 2010;112(4):758–765.
4. Zorro O, Lobato-Polo J, Kano H, et al. Gamma knife radiosurgery for multiple sclerosis-related trigeminal neuralgia. *Neurology.* 2009;73(14):1149–1154.
5. Kondziolka D, Lacomis D, Niranjan A, et al. Histological effects of trigeminal nerve radiosurgery in a primate model: implications for trigeminal neuralgia radiosurgery. *Neurosurgery.* 2000;46(4):971–976; discussion 976–977.
6. Phan C, Mindrum M, Silverman C, et al. Matched-control retrospective study of the acute and late complications in patients with collagen vascular diseases treated with radiation therapy. *Cancer J.* 2003;9(6):461–466.
7. Flickinger JC, Kondziolka D, Lunsford LD. Dose and diameter relationships for facial, trigeminal, and acoustic neuropathies following acoustic neuroma radiosurgery. *Radiother Oncol.* 1996;41(3):215–219.
8. Chopra R, Kondziolka D, Niranjan A, et al. Long-term follow-up of acoustic schwannoma radiosurgery with marginal tumor doses of 12 to 13 Gy. *Int J Radiat Oncol Biol Phys.* 2007;68(3):845–851.
9. Kano H, Kondziolka D, Khan A, et al. Predictors of hearing preservation after stereotactic radiosurgery for acoustic neuroma. *J Neurosurg.* 2009;111(4):863–873.
10. Niranjan A, Mathieu D, Flickinger JC, et al. Hearing preservation after intracanalicular vestibular schwannoma radiosurgery. *Neurosurgery.* 2008;63(6):1054–1062; discussion 1062–1063.
11. Gardner G, Robertson JH. Hearing preservation in unilateral acoustic neuroma surgery. *Ann Otol Rhinol Laryngol.* 1988;97(1):55–66.
12. Huang E, Teh BS, Strother DR, et al. Intensity-modulated radiation therapy for pediatric medulloblastoma: early report on the reduction of ototoxicity. *Int J Radiat Oncol Biol Phys.* 2002;52(3):599–605.
13. Andrews DW, Suarez O, Goldman HW, et al. Stereotactic radiosurgery and fractionated stereotactic radiotherapy for the treatment of acoustic schwannomas: comparative observations of 125 patients treated at one institution. *Int J Radiat Oncol Biol Phys.* 2001;50(5):1265–1278.
14. Meijer OW, Wolbers JG, Baayen JC, et al. Fractionated stereotactic radiation therapy and single high-dose radiosurgery for acoustic neuroma: early results of a prospective clinical study. *Int J Radiat Oncol Biol Phys.* 2000;46(1):45–49.
15. Combs SE, Welzel T, Schulz-Ertner D, et al. Differences in clinical results after LINAC-based single-dose radiosurgery versus fractionated stereotactic radiotherapy for patients with vestibular schwannomas. *Int J Radiat Oncol Biol Phys.* 2010;76(1):193–200.
16. Andrews DW, Werner-Wasik M, Den RB, et al. Toward dose optimization for fractionated stereotactic radiotherapy for acoustic neuromas: comparison of two dose cohorts. *Int J Radiat Oncol Biol Phys.* 2009;74(2):419–426.
17. Chan AW, Black P, Ojemann RG, et al. Stereotactic radiotherapy for vestibular schwannomas: favorable outcome with minimal toxicity. *Neurosurgery.* 2005;57(1):60–70; discussion 60–70.
18. Flickinger JC, Pollock BE, Kondziolka D, et al. Does increased nerve length within the treatment volume improve trigeminal neuralgia radiosurgery? A prospective double-blind, randomized study. *Int J Radiat Oncol Biol Phys.* 2001;51(2):449–454.
19. Tishler RB, Loeffler JS, Lunsford LD, et al. Tolerance of cranial nerves of the cavernous sinus to radiosurgery. *Int J Radiat Oncol Biol Phys.* 1993;27(2):215–221.

20. Morita A, Coffey RJ, Foote RL, et al. Risk of injury to cranial nerves after gamma knife radiosurgery for skull base meningiomas: experience in 88 patients. *J Neurosurg.* 1999;90(1):42–49.

21. Roche PH, Régis J, Dufour H, et al. Gamma knife radiosurgery in the management of cavernous sinus meningiomas. *J Neurosurg.* 2000;93(suppl 3):68–73.

22. Litré CF, Colin P, Noudel R, et al. Fractionated stereotactic radiotherapy treatment of cavernous sinus meningiomas: a study of 100 cases. *Int J Radiat Oncol Biol Phys.* 2009;74(4):1012–1017.

23. Kano H, Niranjan A, Kondziolka D, et al. Stereotactic radiosurgery for trigeminal schwannoma: tumor control and functional preservation Clinical article. *J Neurosurg.* 2009;110(3):553–558.

24. Hamm KD, Gross MW, Fahrig A, et al. Stereotactic radiotherapy for the treatment of nonacoustic schwannomas. *Neurosurgery.* 2008;62(5 suppl):A29–A36; discussion A36.

25. Showalter TN, Werner-Wasik M, Curran WJ Jr, et al. Stereotactic radiosurgery and fractionated stereotactic radiotherapy for the treatment of nonacoustic cranial nerve schwannomas. *Neurosurgery.* 2008;63(4):734–740; discussion 740.

26. Kondziolka D, Lunsford LD, McLaughlin MR, et al. Long-term outcomes after radiosurgery for acoustic neuromas. *N Engl J Med.* 1998;339(20):1426–1433.

27. Kano H, Kondziolka D, Niranjan A, et al. Repeat stereotactic radiosurgery for acoustic neuromas. *Int J Radiat Oncol Biol Phys.* 2010;76(2):520–527.

28. Madhok R, Kondziolka D, Flickinger JC, et al. Gamma knife radiosurgery for facial schwannomas. *Neurosurgery.* 2009;64(6):1102–1105; discussion 1105.

29. Nishioka K, Abo D, Aoyama H, et al. Stereotactic radiotherapy for intracranial nonacoustic schwannomas including facial nerve schwannoma. *Int J Radiat Oncol Biol Phys.* 2009;75(5):1415–1419.

30. Mabanta SR, Buatti JM, Friedman WA, et al. Linear accelerator radiosurgery for nonacoustic schwannomas. *Int J Radiat Oncol Biol Phys.* 1999;43(3):545–548.

31. Martin JJ, Kondziolka D, Flickinger JC, et al. Cranial nerve preservation and outcomes after stereotactic radiosurgery for jugular foramen schwannomas. *Neurosurgery.* 2007;61(1):76–81; discussion 81.

32. Genç A, Bicer A, Abacioglu U, et al. Gamma knife radiosurgery for the treatment of glomus jugulare tumors. *J Neurooncol.* 2010;97(1):101–108.

33. Lin YS, Jen YM, Lin JC. Radiation-related cranial nerve palsy in patients with nasopharyngeal carcinoma. *Cancer.* 2002;95(2):404–409.

34. Delanian S, Porcher R, Balla-Mekias S, Lefaix JL, et al. Randomized, placebo-controlled trial of combined pentoxifylline and tocopherol for regression of superficial radiation-induced fibrosis. *J Clin Oncol.* 2003;21(13):2545–2550.

35. Williamson R, Kondziolka D, Kanaan H, et al. Adverse radiation effects after radiosurgery may benefit from oral vitamin E and pentoxifylline therapy: a pilot study. *Stereotact Funct Neurosurg.* 2008;86(6):359–366.

36. Happold C, Ernemann U, Roth P, et al. Anticoagulation for radiation-induced neurotoxicity revisited. *J Neurooncol.* 2008;90(3):357–362.

37. Torcuator R, Zuniga R, Mohan YS, et al. Initial experience with bevacizumab treatment for biopsy confirmed cerebral radiation necrosis. *J Neurooncol.* 2009;94(1):63–68.

Stefan Rieken
J. Debus

Brainstem

INTRODUCTION

In 1950, 53 years after x-rays had been introduced into clinical application, Boden described 6 patients who—within a group of 24 patients treated with orthovoltage radiation for tumors of the middle ear and nasopharynx—had developed symptoms, typically attributed to brainstem morbidity.[1] As these patients displayed no additional symptoms typical of cerebral lesions, he concluded that the brainstem was more radiosensitive than the cerebrum. Several reports have attempted to define radiation tolerance of the cervical spinal cord since then, but few have focused on tolerance of the brainstem.

In 1971, Holdorff and Schiffter[2] analyzed histopathological changes of brainstem architecture in five patients who had developed lethal encephalopathies between 4 and 30 months after radiation therapy for neoplasms of the skull base. They found vascular pathologies, including vessel wall edema, endothelial hyalinization or perivascular lymphocytosis, and neuroglial alterations such as demyelinization, focal necrosis, and cystic lesions to be associated with cranial nerve palsy including bulbar syndrome, ataxia and further cerebellar dysfunctions, as well as acoustic and visual impairment. Due to its small anatomical size yet high density of important myelinated fiber tracts and numerous neural nuclei, the brainstem was defined to possess an exquisite vulnerability to radiation injury.

More than 25 year later, Debus et al.[3] initiated a study to analyze the long-term incidence of brainstem toxicity in 367 patients treated for skull base tumors with high-dose conformal radiation therapy. Several predisposing factors enhancing the risk of radiation damage to the brainstem were identified, including preexisting metabolic disorders. When predicting the risk for radiation complications, the total volume of tissue irradiated was found to be of greater importance than the maximum doses within the target.

Understanding the mechanisms involved in brainstem damage and precisely establishing guidelines for radiation treatment of tumors within or in close vicinity to the brainstem will contribute to both prevention and treatment of alterations induced by radiation.

THE HUMAN BRAINSTEM

HISTORICAL

In the early 1660s, Thomas Willis (1621–1675), an Oxford physician, published the first work on the anatomy of the brain and is, therefore, today credited with the first detailed description of the brainstem, including the first numbering of those nerves today referred to as the *cranial nerves.*[4,5] Using modern sophisticated approaches to brainstem anatomy and physiology, employing magnetic resonance and positron emission imaging as well as postmortem pathohistological analysis, a great amount of knowledge has been gathered to improve the diagnosis and treatment of brainstem disease.[6]

GROSS ANATOMY

The lower part of the human brain is referred to as the *brainstem* and is located in the posterior fossa of the skull, where it morphologically and structurally adjoins with the spinal cord (Fig. 20.1). Any neurally transducted information from the body to the cerebrum or cerebellum and vice versa must pass through the brainstem. Furthermore, major neuronal stimuli such as parasympathic innervation of the cardiovascular and digestive functions originate from the brainstem.

The brainstem consists of the midbrain (or mesencephalon), pons, and medulla oblongata, which at the decussation—a crossing of motor neurons between the two pyramidal tracts—continuously transits into the spinal cord (Figs. 20.1–20.4). The midbrain is structurally and functionally connected to the diencephalon (thalamus and hypothalamus).

Descending from higher parts of the brain, motor and sensory systems pass through the center of the brainstem, where they may be subjected to dysfunction or damage by disturbances of brainstem integrity. Ten cranial nerves (CN), CN III to XII, emerge from their nuclei within the brainstem and deliver motor, sensory, and vegetative innervation to the head and neck, and to most internal organs. Each cranial nerve originates from at least one nucleus and possesses a transitional zone where the peripheral nerve is formed. The glia surrounding the neuronal cells changes from central oligodendral myelin to peripheral Schwann cell glia. A group of widely spread neurons, known as the reticular formation, is involved in arousal reactions and grade of consciousness.

Blood supply to the brainstem is secured by two vertebral arteries that arise from the subclavian arteries and fuse to form the basilar artery that then proceeds rostrally along the surface of the anterior pons. Medial parts of the brainstem, especially the pons, are perfused via long penetrating paramedian branches that are at particular high risk of hypertensive damage.

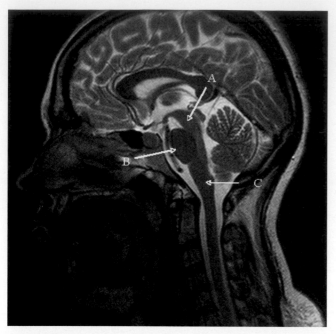

Figure 20.1. T2-weighted fast spin-echo MR image of the three major divisions of the brainstem: (**A**) midbrain; (**B**) pons; and (**C**) medulla oblangata in close proximity to potential targets of radiation therapy such as oro- and nasopharynx, pituitary gland, cervical spine and skull base, supratentorial, and infratentorial brain.

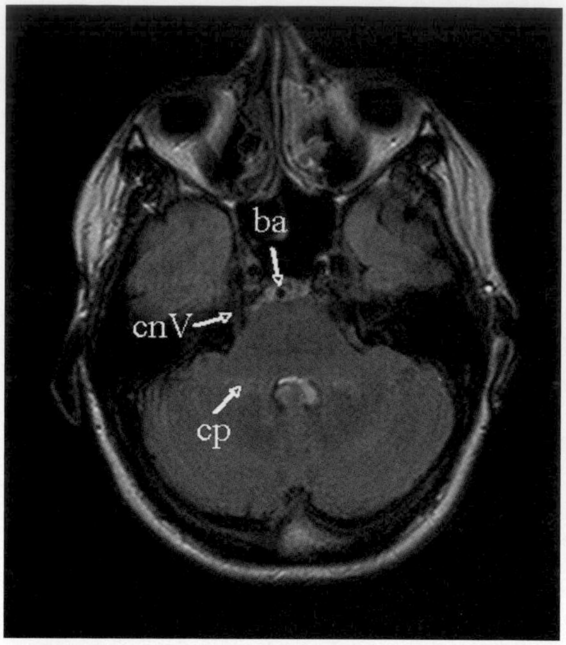

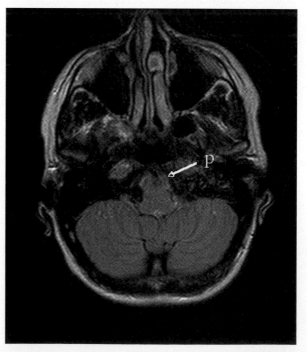

Figure 20.2. Axial FLAIR MR image of the pons through the level of cranial nerve V (cnV), nourished by pontine branches of the rostrally ascending basilar artery (ba) and connecting to the cerebellum via the two medial cerebellar peduncles (cp).

HISTOLOGICAL ANATOMY AND PHYSIOLOGY

The predominant cell types in the brainstem are neurons, glia, and vascular endothelial cells. Resting on the clivus, the basal part of the brainstem consists of major descending tracts, which engage in motor functions and receive additional regulatory input from the cerebellum. Dorsal to these motor tracts, the brainstem tegmentum, including the reticular formation, contains distinct nuclei, each of which possesses an individual

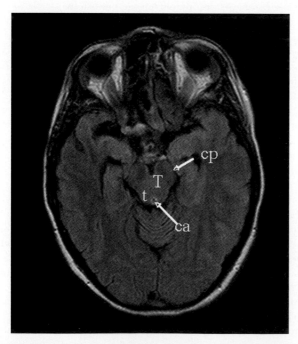

Figure 20.3. Axial FLAIR MR image of the mesencepahlon (midbrain). The mesencephalon consists of two rostral cerebral peduncles (cp), the tegmentum (T) and the tectum (t), which contains the cerebral aqueduct (ca).

Figure 20.4. Axial FLAIR MR image of the medulla oblongata, the lowest of three major brainstem segments that transits into the spinal cord below the level of the ventral decussations of the pyramids (p).

set of chemical, physiological, and anatomic features, such as the noradrenergic locus coeruleus, which is involved in stress response and respiratory regulation. Also, the cranial nerves III to XII arise from these nuclei, receiving somato- and viscero-motor input from more medial nuclei and delivering sensory information to more lateral nuclei, thus resembling spinal cord architecture patterns and, therefore, reminiscent of their common embryonic origin.

The nuclei of the cranial nerves are located in the tegmentum of the brainstem, which itself is located just ventral to the cerebral aqueduct and fourth ventricle. The oculomotor nerves are the first, that is, most superior cranial nerves that exit the brainstem and receive parasympathetic fibers from the Edinger-Westfall nucleus; they run ventrally through the midbrain and exit in the interpeduncular cistern. The trochlear nerves are the only cranial nerves to cross the midline. They course dorsally behind the aqueduct, exit the dorsal midbrain, and run forward in the ambient cisterns to reach the cavernous sinuses. Other major structures within the midbrain include the pyramidal, that is, corticospinal and corticobulbar tracts within the cerebral peduncles, the substantia nigra, the red nuclei, the decussation of the superior cerebellar peduncles, and the superior and inferior colliculi of the quadrigeminal plate.

The pons contains the nuclei for the trigeminal, abducens, facial, and the acoustic cranial nerves. The trigeminal nerves exit the center of the pons ventrolaterally. The spinal tract and the nucleus of the trigeminal nerve extend from the upper pons all the way down into the upper spinal cord. The trochlear nerves exit ventrally at the pontomedullary junction. The facial nerve loops posteriorly around the nucleus of the trochlear nerve and indents the floor of the fourth ventricle (the so-called facial colliculus). The facial and the acoustic nerves exit the inferior pons inferiolaterally, traverse the cerebellopontine cistern, and enter the internal auditory canal. The anterior pons (basis pontis) contains a large number of transverse fibers from the middle cerebellar peduncles and longitudinal, dispersed bundles of the pyramidal tracts.

The medulla contains the remaining cranial nerves. The glossopharyngeal, vagus, and accessory nerves exit laterally just posterior to the olivary nucleus and run through the jugular foramen. The hypoglossal cranial nerve leaves the medulla ventral to the olive and courses ventrally to the hypoglossal canal. The medulla also contains the decussation of the pyramids (corticospinal tracts) ventrally and the inferior cerebellar peduncles posteriorly.

Two other important fiber tracts are the medial longitudinal fasciculus—connecting the oculomotor, abducens, and trochlear nerves nuclei, thus ensuring coordination of eye movement—and the medial lemniscus. The medial longitudinal fasciculus lies in a paramedian position just ventral to the aqueduct and fourth ventricle. Ventrally, the medial lemniscus, the major sensory tract, ascends through the brainstem.

BRAINSTEM IMAGING

Due to the close surrounding of the brainstem by dense skull bones that limit the possibility of exact imaging via computed tomography, MR imaging has an established role in examining structures within the posterior fossa of the skull. The high contrast resolution and multiplanar capabilities of MR make an accurate correlation of clinical findings with the complex anatomy of this region possible (see Fig. 20.1). Gadolinium enhancement is often helpful to identify and characterize lesions.

As for its use in radiation therapy, both preradiation and postradiation examinations have demonstrated that MRI imaging provides additional information, such as precise measurement of diameters and distances, important for treatment planning and follow-up exams, therefore, yielding a significant benefit for those patients who received MRI exams in addition to CT scans. PET-CT exams using various labeled tracers such as [18]FDG or ^{11}C-methionine add important information about tissue vitality for target volume delineation.[7,8]

BRAINSTEM MORBIDITY AND RISK FACTORS

Many diseases affecting the brainstem cause abnormalities of cranial nerve function resulting in auditory, gustatory, and visual disturbances. Also, motor deficits affecting speech and swallowing are typical of brainstem disease and are commonly referred to as "bulbar palsy," because the area of the brainstem that controls the muscles of the throat, tongue, jaw, and face was once known as the "bulb." A progressive paralysis of these muscles was originally described by the renowned French neurologist, G. Duchenne in 1860, when first identifying patients with amyotrophic lateral sclerosis (ALS).

Today, most patients who present with symptoms attributed to the brainstem are diagnosed with comorbidities that are known to cause vascular alterations, such as diabetes mellitus and hypertension. Also patients with autoimmune diseases are at high risk to develop brainstem pathologies. These patients are known to more likely suffer from brainstem damage following radiation therapy and must, therefore, be carefully monitored for adverse events and subjected to strict indication findings.

Diabetic patients carry a greater risk for brainstem morbidity after radiation treatment than do healthy non–diabetic controls. Smith et al. reported on a diabetic patient developing brainstem vascular hyalinization with foci of infarction, edema, and demyelination, yet without diabetic atherosclerotic changes only 3 months after receiving radiation therapy for a nasopharyngeal neoplasm.[9]

While in the 1950s, mesencephalic irradiation was performed in order to treat hypertension,[10] it has become increasingly clear that hypertension may increase the patient's individual risk for complications, as exemplified by studies performed on patients with benign intracranial tumors in close proximity to the skull base. Smith et al. found that in addition to the radiation dose delivered, treated volume, and tumor location, also patient-specific factors such as diabetes and hypertension may significantly increase the risk for treatment toxicity.[11] Furthermore, hypertensive patients suspected of having suffered radiation injury may appear ineligible for precise diagnostic approaches: Patients suffering from hypertension are known to potentially develop brainstem-associated symptoms and may display MRI changes that resemble those alterations seen in patients that received radiation therapy. Lee et al. described hyperintense abnormalities on fluid attenuated inversion recovery (FLAIR) images in pons and midbrain in a patient with malignant hypertension.[12] About 25% of those patients who received radiation doses >50 Gy delivered during IMRT for medulloblastoma will also show increased FLAIR signals after a latency of 6 months.[13]

RADIATION THERAPY

BRAINSTEM TOXICITY FOLLOWING RADIATION

Most radiation toxicity to the brainstem is caused by therapeutic radiation. Several indications of modern radiation oncology impose the risk of radiation exposure of the brainstem onto the patients, including stereotactic radiosurgery, for example, of acoustic neuroma, intensity-modulated radiation therapy (IMRT) of head and neck tumors, and also whole-brain or even total-body irradiation. The radiation doses delivered to tumors that are located centrally within the brainstem, for example, brainstem gliomas, are limited by the close surrounding tissue of the brainstem itself.[14] Tumors that grow outside yet close to the brainstem are treated with modern radiotherapy techniques such as IMRT or image guided radiotherapy, which allow for steep dose gradients and thus make delivery of sufficiently high radiation possible.[15]

Recently evolving treatment modalities such as proton or carbon ion irradiation ensure high target conformity due to characteristic depth dose profiles and achieve promising rates of tumor control. In heavier ions, for example, carbon ions, a higher biological effectiveness is found due to increased linear energy transfers (LET).[16,17] In addition to the LET, the relative biological effectiveness (RBE) is influenced by the number of radiation fractions, the radiation dose, and the tissue irradiated; therefore, models must be created in order to calculate the RBE for individual applications, one of the most important being the local effect model.[18,19] Tumors within or close to the brainstem are ideal targets for particle therapy, which promises increased rates of tumor control without a high risk of toxicity.[20,21]

As part of the informed consent process, patients must be informed about the possibility of brainstem-associated neurological deficits such as cranial nerve palsy, sensomotory paresis, and vision or hearing impairment. During follow-up examinations including imaging, special attention must be paid to morphological changes within the brainstem, which must then be distinguished from artifacts or recurrent tumor.

RADIATION-INDUCED DEFICITS

Based upon its anatomic location, the brainstem may be dose limiting not only in the treatment of central nervous system (CNS) tumors but also in the treatment of head and neck tumors. Depending upon the subregion of the brainstem irradiated, several different patterns of symptomatic disease have been described when observing brainstem injury.

Five cases of radiation-induced brainstem damage after radiotherapy for endocrine orbitopathy, pituitary adenoma,

squamous cell carcinoma of the auditory canal, and cerebellar angioblastoma were described by Holdorff and Schiffter in 1971.[2] Radiation was delivered using high energy photons via two or three fields; one patient with endocrine orbitopathy was irradiated with electrons. Patients became symptomatic with bulbar palsy, ataxia, trigeminal and facial cranial neuropathy, hearing loss, hemianopsia, and hemihypaesthesia. Patients were reported to develop symptoms following an interval of 4 to 30 months after completion of radiation, suffering progression until death within several weeks.[2]

Modern radiation treatment of tumors in close proximity to the brainstem has been known to potentially cause cranial neuropathy. Meeks et al.[22] described the rate of cranial nerve complication in patients treated with stereotactic radiosurgery for acoustic neuroma and found about 15% of all patients to suffer from facial or trigeminal neuropathy. Bhansali et al. described 1 of 114 patients who had received a total dose 45 Gy delivered in 20 fractions for hormone-inactive pituitary tumors to suffer from brainstem necrosis. This patient became symptomatic with cerebellar ataxia almost 9 years after completion of radiotherapy and died after only 3 months.[23]

Debus et al. diagnosed 17 patients within a group of 348 patients treated with conformal radiotherapy for skull base tumors with brainstem symptoms such as motor, sensory, or cerebellar dysfunctions or complex combinations of the above. They found patients with late onset of symptoms after more than 30 months to experience higher grades of toxicity resulting in death in three patients within 6 months of the onset of symptoms.[3]

Carbon ion irradiation of brain tumors was described to cause injury of the surrounding tissue after a longer latency period than does conventional radiation with photons. Also, recovery from carbon ion–induced radiation damage appears more likely than from conventional irradiation because, due to steep dose gradients that are possible with carbon ions, only a smaller volume of surrounding tissue is being irradiated.[24]

IMAGING DIAGNOSIS OF RADIATION TOXICITY

Changes in the central nervous system following radiation therapy have become increasingly evident due to technical progress that was achieved during the past three decades. Once post–radiation brainstem damage is suspected, a thorough clinical neurological examination must be performed; yet, imaging of the brain is indispensable for diagnosis of brainstem toxicity.

Ionizing radiation causes focal necrosis, diffuse white matter injury, atrophy, mineralizing microangiopathy, and large vessel vasculopathy, all of which can be detected by computer-tomography and magnetic resonance imaging.[25] Hyalinization

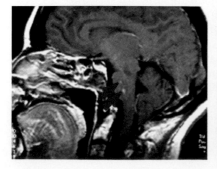 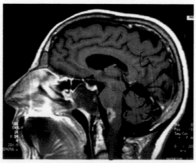

Figure 20.5. Patients after radiation treatment for skull base tumors. Two examples that exhibit radiogenic patchy contrast enhancement of the pons (*left*) and ring-shaped enhancement of the pyramids (*right*).

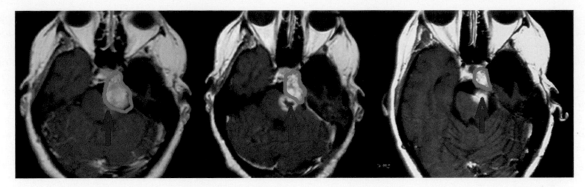

Figure 20.6. Development of contrast enhancement in patients with skull base chondrosarcoma (*blue outline*) with ring enhancement developing 18 months (*left*) and 24 months (*middle*) after irradiation and partial resolution 7 months thereafter (*right*).

and fibrinoid necrosis of the vascular wall result in severe disturbances of the blood-brain barrier and thus enhance contrast signaling within radiation injured tissue.[24,26] A major problem is the diagnosis of radiation injury as opposed to recurrent tumor; focal necrosis, for example, appears as ring-enhancing structures associated with edema and mass effects, hence resembling tumor recurrence (Fig. 20.5). Several follow-up exams including repetitive imagine analysis will help to differentiate typical radiation-associated injuries from relapsing disease (Figs. 20.6 and 20.7). ^{11}C-methionine-PET and magnetic resonance spectroscopy are promising features of modern imaging and will likely contribute to more precise diagnostic approaches.[24] In some cases of radiation injury to the brain, cystic lesions developed outside the radiation field. These cystic lesions possess a thin, faintly enhanced membrane after administering contrast agents and can usually be differentiated from abscesses that have a far thicker and strongly enhanced wall.[24]

MRI analysis of 53 patients who had received IMRT for medulloblastoma revealed that 15% developed FLAIR signal changes in the brainstem after 6 months of latency, in most cases without additional or new neurological deficit.[13] Diffusion tensor imaging (DTI) of patients with small cell lung cancer who received whole-brain irradiation showed increased DTI fractional anisotropy within the brainstem as opposed to other brain regions such as frontal lobe and cerebellum. This may be due to specific damage of crossing fibers leading to increased signaling of coherently oriented fibers. However, patients carrying several vascular risk factors such as diabetes, hypertension, and smoking will display reduced fractional anisotropy even in the brainstem indicating greater damage of any fiber tracts within the brainstem.[27]

CLASSIFICATION OF RADIATION DAMAGE

New agents and techniques are constantly introduced into routine clinical practice of cancer therapy or in clinical trials, requiring thorough monitoring of adverse events and side effects. Usage of common classifications such as "Common Toxicity Criteria" (CTC), "Common Terminology Criteria for Adverse Events," and "Late Effects in Normal Tissues—Subjective, Objective, Management, and Analytic scales" (LENT-SOMA) will help to establish comparability and reproducibility.

According to its timing after radiation treatment, brain injury caused by radiation is classified as acute, early delayed, or late reaction. Acute reactions are known to occur within the first week, usually even within hours after starting radiation, whereas early delayed reactions develop within the first 12 weeks after therapy completion. While both acute and early delayed radiation alterations have shown to be reversible in most cases, late toxicity that develops 12 weeks or even years after finishing a radiation treatment may prove irreversible or even progressive and ultimately fatal.[28]

Acute side effects are based upon alterations in vascular permeability resulting in brain edema and can be treated with steroids in most cases. Data derived from murine models have suggested radiation-induced apoptosis of endothelial cells to be a key player in the pathogenesis of radiation-associated blood brain barrier disturbance. Early delayed reactions are caused by inflammatory reaction, transient demyelinization, and intermittent reduction of oligodendroglia.[29]

Late effects show glial atrophy, demyelination, and necrosis confined to white matter and varying degrees of vascular changes in both white and gray matter.[30] Morphological alterations in

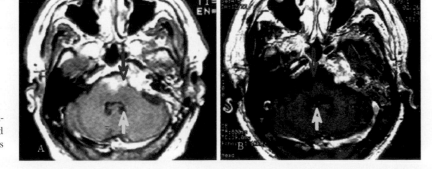

Figure 20.7. Radiation-induced pontine contrast enhancement 23 months after radiation treatment (**A**) and resolution with marked loss of parenchyma after 5 years of follow-up (**B**).

CNS microvessels include telangiectasias, dilatation, vessel wall hyalinization, and thickening with fibrinoid necrosis.[31,32]

Radiation injuries may be classified according to several different classifications: whereas in Western Europe the European Organisation for Research and Treatment of Cancer (EORTC) classified acute and chronic radiation side effects, in the USA the Radiation Therapy Oncology Group (RTOG) criteria were employed to evaluate early and late radiation injury. In 1988, during a consensus conference, the criteria for the most often documented toxicities were summarized and established as the CTC. They consider acute injuries caused by both cytostatics and radiation and may be used for combined—i.e., simultaneous or sequential—therapies. In order to classify late effects, the LENT-SOMA classification was established in 1992, not only addressing subjective patient complaints and objective measurable pathological findings but also recommending diagnostic means and possible therapeutic options.

As for brainstem-specific injuries, it is of special importance to consider adverse events that may be misleading, such as changes in vision, loss of hearing, or even cardiovascular symptoms. Due to its regulatory involvement in most organs and special senses, brainstem injuries may express themselves as impaired vision, disturbances of respiratory or peripheral sensory function—possibly drawing away the investigator's attention from the brainstem and past radiation therapies.

PREDICTIVE MODELS BASED ON DOSE- AND VOLUME-DEPENDENT EFFECTS

Estimates of brainstem tolerance were attempted by Emami et al. based on personal experience at that time.[33] They published brainstem-specific radiation doses that upon radiation of one, two, or three third of brainstem volume yielded a 5% risk of a particular brainstem-specific complication after 5 years, and estimated doses of 50, 53, and 60 Gy (TD 5/5), respectively. Total volume irradiation of the brainstem with 65 Gy or even higher was found to impose a 50% risk for adverse events after a latency period of 5 years.

Detailed quantification of radiation doses that were delivered to the brainstem has shown that the maximum dose does not influence the extent of clinical damage. The tolerance of the brainstem most likely depends on the tissue volume being irradiated during fractionated radiation therapy emphasizing the concept of volume constraints rather than dose constraints in high-dose conformal radiotherapy. The volume of the brainstem receiving more than 60 Cobalt-Gray Equivalents (CGE) was found to be significant in multivariate analysis: the risk for brainstem damage was significantly increased if more 0.9 cc received more than 60 CGE.[3]

When attempting to predict or even calculate the probability of radiation-associated brainstem morbidity, one needs to consider target location in the brain, target histology, and treatment conformality.[22] High precision radiotherapy of acoustic neuroma for example imposes the risk of facial and trigeminal neuropathy due to the close proximity of the radiation target to critical structures from which these cranial nerves emerge, such as the nuclei or transitional zones. The larger the tumor size, the closer its location to the brainstem and the higher the dose applied, the greater the risk for radiation toxicity. Nerves themselves have shown to be rather radiation resistant, as exemplified during radiation treatment for trigeminal neuralgia where doses above 70 Gy need to be administered in order to achieve acceptable analgesic palliation.[34] Therefore, the probability of cranial nerve complication depends upon the radiation dose delivered to the brainstem rather than to the nerve itself. A maximum brainstem dose >16 Gy delivered as a single fraction, for example, is an important risk factor for delayed cranial neuropathy, whereas doses even higher than 16 Gy but delivered outside the brainstem did not increase the risk for cranial nerve complication. Precise techniques for planning and exercising radiation treatment have been associated with lower complication rates, for example, reducing the risk for cranial neuropathy from 34% to 5%.[22,35] Indeed, Meeks et al.[22] have found models for calculating normal tissue complication probability to be unreliable once radiation planning is based upon CT imaging alone instead of additional MRI analysis.

Models employed for predicting or even calculating the risk for brainstem morbidity do not analyze the true radiobiology but rely on the available clinical data and are, thus, based upon phenomenological observations that oftentimes include methods that have already been left or expanded by the time the calculation model is being generated. Meeks et al.[22] have found an α/β-ratio of 2.1 Gy to best fit the clinical data derived from acoustic neuroma radiosurgery.

STRATEGIES FOR AVOIDING TOXICITY

The management of tumors located close to the brainstem such as nasopharyngeal carcinomas and acoustic neuromas remains challenging due to limited surgical access and need for high radiation doses. The best strategy to avoid brainstem toxicity is to clearly avoid radiation exposure to parts of the brainstem that are outside the target volume. Many high precision approaches have been introduced in recent years.

MRI scans should be employed in addition to CT scans since the brainstem is not well defined on CT. Using high tesla magnetic fields in MR imaging will deliver more precise information on histological components of the brainstem, for example, fiber tracts, nuclei, or transitional zones. As exemplified by a typical brainstem disease, ALS, 4.7-T MRI has further established the role of MRI as the leading noninvasive instrument to reveal pathohistological changes in the nervous system. In an animal model, T2-weighted MRI clearly revealed changes in the brains and brainstems of mice. Hyperintensities, indicative of neuropathology, were detectable in several determined areas including the nucleus ambiguus, facial nucleus, trigeminal motor nucleus, rostroventrolateral reticular nucleus, lateral paragigantocellular nucleus, and the substantia nigra. Bioptic histological analysis including neuronal counts of the imaged brains confirmed the T2-weighted MRI findings.[36] Such precise delineation and measurement of constraints will add information essential for both adequately treating tumors and sparing normal tissue. Inversely planning and IMRT have proven to selectively protect critical organs at risk to a great degree—especially in patients with T3/T4 tumors.[37]

In the context of inverse planning, prescription of escalated doses should be effected by the identification and delineation of constraints and simultaneous sufficient target coverage. Delivery of maximum and proportionate doses to defined volumes of the brainstem or other critical structures (V_{max}; V_{20}, V_{50}) must be known to the radiation oncologist for any treatment plan (dose-volume histograms). Controls of patient positioning should be performed via concepts of image guidance that ensure feasibility of treatment plans.[38]

As the human CNS displays high sensitivity to changes in fractionation, modifying the fractionation scheme to fractionated or even hyperfractionated regimens may significantly reduce the incidence of brain necrosis, as was exemplified by the reduced incidence of temporal lobe necrosis after hyperfractionated but not accelerated radiation therapy for nasopharyngeal carcinoma.[39]

Patients with diabetes, hypertension, or other diagnoses that are associated with increased vascular risk and who need radiation therapy that is likely to impose significant radiation doses to their brainstems should be strictly selected and must be carefully monitored for early symptoms of brainstem damage. Also, the number of locoregional surgical procedures must be considered before including a patient into any radiation treatment regimen, as the risk for brainstem toxicity is increased after two or more surgeries to the skull base.[3]

TREATMENT OF INJURY

Acute or delayed subacute radiation damage oftentimes requires steroids in order to reduce brain edema; sometimes, antiepileptic medication will be needed to prevent seizures. Typically in late-onset brainstem toxicity, long-term steroid therapy is commonly necessary. It is recommended to start with an intense short-term therapy with steroids and high osmolar infusions in order to restore normal perfusion in the brainstem and to avoid progression of symptoms due to a vicious circle of reduced perfusion and edema with dying cells. The dose of steroids should then be carefully tapered in order to reduce the risk of cushingoid symptoms. If the risk of aspiration appears high due to bulbar palsy, parenteral nutrition or percutaneous endoscopic gastrostomy feeding tube placement may be necessary. Patients with brainstem toxicity are endangered by pneumonia due to aspiration, which is frequently the final cause of death. In some cases of progressive cystic or necrotizing lesions, neurosurgical intervention or resection will become necessary in order to reduce intracranial pressure or to control topographical symptoms.

Several studies performed in animal models have attempted to focus upon molecular prevention of radiation-induced brain damage including even the use of erythropoietin that was described to inhibit apoptosis and inflammation.[40,41] Also indomethacin was employed to reduce radiation-associated inflammation in microglial environment, exerting its effects via COX-2 inhibition. Other approaches to targeted therapy include kinase blocking drugs and retransplantation of cytokine-inducible brain stem cells, all of which are considered experimental approaches at the time present.[29]

CONCLUSION

Radiation therapy targeting tumors in close vicinity to the brainstem imposes a risk for serious brainstem toxicity. Careful selection of patients and regarding comorbidities such as hypertension and diabetes or previous surgeries close to the skull base are essential. Radiotherapy planning must be based upon modern imaging modalities and should whenever possible allow steep dose gradients along the brainstem surface. After completion of radiation treatment, patients must regularly be monitored for brainstem damage and must be offered adequate therapy once radiation toxicity has occurred.

REFERENCES

1. Boden G. Radiation myelitis of the brainstem. *J Fac Radiol.* 1950;2:79–94.
2. Holdorff B, Schiffter R. Late radiation necrosis of the brain stem, including the hypothalamus after irradiation with ultra hard x-rays and high-speed electrons. Concerning the problem of radiation sensitivity of the brain stem. *Acta Neurochir (Wien).* 1971;25:37–56.
3. Debus J, Hug EB, Liebsch NJ, et al. Brainstem tolerance to conformal radiotherapy of skull base tumors. *Int J Radiat Oncol Biol Phys.* 1997;39:967–975.
4. Grand W. The anatomy of the brain, by Thomas Willis. *Neurosurgery.* 1999;45:1234–1236; discussion 1236–1237.
5. Molnar Z. Thomas Willis (1621–1675), the founder of clinical neuroscience. *Nat Rev Neurosci.* 2004;5:329–335.
6. Cho ZH, Son YD, Kim HK, et al. A fusion PET-MRI system with a high-resolution research tomograph-PET and ultra-high field 7.0 T-MRI for the molecular-genetic imaging of the brain. *Proteomics.* 2008;8:1302–1323.
7. Astnerer ST, Dobrei-Ciuchendea M, Essler M, et al. Effect of (11)C-methionine-positron emission tomography on gross tumor volume delineation in stereotactic radiotherapy of skull base meningiomas. *Int J Radiat Oncol Biol Phys.* 2008;72(4):1161–1167.
8. Weber WA, Grosu AL, Czernin J. Technology Insight: advances in molecular imaging and an appraisal of PET/CT scanning. *Nat Clin Pract Oncol.* 2008;5:160–170.
9. Smith BM, McGinnis W, Cook J, et al. Central nervous system changes complicating the use of radiotherapy for the treatment of a nasopharyngeal neoplasm in a diabetic patient. *Cancer.* 1979;43:2239–2242.
10. Mavrodinov N, Toshkova B, Botev B, et al. Treatment of hypertension by irradiation of the mesencephalon. *Suvr Med (Sofiia).* 1955;6:59–63.
11. Smith MC, Ryken TC, Buatti JM. Radiotoxicity after conformal radiation therapy for benign intracranial tumors. *Neurosurg Clin N Am.* 2006;17:169–180.
12. Lee MS, Tienor BJ. Images in clinical medicine. Changes in the brain stem and fundus in malignant hypertension. *N Engl J Med.* 2008;358:1951.
13. Muscal JA, Jones JY, Paulino AC, et al. Changes Mimicking New Leptomeningeal Disease After Intensity-Modulated Radiotherapy for Medulloblastoma. *Int J Radiat Oncol Biol Phys.* 2009;73(1):214–221.
14. Schulz-Ertner D, Debus J, Lohr F, et al. Fractionated stereotactic conformal radiation therapy of brain stem gliomas: outcome and prognostic factors. *Radiother Oncol.* 2000;57:215–223.
15. Milker-Zabel S, Zabel-du Bois A, Huber P, et al. Fractionated stereotactic radiation therapy in the management of benign cavernous sinus meningiomas: long-term experience and review of the literature. *Strahlenther Onkol.* 2006;182:635–640.
16. Haberer T, Debus J, Eickhoff H, et al. The Heidelberg ion therapy center. *Radiother Oncol.* 2004;73(suppl 2):S186–S190.
17. Schulz-Ertner D, Nikoghosyan A, Thilmann C, et al. Results of carbon ion radiotherapy in 152 patients. *Int J Radiat Oncol Biol Phys.* 2004;58:631–640.
18. Kramer M, Jakel O, Haberer T, et al. Treatment planning for scanned ion beams. *Radiother Oncol.* 2004;73(suppl 2):S80–S85.
19. Scholz M, Kellerer AM, Kraft-Weyrather W, et al. Computation of cell survival in heavy ion beams for therapy. The model and its approximation. *Radiat Environ Biophys.* 1997;36:59–66.
20. Schulz-Ertner D, Karger CP, Feuerhake A, et al. Effectiveness of carbon ion radiotherapy in the treatment of skull-base chordomas. *Int J Radiat Oncol Biol Phys.* 2007a;68:449–457.
21. Schulz-Ertner D, Nikoghosyan A, Hof H, et al. Carbon ion radiotherapy of skull base chondrosarcomas. *Int J Radiat Oncol Biol Phys.* 2007b;67:171–177.
22. Meeks SL, Buatti JM, Foote KD, et al. Calculation of cranial nerve complication probability for acoustic neuroma radiosurgery. *Int J Radiat Oncol Biol Phys.* 2000;47:597–602.
23. Bhansali A, Banerjee AK, Chanda A, et al. Radiation-induced brain disorders in patients with pituitary tumours. *Australas Radiol.* 2004;48:339–346.
24. Kishimoto R, Mizoe JE, Komatsu S, et al. MR imaging of brain injury induced by carbon ion radiotherapy for head and neck tumors. *Magn Reson Med Sci.* 2005;4:159–164.
25. Valk PE, Dillon WP. Radiation injury of the brain. *AJNR Am J Neuroradiol.* 1991;12:45–62.
26. Rabin BM, Meyer JR, Berlin JW, et al. Radiation-induced changes in the central nervous system and head and neck. *Radiographics.* 1996;16:1055–1072.
27. Welzel T, Niethammer A, Mende U, et al. Diffusion tensor imaging screening of radiation-induced changes in the white matter after prophylactic cranial irradiation of patients with small cell lung cancer: first results of a prospective study. *Am J Neuroradiol.* 2008;29:379–383.
28. Henke G, Kucinski T, Simon M, et al. Nebenwirkungen der Therapie von Hirntumoren. *Onkologe.* 2006;12:546–555.
29. Belka C, Budach W, Kortmann RD, et al. Radiation induced CNS toxicity—molecular and cellular mechanisms. *Br J Cancer.* 2001;85:1233–1239.
30. Wong CS, Van der Kogel AJ. Mechanisms of radiation injury to the central nervous system: implications for neuroprotection. *Mol Interv.* 2004;4:273–284.
31. Calvo W, Hopewell JW, Reinhold HS. Time- and dose-related changes in the white matter of the rat brain after single doses of X rays. *Br J Radiol.* 1988;61:1043–1052.
32. Reinhold HS, Calvo W, Hopewell JW, et al. Development of blood vessel-related radiation damage in the fimbria of the central nervous system. *Int J Radiat Oncol Biol Phys.* 1990;18:37–42.
33. Emami B, Lyman J, Brown A, et al. Tolerance of normal tissue to therapeutic irradiation. *Int J Radiat Oncol Biol Phys.* 1991;21:109–122.
34. Foote KD, Friedman WA, Buatti JM, et al. Analysis of risk factors associated with radiosurgery for vestibular schwannoma. *J Neurosurg.* 2001;95:440–449.
35. Mendenhall WM, Friedman WA, Buatti JM, et al. Preliminary results of linear accelerator radiosurgery for acoustic schwannomas. *J Neurosurg.* 1996;85:1013–1019.
36. Zang DW, Yang Q, Wang HX, et al. Magnetic resonance imaging reveals neuronal degeneration in the brainstem of the superoxide dismutase 1 transgenic mouse model of amyotrophic lateral sclerosis. *Eur J Neurosci.* 2004;20:1745–1751.

37. Poon I, Xia P, Weinberg V, et al. A treatment planning analysis of inverse-planned and forward-planned intensity-modulated radiation therapy in nasopharyngeal carcinoma. *Int J Radiat Oncol Biol Phys.* 2007;69:1625–1633.

38. Munter MW, Thilmann C, Hof H, et al. Stereotactic intensity modulated radiation therapy and inverse treatment planning for tumors of the head and neck region: clinical implementation of the step and shoot approach and first clinical results. *Radiother Oncol.* 2003;66:313–321.

39. Jen YM, Hsu WL, Chen CY, et al. Different risks of symptomatic brain necrosis in NPC patients treated with different altered fractionated radiotherapy techniques. *Int J Radiat Oncol Biol Phys.* 2001;51:344–348.

40. Goldman SA, Nedergaard M. Erythropoietin strikes a new cord. *Nat Med.* 2002;8:785–757.

41. Olsen NV. Central nervous system frontiers for the use of erythropoietin. *Clin Infect Dis.* 2003;37(suppl 4):S323–S330.

Arjun Sahgal
C. Shun Wong
Albert J. van der Kogel

Spinal Cord

ANATOMY

The spinal cord is a cylindrical extension of the brain. It is protected by the spinal column and extends from the superior border of the atlas (foramen magnum) to the lumbar vertebrae. The adult human spinal cord typically ends at the junction between the first and second lumbar vertebrae. It is about 45 cm in length in the adult male and 42 cm in the adult female.[25] The spinal cord is bathed in cerebrospinal fluid (CSF), and enclosed by the dura, arachnoid, and pia mater that are separated by the subdural and subarachnoid spaces.

The human spinal cord contains 31 segments, and each segment provides the attachment of the rootlets for a dorsal and ventral root that traverse the dura and unite close to their intervertebral foramina to form spinal nerves.[25,43] The cord gradually tapers craniocaudally except at the level of two enlargements. The cervical enlargement (C3-T2) is the source of large spinal nerves forming the brachial plexus that innervates the upper limbs, and the corresponding nerves from the lumbar enlargement (L1-S3) form the lumbosacral plexus that innervates the lower limbs.[25,43] Nerve roots of the lumbar and sacral segments of the cord form a bundle of roots (known as the *cauda equina*) as they descend to their respective intervertebral foramina.[25,43]

The basic structural organization of the spinal cord consists of central butterfly-shaped gray matter and outer white matter. Ascending tracts of sensory fibers and descending motor tracts are the main components of the white matter that are organized into dorsal, lateral, and ventral funiculi. Gray matter contains the neuronal cell bodies, including those of the large motor and sensory neurons.

The anterior spinal artery and the paired posterior spinal arteries run longitudinally throughout the length of the cord to provide its blood supply. In addition, there are segmental arteries that enter the vertebral canal through the intervertebral foramina that supplement the blood supply to the cord. For specific details regarding anatomy, the reader is directed to neuroanatomy textbooks.

HISTOLOGY AND FUNCTION

The major cell types in the spinal cord are similar to those in the brain and consist of neurons, glia, and vascular endothelial cells. Neurons are the nerve cells responsible for excitation and nerve impulse conduction, whereas the glial cells are the interstitial cells that have important ancillary functions. Neuroglia include oligodendrocytes, astrocytes, microglia, and ependymal cells. Oligodendrocytes are responsible for myelination of axons in the central nervous system (CNS).[70] Myelin sheaths are formed by the wrapping of oligodendrocyte cytoplasmic processes around the axon and are interrupted by the nodes of Ranvier that serve to enhance propagation of action potentials. Myelination thus allows for the propagation of nerve impulses or action potentials. One oligodendrocyte can myelinate several adjacent axons via its cytoplasmic processes. This in contrast to Schwann cells that each myelinates one segment of a peripheral nerve fiber/spinal nerve root. Astrocytes are irregularly shaped glial cells with a large number of branched processes. Many of these processes end in terminal expansions upon the basement membrane of capillaries known as *perivascular feet*. Astrocytes participate in the transmission of neuronal signals as well as in the formation and maintenance of the blood-spinal cord barrier (BSCB). Microglia are small cells that upon activation in response to injury have phagocytic properties. They are thought to be part of the monocyte-macrophage defense system within the CNS.

Similar to the blood-brain barrier, endothelial cells in the spinal cord form a BSCB that severely restricts the passage of most proteins, hydrophilic molecules, and ions in the circulation into the spinal cord. The unusual impermeability of CNS capillaries is attributed to tight junctions between endothelial cells and very limited endothelial vesicular transport. In addition to the specialized endothelium of the spinal cord, other important components of BSCB include the basement membrane, astrocytes, and pericytes in immediate proximity.

It is now recognized that neural progenitors and neural stem cells persist in the adult CNS. Although these cells are generally believed to reside in certain areas of the brain, neural stem cells/progenitors can be isolated from the adult spinal cord.[85]

CLINICAL FEATURES OF RADIATION INJURY TO THE SPINAL CORD

Two distinct clinical syndromes are recognized following radiation injury of the spinal cord. The first is a self-limiting early delayed reaction known as *Lhermitte syndrome*. It occurs after a latent period of 2 to 4 months and is characterized by paresthesia in the back and extremities upon neck flexion or extension. This syndrome typically lasts for a few months followed

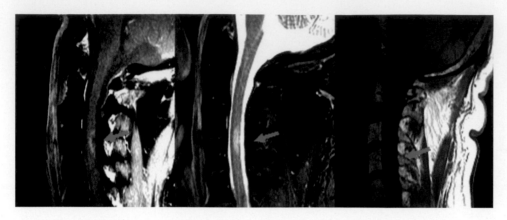

Figure 21.1. This patient developed permanent radiation myelopathy to the C3-4 spinal cord segment and typical MRI imaging findings. On the far left is the T1-post gadolinium sagittal image indicating enhancement at the area of spinal cord necrosis (*green arrow*), on the middle T2-weighted sagittal image the *green arrow* points to the corresponding area of T2 high signal change, and on the right is the lack of signal change apparent at the corresponding spinal cord segment on this T1 sagittal image.

invariably by complete clinical recovery. The pathogenesis of this syndrome remains unknown, although transient demyelination has been postulated to be the underlying mechanism.[18] There is however no correlation of Lhermitte syndrome with the second distinct late effect, permanent radiation myelopathy.

Permanent myelopathy is one of the most devastating late complications of radiotherapy. It generally occurs after a latent time of approximately 1 year but has been reported 3 to 4 years after radiation.[62,91] Clinical symptoms and signs can manifest in various combinations of motor and sensory deficits depending on the anatomic level of cord injury. It can be fatal if the damage occurs at the upper cervical level.[67]

Initial symptoms and signs of radiation myelopathy may be nonspecific and include often a diminished sense of proprioception and/or temperature sensation, minor motor weakness (typically beginning in the legs), and clumsiness. Changes in gait, incontinence, Brown-Sequard syndrome, hyper-reflexia, plegia, paresis, spasticity, and the Babinski sign are examples of more characteristic symptoms and signs that develop as the injury progresses.

Radiation myelopathy is a diagnosis of exclusion. Patients are considered to have the diagnosis based on neurological symptoms and signs of myelopathy that are consistent with the segment of cord irradiated and a clinical course compatible with radiation myelopathy. Evidence of neoplastic disease involving the spinal cord or CNS must be excluded.

The diagnosis of radiation myelopathy is typically supplemented by certain signaling changes of the cord upon magnetic resonance imaging (MRI). The typical MRI findings in the irradiated segment of spinal cord include low or normal signal intensity on T1-weighted images, high signals on T2-weighted images, and focal-to-diffuse contrast enhancement in the irradiated segment of the cord indicating necrosis.[3,84] There may or may not be atrophy of irradiated spinal cord segment.[3] Increased T1 signals in the vertebral bodies are also observed within the volume of spine irradiated. These signaling changes reflect conversion of normal red bone marrow to fatty marrow. Figure 21.1 illustrates typical MRI findings for a patient with radiation myelopathy at the C3-4 spinal cord segment.

Following cranial irradiation to modest doses, increased signals on T2-weighted images in the periventricular areas of the brain are well recognized in asymptomatic patients. In contrast, there are generally no apparent MRI changes in the spinal cord following subclinical damage. In positron emission tomography studies of spinal cord following a subthreshold dose for myelopathy, a temporary increase in [18F]deoxyglucose uptake followed by normalization of standardized uptake values has been reported, as well as [11C]methionine accumulation either normal or diminished.[22,37] Novel imaging techniques using high Tesla magnets, and novel contrast agents such as ultrasmall particles of iron oxide, are currently under investigation, which may allow detection of early or subclinical changes in the spinal cord following radiation.[47]

HISTOPATHOGIC FEATURES OF SPINAL CORD INJURY

In mammalian models of radiation myelopathy, most extensively studied in the rat, the most prominent histopathologic change is necrosis confined to white matter (Fig. 21.2A and B). These lesions consist of randomly distributed areas of cell loss, necrotic debris, swollen axons, and focal-to-extensive demyelination and necrosis (Fig. 21.2C and D). A scant mononuclear infiltrate is occasionally seen.[88] In rat spinal cord, although gross histopathologic changes are not prominent, most white matter lesions have been shown to be invariably preceded by a generalized disruption in vascular permeability or BSCB in white matter (Fig. 21.2E and F).[72]

In rat spinal cord, vascular changes generally occur late, often more than 1 year after irradiation. Vascular changes that have been described include telangiectasia, perivascular fibrosis and inflammation, hyaline degeneration and thickening, edema and fibrin exudation, stagnation and leakage of erythrocytes, and thrombosis with vessel obliteration and hemorrhage.[45,64] Studies that described histopathological changes at lower doses, doses below the threshold of paralysis, or during the latent time prior to the onset of paralysis have not been reported as often. In rat spinal cord following doses of only 5 to 10 Gy paranodal demyelination, nodal widening, and Wallerian-type degeneration of fibers in white matter has been described as early as 2 weeks postradiation followed by remyelination.[40,76] This observation has led to the conclusion that early delayed effects (Lhermitte syndrome) are related to transient demyelination.

In Rhesus monkeys that underwent irradiation to the spinal cord but did not develop myelopathy by 2 years, the histopathology consisted of small mineralized foci in nonmotor tracts, astrocytes that were increased in size and often adjacent to foci of malacia, and microglial cells surrounding flecks of mineral.[65] In addition, vasculopathy of hyaline degeneration

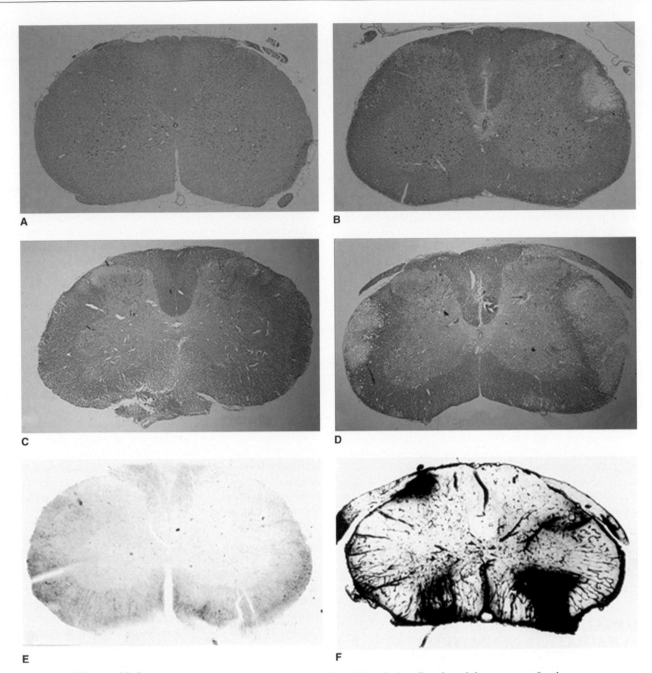

Figure 21.2. Compared to normal cervical rat spinal cord (**A**), the irradiated cord demonstrates focal areas of demyelination and necrosis at 4 months after single doses of radiation exceeding 20 Gy (**B**). Compared to the normal spinal cord (**C**), loss of myelin in white matter is evident upon Luxol blue staining (**D**). These changes are preceded by barrier disruption in white matter at 3½ months using horse radish peroxide as a vascular tracer (**E, F**).

was frequently observed as both an independent process and in close association with lesions of the neuropil.

Histopathologic description of human myelopathy is typically based on case reports or small series where autopsy materials were available. In an analysis of these reports, there were lesions that involved only white matter parenchyma with minor vascular changes, lesions that were mainly vascular, and lesions that demonstrated both white matter and vascular damage.[66] Human studies are limited due to many unknown patient, tumor, treatment, and other confounding factors that may influence the development of damage. In addition, the damage reported typically represented patients with the most severe

damage, such that histologic or autopsy materials were available for examination.

PATHOGENESIS OF INJURY

Largely based on extrapolations of histopathologic changes described above, the oligodendrocyte and the vascular endothelial cell have been implicated as two potential target cells in the mechanism of injury. The "oligodendroglial hypothesis" stems from the observation of demyelination and the presence of lesions confined to white matter. It is further supported by many molecular and cellular events such as changes in oligodendroglial/myelin gene expression, oligodendroglial apoptosis, reduced numbers of oligodendroglial progenitors and oligodendrocytes. However, many of the early and late cellular and molecular events affecting the oligodendroglial population are observed after doses well below the threshold of demyelination and necrosis. This observation suggests that these changes may not be causally associated with the white matter lesions observed after irradiation.[8]

The "vascular hypothesis" is supported by the disruption of the BSCB that precedes, or is invariably associated with, demyelination and white matter lesions, and often prominent vascular changes are observed.[50,69,71,72] Microvessels constitute about 95% of the blood-tissue interface and radiation injury to the microvessels, hence injury to the microvascular endothelial cells, is thought to be critical in the development of damage. Results from a series of experiments in rat spinal cord using boron neutron capture therapy (BNCT) argue strongly for the importance of the microvasculature in the pathogenesis of radiation myelopathy.[17] BNCT with capture agents that did or did not cross the BSCB allowed for selective irradiation of the spinal cord microvasculature. Demyelination and white matter lesions were observed even when BNCT dose was primarily limited to the vascular endothelium. Furthermore, limiting the BNCT dose to the vasculature resulted in significantly higher in vitro clonogenic survival of oligodendrocyte progenitor cells compared to photon irradiation only, despite that all treatments resulted in an equal incidence of white matter necrosis. These results lend support to the critical role of the vasculature rather than clonogenic survival of oligodendrocyte progenitor cells in mediating white matter injury after radiation.

With recent advances in neurobiology, it is recognized that categorizing the pathogenesis separately into a glial and vascular hypothesis is likely too simplistic, and injury is unlikely related to clonogenic cell death of only two target cell types. Therefore, the pathogenesis of spinal cord damage is currently best viewed as a damage continuum culminating in tissue necrosis with eventual clinical manifestation of signs and symptoms of myelopathy.[90]

REGIONAL DIFFERENCES IN CORD RADIATION SENSITIVITY

In rat spinal cord following irradiation, a predominance of dorsal tract lesions in high cervical segments, ventrolateral at mid-cervical levels, and a shift to dorsal lesions in the upper thoracic cord (with greater variability) has been observed.[13,77–80] Despite these differences in distribution of lesions, there was no evidence for a regional difference in radiosensitivity. Similar data in Rhesus monkeys also suggest no difference in radiation sensitivity between the cervical and thoracic cord.[65] Taken together, there is little evidence to support the existence of a significant difference in regional radiosensitivity of the human spinal cord that should affect clinical practice.[66]

In rodents, the lumbar/lumbosacral and cauda equina pathology is markedly different than that for the cervical or thoracic region, and a gradual diminishing severity of cord damage is observed. Below L1/2, damage to the cauda equina was predominantly nerve root necrosis.[77] Similar patterns of radiation response have been reported in both mouse and guinea pig spinal cords.[24,27,34,35,74]

EFFECT OF FRACTIONATION, VOLUME, AND OVERALL TREATMENT TIME

FRACTIONATION

As myelopathy can be objectively determined by the onset of paresis or paralysis, much of what is known about the effect of dose, fractionation, volume, and time on the CNS radiation response has been studied in animal models of radiation myelopathy. This includes the recognition of a high fractionation sensitivity of the CNS based on extensive rodent studies particularly in rat spinal cord whose threshold for induction of paralysis is approximately 20 to 22 Gy after a single dose.[76,88] These fractionation studies also lead to clinical investigations of altered fractionation studies in the 1980s. These studies consisted of alternating the fractionation schedule where the dose per fraction was reduced, and more than a single fraction was given daily in an attempt to improve the therapeutic ratio. For the spinal cord, it was hypothesized that the use of multiple small fractions per day will increase tolerance, but this proved to be not the case clinically.[60,92] Subsequently, a number of extensive experiments involving irradiating the rat cervical cord were performed to determine the kinetics of repair of sublethal damage in spinal cord. Although the results varied from study to study in terms of mathematical models that best described the repair kinetics data, the consistent observation is the lack of complete repair when more than a single fraction was given daily.[32,36,52] Thus, for altered fractionation protocols, it is generally recommended that a reduction of the interfraction interval to 6 to 8 hours is associated with a small but nonetheless significant reduction in spinal cord dose tolerance of 10% to 15%.[4] In summary, the risk of spinal cord injury increases with increasing dose per fraction, total radiation dose, and in the case of multiple daily fractions—shortened interfraction time intervals.

VOLUME EFFECT

As mentioned previously, the tolerance of normal tissues to radiation is unlikely to be dependent solely on the number and radiosensitivity of one or two target cell types. However, the ability of the clonogenic/target cells to maintain a sufficient number of mature cells suitably structured to maintain organ function may still be important. One model that was advanced in the 1980s described functional subunits (FSU), defined as discrete anatomically delineated structures whose relationship to tissue function is clear.[86] Thus, tissue survival may depend on FSU organization, and the proportion of FSU necessary for adequate organ function. However, mathematical models that incorporate parameters for FSU have failed to adequately describe experimental data for the cord.[48,82]

In Rhesus monkeys, a volume effect was not observed when lengths of cord of 4, 8, and 16 cm were treated to a total dose of 70.4 Gy in 2.2 Gy per fraction.[65] Volume dependence only emerged when the data were extrapolated to higher doses and smaller volumes than those used in the experiment. In irradiated pig spinal cord, there was again no evidence of a significant volume effect, and similar ED_{50} values were obtained for irradiated cord lengths of 2.5, 5, and 10 cm, respectively.[75] However, a significant volume effect has been observed in beagle dogs irradiated with 4-Gy fractions to 4- and 20-cm lengths of thoracic spinal cord with greater ED_{50} of 56.9 Gy for 20 cm versus 68.8 Gy for 4-cm fields.[49]

In an early study in rat spinal cord,[30] it was suggested that the effect of volume was complex and might differ depending on the histologic endpoint examined. A greater volume effect was observed using white matter lesions compared to using vascular lesions as endpoints. Some of the limitations of early experiments, such as dosimetric uncertainties and dose inhomogeneity, were addressed recently in a series of experiments using a high precision proton beam to irradiate very short lengths of rat spinal cord.[81]

In a recent series of experiments, four different lengths of the rat spinal cord (2, 4, 8, and 20 mm) were irradiated with single doses of protons (150–190 MeV) using paralysis as functional endpoint. A minor increase in tolerance was observed when the irradiated rat cord length was decreased from 20 mm (ED_{50} = 20.4 Gy) to 8 mm (ED_{50} = 24.9 Gy), whereas a large increase in tolerance was observed when the length was further reduced to 4 mm (ED_{50} = 53.7 Gy) and 2 mm (ED_{50} = 87.8 Gy).[9] These results suggest that for small field lengths there may be a volume effect.

These investigators also addressed the significance of partial volume irradiation and inhomogeneous dose distributions to the cord using a "bath and shower" approach. "Bath" irradiation represents doses to a large volume, whereas "shower" represents doses to a small volume. The effect was compared to homogeneous irradiation of the spinal cord to the same volume. The results indicated that the high ED_{50} values of a small length of 4 mm decreased significantly when the adjacent tissue was irradiated with a bath dose as low as 4 Gy.[12] Furthermore, the effect of a low bath dose appeared to be highest for a shower field of 2 mm, less for 4 mm, and absent for 8 mm (Fig. 21.3).

When an asymmetrical dose distribution was arranged by irradiation of 12 mm (bath) of spinal cord with a dose of 4 Gy, and irradiating only the caudal 2 mm (shower) of the 12-mm bath with variable single doses, the addition of a 4-Gy bath to only one side of a 2-mm field still showed a large effect.[10] Thus, not only is the integral irradiated volume a determining factor for rat cord tolerance, but the shape of the dose distribution may also be of great importance. Interestingly, the low bath doses did not result in any apparent histologic damage. Therefore, the integrity of surrounding tissue around an area of high dose damage may influence repair and may be disabled by doses that on its own would not cause functional deficit.

In another study using grazing proton beams to irradiate the lateral or central parts of the rat cervical spinal cord, a greater sensitivity of the white matter in the lateral cord was observed as compared to the central white and gray matter.[11] The observed difference in radiosensitivity is postulated based on regional sensitivities within the white matter rather than a volume effect. Similar to many previous studies, the gray matter was found to be extremely radioresistant with little or no histopathogic abnormalities observed even after single doses as high as 80 Gy. In a recent study on the tolerance of pig spinal cord using a dedicated radiosurgery linear accelerator, initial results indicate the ED_{50} values for whole cord and hemi-cord irradiation to be approximately 19 Gy.[42]

OVERALL TREATMENT TIME AND REIRRADIATION TOLERANCE

Extensive investigations have been conducted most notably using the rat myelopathy model to characterize the time-dependent long-term recovery of spinal cord damage. Several general conclusions can be drawn from these rodent studies that were done with a view to guide retreatment in the clinic. The consistent observation is the presence of recovery of the radiation-induced damage in rat spinal cord after an interval of 6 to 8 weeks. Hence, the rodent spinal cord can be retreated with doses depending on the size of the initial dose. Other important observations include: (a) shortened latency times to paralysis with increasing doses of reirradiation; (b) shortened latent times to paralysis with increasing size or total doses of the initial treatment; (c) an increase in retreatment tolerance with increasing time intervals between initial treatment and reirradiation; (d) influence of size of initial doses or injury on extent of recovery; (e) lack of a difference in subsequent fractionation sensitivity with retreatment; and (f) lack of complete recovery regardless of time intervals or size of initial injury.[51,52,87–89]

Recovery of occult radiation injury was also observed in a series of experiments in Rhesus monkeys.[50,51] In these experiments, the initial irradiation consisted of 44 Gy in 2.2-Gy daily fractions (approximately 60% of the biologically equivalent dose [BED] for an ED_{50} of 76 Gy) followed by graded reirradiation doses at 2 years (83.6–110 Gy in 2.2-Gy daily fractions). The time interval to retreatment varied from 1 to 3 years. The results indicated substantial (approximately 75% of the initial 44 Gy) recovery at 2 years. There was also evidence for additional recovery between years 1 and 3. Therefore, a large capacity to recover from occult cord radiation injury has been demonstrated in the primate spinal cord. Since human myelopathy has been observed after many years,[62,91] the follow-up period of

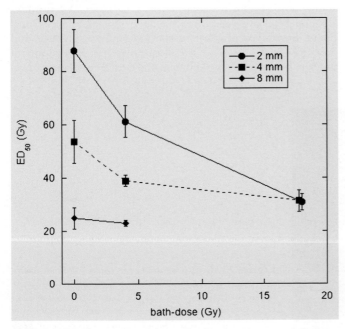

Figure 21.3. Summary of symmetrical bath and shower irradiations of rat spinal cord. The total ED_{50} in the shower volume shown as function of bath dose. (From Bijl HP, van Luijk P, Coppes RP, et al. Regional differences in radiosensitivity across the rat cervical spinal cord. *Int J Radiat Oncol Biol Phys.* 2005;61:543–551; Unexpected changes of rat cervical spinal cord tolerance caused by inhomogeneous dose distributions. *Int J Radiat Oncol Biol Phys.* 2003;57:274–281.)

2 to 3 years postirradiation in the primate experiments does not completely exclude the possibility of a very late occurring injury.

HUMAN CLINICAL DATA FOR RADIATION MYELOPATHY AND GUIDELINES FOR SAFE PRACTICE

Animal data have provided valuable insight into spinal cord tolerance and a number of general conclusions can be made to guide clinical practice:

1. There is a dose threshold above which the risk of radiation myelopathy increases substantially.
2. The risk of cord injury increases with increasing dose per fraction, total dose, and shortened interfractional time intervals when more than a single fraction per day is delivered.
3. There does not seem to be a volume effect for cord lengths ≥1 cm. However, a significant volume effect for <8 mm has been demonstrated in rat spinal cord.[58]
4. There is evidence for long-term time-dependent recovery of injury in various species including rats, pigs, and monkeys.[5,42,87,91]
5. For large single doses to fraction sizes of about 2 Gy given once daily, the linear-quadratic (LQ) model with an α/β value of about 2 Gy provides a satisfactory description of the dose-fractionation response of the cord.[44,58,91]

Given our limited knowledge of human spinal cord tolerance, several additional factors should be considered when applying these general conclusions to the human spinal cord. The fractionation scheme and irradiation techniques are most important factors to consider given that much of what is known about the human cord tolerance is based on myelopathy data following conventional fractionation and techniques. Here, conventional fractionation refers to fraction sizes of ≤5 Gy, and conventional technique refers to a homogeneous irradiation to a long length or volume of spinal cord. These considerations are particularly

relevant in modern radiotherapy as, for example, stereotactic body radiotherapy (SBRT) is increasingly being used. SBRT is defined as high dose per fraction radiotherapy delivered in one to five fractions, and the dose per fraction is typically >5 Gy.[56,73] SBRT requires highly conformal radiotherapy using intensity modulation and image guidance, and allows a high dose to the target while the spinal cord is deliberately spared to a dose thought to be safe.[54–56] An example of an SBRT distribution is shown in Figure 21.4 that highlights the extreme conformality of the dose distribution and dose inhomogeneity within the target and spinal cord.

The LQ model provides a satisfactory description of the dose-fractionation response of the cord and, hence, has been used extensively as a guide to equate dose-fractionation schedules with respect to cord tolerance. It should be pointed out that the applicability of the LQ model with extreme hypofractionated regimens (>5 Gy) has only been demonstrated for rodent spinal cord and should be applied with caution for humans.[26,46,59]

Lastly, reirradiation tolerance is an active field of research, and there is a lack of robust clinical data to help guide safe practice. This is true in both the conventional and the SBRT setting, and the lack of understanding in this area has potential implications for patients who may not be offered reirradiated when further doses can be given safely due to the fear of causing radiation myelopathy.[6]

SPINAL CORD TOLERANCE FOR CONVENTIONAL RADIATION (≤5 Gy/FRACTION) FOR PATIENTS WITH NO PRIOR RADIATION

A 5% risk of myelopathy at 5 years posttreatment with 50 Gy was largely based on expert opinions as summarized by Emami et al.[21] The available human data however suggest that the risk at this dose is approximately 1%.[39,41,61,63] Table 21.1 provides a summary of doses that have resulted in radiation myelopathy in the context of conventional radiotherapy practice, and doses per fraction ≤5 Gy. One must note that the majority of the data are based on two-dimensional treatment planning and

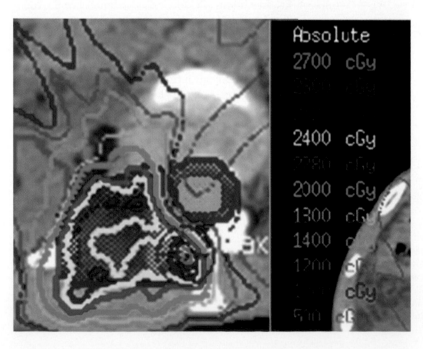

Figure 21.4. This axial slice of a spine SBRT case where the paraspinal target in red color wash is adjacent to the spinal cord and treated with 24 Gy in two fractions (i.e., 12 Gy × 2 fractions). The isodose lines and corresponding doses are shown and the tight conformality of the dose distribution is apparent. The spinal cord is contoured in light blue and the thecal sac in purple color wash. The maximum point dose to the spinal cord was 10.2 Gy in two fractions (BED = 36, nBED = 18) and the maximum point dose to the thecal sac is 14.2 in two fractions (BED = 65, nBED = 32). This practice is in accordance with the proposed guidelines for hypofractionated SBRT.

TABLE 21.1	Absolute Dose and BED/nBED of Known Cases of Radiation Myelopathy in Patients with No Prior History of Radiation with Conventional Radiotherapy Fractionation and Techniques (Dose Per Fraction ≤5 Gy)

Author	*Absolute Dose(Gy)/Fractions*	*Cumulative BED (Gy$_2$)*	*Cumulative nBED (Gy$_{2/2}$)*
Wong et al.[91]	47.0/15	121	60
Wong et al.[91]	20.4/5 + 20.4/5	124	62
Wong et al.[91]	6.4/2 + 30.3/10 + 24/12	141	70.4
Wong et al.[91]	20.5/5 + 20.5/5	125	63
Wong et al.[91]	39.5/15 + 7.0/5	103	52
Wong et al.[91]	55.6/20	133	66
Wong et al.[91]	23.8/5 + 23.6/5	160	80
Wong et al.[91]	29.8/15 + 24.7/10	115	57
Wong et al.[91]	20.6/5 + 20.6/5	126	53
Wong et al.[91]	35/16 + 25/10	130	65
Wong et al.[91]	21.4/5 + 17.1/4 + 1.6/1	124	62
Wong et al.[91]	53.5/15	149	74
Wong et al.[91]	47/20	102	51
Wong et al.[91]	8.9/5 + 45/15	129	65
Wong et al.[91]	21.6/5 + 22.6/5	142	71
Wong et al.[91]	59.8/20	149	75
Eichhorn et al.[20]	66.2/27	147	74
Eichhorn et al.[20]	44.1/18 + 28.4/9	171	86
Abramson et al.[2]	40/10	120	60
Hazra et al.[29]	45/15	120	60
McCunniff et al.[41]	60/30	120	60
Macbeth et al.[38]	39/13	98	49
Dische et al.[19]	50/20	113	56
Jeremic et al.[31]	55/28	109	55
Jeremic et al.[31]	50/30 + 6.7/4	104	52
Atkins et al.[7]	34.8/10	95	48
Atkins et al.[7]	38/12	98	49
Atkins et al.[7]	40/12	107	53
Atkins et al.[7]	52/26	104	52
Atkins et al.[7]	45.5/15	115	57
Atkins et al.[7]	34.8/10	95	48
Abbatucci et al.[1]	54/18	135	68
Abbatucci et al.[1]	51.1/18	124	62
Abbatucci et al.[1]	60/18	160	80
Scruggs et al.[68]	20/5 + 20/8	105	53
Choi et al.[15]	42.9/15	104	52
Hatlevoll et al.[28]	38/8	128	64
Hatlevoll et al.[28]	34/8	106	53
Marcus et al.[39]	46.6/27	87	43
Marcus et al.[39]	49.1/29	91	45
Kim et al.[33]	65/33	129	65
Kim et al.[33]	62/31	124	62
Kim et al.[33]	61.14/33	118	59
Kim et al.[33]	54/23	117	59
Kim et al.[33]	60.55/31	120	60
Eichhorn et al.[20]	69.6/27	159	80
Eichhorn et al.[20]	46.5/18 + 29.9/9	186	93

Note that some of the data represent multiple courses but all patients completed the total radiation intent within 8 weeks from the start of the radiation course.

Note no correction was applied for split course schedules to determine biologic equivalent doses.

the cord doses are less reliable as compared to modern-day computerized dose calculations.[91] To account for the different dose-fractionation schemes resulting in radiation myelopathy, the BED normalized to a 2 Gy-equivalent BED (nBED) using an α/β value of 2 Gy (Gy$_{2/2}$) is calculated. The nBED is also analogous to the EQD2, which refers to the biologically LQ equivalent dose in 2 Gy fractions and an α/β of 2. Based on results listed in Table 21.1, it can be concluded that if the BED is kept below 100 Gy$_2$, or nBED of 50 Gy$_{2/2}$, the risk of myelopathy is negligible. At the 100 to 120 Gy$_2$ (50–60 Gy$_{2/2}$) range, there might be a small risk of radiation myelopathy. Therefore, a nBED of 60 Gy$_{2/2}$ (BED = 120 Gy$_2$) given in conventional fractionation of 1.8 to 2.0 Gy/day using modern CT-based planning may be acceptable depending on the clinical context.

Table 21.1 does not include the myelopathy cases following altered and accelerated fractionation protocols when more than a single fraction is delivered per day. Based on few cases reported following accelerated and hyperfractionated radiation, the total BED for radiation myelopathy cases have been below $100 \, Gy_2$.[60,91] To date, there has not been satisfactory explanation for these myelopathy cases despite using repair kinetics data extrapolated from animal studies to allow for incomplete repair. The important clinical implication is that a reduction of the interfraction interval to 6 to 8 hours is associated with a small but nonetheless significant reduction in spinal cord dose tolerance of 10% to 15%.[4]

In summary, an evidence-based recommendation is that the tolerance dose of the spinal cord in 2-Gy daily fractions is 50 Gy (BED = $100 \, Gy_2$, nBED = $50 \, Gy_{2/2}$), and this represents a very low risk of permanent myelopathy.[60–62] In addition to the caution associated with altered fractionation, one must also note that these recommendations are for patients not treated with concurrent chemotherapy where a more conservative approach is required.

REIRRADIATION SPINAL CORD TOLERANCE AFTER PRIOR CONVENTIONAL RADIATION (≤5 Gy/FRACTION)

Compared to a single course of radiation, there is a lack of data with respect to retreatment tolerance of the human spinal cord. The series by Wong et al. represents the largest series describing reirradiation myelopathy.[91] Table 21.2 summarizes the doses resulting in radiation myelopathy from retreatment cases where the dose per fraction is ≤5 Gy for either course. The total BED of the spinal cord ranged from 129 to $170 \, Gy_2$ (nBED range of $64–85 \, Gy_{2/2}$). Therefore, one could propose a cumulative BED ranging from $≤120 \, Gy_2$ as safe, and this fits well considering in the unirradiated patient that $60 \, Gy_{2/2}$ represents a small, and approximately 5%, risk of radiation myelopathy.[63]

In a subsequent reanalysis of these cases comparing doses to those published retreatment cases without myelopathy, Nieder et al. suggested that a cumulative BED of $135.5 \, Gy_2$ or less could be safe when neither course of radiation exceeds a BED of $98 \, Gy_2$ and the time interval between courses is no shorter

than 6 months.[44] One has to note that the actual dosimetry or treatment records of these controls were not reviewed and based on published data. While the absence of radiation myelopathy in retreatment patients with lower spinal cord doses raised the possibility of the presence of significant long-term recovery in the human spinal cord, the magnitude and kinetics of long-term recovery of radiation damage and its possible dependence on initial damage are unknown in the human. These recommendations again do not represent practice with concurrent chemotherapy or altered fractionation.

SPINAL CORD TOLERANCE WITH HYPOFRACTIONATED RADIATION (>5 Gy/FRACTION) FOR PATIENTS WITH NO PRIOR RADIATION

There have been few cases of radiation myelopathy reported after conventional homogeneous hypofractionated radiotherapy as shown in Table 21.3. The lack of data likely represent the lack of practice with these high-dose fractionation schemes with conventional radiotherapy as accurate cord sparing is not possible with conventional techniques. Important information is learned from these few cases where one can conclude that multiple fractions of homogeneous radiation >8.5 Gy and radical doses in the 30 to 35 Gy in five fractions range are associated with some risk of myelopathy.

The availability of SBRT now permits high dose per fraction radiation delivered accurately to targets (common target doses include 35 Gy in five fractions,[56] 24–27 Gy in three fractions,[14,54] and 16–24 Gy in one fraction[23,53,93]) adjacent to the spinal cord. SBRT poses new challenges to our knowledge and practice regarding cord tolerance as we spare the spinal cord to a hypofractionated dose we regard as "safe." The inhomogeneity of the dose distribution within the spinal cord also poses new challenges to our understanding of spinal cord tolerance as there is the potential for small volumes of spinal cord to receive a high dose while the majority of the spinal cord receives a low dose. The unknown significance of high point doses has resulted in the practice of allowing higher doses to small volumes of spinal cord than we would typically regard as "safe," and has resulted in radiation myelopathy.[56]

TABLE 21.2	Absolute Dose and BED/nBED of Known Reirradiation Cases of Radiation Myelopathy and Conventional Radiotherapy Fractionation and Techniques (Dose Per Fraction ≤5 Gy)			
Author	First Course Absolute Dose(Gy)/Fractions	Second Course Absolute Dose(Gy)/Fractions	Cumulative BED (Gy_2)	Cumulative nBED ($Gy_{2/2}$)
Wong et al.[91]	2.0/1 + 45.9/15	23.6/10	170	85
Wong et al.[91]	23.5/10 + 18.2/5	13.6/5	135	67
Wong et al.[91]	20.6/6	36.4/10	159	79
Wong et al.[91]	20.1/16	14.3/6 + 3.2/2 + 22.6/6 + 2.57	138	69
Wong et al.[91]	24/8 + 24/16	18.1/10	137	69
Wong et al.[91]	24.4/5	17/5	130	65
Wong et al.[91]	31.2/20	30.3/6	163	81
Wong et al.[91]	33.9/10	25.6/10	149	75
Wong et al.[91]	50/20	10.4/10	129	64

The time interval between courses of radiation exceeded 8 weeks in order to be characterized as retreatment.

TABLE 21.3	Absolute Dose and BED/nBED of Known Cases of Radiation Myelopathy in Patients with No Prior Radiation and a Dose Per Fraction >5 Gy using Conventional or SBRT Techniques		
Author	*Absolute Dose(Gy)/ Fractions*	*BED (Gy_2)*	*nBED ($Gy_{2/2}$)*
Sahgal et al.[59] (SBRT)	25.6/2	189	94
Sahgal et al.[59] (SBRT)	30.9/3	190	95
Sahgal et al.[59] (SBRT)	14.8/1	124	62
Sahgal et al.[59] (SBRT)	13.1/1	99	49
Sahgal et al.[59] (SBRT)	10.6/1	67	33
Macbeth et al.[38] (conventional)	17/2	89	45
Dische et al.[19] (conventional)	33.7–35.5/6	128–141	64–70
Atkins et al.[7] (conventional)	19/2	109	55
Atkins et al.[7] (conventional)	23.7/2	164	82
Atkins et al.[7] (conventional)	29.6/3	176	88

The time interval between courses of radiation exceeded 8 weeks in order to be characterized as retreatment.

Sahgal et al. recently reported a detailed dosimetric analysis of five radiation myelopathy cases post-spine SBRT summarized in Table 21.3, and proposed modern guidelines for spinal cord tolerance given hypofractionated radiotherapy. In all patients, dose volume histogram (DVH) data were collected for each case and centrally analyzed,[59] which is unlike prior data where spinal cord dose was extrapolated based on the estimated location of the spinal cord from two-dimensional imaging. In Table 21.3, the doses represent the point maximum dose within the thecal sac for each case.[59] The dose to the thecal sac was chosen as a surrogate for the spinal cord as it provides some margin on the spinal cord (typically 1–2 mm) to account for the potential dosimetric uncertainty effects of intrafractional patient motion, spinal cord motion, and contouring uncertainty.[16,83]

Based on absolute dose and single fraction radiation, the lowest dose causing radiation myelopathy was observed at 10.6 Gy. Overall, the BED of the five cases ranged from 67 to 190 Gy_2 (nBED of 33–95 $Gy_{2/2}$).[59] Sahgal et al. compared this group to a control population treated with spine SBRT (actual DVH data centrally reviewed and analyzed) with no radiation myelopathy, and concluded that a nBED of 30 to 35 $Gy_{2/2}$ as safe with the caveat that single fraction cord dose does not exceed 10 Gy (BED = 60 Gy_2, nBED = 30 $Gy_{2/2}$).

SPINAL CORD TOLERANCE FOR HYPOFRACTIONATED REIRRADIATION (>5 Gy/ FRACTION) IN PATIENTS WITH PRIOR RADIATION

Retreatment with high doses per fraction using SBRT is an emerging practice that is likely to become the standard as it allows the delivery of a second radical course of radiation to the tumor while sparing the spinal cord.[54,56] Radiation myelopathy has been reported and reflects the lack of data to guide safe practice. The data summarized in Table 21.4 consist of four known cases of radiation myelopathy following retreatment with SBRT, and three cases of radiation myelopathy with conventional radiation where at least one course was hypofractionated (>5 Gy). The cumulative nBED resulting in myelopathy ranges from 72 to 153 $Gy_{2/2}$.[57] For the SBRT spinal cord dosimetry, the data represent the point maximum within the thecal sac. At this point, we cannot make any firm recommendations other than a cumulative nBED of >70 $Gy_{2/2}$ has resulted in radiation myelopathy when at least one course is hypofractionated. We are in the process of determining safe SBRT re-treatment doses given common prior external beam radiotherapy practice while respecting a cumulative nBED of 70 $Gy_{2/2}$.[57]

TABLE 21.4	Absolute Dose and BED/nBED of Known Reirradiation Cases of Radiation Myelopathy in Patients Treated with At Least One Course of High Dose Per Fraction (>5 Gy) Radiation and Conventional or SBRT Techniques			
Author	*First Course Absolute Dose(Gy)/Fractions*	*Second Course Absolute Dose(Gy)/Fractions*	*Cumulative BED (Gy_2)*	*Cumulative nBED ($Gy_{2/2}$)*
Sahgal et al.[57] (SBRT)	40/22	20.3/2	199	100
Sahgal et al.[57] (SBRT)	25.2/28	20.9/2	167	83
Sahgal et al.[57] (SBRT)	12.3/1	20/5	148	74
Sahgal et al.[57] (SBRT)	50.2/28	32.6/3	305	153
Wong et al.[91] (conventional)	16.0/5	22.0/3	144	72
Wong et al.[91] (conventional)	20.4/5 + 20.3/5	8.2/1	165	83
Atkins et al.[7] (conventional)	20.4/10	19/2	150	75

TABLE 21.5	Summary of Recommendations for Human Spinal Cord Tolerance Based on Fractionation Scheme		
	BED	*nBED*	*Caveat*
Conventional radiation (≤5 Gy/fraction)	$100\,\mathrm{Gy}_2$	$50\,\mathrm{Gy}_{2/2}$	$60\,\mathrm{Gy}_{2/2}$ may be acceptable for 1.8–2.0 Gy/d fraction sizes under certain clinical circumstances

Conventional reirradiation (neither course exceeds 5 Gy/fraction)	Cumulative BED 100–$120\,\mathrm{Gy}_2$	Cumulative nBED 50–$60\,\mathrm{Gy}_{2/2}$	• BED of up to $135\,\mathrm{Gy}_2$ given that:
			  ○ Time interval of at least 6 months between courses
			  ○ Neither course to exceed BED of $98\,\mathrm{Gy}_2$

Hypofractionated (>5 Gy/fraction)	60–$70\,\mathrm{Gy}_2$ (point maximum within the thecal sac)	30–$35\,\mathrm{Gy}_{2/2}$ (point maximum within the thecal sac)	• Applies to the modern CT based treatment planning and the contoured thecal sac to represent the true spinal cord
			  ○ In a single fraction, an absolute dose of 10 Gy ($30\,\mathrm{Gy}_{2/2}$) is safe to the thecal sac, and for two to five fractions up to $35\,\mathrm{Gy}_{2/2}$
			 • Note nBED of $35\,\mathrm{Gy}_{2/2}$ =
			  ○ 14.5 Gy in 2 fractions
			  ○ 17.5 Gy in 3 fractions
			  ○ 20 Gy in 4 fractions
			  ○ 22 Gy in 5 fractions

Hypofractionated reirradiation (one course >5 Gy/fraction)	Insufficient data at this time	Insufficient data at this time	• A cumulative nBED of $>70\,\mathrm{Gy}_{2/2}$ has resulted in radiation myelopathy

CONCLUSION

Myelopathy represents a devastating late toxicity of radiation treatment. Recent research has provided a better understanding of the tolerance of the mammalian spinal cord and the molecular events associated with this injury, however, human data are sparse. We summarize our evidence-based guidelines in Table 21.5 for safe practice given using conventional fractionation and hypofractionation regimens.

REFERENCES

1. Abbatucci JS, Delozier T, Quint R, et al. Radiation myelopathy of the cervical spinal cord: time, dose and volume factors. *Int J Radiat Oncol Biol Phys.* 1978;4:239–248.
2. Abramson N, Cavanaugh PJ. Short-course radiation therapy in carcinoma of the lung: a second look. *Radiology.* 1973;108:685–687.
3. Alfonso ER, De Gregorio MA, Mateo P, et al. Radiation myelopathy in over-irradiated patients: MR imaging findings. *Eur Radiol.* 1997;7:400–404.
4. Ang KK. Radiation injury to the central nervous system: clinical features and prevention. In: Meyer JL, ed. *Radiation Injury: Advances in Management and Prevention.* Vol 32. Basel: Karger; 1999:145–154.
5. Ang KK, Jiang GL, Feng Y, et al. Extent and kinetics of recovery of occult spinal cord injury. *Int J Radiat Oncol Biol Phys.* 2001;50:1013–1020.
6. Ang KK, Price RE, Stephens LC, et al. The tolerance of primate spinal cord to re-irradiation. *Int J Radiat Oncol Biol Phys.* 1993;25:459–464.
7. Atkins HL, Tretter P. Time-dose considerations in radiation myelopathy. *Acta Radiol Ther Phys Biol.* 1966;3:79–94.
8. Atkinson S, Li YQ, Wong CS. Changes in oligodendrocytes and myelin gene expression after radiation in the rodent spinal cord. *Int J Radiat Oncol Biol Phys.* 2003;57:1093–1100.
9. Bijl HP, van Luijk P, Coppes RP, et al. Dose-volume effects in the rat cervical spinal cord after proton irradiation. *Int J Radiat Oncol Biol Phys.* 2002;52:205–211.
10. Bijl HP, van Luijk P, Coppes RP, et al. Influence of adjacent low-dose fields on tolerance to high doses of protons in rat cervical spinal cord. *Int J Radiat Oncol Biol Phys.* 2006;64:1204–1210.
11. Bijl HP, van Luijk P, Coppes RP, et al. Regional differences in radiosensitivity across the rat cervical spinal cord. *Int J Radiat Oncol Biol Phys.* 2005;61:543–551.
12. Bijl HP, van Luijk P, Coppes RP, et al. Unexpected changes of rat cervical spinal cord tolerance caused by inhomogeneous dose distributions. *Int J Radiat Oncol Biol Phys.* 2003;57:274–281.
13. Bradley WG, Fewings JD, Cumming WJ, et al. Delayed myeloradiculopathy produced by spinal X-irradiation in the rat. *J Neurol Sci.* 1977;31:63–82

14. Chang EL, Shiu AS, Mendel E, et al. Phase I/II study of stereotactic body radiotherapy for spinal metastasis and its pattern of failure. *J Neurosurg Spine.* 2007;7:151–160.
15. Choi NC, Grillo HC, Gardiello M, et al. Basis for new strategies in postoperative radiotherapy of bronchogenic carcinoma. *Int J Radiat Oncol Biol Phys.* 1980;6:31–35.
16. Chuang C, Sahgal A, Lee L, et al. Effects of residual target motion for image-tracked spine radiosurgery. *Med Phys.* 2007;34:4484–4490.
17. Coderre JA, Morris AD, Micca PL, et al. Late effects of radiation on the central nervous system: role of vascular endothelial damage and glial stem cell survival. *Radiat Res.* 2006;166(3):493–503.
18. Delattre JY, Rosenblum MK, Thaler HT, et al. A model of radiation myelopathy in the rat. Pathology, regional capillary permeability changes and treatment with dexamethasone. *Brain.* 1988;111(pt 6):1319–1336.
19. Dische S, Warburton MF, Saunders MI. Radiation myelitis and survival in the radiotherapy of lung cancer. *Int J Radiat Oncol Biol Phys.* 1988;15:75–81.
20. Eichhorn HJ, Lessel A, Rotte KH. Influence of various irradiation rhythms on neoplastic and normal tissue in vivo. *Strahlentherapie.* 1972;143:614–629.
21. Emami B, Lyman J, Brown A, et al. Tolerance of normal tissue to therapeutic irradiation. *Int J Radiat Oncol Biol Phys.* 1991;21:109–122.
22. Esik O, Emri M, Szakall S Jr, et al. PET identifies transitional metabolic change in the spinal cord following a subthreshold dose of irradiation. *Pathol Oncol Res.* 2004;10:42–46.
23. Gerszten PC, Burton SA, Ozhasoglu C, et al. Radiosurgery for spinal metastases: clinical experience in 500 cases from a single institution. *Spine.* 2007;32:193–199.
24. Goffinet DR, Marsa GW, Brown JM. The effects of single and multifraction radiation courses on the mouse spinal cord. *Radiology.* 1976;119:709–713.
25. Gray H. *Anatomy of the Human Body.* Philadelphia, PA: Lea & Febiger; 1918, 2000
26. Guerrero M, Li XA. Extending the linear-quadratic model for large fraction doses pertinent to stereotactic radiotherapy. *Phys Med Biol.* 2004;49:4825–4835.
27. Habermalz HJ, Valley B, Habermalz E. Radiation myelopathy of the mouse spinal cord–isoeffect correlations after fractionated radiation. *Strahlenther Onkol.* 1987;163:626–632.
28. Hatlevoll R, Host H, Kaalhus O. Myelopathy following radiotherapy of bronchial carcinoma with large single fractions: a retrospective study. *Int J Radiat Oncol Biol Phys.* 1983;9:41–44.
29. Hazra TA, Chandrasekaran MS, Colman M, et al. Survival in carcinoma of the lung after a split course of radiotherapy. *Br J Radiol.* 1974;47:464–466.
30. Hopewell JW, Morris AD, Dixon-Brown A. The influence of field size on the late tolerance of the rat spinal cord to single doses of X rays. *Br J Radiol.* 1987;60:1099–1108.
31. Jeremic B, Djuric L, Mijatovic L. Incidence of radiation myelitis of the cervical spinal cord at doses of 5500 cGy or greater. *Cancer.* 1991;68:2138–2141.
32. Kim JJ, Hao Y, Jang D, et al. Lack of influence of sequence of top-up doses on repair kinetics in rat spinal cord. *Radiother Oncol.* 1997;43:211–217.
33. Kim YH, Fayos JV. Radiation tolerance of the cervical spinal cord. *Radiology.* 1981;139:473–478.
34. Knowles JF. The effects of single dose X-irradiation on the guinea-pig spinal cord. *Int J Radiat Biol Relat Stud Phys Chem Med.* 1981;40:265–275.
35. Knowles JF. The radiosensitivity of the guinea-pig spinal cord to X-rays: the effect of retreatment at one year and the effect of age at the time of irradiation. *Int J Radiat Biol Relat Stud Phys Chem Med.* 1983;44:433–442.

36. Landuyt W, Fowler J, Ruifrok A, et al. Kinetics of repair in the spinal cord of the rat. *Radiother Oncol.* 1997;45:55–62.

37. Lengyel Z, Reko G, Majtenyi K, et al. Autopsy verifies demyelination and lack of vascular damage in partially reversible radiation myelopathy. *Spinal Cord.* 2003;41:577–585.

38. Macbeth FR, Wheldon TE, Girling DJ, et al; The Medical Research Council Lung Cancer Working Party. Radiation myelopathy: estimates of risk in 1048 patients in three randomized trials of palliative radiotherapy for non-small cell lung cancer. *Clin Oncol (R Coll Radiol).* 1996;8:176–181.

39. Marcus RB Jr, Million RR. The incidence of myelitis after irradiation of the cervical spinal cord. *Int J Radiat Oncol Biol Phys.* 1990;19:3–8.

40. Mastaglia FL, McDonald WI, Watson JV, et al. Effects of x-radiation on the spinal cord: an experimental study of the morphological changes in central nerve fibres. *Brain.* 1976;99:101–122.

41. McCunniff AJ, Liang MJ. Radiation tolerance of the cervical spinal cord. *Int J Radiat Oncol Biol Phys.* 1989;16:675–678.

42. Medin PM, Foster RD, Follet K, et al. Spinal cord tolerance to radiosurgical dose distributions: a swine model. *Int J Radiat Oncol Biol Phys.* 2007;69:S250–S251.

43. Moore K, Dalley A. *Clinically Oriented Anatomy.* 4th ed. Philadelphia, PA: Williams and Wilkins; 1999.

44. Nieder C, Grosu AL, Andratschke NH, et al. Proposal of human spinal cord reirradiation dose based on collection of data from 40 patients. *Int J Radiat Oncol Biol Phys.* 2005;61:851–855.

45. Okada S, Okeda R. Pathology of radiation myelopathy. *Neuropathology.* 2001;21:247–265.

46. Park C, Papiez L, Zhang S, et al. Universal survival curve and single fraction equivalent dose: useful tools in understanding potency of ablative radiotherapy. *Int J Radiat Oncol Biol Phys.* 2008;70:847–852.

47. Philippens ME, Gambarota G, van der Kogel AJ, et al. Radiation effects in the rat spinal cord: evaluation with apparent diffusion coefficient versus T2 at serial MR imaging. *Radiology.* 2009;250:387–397.

48. Philippens ME, Pop LA, Visser AG, et al. Dose-volume effects in rat thoracolumbar spinal cord; an evaluation of NTCP models. *Int J Radiat Oncol Biol Phys.* 2004;60:578–590.

49. Powers BE, Thames HD, Gillette SM, et al. Volume effects in the irradiated canine spinal cord: do they exist when the probability of injury is low? *Radiother Oncol.* 1998;46:297–306.

50. Rubin P, Gash DM, Hansen JT, et al. Disruption of the blood-brain barrier as the primary effect of CNS irradiation. *Radiother Oncol.* 1994;31:51–60.

51. Ruifrok AC, Kleiboer BJ, van der Kogel AJ. Radiation tolerance and fractionation sensitivity of the developing rat cervical spinal cord. *Int J Radiat Oncol Biol Phys.* 1992;24:505–510.

52. Ruifrok AC, Kleiboer BJ, van der Kogel AJ. Reirradiation tolerance of the immature rat spinal cord. *Radiother Oncol.* 1992;23:249–256.

53. Ryu S, Jin JY, Jin R, et al. Partial volume tolerance of the spinal cord and complications of single-dose radiosurgery. *Cancer.* 2007;109:628–636.

54. Sahgal A, Ames C, Chou D, et al. Stereotactic body radiotherapy is effective salvage therapy for patients with prior radiation of spinal metastases. *Int J Radiat Oncol Biol Phys.* 2009;74:723–731.

55. Sahgal A, Chou D, Ames C, et al. Image-guided robotic stereotactic body radiotherapy for benign spinal tumors: the university of California San Francisco preliminary experience. *Technol Cancer Res Treat.* 2007;6:595–604.

56. Sahgal A, Larson DA, Chang EL. Stereotactic body radiosurgery for spinal metastases: a critical review. *Int J Radiat Oncol Biol Phys.* 2008;71:652–665.

57. Sahgal A, Ma L, Gibbs I, et al. Re-treatment guidelines for spine stereotactic body radiotherapy. *Int J Radiat Oncol Biol Phys.* 2009;75:S239.

58. Sahgal A, Ma L, Gibbs I, et al. Preliminary Guidelines for Avoidance of Radiation Induced Myelopathy Following Spine Stereotactic Body Radiosurgery (SBRS). *Int J Radiat Oncol Biol Phys.* 2008;72:S220.

59. Sahgal A, Ma L, Gibbs I, et al. Spinal cord tolerance for stereotactic body radiotherapy. *Int J Radiat Oncol Biol Phys.* 2010;77:54–552.

60. Saunders MI, Dische S, Hong A, et al. Continuous hyperfractionated accelerated radiotherapy in locally advanced carcinoma of the head and neck region. *Int J Radiat Oncol Biol Phys.* 1989;17:1287–1293.

61. Schultheiss TE. Spinal cord radiation "tolerance": doctrine versus data. *Int J Radiat Oncol Biol Phys.* 1990;19:219–221.

62. Schultheiss TE, Higgins EM, El-Mahdi AM. The latent period in clinical radiation myelopathy. *Int J Radiat Oncol Biol Phys.* 1984;10:1109–1115.

63. Schultheiss TE, Kun LE, Ang KK, et al. Radiation response of the central nervous system. *Int J Radiat Oncol Biol Phys.* 1995;31:1093–1112.

64. Schultheiss TE, Stephens LC. Invited review: permanent radiation myelopathy. *Br J Radiol.* 1992;65:737–753.

65. Schultheiss TE, Stephens LC, Ang KK, et al. Volume effects in rhesus monkey spinal cord. *Int J Radiat Oncol Biol Phys.* 1994;29:67–72.

66. Schultheiss TE, Stephens LC, Maor MH. Analysis of the histopathology of radiation myelopathy. *Int J Radiat Oncol Biol Phys.* 1988;14:27–32.

67. Schultheiss TE, Stephens LC, Peters LJ. Survival in radiation myelopathy. *Int J Radiat Oncol Biol Phys.* 1986;12:1765–1769.

68. Scruggs H, El-Mahdi A, Marks RDJMRD Jr, et al. The results of split-course radiation therapy in cancer of the lung. *Am J Roentgenol Radium Ther Nucl Med.* 1974;121:754–760.

69. Sheline GE, Wara WM, Smith V. Therapeutic irradiation and brain injury. *Int J Radiat Oncol Biol Phys.* 1980;6:1215–1228.

70. Sherman DL, Brophy PJ. Mechanisms of axon ensheathment and myelin growth. *Nat Rev Neurosci.* 2005;6:683–690.

71. Siegal T, Pfeffer MR. Radiation-induced changes in the profile of spinal cord serotonin, prostaglandin synthesis, and vascular permeability. *Int J Radiat Oncol Biol Phys.* 1995;31:57–64.

72. Stewart PA, Vinters HV, Wong CS. Blood-spinal cord barrier function and morphometry after single doses of x-rays in rat spinal cord. *Int J Radiat Oncol Biol Phys.* 1995;32:703–711.

73. Timmerman RD, Kavanagh BD, Cho LC, et al. Stereotactic body radiation therapy in multiple organ sites. *J Clin Oncol.* 2007;25:947–952.

74. Travis EL, Parkins CS, Holmes SJ, et al. Effect of misonidazole on radiation injury to mouse spinal cord. *Br J Cancer.* 1982;45:469–473.

75. van den Aardweg GJ, Hopewell JW, Whitehouse EM. The radiation response of the cervical spinal cord of the pig: effects of changing the irradiated volume. *Int J Radiat Oncol Biol Phys.* 1995;31:51–55.

76. Van der Kogel AJ. Central nervous system radiation injury in small animal models. In: Gutin PH, Leibel SA, Sheline GE, eds. *Radiation Injury to the Nervous System.* New York, NY: Raven Press; 1991:91–111.

77. van der Kogel AJ. *Late Effects of Radiation on the Spinal Cord Dose-Effect Relationships and Pathogenesis.* Rjswijk: Radiobiologic Institute of the Organization for Health Research; 1979.

78. van der Kogel AJ. Mechanisms of late radiation injury in the spinal cord. In: Meyn R, Withers H, eds. *Radiation Biology in Cancer Research.* New York, NY: Raven Press; 1980:461–470.

79. van der Kogel AJ. Radiation-induced nerve root degeneration and hypertrophic neuropathy in the lumbosacral spinal cord of rats: the relation with changes in aging rats. *Acta Neuropathol (Berl).* 1977;39:139–145.

80. van der Kogel AJ. Radiation tolerance of the rat spinal cord: time-dose relationships. *Radiology.* 1977;122:505–509.

81. van Luijk P, Bijl HP, Coppes RP, et al. Techniques for precision irradiation of the lateral half of the rat cervical spinal cord using 150 MeV protons [corrected]. *Phys Med Biol.* 2001;46:2857–2871.

82. van Luijk P, Bijl HP, Konings AW, et al. Data on dose-volume effects in the rat spinal cord do not support existing NTCP models. *Int J Radiat Oncol Biol Phys.* 2005;61:892–900.

83. Wang H, Shiu A, Wang C, et al. Dosimetric effect of translational and rotational errors for patients undergoing image-guided stereotactic body radiotherapy for spinal metastases. *Int J Radiat Oncol Biol Phys.* 2008;71:1261–1271.

84. Wang PY, Shen WC, Jan JS. Serial MRI changes in radiation myelopathy. *Neuroradiology.* 1995;37:374–377.

85. Weiss S, Dunne C, Hewson J, et al. Multipotent CNS stem cells are present in the adult mammalian spinal cord and ventricular neuroaxis. *J Neurosci.* 1996;16:7599–7609.

86. Withers HR, Taylor JM, Maciejewski B. Treatment volume and tissue tolerance. *Int J Radiat Oncol Biol Phys.* 1988;14:751–759.

87. Wong CS, Hao Y. Long-term recovery kinetics of radiation damage in rat spinal cord. *Int J Radiat Oncol Biol Phys.* 1997;37:171–179.

88. Wong CS, Minkin S, Hill RP. Linear-quadratic model underestimates sparing effect of small doses per fraction in rat spinal cord. *Radiother Oncol.* 1992;23:176–184.

89. Wong CS, Poon JK, Hill RP. Re-irradiation tolerance in the rat spinal cord: influence of level of initial damage. *Radiother Oncol.* 1993;26:132–138.

90. Wong CS, Van der Kogel AJ. Mechanisms of radiation injury to the central nervous system: implications for neuroprotection. *Mol Interv.* 2004;4:273–284.

91. Wong CS, Van Dyk J, Milosevic M, et al. Radiation myelopathy following single courses of radiotherapy and retreatment. *Int J Radiat Oncol Biol Phys.* 1994;30:575–581.

92. Wong CS, Van Dyk J, Simpson WJ. Myelopathy following hyperfractionated accelerated radiotherapy for anaplastic thyroid carcinoma. *Radiother Oncol.* 1991;20:3–9.

93. Yamada Y, Bilsky MH, Lovelock DM, et al. High-dose, single-fraction image-guided intensity-modulated radiotherapy for metastatic spinal lesions. *Int J Radiat Oncol Biol Phys.* 2008;71(2):484–490.

Yen-Lin Evelyn Chen
Thomas F. DeLaney

Peripheral Nerves

Radiation-induced peripheral neuropathy is most extensively studied for brachial plexus. Stoll and Andrews' first report of radiation-induced brachial plexopathy in 1966 challenged the long-held notion that adult nervous tissue is radioresistant.[1] Since then, it has been recognized that radiation-induced peripheral neuropathy can result from brachytherapy, intraoperative radiation, and high-dose external beam radiotherapy (EBRT) in the treatment of extremity soft-tissue sarcomas, tumors in the retroperitoneum, pelvis and inguinal region, or paraspinal soft tissue or bone sarcomas around the cauda equinae. Extensive experimental and clinical studies of intraoperative radiotherapy (IORT) suggest that 20 Gy is the tolerance dose for single fraction IORT.[2–10] Emami et al.[11] estimated the TD 5/5 for peripheral neuropathy to be 60 Gy and a TD 50/5 of 75 Gy in standard fractionation when the entire cauda was irradiated. This chapter describes the relevant anatomy of peripheral nerves as well as pathophysiology of radiation-induced peripheral neuropathy and plexopathy other than the brachial plexus, which is addressed in Chapter 23. We describe the clinical presentation, differential diagnoses, workup, risk factors, and treatment of radiation-induced peripheral neuropathy. We draw on experience from intraoperative radiation for retroperitoneal or pelvic tumors, high-dose external beam radiation for lumbosacral spine sarcomas, and external beam/brachytherapy for extremity sarcomas.

ANATOMY OF A PERIPHERAL NERVE

The main functional unit of a peripheral nerve is the nerve fiber, composed of an axon and its associated Schwann cells and myelin. A single Schwann cell covers an internode, or segment, of axon separated by nodes of Ranvier.[12] The peripheral nervous system's main three functions are motor, sensory, and autonomic. For each, the functional unit consists of a neuron, the nerve axon, a neurotransmission junction, and the end organ. For motor function, the lower motor neuron in the anterior horn of the spinal cord gives rise to myelinated and unmyelinated axons, which interface via the neuromuscular junction with the end-organ muscle fibers. For sensation, the dorsal root ganglion cells give rise to axons that junction with end-organ sensory receptors. The autonomic system has sensory fibers to the cord, and motor fibers to the endorgans, such as bladder.[12]

The organization of the peripheral nerve is illustrated in Figure 22-1.

Each nerve fiber consists of an axon, which may be myelinated or nonmyelinated by concentric layers of cytoplasmic membranes from Schwann cells along the length of the myelinated nerve fiber. There are areas between myelinated segments of a nerve fiber called the "nodes of Ranvier" where the cytoplasm of adjacent Schwann cells touches. Nerve impulses are conducted from one node of Ranvier to the next through salutatory conduction along the nerve fiber. The Schwann cells can remyelinate segments of an axon if there is damage.

Nerve fibers, both myelinated and unmyelinated, are grouped by layers of connective tissue and organized into peripheral nerve trunks. The *endoneurium* surrounds individual motor, sensory, or autonomic nerve fibers. Terminal arterioles, contained in the *perineurium*, feed the nerve fibers by sending penetrating branches, or *vasa nervorum*, into the Schwann cells and neurons that comprise nerve fibers. The endothelial cells of the endoneurial capillaries form tight junctions and a blood-nerve barrier throughout the length of the nerve. These fibers are then grouped into fascicles and enclosed by the fibrous *perineurium*. The *epineurium* then encloses all the fascicles that comprise the entire nerve as well as the blood supply to the nerve.[12]

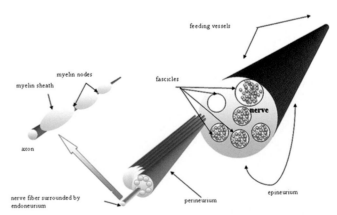

Figure 22.1. Schematic diagram of peripheral nerve. The endoneurium and nervorum envelop nerve fibers. Many nerve fibers form a fascicle surrounded by perineurium. Fascicles are then grouped into nerve by epineurium along with the feeding vessels. (Figure by Chen YL.)

TABLE 22.1	Major Named Nerves, Spinal Nerve Root Levels, and End Function		
Named Nerve	Spinal Nerve Root(s) of Origin	Motor Function	Sensation
Axillary	C5	Deltoid, teres minor, rotator cough	Shoulder
Musculocutaneous	C5,6	Biceps	None
Radial	C5,6	Brachioradialis	
	C6,7	Wrist extensors	
	C7,8	Finger extensors	
	C6,7,8	Triceps	
Median	C6, 7	Wrist flexors	Anterior palm, anterior thumb, index
	C8, T1	Abductor pollicus brevis	finger, and middle finger
Ulnar	C8, T1	Intrinsic muscles of hand	Ring and pinky fingers
Femoral	L2,3,4	Knee extension	Anterior medial thigh
			Medial leg and foot
Obturator	L2,3,4	Thigh adduction	Medial knee and posterior medial thigh
Lateral femoral cutaneous	L2-3	None	Anterior lateral and posterior thigh down to knee
Gluteal nerve	L4-S2	Piriformis, obturator internus, quadratus femoris, gemellus muscles	Upper medial buttock
Sciatic (giving rise to tibial and peroneal nerves	L5,S1	Knee flexion	
Peroneal	L4-5	Ankle dorsiflexion	Web space of 1st toe
			Distal anterior leg and dorsum of foot
Tibial	S1-2	Ankle plantar flexion	Sole of foot, medial heel lateral heel

Motor neuron rootlets mix with dorsal sensory rootlets to form mixed spinal nerves. Based on limb development, the mixed spinal nerves form the brachial plexus (C5-T1), lumbar plexus (L2-4), and sacral plexus (L4-S2). These plexus then give rise to the major peripheral nerves of the arms and legs that may be motor only, sensory only, or mixed (radial, median, ulnar, femoral, and sciatic nerves).[12] Table 22-1 details the major peripheral nerves in the body, the spinal nerve roots of origin, and the end functions of the nerves.

BIOLOGY OF PERIPHERAL NEUROPATHY

In general there are two major mechanisms of peripheral neuropathy depending on the end target of the injury: the Schwann cell or axon. In segmental demyelination, segments of myelin degenerate leaving internodes of denuded axon while the axon itself and the end-organ myocytes remain intact. The denuded axon stimulates remyelination by a population of endoneurium cells that can proliferate and give rise to new Schwann cells. However, the new myelin sheath may be thinner in proportion to the diameter of the axon. Over time, chronic demyelination and remyelination can cause secondary axonal injury.[12]

Sometimes a discrete localized event such as trauma or ischemia or an intrinsic neuron or axon problem can lead directly to axon degeneration. After transection, the distal end of the axon undergoes degeneration within a day and the associated Schwann cells catabolize myelin and engulf fragments of axon. Macrophages are recruited and phagocytose the axon and myelin debris. The associated muscle fibers in the motor unit undergo denervation atrophy, where myosin and actin are down regulated and the fibers become smaller but remain viable.[12]

The mechanism of peripheral nerve recovery has been well studied. First, the proximal stumps of degenerated axons can regenerate at a very slow process, limited by the slow speed of axonal transport (2 mm/d). The surviving axons in the vicinity also sprout connections to the orphaned muscles fibers and reinnervate the muscle fibers. Schwann cells also play a vital role in the regeneration of nerves. In a fully myelinated nerve, Schwann cells do not undergo mitosis.[13] In injured nerves, Schwann cells can proliferate to remyelinate the nerve fibers.[14]

Early studies by Janzen and Warren in rat peripheral nerve in 1942 suggested peripheral nerves were extremely radioresistant.[15] Follow-up time, however, was too short to observe late effects on peripheral nerves. Subsequent studies have observed, both in experimental models and in patient case reports, short-term and long-term histopathological changes in peripheral nerves after radiation.

Initial effects of irradiation on peripheral nerves can appear within a few days. Mendes et al. reported that radiation can cause early bioelectrical alterations, enzyme changes, disrupted microtubule assembly, and increased vascular permeability as early as 2 days after treatment.[16] However, histologic and clinical manifestation of the damage may not appear for much more time. Hassler[17] found that proliferation of Schwann cells after a single dose of 28 Gy to the mouse hind leg decreased early after irradiation, but demyelination was not seen up to 9 months postradiation.

The dose of radiation and subsequent injury to the nerve appear to be important factors for the severity of radiation-induced peripheral neuropathy. Cavanagh irradiated the rat sciatic nerve with 2 to 20 Gy and assessed the proliferation of Schwann cells 7 and 14 days after crush injury. He found a substantial decrease in the number of Schwann cells after 7 days at all doses. However by 14 days post-crush injury, Schwann cell numbers returned to normal levels with higher mitotic rates if the prior dose was 2 or 5 Gy, indicating that there was continued Schwann cell proliferation in response to injury following these radiation doses. After 20 Gy, however, there was only a negligible increase in Schwann cell proliferation at 14 days, reflecting a severely impaired Schwann cell proliferative response at this high dose. After 10 Gy, there was some increase on day 14, but still slightly below normal. Cavanagh suggested that a single dose of 10 Gy may be the threshold for impairing nerve repair in response to crush injury. In contrast, nerves irradiated with 10 Gy that were not crushed showed no morphological abnormality in the nerve fiber or vascular structure when assessed 14 days after radiation.[18]

The effects of radiation on peripheral nerves appear to be long-lasting. Cavanagh found similar Schwann cell proliferation capacity at day 14 after crush injury, whether the radiation (10 Gy) took place 3 weeks, 3, 6, or 9 months prior to the injury. The Schwann cells of these nerves had hyperchromatic, grossly enlarged nuclei, and abnormal mitotic figures. Based on this he concluded there is little cellular replacement in adult peripheral nerves after radiation.[19]

In another early study on radiation peripheral neuropathy, Love administered single doses of 15 or 20 Gy to mouse hind limbs 1 day before the sciatic nerve was crushed or 20 Gy 3 days after the injury and examined the ultrastructural changes in the distal sciatic and posterior tibial nerves up to 120 days after the treatment to answer this question. Irradiation with 15 Gy before crush injury initially reduced proliferation of endoneural cells but after a few weeks the cell numbers recovered to control levels. Remyelination was delayed but not completely impaired. However, when 20 Gy was administered preinjury, the myelin sheaths remained abnormally thin in proportion to axonal size. When 20 Gy was administered postinjury, endoneural cell proliferation was severely reduced and remained reduced for at least 90 days. The number of myelinating cells was insufficient for continuous myelination, and fibers showed thin or segmental demyelination and long intermodal lengths, suggesting that 20 Gy of radiation given pre-injury or postinjury is sufficient to severely impair peripheral nerve repair.[20]

SECONDARY PERIPHERAL NEUROPATHY

Secondary damage to a peripheral nerve can arise from compression due to fibrosis of the connective tissue around the nerve. The endoneurium, perineurium, or epineurium can become hyalinized and progressively lose elasticity, leading to contracture and compression of the nerve. Additional surgical manipulation (neurolysis) can potentially worsen ischemia by devascularizing the nerve.[21] However, separation of nerve from surrounding tissue may prevent fibrosis form entrapping the nerve.[22]

CLINICAL PRESENTATION AND DIAGNOSIS

Peripheral neuropathy may manifest as hypoesthesia, anesthesia, or hyperparesthesia in the affected limb or as monoplegia monoparesis of the affected limb. The risk of neuropathy increases with time, best documented in brachial plexopa-

thy. Powell et al. reported radiation brachial plexus neuropathy from several different fractionated radiation schedules appearing after 10 months.[23] Lumbosacral neuropathy after 20 to 25 Gy single doses of IORT can occur anywhere from 1 to 32 months.[2]

The diagnosis of radiation-induced neuropathy is usually made after CT and/or MRI imaging confirms the absence of tumor recurrence involving the suspected nerve or plexus using CT or MRI in the presence of symptoms, physical exam findings, and/or denervation of affected nerve on electromyography (EMG).

The most common etiology of neuropathy in an oncology patient is tumor involvement or compression. Patients should therefore undergo thorough workup for local tumor progression or metastases involving the affected peripheral nerve or nerve plexus. History should be carefully taken to determine the nature, location, onset, duration, and progression of the neuropathy.[24] It is important to assess whether the symptom consists of pain, paresis, paralysis, paresthesia, and/or anesthesia as well as extent (unilateral, bilateral, proximal, or distal). It is also important to assess whether the patient had the same symptoms on presentation, presurgery or postsurgery and to determine if the neuropathy is new or exacerbation of preexisting neuropathy.

Diagnostic workup includes laboratory tests including complete blood count, sedimentation rate, glucose, chemistry, thyroid function, vitamin B_{12}, folate, rheumatoid factors, hepatitis viral tests, and antinuclear antibodies to rule out other metabolic or nononcologic etiologies of the neuropathy.[24]

EMG may be helpful to evaluate the affected nerve(s) or end motor function. Reduced amplitude, slowed conduction velocity, or increase in latency can be observed and have been reported mostly in cases of brachial plexopathy.[25] However, EMG cannot distinguish between neoplastic and radiation-induced neuropathy.

Imaging studies are essential to determine any neurological involvement by tumor recurrence or treatment changes. This may include CT or MRI. Because of better soft-tissue definition, MRI is the study of choice to differentiate between tumor recurrence and treatment changes.[26] Radiation fibrosis can be low or high in signal intensity on T2 sequences. Biopsy of abnormal tissue around a nerve may be indicated if there is concern of tumor recurrence. Figures 22-2 and 22-3 show EMG and MRI findings in radiation-induced neuropathy.

Lastly, radiation associated tumors may also cause neuropathy, as reported in a case of a patient with progressive ulnar nerve failure 55 years after 22 Gy [226]Ra brachytherapy for hemangioma of the left elbow at 3 months. Workup found an intraneural neurofibroma as well as a nerve sheath ganglion causing nerve compression at the sulcus segment of the ulnar nerve and loss of function. The patient underwent removal of the segment and reconstruction with nerve graft. Therefore radiation-induced benign or malignant tumors need to be kept in the differential diagnosis of neuropathy in an irradiated site.[27]

GRADING OF PERIPHERAL NEUROPATHY

The grading of peripheral neuropathy should take into consideration the impact on sensory, motor units, and pain. This is done in several scoring systems including that used frequently in NCI Cooperative Group studies, the Common Terminology Criteria for Adverse Events (CTCAE version 3) grading scale,

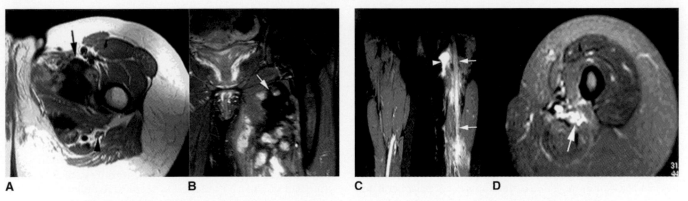

A   B   C   D

Figure 22.2. MRI of a patient with radiation neuropathy of the sciatic nerve. Patient initially underwent resection of fibromatosis followed by 50 Gy of postoperative radiation. The initial MRI (**A,B**) showed the fibromatosis in the vicinity but not involving the sciatic nerve (indicated by large areas of signal void in the MRI; dark and white arrow). One year later, the fibromatosis recurred superior to this area and additional 30 Gy was given, overlapping with the 50-Gy region. Two years later, patient developed progressive numbness and loss of dorsiflexion of the foot. MRI (**C,D**) showed extensive scarring of sciatic nerve. Symptoms improved after neurolysis of fibrotic tissue entrapping the sciatic nerve. (Printed from Gikas PD, Hanna SA, Aston W, et al. Post-radiation sciatic neuropathy: a case report and review of the literature. *World J Surg Oncol.* 2008;6(1):130, with permission.)

where: grade 1 is mild sensory deficits without motor deficit or pain; grade 2 is moderate sensory deficit, mild weakness, but no pain; grade 3 is continuous paresthesia with incomplete motor paresis, and pain requiring analgesics; grade 4 is complete motor paresis, muscle atrophy, excruciating pain. Gillette et al. had also proposed a staging system for peripheral nerves and muscle and soft tissue based on the late effects on normal tissues (LENT system) as well as subjective and objective observations, management, and analytic procedures (SOMA system).[22] Assessment for neuropathy is an important part of long-term follow-up of patients treated with high radiation dose to an area containing nerves with major functions.

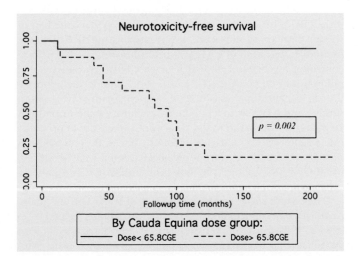

Figure 22.3. Neurotoxicity-free survival in patients treated with high-dose photon/proton radiotherapy to the cauda equina for spinal tumors. There was no lumbosacral neuropathy in patients treated with doses below 65.8 CGE (cobalt-Gy equivalent of protons to photons; assuming RBE of 1.1). Thirteen patients who developed neuropathy had median cauda equina dose of 73.1 CGE. (Reprinted from Pieters RS, Niemierko A, Fullerton BC, et al. Cauda equina tolerance to high-dose fractionated irradiation. *Int J Radiat Oncol Biol Phys.* 2006;64(1):251–257, with permission.)

EXPERIMENTAL AND CLINICAL OBSERVATIONS OF PERIPHERAL NEUROPATHY FROM IORT

A substantial amount of experimental data on dose relationship for peripheral neuropathy come from the work on IORT. IORT generally uses electrons as a method to boost tumor/tumor bed as a supplement to external beam radiation. Advantages for IORT boost include direct visualization of the target and protection of uninvolved tissue and organs by shielding or mobilizing away from the treatment field. Many animal and clinical studies of IORT have found peripheral neuropathy to be the main dose-limiting toxicity.

Kinsella et al. clinically observed five patients with lumbosacral or sciatic neuropathy within 9 months of IORT to a dose of 20 to 25 Gy. Three out of the five had nerve function recovery over several months but two had irreversible near-complete loss of extremity function. To explore this further, the authors created American Foxhound models of IORT and surgically exposed and irradiated the lumbosacral plexus and sciatic nerve with single dose of 20 to 75 Gy. At these doses, 19 of 21 irradiated dogs had clinically evident peripheral nerve injury. The time to onset of paresis ranged from 1 to 19 months in an inverse linear relationship to the dose, with shorter latencies with the larger doses. Histological evaluation found that loss of large myelinated fibers and perineural fibrosis were the main pathological lesions, similar to that observed in humans. They did not observe significant vascular injury.[2] These results suggested peripheral nerve is dose limiting for IORT.

Given the high rate of lumbosacral and sciatic nerve injury with single fractions of 20 to 25 Gy IORT, Kinsella et al. irradiated Foxhounds with 10, 15, or 20 Gy of 9 MeV electrons to assess the threshold for single fraction IORT. The authors shielded the left lumbrosacral plexus and sciatic nerves as internal control in a follow-up study. Neurological exam, EMG, and nerve conduction studies were performed at initially 1 month and then 3-month intervals for 3 years. With follow-up of ≥42 months, no dog receiving 10 or 15 Gy developed peripheral neuropathy, whereas all four dogs receiving 20 Gy had right leg paresis at 8, 9, 9, and 12 months posttreatment.[3]

LeCouteur et al. reported veterinary experience with IORT in beagle dogs 2 years following fractionated irradiation or intraoperative radiation or a combination of the two modalities. The authors performed both neurological examination and electrophysiological examinations to assess the time to onset of peripheral neuropathy. Dogs treated with EBRT alone from 50 to 80 Gy fractionated external beam radiation did not develop any neuropathy. Peripheral neuropathy appeared as early as 6 months after IORT to 35 Gy or more as well as 50 Gy EBRT plus IORT. Peripheral neuropathy increased with IORT doses of 15 Gy or more. Time to development of peripheral neuropathy after IORT alone was around 6 to 18 months with onset in some as late as 24 months. Neuropathy did not resolve in any of the affected animals. Histologically, the damaged nerves showed loss of axons and myelin. Axon and myelin decreased to approximately 60% of normal at 15 Gy of IORT and declined further with doses >15 Gy. The authors also observed increasing fibrosis of endoneurium, perineurium, and epineurium with increasing doses. Furthermore, vascular damage appeared to be important; at most IORT doses there was significant necrosis and hyalination of the media of small arteries and arterioles. The dose for 50% probability of severe vascular damage at the 2-year point was 19.5 Gy IORT alone and 18.7 Gy when combined with EBRT. After EBRT alone, there was minimal axon or myelin loss, and no necrosis or vascular hyalination was seen.[28]

A more recent series of studies by Vujaskovic et al.[5,6,7,29,30] reported 12, 20, 28 Gy single dose of 6-MeV electrons on exposed and isolated right sciatic nerve in beagle dogs with the left sciatic nerve as internal control. As a surgical control another group had surgical exposure of nerve only without radiation. After 12 months, the nerves were evaluated for morphological changes. The authors found threshold dose for severe radiation damage was between 20 and 25 Gy. Morphologically there was direct decrease in Schwann cell population and well decrease in nerve fiber density, especially in the central portion of a nerve in large nerves at doses higher than 20 Gy. On electron microscopy, microtubule and neurofilamaent density is increased within the axons of nerves. They hypothesized a sequence of events leading to peripheral neuropathy starts with radiation-induced vascular damage that causes hypoxia. This ultimately leads to axon damage and nerve fiber dropout. They noted that the volume of irradiated nerve and surrounding tissues including muscle and vasculature or combination of IORT with other treatments can worsen neuropathy. For example, they estimated that the thermal enhancement ratio when IORT is combined with hyperthermia is approximately 1.5 with ED50 for paresis of 15 Gy at 2 years.[7]

Findings from these experimental models were consistent with clinical observation. Kinsella and other reported the neuropathy rates from an NCI randomized trial comparing IORT with 20 Gy using high-energy electrons followed by 35 to 40 Gy postoperative external beam irradiation versus standard therapy of 50 to 55 Gy postoperative external beam irradiation. At median follow-up of 5 years, there were a significant number of patients (4 out of 15) in the IORT arm compared to only 1 out of 20 patients in the standard arm with lumbosacral, femoral, or sciatic neuropathy 6 to 9 months after treatment with symptoms of moderate to severe pain. All had mixed motor/sensory deficits. In two patients, EMG and nerve conduction studies showed reduced motor unit activity and reduced velocity and amplitude of the nerve action potential. All four IORT patients experienced gradual decrease in pain and regained function over several months with conservative measures. The one patient in the control arm had neuropathy directly related to surgery.[2,4] Updates of the NCI study at 10 years of follow-up found two patients (13%) developed mild neuropathy and seven (47%) had moderate or severe neuropathy for a total of 60% with peripheral neuropathy. The high rate was thought to be due to the 20-Gy IORT dose.[9]

Shaw et al. reported on 51 patients treated with IORT as a component of treatment for primary or recurrent pelvic malignancies (colorectal 38 patients) with 30 to 68.9 Gy EBRT (median of 50.4 Gy) followed by surgical debulking and IORT of 10 to 25 Gy (median 17.5 Gy) with 9 to 18 MeV electrons. Fifty patients were evaluable for neurotoxicity. Sixteen (32%) developed peripheral neuropathy. All 16 had pain. Eleven had numbness and tingling, and eight had actual weakness. In 40% of patients, pain, numbness, and tingling resolved. However only one of eight patients with weakness experienced improvement over time. IORT doses 15 Gy or more increased the risk of peripheral neuropathy. External beam dose did not impact incidence of neuropathy, although these results were similarly high as the NCI study that used 20 Gy.[31]

Doses of IORT <20 Gy result in lower neuropathy rate. Gunderson reported in 20 patients with locally advanced or recurrent soft-tissue sarcomas or desmoids primarily in the retroperitoneum treated with 45 to 60 Gy fractionated EBRT and IORT of 10 to 20 Gy, only one patient (5%) developed severe neuropathy.[32] Alektiar et al. reported IORT for retroperitoneal sarcoma using high-dose rate iridium-125 permanent implant to 12 to 15 Gy combined with 45 to 50 Gy EBRT resulted in an acceptable 6% peripheral neuropathy rate.[33]

Petersen et al. reported on the Mayo Clinic experience of intraoperative electron beam radiotherapy in the management of retroperitoneal soft-tissue sarcomas. Eighty-seven patients with either primary or recurrent retroperitoneal or intrapelvic sarcomas were treated with IORT. Median tumor size was 10 cm (2–36 cm). All patients had maximal surgical resection with IORT with doses ranging from 8.75 to 30 Gy (median of 15 Gy). Primary tumors were also treated with EBRT of 45 Gy. At median follow-up of 3.5 years, the author reported 77% local control at 3 years and 59% at 5 years.[34] Thirteen patients had mild peripheral neuropathy (15%), 10 had moderate neuropathy (11%), and 9 patients had severe neuropathy (10%). Both surgery and IORT were felt to be contributory to neuropathy in 16 patients. Compared to the prior two studies, the neuropathy rate was lower.[35] Willett et al.[36] found that in 20 patients with primary or recurrent retroperitoneal sarcoma treated with 40 to 50 Gy EBRT followed by resection and IORT, two patients (10%) developed neuropathy.

The largest series on the late effects of IORT is from Spain. Azinovic et al. reported on 195 out of 739 patients treated from 1984 to 1991 for a number of diagnoses who were alive at least 5 years after IORT using a modified LENT/SOMA scale. With mean follow-up of 94 months in the surviving patients (range 55–162 months), 25% of extremity, 20% of thoracic, and 8% of pelvic IORT patients experienced peripheral neuropathy with median doses of 15 Gy. Patients treated with IORT to large areas of extremities experienced grade 4 neuropathy, including one amputation due to severe neurovascular damage. The author found that treatment intensity (surgery + IORT ± EBRT ± chemotherapy) correlated with severity of toxicity.[37]

As most patients are managed in a multidisciplinary fashion, causes of neuropathy may be multifactorial. Specific analysis including potential contribution of chemotherapy and surgical manipulation is needed to precisely determine the component secondary to IORT. However, based on existing animal and clinical data, the maximal tolerance dose of peripheral nerve to single fraction radiation appears to be 15 Gy, above which neuropathy rate increases significantly. Therefore, the decision to administer IORT should take into consideration proper patient selection with regard to the presence of a critical nerve in the field, the degree of surgical manipulation, and the intensity of other prior/expected adjuvant treatment. When possible, nerves not involved by tumor or at risk for microscopic disease should be shielded from the IORT.

PERIPHERAL NEUROPATHY FROM TREATMENT OF EXTREMITY SARCOMAS

The limb salvage approach to the treatment of extremity sarcoma is well established and for the majority of patients is the preferred local control option. Careful assessment of peripheral nerves involved and expected postoperative function may be one of the most critical factors in determining whether limb conservation is possible, especially in borderline cases. If a tumor abuts but not circumferentially surrounds an essential peripheral nerve, then radiation and epineural dissection may allow salvage of the nerve. However, if the tumor circumferentially involves the tumor, then nerve sacrifice may be necessary for optimal local control. In the latter situation, reconstruction options to preserve limb function are available, including nerve grafting, distal nerve transfer, and tendon transfer. However, completely normal limb function is unlikely. In some cases, amputation and prosthesis may result in better function if there is extensive nerve involvement that is not likely to downstage from preoperative radiotherapy. The orthopedic surgical oncologist plays an important role in this decision.[38]

For patients who are candidates for limb salvage therapy with combined modality therapy (surgery, preoperative vs. postoperative radiotherapy, ± chemotherapy), there is a paucity of reports of radiation-associated peripheral neuropathy in patient with extremity sarcoma treated with radiation and limb conserving surgery. The Canadian randomized trial comparing 50-Gy preoperative radiotherapy versus 60-Gy postoperative radiotherapy reported the 2-year incidence of grade 2 fibrosis (31.5% vs. 48.2%, respectively), joint stiffness (17.8% vs. 23.2%), and edema (15.5% vs. 23.2%). However, no late neuropathy was reported. Two years was likely too early to detect neuropathy.[39]

For patients who have unresected soft-tissue sarcoma, higher doses may be necessary. Kepka et al. reported a series of 112 patients treated with definitive radiotherapy for gross soft-tissue sarcoma, 43% in the extremities, 26% retroperitoneal, 24% in the head and neck, and 7% in the truncal wall for median tumor size of 8 cm to a median dose of 64 Gy (range 25–87.5 Gy). Patients who received doses 63 Gy or greater had higher local control compared to <63 Gy. Four patients developed severe neuropathy: one within a year after 75 Gy at 1.8 Gy BID, one at 10 years after 66 Gy at 2 Gy/fraction, and two with severe fibrosis as well as limb weakness leaving useless leg at 68 Gy at 2 Gy/fraction and 70 Gy (50 Gy with 2 Gy/fraction and 20 Gy IORT) both within 1 year of treatment. The authors

concluded that doses of 63 to 67 Gy resulted in good control without added toxicity while doses >68 Gy were associated with greater complication rate of 26% (including neuropathy, fibrosis, wound complications requiring major surgery, soft tissue and bone necrosis, stenosis) versus 8% ($p = 0.02$).[40]

IORT IN EXTREMITY SOFT-TISSUE SARCOMA

IORT is uncommonly used in extremity soft-tissue sarcoma, likely due to high neuropathy rate from a single large fraction. Azinovic reported on the late effects of 45 patients with extremity soft-tissue sarcoma treated with IORT and moderate-dose postoperative radiotherapy (45–50 Gy). Twenty-six patients had primary tumor and nineteen had isolated local recurrence after prior therapy at the time of treatment. At 5 years, 88% of patients with negative/close margins and 57% of patients with positive margins had local control. Neuropathy developed in five patients (11%). One patient had grade 1 (paresthesia not interfering with daily life). Four patients had grade 3 to 4 neurotoxicity (weakness and/or sensory loss or paresthesia interfering with daily life). No patient had paralysis. Of the five patients, three had nerve included in the IORT field. The neuropathy rate was 25% (3 out of 12) in patients with peripheral nerve included in the IORT field compared to 11% (2 out of 18 patients) if nerve was not included. The time to neurotoxicity was 13 months (range 8–21 months). Three of the five patients recovered (two partially, one completely) 12 months after onset of neuropathy. Two of the patients with grade 3 or 4 neuropathy recovered sufficiently to lead normal daily life while other two had non-reversible neuropathy. The risk factors for neuropathy were tumor size >12 cm and/or IORT doses >15 Gy (in 4/5 patients with neuropathy). Based on these findings, the authors instituted a policy to displace any nerve included in the target. If nerve displacement cannot be accomplished without traction damage or perineural dissection, then 5 Gy is delivered without shielding followed by 10 Gy with shielding using lead layers. If a nerve is inside a low-risk area, on the other hand, it is shielded for the entire procedure.[41]

Beroukas et al. reported 36 patients with soft-tissue sarcoma of the extremities treated with resection, IORT combined with external beam radiation with a median dose of 45 Gy, of whom 12 (33%) had moderate neurotoxicity.[42] These high rates of neuropathy compared to external beam radiation or brachytherapy make single fraction IORT less appealing in the treatment of extremity soft-tissue sarcomas where there is often a critical peripheral nerve in the tumor bed in situations that may warrant a boost (close or positive margin).

BRACHYTHERAPY

In general, brachytherapy appears to be well tolerated with few reported peripheral neuropathies. Zelefsky et al. reported of 299 patients with extremity sarcomas treated with limb-sparing surgery and iridium-192 interstitial implant at Memorial Sloan-Kettering Cancer Center, 15% had locally advanced tumors abutting or encasing major neurovascular structures. Two-thirds of these patients had high-grade lesions and 11% had gross residual disease and another 58% had microscopic disease. A median dose of 44 Gy was delivered. Four patients (9%) developed radiation neuropathy at 6 to 20 months after treatment, all of whom had additional radiation beyond brachytherapy with cumulative doses exceeding 90 Gy to the neurovascular bundle. Eighty-four percent of the patients had preservation of limb function in long-term follow-up.[43]

In a more recent series, Alektiar and others assessed patients with primary high-grade soft-tissue sarcoma of the extremity treated with limb-conserving surgery and adjuvant brachytherapy with remote after loading catheters placed in the tumor bed. Patients were treated to a median dose of 45 Gy delivered over 5 days. The implant dose was prescribed to the median peripheral dose rate using the first and lowest isodose rate line that is continuous to ensure homogeneity and reduce hot spots. The median dose rate was 0.40 Gy/h using iridium-192 in most patients and iridium-125 in patients with adjacent radiosensitive structures such as skin or gonads. With median of 61 months of follow-up, the incidence of grade 3 or worse nerve damage after postoperative radiation was 5%. Neuropathy was twice as common in patients with lower extremity sarcomas.[44] Some of the patients included were drawn from the MSKCC randomized trial of surgery versus surgery and adjuvant brachytherapy. In that trial, the peripheral neuropathy rate was 9% at median follow-up of 100 month in the brachytherapy arm versus 5% in the control (surgical) arm.[45]

Another report described 10 patients treated with interstitial perioperative high-dose rate brachytherapy of 3 Gy/fraction twice daily at 10 mm from plane of sources to 18 to 30 Gy and external beam radiotherapy of 40 to 50 Gy for soft-tissue sarcomas. At median follow-up of 46 months, all 10 patients were locally controlled, and 1 patient had a mild peripheral neuropathy.[46]

A recent report by Kubo and others from Japan described seven patients with STS involving neurovascular bundle treated with limb-preserving surgery and fractionated HDR brachytherapy for negative margin or positive margin using iridium-192 to a total dose of 50 Gy in six patients and 30 Gy plus 20 Gy EBRT in one. With a median follow-up of 4 years, none of the patients developed peripheral neuropathy. The authors performed motor nerve conduction tests of the preserved peripheral nerves in three out of five survivors who were evaluable (sciatic nerve in two and median nerve in one) and found normal conduction velocity 43 to 75 months after brachytherapy.[47] Therefore, it appears that at most standard doses, both LDR and HDR are well tolerated for peripheral nerves; however, most of the reports are limited by relatively short follow-up. Longer follow-up on brachytherapy series would help ascertain these early observations.

SPECIFIC CASE REPORTS ON EXTREMITY PERIPHERAL NEUROPATHY

There are a few detailed case reports of radiation-associated peripheral neuropathy. These case reports describe in depth the patient, tumor, and treatment characteristics as well as the presenting symptoms, differential diagnosis, workup, and management of the neuropathy. These reports illustrate the complex multifactorial nature of neuropathy.

Femoral Neuropathy

The femoral nerve arises from the L2, L3, and L4 and constitute the largest branch of the lumbar plexus. The origins of the femoral nerve is within the psoas major muscle and descends posterolaterally along the pelvis. The femoral nerve crosses the midpoint of the inguinal ligament after which it courses lateral

to the femoral vessels outside the femoral sheath. Distal to the femoral triangle, the femoral nerve divides into terminal branches that supply the anterior thigh muscles as well as cutaneous branches over the anteromedial side of the lower extremity and deep articular branches to the hip and knee joints. The femoral sheath that encloses the proximal portions of the femoral vessels lie within the inguinal ligament but does not enclose the femoral nerve. Traumatic femoral neuropathy is well described.[48] Femoral nerve compression syndrome was first reported from Scandinavia in four patients who had quadriceps paresis 12 to 16 months after treatment due to fibrosis in the inguinal region.[49] The patients were treated with decompression, intradural phenoglycerin injection, cortisone, and oxiphenbutazxone, with three out of four experiencing pain relief.[49]

A more recent report of femoral neuropathy in 1991 described a patient who had been treated for transitional cell carcinoma of the urinary bladder to 2,750 cGy in 12 fractions with cobalt radiation to the bladder using fields directed from the groin bilaterally.[16] Four months post-treatment, the patient developed a fibrotic scar in each side of the groin where he began to have constant pain radiating to the knee. The patient progressed to have paresthesias and burning pain in the medial aspects of the thigh and knee bilaterally and was unable to walk more than 500 m or sit comfortable. Subsequently, patient developed quadriceps weakness. EMG of the quadriceps showed increased motor unit potentials at rest that decreased with maximal muscle activity. At rest, there were fibrillations and positive denervation potentials. The authors concluded this was consistent with fibrosis and entrapment of the nerve. Pelvic traction, anti-inflammatory drugs, and conservative measures failed to alleviate his symptoms. The authors released the femoral nerve operatively on both sides. Endoneurolysis was performed to release fibrotic tissue and decompress the nerve. Immediately postoperatively, the patient had complete sensory and motor paralysis of the right femoral nerve. The paresthesias and pain decreased over 3 months and motor function recovered over 5 months, although not to a preoperative level. After 17 months, EMG showed signs of regeneration in both lower extremities. Ten years after the endoneurolysis, the patient had continued improvement. In this case, the femoral nerves likely received significantly higher dose than 2,750 cGy due to the use of cobalt radiation and relative high dose at superficial depth.[16] This case report illustrates the importance of recognizing fibrosis as a cause of neuropathy and potential effectiveness of endoneurolysis.

Sciatic Neuropathy

The sciatic nerve arises from L4, L5, S1, S2, and S3 nerve roots from two distinct trunks: the lateral peroneal division and the medial tibial division which form the sciatic nerve and divide at midthigh to the distal thigh to form common peroneal and tibial nerves. Sciatic neuropathy is a common orthopedic complaint and can result from focal lesion of the nerve at hip or thigh distal to the lumbosacral plexus but proximal to the distal branches. Most common etiologies are traumatic, compressive, ischemic, or neoplastic from extrinsic tumors or sciatic nerve tumors.[50] Radiation-induced sciatic neuropathy, however, is extremely uncommon. The only reported case of published post-radiation sciatic neuropathy was in 2008.[51] A patient with a left thigh adductor compartment shown on biopsy to have musculoaponeurotic fibromatosis underwent complete excision and postoperative radiotherapy to 50 Gy in 25 fractions over

5 weeks. One-year posttreatment, she developed a recurrence in the postero-medial thigh distal to the previous radiation field and underwent reresection followed by postoperative radiotherapy to 30 Gy in 2 Gy/fraction over 4 weeks with 1 in overlap with the initial treatment field. One year later, the patient developed a recurrence proximal to the initial treatment field for which further excision and Tamoxifen was used. One year later, the patient developed progressive left foot weakness on dorsiflexion associated with pain on the medial aspect of foot and sole. Patient had absent hip adduction and ankle tendon reflex, weak foot and toe extension and eversion, but intact posterior cutaneous sensation indicating an intact sacral plexus but sciatic neuropathy. There was dense scarring in the area of radiation overlap on exam and corresponding edema and swelling of the sciatic nerve. On EMG, there was a non localizing sciatic nerve injury. The patient underwent neurolysis, which halted further deterioration of sciatic nerve function but had persistent weak foot dorsiflexion 5 years after neurolysis.

SACRAL PLEXOPATHY: EXPERIENCE FROM HIGH-DOSE EXTERNAL BEAM RADIATION FOR PARASPINAL SARCOMAS

The lumbar plexus (L2-4) and sacral plexus (L4-S2) arise from the cauda equinae and give rise to the major peripheral nerves of the perineum and lower extremity. Information on the tolerance of lumbosacral plexus comes from high-dose treatment of spine and paraspinal sarcomas.[34]

The most thorough attempt to characterize the tolerance of lumbosacral plexus and cauda equina came from Pieters et al. in 2006. This report provides the first long-term follow-up data on neurotoxicity associated with high-dose radiotherapy to the cauda equine in patients with lumbar, sacral, or retroperitoneal tumors.[52] Fifty-three patients were treated up to 84.6 cobalt-Gray equivalent (CGE) at 2 CGE/fraction for lumbar/sacral chordomas or other retroperitoneal sarcomas with median cauda equinae dose of 65.8 CGE (range 31.9–95.1). At median follow-up of 87 months, 13 patients had neurological toxicity unrelated to tumor recurrence; the median cauda equinae dose of this group was 73.7 CGE. One third of the patients developed severe progressive debility pain of LENT scale grade 4; two thirds had moderate pain that did not exceed LENT grade 2. All grade 4 toxicities occurred at cauda doses exceeding 73 CGE. At doses below the median dose of 65.8 CGE, the risk of cauda equinae toxicity was significantly less likely. The authors noted that these high doses had been given for attempted local control of gross residual neoplasms that required high dose such as chordomas, chondrosarcomas, and osteosarcomas.[52]

The authors differentiated pain or neurological deficits after high-dose radiotherapy from either local recurrence or radiation injury but recognized the difficulty of differentiating tumor regrowth from scar tissue and differentiating between neurological injuries from other causes of pain such as surgical scarring or mechanical stresses from decreased structural integrity of involved vertebrae. Progressive tumors were typically confirmed upon serial imaging and, ultimately, biopsy. In the absence of tumor recurrence, efforts were made to distinguish which symptoms were present at the end of treatment and therefore not considered toxic events versus new or exacerbation of symptoms.

In two patients, sequential CT or MRI imaging leads to diagnosis of local recurrence initially attributed to neurotoxicity.[52]

On multivariate analysis, cauda dose was statistically significant for neurotoxicity ($p = 0.002$). Male gender was also associated with greater toxicity. The estimated TD 5/5 and TD 50/5 were 55 and 72 CGE in males and 67 and 84 CGE in females. Interestingly, it was noted that 7/13 of the neurotoxicities occurred 5 years or more after treatment. TD 5/10 was 8 CGE lower and might continue to decrease with longer follow-up. The probability of neurotoxicity is therefore likely a relatively steep function of dose to the cauda equine with the slope at the gamma 50 (i.e., the dose level producing 50% neuropathy) = 3. The authors cautioned that the gender difference may be related to small numbers and therefore preliminary.[52]

OTHER FACTORS THAT MAY CONTRIBUTE TO RADIATION-ASSOCIATED PERIPHERAL NEUROPATHY

CHEMOTHERAPY

There are insufficient data to conclude whether chemotherapy increases the incidence of peripheral neurotoxicity. The MGH pilot of MAID chemotherapy at 48 months median follow-up did not note any neuropathy, although the follow-up may not be long enough yet.[53] The RTOG phase III trial 9514 on neoadjuvant chemotherapy and radiation therapy in the management of high-risk high-grade soft-tissue sarcomas of the extremities and body wall found local control rate of 82.4%. One percent of patients had grade 3 peripheral neuropathy, none with grade 4.[54] Cassady reported four cases of children receiving radiation therapy with concurrent vincristine who developed severe and prolonged unilateral neuropathy on the side of irradiation, suggesting that vincristine likely enhanced radiation effect on peripheral nerves.[55] Therefore, it is important to consider the contribution of radiosensitization from prior or concurrent adjuvant chemotherapy when evaluating a patient with possible radiation associated peripheral neuropathy.

REIRRADIATION AND NEUROPATHY

Reirradiation resulting in high cumulative dose to peripheral nerve can increase the risk of peripheral neuropathy.[45] The timing of neuropathy after reirradiation may be shorter than primary irradiation and may appear as early as within 2 years. For example, in 74 patients with locally recurrent rectal cancer with 10 to 18 Gy of HDR-IORT plus or minus additional EBRT, the rate of peripheral neuropathy was 16% with only 22 months of follow-up.[56] Reirradiation of patients with recurrent gynecologic tumors with radical resection and HDR-IORT with median dose of 14 Gy (12–15 Gy) resulted in 18% neuropathy with median follow-up of 20 months.[57] Therefore, it is important to consent patients undergoing reirradiation to the higher risk of peripheral neuropathy.

RADIATION PERIPHAL NEUROPATHY IN CHILDREN

While external beam radiation at doses <68 Gy or IORT <20 Gy in adults, children may be more sensitive. Paulino reported the results of 15 children with extremity sarcoma (including Ewings, synovial sarcoma, alveolar rhabdomyosarcoma, and fibrosarcoma in the lower or upper extremities. Doses ranged from 45 to 66 Gy (median dose 55.8 Gy) definitive treatment in 9 children and postoperatively in 6 (41.4–66.4 Gy). Two children (13%) developed peripheral neuropathy. One had received IORT boost of 25 Gy after 41.4 Gy external beam radiation and developed ulnar sensory dysfunction 11 years after RT. Another developed radial nerve palsy 3 years after postoperative radiation.[58] Calvo et al. reported on 38 pediatric patients with localized Ewings or osteosarcoma treated with IORT for either primary disease (90%) or locally recurrent, previously irradiated disease (10%). Doses of 10 to 20 Gy using 6 to 20 MeV electrons were used. At 25 months median follow-up, two patients developed local recurrence. Severe neuropathy was seen in seven patients.[59] Therefore, caution must be used when using high-dose EBRT or IORT in children, who often receive concurrent chemotherapy, which may be radiosensitizing.

TREATMENT OF RADIATION-INDUCED PERIPHERAL NEUROPATHY

Unfortunately, like brachial plexopathy, extremity and lumbosacral peripheral nerve plexopathy can become a permanent and debilitating complication. Treatment of radiation-induced neuropathy and plexopathy included oral medications or release of fibrotic tissue around the peripheral nerves/plexus (neurolysis) with variable results.[16,49,60] Anezaki reported a case of post-irradiation lumbosacral radiculopathy successfully treated with corticosteroid and warfarin.[61] Most reports of treatment approaches are anecdotal. A recent report described two patients with progressive radiation associated lumbosacral polyradiculopathy who experienced a significant clinical improvement over several years in their neurological sensorimotor symptoms with long-term pentoxifylline-tocopherol-clodronate treatment without significant side effects.[62] More research remains to be done to find successful treatments for radiation peripheral neuropathy.

SUMMARY

Peripheral nerves are susceptible to radiation damage. Single-dose tolerance for IORT appears to be around 15 Gy with increasing neuropathy rate at 20 Gy or greater; hence, fraction size is very important. TD 5/5 of lumbosacral nerve appears to be 65 Gy and between 63 and 67 Gy for extremity peripheral nerves, with possible lower thresholds in children or concurrent chemotherapy. Brachytherapy at doses of 45–50 Gy for extremity sarcomas appear to have acceptable peripheral neuropathy rates with attention to peripheral nerve in field. Recognition of fibrosis and compression as treatable causes of radiation associated peripheral neuropathy is important. However, intrinsic peripheral neuropathy can be difficult to manage with variable relief from treatments. Therefore, careful selection of treatment modality, avoidance of hot spots (which result in both focally higher fraction size and total dose), consideration of patient characteristics including age and prior surgical manipulation, chemotherapy treatment or irradiation and appropriate choice of dose fractionation and technique are important to reduce the risk of radiation-induced peripheral neuropathy.

REFERENCES

1. Stoll BA, Andrews JT. Radiation-induced peripheral neuropathy. *Br Med J.* 1966; 1(5491):834.
2. Kinsella TJ, Sindelar WF, DeLuca AM, et al. Tolerance of peripheral nerve to intraoperative radiotherapy (IORT): clinical and experimental studies. *Int J Radiat Oncol Biol Phys.* 1985;11(9):1579–1585.
3. Kinsella TJ, DeLuca AM, Barnes M, et al. Threshold dose for peripheral neuropathy following intraoperative radiotherapy (IORT) in a large animal model. *Int J Radiat Oncol Biol Phys.* 1991;20(4):697–701.
4. Kinsella TJ, Sindelar WF, Lack E, et al. Preliminary results of a randomized study of adjuvant radiation therapy in resectable adult retroperitoneal soft tissue sarcomas. *J Clin Oncol.* 1988;6(1):18.
5. Vujaskovic Z. Structural and physiological properties of peripheral nerves after intraoperative irradiation. *J Peripher Nerv Syst.* 1997;2(4):343–349.
6. Vujaskovic Z, Gillette SM, Powers BE, et al. Intraoperative radiation (IORT) injury to sciatic nerve in a large animal model. *Radiother Oncol.* 1994;30(2):133–139.
7. Vujaskovic Z, Gillette SM, Powers BE, et al. Effects of intraoperative irradiation and intraoperative hyperthermia on canine sciatic nerve: neurologic and electrophysiologic study. *Int J Radiat Oncol Biol Phys.* 1996;34(1):125–131.
8. Sindelar WF, Kinsella TJ. Normal tissue tolerance to intraoperative radiotherapy. *Surg Oncol Clin N Am.* 2003;12(4):925–942.
9. Sindelar WF, Kinsella TJ, Chen PW, et al. Intraoperative radiotherapy in retroperitoneal sarcomas: final results of a prospective, randomized, clinical trial. *Arch Surg.* 1993;128(4): 402–410.
10. Vujaskovic Z, Gillette SM, Powers BE, et al. Ultrastructural morphometric analysis of peripheral nerves after intraoperative irradiation. *Int J Radiat Biol.* 1995;68(1):71.
11. Emami B, Lyman J, Brown A, et al. Tolerance of normal tissue to therapeutic irradiation. *Int J Radiat Oncol Biol Phys.* 1991;21(1):109–122.
12. Kumar V, Robbins SL. *Robbins and Cotran Pathologic Basis of Disease* [Internet]. 8th ed. Philadelphia, PA: Saunders/Elsevier [cited 2009 Dec 2]. Available from: http://nrs.harvard.edu/urn-3:hul.ebook:MDCON_9440183
13. Evans DHL, Vizoso AD. Observations on the mode of growth of motor nerve fibers in rabbits during post-natal development. *J Comp Neurol.* 1951;95(3):429–461.
14. Abercrombie M, Johnson ML. Quantitative histology of Wallerian degeneration: I. Nuclear population in rabbit sciatic nerve. *J Anat.* 1946;80(pt 1):37–50.
15. Janzen A, Warren S. Effect of roentgen rays on the peripheral nerve of the rat. *Radiology.* 1942;38:333–337.
16. Mendes DG, Nawalkar RR, Eldar S. Post-irradiation femoral neuropathy. A case report. *J Bone Joint Surg Am.* 1991;73(1):137–140.
17. Hassler O. Cellular kinetics of the peripheral nerve and striated muscle after a single dose of x-rays: a histological and autoradiographical study, using 3H-thymidine. *Z Zellforsch Mikrosk Anat.* 1968;85(1):62–66.
18. Cavanagh JB. Effects of X-irradiation on the proliferation of cells in peripheral nerve during allerian degeneration in the rat. *Br J Radiol.* 1968;41(484):275–281.
19. Cavanagh J. Prior X-irradiation and the cellular response to nerve crush: duration of effect. *Exp Neurol.* 1968;22(2):253–258.
20. Love S. An experimental study of peripheral nerve regeneration after x-irradiation. *Brain.* 1983;106(1):39.
21. Teixeira MJ, Fonoff ET, Montenegro MC. Dorsal root entry zone lesions for treatment of pain-related to radiation-induced plexopathy. *Spine.* 2007;32(10):E316–E319.
22. Gillette EL, Mahler PA, Powers BE, et al. Late radiation injury to muscle and peripheral nerves. *Int J Radiat Oncol Biol Phys.* 1995;31(5):1309–1318.
23. Powell S, Cooke J, Parsons C. Radiation-induced brachial plexus injury: follow-up of two different fractionation schedules. *Radiother Oncol.* 1990;18(3):213–220.
24. Vasic L. Radiation-induced peripheral neuropathies: etiopathogenesis, risk factors, differential diagnostics, symptoms and treatment. *Arch Oncol.* 2007;15(3–4):81–84.
25. Wadd NJ, Lucraft HH. Brachial plexus neuropathy following mantle radiotherapy. *Clin Oncol (R Coll Radiol).* 1998;10(6):399–400.
26. Hoeller U, Bonacker M, Bajrovic A, et al. Radiation-induced plexopathy and fibrosis. *Strahlenther Onkol.* 2004;180(10):650–654.
27. Lohmeyer JA, Kimmig B, Gocht A, et al. Combined manifestation of a neurofibroma and a nerve sheath ganglion in the ulnar nerve after radiotherapy in early childhood. *J Plast Reconstr Aesthet Surg.* 2007;60(12):1338–1341.
28. LeCouteur RA, Gillette EL, Powers BE, et al. Peripheral neuropathies following experimental intraoperative radiation therapy (IORT). *Int J Radiat Oncol Biol Phys.* 1989;17(3): 583–590.
29. Vujaskovic Z, Gillette SM, Powers BE, et al. Ultrastructural morphometric analysis of peripheral nerves after intraoperative irradiation. *Int J Radiat Biol.* 1995;68(1):71–76.
30. Vujaskovic Z, Powers BE, Paardekoper G, et al. Effects of intraoperative irradiation (IORT) and intraoperative hyperthermia (IOHT) on canine sciatic nerve: histopathological and morphometric studies. *Int J Radiat Oncol Biol Phys.* 1999;43(5):1103–1109.
31. Shaw EG, Gunderson LL, Martin JK, et al. Peripheral nerve and ureteral tolerance to intraoperative radiation therapy: clinical and dose-response analysis. *Radiother Oncol.* 1990;18(3):247–255.
32. Gunderson LL, Nagorney DM, McIlrath DC, et al. External beam and intraoperative electron irradiation for locally advanced soft tissue sarcomas. *Int J Radiat Oncol Biol Phys.* 1993;25(4):647–656.
33. Alektiar KM, Hu K, Anderson L, et al. High-dose-rate intraoperative radiation therapy (HDR-IORT) for retroperitoneal sarcomas. *Int J Radiat Oncol Biol Phys.* 2000;47(1): 157–163.
34. DeLaney TF, Liebsch NJ, Pedlow FX, et al. Phase II study of high-dose photon/proton radiotherapy in the management of spine sarcomas. *Int J Radiat Oncol Biol Phys.* 2009;74(3): 732–739.

35. Petersen IA, Haddock MG, Donohue JH, et al. Use of intraoperative electron beam radiotherapy in the management of retroperitoneal soft tissue sarcomas. *Int J Radiat Oncol Biol Phys.* 2002;52(2):469–475.
36. Willett CG, Suit HD, Tepper JE, et al. Intraoperative electron beam radiation therapy for retroperitoneal soft tissue sarcoma. *Cancer.* 1991;68(2):278–283.
37. Azinovic I, Calvo FA, Puebla F, et al. Long-term normal tissue effects of intraoperative electron radiation therapy (IOERT): late sequelae, tumor recurrence, and second malignancies. *Int J Radiat Oncol Biol Phys.* 2001;49(2):597–604.
38. Ferguson PC. Surgical considerations for management of distal extremity soft tissue sarcomas. *Curr Opin Oncol.* 2005;17(4):366–369.
39. Davis AM, O'Sullivan B, Turcotte R, et al. Late radiation morbidity following randomization to preoperative versus postoperative radiotherapy in extremity soft tissue sarcoma. *Radiother Oncol.* 2005;75(1):48–53.
40. Kepka L, DeLaney TF, Suit HD, et al. Results of radiation therapy for unresected soft-tissue sarcomas. *Int J Radiat Oncol Biol Phys.* 2005;63(3):852–859.
41. Azinovic I, Martinez Monge R, Javier Aristu J, et al. Intraoperative radiotherapy electron boost followed by moderate doses of external beam radiotherapy in resected soft-tissue sarcoma of the extremities. *Radiother Oncol.* 2003;67(3):331–337.
42. Beroukas E, Peponi E, Soulimioti G, et al. Intraoperative electron beam radiotherapy followed by moderate doses of external beam radiotherapy in the treatment of resected soft tissue sarcomas of the extremities. *J BUON.* 2004;9(4):391–398.
43. Zelefsky MJ, Nori D, Shiu MH, et al. Limb salvage in soft tissue sarcomas involving neurovascular structures using combined surgical resection and brachytherapy. *Int J Radiat Oncol Biol Phys.* 1990;19(4):913–918.
44. Alektiar KM, Brennan MF, Singer S. Influence of site on the therapeutic ratio of adjuvant radiotherapy in soft-tissue sarcoma of the extremity. *Int J Radiat Oncol Biol Phys.* 2005;63(1):202–208.
45. Alektiar KM, Zelefsky MJ, Brennan MF. Morbidity of adjuvant brachytherapy in soft tissue sarcoma of the extremity and superficial trunk. *Int J Radiat Oncol Biol Phys.* 2000;47(5):1273–1279.
46. Petera J, Neumanová R, Odrazka K, et al. Perioperative hyperfractionated high-dose rate brachytherapy combined with external beam radiotherapy in the treatment of soft tissue sarcomas. *Tumori.* 2005;91(4):331–334.
47. Kubo T, Sugita T, Shimose S, et al. Nerve tolerance to high-dose-rate brachytherapy in patients with soft tissue sarcoma: a retrospective study. *BMC Cancer.* 2005;5(1):79.
48. Silbert PL, Moore R, Dawson B. Traumatic distal femoral neuropathy. *J Neurol Neurosurg Psychiatr.* 1998;65(4):614.
49. Laurent LE. Femoral nerve compression syndrome with paresis of the quadriceps muscle caused by radiotherapy of malignant tumours: a report of four cases. *Acta Orthop Scand.* 1975;46(5):804–808.
50. Feinberg J, Sethi S. Sciatic neuropathy: case report and discussion of the literature on postoperative sciatic neuropathy and sciatic nerve tumors. *HSS J.* 2006;2(2):181–187.
51. Gikas PD, Hanna SA, Aston W, et al. Post-radiation sciatic neuropathy: a case report and review of the literature. *World J Surg Oncol.* 2008;6(1):130.
52. Pieters RS, Niemierko A, Fullerton BC, et al. Cauda equina tolerance to high-dose fractionated irradiation. *Int J Radiat Oncol Biol Phys.* 2006;64(1):251–257.
53. DeLaney TF, Spiro IJ, Suit HD, et al. Neoadjuvant chemotherapy and radiotherapy for large extremity soft-tissue sarcomas. *Int J Radiat Oncol Biol Phys.* 2003;56(4):1117–1127.
54. Kraybill WG, Harris J, Spiro IJ, et al. Phase II study of neoadjuvant chemotherapy and radiation therapy in the management of high-risk, high-grade, soft tissue sarcomas of the extremities and body wall: Radiation Therapy Oncology Group Trial 9514. *J Clin Oncol.* 2006;24(4):619.
55. Cassady JR, Tonnesen GL, Wolfe LC, et al. Augmentation of vincristine neurotoxicity by irradiation of peripheral nerves. *Cancer Treat Rep.* 1980;64(8–9):963–965.
56. Alektiar KM, Zelefsky MJ, Paty PB, et al. High-dose-rate intraoperative brachytherapy for recurrent colorectal cancer. *Int J Radiat Oncol Biol Phys.* 2000;48(1):219–226.
57. Gemignani ML, Alektiar KM, Leitao M, et al. Radical surgical resection and high-dose intraoperative radiation therapy (HDR-IORT) in patients with recurrent gynecologic cancers. *Int J Radiat Oncol Biol Phys.* 2001;50(3):687–694.
58. Paulino AC. Late effects of radiotherapy for pediatric extremity sarcomas. *Int J Radiat Oncol Biol Phys.* 2004;60(1):265–274.
59. Calvo FA, Ortiz de Urbina D, Sierrasesúmaga L, et al. Intraoperative radiotherapy in the multidisciplinary treatment of bone sarcomas in children and adolescents. *Med Pediatr Oncol.* 1991;19(6):478–485.
60. Jaeckle KA. Neurological manifestations of neoplastic and radiation-induced plexopathies. *Semin Neurol.* 2004;24(4):385–393.
61. Anezaki T, Harada T, Kawachi I, et al. A case of post-irradiation lumbosacral radiculopathy successfully treated with corticosteroid and warfarin. *Rinsho Shinkeigaku.* 1999;39(8).825–829.
62. Delanian S, Lefaix J, Maisonobe T, et al. Significant clinical improvement in radiation-induced lumbosacral polyradiculopathy by a treatment combining pentoxifylline, tocopherol, and clodronate (Pentoclo). *J Neurol Sci.* 2008;275(1–2):164–166.

Brachial Plexus

INTRODUCTION

Radiation-induced brachial plexopathy has been recognized as a possible consequence of treatment since at least the 1950s. It is one of the most disabling complications of radiotherapy. Radiation oncologists must therefore understand how best to avoid such injuries while still accomplishing their therapeutic goals.

This chapter discusses the gross and radiologic anatomy of the brachial plexus; the histologic effects of radiation; the clinical, radiologic, and electrophysiological findings at presentation; the evaluation of patients with suspected radiation brachial plexopathy; the effects of radiation fractionation, treatment volume, and technique on the risk of plexopathy; and the treatment options. Additional reviews of this topic have been published elsewhere.[1–5]

GROSS ANATOMY

The brachial plexus is formed by the union of the ventral rami of the fifth through eighth cervical nerves and the majority of the ventral ramus of the first thoracic nerve.[6,7] The fourth cervical and second thoracic nerves may contribute branches in some individuals. The rami from C4-6 merge at the lateral border of the middle scalene muscle to form the upper trunk of the plexus; the C7 root continues as the middle trunk; and the rami of C8, T1, and (if present) T2 merge behind the anterior scalene muscle to form the lower trunk (Fig. 23.1).[8] The three trunks proceed inferiorly and laterally from the posterior cervical triangle until each splits into an anterior and a posterior division just superior to or posterior to the clavicle. The anterior divisions of the upper and middle trunks unite to form the lateral cord of the plexus, which is located on the lateral aspect of the subclavian artery. The anterior division of the lower trunk (often with additional fibers from C7) forms the medial cord, which passes posterior to and then medial to the subclavian artery. The posterior divisions of all three trunks merge to form the posterior cord, which moves from anterior to the subclavian artery to posterior to the artery as it descends more inferiorly.

The brachial plexus gives rise to nerves responsible for the innervation of the shoulder and the arm. The nerve to the scaleni and longus colli muscles, the dorsal scapular nerve, and the long thoracic nerve arise from the roots of the plexus, prior to their joining into trunks. The suprascapular nerve and the nerve to the subscapularis muscle arise just after the origin of the lateral cord, superior to the clavicle. Inferior to the clavicle, the lateral

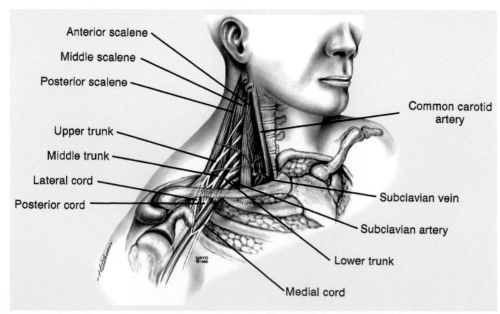

Figure 23.1. Anatomy of the brachial plexus in relation to surrounding structures. (Reprinted from Wittenberg KH, Adkins MC. MR imaging of nontraumatic brachial plexopathies: frequency and spectrum of findings. *Radiographics.* 2000;20:1023–1032, with permission.)

cord gives rise to the lateral pectoral nerve, musculocutaneous nerve, and part of the median nerve. The medial cord gives rise to the medial pectoral nerve, the medial cutaneous nerves of the upper arm and forearm, the ulnar nerve, and part of the median nerve. Finally, the posterior cord gives rise to the upper subscapular, thoracodorsal, lower subscapular, axillary, and radial nerves.

RADIOLOGIC ANATOMY

Modern radiation therapy planning relies on computerized tomography (CT) to delineate areas to be targeted or avoided. Thus, accurately identifying the brachial plexus is potentially important in reducing treatment toxicity. A publication from investigators at the University of Michigan is particularly helpful in this regard.[9] They delineated the brachial plexus in relation to its surrounding structures for use in radiation planning (Fig. 23.2), based on previous work correlating radiologic and gross anatomic findings.[10] Groups at the University of California Davis Cancer Center in Sacramento (Table 23.1 and Fig. 23.3) and at the Princess Margaret Hospital in Toronto (Table 23.2) recently proposed similar, though not identical, guidelines for outlining the brachial plexus.[11,12]

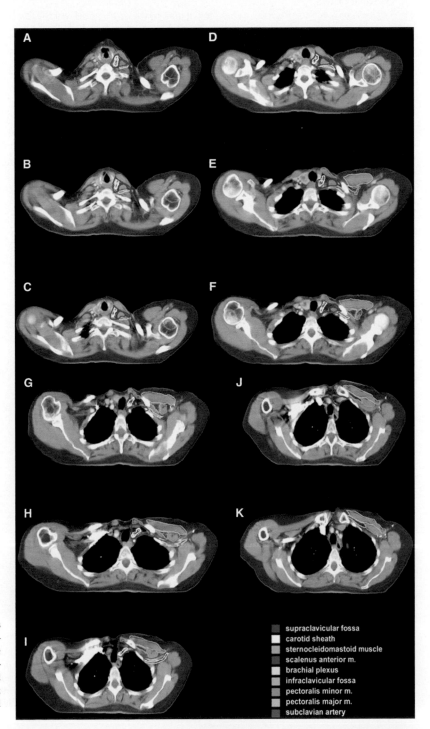

Figure 23.2. Transverse CT sections at 3-mm intervals from the cricothyroid membrane to the base of the clavicular head. (Reprinted from Madu CN, Quint DJ, Normolle DP, et al. Definition of the supraclavicular and infraclavicular nodes: implications for three-dimensional CT-based conformal radiation therapy. *Radiology.* 2001;221:333–339; with permission of the copyright holder, the Radiological Society of North America.)

supraclavicular fossa
carotid sheath
sternocleidomastoid muscle
scalenus anterior m.
brachial plexus
infraclavicular fossa
pectoralis minor m.
pectoralis major m.
subclavian artery

TABLE 23.1	University of California Davis Cancer Center at Sacramento Guidelines for Contouring the Brachial Plexus on Axial Computerized Tomography

1. Identify and contour C5, T1, and T2.
2. Identify and contour the subclavian and axillary neurovascular bundle.
3. Identify and contour anterior and middle scalene muscles from C5 to insertion onto the first rib.
4. To contour the brachial plexus organ-at-risk use a 5-mm diameter paint tool.
5. Start at the neural foramina from C5 to T1; this should extend from the lateral aspect of the spinal canal to the small space between the anterior and middle scalene muscles.
6. For CT slices, where no neural foramen is present, contour only the space between the anterior and middle scalene muscles.
7. Continue to contour the space between the anterior and middle scalene muscles; eventually the middle scalene will end in the region of the subclavian neurovascular bundle.
8. Contour the brachial plexus as the posterior aspect of the neurovascular bundle inferiorly and laterally to one to two CT slices below the clavicular head.
9. The first and second ribs serve as the medial limit of the organ at risk contour.

Source: Adapted from Hall WH, Guiou M, Lee NY, et al. Development and validation of a standardized method for contouring the brachial plexus: preliminary dosimetric analysis among patients treated with IMRT for head and neck cancer. *Int J Radiat Oncol Biol Phys.* 2008;72: 1362–1367.

Breast cancer radiation techniques have traditionally employed an anterior field (sometimes with a supplemental posterior field) prescribed to a depth of 3 or 5 cm to treat the supraclavicular and upper axillary lymph nodes. Hence, the depth of the brachial plexus under the anterior neck and chest wall determines the dose it receives. This depth varies substantially over the course of the plexus, as well as between individuals. In the study from the University of Michigan, the median minimum depth of the plexus in 20 studied patients was 2.3 cm, with a range of 0.5 to 4 cm; its median maximum depth was 6.5 cm, with a range of 3.8 to 9.1 cm.[9] Of note, the median maximum depth of the supraclavicular nodes was 5 cm (range, 3.9–8.3 cm), and the maximum depth of the infraclavicular (or axillary apical) nodes was 5.6 cm (range, 3.3–7.3 cm). The mean depth of the brachial plexus was correlated with the depth of the supraclavicular nodes, though there was substantial variation among individuals in this relationship.

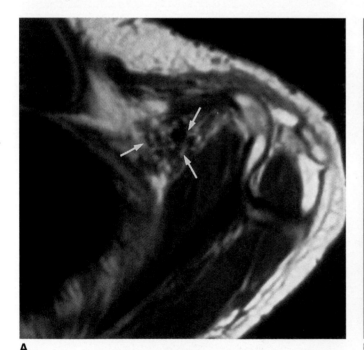

A

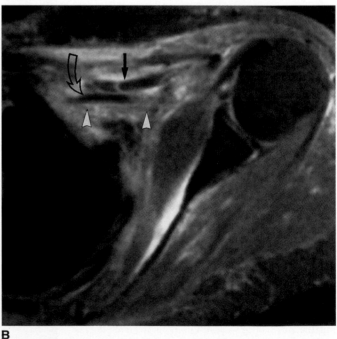

B

Figure 23.3. Oblique sagittal T1-weighted **(A)** and axial fat-saturated gadolinium-enhanced T1-weighted **(B)** images show soft-tissue stranding (*arrows* in **A**) about the brachial plexus (*arrowheads* in **B**) with diffuse gadolinium enhancement. In **(B)**, the solid arrow points to the subclavian vein and the open arrow to the subclavian artery. (Reprinted from Wittenberg KH, Adkins MC. MR imaging of nontraumatic brachial plexopathies: frequency and spectrum of findings. *Radiographics.* 2000;20:1023–1032; with permission of the copyright holder, the Radiological Society of North America.)

TABLE 23.2	Princess Margaret Hospital Guidelines for Contouring the Brachial Plexus on Axial Computerized Tomography

LEVEL 1
Superior: cranial border of the C5 vertebral body.
Inferior: cranial border of the T2 vertebral body.
Anterior: dorsal border of the anterior scalene muscle.
Posterior: ventral border of middle scalene muscle.
Lateral: lateral border of anterior and middle scalene muscles.
Medial: intervertebral foramen.

LEVEL 2
Superior: cranial border of the T2 vertebral body.
Inferior: cranial border of the T3 vertebral body.
Anterior: subclavian artery.
Posterior: ventral border of the serratus anterior muscle.
Lateral: lateral border of the pectoralis major muscle.
Medial: external surface of the ribs.

Source: Adapted from Vakilha M, Phoplunkar W, Chan B, et al. Brachial plexus contouring guidelines assessed with inter observer variability during image guided IMRT for head and neck cancer [abstract 2506]. *Int J Radiat Oncol Biol Phys.* 2008, 72(1 suppl):S395–S396.

HISTOLOGIC EFFECTS OF RADIATION ON THE BRACHIAL PLEXUS

The pathophysiology of brachial plexus injury is thought to be the same as for other peripheral nerves (see Chapter 24). Animal models show changes in action potentials and conduction time within a few days of treatment, accompanied by altered vascular permeability, neurilemmal damage, and anomalies of microtubule assembly.[13–15] As time goes on, extensive fibrosis may develop in the connective tissue surrounding nerves, resulting in decreased vascularity as well as direct pressure on the plexus. In a series from the Royal Marsden Hospital, London, exploration of six patients with brachial plexopathy revealed severe fibrosis in the apex of the axilla, with fibrous bands surrounding the trunks of the plexus. Pathology showed only fibrosis, with biopsies of branch nerves showing thickening of the epineurium and endoneurium, with demyelination in some cases.[16] Others have reported similar findings.[17] Autopsy studies of two patients treated in Melbourne, Australia, who developed severe brachial plexus symptoms showed marked fibrosis surrounding the nerves, with microscopic examination showing varying degrees of fibrous thickening of the neurilemmal sheath, demyelination, and fibrous replacement of some nerve fibrils.[18] One patient with minimal symptoms had fibrosis in the tissues of the anterior aspect of the brachial plexus but no histologic changes of the cords themselves.

CLINICAL AND RADIOLOGIC PRESENTATION

CLINICAL FINDINGS

There appear to be at least two types of radiation-related brachial plexopathy. The classic plexopathy is a chronic, progressive syndrome whose onset is highly variable, from as short as 3 months to as long as 26 years after irradiation.[1] Symptoms can continue to evolve over periods of 30 years or more, at least for those treated to very high doses.[19] Patients usually present with sensory and/or motor symptoms of the ipsilateral limb. Pain can occur but is generally less prominent. For example, in a series of 22 patients with radiation brachial plexopathy seen at Memorial Sloan-Kettering Cancer Center in New York, 55% of patients presented with paresthesia or hypoesthesia; 45% had arm swelling and weakness (predominantly in the distribution of the upper trunks). Severe pain was present in only 19% of patients, compared to 80% of 78 patients with carcinomatous plexopathy.[20] In a study from the Mayo Clinic, 63% of 35 patients with radiation plexopathy had pain (severe in 9%), compared to 93% of 55 patients with neoplastic plexopathy (severe in 22%).[21]

A second, rarer type of radiation plexopathy appears more rapidly (on average) than classic chronic plexopathy and largely resolves spontaneously. This was first described (and termed "paralytic brachial neuritis") in eight patients treated at the Joint Center for Radiation Therapy (JCRT), Boston, between 1968 and 1979.[22] They presented from 1.5 to 14 months after radiation (median, 4.5 months) with hand and forearm paresthesias. Some patients also had mild-to-moderate shoulder and axillary pain or finger weakness. The paresthesias were stable for 3 to 6 months and then resolved, with only minimal residual paresthesias in three patients. Weakness was initially severe in some patients, yet all recovered full strength.

Two cases of brachial plexopathy have been reported due to radiation-related arterial occlusion.[23] This appears to be extremely rare, as no other such reports have appeared.

RADIOLOGIC FINDINGS

Most, but not all, patients with clinical symptoms of classic plexopathy will have increased density on CT consistent with fibrosis.[16,20] The degree of fibrosis is highly variable. The Royal Marsden Hospital group performed contrast-enhanced CT on patients with and without neurologic symptoms suggestive of brachial plexopathy.[16] They defined grade 1 fibrosis as some change in the density of the axillary and subcutaneous fat, with normal vessel outline; grade 2 as greater increase in density of the fat with loss of vessel outlines and a small-to-moderate increase in abnormal axillary soft tissue; and grade 3 as the changes found in grade 2 plus marked abnormal soft tissue in the axilla. Twenty-seven of 28 (96%) patients with neurologic symptoms had some CT changes; the highest level was grade 1 in 10 patients, grade 2 in 9 patients, and grade 3 in 8 patients. Conversely, 5 of 13 patients (38%) without neurologic symptoms had fibrosis, of which 3 were grade 1 and 2 were grade 2.

Magnetic resonance imaging is superior to CT in delineating soft tissue and nerve changes from radiation. Findings generally include diffuse thickening and variable enhancement of the plexus without a focal mass and soft-tissue changes with low signal intensity on both T1- and T2-weighted images (Figs. 23.3 and 23.4).[7,8,24–27] Again, MRI appearances vary substantially among patients.

ELECTROPHYSIOLOGICAL FINDINGS

Electromyography (EMG) has variable findings in patients with classic radiation brachial plexopathy. A study from the Mayo Clinic found that 88% of 35 patients had a conduction block of ulnar F-waves across the plexus with ulnar median nerve

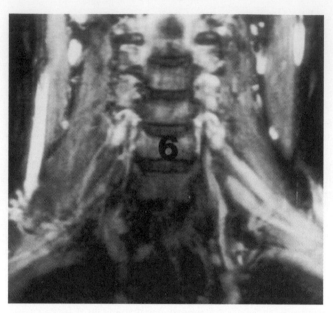

Figure 23.4. Coronal short T-1 inversion recovery (STIR) image of the brachial plexus 2 years after irradiation of the left supraclavicular and axillary nodes, showing enlargement of the roots, trunks, and divisions of the brachial plexus on the left side. Note the uniform and diffuse involvement of all visualized components of the left brachial plexus within the radiation field and the marked difference in size and signal intensity of the structures of the left brachial plexus compared with the right side. (Reprinted from Maravilla KR, Bowen BC. Imaging of the peripheral nervous system: evaluation of peripheral neuropathy and plexopathy. *Am J Neuroradiol.* 1998;19:1011–1023, with permission of the copyright holder, the American Society of Neuroradiology.)

stimulation; this was the only abnormality in five patients.[21] Other common findings include decreased or absent sensory nerve action potentials and abnormalities of fibrillation and fasciculation potential, motor unit potentials, and myokymic discharges on muscle needle examination. Patients with transient subacute plexopathy also show slowed conduction velocity along the thoracic inlet, with improvement seen on serial studies.[22]

EVALUATION

The main goal of evaluating patients with suspected radiation-induced brachial plexopathy is to distinguish it from recurrent tumor or, rarely, radiation-induced sarcomas or other primary cancers.[1,28] Other entities, such as trauma, can usually be eliminated based on history.[26,29] The most useful diagnostic study is MRI. The presence of a mass is the most helpful finding in making this distinction, particularly in individuals presenting with severe pain.[26,30] However, some patients with recurrence may not have a well-defined mass, which may make it difficult to distinguish between the two radiologically. Focal enhancement with gadolinium on MRI suggests the presence of tumor rather than radiation-related fibrosis, but this is not fool-proof.[7,8,25,26] Some patients with an indeterminate MRI may have abnormal uptake of 18-fluoro-deoxyglucose on positron emission tomography, indicating the presence of malignancy.[31] Ultrasound has also been used to assess the brachial plexus, but it does not seem superior to MRI.[32]

Patients with radiation and neoplastic brachial plexopathies may also have similar EMG findings, though certain abnormalities seem more common in one group or another. For example, the Mayo Clinic study found that 23% of 35 patients with radiation plexopathy had fibrillation potentials in cervical paraspinal muscles and 63% had myokymic discharges, compared to incidences of 2% and 4% for these findings, respectively, among 55 patients with carcinomatous plexopathy.[21] However, a more recent study of 11 patients treated in British Columbia did not find myokemia in any patient with radiation plexopathy.[33]

EFFECTS OF RADIATION FRACTIONATION, TREATMENT VOLUME, AND TECHNIQUE

STUDIES IN BREAST CANCER PATIENTS

The great majority of reports of brachial plexopathy and studies of its incidence in the megavoltage treatment era have concerned patients treated for breast cancer. This is due both to its relatively high incidence and its good prognosis, which allows sufficient time for such injuries to manifest themselves.

Table 23.3 lists selected studies of the risk of brachial plexopathy in breast cancer patients receiving nodal irradiation. These series can be broadly divided into two groups: ones that prescribed very large daily fractions (3 Gy or higher) to total doses of 50 Gy or higher; and ones using smaller daily doses and/or lower total doses.

The incidence of plexopathy in series in the first group was generally substantial. For example, one of the earliest reported series, from the Peter MacCallum Clinic in Melbourne, Australia, gave patients 63 Gy in 12 fractions or 57.75 Gy in 11 or 12 fractions, prescribed to the "peak" depth of 4 MV photons.[18] This resulted in minimum doses of 55 or 51 Gy, respectively, at the estimated depth of the brachial plexus at 2 to 4 cm. The crude risk of neurologic symptoms was extremely high in the first group (73%) and still substantial in the second (15%), despite the short maximum follow-up of only 30 months. Patients in the first group of studies also seemed at risk to develop plexopathy for many years after treatment, and their symptoms often continued to evolve over a long time. For example, in a study from Hamburg, Germany, the actuarial risk of plexopathy increased from 4% at 5 years to 25% at 10 years.[35] In a series from Umeå, Sweden, the effect of large fraction sizes and total doses was compounded by a technique resulting in field overlaps.[19] Patients developed brachial plexopathy as long as 19 years after treatment. The severity of patients' symptoms continued to increase for as long as 34 years—resulting in 92% of long-term survivors developing arm paralysis!

In contrast, the incidence of brachial plexopathy was low (0%–5%) in patients receiving doses at the plexus of 50 to 54 Gy in 1.8 to 2 Gy fractions or 40 to 45 Gy in 2.5 to 3 Gy. (The exception was a study of patients participating in trials in Denmark.[37] However, their results are somewhat difficult to compare to other studies, as many eligible patients did not participate in the evaluation.) Although these studies generally had shorter follow-up than the older studies, patients did not appear at risk to develop plexopathies for such a long time. Also, their symptoms were often milder, and many resolved. For example, in the JCRT study, only 4 of the 20 affected patients had severe or permanent injuries.[38] Similarly, in a study from Westmead

| TABLE 23.3 | | | Incidence of Brachial Plexopathy in Selected Series of Patients Treated for Breast Cancer with Megavoltage Radiotherapy | | | | |

Series	Dates	Modality	Prescribed Total Dose/Fraction Size (Gy)	Prescription Point	Estimated Dose/Fraction Size at Plexus (Gy)	Follow-Up (yr)	Incidence
Melbourne[18,a]	1958–1962	4 MV	63/5.25	"Peak"	55/4.6 (2–4 cm)	2.5 (max)	73% (24/33)
			57.75/4.8–5.25	"Peak"	51/4.25–4.6 (2–4 cm)	2.5 (max)	15% (13/84)
Umeå[19,b]	1963–1965	Cobalt-60	44/4	"Peak"	54–57/1.8–5.2 (3 cm)	12	63% (45/71)
							5-yr: 14%
							10-yr: 55%
							20-yr: 65%
DBCG-77 Protocols[34,c]	1977–1982	8 MV	36.6/3	Midplane axilla	43.4/3.6	7.8	35% (28/79)
Hamburg[35]	1980–1993	Cobalt-60	60/3	0.5 cm	52/2.6 (3 cm)	8.2[d]	14% (19/140)
							5-yr: 4%
							10-yr: 25%
Royal Marsden, London[36]	1982–1984	Cobalt-60	51/3.4	[e]	45.9/3.1 (5 cm)	2.7–5.5 (range)	5% (27/388)
			60/2	[e]	54/1.8 (5 cm)	2.7–5.5 (range)	1% (1/111)
DBCG-82 Protocols[37,c]	1982–1990	8 MV	50/2	Midplane axilla	54.25/2.2	4.2	12% (19/161)
JCRT[38]	1968–1985	4–8 MV	50/2	3–5 cm	50/2 (3–5 cm)	6.5	0.2% (20/1117)
Philadelphia[39]	1977–1985	6 MV	46–50/1.8–2	[f]	[f]	[f]	1% (2/231)
British Columbia[40]	1978–1986	Cobalt-60	35/2.2	Midplane axilla	[f]	12.5	0 (0/164)
Westmead[41]	1979–1984	[f]	50/2	1.5 cm	[f]	7.3	1% (5/380)
Edinburgh[42]	1990–1991	4–6 MV	45/2.25	Midplane axilla	[f]	5.7	1% (2/223)
START A Trial[43]	1999–2002	6 MV	50/25	[f]	[f]	5.1	0 (0/122)
			41.6/3.2	[f]	[f]	5.1	1% (1/99)
			39/13	[f]	[f]	5.1	0 (0/97)
START B Trial[44]	1999–2001	6 MV	50/25	[f]	[f]	6.0	0 (0/79)
			40/2.67	[f]	[f]	6.0	0 (0/82)

Median follow-up time listed, unless otherwise noted.

[a]Maximum follow-up, 30 months. Minimum dose at the estimated depth of the plexus of 2 to 4 cm given.

[b]Because of field overlap, the effective daily fraction at the plexus was either 1.8, 3.4, or 5.2 Gy, with a total of 17 fractions given. Cumulative incidence estimated from their Figure 23.1.

[c]Studies included only patients without evidence of recurrence at least 5 years after surgery who were age 70 or younger at time of examination. Median "peak" dose given for brachial plexus dose. Both definite and probable cases of brachial plexopathy included.

[d]Follow-up in disease-free survivors.

[e]Range of follow-up given, but not median. Two different techniques were employed: a "3-field" technique, with the patient changing position between treatment of with separate supraclavicular and tangential fields; and a "4-field" technique with tangential fields, a supraclavicular-axillary-internal mammary field, and a posterior axillary boost, without patient movement during between fields. In the 3-field technique, the supraclavicular field was prescribed to the "maximum dose"; for the 4-field technique, it was prescribed to 2.5 cm. Brachial plexopathy incidences for the large fraction size were 5% (13/250) for the 3-field and 5% (4/88) for the 4-field techniques. For the small fraction size, the incidence of brachial plexopathy in the 3-field group was 1% (1/76) and nil (0/35) for the 4-field group.

[f]Unknown or not stated.

DBCG, Danish Breast Cancer Cooperative Group; JCRT, Joint Center for Radiation Therapy, Boston; max, maximum; MV: megavolt; START: Standardisation of Breast Radiotherapy.

Hospital, in a suburb of Sydney, Australia, all five patients developing plexopathy had complete resolution of symptoms within 30 months.[41]

The use of chemotherapy increased the risk of brachial plexopathy in several studies, whether it was given concurrently or sequentially with radiation.[22,34,37,38] Of note, six of the eight patients in the JCRT series of subacute plexopathies received chemotherapy (melphalan or cyclophosphamide, methotrexate, and 5-fluorouracil) concurrently with or after radiation.[22] The incidence was 0.4% (2/438) for patients not receiving chemotherapy, compared to 5% (6/126) for those receiving it. However, other studies using both nodal irradiation and chemotherapy had no patients who developed plexopathy.[40,45]

The impact of chemotherapy may also vary in relation to radiation dose. In the later JCRT experience, when the axillary dose was 50 Gy or lower, the incidence of plexopathy was 0.4% (3/724) when no chemotherapy was given and 3.4% (10/267) when chemotherapy was employed.[38] When the axillary dose was more than 50 Gy, the incidence of plexopathy was 3% (2/63) when chemotherapy was not used, compared to 8% (5/63) when chemotherapy was given.

A major cause of the high rates of brachial plexopathy seen in early studies was inadequate radiation technique. In the United Kingdom, a group of women who felt they had been so injured formed the "Radiotherapy Action Group Exposure" group in the early 1990s to press for an investigation.[46] A study commissioned by the Royal College of Radiology found that many of the affected patients had been moved from one position to another for different portions of their treatment, which resulted in substantial overlaps of treatment fields.[47,48] This factor also contributed to the high complication rates of other series.[19]

OTHER CANCERS

Both acute[49] and chronic[50–52] brachial plexus neuropathies have been reported in patients treated for Hodgkin disease to doses of 35 to 40 Gy in 1.75 to 2 Gy fractions. However, the risk appears exceedingly low for the treatment regimens commonly used for this disease.

The brachial plexus may receive very high doses (60 Gy or more) when patients are irradiated for head and neck cancers. Investigators at the University of California Davis Cancer Center in Sacramento recently administered a neurological symptom questionnaire to 95 consecutive follow-up patients.[53] They had been treated 6 to 70 months earlier (median, 15 months) to a prescribed dose of 60 to 70 Gy; 31 patients received concurrent chemotherapy. Seven patients had symptoms of brachial plexopathy, but the incidence was 16% (6/38) when patients followed <1 year were excluded. No data were reported on how the actual dose delivered to the plexus or chemotherapy affected this incidence.

Finally, there is no systematic information about the risk of plexopathy in patients with apical lung cancers treated with conventional radiotherapy, although a few such cases have been reported.[54] A recent study from Indiana University identified 7 patients of 36 (19%) with apical lesions who developed brachial plexopathy 6 to 23 months (median, 7 months) after stereotactic body radiotherapy (30–72 Gy in three to four fractions).[55]

TREATMENT OF RADIATION BRACHIAL PLEXOPATHY

Patients with radiation-related plexopathy have often been treated with antiepileptics, tricyclic antidepressants, non-narcotic analgesics, and narcotics, similar to patients with peripheral neuropathic pain of other origin.[1,28,47] However, there are no systematic studies of their effectiveness. Three patients with plexopathy were reported to have reduced symptoms following 3 to 6 months of anticoagulation.[52,56] One patient's symptoms returned when anticoagulation was stopped, but they decreased again when it was resumed.[52] The true success rate and the optimal duration of such treatment are not clear.

Chronic radiation injuries appear due at least in part to an ongoing inflammatory process. Interrupting this process pharmacologically may substantially reverse fibrosis and pain.[57] A group at the Hôpital Saint-Louis in Paris reported dramatic improvement for two patients with late-developing radiation-induced sacral polyneuritis using a combination of pentoxyphylline, vitamin E, and clodronate in alternation with prednisone.[58]

Nonpharmacologic treatment strategies have also been tried. A randomized trial of hyperbaric oxygen performed at the Royal Marsden Hospital in 35 patients showed no evidence of benefit up to 12 months after therapy.[59] Surgical ablation of the dorsal root entry zone successfully relieved pain in six patients in a recent series from São Paulo, Brazil.[60] Finally, surgical removal of scar tissue around the plexus ("neurolysis"), sometimes combined with omentoplasty, has been reported to

benefit some patients, particularly reducing pain.[61–63] However, it is not clear from these studies which patients were most likely to benefit from this approach, nor their risk of having complications from such surgery.

CONCLUSIONS

Radiation-induced brachial plexopathy can have a devastating impact on patients' lives. Fortunately, the risk of this complication with modern techniques that avoid field overlap is likely 1% or smaller when doses of approximately 50 Gy in 2-Gy fractions or 40 Gy in 2.5 to 3 Gy fractions are received by the plexus. Symptoms are usually, though not always, mild and often transient in patients who develop plexopathy at these doses. The risk of plexopathy at higher dose is perhaps 5% to 10% at doses of 55 to 60 Gy in 2-Gy fractions or 45 to 50 Gy in 2.5 to 3 Gy fractions. The risk may be 15% to 20% or higher in patients receiving doses >60 Gy in 2-Gy fractions, and higher yet when such a total dose is given with larger fractions. Chemotherapy appears to increase the risk of plexopathy, though its interactions with radiation are still poorly characterized. Neither imaging studies nor EMG can definitively differentiate between radiation and neoplastic brachial plexopathy in all patients. Exploration may be needed to rule out recurrence by biopsying soft tissue surrounding the plexus. There are only fragmentary data on the management of patients with radiation-related brachial plexopathy, and the true value of specific interventions is unclear. It would certainly seem reasonable to try medical approaches before surgical ones.

REFERENCES

1. Kori SH. Diagnosis and management of brachial plexus lesions in cancer patients. *Oncology (Huntingt).* 1995;9:756–760.
2. Jaeckle KA. Neurological manifestations of neoplastic and radiation-induced plexopathies. *Semin Neurol.* 2004;24:385–393.
3. Galecki J, Hicer-Grzenkowicz J, Grudzien-Kowalska M, et al. Radiation-induced brachial plexopathy and hypofractionated regimens in adjuvant irradiation of patients with breast cancer—a review. *Acta Oncol.* 2006;45:280–284.
4. Johansson S. Radiation induced brachial plexopathies. *Acta Oncol.* 2006;45:253–257.
5. Gosk J, Rutowski R, Reichert P, et al. Radiation-induced brachial plexus neuropathy—aetiopathogenesis, risk factors, differential diagnostics, symptoms and treatment. *Folia Neuropathol.* 2007;45:26–30.
6. Williams PL, Warwick R, eds. *Gray's Anatomy.* 36th British ed. Philadelphia, PA: WB Saunders; 1980.
7. Maravilla KR, Bowen BC. Imaging of the peripheral nervous system: evaluation of peripheral neuropathy and plexopathy. *Am J Neuroradiol.* 1998;19:1011–1023.
8. Wittenberg KH, Adkins MC. MR imaging of nontraumatic brachial plexopathies: frequency and spectrum of findings. *Radiographics.* 2000;20:1023–1032.
9. Madu CN, Quint DJ, Normolle DP, et al. Definition of the supraclavicular and infraclavicular nodes: implications for three-dimensional CT-based conformal radiation therapy. *Radiology.* 2001;221:333–339.
10. Gebarski KS, Glazer GM, Gebarski SS. Brachial plexus: anatomic, radiologic, and pathologic correlation using computed tomography. *J Comput Assist Tomogr.* 1982;6:1058–1063.
11. Hall WH, Guiou M, Lee NY, et al. Development and validation of a standardized method for contouring the brachial plexus: preliminary dosimetric analysis among patients treated with IMRT for head-and-neck cancer. *Int J Radiat Oncol Biol Phys.* 2008;72:1362–1367.
12. Vakilha M, Phoplunkar W, Chan B, et al. Brachial plexus contouring guidelines assessed with inter observer variability during image guided IMRT for head and neck cancer [abstract 2506]. *Int J Radiat Oncol Biol Phys.* 2008;72(1 suppl):S395–S396.
13. Arnold MC, Harrison F, Bonte FJ. The effect of radiation on mammalian nerve. *Radiology.* 1961;77:264–268.
14. Coss RA, Bamburg JR, Dewey WC. The effects of X irradiation on microtubule assembly in vitro. *Radiat Res.* 1981;85:99–115.
15. Gillette EL, Mahler PA, Powers BE, et al. Late radiation injury to muscle and peripheral nerves. *Int J Radiat Oncol Biol Phys.* 1995;31:1309–1318.
16. Cooke J, Powell S, Parsons C. The diagnosis by computed tomography of brachial plexus lesions following radiotherapy for carcinoma of the breast. *Clin Radiol.* 1988;39:602–606.

17. Gosk J, Rutowski R, Urban M, et al. Brachial plexus injuries after radiotherapy—analysis of 6 cases. *Folia Neuropathol.* 2007;45:31–35.

18. Stoll BA, Andrews JT. Radiation-induced peripheral neuropathy. *Br Med J.* 1966;1:834–837.

19. Johansson S, Svensson H, Denekamp J. Timescale of evolution of late radiation injury after postoperative radiotherapy of breast cancer patients. *Int J Radiat Oncol Biol Phys.* 2000;48:745–750.

20. Kori SH, Foley KM, Posner JB. Brachial plexus lesions in patients with cancer: 100 cases. *Neurology.* 1981;31:45–50.

21. Harper CM Jr, Thomas JE, Cascino TL, et al. Distinction between neoplastic and radiation-induced brachial plexopathy, with emphasis on the role of EMG. *Neurology.* 1989;39:502–506.

22. Salner AL, Botnick LE, Herzog AG, et al. Reversible brachial plexopathy following primary radiation therapy for breast cancer. *Cancer Treat Rep* 1981;65:797–802.

23. Gerard JM, Franck N, Moussa Z, et al. Acute ischemic brachial plexus neuropathy following radiation therapy. *Neurology.* 1989;39:450–451.

24. Posniak HV, Olson MC, Dudiak CM, et al. MR imaging of the brachial plexus. *AJR Am J Roentgenol.* 1993;161:373–379.

25. Wouter van Es H, Engelen AM, Witkamp TD, et al. Radiation-induced brachial plexopathy: MR imaging. *Skeletal Radiol.* 1997;26:284–288.

26. Bowen BC, Pattany PM, Saraf-Lavi E, et al. The brachial plexus: normal anatomy, pathology, and MR imaging. *Neuroimaging Clin N Am.* 2004;14:59–85.

27. Todd M, Shah GV, Mukherji SK. MR imaging of brachial plexus. *Top Magn Reson Imaging.* 2004;15:113–125.

28. Royal College of Radiology. Management of radiation-induced brachial plexus neuropathy. *Oncology (Huntingt).* 1996;10:685–698.

29. Mullins GM, O'Sullivan SS, Neligan A, et al. Non-traumatic brachial plexopathies, clinical, radiological and neurophysiological findings from a tertiary centre. *Clin Neurol Neurosurg.* 2007;109:661–666.

30. Moore NR, Dixon AK, Wheeler TK, et al. Axillary fibrosis or recurrent tumor. An MRI study in breast cancer. *Clin Radiol.* 1990;42:42–46.

31. Hathaway PB, Mankoff DA, Maravilla KR, et al. Value of combined FDG PET and MR imaging in the evaluation of suspected recurrent local-regional breast cancer: preliminary experience. *Radiology.* 1999;210:807–814.

32. Graif M, Martinoli C, Rochkind S, et al. Sonographic evaluation of brachial plexus pathology. *Eur Radiol.* 2004;14:193–200.

33. Chung C, Chapman K, Weir L. Radiation-induced brachial plexopathy (RIBP) following locoregional irradiation with short fractionation for breast cancer: neurologic assessment, electrophysiological testing and quality of life (QoL) [abstract 132]. *Radiother Oncol.* 2007;84(2 suppl 2):S38.

34. Olsen NK, Pfeiffer P, Mondrup K, et al. Radiation-induced brachial plexus neuropathy in breast cancer patients. *Acta Oncol.* 1990;29:885–890.

35. Bajrovic A, Rades D, Fehlauer F, et al. Is there a life-long risk of brachial plexopathy after radiotherapy of supraclavicular lymph nodes in breast cancer patients? *Radiother Oncol.* 2004;71:297–301.

36. Powell S, Cooke J, Parsons C. Radiation-induced brachial plexus injury: follow-up of two different fractionation schedules. *Radiother Oncol.* 1990;18:213–220.

37. Olsen NK, Pfeiffer P, Johannsen L, et al. Radiation-induced brachial plexopathy: neurological follow-up in 161 recurrence-free breast cancer patients. *Int J Radiat Oncol Biol Phys.* 1993;26:43–49.

38. Pierce SM, Recht A, Lingos T, et al. Long-term radiation complications following conservative surgery (CS) and radiation therapy (RT) in patients with early stage breast cancer. *Int J Radiat Oncol Biol Phys.* 1992;23:915–923.

39. Fowble BL, Solin LJ, Schultz DJ, et al. Ten year results of conservative surgery and irradiation for stage I and II breast cancer. *Int J Radiat Oncol Biol Phys.* 1991;21:269–277.

40. Ragaz J, Jackson SM, Le N, et al. Adjuvant radiotherapy and chemotherapy in node-positive premenopausal women with breast cancer. *N Engl J Med.* 1997;337:956–962.

41. Chua B, Ung O, Boyages J. Competing considerations in regional nodal treatment for early breast cancer. *Breast J.* 2002;8:15–22.

42. Miller N, Kerr GK, Grant R, et al. Radiation induced brachial plexopathy in early breast cancer [abstract 268]. *Eur J Cancer.* 1998;34(suppl 5):S60.

43. Bentzen SM, Agrawal RK, Aird EG, et al. The UK Standardisation of Breast Radiotherapy (START) Trial A of radiotherapy hypofractionation for treatment of early breast cancer: a randomised trial. *Lancet Oncol.* 2008;9:331–341.

44. Bentzen SM, Agrawal RK, Aird EG, et al. The UK Standardisation of Breast Radiotherapy (START) Trial B of radiotherapy hypofractionation for treatment of early breast cancer: a randomised trial. *Lancet.* 2008;371:1098–1107.

45. Recht A, Come SE, Henderson IC, et al. The sequencing of chemotherapy and radiation therapy after conservative surgery for early-stage breast cancer. *N Engl J Med.* 1996;334:1356–1361.

46. Sikora K. Enraged about radiotherapy. *Br Med J.* 1994;308:188–189.

47. Bates TD, Evans RGB. *Brachial Plexus Neuropathy Following Radiotherapy for Breast Carcinoma.* London: Royal College of Radiologists; 1995.

48. Spittle MF. Brachial plexus neuropathy after radiotherapy for breast cancer: lower does and surgical management of the axilla may be the answer (Editorial). *Br Med J.* 1995;311:1516–1517.

49. Churn M, Clough V, Slater A. Early onset of bilateral brachial plexopathy during mantle radiotherapy for Hodgkin's disease. *Clin Oncol (R Coll Radiol).* 2000;12:289–291.

50. Killer HE, Hess K. Natural history of radiation-induced brachial plexopathy compared with surgically treated patients. *J Neurol.* 1990;237:247–250.

51. Wadd NJ, Lucraft HH. Brachial plexus neuropathy following mantle radiotherapy. *Clin Oncol (R Coll Radiol).* 1998;10:399–400.

52. Soto O. Radiation-induced conduction block: resolution following anticoagulant therapy. *Muscle Nerve.* 2005;31:642–645.

53. Guiou M, Hall WH, Jennelle R, et al. Prospective evaluation of dosimetric variables associated with brachial plexopathy after radiation therapy for head and neck cancer [abstract 2482]. *Int J Radiat Oncol Biol Phys.* 2008;22(1 suppl):S385.

54. Match RM. Radiation-induced brachial plexus paralysis. *Arch Surg.* 1975;110:384–386.

55. Fourquer JA, Fakiris AJ, Timmerman RD, et al. Brachial plexopathy (BP) from stereotactic body radiotherapy (SBRT) in early-stage NSCLC: dose-limiting toxicity in apical tumor sites [abstract 78]. *Int J Radiat Oncol Biol Phys.* 2008;72(1 suppl):S36–S37.

56. Glantz MJ, Burger PC, Friedman AH, et al. Treatment of radiation-induced nervous system injury with heparin and warfarin. *Neurology.* 1994;44:2020–2027.

57. Delanian S, Lefaix JL. Current management for late normal tissue injury: radiation-induced fibrosis and necrosis. *Semin Radiat Oncol.* 2007;17:99–107.

58. Delanian S, Lefaix JL, Maisonobe T, et al. Significant clinical improvement in radiation-induced lumbosacral polyradiculopathy by a treatment combining pentoxifylline, tocopherol, and clodronate (Pentoclo). *Semin Radiat Oncol.* 2007;17(2):99–107.

59. Pritchard J, Anand P, Broome J, et al. Double-blind randomised phase II study of hyperbaric oxygen in patients with radiation-induced brachial plexopathy [abstract 37]. *Radiother Oncol.* 2001;58(suppl 1):S11.

60. Teixeira MJ, Fonoff ET, Montenegro MC. Dorsal root entry zone lesions for treatment of pain-related to radiation-induced plexopathy. *Spine.* 2007;32:E316–E319.

61. Narakas AO. Operative treatment for radiation-induced and metastatic brachial plexopathy in 45 cases, 15 having an omentoplasty. *Bull Hosp Jt Dis Orthop Inst.* 1984;44:354–375.

62. Brunelli G, Brunelli F. Surgical treatment of actinic brachial plexus lesions: free microvascular transfer of the greater omentum. *J Reconstr Microsurg.* 1985;1:197–200.

63. LeQuang C. Postirradiation lesions of the brachial plexus. Results of surgical treatment. *Hand Clin.* 1989;5:23–32.

Cerebral Radionecrosis

INTRODUCTION

The central nervous system (CNS) is exposed to ionizing radiation in a number of clinical situations, predominantly those involving cancer treatment. Radiotherapy remains a major treatment modality for primary and metastatic neoplasms located within the CNS, and exposure of the brain and spinal cord is often unavoidable in the radiotherapeutic management of tumors located close to the CNS such as head and neck cancers. There is also increasing application of radiation in the eradication of arteriovenous malformations (AVMs) and other benign disorders of the brain, such as epilepsy. In each of these situations, the radiation dose that can be administered safely is limited by the potential for injury to normal CNS tissue. Although any type of normal tissue damage is undesirable, the CNS injury that can occur after radiotherapy is associated with a high rate of morbidity and mortality and is especially devastating. Thus, the radioresponse of normal brain and spinal cord has been a subject of considerable research. Radiation-induced CNS injury has been well described in terms of histological and functional criteria as well as radiobiologic parameters,[1-3] though the underlying cellular and biochemical processes remain poorly defined.

Classically, radiation-induced CNS injury has been divided into three categories based on time of expression: acute, early delayed, and late delayed.[1-3] Acute radiation encephalopathy is expressed days to weeks after irradiation and is uncommon under current radiotherapy protocols. Early delayed injury occurs from 1 to 6 months after radiotherapy and can involve transient demyelination with somnolence after brain irradiation or Lhermitte syndrome after spinal irradiation. Acute and early delayed injuries are normally reversible and resolve spontaneously. In contrast, late delayed effects, which occur more than 6 months after irradiation, are not completely reversible and may be progressive, causing the majority of the morbidity and mortality of radiation-induced CNS injury. Late delayed injury is characterized by demyelination, vascular abnormalities, and ultimately necrosis that is generally restricted to the white matter. This classification helps make the important distinction between radiation *injury* (which may be reversible) versus radiation *necrosis* (an irreversible late effect involving tissue death). This chapter reviews the dose dependence, latency, incidence, histopathologic features, pathophysiology, diagnosis, and treatment of radiation-induced brain necrosis.

HISTORICAL PERSPECTIVE

Brain radiation necrosis has been recognized as a potential complication of radiation therapy for cancer for at least five decades. Some of the earliest experiments demonstrating radiation necrosis in the CNS were performed in primates and small animals.[4,5] In 1950, Lowenberg-Scharenberg and Bassett described amyloid degeneration of the human brain following x-ray therapy.[6] Subsequently, multiple instances of cerebral radiation necrosis were reported.[7-9] It soon became apparent that this pathology could simulate the disease originally treated with radiation, a dilemma that is still a common clinical problem.[10,11] In many cases, pathologic examination of surgical or autopsy specimens was, and still is, necessary for definitive diagnosis.

DOSE AND VOLUME DEPENDENCE

The radiation tolerance of normal tissues depends on total dose, dose per fraction, total time of exposure, volume, radiation quality, and adjunctive therapies such as chemotherapy. In 1980, Sheline et al.[3] published a pioneering study on brain radiation tolerance based on dose and fraction size. They created a log-log plot of megavoltage dose versus number of treatment fractions from 80 published cases of brain radionecrosis and determined an isoeffect line below which few cases of necrosis were observed (Fig. 24.1). They then modified the existing equivalent dose formula of the era, the Ellis formula for nominal standard dose in "ret," to create a formula for brain tolerance in "neuret" where

$$\text{neuret} = D \times N^{-0.44} \times T^{-0.06},$$

with D, total radiation dose in rad (cGy); N, number of radiation fractions; and T, total time in days.[3] Of note, the exponents indicate that fraction size is much more important to brain radiation tolerance than is treatment time. The threshold for necrosis was about 1,000 to 1,100 neuret.

The influence of fraction size was also assessed by Lee et al.[12] using a product of total dose (D) and fraction size (d) in Gy^2. The product (Dd) was found to be the most significant predictive factor for necrosis in a multivariate analysis of seven treatment parameters.[12,13] A study by Ruben et al.[14] confirms the significance of Dd and also demonstrates that average fraction size ≥ 2.25 Gy is a significant independent risk factor. Shorter overall

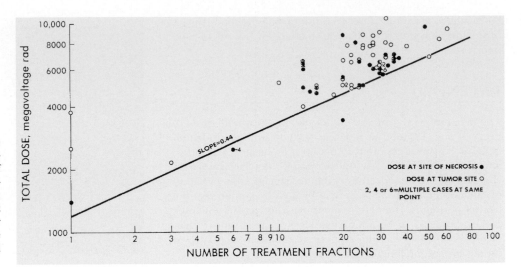

Figure 24.1. Megavoltage dose equivalent in rad (cGy) versus number of treatment fractions for cases of brain radionecrosis from the 1980 publication by Sheline, Wara, and Smith describing the neuret formula. Most cases of radiation necrosis occurred for dose/fraction combinations above the line with a slope of 0.44. (Reproduced with permission.)

treatment time from giving twice-daily radiation treatment was also found to be a significant risk factor the study by Lee et al.[12]

In the 1970s, a linear quadratic model was developed to describe cell survival after exposure to ionizing radiation, where the surviving fraction of cells S after exposure to a dose *D* is represented by

$$S = e^{-(\alpha D + \beta D^2)}.$$

The constant α describes the initial slope of the survival curve at low doses and β describes the quadratic component of cell killing.[15] A common related formula first introduced in the early 1980s[16] is for biologically effective dose (BED):

$$BED = D\left[1 + \frac{d}{(\alpha/\beta)}\right]$$

where *D* is the total dose and *d* is the size of a single radiation fraction in Gy. The ratio of α/β is in units of dose in Gy and tends to be in the range of 2 to 3 for late effects such as lung fibrosis or CNS injury versus around 8 to 10 for acute-responding tissues such as hair follicles, mucosa, and rapidly dividing tumor cells. As an example, BED = 100 for 50 Gy given at 2 Gy per daily fraction, assuming α/β = 2. A biologically equivalent dose for late effects given at 3 Gy/fraction can be determined by solving the formula 100 = D(1 + 3/2) = D × 2.5, which gives D = 100/2.5 = 40. Thus, 39 Gy at 3 Gy/fraction is approximately equivalent to 50 Gy at 2 Gy/fraction in terms of late effects.

Useful tolerance parameters are the 5% and 50% probabilities of brain injury at 5 years ($TD_{5/5}$ and $TD_{50/5}$, respectively). At "standard" fractionation of 1.8 to 2.0 Gy per daily treatment, the $TD_{5/5}$ is estimated to be 50 ± 10 Gy for the whole brain, 60 ± 10 Gy for a portion of the brain, and 45 to 50 Gy for a 10-cm segment of spinal cord.[17,18] Thresholds of 54 Gy[19] and 57.6 Gy[1] have been reported for cerebral radiation necrosis, but it is apparent that radionecrosis may occur below these limits with conventional therapeutic radiation.[3,20] In the North Central Cancer Treatment Group low-grade glioma trial, patients who received 60.8 Gy with conventionally fractionated radiation had a significantly higher actuarial incidence of necrosis than those who received 50.4 Gy, and only one patient treated with

50.4 Gy in 28 fractions developed radionecrosis.[20] In a report by Marks et al.,[19] also only one patient developed necrosis in an area irradiated to <50 Gy in 27 fractions. In the study by Sheline et al.,[3] only 20 of 80 cases of brain radionecrosis were in patients receiving doses ≤50 Gy, but of these, 17 (81%) received fraction sizes ≥2.5 Gy.

In single-fraction radiosurgery, the risk of brain necrosis increases rapidly above 12 or 13 Gy, and there is a higher risk with larger volume encompassed by the 12-Gy isodose line, particularly over 10 mL.[21,22] A dose-finding protocol, Radiation Therapy Oncology Group 90-05, found a similar relationship between higher risk of CNS toxicity from single-fraction radiosurgery and larger tumor volume, with lower "maximum tolerated doses" for larger tumors.[23] Modern radiotherapeutic management of brain tumors relies heavily on data such as these as physicians attempt to balance the risk of increased injury with potentially increased tumor control associated with higher radiation doses.

RETREATMENT TOLERANCE

Although there is substantial evidence for the safety of spinal cord reirradiation,[24,25] there is much less information about brain reirradiation. To study this question, Mayer and Sminia[26] reviewed 21 clinical series on reirradiation of glioma patients published from 1996 to 2006. They converted radiation doses from the first and second courses of treatment into BED assuming an α/β ratio of 2 and determined normalized total dose (NTD) in 2-Gy fractions. They noted that the cumulative NTD tended to be lowest when retreatment was accomplished with conventional radiotherapy (range, 81.6–101.9 Gy), intermediate for fractionated stereotactic radiosurgery (range, 90–133.9 Gy), and highest for radiosurgery (range, 111.6–137.2 Gy). There was a correlation between cumulative NTD and reirradiation volume (p = 0.0116), with smaller volumes receiving higher dose. Brain necrosis was found to occur at cumulative NTD > 100 Gy, with two exceptions when necrosis occurred at cumulative NTD < 90 Gy: one hyperfractionation study (perhaps indicating inadequate repair of radiation injury in the 6-hour interfraction interval) and one concurrent hyperbaric oxygen (HBO) study (perhaps indicating radiosensitization by HBO).

Surprisingly, the interval between the first and second courses of treatment appeared to have little effect on the risk of radionecrosis.[26]

LATENCY

The mean interval from the end of radiotherapy until onset of necrosis was 11.6 months in a recent study,[14] though radiation necrosis has been reported to manifest as early as 3 months[27] and as late as 47 years after radiotherapy.[28] Peritumoral parenchyma seems to be more vulnerable to damage from radiation or chemotherapy as was suggested by the observation that the latency period for the development of radionecrosis in glioma patients appears to be approximately five times shorter than in other patients receiving equivalent radiation dose, such as those with nasopharyngeal carcinoma.[3,12,19,29,30]

INCIDENCE

The incidence of cerebral radiation necrosis after conventional radiotherapy for primary brain tumors in modern radiation oncology practice is poorly defined. This is partially due to limited data on radiation dose-fractionation schedules and lack of both the numerator and the denominator for patient populations within which cases of radiation necrosis are described.[3] Additional barriers relate to the difficulty of distinguishing necrosis from tumor recurrence by neuroimaging and the low rates of reoperation and autopsy in these patients[27] and to limited survival time in patients with malignant brain tumors. Despite advances in magnetic resonance imaging (MRI) and functional imaging, necrosis or necrosis combined with tumor is still probably frequently mistaken for tumor progression alone, likely resulting in underestimation of the true incidence of brain radionecrosis.

A recent review of 426 patients treated for glioma and followed until death or for at least 3 years identified 21 patients with cerebral radionecrosis.[14] Most patients were treated with conventional radiotherapy along with chemotherapy, but ten of the patients who developed radionecrosis had additional boost or salvage stereotactic radiation, usually 18 Gy in three fractions. The crude radionecrosis incidence was 4.9% and the actuarial incidence was 2.9%, 5.1%, 9.3%, and 13.3% at 6, 12, 24, and 36 months posttreatment, respectively.[14] When analysis was restricted to patients treated with a radiation dose biologically equivalent to at least 45 Gy in 25 fractions, the crude incidence of radionecrosis increased to 6%.[14]

The use of radiosurgery or interstitial radiation after conventional radiotherapy clearly increases the risk of radionecrosis, though technique variability and patient population heterogeneity complicate estimation of the rate of radionecrosis, which ranges from 2.6% to 56% in reported series.[31–35]

It is important to note that many studies of brain radionecrosis include patients treated with chemotherapy in addition to radiotherapy. Although some investigators have suggested that injury is more often related to radiation than chemotherapy,[36] others reported changes similar to "radiation" necrosis from treatment with chemotherapy *only* for extracranial malignancies.[37] It is now widely accepted that both treatment modalities are injurious to normal brain, with the risk of necrosis increasing when they are used together.

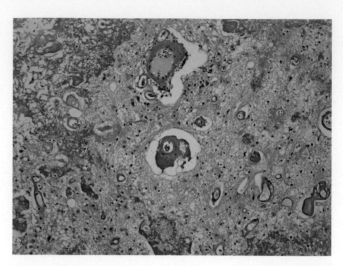

Figure 24.2. Histopathologic appearance of radiation necrosis, courtesy of Dr Tarik Tihan. Radiation necrosis most commonly induces changes within the cerebral blood vessels such as hyalinization, mural thickening, and fibrinoid necrosis. These changes can occur anywhere in the radiation field but typically affect the white matter. Areas of coagulative necrosis in association with blood vessels and scattered chronic inflammatory cells are also commonly observed.

HISTOPATHOLOGIC FEATURES

The end point of irreversible radiation injury in the brain is necrosis that may develop months to years after the completion of radiation therapy.[1,7] Radiation necrosis occurs most commonly around blood vessels within white matter. The most frequent histopathologic feature is fibrinoid necrosis of blood vessel walls with surrounding perivascular parenchymal coagulative necrosis (Fig. 24.2).[38] Focal radiation necrosis may be peritumoral or distant, as well as unifocal or multifocal.[39] Extension and confluence of multiple perivascular foci of necrosis result in large serpentine or confluent zones of parenchymal necrosis.[1,40] Over time, dystrophic calcifications can develop in these necrotic areas. An additional vascular lesion that is often observed consists of clusters of abnormally dilated, thin-walled telangiectasias. Late vascular changes include vessel wall thickening caused by hyalinization, with resultant luminal narrowing. White matter changes may also be focal or diffuse; in the diffuse pattern, widespread periventricular demyelination is seen.[7]

PATHOPHYSIOLOGY

Various hypotheses have been advanced regarding the primary cell population within the CNS whose death or inactivation after irradiation results in white matter necrosis. Because vascular abnormalities and demyelination dominate the histological presentation of radiation injury in the CNS, considerable effort has been focused on the radioresponse of the vasculature and cells of oligodendrocytic lineage.[40]

VASCULAR HYPOTHESIS

According to this hypothesis, white matter necrosis is considered to be a secondary response to ischemia. Substantial data are available describing radiation-induced vascular abnormalities including slowly evolving vessel wall thickening, vessel dilation, and nuclear enlargement in endothelial cells, which are presumed to be the result of endothelial cell damage.[41–44] Time- and dose-related reductions in blood vessel density (so-called vascular drop-out) and variable loss of endothelial cells have been reported prior to the development of necrosis in the white matter.[41,42] Interestingly, newer physiologic MRI methods that enable hemodynamic measurements within regions of interest in the brain have been used to differentiate recurrent tumor from radiation necrosis in the clinical setting.[45]

Other findings argue against vascular damage as the sole etiology of brain necrosis. Radiation-induced necrosis has sometimes been reported in the absence of vascular changes. Furthermore, the vascular hypothesis assumes that ischemia is ultimately responsible for necrosis, but the cell type most sensitive to oxygen deprivation is the neuron,[46] which is located in the gray matter, a relatively radioresistant region. Although the differences in blood flow between gray and white matter may be involved,[46] the predilection of radiation-induced necrosis for periventricular white matter is inconsistent with a solely vascular basis. Thus, although it seems unlikely that radiation injury can be attributed to a singular target, there is little doubt that vascular damage and endothelial cell loss play significant roles in the expression of white matter necrosis.

OLIGODENDROCYTE HYPOTHESIS

In addition to vascular abnormalities, the histologic presentation of radiation-induced CNS injury is typically dominated by demyelination, which implies oligodendrocytes as a target cell population. These terminally differentiated cells provide the myelin sheath for neurons, and their loss is an obvious source of demyelination. This hypothesis gained momentum in the 1980s with the identification of the O-2A progenitor cell, which serves as the precursor and source of new oligodendrocytes.[47] With the development of an in vivo/in vitro assay, van der Kogel et al.[48–50] demonstrated that irradiation results in the loss of reproductive capacity of the O-2A progenitor cells in both the brain and spinal cord of adult rats, which then results in the loss of reparative function or the failure to replace normally turned-over oligodendrocytes. The eventual outcome of this sequence of events is demyelination. The strength of this hypothesis is that it accounts for the white matter selectivity of radiation-induced CNS injury and is consistent with the established concept of stem cells as a source of functional, terminally differentiated oligodendrocytes. Furthermore, an acute loss of O-2A progenitors can be detected after irradiation, with their recovery being dependent on time and dose.[51–53]

However, there are inconsistencies that argue against oligodendrocytes as the source of radiation-induced white matter necrosis. In other demyelinating disorders such as multiple sclerosis, the degeneration of denuded axons is not a general finding, strongly suggesting that loss of oligodendrocytes alone is not sufficient for necrosis.[54] Additionally, whereas the kinetics of oligodendrocyte loss is consistent with the relatively early transient demyelination detected after irradiation, it is not consistent with the late onset of necrosis.[55,56] Furthermore, depletion of glial cells has been detected in rat, dog, and human brain after relatively low radiation doses that are not associated with significant risk of necrosis.[1,57,58] Thus, although there is detectable loss of O-2A cells and eventually oligodendroglia after irradiation, it appears that additional factors are required to cause late delayed white matter necrosis.

NEURAL STEM CELL HYPOTHESIS

The subventricular zone (SVZ) is the main source of neurons, astrocytes, and oligodendrocytes in the late embryonic forebrain of mammals. These SVZ cells migrate tangentially into the olfactory lobe, where they differentiate into neurons, and radially into neighboring structures such as the striatum, corpus callosum, and neocortex, where they differentiate into glia.[59–61] The SVZ persists into adulthood as a mitotically active area[62–64] and cells isolated from the SVZ of adult mice were found to have an extended ability to generate multilineage cell types (e.g., neurons and glia), thus meeting the criteria of stem cells.[65,66] Not all regions of the SVZ are equal in terms of proliferative activity, with mitotic activity varying with respect to rostrocaudal level within the SVZ.[67,68] Furthermore, these postnatal neural stem cells in different regions of the SVZ produce different types of neurons, suggesting that rather than being plastic and homogeneous, neural stem cells are a restricted and diverse population of progenitors.[69]

Based on their multipotential properties, it has been suggested that neural stem cells act as a reserve population of undifferentiated cells that can be recruited after tissue injury. Recent studies have shown that in response to chemical or physical injury in mouse brain, cells from the SVZ are capable of proliferating, migrating to the site of injury, and differentiating into various glial or neuronal cells.[70–72] The behavior of neural stem cells is under complex control of various growth factors and chemokines, but as of yet, it is incompletely understood.[73]

Hopewell and colleagues first suggested that the depletion of the SVZ cells (or subependymal plate cells, in early studies) could play a role in radiation-induced late delayed effects, contending that if the restorative response observed in SVZ should fail, a gradual decline in number of glial cells in the brain ultimately would lead to necrosis.[74–76] In spite of interesting correlative data, a cause-and-effect relationship between the radiation response of the SVZ and late effects has not been established. However, there are numerous recent publications that continue to explore the impact of x-ray irradiation on the SVZ cells and cerebral homeostasis.[71,72,77,78] This is an area of active research.[79,80]

CHRONIC INFLAMMATION HYPOTHESIS

Radiation directly induces a certain level of acute cell death. This has been demonstrated after in vivo irradiation in O-2A progenitors, SVZ neural stem cells, and oligodendrocytes.[48,49,81–83] Radiation also activates molecular and biochemical cascades that generate a persistent oxidative stress, which ultimately contributes to tissue injury.[84] Oxidative stress is a deleterious process that results from the production of free radicals in excess of the ability of a cell or tissue to defend against them.[85] The CNS is particularly susceptible to the development of oxidative stress;[86–88] it has a relatively high rate of oxidative metabolism, with approximately 2% to 5% of the consumed oxygen converted to superoxide and other reactive oxygen species (ROS) through mitochondrial electron transport.[89] Furthermore, because of the limited capacity of the CNS to perform anaerobic glycolysis, the mitochondrial production of ROS is substantially increased under hypoxic conditions.[90] In addition to the high rates of oxygen use and production of ROS, the CNS has relatively low levels of antioxidant defenses, especially in oligodendrocytes, neurons, and endothelial cells.[86,91,92] Thus, not only is the CNS environment conducive to the development of oxidative stress, it is also inherently more susceptible to oxidative injury.

Oxidative stress has been detected in and is considered to contribute to expression of CNS injury after ischemic, traumatic, and excitotoxic insults.[93–96] Additionally, it has been implicated as playing a causative role in various neurodegenerative conditions such as Alzheimer and Parkinson diseases.[94,97] The susceptibility of the myelin membrane to oxidative damage may account for the predilection of injury for white matter.[98] It is well established that exposure of cells to ionizing radiation results in the generation of short-lived ROS.[99] However, several studies now demonstrate presence and persistence of chronic inflammation in both in vitro and in vivo models for many weeks after exposure to ionizing radiation.[40,100–104] Whether the persistent oxidative stress induced by radiation contributes to normal tissue injury remains to be determined.

DIAGNOSIS

Radiation necrosis should be in the differential diagnosis for any patient with progressive neurological symptoms or a new or enlarging enhancing brain lesion with a history of intracranial radiation therapy several months or more previously to the equivalent of at least 12 Gy in a single dose (Fig. 24.3) or 50 Gy with at 1.8 to 2.0 Gy per daily fraction. A major dilemma in the diagnosis of radiation necrosis is differentiating it from recurrent or persistent tumor. Metastatic tumor recurrence

and radiation necrosis often have a similar appearance on conventional contrast-enhanced MRI.[105,106] Because of this, it is often difficult to distinguish which entity is responsible for the appearance of an enlarging lesion. Traditionally, a patient's clinical course, biopsy, and serial imaging for several months have been used to try to distinguish between tumor recurrence and radionecrosis.[105–107] Any investigation short of extensive tissue examination lacks diagnostic sensitivity and specificity. Anatomic and physiologic MRI, positron emission spectroscopy (PET), and thallium single photon emission computed tomography (SPECT) imaging have all been used in an attempt to define the best noninvasive method to diagnose radiation necrosis, though there is no evidence to date that any of these investigations is clearly superior to the other modalities.

ANATOMIC MAGNETIC RESONANCE IMAGING

Radiation necrosis can closely resemble recurrent tumor on anatomic ("conventional") MRI because of the following shared features: (a) focus at or close to the original tumor site, which is commonly the site of maximum radiation dose, (b) contrast enhancement, (c) progressive enlargement, at least over several months, (d) surrounding edema, and (e) exertion of mass effect. On MRI, brain necrosis usually consists of a somewhat irregular rim-enhancing mass with a central area of low signal on T1-weighted images (Fig. 24.3, upper center). The contrast enhancement of these lesions is thought to be secondary to radiation-induced endothelial damage resulting in breakdown of the blood-brain barrier. On T2-weighted images, the surrounding edema has high signal intensity, the solid portion of

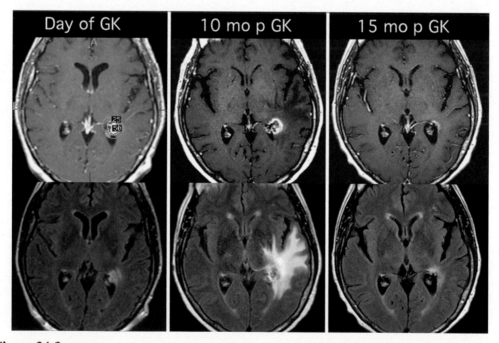

Figure 24.3. MRI T1-weighted postgadolinium images (*upper panels*) and T2-FLAIR images (*lower panels*) for a patient with a metastasis from breast cancer treated with 18-Gy single-fraction stereotactic radiosurgery at the 50% isodose contour (*upper left*). Symptomatic radiation necrosis developed 10 months later (*center*). Note the somewhat irregular rim enhancement around a central low signal intensity region on the T1-weighted image (*upper center*) and the extensive surrounding edema best seen as high signal on the T2-FLAIR sequence (*lower center*). Five months after onset of necrosis, following a two-month long course of dexamethasone, there was significant improvement in the imaging appearance (*upper and lower right*). Symptoms had resolved quickly on steroids and did not recur after discontinuance of steroids.

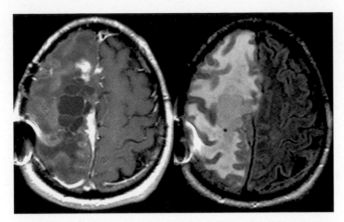

Figure 24.4. Example of late cyst formation after two courses of external beam radiotherapy and multiple treatments with single-fraction radiosurgery for multiple atypical meningiomas over 13 years, seen on brain MRI T1-weighted post-gadolinium sequence (*left*) and T2-FLAIR sequence (*right*).

defined a radiographic feature, the lesion quotient, which is the ratio of the nodule as seen on T2 imaging to the total enhancing area on T1 imaging, and suggested that a lesion quotient ≥0.6 correlates with recurrent tumor, whereas a quotient of ≤0.3 correlates with radionecrosis. The examined radiographic features, taken together, achieved 80% or greater predictive value but had either low sensitivity or low specificity.[108] In an older study, Kumar et al.[39] cite two radiographic features that are consistent with radiation necrosis, the "Swiss cheese" pattern and the "soap bubble" pattern. The first pattern is characterized by diffuse areas of enhancement affecting the cortex and white matter and intermixed with necrotic areas. The soap bubble appearance refers to smaller lesions with heterogeneously enhancing necrotic cores.[39]

The key point is that radiation necrosis should be included high in the differential diagnosis if some of the described imaging features or patterns are recognized. However, no radiographic pattern is pathognomonic for radiation necrosis and as such, supplementary functional imaging is often necessary and even then, surgical excision may still be required.

the radionecrotic lesion has low signal intensity, and the central necrotic component shows increased signal intensity (Fig. 24.3, lower center). Later, focal brain atrophy develops, and sometimes large cysts develop (Fig. 24.4). The arcuate fibers in white matter are relatively resistant to radiation necrosis and are usually involved late in the disease process. The predilection for periventricular white matter involvement in radiation necrosis may, on some occasions, mimic multiple sclerosis. Multiple lesions can resemble multiple metastases and radiation-induced necrotic lesions can also spread subependymally and mimic subependymal tumor spread.

Despite the many commonalities in radiographic appearance between tumor and necrotic tissue, several investigators have attempted to define patterns of radiation necrosis on conventional MRI with the aim of distinguishing tumor from necrosis. A recent study of 59 patients treated with radiosurgery for metastatic brain tumors who underwent subsequent craniotomy for symptomatic lesion enlargement analyzed the following features: (a) arteriovenous shunting, (b) gyriform lesion or edema distribution, (c) perilesional edema, (d) cyst formation, and (e) pattern of enhancement.[108] The authors also

MAGNETIC RESONANCE SPECTROSCOPY

Magnetic resonance spectroscopy (MRS) has been explored as a noninvasive means of diagnosing radiation necrosis and distinguishing it from tumor recurrence. The technique allows metabolites from an area of interest to be quantified and compared with those of surrounding normal tissue.[109] Metabolites such as *N*-acetyl aspartate (NAA), phosphorylcholine/glycerophosphorylcholine (Cho), creatine (Cr), lactate (Lac), and mobile lipids (Lip) provide different spectra in tumors compared with normal brain or radiation necrosis. Elevated levels of choline compounds have been repeatedly reported in the "peritumoral region" for gliomas[110–114] but not metastases.[111]

In general, regions of tumor are characterized by NAA/Cho ratio <1 and Lip/Cho ratio <3. In contrast, Lip/Cho ratio >3 or significant decrease of all metabolite levels within the lesion or surrounding brain are considered characteristic of radiation-induced necrosis (Fig. 24.5).[115] The technique has evolved significantly from single-voxel, low-resolution studies to multivoxel acquisitions that have a much higher resolution.[115,116]

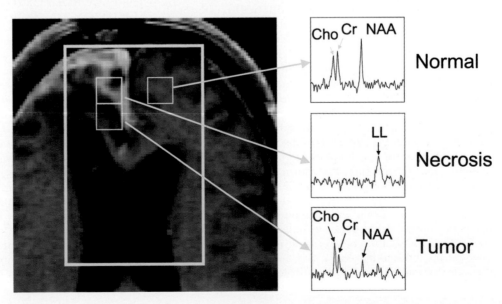

Figure 24.5. MRS appearance of normal brain tissue, necrosis, and tumor voxels in a patient with recurrent glioblastoma. Note the increased ratio of the choline (Cho)/creatine (Cr) to NAA in the tumor spectrum compared to the normal brain spectrum, and the depression of Cho, Cr, and NAA in the area of necrosis along with appearance of a lactate/lipid (LL) peak. (Modified and reproduced with permission, Chan et al., Proton Magnetic Resonance Spectroscopic Imaging as a tool for evaluating grade IV glioma patients undergoing gamma knife radiosurgery. *J Neurosurg.* 2004;101(3):467–475.)

In practice, MRS has been used alone in an attempt to reduce the need to biopsy new enhancing lesions on MRI[117,118] and in combination with biopsy to help guide sampling and improve diagnostic yield.[119,120]

DIFFUSION-WEIGHTED IMAGING

Diffusion-weighted imaging (DWI) is another interesting approach for utilizing MR technology to diagnose radiation necrosis. The technique depends on the diffusion of water molecules within the tissue under study and generates an apparent diffusion coefficient (ADC) map.[109] Areas with high ADC appear dark on DWI whereas low ADC areas produce increased signal. The differences in ADC in various tissues are thought to result from both changes in the balance between intracellular and extracellular water and changes in the structure of the two compartments. In theory, areas of radiation necrosis should have higher (or better) diffusion coefficients than areas of hypercellular tumor so that the technique could be used to differentiate the two conditions. This explanation represents a gross simplification of the biologic milieu of both tumor and necrosis, but high diffusion on ADC has been reported in cerebral radiation necrosis caused by treatment of brain tumors.[121–124]

Previous studies applied this technique to evaluate cellularity in gliomas with the aim of determining tumor grade noninvasively.[125] Signal intensity and ADCs in neoplastic tissue, peritumoral edema, and normal brain tissue have been reported for low- and high-grade gliomas, meningiomas, and brain metastases.[126] Necrotic brain tissue in the temporal lobe after radiation therapy for nasopharyngeal carcinoma has been characterized using DWI as well.[127] Previously reported ADC values for high-grade glial tumors vary from 1.1 to $1.37 \times 10^{-3}\,mm/s^2$.[125,128,129] ADCs in peritumoral edema or temporal lobe necrosis were reported as 1.29 and $2.88 \times 10^{-3}\,mm/s^2$ in two notable studies.[127,130] Although ADC maps can provide useful information that may help distinguish tumor from necrosis, DWI has not been studied sufficiently to permit unequivocal diagnosis. Presently, DWI is primarily used as an adjunct to other studies.

PERFUSION MRI

Dynamic, contrast-enhanced perfusion MRI (pMRI) of the brain provides hemodynamic information that complements the anatomic information available from conventional MRI. Contrast-enhanced pMRI methods exploit signal changes that accompany the passage of a paramagnetic contrast agent (gadolinium) through the cerebrovascular system to derive relative blood volume and flow information.[131,132] Analysis of dynamic data from pMRI yields quantitative estimates of the relative cerebral blood volume (rCBV) of the lesion versus other regions of interest such as surrounding tissue or contralateral normal tissue. For CBV measurements, a series of images is acquired at intervals of approximately 1 second before, during, and after bolus injection of the contrast agent. Rapid gradient-echo or echo-planar imaging is generally used to acquire multiple T1-weighted slices at each time point during the imaging interval. When a paramagnetic contrast agent passes through the cerebral vascular system, it induces differences in local magnetic susceptibility between the intravascular space and the surrounding normal tissue, with a transient and differential loss of relaxation signal. This enables calculation of the contrast concentration-time

curve, and rCBV can then be estimated from the area under this curve and corrected for contrast leakage using a reference measurement in the contralateral, unaffected centrum semiovale white matter.

Sugahara et al.[133] were among the first to propose that this technique should be utilized when it is necessary to differentiate tumor recurrence from radiation necrosis.[133] In a series of 20 cases, these authors found that a normalized rCBV of 2.6 or higher indicated tumor recurrence and a ratio of 0.6 or less was suggestive of nonneoplastic contrast-enhancing tissue.[133]

A more recent approach, described by Barajas et al., uses three hemodynamic variables to describe the shape of the signal intensity-time curve obtained from dynamic susceptibility contrast pMRI: rCBV, relative peak height, and percentage of signal-intensity recovery; among 27 patients with necrosis or tumor recurrence or progression after single-fraction radiosurgery for brain metastases, rCBV and relative peak height were significantly higher and the percentage of signal intensity recovery was significantly lower for tumor versus necrosis (Fig. 24.6).[45,134] Relative CBV is the most widely used hemodynamic variable derived from pMRI and has been shown to correlate with tumor grade and tumor microvascular attenuation.[111,133–140] Relative peak height, which represents the maximal change in signal intensity during the passage of contrast agent, has been shown to correlate with rCBV measurements and tumor capillary blood volume.[111,135,136] Finally, percentage of signal-intensity recovery, an indicator of the blood-brain barrier integrity, reflects the degree of contrast agent leakage through tumor microvasculature and provides insight into the alteration of capillary permeability.[111,135,136]

Several important limitations are associated with dynamic, contrast-enhanced pMRI. Because the technique is susceptibility weighted, it is extremely sensitive to structures or lesions that induce strong magnetic field inhomogeneities such as blood products, calcium, melanin, metals, or lesions near brain-bone-air interfaces such as the skull base. When there is a large amount of susceptibility artifact, pMRI fails to provide any meaningful information.[141] Also, the calculation of rCBV can be grossly inaccurate in lesions with a severe breakdown or absence of the blood-brain barrier.

^{18}F-FLUORODEOXYGLUCOSE POSITRON EMISSION TOMOGRAPHY

Positron emission tomography (PET) can be used to measure the metabolism of glucose labeled with an ^{18}F analog. Because radiation necrosis should be characterized by low glucose consumption, ^{18}F-fluorodeoxyglucose (FDG) is often used in PET studies to provide contrast with areas of tumor, which should have higher uptake. Early studies reported that ^{18}F-FDG-PET had a sensitivity of 81% to 86% and a specificity of 40% to 94% for distinguishing between radiation necrosis and tumor.[142]

There are multiple limitations to the usefulness of PET in the brain. Tumor glucose metabolism is highly variable, and the overlap of ^{18}F-FDG uptake between radiation necrosis and tumor can be considerable.[143–145] In addition, tumor glucose metabolism is frequently lower than that of normal brain tissue; thus, tumor uptake may be difficult to appreciate amid the background of highly metabolically active normal brain tissue or of treated brain tissue, which tends to have lower glucose metabolism than untreated brain and may also have a wide range of metabolic activity (Fig. 24.7). Also, high ^{18}F-FDG

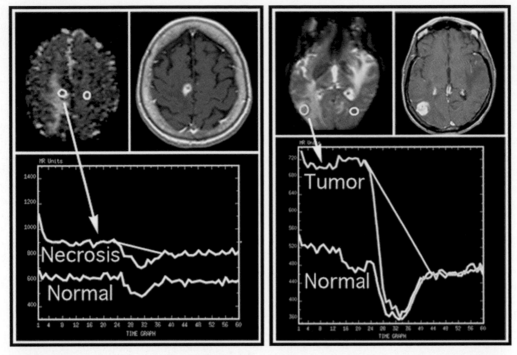

Figure 24.6. Perfusion/blood volume MRI examples showing necrosis (*left panels*) versus tumor (*right panels*). A bolus of contrast is given at time zero, and images are obtained every second for one minute to capture the first pass of contrast through the brain circulation. Magnetic resonance signal is plotted versus time for one or more regions of interest placed in normal white matter (*circles without arrows*) and in the lesion to be evaluated (*circles with arrows*). In areas of necrosis, the drop in signal (relative peak height) is similar to less than that within the normal region, and there is usually good signal intensity recovery toward the baseline level. In tumor, the drop in signal is greater, indicating elevated blood flow, and there is often less signal intensity recovery because of the increased leakiness of tumor vasculature.

uptake can occur from inflammation that may be associated with necrosis, resulting in misinterpretation. In general, it has not been possible to define a reliable cutoff of standardized uptake values to distinguish between tumor and necrosis. Strategies to improve predictive value include comparing the ratio of the lesion to contralateral normal white or gray matter or determining whether lesion activity is above the expected background activity in adjacent brain tissue;[146-148] in either

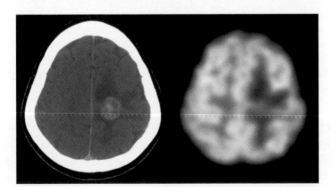

Figure 24.7. CT image (*left*) and corresponding ^{18}F-FDG PET image (*right*) of a left frontal metastasis from ovarian cancer. The lesion initially shrank after single-fraction radiosurgery with 17.5 Gy, but then increased in size 7 months later. PET showed markedly reduced FDG uptake surrounding the treated lesion and mildly abnormal FDG uptake within the lesion, intermediate between that of normal white matter and normal gray matter. Based on this finding, tumor progression was considered to be more likely than radiation necrosis.

case, it can be helpful to have the anatomic information from co-registration with MRI.[149,150]

AMINO ACID PET

Amino acid PET tracers and amino acid analog PET tracers constitute another class of tumor imaging agents.[151,152] These are particularly attractive for imaging brain tumors because of the high uptake in tumor tissue and low uptake in normal brain tissue; amino acids are transported into the cell via carrier-mediated processes,[152] and amino acid transport is generally increased in malignant cells.[153,154]. The most extensively studied amino acid tracer is ^{11}C-methionine.[155] Because of the short half-life of [11]C (approximately 20 minutes), ^{18}F-labeled aromatic amino acid analogs (with a half-life of approximately 109 minutes) have been developed for tumor imaging.[156]

Because amino acid tracers appear more sensitive than ^{18}F-FDG-PET in visualizing tumor, they also have potentially better diagnostic accuracy in evaluating radiation necrosis. However, the degree of amino acid uptake in radiation necrosis lesions is not known. ^{11}C-methionine has been available for about two decades, but few studies have been published on its performance in differentiating radiation necrosis from brain tumor recurrence.[147] In a study of 21 patients with brain metastases treated with stereotactic radiosurgery, ^{11}C-methionine correctly identified seven of nine recurrences and 10 of 12 radiation injury lesions.[157]

In rats, uptake of ^{18}F-FET (^{18}F-fluoroethyl-L-tyrosine), ^{18}F-FDG, and ^{18}F-choline has been compared in acute lesions caused by cerebral irradiation and cryotherapy.[158] Both ^{18}F-FDG and ^{18}F-choline accumulated in macrophages, a common inflammatory cell type in radiation necrosis, but ^{18}F-FET uptake was absent from macrophages. Moreover, the ratio of ^{18}F-FET uptake in radiation necrosis to that in normal cortex was much lower than the corresponding ratios for ^{18}F-FDG and ^{18}F-choline, suggesting that ^{18}F-FET may be able to differentiate radiation necrosis from tumor recurrence. Absence of ^{18}F-FET uptake in a case of radiation necrosis has been reported.[159] Although these results are promising, larger systematic studies are needed to evaluate the diagnostic performance of these tracers.

SINGLE PHOTON EMISSION COMPUTED TOMOGRAPHY

SPECT relies on the injection of a radionuclide such as [201]Tl (Thallium-201) or [99m]Tc (Technetium-99) and the use of a gamma camera and computed tomography (CT) to detect its distribution in the brain. Uptake of the radionuclide is greater in tumor cells than in normal tissue and inflammatory cells, and depends on Na/K-ATPase pump activity.[160] Because uptake requires a viable cell, it is correspondingly low in necrotic areas. This technique is much less expensive and more widely available than PET but has disadvantages with regard to limited breadth of molecular processes that are accessible, quantitation accuracy, and spatial resolution.[160]

High-grade tumors have a higher thallium index than low-grade tumors. In a series of 15 biopsy-proven cases, Schwartz et al.[161] found an excellent correlation between imaging and histology (14/15 cases) using dual-isotope SPECT scanning with ^{201}Tl and ^{99m}Tc-hexamethylpropylene amine oxime (HMPAO).[161] A subsequent study revealed a high ^{201}Tl uptake in recurrent tumor and low uptake in radiation necrosis. In cases with intermediate uptake, ^{99m}Tc-HMPAO uptake helped to differentiate tumor recurrences from radiation necrosis by showing increased perfusion in tumor.[161] After these initial exciting reports of sensitivities in excess of 90% for detecting tumor recurrence with specificity approximately 60%,[162] other reports citing concerns about the diagnostic accuracy of the technique for distinguishing recurrent tumor from radiation necrosis began to surface, including cases of thallium-avid radiation necrosis.[163–165]

More recently, Alexiou et al.[166] substantiated a potential superiority of ^{99m}Tc-tetrofosmin (^{99m}Tc-TF) over ^{99m}Tc-sestamibi, a commonly used imaging agent, for brain tumor imaging, owing to the fact that ^{99m}Tc-TF accumulation is independent of the multidrug-resistance phenotype of some glioma cells.[167,168] ^{99m}Tc-TF is a tumor-seeking diphosphine that does not cross the intact blood-brain barrier, and uptake is dependent on regional blood flow and cell membrane integrity, thus reflecting cellular metabolic status and viability. Alexiou et al. also reported that ^{99m}Tc-TF could successfully differentiate tumor recurrence from radiation injury.[166,169] These results have yet to be confirmed by other groups.

HISTOLOGIC EXAMINATION

Given the limitations of the various imaging techniques, a definitive diagnosis of radiation necrosis may require pathologic examination of surgical specimens. Because of the potential for sampling error with biopsy alone, total resection is preferred. Resection also improves edema and mass effect associated with radiation necrosis and/or active tumor. If resection is not safe or feasible, the imaging modalities described above may be used to guide biopsies, so that the region most suspicious for active tumor can be sampled to maximize diagnostic yield.

TREATMENT

While the finding of radiation necrosis, or "treatment effect," is often met with relief that the changes seen on imaging do not represent tumor growth, patients and their families and health care providers need to understand the implication of this condition. Radiation necrosis can produce symptoms that are as disabling as tumor recurrence. Most patients with radiation necrosis present with focal neurologic deficits related to the necrotic lesion as well as headaches as a result of mass effect from reactive vasogenic edema. Some cases stabilize or improve with the treatments described below or with the passage of time, but some cases may be relentlessly progressive.

STEROIDS

Steroids are frequently used to treat radiation-induced edema and necrosis. Animal models of radiation-induced CNS necrosis demonstrate that edema precedes the development of necrosis and that the antiinflammatory effect of dexamethasone, when provided early, can modify subsequent vascular and inflammatory changes to reduce and delay the development of subsequent necrosis.[170–172] Thus, controlling edema after irradiation or in the early stages of necrosis may limit the subsequent development or course of necrosis (Fig. 24.3, right). Among patients with temporal lobe necrosis after radiotherapy for nasopharyngeal cancer, dexamethasone given at the onset of radiation necrosis, during which there was marked reactive edema, resulted in significant objective improvement of necrosis in 38% of patients, whereas none of the patients with cystic necrosis improved.[173]

The optimal dose and timing of the corticosteroids have not been prospectively studied; however, it appears that administration early in the course of radionecrosis is more effective than one that is delayed, and the doses given must be adequate to control clinical symptoms. After symptoms improve, the steroid dose should be tapered as tolerated. Some patients become symptomatic when steroid treatment is discontinued and thus require long-term treatment over many weeks or up to approximately 6 to 8 months. Attention must then be directed toward minimizing the medical complications associated with steroid treatment, such as steroid myopathy, glucose intolerance, and osteopenia.

SURGICAL RESECTION

Radiation-induced necrosis is clearly a dynamic process. Cases have been documented in which necrosis spontaneously resolves, remains stable, or progressively enlarges to produce a space-occupying lesion that becomes increasingly symptomatic. When steroid therapy is poorly tolerated or when radiation necrosis becomes progressively larger and symptomatic despite the use of steroids, surgical excision of the necrotic mass is indicated.[1,172,174] In general, surgical treatment is an effective therapy for well-circumscribed areas of necrosis and much less effective for diffusely necrotic lesions.[174] It is presumed that removal of the necrotic nidus, a source of inflammation,

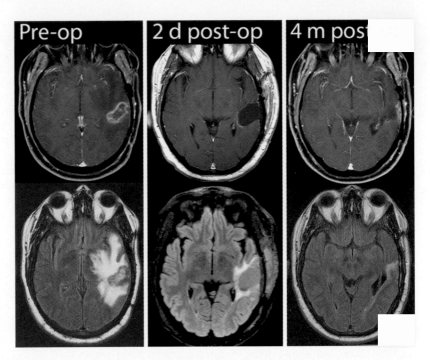

Figure 24.8. Preoperative T1-weighted (*upper left*) and T2-FLAIR (*lower left*) MRI sequences, 2-day postoperative postgadolinium T1-weighted (*upper center*) and T2-FLAIR (*lower center*) MRI sequences, and 4-month postoperative postgadolinium T1-weighted (*upper right*) and T2-FLAIR (*lower right*) MRI sequences showing marked improvement in enhancement, edema, and mass effect after surgical resection of a necrotic lesion.

reduces the associated edema and thereby, secondary mass effect (Fig. 24.8). Surgery thus provides an immediate relief of symptoms and frequently enables patients to be rapidly tapered off steroids.

HYPERBARIC OXYGEN

HBO therapy is the inhalation of 100% oxygen at an elevated pressure, usually over 1.5 times the atmospheric pressure, in a controlled and monitored environment. When used after radiation therapy, HBO has been shown to increase tissue oxygenation and angiogenesis and improve capillary bed function.[175] HBO has been used in the treatment and prevention of late complications after radiotherapy in different sites, and many papers have been published reporting its use.[176] Hulshof et al.[177] prospectively evaluated HBO in patients with cognitive problems following cerebral radiotherapy and found that only one out of seven patients experienced a significant improvement. Leber et al.[178] reported two cases of successful HBO therapy for radiation damage following gamma knife radiosurgery for AVMs, with marked improvement in necrotic lesions on imaging without the use of corticosteroids. Given the scarcity of evidence and lack of controlled trials, there is considerable uncertainty on the place of HBO in the management of late neurological sequelae of radiation therapy.

ANTICOAGULANTS

Because it is thought that radiation necrosis results mainly from vascular changes associated with ischemia, anticoagulants (heparin and warfarin [*Coumadin*]) and antiplatelet medications such as Pentoxifylline (*Trental*), aspirin, and ticlopidine (*Ticlid*) have been used to attempt to halt its progression. Five of eight patients with cerebral radiation necrosis unresponsive to steroids had clinical improvement on anticoagulation with heparin (*Heparin*) and warfarin (*Coumadin*).[179] The potential risk of bleeding from these agents must be weighed against any

expected benefit, and these patients must be closely monitored for consumptive coagulopathies, especially in the setting of concurrent chemotherapy. Definitive conclusions are not available owing to the small numbers of patients studied. However, in cases where radiation necrosis is progressive and symptomatic, full anticoagulation is reasonable assuming there are no contraindications. There are no published comparisons for antiplatelet versus anticoagulant agents.

ANTIOXIDANT THERAPY

Oral pentoxifylline (Trental) and tocopherol (vitamin E) combination therapy has been reported to benefit patients with skin and chest wall radionecrosis as well as mandibular osteoradionecrosis.[180] Pentoxifylline is thought to reverse radiation damage primarily through its ability to increase locoregional blood flow; it improves red blood cell deformability and promotes laminar blood flow by inhibiting intercellular adhesion molecule expression, resulting in decreased adhesion between endothelial cells and leukocytes. Pentoxifylline also decreases plasma fibrinogen while increasing fibrinolytic activity,[181] and it is a nonspecific inhibitor of many inflammatory cytokines.[180] Tocopherol is an antioxidant compound that scavenges ROS generated during oxidative stress and protects lipid membranes against lipid peroxidation.[182] Williamson et al.[183] reported on 11 patients with delayed adverse radiation effects after treatment with gamma knife radiosurgery for various benign and malignant disorders who were treated with pentoxifylline (400 mg orally twice daily) and tocopherol (400 IU orally twice daily). The edema volume measured on serial FLAIR-MRI improved in 10 of 11 patients, with an average volume decrease of 72.3 mL.[183] The only patient without improvement was found to have tumor recurrence. The authors concluded that pentoxifylline and tocopherol may be of benefit for treatment of adverse radiation effects. Further studies are needed to determine the efficacy of this regimen for the treatment of brain radionecrosis.

VASCULAR ENDOTHELIAL GROWTH FACTOR INHIBITORS

The premise for the use of bevacizumab (*Avastin*) for radiation necrosis came from observations of radionecrosis-associated endothelial cell dysfunction and hypoxia with liberation of vasoactive compounds, including vascular endothelial growth factor (VEGF). Bevacizumab is a humanized murine monoclonal antibody against the VEGF molecule. It blocks VEGF from reaching its capillary targets and is currently being used in the treatment of several solid tumors. Gonzalez et al.[184] retrospectively evaluated 15 patients treated with bevacizumab or bevacizumab combined with chemotherapy after radiation for malignant brain tumors. Radiation necrosis was diagnosed in eight patients, all of whom underwent therapy with bevacizumab on either a 5 mg/kg/2-wk or 7.5 mg/kg/3-wk schedule. Posttreatment MRI scans, performed approximately 8 weeks after therapy, demonstrated measurable improvements in all patients. The imaging findings correlated with clinical improvement as evaluated by the average reduction in daily dexamethasone requirement by 8.6 mg. The authors of this study concluded that bevacizumab, alone or in combination with other agents, can reduce radiation necrosis by decreasing capillary leakage and the associated brain edema.[184] Torcuator et al.[185] reported on six glioma patients with biopsy-proven brain radionecrosis treated with bevacizumab at 10 mg/kg every other week, combined with irinotecan in two cases of suspected tumor cells in addition to necrosis. Compared with prebevacizumab imaging, the mean decrease in volume of contrast enhancement was 79% and the mean decrease in T2-FLAIR volume was 49%.[185] Similar results were published in a recent case report of bevacizumab at 5 mg/kg every other week for temporal lobe necrosis that developed 2 years after aggressive radiotherapy with chemotherapy for nasopharyngeal carcinoma[186] and in three of four children with pontine gliomas suspected of having radiation necrosis.[187] Recently, Gutin et al.[188] reported no cases of radionecrosis among 25 patients with recurrent malignant gliomas treated with fractionated stereotactic reirradiation to 30 Gy in six fractions along with bevacizumab, 10 mg/kg every 2 weeks. Optimal dosing, duration of treatment, and efficacy of bevacizumab (or similar agents) need further evaluation in prospective trials.

REHABILITATION

Depending on the symptoms and clinical deficits caused by radiation necrosis, patients may benefit from physical, occupational, or speech therapy.

CONCLUSION

Brain necrosis is associated with a significant degree of morbidity and sometimes mortality. It has been recognized as a potential complication of brain radiation therapy for at least five decades, with higher risk for larger volumes, higher total dose, and higher dose per fraction, especially above about 50 Gy at 1.8 to 2.0 Gy per daily fraction or 12 Gy in one fraction. The latency period is highly variable, but the minimum latency is about 3 months after radiation exposure. The pathophysiology is not completely understood; contributing factors appear to include injury to vasculature, oligodendrocytes, and/or neural stem cells and chronic inflammation. It may be difficult to distinguish radiation necrosis from progressive or recurrent tumor following treatment for primary or metastatic brain tumors. Techniques that have been used include MRI, MRS, PET, and SPECT, short of surgical biopsy or resection for a histopathologic diagnosis. The symptoms of radiation necrosis may be mild or reversible, but are sometimes significant or progressive, warranting treatment with steroids and/or surgical resection. Less well-proven but possibly effective interventions include HBO therapy, anticoagulation, antioxidant therapy, and therapy with VEGF inhibitors. The diagnosis and management of each patient requires a thoughtful clinical approach, and further investigations are needed to allow better avoidance or prevention and to optimize diagnosis and treatment of brain necrosis.

REFERENCES

1. Gutin PH, Leibel SA, Sheline GE. *Radiation injury to the nervous system.* New York, NY: Raven Press; 1991.
2. Hopewell JW, Wright EA. The nature of latent cerebral irradiation damage and its modification by hypertension. *Br J Radiol.* 1970;43:161–167.
3. Sheline GE, Wara WM, Smith V. Therapeutic irradiation and brain injury. *Int J Radiat Oncol Biol Phys.* 1980;6:1215–1228.
4. Arnold A, Bailey P. Alterations in the glial cells following irradiation of the brain in primates. *AMA Arch Pathol.* 1954;57:383–391.
5. Russell DS, Wilson CW, Tansley K. Experimental radio-necrosis of the brain in rabbits. *J Neurol Neurosurg Psychiatry.* 1949;12:187–195.
6. Lowenberg-Scharenberg K, Bassett RC. Amyloid degeneration of the human brain following X-ray therapy. *J Neuropathol Exp Neurol.* 1950;9:93–102, illust.
7. Lampert P, Tom MI, Rider WD. Disseminated demyelination of the brain following Co60 (gamma) radiation. *Arch Pathol.* 1959;68:322–330.
8. Nielsen SL, Kjellberg RN, Asbury AK, et al. Neuropathologic effects of proton-beam irradiation in man. I. Dose-response relationships after treatment of intracranial neoplasms. *Acta Neuropathol.* 1972;20:348–356.
9. Pennybacker J, Russell DS. Necrosis of the brain due to radiation therapy; clinical and pathological observations. *J Neurol Neurosurg Psychiatry.* 1948;11:183–198.
10. Eyster EF, Nielsen SL, Sheline GE, et al. Cerebral radiation necrosis simulating a brain tumor. Case report. *J Neurosurg.* 1974;40:267–271.
11. Ghatak NR, White BE. Delayed radiation necrosis of the hypothalamus. Report of a case simulating recurrent craniopharyngioma. *Arch Neurol.* 1969;21:425–430.
12. Lee AW, Kwong DL, Leung SF, et al. Factors affecting risk of symptomatic temporal lobe necrosis: significance of fractional dose and treatment time. *Int J Radiat Oncol Biol Phys.* 2002;53:75–85.
13. Lee AW, Foo W, Chappell R, et al. Effect of time, dose, and fractionation on temporal lobe necrosis following radiotherapy for nasopharyngeal carcinoma. *Int J Radiat Oncol Biol Phys.* 1998;40:35–42.
14. Ruben JD, Dally M, Bailey M, et al. Cerebral radiation necrosis: incidence, outcomes, and risk factors with emphasis on radiation parameters and chemotherapy. *Int J Radiat Oncol Biol Phys.* 2006;65:499–508.
15. Douglas BG, Fowler JR. Fractionation schedules and a quadratic-dose effect relationship. *Br J Radiol (Letter).* 1975;48:502–504.
16. Barendsen GW. Dose fractionation, dose rate, and isoeffect relationships for normal tissue responses. *Int J Radiat Oncol Biol Phys.* 1982;8:1981–1997.
17. Hall EJ, Giaccia AJ. *Radiobiology for the Radiologist.* 6th ed. Philadelphia, PA: Lippincott Williams & Wilkins; 2006.
18. Milano MT, Constine LS, Okunieff P. Normal tissue tolerance dose metrics for radiation therapy of major organs. *Semin Radiat Oncol.* 2007;17:131–140.
19. Marks JE, Baglan RJ, Prassad SC, et al. Cerebral radionecrosis: incidence and risk in relation to dose, time, fractionation and volume. *Int J Radiat Oncol Biol Phys.* 1981;7:243–252.
20. Shaw E, Arusell R, Scheithauer B, et al. Prospective randomized trial of low- versus high-dose radiation therapy in adults with supratentorial low-grade glioma: initial report of a North Central Cancer Treatment Group/Radiation Therapy Oncology Group/Eastern Cooperative Oncology Group study. *J Clin Oncol.* 2002;20:2267–2276.
21. Flickinger JC, Kondziolka D, Pollock BE, et al. Complications from arteriovenous malformation radiosurgery: multivariate analysis and risk modeling. *Int J Radiat Oncol Biol Phys.* 1997;38:485–490.
22. Korytko T, Radivoyevitch T, Colussi V, et al. 12 Gy gamma knife radiosurgical volume is a predictor for radiation necrosis in non-AVM intracranial tumors. *Int J Radiat Oncol Biol Phys.* 2006;64:419–424.
23. Shaw E, Scott C, Souhami L, et al. Single dose radiosurgical treatment of recurrent previously irradiated primary brain tumors and brain metastases: final report of RTOG protocol 90–05. *Int J Radiat Oncol Biol Phys.* 2000;47:291–298.
24. Ang KK, Jiang GL, Feng Y, et al. Extent and kinetics of recovery of occult spinal cord injury. *Int J Radiat Oncol Biol Phys.* 2001;50:1013–1020.
25. Nieder C, Grosu AL, Andratschke NH, et al. Update of human spinal cord reirradiation tolerance based on additional data from 38 patients. *Int J Radiat Oncol Biol Phys.* 2006;66:1446–1449.

26. Mayer R, Sminia P. Reirradiation tolerance of the human brain. *Int J Radiat Oncol Biol Phys.* 2008;70:1350–1360.

27. Gilbert HA, Kagan AR. *Radiation Damage to the Nervous System: A Delayed Therapeutic Hazard.* New York, NY: Raven Press; 1980.

28. Babu R, Huang PP, Epstein F, et al. Late radiation necrosis of the brain: case report. *J Neurooncol.* 1993;17:37–42.

29. Soffietti R, Sciolla R, Giordana MT, et al. Delayed adverse effects after irradiation of gliomas: clinicopathological analysis. *J Neurooncol.* 1985;3:187–192.

30. Woo E, Lam K, Yu YL, et al. Temporal lobe and hypothalamic-pituitary dysfunctions after radiotherapy for nasopharyngeal carcinoma: a distinct clinical syndrome. *J Neurol Neurosurg Psychiatry.* 1988;51:1302–1307.

31. Kreth FW, Faist M, Warnke PC, et al. Interstitial radiosurgery of low-grade gliomas. *J Neurosurg.* 1995;82:418–429.

32. Scharfen CO, Sneed PK, Wara WM, et al. High activity iodine-125 interstitial implant for gliomas. *Int J Radiat Oncol Biol Phys.* 1992;24:583–591.

33. Shrieve DC, Alexander E, Black PM, et al. Treatment of patients with primary glioblastoma multiforme with standard postoperative radiotherapy and radiosurgical boost: prognostic factors and long-term outcome. *J Neurosurg.* 1999;90:72–77.

34. Sneed PK, McDermott MW, Gutin PH. Interstitial brachytherapy procedures for brain tumors. *Semin Surg Oncol.* 1997;13:157–166.

35. Wowra B, Schmitt HP, Sturm V. Incidence of late radiation necrosis with transient mass effect after interstitial low dose rate radiotherapy for cerebral gliomas. *Acta Neurochir (Wien).* 1989;99:104–108.

36. Imperato JP, Paleologos NA, Vick NA. Effects of treatment on long-term survivors with malignant astrocytomas. *Ann Neurol.* 1990;28:818–822.

37. Burger PC, Kamenar E, Schold C, et al. Encephalomyelopathy following high-dose BCNU therapy. *Cancer.* 1981;48:1318–1327.

38. Schultheiss TE, Stephens LC, Maor MH. Analysis of the histopathology of radiation myelopathy. *Int J Radiat Oncol Biol Phys.* 1988;14:27–32.

39. Kumar AJ, Leeds NE, Fuller GN, et al. Malignant gliomas: MR imaging spectrum of radiation therapy- and chemotherapy-induced necrosis of the brain after treatment. *Radiology.* 2000;217:377–384.

40. Yoshii Y. Pathological review of late cerebral radionecrosis. *Brain Tumor Pathol.* 2008;25:51–58.

41. Calvo W, Hopewell JW, Reinhold HS, et al. Time- and dose-related changes in the white matter of the rat brain after single doses of X rays. *Br J Radiol.* 1988;61:1043–1052.

42. Reinhold HS, Calvo W, Hopewell JW, et al. Development of blood vessel-related radiation damage in the fimbria of the central nervous system. *Int J Radiat Oncol Biol Phys.* 1990;18:37–42.

43. Schultheiss TE, Stephens LC. The pathogenesis of radiation myelopathy: widening the circle. *Int J Radiat Oncol Biol Phys.* 1992;23:1089–1091; discussion 1093–4.

44. Schultheiss TE, Stephens LC. Invited review: permanent radiation myelopathy. *Br J Radiol.* 1992;65:737–753.

45. Barajas RF, Chang JS, Sneed PK, et al. Distinguishing recurrent intra-axial metastatic tumor from radiation necrosis following gamma knife radiosurgery using dynamic susceptibility-weighted contrast-enhanced perfusion MR imaging. *Am J Neuroradiol.* 2009;30(2):367–372.

46. Lutz PL. Mechanisms for anoxic survival in the vertebrate brain. *Annu Rev Physiol.* 1992;54:601–618.

47. Raff MC, Miller RH, Noble M. A glial progenitor cell that develops in vitro into an astrocyte or an oligodendrocyte depending on culture medium. *Nature.* 1983;303:390–396.

48. van der Maazen RW, Kleiboer BJ, Verhagen I, et al. Irradiation in vitro discriminates between different O-2A progenitor cell subpopulations in the perinatal central nervous system of rats. *Radiat Res.* 1991;128:64–72.

49. van der Maazen RW, Verhagen I, Kleiboer BJ, et al. Radiosensitivity of glial progenitor cells of the perinatal and adult rat optic nerve studied by an in vitro clonogenic assay. *Radiother Oncol.* 1991;20:258–264.

50. van der Maazen RW, Kleiboer BJ, Verhagen I, et al. Repair capacity of adult rat glial progenitor cells determined by an in vitro clonogenic assay after in vitro or in vivo fractionated irradiation. *Int J Radiat Biol.* 1993;63:661–666.

51. van der Maazen RW, Verhagen I, Kleiboer BJ, et al. Repopulation of O-2A progenitor cells after irradiation of the adult rat optic nerve analyzed by an in vitro clonogenic assay. *Radiat Res.* 1992;132:82–86.

52. Philippo H, Winter EA, van der Kogel AJ, et al. Recovery capacity of glial progenitors after in vivo fission-neutron or X irradiation: age dependence, fractionation and low-dose-rate irradiations. *Radiat Res.* 2005;163:636–643.

53. Belka C, Budach W, Kortmann RD, et al. Radiation induced CNS toxicity—molecular and cellular mechanisms. *Br J Cancer.* 2001;85:1233–1239.

54. Franklin RJ, Ffrench-Constant C. Remyelination in the CNS: from biology to therapy. *Nat Rev Neurosci.* 2008;9:839–855.

55. Mastaglia FL, McDonald WI, Watson JV, et al. Effects of x-radiation on the spinal cord: an experimental study of the morphological changes in central nerve fibres. *Brain.* 1976;99:101–122.

56. Hornsey S, Myers R, Coultas PG, et al. Turnover of proliferative cells in the spinal cord after X irradiation and its relation to time-dependent repair of radiation damage. *Br J Radiol.* 1981;54:1081–1085.

57. Fike JR, Cann CE, Turowski K, et al. Radiation dose response of normal brain. *Int J Radiat Oncol Biol Phys.* 1988;14:63–70.

58. Asai A, Matsutani M, Kohno T, et al. Subacute brain atrophy after radiation therapy for malignant brain tumor. *Cancer.* 1989;63:1962–1974.

59. Lois C, Alvarez-Buylla A. Proliferating subventricular zone cells in the adult mammalian forebrain can differentiate into neurons and glia. *Proc Natl Acad Sci U.S.A.* 1993;90:2074–2077.

60. Luskin MB. Restricted proliferation and migration of postnatally generated neurons derived from the forebrain subventricular zone. *Neuron.* 1993;11:173–189.

61. Levison SW, Chuang C, Abramson BJ, et al. The migrational patterns and developmental fates of glial precursors in the rat subventricular zone are temporally regulated. *Development.* 1993;119:611–622.

62. Schultze B, Korr H. Cell kinetic studies of different cell types in the developing and adult brain of the rat and the mouse: a review. *Cell Tissue Kinet.* 1981;14:309–325.

63. Privat A, Leblond CP. The subependymal layer and neighboring region in the brain of the young rat. *J Comp Neurol.* 1972;146:277–302.

64. Lewis PD. A quantitative study of cell proliferation in the subependymal layer of the adult rat brain. *Exp Neurol.* 1968;20:203–207.

65. Gritti A, Parati EA, Cova L, et al. Multipotential stem cells from the adult mouse brain proliferate and self-renew in response to basic fibroblast growth factor. *J Neurosci.* 1996;16:1091–1100.

66. Gage FH, Ray J, Fisher LJ. Isolation, characterization, and use of stem cells from the CNS. *Annu Rev Neurosci.* 1995;18:159–192.

67. Morshead CM, Reynolds BA, Craig CG, et al. Neural stem cells in the adult mammalian forebrain: a relatively quiescent subpopulation of subependymal cells. *Neuron.* 1994;13:1071–1082.

68. Morshead CM, Craig CG, van der Kooy D. In vivo clonal analyses reveal the properties of endogenous neural stem cell proliferation in the adult mammalian forebrain. *Development.* 1998;125:2251–2261.

69. Merkle FT, Mirzadeh Z, Alvarez-Buylla A. Mosaic organization of neural stem cells in the adult brain. *Science.* 2007;317:381–384.

70. Parent JM. Injury-induced neurogenesis in the adult mammalian brain. *Neuroscientist.* 2003;9:261–272.

71. Monje ML, Toda H, Palmer TD. Inflammatory blockade restores adult hippocampal neurogenesis. *Science.* 2003;302:1760–1765.

72. Monje ML, Mizumatsu S, Fike JR, et al. Irradiation induces neural precursor-cell dysfunction. *Nat Med.* 2002;8:955–962.

73. Moyse E, Segura S, Liard O, et al. Microenvironmental determinants of adult neural stem cell proliferation and lineage commitment in the healthy and injured central nervous system. *Curr Stem Cell Res Ther.* 2008;3:163–184.

74. Cavanagh JB, Hopewell JW. Mitotic activity in the subependymal plate of rats and the long-term consequences of X-irradiation. *J Neurol Sci.* 1972;15:471–482.

75. Hopewell JW, Cavanagh JB. Effects of X irradiation on the mitotic activity of the subependymal plate of rats. *Br J Radiol.* 1972;45:461–465.

76. Hubbard BM, Hopewell JW. Quantitative changes in the cellularity of the rat subependymal plate after X-irradiation. *Cell Tissue Kinet.* 1980;13:403–413.

77. Mizumatsu S, Monje ML, Morhardt DR, et al. Extreme sensitivity of adult neurogenesis to low doses of X-irradiation. *Cancer Res.* 2003;63:4021–4027.

78. Monje ML, Palmer T. Radiation injury and neurogenesis. *Curr Opin Neurol.* 2003;16:129–134.

79. Barani IJ, Benedict SH, Lin PS. Neural stem cells: implications for the conventional radiotherapy of central nervous system malignancies. *Int J Radiat Oncol Biol Phys.* 2007;68:324–333.

80. Fike JR, Rola R, Limoli CL. Radiation response of neural precursor cells. *Neurosurg Clin N Am.* 2007;18:115–127.

81. Li YQ, Jay V, Wong CS. Oligodendrocytes in the adult rat spinal cord undergo radiation-induced apoptosis. *Cancer Res.* 1996;56:5417–5422.

82. Tada E, Yang C, Gobbel GT, et al. Long-term impairment of subependymal repopulation following damage by ionizing irradiation. *Exp Neurol.* 1999;160:66–77.

83. Andres-Mach M, Rola R, Fike JR. Radiation effects on neural precursor cells in the dentate gyrus. *Cell Tissue Res.* 2008;331:251–262.

84. Zhao W, Diz DI, Robbins ME. Oxidative damage pathways in relation to normal tissue injury. *Br J Radiol.* 2007;80(Spec No 1):S23–S31.

85. Simonian NA, Coyle JT. Oxidative stress in neurodegenerative diseases. *Annu Rev Pharmacol Toxicol.* 1996;36:83–106.

86. Smith KJ, Kapoor R, Felts PA. Demyelination: the role of reactive oxygen and nitrogen species. *Brain Pathol.* 1999;9:69–92.

87. Mhatre M, Floyd RA, Hensley K. Oxidative stress and neuroinflammation in Alzheimer's disease and amyotrophic lateral sclerosis: common links and potential therapeutic targets. *J Alzheimers Dis.* 2004;6:147–157.

88. Floyd RA, Hensley K. Oxidative stress in brain aging. Implications for therapeutics of neurodegenerative diseases. *Neurobiol Aging.* 2002;23:795–807.

89. Tofilon PJ, Fike JR. The radioresponse of the central nervous system: a dynamic process. *Radiat Res.* 2000;153:357–370.

90. Bast A, Haenen GR, Doelman CJ. Oxidants and antioxidants: state of the art. *Am J Med.* 1991;91:2S-13S.

91. Bolanos JP, Almeida A, Stewart V, et al. Nitric oxide-mediated mitochondrial damage in the brain: mechanisms and implications for neurodegenerative diseases. *J Neurochem.* 1997;68:2227–2240.

92. Peuchen S, Bolanos JP, Heales SJ, et al. Interrelationships between astrocyte function, oxidative stress and antioxidant status within the central nervous system. *Prog Neurobiol.* 1997;52:261–281.

93. Wilson JX. Antioxidant defense of the brain: a role for astrocytes. *Can J Physiol Pharmacol.* 1997;75:1149–1163.

94. Beal MF. Aging, energy, and oxidative stress in neurodegenerative diseases. *Ann Neurol.* 1995;38:357–366.

95. Love S. Oxidative stress in brain ischemia. *Brain Pathol.* 1999;9:119–131.

96. Juurlink BH, Paterson PG. Review of oxidative stress in brain and spinal cord injury: suggestions for pharmacological and nutritional management strategies. *J Spinal Cord Med.* 1998;21:309–334.

97. Forster MJ, Dubey A, Dawson KM, et al. Age-related losses of cognitive function and motor skills in mice are associated with oxidative protein damage in the brain. *Proc Natl Acad Sci U S A.* 1996;93:4765–4769.

98. Bongarzone ER, Pasquini JM, Soto EF. Oxidative damage to proteins and lipids of CNS myelin produced by in vitro generated reactive oxygen species. *J Neurosci Res.* 1995;41:213–221.

99. Hall E. *Radiobiology for the Radiobiologist.* 4th ed. Philadelphia, PA: J.B. Lippincott Company; 1994.
100. Limoli CL, Hartmann A, Shephard L, et al. Apoptosis, reproductive failure, and oxidative stress in Chinese hamster ovary cells with compromised genomic integrity. *Cancer Res.* 1998;58:3712–3718.
101. Rola R, Fishman K, Baure J, et al. Hippocampal neurogenesis and neuroinflammation after cranial irradiation with (56)Fe particles. *Radiat Res.* 2008;169:626–632.
102. Rola R, Sarkissian V, Obenaus A, et al. High-LET radiation induces inflammation and persistent changes in markers of hippocampal neurogenesis. *Radiat Res.* 2005;164:556–560.
103. Kyrkanides S, Moore AH, Olschowka JA, et al. Cyclooxygenase-2 modulates brain inflammation-related gene expression in central nervous system radiation injury. *Brain Res Mol Brain Res.* 2002;104:159–169.
104. Dheen ST, Kaur C, Ling EA. Microglial activation and its implications in the brain diseases. *Curr Med Chem.* 2007;14:1189–1197.
105. Tsuruda JS, Kortman KE, Bradley WG, et al. Radiation effects on cerebral white matter: MR evaluation. *AJR Am J Roentgenol.* 1987;149:165–171.
106. Dooms GC, Hecht S, Brant-Zawadzki M, et al. Brain radiation lesions: MR imaging. *Radiology.* 1986;158:149–155.
107. Mintz A, Perry J, Spithoff K, et al. Management of single brain metastasis: a practice guideline. *Curr Oncol.* 2007;14:131–143.
108. Dequesada IM, Quisling RG, Yachnis A, et al. Can standard magnetic resonance imaging reliably distinguish recurrent tumor from radiation necrosis after radiosurgery for brain metastases? A radiographic-pathological study. *Neurosurgery.* 2008;63:898–903; discussion 904.
109. Kang TW, Kim ST, Byun HS, et al. Morphological and functional MRI, MRS, perfusion and diffusion changes after radiosurgery of brain metastasis. *Eur J Radiol.* 2009;72(3):370–380.
110. Fan G, Sun B, Wu Z, et al. In vivo single-voxel proton MR spectroscopy in the differentiation of high-grade gliomas and solitary metastases. *Clin Radiol.* 2004;59:77–85.
111. Law M, Cha S, Knopp EA, et al. High-grade gliomas and solitary metastases: differentiation by using perfusion and proton spectroscopic MR imaging. *Radiology.* 2002;222:715–721.
112. Moller-Hartmann W, Herminghaus S, Krings T, et al. Clinical application of proton magnetic resonance spectroscopy in the diagnosis of intracranial mass lesions. *Neuroradiology.* 2002;44:371–381.
113. Nelson SJ, McKnight TR, Henry RG. Characterization of untreated gliomas by magnetic resonance spectroscopic imaging. *Neuroimaging Clin N Am.* 2002;12:599–613.
114. Sabatier J, Gilard V, Malet-Martino M, et al. Characterization of choline compounds with in vitro 1H magnetic resonance spectroscopy for the discrimination of primary brain tumors. *Invest Radiol.* 1999;34:230–235.
115. Chernov MF, Hayashi M, Izawa M, et al. Multivoxel proton MRS for differentiation of radiation-induced necrosis and tumor recurrence after gamma knife radiosurgery for brain metastases. *Brain Tumor Pathol.* 2006;23:19–27.
116. Fayed N, Davila J, Medrano J, et al. Malignancy assessment of brain tumours with magnetic resonance spectroscopy and dynamic susceptibility contrast MRI. *Eur J Radiol.* 2008;67:427–433.
117. Wald LL, Nelson SJ, Day MR, et al. Serial proton magnetic resonance spectroscopy imaging of glioblastoma multiforme after brachytherapy. *J Neurosurg.* 1997;87:525–534.
118. Lin A, Bluml S, Mamelak AN. Efficacy of proton magnetic resonance spectroscopy in clinical decision making for patients with suspected malignant brain tumors. *J Neurooncol.* 1999;45:69–81.
119. Dowling C, Bollen AW, Noworolski SM, et al. Preoperative proton MR spectroscopic imaging of brain tumors: correlation with histopathologic analysis of resection specimens. *Am J Neuroradiol.* 2001;22:604–612.
120. Hall WA, Martin A, Liu H, et al. Improving diagnostic yield in brain biopsy: coupling spectroscopic targeting with real-time needle placement. *J Magn Reson Imaging.* 2001;13:12–15.
121. Tsui EY, Chan JH, Leung TW, et al. Radionecrosis of the temporal lobe: dynamic susceptibility contrast MRI. *Neuroradiology.* 2000;42:149–152.
122. Asao C, Korogi Y, Kitajima M, et al. Diffusion-weighted imaging of radiation-induced brain injury for differentiation from tumor recurrence. *Am J Neuroradiol.* 2005;26:1455–1460.
123. Nowinski WL, Prakash B, Volkau I, et al. Rapid and automatic calculation of the midsagittal plane in magnetic resonance diffusion and perfusion images. *Acad Radiol.* 2006;13: 652–663.
124. Park SH, Chang KH, Song IC, et al. Diffusion-weighted MRI in cystic or necrotic intracranial lesions. *Neuroradiology.* 2000;42:716–721.
125. Lam WW, Poon WS, Metreweli C. Diffusion MR imaging in glioma: does it have any role in the pre-operation determination of grading of glioma? *Clin Radiol.* 2002;57:219–225.
126. Kono K, Inoue Y, Nakayama K, et al. The role of diffusion-weighted imaging in patients with brain tumors. *Am J Neuroradiol.* 2001;22:1081–1088.
127. Tsui EY, Chan JH, Ramsey RG, et al. Late temporal lobe necrosis in patients with nasopharyngeal carcinoma: evaluation with combined multi-section diffusion weighted and perfusion weighted MR imaging. *Eur J Radiol.* 2001;39:133–138.
128. Sugahara T, Korogi Y, Kochi M, et al. Usefulness of diffusion-weighted MRI with echoplanar technique in the evaluation of cellularity in gliomas. *J Magn Reson Imaging.* 1999;9:53–60.
129. Krabbe K, Gideon P, Wagn P, et al. MR diffusion imaging of human intracranial tumours. *Neuroradiology.* 1997;39:483–489.
130. Castillo M, Smith JK, Kwock L, et al. Apparent diffusion coefficients in the evaluation of high-grade cerebral gliomas. *Am J Neuroradiol.* 2001;22:60–64.
131. Rosen BR, Belliveau JW, Vevea JM, et al. Perfusion imaging with NMR contrast agents. *Magn Reson Med.* 1990;14:249–265.
132. Potchen EJ. *Magnetic Resonance Angiography: Concepts and Applications.* St. Louis, MO: Mosby-Year Book; 1993.
133. Sugahara T, Korogi Y, Tomiguchi S, et al. Posttherapeutic intraaxial brain tumor: the value of perfusion-sensitive contrast-enhanced MR imaging for differentiating tumor recurrence from nonneoplastic contrast-enhancing tissue. *Am J Neuroradiol.* 2000;21:901–909.
134. Cha S, Lu S, Johnson G, et al. Dynamic susceptibility contrast MR imaging: correlation of signal intensity changes with cerebral blood volume measurements. *J Magn Reson Imaging.* 2000;11:114–119.
135. Cha S, Lupo JM, Chen MH, et al. Differentiation of glioblastoma multiforme and single brain metastasis by peak height and percentage of signal intensity recovery derived from dynamic susceptibility-weighted contrast-enhanced perfusion MR imaging. *Am J Neuroradiol.* 2007;28:1078–1084.
136. Lupo JM, Cha S, Chang SM, et al. Dynamic susceptibility-weighted perfusion imaging of high-grade gliomas: characterization of spatial heterogeneity. *Am J Neuroradiol.* 2005;26:1446–1454.
137. Essig M, Waschkies M, Wenz F, et al. Assessment of brain metastases with dynamic susceptibility-weighted contrast-enhanced MR imaging: initial results. *Radiology.* 2003;228: 193–199.
138. Sugahara T, Korogi Y, Kochi M, et al. Correlation of MR imaging-determined cerebral blood volume maps with histologic and angiographic determination of vascularity of gliomas. *AJR Am J Roentgenol.* 1998;171:1479–1486.
139. Lev MH, Ozsunar Y, Henson JW, et al. Glial tumor grading and outcome prediction using dynamic spin-echo MR susceptibility mapping compared with conventional contrast-enhanced MR: confounding effect of elevated rCBV of oligodendrogliomas [corrected]. *Am J Neuroradiol.* 2004;25:214–221.
140. Aronen HJ, Gazit IE, Louis DN, et al. Cerebral blood volume maps of gliomas: comparison with tumor grade and histologic findings. *Radiology.* 1994;191:41–51.
141. Young IR, Cox IJ, Coutts GA, et al. Some considerations concerning susceptibility, longitudinal relaxation time constants and motion artifacts in vivo human spectroscopy. *NMR Biomed.* 1989;2:329–339.
142. Langleben DD, Segall GM. PET in differentiation of recurrent brain tumor from radiation injury. *J Nucl Med.* 2000;41:1861–1867.
143. Hustinx R, Smith RJ, Benard F, et al. Can the standardized uptake value characterize primary brain tumors on FDG-PET? *Eur J Nucl Med.* 1999;26:1501–1509.
144. Spence AM, Mankoff DA, Muzi M. Positron emission tomography imaging of brain tumors. *Neuroimaging Clin N Am.* 2003;13:717–739.
145. Wong TZ, van der Westhuizen GJ, Coleman RE. Positron emission tomography imaging of brain tumors. *Neuroimaging Clin N Am.* 2002;12:615–626.
146. Henze M, Mohammed A, Schlemmer HP, et al. PET and SPECT for detection of tumor progression in irradiated low-grade astrocytoma: a receiver-operating-characteristic analysis. *J Nucl Med.* 2004;45:579–586.
147. Hustinx R, Pourdehnad M, Kaschten B, et al. PET imaging for differentiating recurrent brain tumor from radiation necrosis. *Radiol Clin North Am.* 2005;43:35–47.
148. Ricci PE, Karis JP, Heiserman JE, et al. Differentiating recurrent tumor from radiation necrosis: time for re-evaluation of positron emission tomography? *Am J Neuroradiol.* 1998;19:407–413.
149. Chao ST, Suh JH, Raja S, et al. The sensitivity and specificity of FDG PET in distinguishing recurrent brain tumor from radionecrosis in patients treated with stereotactic radiosurgery. *Int J Cancer.* 2001;96:191–197.
150. Wang SX, Boethius J, Ericson K. FDG-PET on irradiated brain tumor: ten years' summary. *Acta Radiol.* 2006;47:85–90.
151. Ishiwata K, Kubota K, Murakami M, et al. Re-evaluation of amino acid PET studies: can the protein synthesis rates in brain and tumor tissues be measured in vivo? *J Nucl Med.* 1993;34:1936–1943.
152. Jager PL, Vaalburg W, Pruim J, et al. Radiolabeled amino acids: basic aspects and clinical applications in oncology. *J Nucl Med.* 2001;42:432–445.
153. Isselbacher KJ. Sugar and amino acid transport by cells in culture–differences between normal and malignant cells. *N Engl J Med.* 1972;286:929–933.
154. Busch H, Davis JR, Honig GR, et al. The uptake of a variety of amino acids into nuclear proteins of tumors and other tissues. *Cancer Res.* 1959;19:1030–1039.
155. Herholz K, Holzer T, Bauer B, et al. 11C-methionine PET for differential diagnosis of low-grade gliomas. *Neurology.* 1998;50:1316–1322.
156. Laverman P, Boerman OC, Corstens FH, et al. Fluorinated amino acids for tumour imaging with positron emission tomography. *Eur J Nucl Med Mol Imaging.* 2002;29:681–690.
157. Tsuyuguchi N, Sunada I, Iwai Y, et al. Methionine positron emission tomography of recurrent metastatic brain tumor and radiation necrosis after stereotactic radiosurgery: is a differential diagnosis possible? *J Neurosurg.* 2003;98:1056–1064.
158. Spaeth N, Wyss MT, Weber B, et al. Uptake of 18F-fluorocholine, 18F-fluoroethyl-L-tyrosine, and 18F-FDG in acute cerebral radiation injury in the rat: implications for separation of radiation necrosis from tumor recurrence. *J Nucl Med.* 2004;45:1931–1938.
159. Weber WA, Wester HJ, Grosu AL, et al. O-(2-[18F]fluoroethyl)-L-tyrosine and L-[methyl-11C]methionine uptake in brain tumours: initial results of a comparative study. *Eur J Nucl Med.* 2000;27:542–549.
160. Schillaci O, Filippi L, Manni C, et al. Single-photon emission computed tomography/computed tomography in brain tumors. *Semin Nucl Med.* 2007;37:34–47.
161. Schwartz RB, Carvalho PA, Alexander Er, et al. Radiation necrosis vs high-grade recurrent glioma: differentiation by using dual-isotope SPECT with 201Tl and 99mTc-HMPAO. *Am J Neuroradiol.* 1991;12:1187–1192.
162. Kline JL, Noto RB, Glantz M. Single-photon emission CT in the evaluation of recurrent brain tumor in patients treated with gamma knife radiosurgery or conventional radiation therapy. *Am J Neuroradiol.* 1996;17:1681–1686.
163. Moody EB, Hodes JE, Walsh JW, et al. Thallium-avid cerebral radiation necrosis. *Clin Nucl Med.* 1994;19:611–613.
164. Yoshii Y, Moritake T, Suzuki K, et al. Cerebral radiation necrosis with accumulation of thallium 201 on single-photon emission CT. *Am J Neuroradiol.* 1996;17:1773–1776.
165. de Vries B, Taphoorn MJ, van Isselt JW, et al. Bilateral temporal lobe necrosis after radiotherapy: confounding SPECT results. *Neurology.* 1998;51:1183–1184.
166. Alexiou GA, Fotopoulos AD, Papadopoulos A, et al. Evaluation of brain tumor recurrence by (99m)Tc-tetrofosmin SPECT: a prospective pilot study. *Ann Nucl Med.* 2007;21: 293–298.

167. Le Jeune N, Perek N, Denoyer D, et al. Influence of glutathione depletion on plasma membrane cholesterol esterification and on Tc-99m-sestamibi and Tc-99m-tetrofosmin uptakes: a comparative study in sensitive U-87-MG and multidrug-resistant MRP1 human glioma cells. *Cancer Biother Radiopharm.* 2004;19:411–421.

168. Le Jeune N, Perek N, Denoyer D, et al. Study of monoglutathionyl conjugates TC-99M-sestamibi and TC-99M-tetrofosmin transport mediated by the multidrug resistance-associated protein isoform 1 in glioma cells. *Cancer Biother Radiopharm.* 2005;20:249–259.

169. Alexiou GA, Tsiouris S, Kyritsis AP, et al. Brain SPECT by 99mTc-tetrofosmin for the differentiation of tumor recurrence from radiation injury. *J Nucl Med.* 2008;49:1733–1734; author reply 1734.

170. Delattre JY, Rosenblum MK, Thaler HT, et al. A model of radiation myelopathy in the rat. Pathology, regional capillary permeability changes and treatment with dexamethasone. *Brain.* 1988;111:1319–1336.

171. Tada E, Matsumoto K, Kinoshita K, et al. The protective effect of dexamethasone against radiation damage induced by interstitial irradiation in normal monkey brain. *Neurosurgery.* 1997;41:209–217; discussion 217–219.

172. Martins AN, Severance RE, Henry JM, et al. Experimental delayed radiation necrosis of the brain. Part 1: Effect of early dexamethasone treatment. *J Neurosurg.* 1979;51:587–596.

173. Lee AW, Ng SH, Ho JH, et al. Clinical diagnosis of late temporal lobe necrosis following radiation therapy for nasopharyngeal carcinoma. *Cancer.* 1988;61:1535–1542.

174. Lorenzo ND, Nolletti A, Palma L. Late cerebral radionecrosis. *Surg Neurol.* 1978;10:281–290.

175. Marx RE, Ehler WJ, Tayapongsak P, et al. Relationship of oxygen dose to angiogenesis induction in irradiated tissue. *Am J Surg.* 1990;160:519–524.

176. Pasquier D, Hoelscher T, Schmutz J, et al. Hyperbaric oxygen therapy in the treatment of radio-induced lesions in normal tissues: a literature review. *Radiother Oncol.* 2004;72:1–13.

177. Hulshof MC, Stark NM, van der Kleij A, et al. Hyperbaric oxygen therapy for cognitive disorders after irradiation of the brain. *Strahlenther Onkol.* 2002;178:192–198.

178. Leber KA, Eder HG, Kovac H, et al. Treatment of cerebral radionecrosis by hyperbaric oxygen therapy. *Stereotact Funct Neurosurg.* 1998;70(suppl 1):229–236.

179. Glantz MJ, Burger PC, Friedman AH, et al. Treatment of radiation-induced nervous system injury with heparin and warfarin. *Neurology.* 1994;44:2020–2027.

180. Delanian S, Lefaix JL. Current management for late normal tissue injury: radiation-induced fibrosis and necrosis. *Semin Radiat Oncol.* 2007;17:99–107.

181. Okunieff P, Augustine E, Hicks JE, et al. Pentoxifylline in the treatment of radiation-induced fibrosis. *J Clin Oncol.* 2004;22:2207–2213.

182. Delanian S, Porcher R, Balla-Mekias S, et al. Randomized, placebo-controlled trial of combined pentoxifylline and tocopherol for regression of superficial radiation-induced fibrosis. *J Clin Oncol.* 2003;21:2545–2550.

183. Williamson R, Kondziolka D, Kanaan H, et al. Adverse radiation effects after radiosurgery may benefit from oral vitamin E and pentoxifylline therapy: a pilot study. *Stereotact Funct Neurosurg.* 2008;86:359–366.

184. Gonzalez J, Kumar AJ, Conrad CA, et al. Effect of bevacizumab on radiation necrosis of the brain. *Int J Radiat Oncol Biol Phys.* 2007;67:323–326.

185. Torcuator R, Zuniga R, Mohan YS, et al. Initial experience with bevacizumab treatment for biopsy confirmed cerebral radiation necrosis. *J Neurooncol.* 2009;94:63–68.

186. Wong ET, Huberman M, Lu XQ, et al. Bevacizumab reverses cerebral radiation necrosis. *J Clin Oncol.* 2008;26:5649–5650.

187. Liu AK, Macy ME, Foreman NK. Bevacizumab as therapy for radiation necrosis in four children with pontine gliomas. *Int J Radiat Oncol Biol Phys.* 2009;75:1148–1154.

188. Gutin PH, Iwamoto FM, Beal K, et al. Safety and efficacy of bevacizumab with hypofractionated stereotactic irradiation for recurrent malignant gliomas. *Int J Radiat Oncol Biol Phys.* 2009;75:156–163.

Nicola Rosenfelder
Fiona Stewart
Michael Brada

Vascular Effect of Radiation in the Central Nervous System

INTRODUCTION

Vascular injury is a recognized side effect of radiotherapy and vessels of all calibers may be affected.[1–8] Radiation sequelae in large arteries include atherosclerotic changes, stenosis, occlusion, thromboembolism, rupture, aneurysm, and fistula formation. In the microvasculature, early inflammatory, permeability and thrombotic changes are followed by focal capillary loss, leading to ischemic necrosis.

The effect of radiotherapy on vascular tissue was recognized over 65 years ago, when irradiated arteries were shown to exhibit atherosclerotic changes with plaque-like thickening of the intimae and a cellular infiltrate between the intimae and the internal elastic membrane.[1] The first case report of a cerebrovascular accident (CVA) due to thrombotic occlusion only a few months after completing treatment for Hodgkin disease was published in 1975,[9] and 3 years later Silverberg et al.[10] described "radiation-induced carotid disease as a clinical entity."

Both direct and indirect effects of radiation induced vascular toxicity have been recognized in the central nervous system (CNS). With improved understanding of the pathogenesis of vascular injury and its role in the development of radiation toxicity, it may be possible to explore methods to protect against it, allowing for safer delivery of radiation in patients with good long-term prognosis and for potential dose escalation in patients with CNS malignancies where the outcome is currently poor.

PATHOLOGY OF RADIATION INJURY TO BLOOD VESSELS

RADIATION EFFECTS ON EXTRACRANIAL BLOOD VESSELS

Radiation damage in vessels has been best described in the carotid artery following radiotherapy to the neck for Hodgkin disease, non-Hodgkin lymphoma,[11] and tumors of the head and neck.[12–14] Vascular damage may lead to vessel occlusion causing hypoxic and ischemic parenchymal injuries and subsequent necrosis and fibrosis. The understanding of vascular damage outside the CNS is used as an analogy for radiation sequelae within the CNS.

STENOSIS AND STROKE AFTER RADIOTHERAPY TO THE NECK

Clinical Evidence

Both prospective and retrospective studies following radiotherapy to the head and neck reported higher incidence of carotid artery stenosis than would be expected in the normal population.[15–19] The incidence of stenotic lesions occupying more than 50% of the vessel wall was tenfold higher 5 years after radiotherapy for head and neck tumors than in asymptomatic control subjects (38% vs. 4%).[20] In patients with nasopharyngeal carcinoma, the incidence of carotid artery stenosis rose from 22% before treatment to 79% following treatment.[17] This effect is also seen in younger people (aged 18–37 years) where asymptomatic carotid artery stenosis was reported in 26% of irradiated patients compared to 3% in a control group ($p < 0.01$).[21] Stenotic lesions following radiotherapy also have a more aggressive behavior than those arising in unirradiated vessels[15,17,22–24] with a higher annual rate of progression to more severe stenosis (15.4% vs. 4.8%).[23]

Since risk factors for cerebrovascular disease such as age, smoking, and male sex overlap with factors associated with the development of head and neck tumors, the independent contribution of radiotherapy to the increased risk of cerebrovascular disease is difficult to determine, particularly as healthy people rather than unirradiated patients with head and neck tumors are often used as controls. However, in a prospective cross-sectional study in which consecutive head and neck cancer patients who underwent radiotherapy were compared with unirradiated patients,[18] carotid artery stenosis scores correlated not only with age and hyperlipidemia but also with the use of radiotherapy.

Patients treated with radiotherapy to the neck are at increased risk of stenosis and stroke. After radiation to the head and neck, the relative risk (RR) of ischemic stroke is 2 to 9 following doses of 60 to 70 Gy,[13,19,25] and the RR may increase with time.[13] A systematic review of 6,908 patients from institutional series or cohort analyses reported an increased risk of stroke (RR: 9.0; 95% CI: 4.9–16.7) after neck and supraclavicular radiotherapy compared to nonirradiated patients.[19] The risk of stroke in adults irradiated for Hodgkin lymphoma was also increased with standardized incidence ratio (SIR) of 2.2 for clinically verified stroke (95%CI: 1.7–2.8) and SIR of 3.1 for transient ischemic attack (TIA) (95%CI: 2.2–4.4). The risk was higher in those treated below the age of 20 with an SIR of 3.8 (95%CI: 1.6–7.4) for stroke and 7.6 (95%CI: 2.4–17) for TIA.

The risk of stroke is also increased in children who have undergone radiotherapy to the neck. The incidence of self-reported stroke in a multi-institutional cohort of survivors of childhood Hodgkin lymphoma (treated to a median dose 40 Gy at a mean age of 14 years)[11] was increased with an RR of 4.3 (95%CI: 2.0–9.3) compared to sibling controls. However, the RR of stroke following cranial irradiation in childhood may be even greater than after neck irradiation with a RR of 38 reported after treatment for childhood brain tumors with a cranial dose of 30 Gy or more.[26]

Pathogenesis

The apparent aggressive behavior of radiation-induced atherosclerotic lesions has led to investigations comparing the pathogenesis of radiation-induced atherosclerosis and spontaneous atherosclerosis in unirradiated vessels. Atherosclerosis in unirradiated vessels usually begins with injury to the vascular endothelium, which causes local macrophages and circulating monocytes to migrate into the intimae where they take up low-density lipoprotein (LDL) cholesterol, forming foam cells. High LDL levels overwhelm the antioxidant properties of endothelium and resulting oxidized LDL cholesterol causes free radical formation, decreased nitric oxide, and a procoagulant environment, leading to accumulation of serum lipoproteins in the intimae causing the fatty streak, within which are lipid-laden macrophages and T lymphocytes. Under the influence of growth factors, smooth muscle cells proliferate and produce collagen, elastin, and proteoglycans. This results in the formation of atheromas that progress from being lipid-rich early lesions to unstable thrombotic lesions prone to rupture, or to advanced atherosclerotic fibrous plaque.[27–29] Radiation-induced plaques in mice appear to be macrophage rich and lipid filled rather than the macrophage-poor, collagenous type seen in nonirradiated controls.[30–32]

An atherosclerosis-prone (ApoE knockout) mouse model was used to compare the phenotype of radiation-induced atherosclerosis with age-related atherosclerosis. Although the burden of plaque was not significantly higher following radiation, the plaques were frequently macrophage containing and grew to large sizes without progressing to the fibrous lesions seen in classic atherosclerosis.[32] Intraplaque hemorrhages and erythrocyte-containing macrophages were only seen in irradiated arteries. These histological differences may account for the more aggressive phenotype identified in patients with radiation-induced stenosis.

ANEURYSM, RUPTURE, AND FISTULAE FOLLOWING RADIOTHERAPY

Radiotherapy has been linked with aneurysm formation, vessel rupture, and fistula formation. Aneurysms have been reported following radiotherapy at both intracranial and extracranial sites including the internal carotid, posterior cerebral,[33] vertebral,[34] and femoral[35] arteries. Vessel rupture, ascribed to necrosis in the ruptured vessel wall, has also been reported in large and medium-sized vessels, including the aorta, carotid and femoral arteries.[36–39] Fistulae arising as a consequence of radiotherapy can be associated with accelerated atherosclerosis, hyaline necrosis in the irradiated vessels of the fistula tract,[40,41]

and inflammation of the vasa vasorum and necrosis of the vessel wall.[42] Aortoenteric fistulae have been reported many years after radiotherapy.[40,42–46]

THE EFFECT OF DOSE FRACTIONATION

The arterial sequelae of different dose fractionation schedules have been studied in animal models of intraoperative radiotherapy (IORT) and following fractionated external beam radiotherapy (EBRT) at extracranial sites.[47,48] Fractionated EBRT and lower single IORT doses to the paraaortic region of dogs predominantly cause fibroelastic proliferation, thickening of the tunica intimae, and severe luminal narrowing. Large single intraoperative doses either alone or combined with EBRT result in mild subendothelial proliferation but caused a significant risk of aneurysm or large thrombus formation 4 to 5 years after radiotherapy with subsequent risk of vessel rupture.[49]

These studies have shown the different radiation effects on vasculature with increasing dose per fraction. Large doses per fraction appear to cause intimal cell death or loss of reproductive capability, which over time may result in rupture, aneurysm, or fissure formation. Small doses per fraction allow cellular proliferation to continue but increase vascular endothelial damage with intimal thickening with fibroelastic proliferation. Following radiotherapy at single doses <20 Gy, and after all fractionated doses, the intimal area increases, suggestive of proliferation; after doses >20 Gy, intimal proliferation tends to be inhibited.[50] Adventitial fibrosis increases with increasing dose and may contribute to late vascular remodeling.

THE EFFECT OF RADIATION ON THE CNS VASCULATURE

With the exception of the subependymal plate, cells in the CNS have long turnover times and are usually quiescent. Neurons are highly differentiated and lose their capacity to proliferate shortly after birth. Glial cells (astrocytes, oligodendrocytes) retain their capacity to divide in response to injury, although cell turnover is normally very slow (>200 days in adults).[51,52] A transient, dose-dependent increase in cellular proliferation of oligodendrocytes occurs during the first 1 to 2 months after spinal cord irradiation. This is followed by a sharp decline in cell number immediately prior to the onset of necrosis (at 3–4 months after irradiation), with a second wave of proliferation after the onset of necrosis.[52] The early wave of proliferation is probably in response to apoptotic cell loss and segmental demyelination after radiation, whereas the second proliferative burst occurs in response to white matter necrosis.

The dominant features of late radiation damage to the nervous system include glial atrophy, demyelination, and necrosis confined to white matter and various vascular changes in both the white and the gray matter.[53–55] These findings have been identified in humans with severe radiation injury,[56] but evidence from humans in less severe cases is limited by the risks associated with tissue biopsy in the CNS. Therefore, data for patients with milder symptoms are sparse.

Animal studies have been used to help define the effect of dose and fractionation on the CNS. These studies show that the spinal cord has a high capacity for repair of sublethal damage, with α/β ratios of about 2 Gy for cervical cord and 3 to 5 Gy for lumbar cord.[52,57–60] The size of the dose per fraction is therefore of great importance in determining the acceptable total dose of spinal cord radiation, with high doses per fraction resulting in much greater damage and lower tolerance doses. This is entirely consistent with more limited clinical data, indicating a high risk of myelitis using doses per fraction of 4 to 6 Gy to the spinal cord, even for relatively low total doses of 35 to 40 Gy.[61] The current estimate for α/β ratio for human cervical cord is <1 Gy.[62] These α/β ratio calculations describe the response of the spinal cord to a variety of dose-fractionation schedules, and are therefore likely to reflect, in part, the effect of dose on the vasculature, incorporating the consequences of vascular injury on the neuronal cell population.

Similar dose-fractionation effects occur in the CNS vasculature as in extracranial vessels. Demyelination and vascular toxicity occur with large fractions but not with low doses per fraction. From about 4 to 6 months after high-dose radiation (>20 Gy single dose), focal demyelination of the spinal cord occurs with the latency inversely related to the dose. This may progress to tissue necrosis. Vascular lesions, including edema, thrombosis, and hemorrhage, are features of late damage to CNS particularly with large doses and may be responsible for the development of necrosis.[52] After delivery of lower doses, vascular changes including telangiectasia and hemorrhagic infarcts are seen at 1 to 2 years.[52]

Cognitive impairment may result from low-dose radiotherapy to the brain, and this is thought to be related to impairment of neurogenesis in the subgranular zone of the dentate gyrus.[63–66] Radiation-related impairment of neurogenesis is associated with disruption of the dentate gyrus microvasculature in the rat. Administration of the anti-inflammatory drug indomethacin can partially restore this neurogenesis,[67] suggesting that reducing the inflammation from the vascular endothelium dysfunction may represent a useful method to preserve cognition following radiotherapy. Cognitive impairment, after whole brain irradiation of rats, is associated with alterations in the *N*-methyl-D-aspartic acid receptor subunits, important for synaptic transmission, and these changes can occur in the absence of neural degeneration. Other behavioral studies in mice suggest that impaired memory and motor activities are related to cerebral oxidative stress[68] and impairment of hippocampal neurogenesis in young mice.[69] Studies in rats showed that the memory defects at 9 months after 40 Gy in 5-Gy fractions were preceded by a significant decrease in capillary density, suggesting that the cognitive impairment may be a form of vascular dementia.[70]

TARGETS FOR RADIATION INJURY IN THE CNS

With white matter and vascular injuries dominating the pathological response of the CNS, oligodendrocyte and vascular endothelial cell populations are the principal suspects for injury. Elucidating whether the vascular endothelial or oligodendrocyte cell population is the target cell responsible for late radiation changes in the CNS has been the subject of much research, and both "vascular hypotheses" and "glial hypotheses" have been proposed supporting the role of each cell population, respectively[71]

THE VASCULAR HYPOTHESIS

Endothelial cells appear to play a critical role in the development of radiation-induced vascular lesions. Documented associations between disruption of the blood-brain barrier (BBB) and spinal cord-brain barrier and both acute and late radiation toxicity suggest that the endothelial cells play an important role in the development of these side effects.[72,73] Studies on the rat brain have shown a decline in vascular endothelial cells by up to 15% within 24 hours of radiation with doses between 5 and 200 Gy.[74,75] Early apoptotic cell loss continued for up to 1 month and was subsequently followed by a slower, dose-independent decline in cell density for up to 6 months.[74] When the cell population reached approximately 65% of the baseline value, an attempt at repopulation was made in those receiving 25 to 40 Gy, but improvement was transient and further endothelial cell loss subsequently occurred, with brain necrosis following shortly after. This transient rise was not seen in rats exposed to higher doses of radiation (40–60 Gy). The initial depletion of up to 15% of cells suggests a particularly sensitive subpopulation of endothelial cells that perhaps play a particular role in vessel function or health. Pretreatment delivery of a radioprotector, which localizes in vascular endothelial cells (Hoechst 33342), protects against the initial endothelial cell depletion in the 24 hours.[76]

Alpha particle radiation has been used to examine direct effects of radiotherapy on endothelial cells.[77] Boron-containing compounds that cannot cross the BBB allow the study of selective microvascular irradiation, as α particles released from the boron neutron capture reaction exert their influence within the range of the vascular endothelial cells but outside the range of the parenchymal cells. Selective intravascular endothelial irradiation caused significant demyelination and necrosis of white matter supporting the role of endothelial cells in the pathogenesis of white matter necrosis following radiotherapy. In another study, a single 25-Gy fraction was delivered to the brain of rats. Administration preradiotherapy of a radioprotector that selectively protects vascular endothelial cells and does not cross the BBB reduced endothelial cell decline after 24 hours, such that cell loss in the radioprotector group was insufficient to produce the repopulation attempt demonstrated between weeks 26 and 52 in those receiving radiotherapy alone.[78] Histological examination showed considerably lower rates of vessel damage (mainly telangiectasia) at 39 weeks and necrosis at 52 weeks in the group receiving the radioprotector (<10% vs. >75% and <10% vs. 55%, respectively). As expected, both vascular abnormalities and necrotic damage were found predominantly in the white matter.

Thus, white matter necrosis, arising as a late effect of CNS radiation, may occur as a secondary consequence of ischemia.[71] Radiation causes thickening of the vessel wall, vessel dilatation, and enlargement of endothelial cell nuclei in the vasculature of the CNS[79–81]; and reduction in blood vessel density and mild endothelial loss have been demonstrated prior to the development of necrosis.[79,80]

A number of factors suggest that vascular injury does not entirely account for subsequent damage. In particular, radiation effects can occur in the absence of apparent injury to the vasculature suggesting a role for other contributory factors.[71,81,82] Furthermore, it would be reasonable to expect the greatest injury to the cells most susceptible to ischemia, that is, the neurons located in the gray matter. However, gray matter appears to be relatively radioresistant. Although variations in the blood flow between the white and gray matter exist, it seems likely that the differential damage is due to factors other than vascular density difference.

In summary, animal studies demonstrate the effect of radiotherapy on blood vessels and in particular endothelial cell population. However, this is unlikely to be the sole cause of subsequent histopathological changes responsible for the clinical effects of radiation. It is also important to consider that most of the existing animal data are from studies in which single large fractions were investigated and these may be less relevant to clinical practice.

THE GLIAL HYPOTHESIS

Demyelination, together with vascular changes, dominates the histological appearances of radiation-induced CNS injury. The glial hypothesis concentrates on the effect of radiation on oligodendrocytes, as these cells are responsible for the production of myelin.[78] Oligodendrocytes have been shown to be the glial cell most sensitive to radiation, and relatively low doses are sufficient to cause apoptotic cell death within 2 weeks.[83,84] This cell loss is followed by two waves of stimulated proliferation.

The progenitor cell of the oligodendrocytes, the oligodendrocyte type 2 Astrocyte (O-2A), replenishes the population of oligodendrocytes.[85] Evidence that irradiation reduces the reproductive effect of O-2A cells in the spinal cord and brain of the adult rat supports the role of the oligodendrocytes in radiation injury.[86–89] Repopulation of O-2A cells was initiated almost immediately after irradiation in the adult rat optic nerve and continued for up to 6 months. However, after higher doses (>12 Gy), there was a sustained reduction in the O-2A population as well as a sustained reduction in the number of offspring. This effect was increased in older rats. This consequence of radiation on the progenitor cells provided evidence to account for delayed demyelination, while the damage to the existing mature oligodendrocyte population by radiation, with an immediate drop in mature oligodendrocyte population, can account for the early delayed demyelination. The lost oligodendrocytes cannot be replenished due to the damage of the O-2A cells. An acute loss of O-2A cells can be detected after irradiation, with time- and dose-dependent recovery.

As with the endothelial cells, it is unlikely that the effect on oligodendrocytes is solely responsible for radiation-induced neurological damage.[71] First, although the time of early loss of oligodendrocytes is consistent with early transient demyelination, the later loss of O-2A cells is not entirely consistent with the late onset of necrosis.[82,90] Furthermore, small doses of radiation may be sufficient to cause loss of oligodendrocytes but not necrosis. In other demyelinating conditions, such as multiple sclerosis, demyelinated axons do not undergo necrosis, suggesting another factor is causing the necrosis in radiation-induced injury. It is likely, therefore, that an additional pathology is responsible for the progression to necrosis.[71]

THE ROLE OF OTHER CELLS WITHIN THE CNS

Other cells in the CNS such as neurons, astrocytes, and microglia may also be important in the pathogenesis of vascular and parenchymal injury in response to radiation. Cell-cell interactions in the CNS can affect the vasculature and oligodendrocytes cells either directly or indirectly. In particular, astrocytes maintain the BBB and produce a number of growth factors and cytokines such as PDGF, FGF2, NT3, and CNTF that are involved in proliferation and differentiation of O2-A cells. In addition, they produce vascular endothelial growth factor (VEGF) and angiotensinogen that regulate vascular permeability and angiogenesis.[91,92] After moderate doses of radiation (20–25 Gy), an increase in number of astrocytes was observed in the fimbria of rats.[79]

MOLECULAR UNDERSTANDING OF BLOOD VESSEL RADIATION INJURY

With increasing understanding of the molecular effects of radiation, there has been a shift away from the hypotheses of clonogenic cell death of "target cells" (the glial or vascular hypothesis). Instead, the CNS response to radiation is thought to be "a continuous and *interacting*/interactive process"[55] mediated by apoptotic cell death and secondary damage from cytokine release and the stress response.

Cytokines

Increased expression of a number of proinflammatory genes is seen in the rat brain within hours of radiotherapy[93–96] including nuclear factor-κ B, tumor necrosis factor-α (TNF-α), interleukin-1β (IL-1β).[93,95,97,71] Rises in the levels of TNF-α and IL-1β precede acute segmental white matter demyelination due to oligodendrocyte loss,[52,82] and both have been implicated in this demyelination.[98] Furthermore, TNF-α mediates intercellular adhesion molecule-1 (ICAM-1) and increased levels of ICAM-1 occur in the mouse brain and rat spinal cord within 24 hours of radiotherapy. Hem-oxygenase 1 (HO-1), a marker of oxidative stress, increases after radiation in the mouse brain and can modulate the expression of proinflammatory genes associated with endothelial cell activation.[99] Together with ICAM-1, HO-1 may protect against the early BBB disruption and neuronal cell loss.

Reactive Oxygen Species

Reactive oxygen species (ROS), which include oxygen ions, free radicals, and inorganic and organic peroxides, are produced continually in most healthy tissue and have a role in cell signaling. The healthy brain is metabolically very active and produces ROS continually in the mitochondria. Protective antioxidants such as superoxide dismutase (SOD), catalase, and glutathione peroxidase usually protect tissues from oxidative damage by these ROS but during times of stress, tissue hypoxia or following injury, ROS levels may be increased such that the antioxidants are overwhelmed and significant damage may result from the high ROS.[100–102] Glial cells and neurons contain relatively low level of antioxidants such as SOD, glutathione, etc.,[103] and as myelin contains high level of peroxidizable fatty acids, they are particularly susceptible to ROS.[102,104] Higher levels of ROS following injury will make the brain (and oligodendrocytes in particular) susceptible to damage. Antioxidants have been used to attempt to ameliorate the effects of radiation by reducing the effect of the ROS produced by proinflammatory cytokines; total antioxidant reduction in response to radiation was reduced in rodents fed antioxidants.[105] This may be attractive as a method to reduce toxicity in humans.[102]

Additionally, increased reactive astrocytes (gliosis) and microglia in the region of radionecrosis[95,106] produce ROS, cytokines, and growth factors that may mediate progressive inflammatory injury.[94,107,108] Excessive generation of ROS from injured or proinflammatory cells has been implicated in the development of late radiation effects, as part of a continuous, ongoing process.[102] The ensuing pathologies are thought to be as a consequence of processes and interactions cells including vascular endothelial cells and the production of ROS.

VEGF and Angiotensinogen

Upregulation of VEGF occurs early in the pathogenesis associated with late side effects and occurs with white matter necrosis[78,109] prior to the development of tissue pathology.[110] With the early loss of vascular endothelial cells and subsequent breakdown of the BBB, vasogenic edema occurs causing hypoxia in the nearby tissues. In response, HIF-1α (hypoxia induced factor) and VEGF are produced[107,109,111]; the latter exacerbates the vascular permeability increasing the disruption of the BBB causing further production of VEGF, etc. Eventually, the level of VEGF rises sufficiently to stimulate angiogenesis. Although this angiogenic response persists for up to 20 weeks, it is insufficient to repair the BBB and a sharp fall in endothelial cell number occurs, leading to white matter necrosis. Kim et al.[102] suggest that as anti-VEGF therapy may be able to normalize BBB function in microvessels damaged during surgery, the same approach may reduce the damage from radiation. This observation has led to clinical trials using Bevacizumab, a monoclonal antibody against VEGF after brain irradiation. Significant reductions in brain edema have been reported, albeit in small numbers of patients.[112,113]

APOPTOSIS

Apoptosis is seen within 24 hours of radiation in endothelial cells, oligodendrocytes, subependymal cells, and some neurons. Dose-dependent endothelial cell apoptosis occurs in the rat spinal cord[75] with the peak loss occurring at 12 hours[114] and is mediated by the acid sphingomyelinase (ASMase).[115] Irradiation of ASMase knockout mice with a dose of 50 Gy did not result in endothelial cell apoptosis or disruption of the blood-spinal cord barrier (BSCB), whereas disruption was present in p53 knockout mice.[115] Apoptotic reduction in oligodendrocytes also occurs within 24 hours of irradiation in the spinal cord after radiation[116,117] and is followed by a dramatic loss of progenitor cells at 2 to 4 weeks.[118] Recovery to 40% to 80% may occur by 3 months but with very high doses (>23 Gy) a secondary decline in the oligodendrocytes progenitor pool occurs 4 to 5 months after radiotherapy.[84] In contrast to apoptosis of endothelial cells, apoptosis of oligodendrocytes is p53, and not ASMase dependent.[117,119] It is therefore thought that apoptosis of endothelial cells, rather than of oligodendrocytes, is responsible for disruption of the BSCB after radiation and that the likely trigger is inflammatory cell expression and oxidative stress. Accordingly, oligodendrocytes apoptosis and focal demyelination occur as a secondary reaction to this.[84]

The relationship between early gene expression and early endothelial or oligodendrocytes cell loss and later tissue injury is not yet known.

CLINICAL EFFECTS OF HIGH-DOSE RADIATION

Clinical effects related to vascular injury of CNS radiotherapy may be either due to the direct effect of radiation on blood vessels or as a secondary effect following either parenchymal damage or as a result of changes in endocrine status affecting lipid metabolism. Most of the clinical data are descriptive without pathological information. While it is possible on the basis of imaging and clinical presentation to separate vascular events into occlusive and blood vessel rupture, the mechanism of vascular damage is not fully defined and is largely presumptive.

DIRECT VASCULAR PATHOLOGY

CNS radiotherapy can cause a number of direct vascular events including blood vessel occlusion, large vessel vasculopathy, Moyamoya disease,[120–122] blood vessel rupture, telangiectasia,

formation of cavernous angioma, aneurysm formation, and mineralizing microangiopathy. However, they are relatively uncommon and the consequence in terms of occlusion and hemorrhage is likely to have a multifactorial etiology. The most common clinical event is (CVA/stroke) or, in case of aneurysm, formation subarachnoid, or intracranial hemorrhage.

ARTERIAL STENOSIS, STROKE, AND TRANSIENT ISCHEMIC ATTACKS

Most of the published data on arterial stenosis come from the effects of neck irradiation on the carotid artery as well as the effect of irradiation for brain and nasopharyngeal tumors on intracranial blood vessels.[17,22,24,38,123–130]

Large vessel irradiation results in proliferation of small blood vessels, hyalinization, and fibrinoid necrosis of vessel walls and proliferation of the endothelial lining resulting in luminal narrowing, which can lead to ischemia and infarction.

The RR of CVA in a cohort of patients with pituitary adenoma treated with radiotherapy was 4 and the predisposing factors included gender, the extent of surgery, and RT dose.[131] The RR was independent of age but as would be expected is higher in patients with endocrinopathy known to be associated with vascular disorders, such as seen in acromegaly and Cushing disease.

While radiotherapy is likely to be a contributing factor, the higher incidence of stroke in women suggests further endocrine influence, such as premature menopause that is known to be a risk factor in general population and is likely to occur following irradiation of the hypothalamic pituitary axis. Higher risks in patients undergoing surgery also suggest involvement of surgically induced, perhaps latent, vascular damage. Factors that may contribute to the higher risk of stroke in patients with pituitary adenoma are summarized in Figure 25.2. The increased incidence of stroke in this patient population is accompanied by increased CVA mortality.[126]

Moyamoya is a progressive disease of the distal internal carotid arteries and their major branches with vessel occlusion due to intimal proliferation. A collateral network of blood vessels at the base of the brain leads to the characteristic angiographic appearances described as a "puff of smoke" (Fig. 25.1). Moyamoya has been reported in both adults and children as

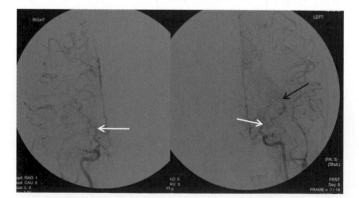

Figure 25.1. Carotid angiograms of the right and left arterial system show occluded middle cerebral arteries bilaterally (*white arrow*) with reconstitution of the left MCA vessel with collateral vasculature (*red arrow*) diagnostic of Moyamoya. (Courtesy of Dr Philip Rich.)

a consequence of radiation therapy in the CNS particularly involving the Circle of Willis[132–136] and is often associated with a background history of neurofibromatosis type 1 (NF1)[137] particularly after radiotherapy for optic nerve gliomas (see "Irradiation in Children").

INTRACRANIAL HAEMORRHAGE

Intracranial hemorrhage is an uncommon presumed late effect of CNS radiotherapy in children and adults.[138–144] The average time to occurrence is in the region of 8 years[138,143] but can be as long as 20 to 30 years.[138,144] There is no clear relationship to radiation dose, use of chemotherapy, and age at treatment. Presumed mechanisms of intracranial hemorrhage include the presence of abnormal blood vessels, with proliferation of large thin-walled new vessels and telangiectatic histological pattern on a background of gliosis and fibrinoid necrosis[143] or the development of either cavernous angiomas[138] or aneurysms.[145,146] As radiological features may suggest a space-occupying lesion, differentiating recurrent disease from hemorrhage is of importance.[144] The incidence and mortality from subarachnoid hemorrhage is most likely due to the presence of aneurysms presumed to be at least in part related to radiotherapy.[126]

INTRACRANIAL ANEURYSM, TELANGIECTASIA AND MINERALIZING MICROANGIOPATHY

While published case reports record potential association of new and occasionally multiple aneurysms with previous irradiation for intracranial tumors,[33,145–149] the incidence is not known. Histopathological findings at autopsy from three patients who died from rupture of saccular aneurysms following radiotherapy for cerebellar medulloblastoma, revealed histopathological features not typical of congenital saccular aneurysms, on the background of widespread radiation-induced vasculopathy.[148] Aneurysm formation and/or rupture generally occur years after radiation but have been reported as early as 10 months after radiotherapy.[149]

Telangiectasia formation with development of collateral vessels due to radiation-induced small vessel thrombosis may also cause subclinical or clinical hemorrhage and has been described more frequently in children than adults.[138,150,151] While mineralizing microangiopathy due to calcium deposition in small vessel wall is a frequent finding on imaging in children,[151–154] it is usually asymptomatic.

SECONDARY PARENCHYMAL DAMAGE

Acute, early delayed, and late delayed side effects of CNS irradiation,[71,77] while primarily described as parenchymal, have an important vascular component. Acute effects, presumed in part to be due to edema, involve a component of BBB disruption. They are rarely seen following conventional fractionated radiotherapy with fraction sizes under 7 Gy.[155,156] Early delayed injury does not have a clear vascular component.

The hallmarks of late delayed effects are demyelination and vascular abnormalities[71,102,157] ultimately leading to necrosis, which is usually confined to white matter. Necrosis can be accompanied by edema most likely due to the disruption of the BBB. Late damage to the spinal cord in the form of myelopathy, as a consequence of irradiation beyond tolerance doses, is associated with the same vascular and parenchymal pathological

changes as late radiation injury to the brain with telangiectasia, hyaline degeneration, perivascular fibrosis, vasculitis, fibrinoid necrosis, thrombosis, and hemorrhage.[54]

Vascular damage causing ischemia not resulting in necrosis may lead to white matter injury and CNS atrophy, which may in part be due to injury to deep perforating arteries.[151] Radiation-induced vasculopathy causing hemorrhage and gliosis is considered one of the main causes of radiation optic neuropathy.[120,158]

VASCULOPATHY DUE TO ENDOCRINE DISTURBANCES

Radiation-induced hypopituitarism (RIH) is a common consequence of radiation for intracranial tumors and as part of cranial prophylaxis in leukemia.[159] The characteristic pattern of evolution of RIH is initial growth hormone (GH) and gonadotrophin deficiency with a later appearance of corticotroph and thyrotroph insufficiency.[160] The effects of hormonal derangement vary with age of irradiation.

GH deficiency is the most common consequence of cranial irradiation and is dose dependent. In adults, it leads to changes in lipid metabolism with increased total and LDL cholesterol levels and decreased high-density lipoprotein (HDL) cholesterol,[161] with increased predisposition to atheromatous vascular disease. Hypopituitarism is an independent risk factor for increased mortality, which is assumed to be principally due to cerebrovascular causes.[126,162–166]

IRRADIATION IN CHILDREN

Despite improved survival of children with malignant disease, almost 30% develop a severe or life-threatening condition in adult life.[167] Increased risk of cerebrovascular disease is seen where radiation is considered one of the predisposing factors,[168] with a suggestion of dose-response relationship.[169,170]

Age at the time of radiotherapy delivery may affect the pathological response; the time to develop late vascular complication following fractionated radiotherapy is longer in children than in adults. This is ascribed to accelerated progression of preexisting vascular disease in adults, while in children the longer latency may represent radiation-induced cell loss.[171] The use of smaller doses per fraction in children may also contribute to the longer latency.

CEREBROVASCULAR DISEASE IN CHILDREN

As in adults, the RR of developing cerebrovascular disease is increased following cranial radiation in children. Intracranial steno-occlusive disease after childhood cranial radiotherapy develops with a median latency of 3 years.[169,172] Although the incidence is not defined, the risk appears to be higher following radiotherapy for suprasellar and/or chiasmatic lesions, optic gliomas and germ cell tumors, adjacent to the Circle of Willis.[173,169]

The RR of stroke in survivors of all childhood cancers is nearly ten times higher than in sibling control groups.[167] The risk of stroke is also increased in long-term survivors of childhood leukemia (RR 5.9; 2.6–13.4) and survivors of brain tumors treated with cranial doses of 30 Gy or more (RR 38, 17.6–79.9).[26] As in adults, it is difficult to separate the effect of cranial irradiation from other predisposing factors, which include the brain tumor itself, surgery, endocrine sequelae

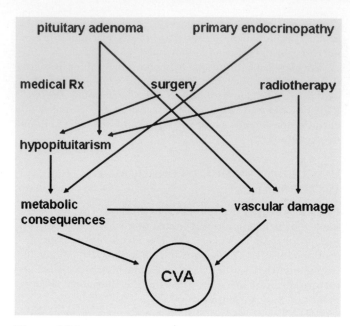

Figure 25.2. Factors contributing to the risk of CVA in patients with pituitary adenoma.

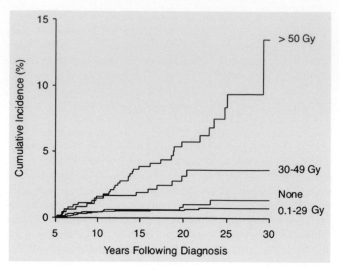

Figure 25.4. The actuarial cumulative incidence of stroke in 5-year survivors of childhood leukemia and brain tumors who received CRT to the temporal lobe, hypothalamus, and circle of Willis comparing no radiation related to the maximum dose of cranial radiation therapy (*no radiation vs. 0.1 to 29 Gy [p= 0.38], 0.1 to 29 vs. 30 to 49 Gy [p < 0.001], and 30 to 49 vs. 50 Gy [p < 0.02]*). (Reprinted from Bowers D, et al. Late-occurring stroke among long-term survivors of childhood leukemia and brain tumors: a report from the Childhood Cancer Survivor Study. *J Clin Oncol.* 2006;24:5277–5282, with permission. © 2008 American Society of Clinical Oncology. All rights reserved.)

of the disease, and other treatments including chemotherapy (Fig. 25.2). The risk of stroke is dose related (Fig. 25.3).

The risk of developing Moyamoya is higher in children than in adults and has been particularly noted following radiotherapy that includes the Circle of Willis[132–136] and in children with NF1. This latter group may develop vasculopathy sooner, after lower radiation doses (18–39 Gy).[136,137,169,174,175] Two of twenty-three children without NF1 (9%) who received radiation for optic pathway glioma compared to three of five patients with NF1 (60%) developed Moyamoya.[136] In a separate review assessing the risk factors for the development of Moyamoya in children, 12 of 345 patients developed Moyamoya (3.5%) with a more rapid onset in patients with NF1 (median: 38 vs. 55 months) and for patients receiving >50 Gy (median: 42 vs. 67 months). The estimate is a 7% increase in the risk of developing Moymoya

(HR = 1.07, 95% CI: 1.02–1.13, p = 0.01) for each 1-Gy increase in radiation dose with a threefold higher risk in the presence of NF1 (HR = 3.07, 95% CI: 0.90–10.46, p = 0.07)[174] (Fig. 25-4).

Current guidelines suggest annual neurological examination in patients who received ≥18 Gy cranial radiation, with those who received ≥50 Gy at greatest risk. If clinical suspicion of neurovascular sequelae arises, a brain MRI with diffusion-weighted imaging and MR angiography is recommended. Stroke prevention strategies may be instituted although antiplatelet prophylaxis has not shown to be of benefit in Moyamoya or postradiation occlusive disease. Surgical revascularization has also been used but developmental and functional data are not available.[169,176]

Vascular Malformations in Children

Vascular malformations after radiation in children include venous malformations (including cavernomas), telangiectasia, and aneurysms. As with steno-occlusive disease, evidence largely comes from case reports and retrospective series and may be detected as incidental finding on imaging.

Cavernoma was reported in 3% of children treated for brain tumors at a median of 37 months after radiotherapy.[177] Higher doses (>30 Gy) were associated with shorter latency.[178] Telangiectasia was identified in 20% of patients after radiation for leukemia or brain tumors regardless of dose.[179] Intracranial aneurysms may occur as early as 10 months and as late as decades after radiation with no clear relationship between dose and latency.[148,149]

Mineralizing microangiopathy is a frequent neuroradiologic finding in children after radiotherapy. It is a distinctive pathological process affecting small vessels of previously irradiated cerebral and cerebellar parenchyma, leading to calcification of the basal ganglia, and may occur after doses as low as 15 Gy.[151,180] Although it can occur after radiation alone, it is more common

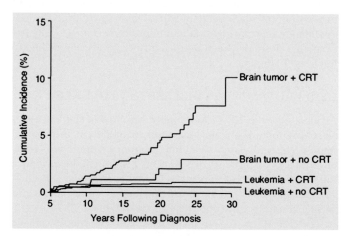

Figure 25.3. The actuarial cumulative incidence of stroke in 5-year survivors of childhood leukemia and brain tumors with and without cranial radiation therapy (CRT). (Reprinted from Bowers D, et al. Late-occurring stroke among long-term survivors of childhood leukemia and brain tumors: a report from the Childhood Cancer Survivor Study. *J Clin Oncol.* 2006;24:5277–5282, with permission. © 2008 American Society of Clinical Oncology. All rights reserved.)

after combined treatment with chemotherapy. In an autopsy series, mineralizing microangiopathy was detected in 17% of children who had undergone radiotherapy for leukemia and was detected as early as 10 months after completion of radiotherapy.[181] The relationship between radiologic appearance and clinical symptoms is unclear.[152]

VASCULAR EFFECTS OF LOW-DOSE IRRADIATION

Low-Dose Irradiation in Children

Late effects of low-dose cranial irradiation in the form of neurocognitive and psychiatric disorders are considered, at least in part, to be of vascular etiology (see earlier). Between the years 1940 and 1960, irradiation of the scalp was extensively used in treatment of children with tinea capitis (ringworm). Brain doses were in the range 0.7 to 1.75 Gy. Several epidemiological and functional studies have been carried out on these subjects to investigate the long-term effects of low-dose cerebral irradiation on mental function. Long-term follow-up (average: 20 years) of 2,215 irradiated subjects and 1,395 nonirradiated subjects treated for tinea capitis at New York University hospital demonstrated a 40% excess of treated psychiatric disorders in the irradiated white American patients, but no difference among black Americans.[170] Psychiatric and psychometric analysis of a subgroup of 177 irradiated and 68 unirradiated subjects confirmed an increase in psychiatric symptoms and more deviant scores in the irradiated white group, although the overall rating of psychiatric status showed only borderline differences.[182]

In a larger study on 11,000 irradiated Israeli subjects and 11,000 population controls, the irradiated children (mean brain doses of 1.3 Gy) were also found to have lower IQ and psychological scores and a slightly higher incidence of mental retardation.[183] A separate analysis of visual evoked responses on 44 irradiated and 57 controls also showed significant differences between the groups.[184]

An analysis of adult survivors of childhood cancers of the CNS ($n = 1,877$) demonstrated significantly elevated risks of neurocognitive impairment and reduced socioeconomic outcomes compared with sibling controls ($n = 3,899$).[185] Survivors had significantly impaired attention spans and memory, as well as problems with organization and emotional regulation. These impairments were related to the cranial radiation doses (no cranial radiation, <50 Gy, >50 Gy total fractionated dose) for treatment of astrocytoma, glial tumors, or ependymoma, but there was no clear dose-response relationship for medulloblastoma.

A population-based cohort study of 3,094 men who were irradiated for cutaneous hemangioma before age 18 months showed that intellectual development was adversely affected by radiation doses >100 mGy.[186] The proportion of boys attending high school decreased with increasing dose of radiation, from 32% among those not irradiated to 17% in those who received >250 mGy. For irradiation to the frontal part of the brain, the multivariate odds ratio was 0.47 (0.26–0.85), and for the posterior brain, it was 0.59 (0.23–1.46). Taken together, the results of these studies indicate that low-dose irradiation (<1–2 Gy) to the immature developing brain can cause long-term cognitive and behavioral defects.

Low-Dose Irradiation in Adults

The effects of low-dose irradiation have been studied in nuclear plant workers, cohorts accidentally exposed to radiation, Chernobyl survivors, and atomic bomb survivors and all suggest that even low-dose irradiation is associated with cerebrovascular morbidity.

In a large cohort of atomic bomb survivors followed for more than 50 years, the excess relative risk (ERR) of mortality per Gy was 14% (6%–23%, $p < 0.001$) for heart disease and 9% (1%–17%, $p = 0.02$) for stroke[187] with a suggestion of a dose-response relationship. The ERR for stroke was higher in people exposed before the age of 60. The study suggests that exposure to low-dose irradiation up to 4 Gy increases the risk of stroke (and heart disease), and this has also been demonstrated by others.[188–190]

The population exposed to radiation through the Chernobyl Nuclear Power plant accident in 1986 had an increased risk of cardiovascular and cerebrovascular disease. The ERR per Gy for ischemic heart disease, essential hypertension, and cerebrovascular disease were 1.41 (95% CI: 0.05–0.78), 0.36 (0.005–0.71), and 0.45 (0.11–0.80), respectively.[191,192] Nuclear power plant workers do not have increased risk of cerebrovascular or cardiovascular disease.[193,194]

CONCLUSION

Late effects of radiation on blood vessels in the central nervous system result in ischemic and hemorrhagic injury of potentially devastating consequences to the patient. With longer survival following cranial radiotherapy in both children and adults and with more frequent use of radiation for benign intracranial disease, delayed effects of radiation are increasingly recognized and gain greater importance as determinants of survival and quality of life. Better understanding of the cellular and molecular mechanisms of blood vessel injury may lead to selective vascular protection although attempts at molecular manipulation of radiation injury to normal tissues have so far met with limited success. Recognizing genetic predisposition to blood vessel injury may lead to use of treatments not employing radiation, particularly in children. In the absence of modifiable biological factors it remains important to employ modern techniques of radiation that localize the delivery of ionizing radiation and avoid dose fractionation schemes associated with a high risk of injury. It is also important to continue long-term follow up of patients receiving cranial irradiation and ensure that known medical predisposing factors to cerebrovascular disease are appropriately treated ideally before the consequences become clinically apparent. As in other disease sites this may require establishing long-term surveillance clinics both treating and documenting late radiation injury.

REFERENCES

1. Sheehan JF. Foam cell plaques in the intima of irradiated small arteries (one hundred to five hundred microns in external diameter). *Arch Pathol.* 1944;37:297–307.
2. Sams A. Histological changes in the larger blood vessels of the hind limb of the mouse after x-irradiation. *Int J Radiat Biol Relat Stud Phys Chem Med.* 1965;9:165–174.
3. Lawson JA. Surgical treatment of radiation induced atherosclerotic disease of the iliac and femoral arteries. *J Cardiovasc Surg (Torino).* 1985;26(2):151–156.
4. McCready RA, Hyde GL, Bivins BA, et al. Radiation-induced arterial injuries. *Surgery.* 1983;93(2):306–312.
5. Thomas E, Forbus WD. Irradiation injury to the aorta and the lung. *AMA Arch Pathol.* 1959;67(3):256–263.
6. Adams MJ, Lipshultz SE. Pathophysiology of anthracycline- and radiation-associated cardiomyopathies: implications for screening and prevention. *Pediatr Blood Cancer.* 2005;44(7):600–606.
7. Stewart JR, Fajardo LF, Gillette SM, et al. Radiation injury to the heart. *Int J Radiat Oncol Biol Phys.* 1995;31(5):1205–1211.
8. Veinot JP, Edwards WD. Pathology of radiation-induced heart disease: a surgical and autopsy study of 27 cases. *Hum Pathol.* 1996;27(8):766–773.

9. Conomy JP, Kellermeyer RW. Delayed cerebrovascular consequences of therapeutic radiation. A clinicopathologic study of a stroke associated with radiation-related carotid arteriopathy. *Cancer.* 1975;36(5):1702–1708.
10. Silverberg GD, Britt RH, Goffinet DR. Radiation-induced carotid artery disease. *Cancer.* 1978;41(1):130–137.
11. Bowers DC, McNeil DE, Liu Y, et al. Stroke as a late treatment effect of Hodgkin's Disease: a report from the Childhood Cancer Survivor Study. *J Clin Oncol.* 2005;23(27):6508–6515.
12. Muzaffar K, Collins SL, Labropoulos N, et al. A prospective study of the effects of irradiation on the carotid artery. *Laryngoscope.* 2000;110(11):1811–1814.
13. Dorresteijn LD, Kappelle AC, Boogerd W, et al. Increased risk of ischemic stroke after radiotherapy on the neck in patients younger than 60 years. *J Clin Oncol.* 2002;20(1):282–288.
14. Martin JD, Buckley AR, Graeb D, et al. Carotid artery stenosis in asymptomatic patients who have received unilateral head-and-neck irradiation. *Int J Radiat Oncol Biol Phys.* 2005;63(4):1197–1205.
15. Carmody BJ, Arora S, Avena R, et al. Accelerated carotid artery disease after high-dose head and neck radiotherapy: is there a role for routine carotid duplex surveillance? *J Vasc Surg.* 1999;30(6):1045–1051.
16. Steele SR, Martin MJ, Mullenix PS, et al. Focused high-risk population screening for carotid arterial stenosis after radiation therapy for head and neck cancer. *Am J Surg.* 2004;187(5):594–598.
17. Lam WW, Leung SF, So NM, et al. Incidence of carotid stenosis in nasopharyngeal carcinoma patients after radiotherapy. *Cancer.* 2001;92(9):2357–2363.
18. Chang YJ, Chang TC, Lee TH, et al. Predictors of carotid artery stenosis after radiotherapy for head and neck cancers. *J Vasc Surg.* 2009;50(2):280–285.
19. Scott AS, Parr LA, Johnstone PA. Risk of cerebrovascular events after neck and supraclavicular radiotherapy: a systematic review. *Radiother Oncol.* 2009;90(2):163–165.
20. Dubec JJ, Munk PL, Tsang V, et al. Carotid artery stenosis in patients who have undergone radiation therapy for head and neck malignancy. *Br J Radiol.* 1998;71(848):872–875.
21. King LJ, Hasnain SN, Webb JA, et al. Asymptomatic carotid arterial disease in young patients following neck radiation therapy for Hodgkin lymphoma. *Radiology.* 1999;213(1):167–172.
22. Cheng SW, Ting AC, Lam LK, et al. Carotid stenosis after radiotherapy for nasopharyngeal carcinoma. *Arch Otolaryngol Head Neck Surg.* 2000;126(4):517–521.
23. Cheng SW, Ting AC, Ho P, et al. Accelerated progression of carotid stenosis in patients with previous external neck irradiation. *J Vasc Surg.* 2004;39(2):409–415.
24. Lam WW, Liu KH, Leung SF, et al. Sonographic characterisation of radiation-induced carotid artery stenosis. *Cerebrovasc Dis.* 2002;13(3):168–173.
25. Haynes JC, Machtay M, Weber RS, et al. Relative risk of stroke in head and neck carcinoma patients treated with external cervical irradiation. *Laryngoscope.* 2002;112(10):1883–1887.
26. Bowers DC, Liu Y, Leisenring W, et al. Late-occurring stroke among long-term survivors of childhood leukemia and brain tumors: a report from the Childhood Cancer Survivor Study. *J Clin Oncol.* 2006;24(33):5277–5282.
27. Munro JM, Cotran RS. The pathogenesis of atherosclerosis: atherogenesis and inflammation. *Lab Invest.* 1988;58(3):249–261.
28. Schwartz CJ, Valente AJ, Sprague EA, et al. The pathogenesis of atherosclerosis: an overview. *Clin Cardiol.* 1991;14(2 suppl 1):I1– I16.
29. Wissler RW. Update on the pathogenesis of atherosclerosis. *Am J Med.* 1991;91(1B):3S–9S.
30. Schiller NK, Kubo N, Boisvert WA, et al. Effect of gamma-irradiation and bone marrow transplantation on atherosclerosis in LDL receptor-deficient mice. *Arterioscler Thromb Vasc Biol.* 2001;21(10):1674–1680.
31. Pakala R, Leborgne L, Cheneau E, et al. Radiation-induced atherosclerotic plaque progression in a hypercholesterolemic rabbit: a prospective vulnerable plaque model? *Cardiovasc Radiat Med.* 2003;4(3):146–151.
32. Stewart FA, Heeneman S, Te Poele J, et al. Ionizing radiation accelerates the development of atherosclerotic lesions in ApoE−/− mice and predisposes to an inflammatory plaque phenotype prone to hemorrhage. *Am J Pathol.* 2006;168(2):649–658.
33. Moriyama T, Shigemori M, Hirohata Y, et al. Multiple intracranial aneurysms following radiation therapy for pituitary adenoma; a case report. *No Shinkei Geka.* 1992;20(4):487–492.
34. Martinez Del Pero M, Majumdar S, Coley SC, et al. Near fatal haemorrhage 35 years after radiation for laryngeal cancer: emergency embolisation of a vertebral artery aneurysm. *Emerg Med J.* 2006;23(4):e26.
35. Ross HB, Sales, JE. Post-irradiation femoral aneurysm treated by iliopopliteal by-pass via the obturator foramen. *Br J Surg.* 1972;59(5):400–405.
36. Fajardo LF, Lee, A. Rupture of major vessels after radiation. *Cancer.* 1975;36(3):904–913.
37. von Rahden BH, Stein HJ, Reiter R, et al. Delayed aortic rupture after radiochemotherapy and esophagectomy for esophageal cancer. *Dis Esophagus.* 2003;16(4):346–349.
38. Lam HC, Abdullah VJ, Wormald PJ, et al. Internal carotid artery hemorrhage after irradiation and osteoradionecrosis of the skull base. *Otolaryngol Head Neck Surg.* 2001;125(5):522–527.
39. Okamura HO, Kamiyama R, Takiguchi Y, et al. Histopathological examination of ruptured carotid artery after irradiation. *ORL J Otorhinolaryngol Relat Spec.* 2002;64(3):226–228.
40. Drognitz O, Pfeiffenberger J, Schareck W, et al. Primary aortoduodenal fistula as a late complication of para-aortic radiation therapy. A case report. *Der Chirurg.* 2002;73(6):633–637.
41. Fukasawa H, Okamoto M, Narushima M, et al. A case of aortoduodenal fistula following radiotherapy of retroperitoneal metastatic disease. *Gan To Kagaku Ryoho.* 1991;18(1):119–122.
42. Gabrail NY, Harrison BR, Sunwoo YC. Chemo-irradiation induced aortoesophageal fistula. *J Surg Oncol.* 1991;48(3):213–215.
43. Sivaraman SK, Drummond R. Radiation-induced aortoesophageal fistula: an unusual case of massive upper gastrointestinal bleeding. *J Emerg Med.* 2002;23(2):175–178.
44. Estrada FP, Tachovsky TJ, Orr RM Jr, et al. Primary aortoduodenal fistula following radiotherapy. *Surg Gynecol Obstet.* 1983;156(5):646–650.
45. Kalman DR, Barnard GF, Massimi GJ, et al. Primary aortoduodenal fistula after radiotherapy. *Am J Gastroenterol.* 1995;90(7):1148–1150.
46. Perera GB, Wilson SE, Barie PS, et al. Duodenocaval fistula: a late complication of retroperitoneal irradiation and vena cava replacement. *Ann Vasc Surg.* 2004;18(1):52–58.
47. Hoopes PJ, Gillette EL, Withrow SJ. Intraoperative irradiation of the canine abdominal aorta and vena cava. *Int J Radiat Oncol Biol Phys.* 1987;13(5):715–722.
48. Gillette EL, Powers BE, McChesney SL, et al. Response of aorta and branch arteries to experimental intraoperative irradiation. *Int J Radiat Oncol Biol Phys.* 1989;17(6):1247–1255.
49. Gillette EL, Powers BE, McChesney SL, et al. Aortic wall injury following intraoperative irradiation. *Int J Radiat Oncol Biol Phys.* 1988;15(6):1401–1406.
50. Powers BE, Thames HD, Gillette EL. Long-term adverse effects of radiation inhibition of restenosis: radiation injury to the aorta and branch arteries in a canine model. *Int J Radiat Oncol Biol Phys.* 1999;45(3):753–759.
51. Schultze B, Korr H. Cell kinetic studies of different cell types in the developing and adult brain of the rat and the mouse: a review. *Cell Tissue Kinet.* 1981;14(3):309–325.
52. van der Kogel AJ. Radiation-induced damage in the central nervous system: an interpretation of target cell responses. *Br J Cancer Suppl.* 1986;7:207–217.
53. Nieder C, Andratschke N, Astner ST. Experimental concepts for toxicity prevention and tissue restoration after central nervous system irradiation. *Radiat Oncol.* 2007;2:23.
54. Schultheiss TE, Kun LE, Ang KK, et al. Radiation response of the central nervous system. *Int J Radiat Oncol Biol Phys.* 1995;31(5):1093–1112.
55. Wong CS, Van der Kogel AJ. Mechanisms of radiation injury to the central nervous system: implications for neuroprotection. *Mol Interv.* 2004;4(5):273–284.
56. Schultheiss TE, Stephens LC, Maor MH. Analysis of the histopathology of radiation myelopathy. *Int J Radiat Oncol Biol Phys.* 1988;14(1):27–32.
57. Ang KK, van der Kogel AJ, van der Schueren E. The effect of small radiation doses on the rat spinal cord: the concept of partial tolerance. *Int J Radiat Oncol Biol Phys.* 1983;9(10):1487–1491.
58. Thames HD, Ang KK, Stewart FA, et al. Does incomplete repair explain the apparent failure of the basic LQ model to predict spinal cord and kidney responses to low doses per fraction? *Int J Radiat Biol.* 1988;54(1):13–19.
59. White A, Hornsey S. Radiation damage to the rat spinal cord: the effect of single and fractionated doses of X rays. *Br J Radiol.* 1978;51(607):515–523.
60. Wong CS, Hao Y, Hill RP. Response of rat spinal cord to very small doses per fraction: lack of enhanced radiosensitivity. *Radiother Oncol.* 1995;36(1):44–49.
61. Abramson N, Cavanaugh PJ. Short-course radiation therapy in carcinoma of the lung. A second look. *Radiology.* 1973;108(3):685–687.
62. Schultheiss TE. The radiation dose-response of the human spinal cord. *Int J Radiat Oncol Biol Phys.* 2008;71(5):1455–1459.
63. Raber J, Rola R, LeFevour A, et al. Radiation-induced cognitive impairments are associated with changes in indicators of hippocampal neurogenesis. *Radiat Res.* 2004;162(1):39–47.
64. Madsen TM, Kristjansen PE, Bolwig TG, et al. Arrested neuronal proliferation and impaired hippocampal function following fractionated brain irradiation in the adult rat. *Neuroscience.* 2003;119(3):635–642.
65. Fike JR, Rola R, Limoli CL. Radiation response of neural precursor cells. *Neurosurg Clin N Am.* 2007;18(1):115–127, x.
66. Mizumatsu S, Monje ML, Morhardt DR, et al. Extreme sensitivity of adult neurogenesis to low doses of X-irradiation. *Cancer Res.* 2003;63(14):4021–4027.
67. Monje ML, Palmer T. Radiation injury and neurogenesis. *Curr Opin Neurol.* 2003;16(2):129–134.
68. Manda K, Ueno M, Moritake T, et al. Radiation-induced cognitive dysfunction and cerebellar oxidative stress in mice: protective effect of alpha-lipoic acid. *Behav Brain Res.* 2007;177(1):7–14.
69. Rola R, Raber J, Rizk A, et al. Radiation-induced impairment of hippocampal neurogenesis is associated with cognitive deficits in young mice. *Exp Neurol.* 2004;188(2):316–330.
70. Brown WR, Blair RM, Moody DM, et al. Capillary loss precedes the cognitive impairment induced by fractionated whole-brain irradiation: a potential rat model of vascular dementia. *J Neurol Sci.* 2007;257(1–2):67–71.
71. Tofilon PJ, Fike JR. The radioresponse of the central nervous system: a dynamic process. *Radiat Res.* 2000;153(4):357–370.
72. Nordal RA, Wong CS. Molecular targets in radiation-induced blood-brain barrier disruption. *Int J Radiat Oncol Biol Phys.* 2005;62(1):279–287.
73. Rubin P, Gash DM, Hansen JT, et al. Disruption of the blood-brain barrier as the primary effect of CNS irradiation. *Radiother Oncol.* 1994;31(1):51–60.
74. Ljubimova NV, Levitman MK, Plotnikova ED, et al. Endothelial cell population dynamics in rat brain after local irradiation. *Br J Radiol.* 1991;64(766):934–940.
75. Li YQ, Chen P, Jain V, et al. Early radiation-induced endothelial cell loss and blood-spinal cord barrier breakdown in the rat spinal cord. *Radiat Res.* 2004;161(2):143–152.
76. Lyubimova NV, Coultas PG, Yuen K, et al. In vivo radioprotection of mouse brain endothelial cells by Hoechst 33342. *Br J Radiol.* 2001;74(877):77–82.
77. Coderre JA, Morris GM, Micca PL, et al. Late effects of radiation on the central nervous system: role of vascular endothelial damage and glial stem cell survival. *Radiat Res.* 2006;166(3):495–503.
78. Lyubimova N, Hopewell JW. Experimental evidence to support the hypothesis that damage to vascular endothelium plays the primary role in the development of late radiation-induced CNS injury. *Br J Radiol.* 2004;77(918):488–492.
79. Calvo W, Hopewell JW, Reinhold HS, et al. Time- and dose-related changes in the white matter of the rat brain after single doses of X rays. *Br J Radiol.* 1988;61(731):1043–1052.
80. Reinhold HS, Calvo W, Hopewell JW, et al. Development of blood vessel-related radiation damage in the fimbria of the central nervous system. *Int J Radiat Oncol Biol Phys.* 1990;18(1):37–42.
81. Schultheiss TE, Stephens LC. Invited review: permanent radiation myelopathy. *Br J Radiol.* 1992;65(777):737–753.
82. Mastaglia FL, McDonald WI, Watson JV, et al. Effects of x-radiation on the spinal cord: an experimental study of the morphological changes in central nerve fibres. *Brain.* 1976;99(1):101–22.

83. Vrdoljak E, Bill CA, Stephens LC, et al. Radiation-induced apoptosis of oligodendrocytes in vitro. *Int J Radiat Biol.* 1992;62(4):475–480.

84. Hopewell JW, van der Kogel AJ. Pathophysiological mechanisms leading to the development of late radiation-induced damage to the central nervous system. *Front Radiat Ther Oncol.* 1999;33:265–275.

85. Raff MC, Miller RH, Noble M. A glial progenitor cell that develops in vitro into an astrocyte or an oligodendrocyte depending on culture medium. *Nature.* 1983;303(5916):390–396.

86. van der Maazen RW, Verhagen I, Kleiboer BJ, et al. Radiosensitivity of glial progenitor cells of the perinatal and adult rat optic nerve studied by an in vitro clonogenic assay. *Radiother Oncol.* 1991;20(4):258–264.

87. van der Maazen RW, Kleiboer BJ, Verhagen I, et al. Irradiation in vitro discriminates between different O-2A progenitor cell subpopulations in the perinatal central nervous system of rats. *Radiat Res.* 1991;128(1):64–72.

88. van der Maazen RW, Verhagen I, Kleiboer BJ, et al. Repopulation of O-2A progenitor cells after irradiation of the adult rat optic nerve analyzed by an in vitro clonogenic assay. *Radiat Res.* 1992;132(1):82–86.

89. van der Maazen RW, Kleiboer BJ, Verhagen I, et al. Repair capacity of adult rat glial progenitor cells determined by an in vitro clonogenic assay after in vitro or in vivo fractionated irradiation. *Int J Radiat Biol.* 1993;63(5):661–666.

90. Hornsey S, Myers R, Coultas PG, et al. Turnover of proliferative cells in the spinal cord after X irradiation and its relation to time-dependent repair of radiation damage. *Br J Radiol.* 1981;54(648):1081–1085.

91. Hong-Brown LQ, Brown CR. Cytokine and insulin regulation of alpha 2 macroglobulin, angiotensinogen, and hsp 70 in primary cultured astrocytes. *Glia.* 1994;12(3):211–218.

92. Ijichi A, Sakuma S, Tofilon PJ. Hypoxia-induced vascular endothelial growth factor expression in normal rat astrocyte cultures. *Glia.* 1995;14(2):87–93.

93. Hong JH, Chiang CS, Campbell IL, et al. Induction of acute phase gene expression by brain irradiation. *Int J Radiat Oncol Biol Phys.* 1995;33(3):619–626.

94. Chiang CS, Hong JH, Stalder A, et al. Delayed molecular responses to brain irradiation. *Int J Radiat Biol.* 1997;72(1):45–53.

95. Raju U, Gumin GJ, Tofilon PJ. Radiation-induced transcription factor activation in the rat cerebral cortex. *Int J Radiat Biol.* 2000;76(8):1045–1053.

96. Kyrkanides S, Moore AH, Olschowka JA, et al. Cyclooxygenase-2 modulates brain inflammation-related gene expression in central nervous system radiation injury. *Brain Res Mol Brain Res.* 2002;104(2):159–169.

97. Gaber MW, Sabek OM, Fukatsu K, et al. Differences in ICAM-1 and TNF-alpha expression between large single fraction and fractionated irradiation in mouse brain. *Int J Radiat Biol.* 2003;79(5):359–366.

98. Palma JP, Kwon D, Clipstone NA, et al. Infection with Theiler's murine encephalomyelitis virus directly induces proinflammatory cytokines in primary astrocytes via NF-kappaB activation: potential role for the initiation of demyelinating disease. *J Virol.* 2003;77(11):6322–6331.

99. Soares MP, Seldon MP, Gregoire IP, et al. Heme oxygenase-1 modulates the expression of adhesion molecules associated with endothelial cell activation. *J Immunol.* 2004;172(6):3553–3563.

100. Simonian NA, Coyle JT. Oxidative stress in neurodegenerative diseases. *Annu Rev Pharmacol Toxicol.* 1996;36:83–106.

101. Ehara S, Ueda M, Naruko T, et al. Elevated levels of oxidized low density lipoprotein show a positive relationship with the severity of acute coronary syndromes. *Circulation.* 2001;103(15):1955–1960.

102. Kim JH, Brown SL, Jenrow KA, et al. Mechanisms of radiation-induced brain toxicity and implications for future clinical trials. *J Neurooncol.* 2008;87(3):279–286.

103. Dringen R, Gutterer JM, Hirrlinger J. Glutathione metabolism in brain metabolic interaction between astrocytes and neurons in the defense against reactive oxygen species. *Eur J Biochem.* 2000;267(16):4912–4916.

104. Smith KJ, Kapoor R, Felts PA. Demyelination: the role of reactive oxygen and nitrogen species. *Brain Pathol.* 1999;9(1):69–92.

105. Guan J, Stewart J, Ware JH, et al. Effects of dietary supplements on the space radiation-induced reduction in total antioxidant status in CBA mice. *Radiat Res.* 2006;165(4):373–378.

106. Belka C, Budach W, Kortmann RD, et al. Radiation induced CNS toxicity–molecular and cellular mechanisms. *Br J Cancer.* 2001;85(9):1233–1239.

107. Tsao MN, Li YQ, Lu G, et al. Upregulation of vascular endothelial growth factor is associated with radiation-induced blood-spinal cord barrier breakdown. *J Neuropathol Exp Neurol.* 1999;58(10):1051–1060.

108. Logan A, Berry M. Transforming growth factor-beta 1 and basic fibroblast growth factor in the injured CNS. *Trends Pharmacol Sci.* 1993;14(9):337–342.

109. Li YQ, Ballinger JR, Nordal RA, et al. Hypoxia in radiation-induced blood-spinal cord barrier breakdown. *Cancer Res.* 2001;61(8):3348–3354.

110. Schuller BW, Binns PJ, Riley KJ, et al. Selective irradiation of the vascular endothelium has no effect on the survival of murine intestinal crypt stem cells. *Proc Natl Acad Sci USA.* 2006;103(10):3787–3792.

111. Nordal RA, Nagy A, Pintilie M, et al. Hypoxia and hypoxia-inducible factor-1 target genes in central nervous system radiation injury: a role for vascular endothelial growth factor. *Clin Cancer Res.* 2004;10(10):3342–3353.

112. Gonzalez J, Kumar AJ, Conrad CA, et al. Effect of bevacizumab on radiation necrosis of the brain. *Int J Radiat Oncol Biol Phys.* 2007;67(2):323–326.

113. Torcuator R, Zuniga R, Mohan YS, et al. Initial experience with bevacizumab treatment for biopsy confirmed cerebral radiation necrosis. *J Neurooncol.* 2009;94(1):63–68.

114. Pena LA, Fuks Z, Kolesnick RN. Radiation-induced apoptosis of endothelial cells in the murine central nervous system: protection by fibroblast growth factor and sphingomyelinase deficiency. *Cancer Res.* 2000;60(2):321–327.

115. Li YQ, Chen P, Haimovitz-Friedman A, et al. Endothelial apoptosis initiates acute blood-brain barrier disruption after ionizing radiation. *Cancer Res.* 2003;63(18):5950–5956.

116. Atkinson S, Li YQ, Wong CS. Changes in oligodendrocytes and myelin gene expression after radiation in the rodent spinal cord. *Int J Radiat Oncol Biol Phys.* 2003;57(4):1093–1100.

117. Li YQ, Jay V, Wong CS. Oligodendrocytes in the adult rat spinal cord undergo radiation-induced apoptosis. *Cancer Res.* 1996;56(23):5417–5422.

118. Chari DM, Huang WL, Blakemore WF. Dysfunctional oligodendrocyte progenitor cell (OPC) populations may inhibit repopulation of OPC depleted tissue. *J Neurosci Res.* 2003;73(6):787–793.

119. Chow BM, Li YQ, Wong CS. Radiation-induced apoptosis in the adult central nervous system is p53-dependent. *Cell Death Differ.* 2000;7(8):712–720.

120. Tartaglino LM, Rao VM, Markiewicz DA. Imaging of radiation changes in the head and neck. *Semin Roentgenol.* 1994;29(1):81–91.

121. Brant-Zawadzki M, Anderson M, DeArmond SJ, et al. Radiation-induced large intracranial vessel occlusive vasculopathy. *Am J Roentgenol.* 1980;134(1):51–55.

122. Foreman NK, Laitt RD, Chambers EJ, et al. Intracranial large vessel vasculopathy and anaplastic meningioma 19 years after cranial irradiation for acute lymphoblastic leukaemia. *Med Pediatr Oncol.* 1995;24(4):265–268.

123. Beyer RA, Paden P, Sobel DF, et al. Moyamoya pattern of vascular occlusion after radiotherapy for glioma of the optic chiasm. *Neurology.* 1986;36(9):1173–1178.

124. Grenier Y, Tomita T, Marymont MH, et al. Late postirradiation occlusive vasculopathy in childhood medulloblastoma. Report of two cases. *J Neurosurg.* 1998;89(3):460–464.

125. Maher CO, Raffel C. Early vasculopathy following radiation in a child with medulloblastoma. *Pediatr Neurosurg.* 2000;32(5):255–258.

126. Brada M, Ashley S, Ford D, et al. Cerebrovascular mortality in patients with pituitary adenoma. *Clin Endocrinol (Oxf).* 2002;57(6):713–717.

127. Hasegawa S, Hamada J, Morioka M, et al. Radiation-induced cerebrovasculopathy of the distal middle cerebral artery and distal posterior cerebral artery—case report. *Neurol Med Chir (Tokyo).* 2000;40(4):220–223.

128. Katoh M, Kamiyama H, Abe H, et al. Complete occlusion of right middle cerebral artery by radiation therapy after removal of pituitary adenoma: case report. *No Shinkei Geka.* 1990;18(9):855–859.

129. Kyoi K, Kirino Y, Sakaki T, et al. Therapeutic irradiation of brain tumor and cerebrovasculopathy. *No Shinkei Geka.* 1989;17(2):163–170.

130. Maffei P, Albano I, Martini C, et al. Middle cerebral artery occlusion 25 years after cranial radiation therapy in acromegaly: a case report. *J Thromb Thrombolysis.* 2009;28(3):358–361.

131. Brada M, Burchell L, Ashley S, et al. The incidence of cerebrovascular accidents in patients with pituitary adenoma. *Int J Radiat Oncol Biol Phys.* 1999;45(3):693–698.

132. Servo A, Puranen M. Moyamoya syndrome as a complication of radiation therapy. Case report. *J Neurosurg.* 1978;48(6):1026–1029.

133. Rajakulasingam K, Cerullo LJ, Raimondi AJ. Childhood moyamoya syndrome. Postradiation pathogenesis. *Childs Brain.* 1979;5(5):467–475.

134. Ishiyama K, Tomura N, Kato K, et al. A patient with Moyamoya-like vessels after radiation therapy for a tumor in the basal ganglia. *No To Shinkei.* 2001;53(10):969–973.

135. Maruyama K, Mishima K, Saito N, et al. Radiation-induced aneurysm and moyamoya vessels presenting with subarachnoid haemorrhage. *Acta Neurochir (Wien).* 2000;142(2):139–143.

136. Kestle JR, Hoffman HJ, Mock AR. Moyamoya phenomenon after radiation for optic glioma. *J Neurosurg.* 1993;79(1):32–35.

137. Serdaroglu A, Simsek F, Gucuyener K, et al. Moyamoya syndrome after radiation therapy for optic pathway glioma: case report. *J Child Neurol.* 2000;15(11):765–767.

138. Poussaint TY, Siffert J, Barnes PD, et al. Hemorrhagic vasculopathy after treatment of central nervous system neoplasia in childhood: diagnosis and follow-up. *Am J Neuroradiol.* 1995;16(4):693–699.

139. Allen JC, Miller DC, Budzilovich GN, et al. Brain and spinal cord hemorrhage in long-term survivors of malignant pediatric brain tumors: a possible late effect of therapy. *Neurology.* 1991;41(1):148–150.

140. Chung E, Bodensteiner J, Hogg JP. Spontaneous intracerebral hemorrhage: a very late delayed effect of radiation therapy. *J Child Neurol.* 1992;7(3):259–263.

141. Tamura M, Ono N, Zama A, et al. Delayed brain hemorrhage associated with prophylactic whole brain irradiation for pediatric malignant brain tumor: a case report. *Childs Nerv Syst.* 1993;9(5):300–301.

142. Woo E, Chan YF, Lam K, et al. Apoplectic intracerebral hemorrhage: an unusual complication of cerebral radiation necrosis. *Pathology.* 1987;19(1):95–98.

143. Cheng KM, Chan CM, Fu YT, et al. Acute hemorrhage in late radiation necrosis of the temporal lobe: report of five cases and review of the literature. *J Neurooncol.* 2001;51(2):143–150.

144. Lee JK, Chelvarajah R, King A, et al. Rare presentations of delayed radiation injury: a lobar hematoma and a cystic space-occupying lesion appearing more than 15 years after cranial radiotherapy: report of two cases. *Neurosurgery.* 2004;54(4):1010–1013; discussion 1013–1014.

145. Azzarelli B, Moore J, Gilmor R, et al. Multiple fusiform intracranial aneurysms following curative radiation therapy for suprasellar germinoma. Case report. *J Neurosurg.* 1984;61(6):1141–1145.

146. Casey AT, Marsh HT, Uttley D. Intracranial aneurysm formation following radiotherapy. *Br J Neurosurg.* 1993;7(5):575–579.

147. Sciubba DM, Gallia GL, Recinos P, et al. Intracranial aneurysm following radiation therapy during childhood for a brain tumor. Case report and review of the literature. *J Neurosurg.* 2006;105(2 Suppl):134–139.

148. Benson PJ, Sung JH. Cerebral aneurysms following radiotherapy for medulloblastoma. *J Neurosurg.* 1989;70(4):545–550.

149. Jensen FK, Wagner A. Intracranial aneurysm following radiation therapy for medulloblastoma. A case report and review of the literature. *Acta Radiol.* 1997;38(1):37–42.

150. Gaensler EH, Dillon WP, Edwards MS, et al. Radiation-induced telangiectasia in the brain simulates cryptic vascular malformations at MR imaging. *Radiology.* 1994;193(3):629–636.

151. Rabin BM, Meyer JR, Berlin JW, et al. Radiation-induced changes in the central nervous system and head and neck. *Radiographics.* 1996;16(5):1055–1072.

152. Valk PE, Dillon WP. Radiation injury of the brain. *Am J Neuroradiol.* 1991;12(1):45–62.

153. Ball WS Jr, Prenger EC, Ballard ET. Neurotoxicity of radio/chemotherapy in children: pathologic and MR correlation. *Am J Neuroradiol.* 1992;13(2):761–776.

154. Rowley HA, Dillon WP. Iatrogenic white matter diseases. *Neuroimaging Clin N Am.* 1993; 3:379–404.

155. Young DF, Posner JB, Chu F, et al. Rapid-course radiation therapy of cerebral metastases: results and complications. *Cancer.* 1974;34(4):1069–1076.

156. Sheline GE, Wara WM, Smith V. Therapeutic irradiation and brain injury. *Int J Radiat Oncol Biol Phys.* 1980;6(9):1215–1228.

157. Brown WR, Thore CR, Moody DM, et al. Vascular damage after fractionated whole-brain irradiation in rats. *Radiat Res.* 2005;164(5):662–668.

158. Hudgins PA, Newman NJ, Dillon WP, et al. Radiation-induced optic neuropathy: characteristic appearances on gadolinium-enhanced MR. *Am J Neuroradiol.* 1992;13(1):235–238.

159. Fernandez A, Brada M, Zabuliene L, et al. Radiation-induced hypopituitarism. *Endocr Relat Cancer.* 2009;16(3):733–772.

160. Littley MD, Shalet SM, Beardwell CG, et al. Hypopituitarism following external radiotherapy for pituitary tumours in adults. *Q J Med.* 1989;70(262):145–160.

161. Bengtsson BA, Johannsson G. Effect of growth-hormone therapy on early atherosclerotic changes in GH-deficient adults. *Lancet.* 1999;353(9168):1898–1899.

162. Rosen T, Bengtsson BA. Premature mortality due to cardiovascular disease in hypopituitarism. *Lancet.* 1990;336(8710):285–288.

163. Bates AS, Van't Hoff W, Jones PJ, et al. The effect of hypopituitarism on life expectancy. *J Clin Endocrinol Metab.* 1996;81(3):1169–1172.

164. Bulow B, Hagmar L, Mikoczy Z, et al. Increased cerebrovascular mortality in patients with hypopituitarism. *Clin Endocrinol.* 1997;46(1):75–81.

165. Bates AS, Bullivant B, Sheppard MC, et al. Life expectancy following surgery for pituitary tumours. *Clin Endocrinol (Oxf).* 1999;50(3):315–319.

166. Tomlinson JW, Holden N, Hills, RK et al. Association between premature mortality and hypopituitarism. West Midlands Prospective Hypopituitary Study Group. *Lancet.* 2001;357(9254):425–431.

167. Oeffinger KC, Mertens AC, Sklar CA, et al. Chronic health conditions in adult survivors of childhood cancer. *N Engl J Med.* 2006;355(15):1572–1582.

168. Smith GL, Smith BD, Buchholz TA, et al. Cerebrovascular disease risk in older head and neck cancer patients after radiotherapy. *J Clin Oncol.* 2008;26(31):5119–5125.

169. Morris B, Partap S, Yeom K, et al. Cerebrovascular disease in childhood cancer survivors: A Children's Oncology Group Report. *Neurology.* 2009;73(22):1906–1913.

170. Shore RE, Albert RE, Pasternack BS. Follow-up study of patients treated by X-ray epilation for Tinea capitis; resurvey of post-treatment illness and mortality experience. *Arch Environ Health.* 1976;31(1):21–28.

171. Hull MC, Morris CG, Pepine CJ, et al. Valvular dysfunction and carotid, subclavian, and coronary artery disease in survivors of Hodgkin lymphoma treated with radiation therapy. *JAMA.* 2003;290(21):2831–2837.

172. Painter MJ, Chutorian AM, Hilal SK. Cerebrovasculopathy following irradiation in childhood. *Neurology.* 1975;25(2):189–194.

173. Keene DL, Johnston DL, Grimard L, et al. Vascular complications of cranial radiation. *Childs Nerv Syst.* 2006;22(6):547–555.

174. Ullrich NJ, Robertson R, Kinnamon DD, et al. Moyamoya following cranial irradiation for primary brain tumors in children. *Neurology.* 2007;68(12):932–938.

175. Kikuchi A, Maeda M, Hanada R, et al. Moyamoya syndrome following childhood acute lymphoblastic leukemia. *Pediatr Blood Cancer.* 2007;48(3):268–272.

176. Fung LW, Thompson D, Ganesan V. Revascularisation surgery for paediatric moyamoya: a review of the literature. *Childs Nerv Syst.* 2005;21(5):358–364.

177. Burn S, Gunny R, Phipps K, et al. Incidence of cavernoma development in children after radiotherapy for brain tumors. *J Neurosurg.* 2007;106(5 Suppl):379–383.

178. Heckl S, Aschoff A. Kunze S. Radiation-induced cavernous hemangiomas of the brain: a late effect predominantly in children. *Cancer.* 2002;94(12):3285–3291.

179. Koike S, Aida N, Hata M, et al. Asymptomatic radiation-induced telangiectasia in children after cranial irradiation: frequency, latency, and dose relation. *Radiology.* 2004; 230(1):93–99.

180. Shanley DJ. Mineralizing microangiopathy: CT and MRI. *Neuroradiology.* 1995;37(4): 331–333.

181. Price RA, Birdwell DA. The central nervous system in childhood leukemia. III. Mineralizing microangiopathy and dystrophic calcification. *Cancer.* 1978;42(2):717–728.

182. Omran AR, Shore RE, Markoff RA, et al. Follow-up study of patients treated by X-ray epilation for tinea capitis: psychiatric and psychometric evaluation. *Am J Public Health.* 1978; 68(6):561–567.

183. Ron E, Modan B, Floro S, et al. Mental function following scalp irradiation during childhood. *Am J Epidemiol.* 1982;116(1):149–160.

184. Yaar I, Ron E, Modan M, et al. Long-term cerebral effects of small doses of x-irradiation in childhood as manifested in adult visual evoked responses. *Ann Neurol.* 1980;8(3):261–268.

185. Armstrong GT, Liu Q, Yasui Y, et al. Long-term outcomes among adult survivors of childhood central nervous system malignancies in the Childhood Cancer Survivor Study. *J Natl Cancer Inst.* 2009;101(13):946–958.

186. Hall P, Adami HO, Trichopoulos D, et al. Effect of low doses of ionising radiation in infancy on cognitive function in adulthood:Swedish population based cohort study. *BMJ.* 2004;328(7430):19.

187. Heckl S, Kodama K, Nishi N, et al. Radiation exposure and circulatory disease risk: Hiroshima and Nagasaki atomic bomb survivor data, 1950–2003. *BMJ.* 2010;340:b5349.

188. Preston DL, Shimizu Y, Pierce DA, et al. Studies of mortality of atomic bomb survivors. Report 13:Solid cancer and noncancer disease mortality:1950–1997. *Radiat Res.* 2003;160(4):381–407.

189. Shimizu Y, Kato H, Schull WJ, et al. Studies of the mortality of A-bomb survivors. 9. Mortality, 1950–1985: Part 3. Noncancer mortality based on the revised doses (DS86). *Radiat Res.* 1992;130(2):249–266.

190. Shimizu Y, Pierce DA, Preston DL, et al. Studies of the mortality of atomic bomb survivors. Report 12, part II. Noncancer mortality:1950–1990. *Radiat Res.* 1999;152(4):374–389.

191. Ivanov VK, Maksioutov MA, Chekin SY, et al. The risk of radiation-induced cerebrovascular disease in Chernobyl emergency workers. *Health Phys.* 2006;90(3):199–207.

192. Ivanov VK. Late cancer and noncancer risks among Chernobyl emergency workers of Russia. *Health Phys.* 2007;93(5):470–479.

193. Howe GR, Zablotska LB, Fix JJ, et al. Analysis of the mortality experience amongst U.S. nuclear power industry workers after chronic low-dose exposure to ionizing radiation. *Radiat Res.* 2004;162(5):517–526.

194. McGeoghegan D, Binks K, Gillies M, et al. The non-cancer mortality experience of male workers at British Nuclear Fuels plc, 1946–2005. *Int J Epidemiol.* 2008;37(3):506–518.

Michael D. Chan
Mike E. Robbins, Carsten Nieder
Edward G. Shaw

Treatment of Radiation Injury in the Central Nervous System

INTRODUCTION

Neoplasms of the central nervous system (CNS) are a pathologically diverse group of benign and malignant tumors for which a variety of management strategies, including observation, surgery, radiation therapy, and/or chemotherapy are employed. Shown in Table 26.1 are the usual radiation doses used to treat primary and metastatic brain and spinal cord tumors, which span a broad range of total doses and doses per fraction. Regardless of the type of CNS tumor treated, what usually limits the dose of radiation that can be utilized and therefore what typically determines the local control and cure rate of that tumor are the tolerance doses of the adjacent or underlying normal tissues in and around the CNS. This chapter (i) outlines the biologic and clinical principles of CNS radiation tolerance, (ii) reviews the growing body of preclinical data indicating that radiation-induced late effects in the CNS can be ameliorated or prevented, and (iii) outlines the clinical management of radiation-induced CNS injury. Although the vast majority of studies investigating radiation-induced CNS morbidity utilize therapeutic doses of radiation, the effects of nontherapeutic radiation exposure resulting from accidents or from intentional detonation of nuclear devices have received renewed interest with the events of September 11, 2001, and the increased risk of radiological terrorist events, and thus these will also be reviewed, albeit briefly.

RADIATION-INDUCED CNS INJURY

Nontherapeutic radiation: Exposure to high doses of radiation (>20 Gy) resulting from nuclear accidents or detonation of nuclear weapons leads to the cerebrovascular syndrome.[5] Only a few instances of accidental human exposure have involved doses great enough to produce this effect. Individuals receiving supralethal doses present with fever, hypotension, and major impairment of cognitive function. The ensuing complications of hypotension, cerebral edema, increased intracranial pressure and cerebral anoxia result in death within 2 days.

Studies of prenatally exposed atomic-bomb survivors in Japan have shown that radiation exposure during gestation has harmful effects on the developing human brain.[6] Severe mental retardation and microcephaly is observed in individuals exposed at 8 to 15 weeks gestational age, with a threshold dose of approximately 0.15 to 0.25 Gy. Exposure at 16 to 25 weeks gestational age is associated with mental retardation alone; the threshold dose is in the range of 0.25 to 0.28 Gy.[7] The biological mechanisms involved in these abnormalities remain unclear. Magnetic resonance imaging (MRI) of brains from a cohort of mentally retarded survivors revealed a region of abnormally situated gray matter, suggesting a defect in neuronal migration. The radiation-induced microcephaly appears related to generalized growth retardation.[7] Neuropsychological assessment of adult A-bomb survivors suggests that exposure to atomic-bomb radiation had no apparent effect on cognitive function.[8]

Therapeutic radiation: Based on the time of clinical expression, radiation-induced brain injury is described in terms of acute, early delayed, and late delayed reactions.[9] Acute injury (acute radiation encephalopathy), expressed in days to weeks after irradiation, is rare under current radiation therapy regimens. Early delayed injury occurs from 1 to 6 months postirradiation and can involve transient demyelination with somnolence after brain irradiation or Lhermitte syndrome after spinal cord irradiation. While both these early injuries can result in severe reactions, they are normally reversible and resolve spontaneously. In contrast, late delayed effects, characterized histopathologically by demyelination, vascular abnormalities, and ultimate white matter necrosis,[10] are observed >6 months postirradiation and have been viewed as irreversible and progressive. In addition to these histopathologic endpoints, there is a growing awareness of intellectual deterioration in patients receiving brain irradiation.[11] Cognitive impairment, including dementia, induced by partial or whole-brain irradiation (WBI) is reported to occur in up to 50% of adult brain tumor patients who are long-term survivors (>6 months postirradiation).[11-14] The resultant impact on quality of life (QOL) has become an extremely important concern for long-term survivors, and QOL is now recognized as one of the most important measurements of cancer therapy outcomes, second only to survival in clinical trials.[15]

PATHOGENESIS OF RADIATION-INDUCED CNS INJURY

Vascular abnormalities and demyelination are the predominant histological changes seen in radiation-induced CNS injury.

TABLE 26.1	Radiation Treatment Recommendations for Primary CNS Tumors		
Pathologic Type	*Gross Tumor Volume (GTV)*	*Clinical Tumor Volume*	*Total Dose (Gy per No. of Fractions)*
Glioblastoma (WHO IV), anaplastic astrocytoma (WHO III)[a]			60/30 or 64.8/36
Initial field	Edema and enhancing tumor	GTV + 2–3 cm margin	46/23 or 50.4/28
Boost field	Enhancing tumor	GTV + 2–2.5 cm margin	14/7 or 14.4/8
Astrocytoma (WHO II)[b,c]	Edema (and enhancing tumor if present)	GTV + 1–2 cm margin[c]	50.4/28 to 59.4/33
Pilocytic astrocytoma (WHO I)	Enhancing tumor	GTV + 1–2 cm margin[c]	50.4/28 to 55.8/31
Meningioma[d]	Enhancing tumor	GTV + 1–2 cm margin[c]	50.4/28 to 59.4/33
Medulloblastoma and anaplastic ependymoma			55.2/34 to 55.8/35
Initial volume	Entire brain and spine	GTV + 1–2 cm margin[e]	30.6/17 to 36/24
Boost volume	Enhancing tumor	GTV + 1–2 cm margin	19.8/11 to 25.2/14
Ependymoma	Enhancing tumor	GTV + 1–2 cm margin[c]	50.4/28 to 59.4/33

[a]For anaplastic astrocytomas that are nonenhancing, plan similar to a low-grade diffuse astrocytoma.

[b]Most astrocytomas (WHO I) are nonenhancing. The tumor (i.e., edema) is best seen on the T2-weighted MRI. If there is enhancing tumor, plan similar to a glioblastoma multiforme.

[c]Reduce to a 1-cm margin after 50.4 Gy if total dose exceeds 50.4 Gy.

[d]Malignant meningiomas should be planned similar to glioblastoma multiforme. For meningeal hemangiopericytoma, the CTV should include the GTV + 2 to 3 cm margin.

[e]Margin at skull base should be about 1 cm, including cribriform plate. Margin on spinal canal should be 1.5 to 2 cm except inferior border of lower spine field, which should be at bottom of S3.

Source: Data from Levin VA, Leibel SA, Gutin PH. Neoplasms of the central nervous system. In: DeVita VT, Hellman S, Rosenberg SA, eds. *Cancer—Principles and Practice of Oncology*. Philadelphia, PA: Lippincott Williams and Wilkins; 2001; Scally LT, Lin C, Beriwal S, et al. Brain, brain stem, and cerebellum. In: Perez CA, Brady LW, Halperin EC, Schmidt-Ulrich RKA, eds. *Principles and Practice of Radiation Oncology*. Philadelphia, PA: Lippincott Williams and Wilkins; 2004; Kun LE. The brain and spinal cord. In: Cox JD, ed. *Moss' Radiation Oncology—Rationale, Technique, Results*. St. Louis, MO: Mosby, Year Book, Inc.; 1994; and Halperin EC, Constine LS, Tarbell NJ, et al., eds. *Pediatric Radiation Oncology*. 2nd ed. New York, NY: Raven Press; 1994.

Classically, late delayed injury was viewed as due solely to a reduction in the number of surviving clonogens of either parenchymal, that is, oligodendrocyte[16] or vascular, that is endothelial[17] target cell populations leading to white matter necrosis.

Vascular hypothesis: Proponents of the vascular hypothesis argued that vascular damage led to ischemia with secondary white matter necrosis. In support of this hypothesis is the large amount of data describing radiation-induced vascular changes including vessel wall thickening, vessel dilation, and endothelial cell nuclear enlargement.[10,17,18] Quantitative studies in the irradiated rat brain noted time- and dose-related reductions in the number of endothelial cell nuclei and blood vessels prior to the development of necrosis.[18] Further, recent boron neutron capture studies in which radiation was delivered essentially to the vasculature alone, still led to the development of white matter necrosis.[19] In contrast, radiation-induced necrosis has been reported in the absence of vascular changes.[10] Moreover, while the vascular hypothesis argues that ischemia is responsible for white matter necrosis, the most sensitive component of the CNS to oxygen deprivation, the neuron, is located in the gray matter, a relatively radioresistant region. Thus, radiation injury to the CNS is not due solely to damage to the vasculature alone.

Parenchymal hypothesis: The parenchymal hypothesis for radiation-induced CNS injury focused on the oligodendrocyte, required for the formation of myelin sheaths. The key cell for the generation of mature oligodendrocytes is the oligodendrocyte type 2 astrocyte (O-2A) progenitor cell.[20] Irradiation results in the loss of reproductive capacity of the O-2A progenitor cells in the rat CNS.[21,22] It was hypothesized that radiation induced loss of O2-A progenitor cells, leading to a failure to replace oligodendrocytes and subsequent demyelination. However, a mechanistic link between loss of oligodendrocytes and demyelination has not been established. Further, while the kinetics of oligodendrocytes is consistent with the early transient demyelination seen in the early delayed reactions, it is inconsistent with the late onset of white matter necrosis.[23] Thus, it is unlikely that loss of O2-A progenitor cells and oligodendrocytes alone can lead to late radiation injury.

Current model of dynamic interactions between multiple cell types: The classic model of late delayed injury to the CNS was associated with the concept that radiation-induced late normal tissue injury was inevitable, progressive, and untreatable. In the last decade or so, a growing body of data suggests that this hypothesis is no longer tenable. Radiation-induced late effects are now viewed in terms of dynamic interactions between multiple cell types that can be modulated[24,25] within a particular organ.[26–29] In the brain, these include not only the oligodendrocytes and endothelial cells but also the astrocytes, microglia, and neurons.[9] These now are viewed not as passive bystanders, merely dying as they attempt to divide, but rather as active participants in an orchestrated response to injury. We will briefly review the radiation response of each of these cell types below.

Astrocytes constitute approximately 50% of the total glial cell population in the brain and outnumber the neurons nine to one in the mammalian CNS.[30] Once viewed as playing a mere supportive role in the CNS, astrocytes have now been recognized as a heterogeneous class of cells that perform diverse functions in the CNS including modulation of synaptic transmission and secretion of neurotrophic factors such as basic fibroblast growth factor to promote neurogenesis.[31,32] Astrocytes have been shown to protect endothelial cells and neurons from oxidative injury.[33] Also, juxtacrine signaling between astrocytes and endothelial cells is critical for generation and maintenance of a functional blood-brain barrier (BBB), a structure that restricts the entry of blood-borne elements into the CNS.[34] In response to injury, astrocytes undergo proliferation, exhibit heterotrophic nuclei and cell bodies, and show increased expression of glial fibrillary acidic protein, GFAP.[31,35] These reactive astrocytes secrete a host of proinflammatory mediators such as cyclooxygenase (Cox)-2 and intercellular adhesion molecule (ICAM)-1, which may aid in the infiltration of leukocytes into the brain via BBB breakdown.[36] Irradiating the rat and mouse brain increases the GFAP protein levels both acutely (24 hours) and chronically (4–5 months).[37,38] In vitro, conditioned media from irradiated microglial cells has been shown to induce astrogliosis, which might contribute to radiation-induced edema.[39] However, the exact role of astrocytes in the pathogenesis of radiation-induced brain injury is still unknown.

Microglia are the immune cells of the brain, representing about 12% of the total cells in the CNS.[40] In the adult brain, the microglia exist as cells with an elongated soma-bearing processes extending from both poles of the cell, the ramified or resting microglia.[41] Ramified microglia are not passive but rather actively survey and maintain a homeostatic environment in the CNS. Their density is highest in the hippocampus, olfactory telencephalon, basal ganglia, and substantia nigra.[42] They express neurotropins that selectively regulate microglial function and proliferation and secrete neurotrophic factors such as neuronal growth factor that promote neuronal survival.[43] However, following brain injury, the microglial cells become activated, a change characterized by retraction of cell processes, rounding of cell body, proliferation, upregulation of surface molecules, cytokines, reactive oxygen species, and chemokines.[41,44] Microglial activation plays an important role in phagocytosis of dead cells in the CNS, but protracted activation leads to a sustained inflammatory status, and has been implicated in acute and chronic neurodegenerative diseases, as well as radiation-induced brain injury.[45,46] Indeed, irradiation of the CNS has been shown to result in increased numbers of microglia in areas of tissue injury, and can occur during the latent period before the clinical expression of injury.[47,48]

In vitro studies suggest that irradiating microglia leads to a marked increase in expression of proinflammatory genes including tumor necrosis factor-α (TNF-α), interleukin 1 beta (IL-1β), IL-6, and Cox-2.[39,49] Radiation-induced expression of microglial TNF-α and IL-1β has been shown to enhance ICAM-1 expression in nonirradiated astrocytes.[49] More importantly, animal studies and human tissue sample analysis suggest that the detrimental effect of brain irradiation on hippocampal neurogenesis and cognitive function is associated with a significant increase in microglial activation.[50–52] Further, administration of the anti-inflammatory drug indomethacin decreased radiation-induced microglial activation and partially restored neurogenesis.[53] Together, these data suggest that altered neurogenesis as a result of oxidative stress and/or neuroinflammation is one of the primary mechanisms of radiation-induced brain injury.

Neurons, once considered to be a radioresistant population due to their postmitotic nature, have recently been demonstrated to be sensitive to radiation. In vivo and in vitro experimental studies have shown radiation-induced changes in hippocampal cellular activity, synaptic efficiency, and spike generation,[54] and in neuronal gene expression.[55] More recently, it has been demonstrated that WBI-induced cognitive impairment is associated with alterations in the *N*-methyl-D-aspartic acid (NMDA) receptor subunits important for synaptic transmission and/or plasticity.[56] Interestingly, these changes appeared in the absence of any alteration in the total number of neurons following WBI.[57] Therefore, radiation appears to impair neuronal function by subtle cellular and molecular changes that do not lead to overt neurodegeneration. An additional and important component of radiation injury is the relatively recent observation that irradiation can inhibit hippocampal neurogenesis.

Radiation-induced changes in neurogenesis and cognitive function: The hippocampus is central to short-term declarative memory and spatial information processing. It consists of the dentate gyrus (DG), CA3, and CA1 regions. Resident in the hippocampus are neural stem cells, self-renewing cells capable of generating neurons, astrocytes, and oligodendrocytes.[58,59] Neurogenesis depends on the presence of a specific neurogenic microenvironment; both endothelial cells and astrocytes can promote/regulate neurogenesis.[32,60] Experimental studies have indicated that brain irradiation results in increased apoptosis,[61] decreased cell proliferation, and a decreased stem/precursor cell differentiation into neurons within the neurogenic region of the hippocampus.[50,62,63] Rats irradiated with a single dose of 10 Gy produce only 3% of the new hippocampal neurons formed in control animals.[50] Of note, these changes were observed after doses of radiation that failed to produce demyelination and/or white matter necrosis of the rat brain. Further evidence demonstrating the importance of the microenvironment for successful neurogenesis comes from studies showing that nonirradiated stem cells transplanted into the irradiated hippocampus failed to generate neurons; this may reflect a pronounced microglial inflammatory response, since neuroinflammation is a strong inhibitor of neurogenesis.[53] In contrast to the reduction in neurogenesis, gliogenesis appears to be preserved following irradiation.

Several experimental findings suggest that the detrimental effect of WBI on adult hippocampal neurogenesis is a key contributing factor to radiation-induced cognitive impairment. In vitro, irradiation leads to a loss of proliferative capacity of the neuronal precursor cells.[50] In vivo, WBI of the mouse and rat brain leads to a significant decrease in the number of newborn mature and immature neurons in the DG.[50,51,64]

This radiation-induced decrease in hippocampal neurogenesis is associated with hippocampal-dependent spatial learning and memory impairments in adult mice 3 months after a single dose of 10 Gy to the bilateral hippocampus and cortex.[52] Radiation-induced impairment in hippocampal-dependent cognitive function has also been observed after fractionated WBI of the rat brain. Lamproglou et al.[65] demonstrated a progressive deterioration of memory function over a 7-month period following fractionated WBI in aged rats using avoidance and water maze tasks. A similar late onset of cognitive impairment has been observed in adult rats that were 4 to 12 months old at the start of the fractionated WBI.[56,66,67] This radiation-induced cognitive impairment is observed in the absence of gross histological alterations, suggesting that cognitive impairment precedes detectable radiation-induced morphological changes in the brain or that cognitive impairment can arise without them.[68] Using a recently characterized rat model,[66] Robbins et al. have used the non–hippocampal-dependent novel object recognition task to assess recognition memory; this is significantly impaired by 6 months postirradiation and gets worse over the next 6 months.[68] Thus, fractionated WBI leads to a significant and progressive reduction in both hippocampal- and non–hippocampal-dependent cognitive function, suggesting that multiple regions of the brain play a role in radiation-induced cognitive impairment. Although there is no clearly identified pathogenic mechanism to account for these findings, experimental evidence supports the idea that the radiation-induced decrease in hippocampal neurogenesis is associated with an altered brain microenvironment characterized by oxidative stress and neuroinflammation.

Radiation-induced oxidative stress and inflammation: A growing body of evidence supports the hypothesis that radiation-induced late normal tissue injury, including that seen in the brain, is driven in part by acute and chronic oxidative stress and inflammatory responses.[69,70] An acute molecular response characterized by increased expression of proinflammatory molecules such as TNF-α, IL-1β, ICAM-1, and Cox-2 as well as activation of proinflammatory transcription factors such as nuclear factor κB has been observed within hours of irradiating the rodent brain.[36,49,71,72] In addition, a chronic elevation of TNF-α has been observed in the mouse brain up to 6 months postirradiation.[37] The radiation-induced inhibition of hippocampal neurogenesis discussed is associated with neuroinflammation, evidenced as a marked increase in the number of activated microglia present in the neurogenic zone[50]; inhibiting microglial activation using indomethacin partially restores neurogenesis.[53]

Direct experimental evidence for radiation-induced oxidative/nitrosative stress has been obtained from studies using neonatal and adult rats and mice. Irradiating one hemisphere of postnatal day 8 rats or of postnatal day 10 mice with a single dose of 4 to 12 Gy of 4 MV x-rays led to time-dependent increases in nitrotyrosine in the subventricular zone and the granular cell layer of the DG 2 to 12 h postirradiation.[73] An oxidative stress, evidenced as a significant increase in lipid peroxidation was noted in the adult male mouse hippocampus 2 weeks after brain irradiation with a single dose of 10 Gy.[74] More recently, Rola et al.[75] reported a chronic inflammatory response in the mouse subgranular zone 9 months following high-linear energy transfer (LET) brain irradiation; expression of the CCR2 receptor, important in neuroinflammation,[76,77] increased in the irradiated brains as compared to the sham-irradiated control brains. Persistent microglial activation in the rat brain has also been observed after fractionated WBI.[78] These findings provide the rationale

for applying proven anti-inflammatory-based interventions to prevent or ameliorate the severity of late radiation-induced brain injury as discussed below.

LABORATORY STUDIES OF THERAPEUTIC INTERVENTIONS FOR RADIATION-INDUCED SPINAL CORD INJURY

As noted earlier, radiation-induced CNS injury has been well characterized in terms of histological criteria. In contrast, details of the molecular, cellular, and biochemical processes responsible for the expression and progression of radiation-induced CNS injury have only recently started to be elucidated. Thus, initial interventional procedures directed at reducing the severity of late radiation injury utilized several pragmatic but unspecific approaches (Table 26.2).

Intrathecal administration of the classic radioprotector WR-2721 (amifostine) before spinal cord irradiation resulted in a dose-modifying factor of 1.3 and a prolongation of median latency to myelopathy by 63% at the ED_{50}.[79] Fike et al.[80] observed that the polyamine synthesis inhibitor α-difluoromethylornithine reduced the volume of radionecrosis and contrast enhancement in the irradiated dog brain; a delayed increase in microglia was also noted.[81] Hornsey et al.[82] hypothesized that treating rats with the iron-chelating agent desferrioxamine would reduce hydroxyl-mediated reperfusion-related injury in the irradiated spinal cord. Rats were fed a low-iron diet from 85 days after local spinal cord irradiation and received desferrioxamine (30 mg in 0.3 mL, sc, three times per week) from day 120, the time at which changes in vascular permeability were noted. The onset of ataxia due to white matter necrosis was delayed and the incidence of lesions was reduced after single doses of 25 and 27 Gy. Dexamethasone also delayed the development of radiation-induced ataxia along with a reduction in regional capillary permeability. In contrast, indomethacin did not appear to affect any of these endpoints. In the pig, administration of the polyunsaturated fatty acids γ-linolenic acid (GLA; 18C:3n-6) and eicosapentaenoic acid (EPA; 20C:5n-3), starting the day after spinal cord irradiation, was associated with a reduced incidence of paralysis, from 80% down to 20%.[83] Prophylactic hyperbaric oxygen (HBO) has also been tested for its ability to prevent radiation-induced myelopathy in a rat model. Using a dose of 65 Gy in ten fractions with or without 30 HBO treatments following the irradiation, Sminia et al.[84] did not demonstrate any

TABLE 26.2	Possible Preventive and Therapeutic Interventions for Radiation-Induced Brain Injury
Intervention	*Reference*
Amifostine (WR2721)	Spence et al[79]
α-difluoromethylornithine	Fike et al[80]; Nakagawa et al[81]
Desferrioxamine	Hornsey et al[82]
Polyunsaturated Fatty Acids	Hopewell et al[83]
Hyperbaric Oxygen	Sminia et al[84]
ACE Inhibitors and AT₁RA	Kim et al[106]; Robbins et al[105]
Indomethacin	Monje et al[53]
PDGF, IGF-1, VEGF, bFGF	Andratschke et al[87]
Pioglitazone	Zhao et al[95]

ACE Angiotensin Converting Enzyme, *AT1RA* Angiotensin Type 1 Receptor Antagonist, *bFGF* Basic Fibroblast Growth Factor, *IGF-1* Insulin-like Growth Factor-1, *PDGF* Platelet Derived Growth Factor, *VEGF* Vascular Endothelial Growth Factor.

preventive value to HBO. In fact, there was a "tendency toward radiosensitization" in the HBO-treated rats.

Treatment with insulin-like growth factor-1 for a few days concomitantly with irradiation significantly increased the latent time to development of spinal cord necrosis.[85] When combined with intrathecal basic fibroblast growth factor or amifostine, improved efficacy was noted.[86] Dose-effect curves suggested a modest 7% increase in the long-term radiation tolerance following single dose irradiation. Additional studies in the spinal cord indicate that platelet-derived growth factor can increase long-term radiation tolerance by approximately 5%.[87]

Studies in the adult rat have implicated a role for vascular endothelial growth factor (VEGF) in radiation-induced spinal cord injury. A marked, dose-dependent increase in the number of VEGF-expressing cells was noted 16 weeks after single doses of 17 to 25 Gy; this increase preceded the onset of radiation-induced paralysis and white matter necrosis.[88] Subsequent studies provided evidence for a dose-dependent temporal and spatial association of hypoxia, increased VEGF expression, and radiation-induced dysfunction of the blood spinal cord barrier.[89] Transgenic mice with reduced VEGF expression exhibited protection and had a longer median time to development of ataxia and paralysis following spinal cord irradiation as compared with wild-type mice and transgenic mice overexpressing VEGF.[90] These data suggest a causal role for VEGF in the development of radiation myelopathy and provide clear targets for intervention. Indeed, as discussed below, these observations have been translated to clinical trials using Bevacizumab, a monoclonal antibody to VEGF.

LABORATORY STUDIES OF THERAPEUTIC INTERVENTIONS FOR RADIATION-INDUCED BRAIN INJURY

The growing body of evidence linking radiation-induced brain injury with oxidative stress and/or inflammation described above has provided the rationale for applying proven anti-inflammatory-based interventions to prevent or ameliorate the severity of radiation-induced cognitive impairment. Recent studies have tested drugs that can either attenuate inflammation or reduce chronic oxidative stress, namely peroxisome proliferator-activated receptor (PPAR) agonists and renin angiotensin system (RAS) blockers.

PPARs (α, δ, and γ) are members of the nuclear hormone receptor superfamily of ligand-activated transcription factors that heterodimerize with the retinoid X receptor to regulate gene expression.[91] PPARs display distinct physiological and pharmacological functions depending on their target genes and tissue distribution.[92] A growing body of evidence suggests that PPARs regulate inflammatory signaling and are neuroprotective in a variety of CNS diseases.[93,94] Given the putative role of oxidative stress/inflammation in radiation-induced brain injury,[70] Zhao et al. tested the hypothesis that administration of the PPARγ agonist, pioglitazone (Pio), would mitigate the severity of radiation-induced cognitive impairment. Indeed, administering Pio to young adult male rats starting prior to, during, and for 4 or 54 weeks after the completion of fractionated WBI, prevented the radiation-induced cognitive impairment measured 52 weeks postirradiation.[95] However, administration of Pio for 54 weeks starting after the completion of fractionated WBI did not significantly modulate the radiation-induced cognitive impairment.

One of the most effective approaches to modulate radiation-induced late effects has been blockade of the RAS.[96] Angiotensin-converting enzyme inhibitors (ACEI) or angiotensin type 1 receptor antagonists (AT$_1$RA) have proved highly effective in the treatment and prevention of experimental radiation nephropathy[97] and pneumopathy.[98] The RAS has been classically viewed as a complex systemic hormonal system. More recently, a number of intraorgan RASs have been identified, including a brain RAS,[99] involved in brain-specific functions, including modulation of the BBB, stress, memory, and cognition.[100,101] Beneficial effects of RAS blockade have been observed both experimentally[102] and clinically,[103] suggesting an important role for the brain RAS in normal cognitive function and potentially in the treatment of dysfunctional memory disease states.[104] Based on these observations, Robbins et al. hypothesized that blocking the brain RAS with the AT$_1$RA, L-158,809, would prevent or ameliorate radiation-induced cognitive impairment. As hypothesized, administering L-158,809 before, during, and for 28 or 54 weeks after fractionated WBI prevented or ameliorated the radiation-induced cognitive impairment observed 26 and 52 weeks postirradiation. Moreover, giving L-158,809 before, during, and for only 5 weeks postirradiation ameliorated the significant cognitive impairment seen 26 weeks postirradiation.[105]

Modulation of the RAS has been shown previously to mitigate the severity of radiation-induced CNS injury.[106,107] Chronic administration of the ACEI ramipril, initiated 2 weeks after stereotactic irradiation of the rat brain with a single dose of 30 Gy, was associated with a reduction in the severity of functional and histopathologic markers of optic neuropathy assessed 6 months postirradiation.[106] However, delaying the start of ramipril treatment to 4 weeks after irradiation resulted in a failure to reduce the severity of the radiation injury.[107]

Thus, data from the Pio and L-158,809 studies indicate, at least in the young adult male rat, that prevention or amelioration of radiation-induced cognitive impairment appears to require administration of the drug before, during, and perhaps for only 4 to 5 weeks after WBI. Concomitant administration of these drugs with fractionated WBI raises concerns as to the potential for protecting the tumor against radiation-induced injury. A review of the literature suggests that such concerns are unwarranted. PPARγ agonists have antineoplastic properties in humans, animal models, and a variety of tumor cell lines, including gliomas.[108,109] Similarly, AT$_1$RAs exhibit antitumor effects[110] suggesting that their use in combination with ionizing radiation would likely lead to an increased, rather than a decreased, therapeutic window. Moreover, since both Pio and AT$_1$RAs are routinely prescribed for the treatment of type 2 diabetes[111] and hypertension,[112] respectively, and are well-tolerated, they offer the promise of improving the QOL of brain tumor patients who receive partial or WBI.

CLINICAL ASPECTS OF CNS RADIATION TOLERANCE

The radiation tolerance of the CNS is dependent on a number of factors, including total dose, dose per fraction, total time, volume, host factors, radiation quality (LET), adjunctive therapies, and the clinical endpoint being evaluated. The classic clinical endpoint evaluated in the CNS is radionecrosis. Table 26.3 defines the role of factors in radiation tolerance and

TABLE 26.3	Factors Associated with Radiation Tolerance of the Normal CNS Tissues	
Factor[a]	*Factors for Increased Risk of Injury*	*Tolerance Increased By*
Total dose	Higher total dose	Decreasing total dose, hyperfractionation[b], radiosensitizers
Dose per fraction	Dose per fraction >180–200 cGy	Decreasing dose per fraction to ≤180–200 cGy
Volume	Increased volume, e.g., whole-organ radiation	Decreasing volume, e.g., partial-organ radiation
Host factors	Medical illness, e.g., hypertension, diabetes	Unknown, possibly radioprotectors
Beam quality	High LET radiation beams, e.g., neutrons	Low LET beams, e.g., photons
Adjunctive therapy	Concomitant use of CNS toxic drugs, e.g., methotrexate	Avoid concomitant use of CNS toxic drugs, or use sequentially

[a]Total time is not a major determinant of normal CNS tissue tolerance.
[b]Defined as multiple daily fractions, usually two with doses per fraction of ≤180 to 200 cGy, usually 100 to 120 cGy, separated by 4 to 8 hours, to total doses higher than those given with "standard" fractionation.
Source: Data from Leibel and Sheline,[113] and Schultheiss et al.[114]

injury to the brain to the endpoint of radionecrosis.[113–115] The paradigm of using radionecrosis as the clinical endpoint of radiation-induced brain toxicity comes from the fact that radiation therapy has classically been used to treat patients with poor prognosis and compromised neurocognitive status. As such, an endpoint such as radionecrosis to define the threshold dose of radiation tolerance and toxicity was appropriate because it was an endpoint with sufficient severity to cause either death, surgical intervention, or a significant decline in QOL.

There is emerging evidence that radiation-induced cognitive decline is a phenomenon that can be seen even in the patient population with malignant brain tumors and brain metastases that have a limited prognosis. Moreover, there is a population of patients with low-grade glioma, meningioma, and pituitary tumors with a more protracted life expectancy that have indications for brain radiotherapy. While the radiation doses for such low-grade or benign brain tumors are often below the threshold necessary to induce radionecrosis, they are clearly sufficient to cause late toxicities such as short-term memory loss and impairment in learning of new skills. These late sequelae are also seen in the absence of radiographic or clinical radiation necrosis.

While satisfactory statistical models are unavailable to predict the likelihood of radiation-induced cognitive decline, a mathematical model has been described by Sheline et al.[115] to predict the likelihood of radiation-induced brain necrosis:

$$\text{Neuret} = (D)\ (N^{-0.41})\ (T^{-0.03})$$

where D is the total dose, N the number of fractions, and T the time.

The linear quadratic model links the response of fractionated irradiation to the fractional reproductive survival of clonogenic target cells. Fractionated data can be analyzed using the formula:

$$E = n(\alpha d + \beta d^2)$$

where the effect (E) is a linear and quadratic function of the dose per fraction (d) and a function of the fraction number (n). This equation allows determination of the α/β ratio, a measure of the "bendiness" of the underlying putative target cell survival curve. For brain and spinal cord, an average α/β ratio of 2 Gy appears appropriate.[116]

Table 26.4 shows partial- and whole-organ tolerance doses for the brain and spinal cord, and includes doses predicted to result in a 5% and 50% probability of injury 5 years following treatment with radiation (TD 5/5 and TD 50/5, respectively).[117,118] Based on various models, the TD 5/5 for the whole brain and for part of the brain is 50 ± 10 Gy and 60 ± 10 Gy, respectively. For a 10-cm segment of spinal cord the TD 5/5 is 45 to 50 Gy (Table 26.4). Although the TD 50/5 value for spinal cord is lower than that of brain, there are not good data to support this difference. Rather, the sequelae of spinal cord radiation injury are perceived as greater than those of brain injury; therefore, tolerance doses have been arbitrarily lowered. In clinical practice, TD 5/5 and 1/5 values of 60 to 65 and 50 to 55 Gy for partial brain irradiation and TD 5/5 and 1/5 values of 55 to 60 and 45 to 50 Gy for a limited segment of spinal cord are commonly used. Clinical data have borne out these somewhat empiric dose ranges. In a study of 203 adults with supratentorial low-grade glioma, patients were randomized to partial brain treatment fields with either 50.4 Gy in 28 fractions of 1.8 Gy each or 64.8 Gy in 36 fractions of 1.8 Gy.[119] Radiation necrosis developed in 1% of patients who received 50.4 Gy and 5% of those who had 64.8 Gy.

The evidence for radiation-induced cognitive decline continues to evolve. The reports in the literature are somewhat controversial as the populations used to describe this clinical phenomenon are often pretreated with chemotherapy, or have parenchymal brain tumors and cognitive deficits prior to radiotherapy. It is thought that the factors that predispose to radiation necrosis are the same factors that will predispose to other radiation-induced brain injury: fraction size, total dose, preexisting vascular disease, and the use of concurrent chemotherapy. The target structures of radiation-induced cognitive decline, as well as the dose thresholds have yet to be fully elucidated. The hippocampus and neural stem cell niche in the periventricular regions are attractive target structures of radiation damage. However, like stem cells found in other organ systems, they are thought to be exquisitely sensitive to ionizing radiation with estimated toxicity thresholds in the range of 2 to 6 Gy.[120,121] An analysis of functional outcomes of patients with low-grade glioma supports this hypothesis as patients receiving fraction sizes of 2 Gy or greater have been found to have worsened neurocognitive outcomes.[122] Ultimately, because of the multifactorial nature of radiation-induced cognitive dysfunction, it is likely that normal tissue complication probability (NTCP) models will be necessary to help predict for neurocognitive decline and help to dictate treatment planning techniques for brain radiotherapy.

TABLE 26.4	Tolerance Doses for Normal CNS Tissues[a]			
CNS Tissue	TD 5/5 (Gy)	TD 50/5 (Gy)	End Point	
Rubin and Casarett[117]				
Brain			Infarction, necrosis	
Whole	60	70		
Partial (25%)	70	80		
Spinal cord			Infarction, necrosis	
Partial (10-cm length)	45	55		
Emami et al.[118]				
Brain			Infarction, necrosis	
One third	60	75		
Two thirds	50	65		
Whole	40	60		
Brainstem			Infarction, necrosis	
One third	60	—		
Two thirds	53	—		
Whole	50	65		
Spinal cord			Myelitis, necrosis	
5 cm	50	70		
10 cm	50	70		
20 cm	47	—		
Cauda equine	60	75	Clinically apparent nerve damage	
Brachial plexus			Clinically apparent nerve damage	
One third	62	77		
Two thirds	61	76		
Whole	60	75		

[a]Assumes 2 Gy/fraction, 5 d/wk.
Source: Data from Rubin and Casarett[117] and Emami et al.[118]

In a retrospective study of 53 head and neck cancer patients undergoing typical posterior cervical treatment fields including the cervical spinal cord to doses of 56 to 60 Gy in fraction sizes of ≤2 Gy, the incidence of radiation myelopathy was 1.9%.[123] In a subsequent study of 1,048 lung cancer patients treated with thoracic radiation on three Medical Research Council Lung Cancer Working Party clinical trials, the only patients who developed radiation myelopathy were those treated with 3-Gy fractions or larger. The 2-year risk of radiation myelopathy was 2.2% to 2.5% among patients receiving thoracic spinal cord doses of 17 Gy in 2 fractions or 39 Gy in 13 fractions. The authors concluded that a total cord dose of 48 Gy given in 2-Gy fractions was safe.[124]

For primary CNS tumor patients being treated with curative intent, fraction size should rarely exceed 200 cGy daily, and in most situations, should be 180 to 200 cGy (including areas or volumes of "hot spots" on three-dimensional conformal or intensity-modulated radiation therapy treatment plans). Fraction sizes >200 cGy daily (usually 250–300 cGy) are commonly used for palliation of brain metastases and spinal cord compression, but only because such patients are not expected to live long enough to manifest normal tissue injury. Table 26.5 shows the tolerance doses for other normal tissues of the CNS, including the brainstem, eye, ear, optic chiasm, optic nerve, and pituitary gland. The clinical manifestations of severe injury to these structures are listed.[118,125–127]

QUANTITATIVE SCORING OF CNS TOXICITY

Clinically, radiation-induced toxicities are usually graded as mild, moderate, severe, life threatening, or fatal, and are

TABLE 26.5	Tolerance Doses for Miscellaneous Normal Tissues of the Cranium		
Normal Tissue	TD 5/5 (Gy)	TD 50/5 (Gy)	Manifestations of Severe Injury
Ear (middle/external)	30–55	40–65	Acute or chronic serous otitis
Eye			
Retina	45	65	Blindness
Lens	10	18	Cataract formation
Optic nerve or chiasm	50	65	Blindness

Source: Data from Emami et al.,[118] Sklar and Constine,[125] Gordon et al.,[126] and Cooper et al.[127]

TABLE 26.6	RTOG and EORTC CNS Toxicity Tables			
	Grade			
	1	*2*	*3*	*4*
ACUTE TOXICITY, BRAIN	Fully functional status (i.e., able to work) with minor neurological findings; no medication needed	Neurological findings sufficient to require home care; nursing assistance may be required; medications including steroids and antiseizure agents may be required	Neurological findings requiring hospitalization for initial management	Serious neurological impairment that includes paralysis, coma, or seizures >3/wk despite medication and/or hospitalization required
CHRONIC TOXICITY, BRAIN	Mild headache; slight lethargy	Moderate headache; great Lethargy	Severe headaches; severe CNS dysfunction (partial loss of power or dyskinesia)	Seizure or paralysis; coma
CHRONIC TOXICITY, SPINAL CORD	Mild Lhermitte syndrome	Severe Lhermitte syndrome	Objective neurological findings at or below cord level treated	Monoplegia, paraplegia, or quadriplegia

Grade 0 toxicity, none; grade 1, mild; grade 2, moderate; grade 3, severe; grade 4, life threatening; grade 5, fatal.
Source: Data from Cox et al.[128]

defined in an organ-specific manner. These toxicities are generally described in terms of the time course over which they are observed. Acute injury occurs during the course of radiotherapy, while early delayed reactions occur weeks to months after radiotherapy has been completed. Late reactions of radiotherapy occur months following treatment. Table 26.6 shows the toxicity tables used for brain tumor clinical research protocols by the Radiation Therapy Oncology Group (RTOG) and its European counterpart, the European Organization for the Research and Treatment of Cancer (EORTC).[128] Alternatively, the National Cancer Institute Common Terminology Criteria for Adverse Events version 3.0 can be used (http://ctep.cancer.gov/reporting/ctc.html). To measure QOL in brain tumor patients undergoing combined modality therapy including brain radiation, the Functional Assessment of Cancer Therapy scale is used, including the brain subscale.[129]

The quantitative analysis of radiation-induced cognitive dysfunction is more complex than for radionecrosis or myelopathy. The complexity stems from the fact that radiotherapy can affect multiple domains of neurocognitive function including verbal and spatial memory, as well as analytic and abstract thinking. While there are specific neurocognitive tests for such domains as intelligence, perception, psychomotor speed, memory and attention, such an intense battery of testing on each patient prior to and after radiotherapy is not practical. Simpler tests such as the mini-mental status examination (MMSE) are not sensitive enough to detect the subtle differences in function that may be caused by radiotherapy over time. The RTOG is currently accruing for a trial in which neurocognitive outcomes are major endpoints. In its 0614 trial, the RTOG is using a combination of the MMSE along with tests for memory, visual-motor scanning speed, executive function, verbal fluency, and cognitive function. While the RTOG has estimated that the evaluation time for neurocognitive testing will be approximately 30 minutes, a factor that will continue to confound future data is the fact that as patients become more ill, they will be less likely to participate in such a battery of testing.

MANAGEMENT OF RADIATION-INDUCED CNS INJURY

ACUTE REACTIONS

The most common acute reactions associated with brain radiation include fatigue, hair loss, and skin erythema. The onset of fatigue is generally several weeks after the first radiation treatment. It is usually mild to moderate in severity. Typically, the fatigue persists for several months after the completion of treatment but may be chronic in a small percentage of patients. One characteristic of the fatigue associated with radiation therapy is a lack of improvement by rest. Methylphenidate (*Ritalin*) and modafinil (*Provigil*) have been used in the treatment of radiation-induced fatigue.[130,131] The usual dose of methylphenidate is 10 mg bid, escalating to 30 mg bid in 1 to 2 week increments as tolerated. The dose-limiting toxicities are anxiety and insomnia. Modafinil is generally used at a dose of 200 mg qd, escalating to 400 mg qd if necessary. Headache, insomnia, and dizziness have been reported at these doses for modafinil. In a pilot study presented at ASCO in 2006, modafinil appeared to improve fatigue levels, and even depression symptoms and some neurocognitive outcomes 8 weeks after drug initiation.[131]

LATE DELAYED REACTIONS

Although edema and necrosis of the white matter are classified as late delayed reactions, edema of the brain and spinal cord can occur as an early or a late effect of radiation. The treatment of radiation-induced edema is more of an art than a science and typically involves the use of corticosteroid medications. Oral dexamethasone is usually used in initial doses of 4 mg bid for mild symptoms and 4 mg qid for moderate to severe symptoms. Doses in excess of 10 mg qid (40 mg daily) do not increase the likelihood of clinical benefit. The initial dexamethasone dose is usually maintained during the course of radiation, with a slow taper (2–4 mg every 5–7 days) as tolerated thereafter. For life-threatening edema, intravenous dexamethasone is used, 10 to 25 mg as a bolus followed by 4 to 10 mg qid. If these patients do not respond to dexamethasone, intravenous mannitol may be required. Patients on dexamethasone should receive gastritis prophylaxis (with ranitidine, omeprazole, or an equivalent medication), appropriate treatments for hyperglycemia (oral hypoglycemic agents or insulin), and oral thrush (fluconazole 200 mg day 1 then 100 mg daily for 6 days) should they arise.

Because of the vascular and inflammatory components of late radiation damage to the CNS, the combination of vitamin E and pentoxifylline (PTX) has been seen as an attractive therapeutic regimen. A recent pilot study of 11 patients with radiation-induced edema treated with 400 IU vitamin E and 400 mg PTX, p.o. twice a day showed a radiographic decrease in edema volume in the majority of patients.[132] Bevacizumab, a monoclonal antibody to VEGF-A, has also recently been reported to reduce edema in patients with radionecrosis. In one series from the MD Anderson Cancer Center, eight of eight patients with biopsy-proven radionecrosis showed a radiographic decrease in edema volume on posttreatment MRI.[133] A second study from Henry Ford demonstrated a response in six of six patients with an average reduction in edema volume of 79% in the postgadolinium studies.[134]

There are several ongoing research studies for the treatment or prevention of radiation-induced cognitive dysfunction. The Comprehensive Cancer Center of Wake Forest University Community Clinical Oncology Program Research Base has an open trial randomizing 6 month or greater survivors of partial- or WBI to either the reversible acetylcholinesterase inhibitor donepezil (Aricept), 5 to 10 mg/d for 6 months, or placebo. The study is based on a phase 2 open-label study of donepezil in the same patient population showing significant improvements in energy level, mood, and cognitive function.[135] The RTOG is currently conducting a randomized placebo-controlled trial evaluating the efficacy of memantine, an NMDA receptor antagonist that has been shown to be effective in vascular dementia. It is hypothesized that blocking this receptor would block ischemia-induced NMDA excitation and be neuroprotective in the setting of radiation-induced ischemia. Other potential agents currently under investigation as cytoprotective agents against radiation-induced neurocognitive decline include PPAR agonists and ACE inhibitors.

CONCLUSION

While pharmaceutical prophylaxis may hold a future in prevention of radiation-induced cognitive dysfunction, advancements in radiation therapy treatment planning will also likely play a role in the prevention of the late sequelae of brain radiotherapy. NTCP modeling and the identification of radiation dose thresholds of the target structures within the brain will allow for selective sparing of structures in the brain such as the subventricular stem cell niches, the hippocampus, and the dominant temporal lobe. Functional imaging will also likely play a role in the more precise localization of critical structures to memory and learning. Once these structures and their dose tolerances are identified, treatment modalities such as tomotherapy, radiosurgery, and proton beam radiotherapy will ultimately allow for their selective sparing.

REFERENCES

1. Levin VA, Leibel SA, Gutin PH. Neoplasms of the central nervous system. In: DeVita VT, Hellman S, Rosenberg SA, eds. *Cancer—Principles and Practice of Oncology*. Philadelphia, PA: Lippincott Williams and Wilkins; 2001.
2. Scally LT, Lin C, Beriwal S, et al. Brain, brain stem, and cerebellum. In: Perez CA, Brady LW, Halperin EC, Schmidt-Ulrich RKA, eds. *Principles and Practice of Radiation Oncology*. Philadelphia, PA: Lippincott Williams and Wilkins; 2004.
3. Kun LE. The brain and spinal cord. In: Cox JD, ed. *Moss' Radiation Oncology—Rationale, Technique, Results*. St. Louis, MO: Mosby, Year Book, Inc.; 1994.
4. Halperin EC, Constine LS, Tarbell NJ, et al., eds. *Pediatric Radiation Oncology*. 2nd ed. New York, NY: Raven Press; 1994.
5. Waselenko JK, MacVittie TJ, Blakely WF, et al. Medical management of the acute radiation syndrome: recommendations of the strategic national stockpile radiation working group. *Ann Int Med.* 2004;140:1037–1051.
6. Otake M, Schull WJ, Lee S. Threshold for radiation-related severe mental retardation in prenatally exposed A-bomb survivors: a re-analysis. *Int J Radiat Biol.* 1996;70:755–763.
7. Otake M, Schull WJ. Radiation-related brain damage and growth retardation among the prenatally exposed atomic bomb survivors. *Int J Radiat Biol.* 1998;74:159–171.
8. Yamada M, Sasaki H, Kasagi F, et al. Study of cognitive function among the Adult Health Study (AHS) population in Hiroshima and Nagasaki. *Radiat Res.* 2002;158:236–240.
9. Tofilon PJ, Fike JR. The radioresponse of the central nervous system: a dynamic process. *Radiat Res.* 2000;153:357–370.
10. Schultheiss TE, Stephens LC. Permanent radiation myelopathy. *Br J Radiol.* 1992;65:737–753.
11. Crossen JR, Garwood D, Glatstein E, et al. Neurobehavioral sequelae of cranial irradiation in adults: a review of radiation-induced encephalopathy. *J Clin Oncol.* 1994;12:627–642.
12. Johannesen TB, Lien HH, Hole KH, et al. Radiological and clinical assessment of long-term brain tumour survivors after radiotherapy. *Radiother Oncol.* 2003;69:169–176.
13. Giovagnoli AR, Boiardi A. Cognitive impairment and quality of life in long-term survivors of malignant brain tumors. *Ital J Neurol Sci.* 1994;15:481–488.
14. Meyers CA, Brown PD. Role and relevance of neurocognitive assessment in clinical trials of patients with CNS tumors. *J Clin Oncol.* 2006;24:1305–1309.
15. Frost MH, Sloan JA. Quality of life measurements: a soft outcome-or is it? *Am J Manag Care.* 2002;8:S574–S579.
16. van der Maazen RWM, Kleiboer BJ, Berhagen I, et al. Repair capacity of adult rat glial progenitor cells determined by an in vitro clonogenic assay after in vitro or in vivo fractionated irradiation. *Int J Radiat Biol.* 1993;63:661–666.
17. Calvo W, Hopewell JW, Reinhold HS, et al. Time-and dose-related changes in the white matter of the rat brain after single doses of X rays. *Br J Radiol.* 1988;61:1043–1052.
18. Reinhold HS, Calvo W, Hopewell JW, et al. Development of blood vessel-related radiation damage in the fimbria of the central nervous system. *Int J Radiat Oncol Biol Phys.* 1990;18:37–42.
19. Morris GM, Coderre JA, Bywaters A, et al. Boron neutron capture irradiation of the rat spinal cord: histopathological evidence of a vascular-mediated pathogenesis. *Radiat Res.* 1996;146:313–320.
20. Raff MC, Miller RH, Noble M. A glial progenitor cell that develops in vitro into an astrocyte or an oligodendrocyte depending on culture medium. *Nature.* 1983;303:390–396.
21. van der Maazen RWM, Kleiboer BJ, Verhagen I, et al. Irradiation in vitro discriminates between different O-2A progenitor cell subpopulations in the perinatal central nervous system of rats. *Radiat Res.* 1991;128:64–72.
22. van der Maazen RWM, Verhagen I, Kleiboer BJ, et al. Radiosensitivity of glial progenitor cells of the perinatal and adult rat optic nerve studies by an in vitro clonogenic assay. *Radiother Oncol.* 1991;20:258–264.
23. Hornsey S, Myers R, Coultas PG, et al. Turnover of proliferative cells in the spinal cord after irradiation and its relation to time dependent repair of radiation damage. *Br J Radiol.* 1981;54:1081–1085.
24. Stone HB, McBrideWH, Coleman CN. Modifying normal tissue damage postirradiation. *Radiat Res.* 2002;157:204–223.
25. Bentzen SM. Preventing or reducing late side effects of radiation therapy: radiobiology meets molecular pathology. *Nat Rev Cancer.* 2006;6:702–713.
26. Kim JH, Brown SL, Jenrow KA, et al. Mechanisms of radiation-induced brain toxicity and implications for future clinical trials. *J Neurooncol.* 2008;87:279–286.
27. Moulder JE, Fish BL, Cohen EP. Treatment of radiation nephropathy with ACE inhibitors and AII type-1 and type-2 receptor antagonists. *Curr Pharm Des.* 2007;13:1317–1325.
28. Rubin P, Finkelstein J, Shapiro D. Molecular biology mechanisms in the radiation induction of pulmonary injury syndromes: interrelationship between the alveolar macrophages and the septal fibroblast. *Int J Radiat Oncol Biol Phys.* 1992;24:93–101.
29. Hauer-Jensen M, Wang J, Boerma M, et al. Radiation damage to the gastrointestinal tract: mechanisms, diagnosis, and management. *Curr Opin Support Palliat Care.* 2007;1:23–29.
30. Hansson E. Astroglia from defined brain regions as studied with primary cultures. *Prog Neurobiol.* 1988;30:369–397.
31. Seth P, Koul N. Astrocyte, the star avatar: redefined. *J Biosci.* 2008;33:405–421.
32. Song H, Stevens CF, Gage FH. Astroglia induce neurogenesis from adult neural stem cells. *Nature.* 2002;417:39–44.
33. Wilson JX. Antioxidant defense of the brain: a role for astrocytes. *Can J Physiol Pharmacol.* 1997;75:1149–1163.
34. Janzer RC, Raff MC. Astrocytes induce blood-brain barrier properties in endothelial cells. *Nature.* 1987;325:253–257.
35. Seifert G, Schilling K, Steinhauser C. Astrocyte dysfunction in neurological disorders: a molecular perspective. *Nat Rev Neurosci.* 2006;7:94–206.
36. Kyrkanides S, Olschowka JA, Williams JP, et al. TNF alpha and IL-1beta mediate intercellular adhesion molecule-1 induction via microglia-astrocyte interaction in CNS radiation injury. *J Neuroimmunol.* 1999;95:95–106.

37. Hong JH, Chiang CS, Campbell IL, et al. Induction of acute phase gene expression by brain irradiation. *Int J Radiat Oncol Biol Phys.* 1995;33:619–626.
38. Chiang CS, McBride WH, Withers HR. Radiation-induced astrocytic and microglial responses in mouse brain. *Radiother Oncol.* 1993;29:60–68.
39. Hwang SY, Jung JS, Kim TH, et al. Ionizing radiation induces astrocyte gliosis through microglia activation. *Neurobiol Dis.* 2006;21:457–467.
40. Gebicke-Haerter PJ. Microglia in neurodegeneration: molecular aspects. *Microsc Res Tech.* 2001;54:47–58.
41. Kreutzberg GW. Microglia: a sensor for pathologic events in the CNS. *Trends Neurosci.* 1996;19:312–318.
42. Lawson LJ, Perry VH, Dri PGS. Heterogeneity in the distribution and morphology of microglia in the normal adult mouse brain. *Neuroscience.* 1990;39:51–170.
43. Elkabes S, DiCicco-Bloom EM, Black IB. Brain microglia/macrophages express neurotropins that selectively regulate microglial proliferation and function. *J Neurosci.* 1996;16:2508–2521.
44. Block ML, Zecca L, Hong JS. Microglia-mediated neurotoxicity: uncovering the molecular mechanisms. *Nat Rev Neurosci.* 2007;8:57–69.
45. Lucas S-M, Rothwell NJ, Gibson RM. The role of inflammation in CNS injury and disease. *Br J Pharamcol.* 2006;147:S232–S240.
46. Pocock J, Liddle AC. Microglial signalling cascades in neurodegenerative diseases. *Prog Brain Res.* 2001;132:555–565.
47. Price RE, Langford LA, Jackson EF, et al. Radiation-induced morphologic changes in the rhesus monkey (*Macaca mulatta*) brain. *J Med Primatol.* 2003;30:81–87.
48. Mildenberger M, Beach TG, McGeer EG, et al. An animal model of prophylactic cranial irradiation: histologic effects at acute, early and delayed stages. *Int J Radiat Oncol Biol Phys.* 1990;18:1051–1060.
49. Kyrkanides S, Moore AH, Olschowka JA, et al. Cyclooxygenase-2 modulates brain inflammation-related gene expression in central nervous system radiation-injury. *Brain Res Mol Brain Res.* 2002;104:159–169.
50. Monje ML, Mizumatsu S, Fike JR, et al. Irradiation induced neural precursor-cell dysfunction. *Nat Med.* 2002;8:955–961.
51. Raber J, Rola R, LeFevour A, et al. Radiation-induced cognitive impairments are associated with changes in indicators of hippocampal neurogenesis. *Radiat Res.* 2004;162:39–47.
52. Monje ML, Vogel H, Masek M, et al. Impaired human hippocampal neurogenesis after treatment for central nervous system malignancies. *Ann Neurol.* 2007;62:515–520.
53. Monje ML, Toda H, Palmer TD. Inflammatory blockade restores adult hippocampal neurogenesis. *Science.* 2003;302:1760–1765.
54. Pellmar TC, Lepinski DL. Gamma radiation (5–10 Gy) impairs neuronal function in the guinea pig hippocampus. *Radiat Res.* 1993;136:255–261.
55. Noel F, Gumin GJ, Raju U, et al. Increased expression of prohormone convertase-2 in the irradiated rat brain. *FASEB J.* 1998;12:1725–1730.
56. Shi L, Adams MM, Long A, et al. Spatial learning and memory deficits after whole-brain irradiation are associated with changes in NMDA receptor subunits in the hippocampus. *Radiat Res.* 2006;166:892–899.
57. Shi L, Molina DP, Robbins ME, et al. Hippocampal neuron number is unchanged 1 year after fractionated whole-brain irradiation at middle age. *Int J Radiat Oncol Biol Phys.* 2008;71:526–532.
58. Gage FH, KempermannG, Palmer TD, et al. Multipotent progenitor cells in the adult dentate gyrus. *J Neurobiol.* 1998;36:249–266.
59. Palmer TD, Takahashi J, Gage FH. The adult rat hippocampus contains primordial neural stem cells. *Mol Cell Neurosci.* 1997;8:389–404.
60. Palmer TD, Willhoite AR, Gage FH. Vascular niche for adult hippocampal neurogenesis. *J Comp Neurol.* 2000;425:479–494.
61. Bellinzona M, Gobbel GT, Shinohara C, et al. Apoptosis is induced in the subependyma of young adult rats by ionizing irradiation. *Neurosci Lett.* 1996;208:163–166.
62. Snyder JS, Kee N, Wojtowicz JM. Effects of adult neurogenesis on synaptic plasticity in the rat dentate gyrus. *J Neurophysiol.* 2003;85:2423–2431.
63. Mizumatsu S, Monje ML, Morhardt DR, et al. Extreme sensitivity of adult neurogenesis to low doses of X-irradiation. *Cancer Res.* 2003;63:4021–4027.
64. Rola R, Raber J, Rizk A, et al. Radiation-induced impairment of hippocampal neurogenesis is associated with cognitive deficits in young mice. *Exp Neurol.* 2004;188:316–330.
65. Lamproglou I, Chen QM, Boisserie G, et al. Radiation-induced cognitive dysfunction: an experimental model in the old rat. *Int J Radiat Oncol Biol Phys.* 1995;31:65–70.
66. Brown WR, Blair RM, Moody DM, et al. Capillary loss precedes cognitive impairment induced by fractionated whole-brain irradiation. *J Neurol Sci.* 2007;257:67–71.
67. Yoneoka Y, Satoh M, Akiyama K, et al. An experimental study of radiation-induced cognitive dysfunction in an adult rat model. *Br J Radiol.* 1999;72:1196–1201.
68. Atwood T, Payne VS, Zhao W, et al. Quantitative magnetic resonance spectroscopy reveals a potential relationship between radiation-induced changes in rat brain metabolites and cognitive impairment. *Radiat Res.* 2007;168:574–581.
69. Robbins MEC, Zhao W. Chronic oxidative stress and radiation-induced late normal tissue injury: a review. *Int J Radiat Biol.* 2004;80:251–259.
70. Zhao W, Diz DI, Robbins ME. Oxidative damage pathways in relation to normal tissue injury. *Br J Radiol.* 2007;80:S23–S31.
71. Chiang C-S, Hong J-H, Stalder A, et al. Delayed molecular responses to brain irradiation. *Int J Radiat Biol.* 1997;72:45–53.
72. Raju U, Gumin GJ, Tofilon PJ. NFkB activity and target gene expression in the rat brain after one or two exposures to ionizing radiation. *Radiat Oncol Invest.* 1999;7:145–152.
73. Fukuda H, Fukuda A, Zhu C, et al. Irradiation-induced progenitor cell death in the developing brain is resistant to erythropoietin treatment and caspase inhibition. *Cell Death Differ.* 2004;11:1166–1178.
74. Limoli CL, Rola R, Giedzinski E, et al. Cell-density-dependent regulation of neural precursor cells function. *PNAS.* 2004;101:16052–16057.
75. Rola R, Sarkissian V, Obenaus A, et al. High-LET radiation induces inflammation and persistent changes in markers of hippocampal neurogenesis. *Radiat Res.* 2005;164:556–560.
76. Gerard C, Rollins BJ. Chemokines and disease. *Nat Immunol.* 2001;2:108–115.
77. Banisadr G, Queraud-Lesaux F, Boutterin MC, et al. Distribution, cellular localization and functional role of CCR2 chemokine receptors in adult rat brain. *J Neurochem.* 2002;81:257–269.
78. Schindler MK, Forbes ME, Robbins ME, et al. Aging-dependent changes in the radiation response of the adult rat brain. *Int J Radiat Oncol Biol Phys.* 2008;70:826–834.
79. Spence AM, Krohn KA, Edmonson SW, et al. Radioprotection in rat spinal cord with WR-2721 following cerebral lateral intraventricular injection. *Int J Radiat Oncol Biol Phys.* 1986;12:1479–1482.
80. Fike JR, Goebbel GT, Martob LJ, et al. Radiation brain injury is reduced by the polyamine inhibitor alpha-difluoromethylornithine. *Radiat Res.* 1994;138:99–106.
81. Nakagawa M, Bellinzona M, Seilhan TM, et al. Microglial responses after focal radiation-induced injury are affected by alpha-difluormethylornithine. *Int J Radiat Oncol Biol Phys.* 1996;36:113–123.
82. Hornsey S, Myers R, Jenkinson T. The reduction of radiation damage to the spinal cord by postirradiation administration of vasoactive drugs. *Int J Radiat Oncol Biol Phys.* 1990;18:1437–1442.
83. Hopewell JW, van den Aardweg GJMJ, Morris GM, et al. Unsaturated lipids as modulators of radiation damage in normal tissues. In: Horrobin DF, ed. *New Approaches in Cancer Treatment.* London: Churchill Communications Europe; 1993;88–106.
84. Sminia P, van der Kleij AJ, Carl UM, et al. Prophylactic hyperbaric oxygen treatment and rat spinal cord irradiation. *Cancer Lett.* 2003;191:59–65.
85. Nieder C, Andratschke N, Price RE, et al. Evaluation of insulin-like growth factor-1 for prevention of radiation-induced myelopathy. *Growth Factors.* 2005;23:5–18.
86. Nieder C, Price E, Rivera B, et al. Effects of insulin-like growth factor-1 and amifostine in spinal cord re-irradiation. *Strahlenther Oncol.* 2005;181:691–695.
87. Andratschke N, Nieder C, Price RE, et al. Modulation of rat spinal cord radiation tolerance by administration of platelet-derived growth factor. *Int J Radiat Oncol Biol Phys.* 2004;60:1257–1263.
88. Tsao MN, Li YQ, Lu G, et al. Upregulation of vascular endothelial growth factor is associated with radiation-induced blood-spinal cord barrier breakdown. *J Neuropathol Exp Neurol.* 1999;58:1051–1060.
89. Li YQ, Ballinger JR, Nordal RA, et al. Hypoxia in radiation-induced blood-spinal cord barrier breakdown. *Cancer Res.* 2001;61:3348–3354.
90. Nordal RA, Nagy A, Pintilie M, et al. Hypoxia and hypoxia inducible factor-1 target genes in central nervous system radiation injury: a role for vascular endothelial growth factor. *Clin Cancer Res.* 2004;10:3342–3353.
91. Blumberg B, Evans RM. Orphan nuclear receptors-new ligands and new possibilities. *Genes Dev.* 1998;12:3149–3155.
92. Michalik L, Wahli W. Involvement of PPAR nuclear receptors in tissue injury and wound repair. *J Clin Invest.* 2006;116:598–606.
93. Bright JJ, Kanakasabai S, Chearwae W, et al. PPAR regulation of inflammatory signaling in CNS diseases. *PPAR Res.* 2008;2008:658520.
94. Stahel PF, Smith WR, Bruchis J, et al. Peroxisome proliferator-activated receptors: "Key" regulators of neuroinflammation after traumatic brain injury. *PPAR Res.* 2008;2008:538141.
95. Zhao W, Payne V, Tommasi E, et al. Administration of the peroxisomal proliferator-activated receptor (PPAR)γ agonist pioglitazone during fractionated brain irradiation prevents radiation-induced cognitive impairment. *Int J Radiat Oncol Biol Phys.* 2007;67:6–9.
96. Robbins ME, Diz DI. Pathogenic role of the renin-angiotensin system in modulating radiation-induced late effects. *Int J Radiat Oncol Biol Phys.* 2006;64:6–12.
97. Moulder JE, Fish BL, Cohen EP. ACE inhibitors and AII receptor antagonists in the treatment and prevention of bone marrow transplant nephropathy. *Curr Pharm Des.* 2003;9:737–749.
98. Molteni A, Moulder JE, Cohen EP, et al. Control of radiation-induced pneumopathy and lung fibrosis by angiotensin-converting enzyme inhibitors and an angiotensin II type 1 receptor blocker. *Int J Radiat Biol.* 2000;76:523–532.
99. Davisson RL. Physiological genomic analysis of the brain renin-angiotensin system. *Am J Physiol Regul Integr Comp Physiol.* 2003;285:R498–R511.
100. McKinley MJ, Albiston AL, Allen AM, et al. The brain renin-angiotensin system: location and physiological roles. *Int J Biochem Cell Biol.* 2003;35:901–918.
101. Gard PR. The role of angiotensin II in cognition and behaviour. *Eur J Pharmacol.* 2002;438:1–14.
102. Basso N, Paglia N, Stella I, et al. Protective effect of the inhibition of the renin-angiotensin system on aging. *Regul Pept.* 2005;128:247–252.
103. Tedesco MA, Ratti G, Di Salvo G, et al. Does the angiotensin II receptor antagonist losartan improve cognitive function? *Drugs Aging.* 2002;19:723–732.
104. Wright JW, Harding JW. The brain angiotensin system and extracellular matrix molecules in neuralplasticity, learning, and memory. *Prog Neurobiol.* 2004;72:263–293.
105. Robbins ME, Payne V, Tommasi E, et al. The AT_1 receptor antagonist, L-158,809, prevents or ameliorates fractionated whole-brain irradiation-induced cognitive impairment. *Int J Radiat Oncol Biol Phys.* 2009;73:499–505.
106. Kim JH, Brown SL, Kolozsvary A, et al. Modification of radiation injury by ramipril, inhibitor of angiotensin-converting enzyme, on optic neuropathy in the rat. *Radiat Res.* 2004;161:137–142.
107. Ryu S, Kolozsvary A, Jenrow KA, et al. Mitigation of radiation-induced optic neuropathy in rats by ACE inhibitor ramipril: importance of ramipril dose and treatment time. *J Neurooncol.* 2007;82:119–124.
108. Grommes C, Landreth GE, Sastre M, et al. Inhibition of in vivo glioma growth and invasion by peroxisome proliferator-activated receptor γ agonist treatment. *Mol Pharmacol.* 2006;70:1524–1533.
109. Grommes C, Landreth GE, Heneka MT. Antineoplastic effects of peroxisome proliferator-activated receptor gamma agonists. *Lancet Oncol.* 2004;5:419–429.
110. Molteni A, Ward WF, Ts'ao C, et al. Cytostatic properties of some angiotensin I converting enzyme inhibitors and of angiotensin II type I receptor antagonists. *Curr Pharm Des.* 2003;9:751–761.

111. Molavi B, Rassouli N, Bagwe S, et al. A review of thiazolidinediones and metformin in the treatment of type 2 diabetes with focus on cardiovascular complications. *Vasc Health Risk Manag.* 2007;3:967–973.

112. Ribeiro AB. Angiotensin II antagonists-therapeutic benefits spanning the cardiovascular disease cintinuum from hypertension to heart failure and diabetic nephropathy. *Curr Med Res Opin.* 2006;22:1–16.

113. Leibel SA, Sheline GE. Tolerance of the brain and spinal cord to conventional irradiation. In: Gutin P, Liebel SA, Sheline GE, eds. *Radiation Injury to the Nervous System.* 1st ed. New York, NY: Raven Press; 1991:211–238.

114. Schultheiss TE, Kun LE, Ang KK, et al. Radiation response of the central nervous system. *Int J Radiat Oncol Biol Phys.* 1995;31:1093–1112.

115. Sheline GE, Wara WM, Smith V. Therapeutic irradiation and brain injury. *Int J Radiat Oncol Biol Phys.* 1980;6:1215–1218.

116. Fowler J. Brief summary of radiobiological principles in fractionated radiotherapy. *Semin Radiat Oncol.* 1992;2:6–24.

117. Rubin P, Casarett GW. *Clinical Radiation Pathology.* Vols 1 and 2. Philadelphia, PA: WB Saunders; 1968.

118. Emami B, Lyman J, Brown A, et al. Tolerance of normal tissue to therapeutic irradiation. *Int J Radiat Oncol Biol Phys.* 1991;21:109–122.

119. Shaw E, Arusell R, Scheithauer B, et al. A prospective randomized trial of low-versus high-dose radiation therapy in adults with supratentorial low-grade glioma: initial report of a NCCTG-RTOG-ECOG study. *J Clin Oncol.* 2002;20:2267–2276.

120. Barani IJ, Benedict SH, Lin PS. Neural stem cells: implications for the conventional radiotherapy of central nervous system malignancies. *Int J Radiat Oncol Biol Phys.* 2007;68:324–333.

121. Gutierrez AN, Westerly DC, Tome WA, et al. Whole brain radiotherapy with hippocampal avoidance and simultaneously integrated brain metastases boost: a planning study. *Int J Radiat Oncol Biol Phys.* 2007;69:589–597.

122. Klein M, Heimans JJ, Aaronson NK, et al. Effect of radiotherapy and other treatment-related factors on mid-term to long-term cognitive sequelae in low-grade gliomas: a comparative study. *Lancet.* 2002;360:1361–1368.

123. McCunniff AJ, Liang AJ. Radiation tolerance of the cervical spinal cord. *Int J Radiat Oncol Biol Phys.* 1989;16:675–678.

124. Macbeth FR, Wheldon TE, Girling DJ, et al. The Medical Research Council Lung Cancer Working Party. Radiation myelopathy: estimates of risk in 1048 patients in three randomized trials of palliative radiotherapy for non-small cell lung cancer. *Clin Oncol (R Coll Radiol).* 1996;8:176–181.

125. Sklar CA, Constine LS. Chronic neuroendocrinological sequelae of radiation therapy. *Int J Radiat Oncol Biol Phys.* 1995;31:1113–1122.

126. Gordon KB, Char DH, Sagerman RH. Late effects of radiation on the eye and ocular adnexa. *Int J Radiat Oncol Biol Phys.* 1995;31:1123–1140.

127. Cooper JS, Fu K, Marks J, et al. Late effects of radiation in the head and neck region. *Int J Radiat Oncol Biol Phys.* 1995;31:1141–1164.

128. Cox JD, Stetz J, Pajak TF. Toxicity criteria of the Radiation Therapy Oncology Group and the European Organization for Research and Treatment of Cancer. *Int J Radiat Oncol Biol Phys.* 1995;31:1341–1346.

129. Weitzner MA, Meyers CA, Gelke CK, et al. The Functional Assessment of Cancer Therapy (FACT) scale: development of a brain subscale and revalidation of the general version (FACT-G) in patients with primary brain tumors. *Cancer.* 1995;75:1151–1161.

130. Weitzner MA, Meyers CA, Valentine AD. Methylphenidate in the treatment of neurobehavioral slowing associated with cancer and cancer treatment. *J Neuropsyc Clin Neurosci.* 1995;7:347–350.

131. Kaleita TA, Wellisch DK, Graham CA, et al. Pilot study of modafinil for treatment of neurobehavioral dysfunction and fatigue in adult patients with brain tumors [abstract]. *J Clin Oncol.* 2006;ASCO Meeting:1503.

132. Williamson R, Kondziolka D, Kanaan H, et al. Adverse radiation effects after radiosurgery may benefit from oral vitamin E and pentoxifylline therapy: a pilot study. *Stereotact Funct Neurosurg.* 2008;86:359–366.

133. Gonzalez J, Kumar AJ, Conrad CA, et al. Effect of bevacizumab on radiation necrosis of the brain. *Int J Radiat Oncol Biol Phys.* 2007;67:323–326.

134. Torcuator R, Zuniga R, Mohan YS, et al. Initial experience with bevacizumab treatment for biopsy confirmed cerebral radiation necrosis. *J Neurooncol.* 2009;online Feb 3.

135. Shaw EG, Rosdahl R, D'Agostino RB Jr, et al. A phase II study of donepezil in irradiated brain tumor patients: effect on cognitive function, mood, and quality of life. *J Clin Oncol.* 2006;24:1415–1420.

Andrew Kee
Robert L. Foote

Head and Neck

INTRODUCTION

Treatment of primary head and neck malignancies is challenging as patients suffer many treatment-related toxicities due to the presence of multiple critical organs in this anatomic location. Manifestations of these toxicities include both temporary and permanent alterations in normal organ function. The economic costs associated with treatment of these complications can be significant.[1] This chapter discusses the etiology, risk factors, prevention, and treatment of common radiation-related toxicities in the head and neck region.

TASTE

Many patients undergoing radiotherapy to the head and neck region experience ageusia (complete loss of taste), hypogeusia (partial loss), or dysgeusia (altered taste). Changes in taste can occur rapidly during the course of treatment. Altered taste poses a significant risk to a patient's nutritional status and quality of life especially during a time when it is essential to their recovery from treatment. Taste is a sensation mediated by cranial nerves VII (anterior tongue) and IX (posterior tongue). Found in the fungiform, foliate, and circumvallate papillae, taste buds contain 50 to 100 taste cells that produce all four taste sensations (sweet, sour, bitter, and salty). Each taste bud has a pore in which molecules and ions are collected and transported to receptors on the taste cells that initiate a signal transmitted by the cranial nerve. Taste sensation may be tested by using four suprathreshold stimulant solutions (sucrose, sodium chloride, citric acid, and caffeine) administered by micropipettes to four tongue regions, anterior right and left, and posterior right and left. Direct radiation damage to taste nerves may affect their trophic function leading to taste bud atrophy. Taste perception and sensitivity is related to the number and density of taste buds. In addition, radiation may cause taste cell membrane damage. Saliva production also plays an important role in taste sensation in breaking down and transporting the molecules and ions to the taste buds for sensory reception.

In a prospective longitudinal study performed by Mirza et al.,[2] patients undergoing radiotherapy for head and neck malignancies underwent regional taste tests of the lingual region prior to and after radiotherapy. In addition, the authors used video microscopy to capture and store images of the number and location of taste pores and lingual papillae during the course of the study. They found that some patients suffered from taste dysfunction even prior to radiotherapy. They also documented a significant reduction in the number of taste pores and a decreased ability to taste (mainly sour) in patients undergoing radiotherapy in comparison to a control group. Recovery of taste as well as the number of pores was seen at 6 months following radiotherapy. Irradiation of rat tongues has also been shown to result in acute changes including a significant decline in the number of taste buds followed by a gradual recovery with time after irradiation.[3]

Yamashita et al.[4] were able to show that patients' taste sensation gradually declined during radiotherapy by performing taste tests weekly during radiotherapy and determining that significant impairment occurred three weeks into treatment. No dose response for taste loss was seen in patients who received either low dose (≤20 Gy) or high hose (>20 Gy) to the majority of the tongue. Patients in whom the anterior portion of the tongue was not in the treatment volume did not suffer taste loss. No difference in tasting ability was seen in patients who underwent concurrent chemotherapy. Taste recovery was seen 4 months after completing treatment. Minimizing the volume of tongue exposed to radiation in order to preserve taste was also seen reported in a study by Fernando et al.[5]

Halyard et al. performed a phase III, double-blinded, and placebo-controlled clinical trial to determine if zinc sulfate (45 mg) administered three times a day during radiotherapy and for a month following radiotherapy would reduce the incidence and duration of radiation-induced alterations in taste in patients receiving ≥20 Gy to ≥30% of the oral cavity. They found that zinc sulfate, as administered in this trial to this patient population, did not prevent taste alterations or favorably affect the interval to taste recovery.[6]

These studies suggest that the acute effects of radiotherapy on taste pores occur early in the course of treatment and that loss of taste cells and cellular function within the pores is the primary cause of altered taste during treatment. Methods to minimize loss of taste sensation appear to include minimizing radiation dose to the tongue without compromising treatment of the target volume. This can be accomplished using either intensity-modulated radiotherapy (IMRT) with the anterior tongue as an avoidance structure or intraoral stents that displace the tongue out of the treatment volume or both in patients with appropriately selected nasal cavity and paranasal sinus cancers, oral cavity cancers (non-tongue, well lateralized), nasopharyngeal carcinoma, selected tonsil and tongue base cancers, pharyngeal wall cancers, laryngeal and hypopharyngeal cancers, and salivary gland cancers.

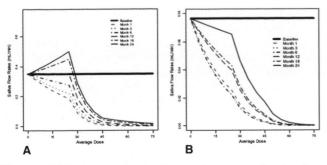

A **B**

Figure 27.1. A: Stimulated saliva production predicted at baseline and 1, 3, 6, 12, 18, and 24 months after radiation therapy. **B:** Unstimulated saliva production predicted at baseline and 1, 3, 6, 12, 18, and 24 months after radiation therapy. (Reprinted from Li Y. The impact of dose on parotid salivary recovery in head and neck cancer patients treated with radiation therapy. *Int J Radiat Oncol Biol Phys.* 2007;67(3):660–669, with permission.)

SALIVARY GLANDS

The major salivary glands (parotid, submandibular, and sublingual) produce up to 80% of the salivary secretions with the rest supplied by the minor salivary glands in the oral cavity. The saliva is important in maintaining oral health as the fluid provides antibacterial activity, alkaline pH, lubrication, maintenance of teeth, and solubilization of solid foods for taste and aids in digestion and speech. The submandibular glands produce saliva during a resting state, while the parotid glands are the main contributors under a stimulated state.

Radiation injury to the major salivary glands can be seen in the first 1 to 2 weeks of a course of radiotherapy. The serous-producing cells appear to be more sensitive than the mucinous-producing cells as the saliva becomes more mucinous, thick, ropey, and sticky. Patients commonly present with changes in physical properties of their saliva as well as reduction in baseline and stimulated flow. Interphase death of serous cells occurs resulting in atrophy of the cells without inflammation suggesting apoptosis plays a role during this phase. Progressive reduction in flow rates, pH, and secretory immunoglobulin A is observed as the radiation dose increases.

The TD 50/5 for the parotid gland (uniform dose resulting in a 50% complication probability at 5 years) is 38 to 46 Gy with gradual improvement in parotid flow after radiotherapy.[6] There is a linear correlation with 5% loss of function per 1 Gy of mean dose to the parotid with no threshold dose. The incidence of xerostomia is significantly reduced when the mean dose of at least one parotid gland is kept ≤26 Gy and may return back to pretreatment levels when the mean dose is <25 to 30 Gy.[7,8] Figure 27.1 illustrates the mean stimulated and unstimulated saliva production predicted by a model designed by Li et al. at the University of Michigan. Patients continue to have recovery of salivary function during the 2 years following irradiation with diminished recovery in glands receiving >30 Gy. Reduced baseline saliva production occurs more or less in a linear fashion with dose. For complete salivary production recovery after 24 months, the volume of the contralateral parotid gland receiving >40 Gy should be <33%.[11]

The same University of Michigan group was able to perform dose modeling for the submandibular gland and found that it is more radioresistant in comparison to the parotid gland.[9] They observed that stimulated and unstimulated flow rates recovered at two years post treatment when the mean dose did not exceed 39 Gy. Both stimulated and unstimulated salivary flow rates

decreased exponentially with dose with a more precipitous drop in the unstimulated salivary function (Fig. 27.2).

A prospective study done by Jellema et al.[10] observed a correlation between xerostomia and its negative impact on quality of life especially in younger patients who generally lead more active lives. Meirovitz et al.[11] found that patient self-reported xerostomia correlated better with quality of life compared to observer-based scores as this underestimated the quality-of-life impact of xerostomia. Therefore, reducing dose to the salivary glands should translate into objective and subjective improvement of xerostomia and quality of life in patients undergoing head and neck radiotherapy.

IMRT has been shown in prospective uncontrolled and in phase III controlled clinical trials to preserve parotid salivary flow and improve quality of life by reducing parotid dose.[12–17] Braam et al. were able to show significant reduction in parotid dose with IMRT compared to 3D conformal radiotherapy (Fig. 27.3). The authors reported a parotid mean dose reduction from 48 to 34 Gy with IMRT. IMRT was also able to preserve flow rate with the proportion of patients having compromised stimulated salivary function reduced from 81% to 56%.[12] Pow et al. were able to show in a randomized

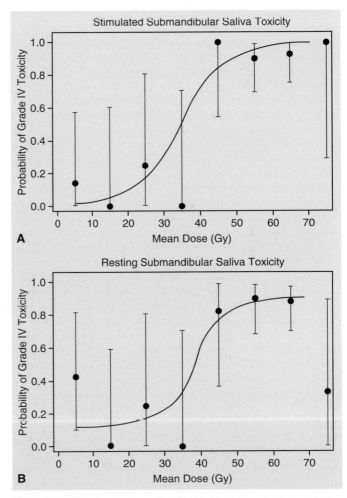

A **B**

Figure 27.2. Mean submandibular dose versus grade IV toxicity for **(A)** stimulated and **(B)** unstimulated submandibular gland. The bars represent 95% CI. (Reprinted from Murdoch-Kinch CA, et al. Dose-effect relationships for the submandibular salivary glands and implications for their sparing by intensity modulated radiotherapy. *Int J Radiat Oncol Biol Phys.* 2008;72(2):373–382, with permission.)

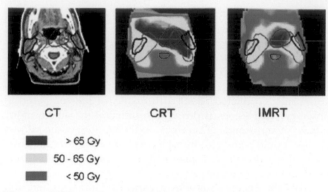

Figure 27.3. Dose distribution (*red*, *yellow*, and *green* color wash) achieved with 3D conformal radiotherapy (CRT) compared to IMRT for the same patient at the same axial computed tomography (CT) slice (tumor bed (*blue*), parotid (*black*), spinal cord (*red*), and lymph nodes (*purple*). (Reprinted from Braam PM, et al. Intensity-modulated radiotherapy significantly reduces xerostomia compared to conventional radiotherapy. *Int J Radiat Oncol Biol Phys.* 2006;66(4):975–980, with permission.)

controlled trial the superiority of IMRT over conformal radiotherapy (CRT) in salivary production preservation and quality of life. In this study, 83% of the patients in the IMRT group were able to achieve at least 25% of their preradiotherapy parotid flow versus 10% of those randomized to CRT.[13] Patients also reported better quality-of-life scores with the preservation of salivary function. As an alternative, Portaluri et al.[18] reported a cost-effective 3D CRT method for reducing parotid dose and xerostomia prevention. The authors were able to preserve salivary function by achieving a mean dose between 30 and 38 Gy (depending on the primary tumor site) to the contralateral parotid using a single isocenter with 10 to 14 fields.

Amifostine appears to reduce radiation-induced xerostomia and may prove to be helpful in preventing or minimizing the effects of xerostomia and loss of taste.[19–24] In a retrospective study by Münter in patients undergoing head and neck radiotherapy with either IMRT or CRT with and without amifostine, IMRT and its ability to lower dose to the parotid glands was the largest contributor to salivary preservation. The authors found that amifostine prevented reduced salivary gland function only when the dose to the parotid was <40.6 Gy in CRT patients.[25] In patients receiving concurrent chemoradiotherapy, a multicenter phase III randomized trial from Germany and Austria did not demonstrate a benefit in salivary function preservation associated with amifostine. All patients in this trial received CRT with definitive or postoperative doses ranging from 60 to 70 Gy.[26] In addition, more adverse events requiring study drug discontinuation were reported in the amifostine arm (30% vs. 11% in placebo; $p = 0.009$). Jellema et al.[20] also reported 28% of their patients discontinuing amifostine before the end of therapy secondary to increased nausea and emesis. Although there is a subcutaneous formulation of amifostine that is suggested to cause less severe nausea, emesis, and hypotension than the IV formulation, the efficacy of preserving salivary function in the era of IMRT is limited.[27]

The parotid glands have been shown to decrease in size (volume) by about 5%/wk during a course of radiotherapy. This results in a shift of the lateral superficial lobe medially by about 0.85 mm/wk during treatment. So with the use of IMRT, the parotid glands are shrinking and shifting during treatment from

the low-dose region into the high-dose region. This results in a 15% increase in dose over what was originally planned (range 6%–42%).[31,32] The use of image-guided adaptive radiotherapy with weekly replanning may allow further dose reduction to the parotid glands with better sparing of salivary production.

Three large randomized, double-blind, placebo-controlled, multicenter clinical trials have documented the efficacy of oral pilocarpine (5.0 mg given orally three times a day) and cevimeline (30–45 mg given orally three times a day) in relieving oral dryness; improving salivary flow, mouth comfort, and ability to speak; and reducing the need for oral comfort agents after head and neck irradiation. Adverse reactions are minimal, with the most common being mild to moderate sweating, which is dose related. Best results may require continuous treatment for more than 8 weeks.[33–36] Most patients report significant relief of symptoms of xerostomia and improvement in quality of life that do not appear to be dependent on previous radiotherapy dose/volume parameters, suggesting that oral pilocarpine acts primarily by stimulating ectopic salivary glands and can be of benefit for a whole range of patients with xerostomia of varying severity. Topical pilocarpine administration has shown results similar to those achieved with systemic treatment but with improved patient tolerance.[28]

One small retrospective trial and two small double-blind, placebo-controlled, randomized trials suggested that pilocarpine (5.0 mg given orally four times a day), started the day before or on the same day as radiation therapy, given concurrently with radiation therapy and for 3 months after radiation therapy, results in a lower frequency of oral symptoms and xerostomia during treatment and afterward. It may not be necessary to continue the use after 3 months to maintain the benefit.[29–31] Two large placebo-controlled clinical trials conducted by Princess Margaret Hospital and the RTOG, nonetheless, failed to confirm these initial findings and did not demonstrate any reduction in the incidence or severity of radiation-induced xerostomia with prophylactic use of pilocarpine 3 days before radiation therapy, during radiation therapy, and for 3 months after completion of radiation therapy.[32,33]

DENTAL HEALTH

Patients undergoing radiotherapy to the oral cavity have an increased risk of dental caries. The changes in saliva quality and production can lead to more cariogenic flora. Mucositis, dryness, and the associated oral discomfort often result in changes in a patient's diet to sugar-containing drinks and softer foods that can further increase the risk of rampant cavity formation. In addition, radiotherapy-induced oral discomfort can lead to reduction in brushing and flossing, thus increasing the risk of dental caries, which can lead to extraction, soft tissue necrosis, bone exposure, and osteoradionecrosis. Poor dental status has been found to have a persistent impact on a patient's quality of life for many years after radiotherapy is completed.[34] Children who receive ≥20 Gy to the dentition have a significantly higher risk of developing one or more dental abnormalities including microdontia, hypodontia, root abnormalities, abnormal enamel, tooth loss, severe gingivitis, and xerostomia.[35]

PREVENTION

All patients should undergo thorough dental evaluation and cleaning prior to initiating head and neck radiotherapy.

Edentulous patients should be evaluated for retained root tips, abscesses, bone loss, and assessment of oral hygiene. Dentures should be checked for fit and patients should be discouraged from wearing them until the mucosa is healed from the effects of radiotherapy. Although extraction of healthy or restorable teeth is discouraged, removal of nonsalvageable teeth prior to radiotherapy will reduce the risk of osteoradionecrosis.[36-37] Patients should have custom-made fluoride carriers and apply a neutral 1.1% sodium fluoride gel to the teeth once a day at the initiation of radiation therapy. After treatment is complete, depending on the patient's dental status and salivary production recovery, application of fluoride can be reduced to twice-weekly indefinitely or discontinued. The dosage and frequency should be modified based on the patient's history of caries and oral hygiene status. Patients can also use amorphous calcium phosphate (ACP) rinse after fluoride treatments. ACP can prevent future caries and repair existing small caries by dissolving in enamel fluids. The calcium and the phosphate ions precipitate and recrystallize to repair small existing cavities.

TREATMENT OF DENTAL CARIES

After radiotherapy, patients should initially have dental evaluations every 3 months. Routine dental procedures can be performed without precautions. If extractions are required, removal of teeth one at a time while minimizing trauma to adjacent soft tissue and performing an alveoplasty as indicated will allow time for the soft tissues to heal before the next procedure and reduce the chance of osteoradionecrosis. Prophylactic antibiotic coverage should be started 1 day prior to any radical periodontal treatment or extractions and continued until the site is healed. Although some institutions are routinely offering hyperbaric oxygen prior to extractions, there is insufficient evidence that this added treatment will prevent osteoradionecrosis.[38,39]

SWALLOW FUNCTION

Swallowing involves a series of coordinated voluntary and involuntary events involving six cranial nerves and more than 30 pairs of muscles.[40] Coordination of the sensory and motor functions is required for effective and efficient swallowing. With improved tumor control rates reported in altered fractionation and concurrent chemoradiotherapy trials, quality-of-life outcomes are increasingly becoming important issues in head and neck cancer treatment. The patient's ability to eat has direct correlation with better quality-of-life scores.[41-44] Multiple abnormalities can be seen in the organs involved in swallowing after head and neck radiotherapy.[45,46]

Pretreatment Evaluation

Up to 66% of head and neck cancer patients have varying degrees of dysphagia and 53% have aspiration at presentation.[47,48] A comprehensive multidisciplinary approach with use of videofluoroscopic examination and involvement of speech pathologists is essential to recognizing preexisting swallowing dysfunction and deterioration due to treatment. Early diagnosis allows initiation of early intervention. Whether it is treatment or tumor related or both, dysphagia can lead to many problems including aspiration, malnutrition, and decline in quality of life. Early preventative measures such as pretreatment swallowing exercises have shown improvement in posttreatment swallowing

function as measured by videofluoroscopy.[49] In addition, there is also a suggestion that quality of life is improved in patients who underwent preradiotherapy exercises.[50]

The extent of pretreatment tumor volume, location, extension, invasion, and discomfort are contributing factors to posttreatment swallowing impairment. Patients with hypopharyngeal and laryngeal carcinomas have a higher rate of pretreatment functional impairment. Evaluation of swallow function in 79 consecutive head and neck cancer patients at the University of Chicago revealed significantly higher rates of aspiration and severe esophageal and pharyngeal impairment in laryngeal and hypopharyngeal cancer patients in comparison to patients with oral or oropharyngeal carcinoma. In their series, 80% of patients with hypopharyngeal and 67% of laryngeal carcinoma patients had aspiration at presentation.[47] Although lower rates of aspiration are seen in patients with oral cavity and oropharyngeal carcinomas, patients who have had free flap reconstruction for treatment of these two subsites were found to have an increased incidence of postsurgical aspiration when more than half of the tongue base was removed or when the patient had previous radiotherapy.[51] As a result, all head and neck patients should have a video swallow examination prior to initiating radiotherapy.

A study by Eisbruch et al. prospectively evaluated swallowing function using videofluoroscopy, direct endoscopy, and CT. They observed that damage to the pharyngeal constrictors, glottis, and supraglottic larynx results in impaired bolus movement and aspiration. The same group later reported significant dose-volume relationships between superior constrictors and aspiration and dysphagia. The lateral but not medial retropharyngeal (RP) nodes are considered to be at risk for harboring subclinical metastases, which may allow sparing of the medial constrictor muscles (Fig. 27.4).[52,53] Teguh et al. observed

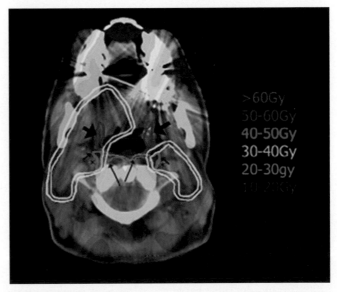

Figure 27.4. IMRT isodose plan. The CTV and PTV (*yellow*) encompasses the lateral RP nodes (*green, small arrows*, medial to carotid artery [*asterisks*]). The medial RP nodes (*blue, long arrows*) are not included in the CTV. *Yellow*, CTV and PTV; *red*, Pharyngeal constrictor (*thick arrows*), *green*, Lateral RP nodes; *blue*, Medial RP nodes. (Reprinted from Feng FY, et al. Intensity-modulated radiotherapy of head and neck cancer aiming to reduce dysphagia: early dose-effect relationships for the swallowing structures. *Int J Radiat Oncol Biol Phys.* 2007;68(5):1289–1298, with permission.)

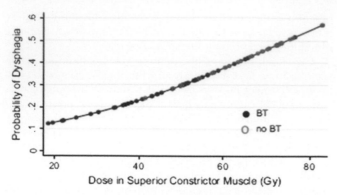

Figure 27.5. Dose-effect relationship for the probability of having dysphagia (Performance Status Scale for normalcy of diet) and dose (Gy) to the superior constrictor muscle. BT, brachytherapy). (Reprinted from Teguh DN, et al. Treatment techniques and site considerations regarding dysphagia-related quality of life in cancer of the oropharynx and nasopharynx. *Int J Radiat Oncol Biol Phys.* 2008;72(4):1119–1127, with permission.)

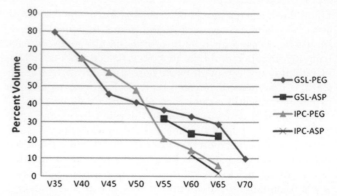

Figure 27.6. Threshold dose-volume histogram for PEG tube dependence and aspiration (ASP). GSL, larynx; IPC, inferior pharyngeal constrictor; V_x, volume receiving x dose. (Reprinted from Caudell JJ, et al. Dosimetric factors associated with long-term dysphagia after definitive radiotherapy for squamous cell carcinoma of the head and neck. *Int J Radiat Oncol Biol Phys.* 2010;76(2):403–409, with permission.)

site-dependent dysphagia after treatment of a variety of head and neck cancers. They observed that the prevalence of severe dysphagia was higher in patients with base of tongue cancers in comparison to nasopharyngeal cancer patients. A dose relationship between the constrictor muscles and the probability of dysphagia was determined based on location of the primary cancer (Fig. 27.5).[54] A similar relationship was found by investigators at Dana-Faber Cancer Center where the mean dose to the inferior constrictor and larynx and the volume of larynx receiving ≥50 Gy were found to be the most significant predictors of both aspiration and stricture formation. The authors reported no aspiration or stricture formation when <21% of the larynx received >50 Gy and when <51% of the inferior constrictor received >50 Gy.[55] Investigators from Peter MacCallum Cancer Center reported a direct correlation between dose to the pharyngoesophageal axis and the need for a feeding tube in nasopharyngeal cancer patients. The mean dose to the esophagus and larynx below the hyoid was 55.2 Gy using IMRT for the entire head and neck field compared to 27.3 Gy when IMRT is used to treat only the nasopharynx and upper neck nodes while using a single anterior beam for the lower neck. This correlated with a feeding tube rate of 95% and 63%, respectively, with a shortened duration of needing a feeding tube when the dose to the pharyngoesophageal axis is lowered.[56] Caudell et al. from the University of Alabama at Birmingham have reported that a mean dose > 41 Gy and V_{60} > 24% to the larynx were significantly associated with percutaneous endoscopic gastrostomy (PEG) tube dependence and aspiration. These authors also found that a V_{60} > 12% to the inferior pharyngeal constrictor was also significantly associated with increased PEG tube dependence and aspiration. In addition, they found that a V_{65} > 33% to the superior pharyngeal constrictor or >75% to the middle pharyngeal constrictor was associated with pharyngoesophageal stricture requiring dilation (Fig. 27.6).[57]

Posttreatment functional outcomes are dependent on several factors including stage and location of the primary cancer, type of treatment, and extent of rehabilitation. Several studies report superior organ preservation rates with concurrent chemoradiotherapy when compared to radiotherapy alone for various subsites of head and neck cancers. Unfortunately, preservation

of organ anatomy does not always equate to preservation of organ function. Twenty-three percent of patients treated on the RTOG 91-11 concurrent chemoradiotherapy arm for larynx cancer could only swallow soft food or liquid at 1 year.[58] The GORTEC 94-01 clinical trial reported a feeding tube rate of 37% in patients with oropharyngeal cancer treated on the concurrent chemoradiotherapy arm.[59] Observed posttreatment functional changes include impaired intraoral sensation, difficulty in discrimination of food texture, reduced tongue base retraction, delayed laryngeal closure, reduced cricopharyngeal opening, and reduced laryngeal elevation.[60–62] Interestingly, investigators at the University of Chicago observed that patients with advanced primaries (T3 and T4) have better swallowing ability following treatment in comparison to pretreatment baseline as measured by video swallow studies.[63]

Due to the close proximity of the primary cancer to swallowing structures, patients with larynx and hypopharynx cancers have worse functional outcome after therapy in comparison to other subsites of the head and neck. These patients have a higher rate of baseline dysfunction prior to therapy. Investigators at the University of Chicago reported a higher rate of aspiration for patients with larynx and hypopharyngeal cancers with 79% and 71% of patients, respectively, having aspiration prior to treatment. Of patients found to experience aspiration, 75% were found to have silent aspiration.[48] The clinical significance is unclear as these patients are not usually diagnosed with complications from aspiration such as recurrent pneumonia. In a series by Lee et al. at Cleveland Clinic, the highest percentage of patients suffering esophageal stricture occurred in patients with hypopharyngeal primaries. Thirty-one percent of hypopharyngeal patients were found to have a stricture of the esophagus.[64] Investigators at Memorial Sloan-Kettering Cancer Center observed a 31% and 15% PEG tube dependency at 2 years in advanced hypopharyngeal and laryngeal cancers, respectively, treated with IMRT.[65] The same group reported a 4% PEG tube dependency rate at 2 years for advanced oropharyngeal carcinomas treated with IMRT.[66] Chen et al. found that in a group of 211 patients treated with radiation therapy for head and neck cancer, the incidence of grade 3 or higher esophageal toxicity at 3 and 6 months following treatment was 30% and 19%, respectively. The rate of gastrostomy-tube dependence at 3 and

6 months was 20% and 11%, respectively. These authors found that hypopharyngeal and unknown primary site, T4 disease, and the use of concurrent chemotherapy were associated with severe or greater esophageal toxicity and stricture formation.[67]

It appears that patients treated with IMRT have better swallowing function in comparison to patients treated with 3D conformal radiotherapy (CRT). A quality-of-life study performed at the University of Iowa showed better quality-of-life scores for patients treated with IMRT. At 1 year post definitive radiotherapy or chemoradiotherapy, 48% of the patients treated with CRT had a diet that consisted of mostly soft foods, liquids, or had no oral intake compared to 16% in the IMRT group. Over 90% of the IMRT group were treated with combined chemotherapy while approximately 50% received chemotherapy in the CRT group.[41] A retrospective comparison by Lee et al.[66] reported a 21% PEG tube rate with CRT versus 4% with IMRT at two years posttreatment for oropharyngeal carcinomas.

Patients should be encouraged to maintain as much of their nutritional needs via oral intake as possible to continue to exercise the swallowing mechanism. Even when a PEG tube is required, oral supplements are recommended to prevent mucosal adhesions, which often require endoscopic recanalization. Other post-treatment sequelae such as fibrosis and/or atrophy of the swallowing muscles can occur, which require early identification and management through intensive rehabilitation. Routine placement of PEG tube is discouraged as patients may cease all efforts to maintain oral swallowing efforts. Early recognition and intervention of dysphagia will lead to improvement in quality of life and reduce the chance of permanent PEG tube dependency.[43] Some patients may require frequently repeated esophageal dilatation to maintain oral nutritional intake.

TRISMUS

Trismus, or the restriction of mouth opening, occurs secondary to fibrosis of the muscles of mastication secondary to surgery, radiotherapy, and/or advanced carcinomas involving the pterygoid and/or masseter musculature. Fibrosis of the pterygoid (medial and lateral), temporalis, and masseter muscles leading to trismus is gradual, painless, and can be difficult to treat.[68] Trismus can impact quality of life as patient's nutritional needs, dental hygiene, and phonation can be compromised. A commonly used functional definition of reduced mouth opening is an interincisor distance of ≤35 mm. Severe limitation is defined as distances of 18 to 20 mm.[69,70] The rate of trismus after radiotherapy varies from published series and ranges from 5% to 38%.[69–71] In a prospective single arm study by Wang et al., patients with nasopharyngeal carcinoma treated with 3D conformal radiotherapy were followed with serial measurements of the maximal interincisor distance (MID). The authors observed a rapid decline in MID of 2.4%/mo during the first 9 months following radiotherapy with continued decline at 0.2%/mo during years 1 to 2 and 0.1%/mo for years 2 to 4 postradiotherapy. The mean decline from the initial interincisor distance was found to be 32% at 4 years after radiotherapy.[71]

Prevention and Treatment

The severity of trismus can be lessened with the use of improved radiotherapy techniques, exercises, and medications. Sophisticated radiotherapy plans can reduce the rate and severity of

Right temporalis muscle	Left Coronoid process
Left temporalis muscle	Right Mandibular condyl
Right lateral pterygoid muscle	Left Mandibular condyl
Right medial pterygoid muscle	Right parotid gland superficial lobe
Left lateral pterygoid muscle	Left parotid gland superficial lobe
Left medial pterygoid muscle	Right parotid gland deep lobe
Right masseter muscle	Left parotid gland deep lobe
Left masseter muscle	Oral mucosa
Right Coronoid process	

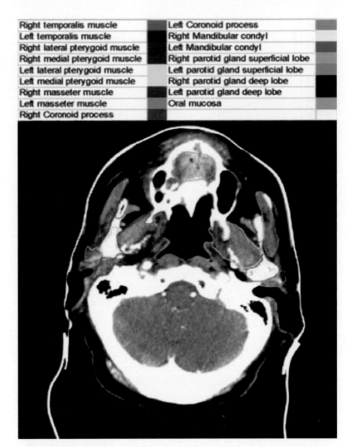

Figure 27.7. Schematic diagram of the delineated structures of the mastication apparatus. (Reprinted from Teguh DN, et al. Trismus in patients with oropharyngeal cancer: relationship with dose in structures of mastication apparatus. *Head Neck.* 2008;30:622–630, with permission.)

trismus. Teguh et al. studied a cohort of 81 oropharynx cancer patients treated with radiotherapy and evaluated mean dose to the mastication apparatus as seen in Figure 27.7. The authors observed a 24% increase in the probability of trismus for every 10 Gy after 40 Gy to the pterygoid muscles. Using IMRT and placing constraints on the masseter and pterygoid muscles significantly decreased the dose to these structures (Fig. 27.8).[72] Unlike the Wang series in which the dramatic onset of trismus was observed with parallel opposed fields in patients with nasopharyngeal carcinoma, Hsiung observed that patients maintained 98.1% of their pretreatment MID at 12 months with the use of IMRT.[71,73] The IMRT planning did not involve specific dose constraints to the pterygoids or masseter muscles but involved parotid sparing, which lead to lower doses to the pterygoid and masseter musculature.

A consultation with the physical medicine and rehabilitation team including a speech therapist should be considered in high-risk patients such as those with tumor involvement of the muscles of mastication and/or those treated with combined surgery and postoperative radiotherapy. Daily jaw-stretching exercises and commercially available jaw-stretching tools are available for patients exhibiting early signs of trismus. Tapered corks or stacked tongue blades can be used as well as elaborate dynamic opening systems (Therabite). These devices are inserted between the teeth, and the interincisor distance is increased until the patient experiences slight pain and then held for 30 seconds.

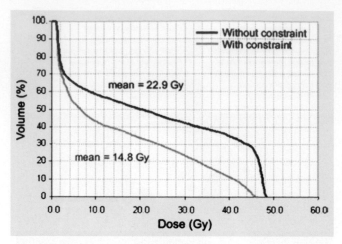

Figure 27.8. Dose–volume histogram for the left masseter muscle with and without a constraint placed on the muscle. (Reprinted from Teguh DN, et al. Trismus in patients with oropharyngeal cancer: relationship with dose in structures of mastication apparatus. *Head Neck.* 2008;30:622–630, with permission.)

Every few days, the interincisor distance can be increased. Application of localized moist heat may also be helpful.

Pharmacotherapy may also help patients suffering from trismus. Baclofen, cyclobenzaprine, tizanidine, and clonazepam have been used. Pentoxifylline, a methylxanthine derivative, improves microcirculation and tissue oxygenation. Pentoxifylline combined with alpha-tocopherol (a vitamin E derivative and scavenger of reactive oxygen species, ROS) was initially reported to reduce the severity of radiation-induced fibrosis in animal models and patients.[74–76] In a small pilot study, patients deemed to have severe trismus (interincisor distance ≤ 25 mm) had a mean improvement of 4 mm after an 8-week course of pentoxifylline therapy.[77] For more severe cases, Botox injections or surgical intervention may be indicated.

MUCOSITIS

Mucositis is a common acute side effect secondary to radiotherapy or chemotherapy in which patients suffer pain due to inflammation and ulceration of the mucosa. Mucositis is the result of a complex series of events that leads to damage of the oral mucosal barrier. Both chemotherapy and radiotherapy directly damage DNA and stimulate secondary mediators of apoptosis through ROS. ROS also stimulate secondary mediators such as NF-αB, which results in gene upregulation for proteins involved in proinflammatory cytokines (IL-1β, IL-6) leading to tissue injury and apoptosis of cells in the mucosa (Fig. 27.9). Eventually, loss of mucosal integrity results in painful lesions and allows for secondary bacterial colonization.[78] Head and neck cancer patients often receive concurrent chemotherapy and radiotherapy leading to more pronounced mucositis than is caused by either agent alone.

A dose-response relationship for oral mucositis was suggested in a prospective study of 12 patients where a cumulative point dose of 39.1 Gy resulted in 3 or more weeks of oral mucositis. A cumulative point dose of <32 Gy resulted in mild mucositis ≤grade 1 lasting ≤ 1 week.[2] In a retrospective review of over 200 head and neck cancer patients treated with radiotherapy at MD Anderson, 66% of the patients had either grade 3 or 4 mucositis per CTC version 2.0. Patients who were treated with concurrent chemotherapy or altered fractionation radiotherapy, or who had an oral cavity, nasopharynx, or oropharynx primary cancer had a higher rate of mucositis. Patients had higher levels of pain, weight loss, and higher costs associated with their treatment when mucositis was present.[1,79] The severity of mucositis is also determined by dose (daily and cumulative) and volume of irradiated tissue. Cumulative doses above 5,000 cGy are associated with higher rates of mucositis.[79] With standard daily fraction sizes of 180 to 200 cGy, patients usually present with erythematous mucosa after 1 or 2 weeks of radiotherapy. This will transition into white patchy ulcers or pseudomembranous lesions, which eventually coalesce into

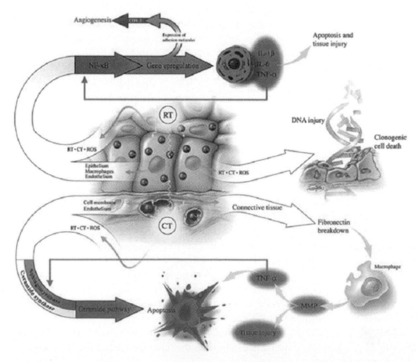

Figure 27.9. Radiotherapy (RT) and chemotherapy (CT) generate ROS resulting in direct DNA injury as well as stimulation of secondary mediators leading to apoptosis. Other genes are also up regulated leading to angiogenesis. (Reprinted from Sonis ST, et al. Perspectives on cancer therapy-induced mucosal injury: pathogenesis, measurement, epidemiology, and consequences for patients. *Cancer.* 2004;100:1995–2025, with permission.)

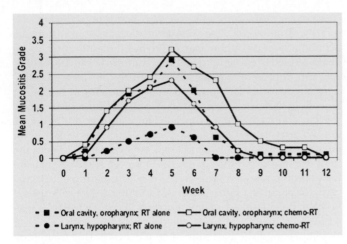

Figure 27.10. Mean grade of mucositis during 6 weeks of radiotherapy and 6 weeks of follow-up for each head and neck site. CTC version 2.0 grade 0 to 4 scale. Reprinted from Elting LS, et al. Risk, outcomes, and costs of radiation-induced oral mucositis among patients with head-and-neck malignancies. *Int J Radiat Oncol Biol Phys.* 2007;68(4):1110–1120, with permission.)

confluent pseudomembranes and/or ulceration that can easily bleed with minor trauma. Figure 27.10 shows the distribution of mucositis during a 6-week course of radiotherapy.[1] In a minority of cases, patients may present with spontaneous bleeding requiring interruption of their scheduled treatment. Interruption of radiotherapy is discouraged, as a protracted treatment course is known to decrease local tumor control and curability.[80,81]

Patients suffering from mucositis frequently report pain, which can lead to compromised nutrition, hydration, and oral hygiene. Pain secondary to mucositis is a common complaint during therapy. Figure 27.11 shows the progression of pain during and after radiotherapy for each head and neck sub-site.[1] Odynophagia and dysphagia caused by combined esophagitis and oral and/or pharyngeal mucositis often lead

to a requirement for IV hydration. Eventually, many patients require nutritional support via a feeding tube during their course of radiotherapy. Dead surface epithelium, fibrin, and polymorphonuclear leukocytes on a moist background provide a favorable environment for opportunistic infections such as candidiasis, which in some series account for up to 70% of oral infections.[82] Nystatin suspension, clotrimazole troches, or oral fluconazole are common agents used to treat candidiasis with resistant infections requiring prolonged fluconazole therapy at higher doses and/or for extended periods.[83]

Prevention and Treatment

A comprehensive oral examination by a multidisciplinary team, including head and neck surgeon, radiation oncologist, and dental professionals (prosthodontist and oral surgeon), is required prior to initiation of radiotherapy. A team of physicians and nurses should assess oral pain, oral health, and hygiene prior to and during therapy. Dental professionals are vital throughout treatment and during follow-up visits.

Despite the postulated role of infection in the pathogenesis of mucositis, several clinical trials evaluating the use of nonabsorbable antibiotics (polymyxin, tobramycin, and amphotericin B or bacitracin, clotrimazole, and gentamicin) showed no improvement in the incidence or severity of mucositis.[84,85] Topical coating agents such as sucralfate have also proven to be ineffective in reducing the severity of radiation induced mucositis.[86] Use of chlorhexidine mouthwash to alleviate mucositis is discouraged due to increased toxicity during therapy.[87, 88]

Controlling mucositis pain is important to maintain a patient's sense of well-being and minimize the potential for prolongation of therapy. A comprehensive nursing intervention during therapy with prompt changes in pain medication when needed has shown improved pain management.[89] Topical analgesics such as viscous 2% lidocaine provide temporary relief and require frequent administration. Mild mucositis-related discomfort can be treated with "Haddad's Maalox Mixture," which is a

Figure 27.11. Mean pain score during 6 weeks of radiotherapy and 6 weeks of follow-up by site. Pain scale 0 to 10 with 10 being the worst pain possible. (Reprinted from Elting LS, et al. Risk, outcomes, and costs of radiation-induced oral mucositis among patients with head and neck malignancies. *Int J Radiat Oncol Biol Phys.* 2007;1110–1120, with permission.)

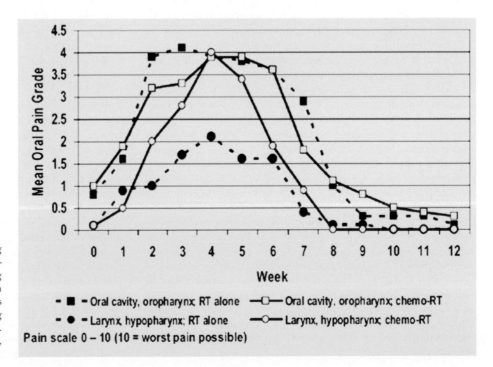

mixture of equal parts 2% viscous lidocaine, diphenhydramine, and magnesium aluminum hydroxide (Maalox). Patients may swish and swallow 10 to 15 mL every 4 to 6 hours, or swish and expectorate more frequently. Morphine sulfate mouthwash is an alternative that has been found to provide more effective pain relief. Morphine sulfate is diluted in water, used as an oral rise for 2 minutes, and then expectorated.[90] Liquid morphine sulfate and oxycodone are common oral pain medications used to treat painful mucositis with fentanyl dermal patches reserved for patients who cannot swallow. Capsaicin lozenges and tricyclic antidepressants have also shown efficacy in pain management as an alternative to patients with contraindications to opioids.[91,92] These alternatives unfortunately have provided mixed results providing only temporary relief with many patients eventually requiring opioids.

Amifostine, an organic thiophosphate, used as a normal tissue protector during radiotherapy, has been studied in the prevention of radiation-induced mucositis. Significant toxicity such as nausea, vomiting, hypotension, and allergic reactions along with questionable efficacy has led to ASCO clinic practice guidelines not recommending amifostine for the prevention of mucositis.[19,21,26,93]

Low-energy He/Ne laser has been studied in the prevention of radiation-induced mucositis in a multicenter phase III randomized study. Grade 3 mucositis was reduced when compared to placebo (light therapy) from 35% to 8%. Grade 3 pain was also reduced from 24% to 2% with control of the pain throughout radiotherapy.[94] Although the results are encouraging, universal application cannot be advocated based upon the results of this small 30-patient trial. Other investigational agents include Palifermin, a recombinant human keratinocyte growth factor, which stimulates the proliferation and differentiation of mucosal epithelium. Given once weekly, Brizel et al. tested the drug in a phase II trial. Although patients were found to have shorter duration of grade 2 or higher mucositis, the difference did not reach statistical significance. The authors acknowledged the limitations of the trial, which included a 12-week cut-off for assessment of mucositis noting that nearly 50% of the patients continued to have mucositis beyond 12 weeks post therapy. In addition, grading of mucositis was not standardized among the 18 institutions that participated in the study.[95] Benzydamine oral rinse is a topical agent with analgesic, antimicrobial, and anti-inflammatory activity that has shown encouraging results in a double-blind, placebo-controlled trial with reduction in erythema and ulceration by 30% compared to placebo.[96] However, this drug is not approved for use in United States at this time. Other experimental agents that have shown promising results in small clinical trials include IV L-alanyl-L-glutamine, oral zinc sulfate, alpha-tocopherol, and recombinant human epidermal growth factor.[97–99] Their role in the treatment of mucositis is uncertain until confirmatory trials support their use. An example of a promising drug that later proved to be ineffective in reducing mucositis is granulocyte-macrophage colony stimulating factor (GM-CSF). Delivered topically or subcutaneously, the drug initially showed promising results in pilot studies.[100,101] Subsequent clinical trials have shown no evidence that GM-CSF reduces the severity of radiation-induced mucositis.[102–104] A phase III clinical trial suggested that there may be a slight advantage in reducing oral mucositis pain by delivering the dose of radiation therapy in the morning as opposed to the evening based on the circadian rhythm of the cell cycle of normal mucosal cells.[105]

Modern radiation tools can also assist in reducing the severity of mucositis. The volume of normal tissue within the planning target volume can be reduced significantly using image-guided treatment planning, conformal radiation therapy, and devices to exclude uninvolved tissues from the planning target volume.[106] Intraoral stents are useful in excluding mucosa in the oral cavity. For example, an intraoral stent will support and move the hard palate and a portion of the buccal mucosa away from the irradiated tissue in patients with floor of mouth, oral tongue, or mandibular gingival cancer. The same stent can also move the tongue and floor of mouth away from the planning target volume in patients with hard palate, nasal cavity, or paranasal sinus cancers. Moistened dental rolls placed between dental amalgam and mucosa will reduce electron scatter in the mucosa and lessen the degree of mucositis. This can also be accomplished with use of dental trays during treatment, which can separate the tongue and buccal mucosa from the amalgam. Lastly, IMRT with dose constraints on the mucosa can significantly reduce the dose to the mucosa outside the planning target volume.[107] Placing oral cavity constraints during the IMRT planning process will significantly reduce mean dose to the mucosa of the oral cavity and minimize "hot spots" within the normal tissue outside the target volume.

Mucositis and its associated pain have a great impact on a patient's quality of life during and after radiotherapy. There is currently no standard effective preventative or therapeutic treatment. The treating physician should follow a model similar to Janjan et al. in which a team of radiation therapy nurses and physicians intervene frequently on an as-needed basis in dispensing appropriate pain medications and laxatives, monitoring oral intake, and evaluating the well-being of the patient throughout their treatment.[89] Oral health should be evaluated by a comprehensive team including dental professionals. The radiation oncologist should monitor the oral health at least once a week during treatment.

LARYNX

Radiotherapy has been proven to be a safe and effective treatment for both advanced- and early-stage larynx cancer. Multiple clinical trials have proven the efficacy of chemoradiotherapy in preserving the larynx.[58,108,109] Although larynx preservation rates are over 80% with concurrent chemoradiotherapy, limited information exists from these prospective trials regarding the functional status of the larynx in terms of speech, swallowing, and respiration. Emphasis has been placed on laryngectomy free and overall survival rates. A small study by Carrara-de Angelis et al.[110] reported moderate to severe dysphonia in 10 of 15 patients who underwent larynx preservation with concurrent chemoradiotherapy. In a long-term follow-up quality-of-life survey of patients enrolled in the randomized VA Laryngeal Cancer Study, patients with an intact larynx had better quality-of-life scores in the mental health domain and better head and neck quality of life (HNQOL) pain scores than patients undergoing a total laryngectomy. Surprisingly, speech scores were similar for the total laryngectomy and the induction chemotherapy and radiotherapy patients, leading the authors to question if patients undergoing larynx preserving nonsurgical treatment have substantial problems with voice or if the total laryngectomy patients adapt to an artificial voice. The authors recognized the limitations of this study with the small sample size. Over one third of the patients either did not complete the survey or could

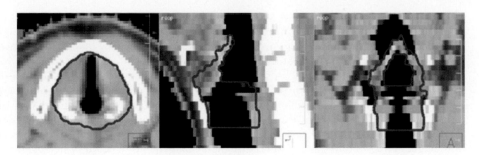

Figure 27.12. Larynx delineation as defined by Sanguineti et al. (Reprinted from Sanguineti et al. Dosimetric predictors of laryngeal edema. *Int J Radiat Oncol Biol Phys.* 2007;68:741–749, with permission.)

not be reached leading to potential selection bias.[111] However, when function was measured as intelligibility of speech, reading rate, and Communication Profile, patients with larynx preservation displayed the highest scores for all three measures. These patients also required less voice and speech therapy. In contrast, there were few significant differences between treatment groups in terms of swallowing and eating-related function. Patients with laryngeal preservation did have significantly better taste function but more dry mouth. Finally, there was no difference in employment status.[111] Thus, limited information exists on the functional outcome of patients who undergo larynx-preserving radiotherapy for locally advanced larynx cancer.

There are multiple treatment options available for early stage larynx cancer with definitive radiotherapy having excellent local control and voice quality compared to cordectomy or partial laryngectomy.[111–114] Fifty percent of patients who have poor voice quality prior to radiotherapy have voice characteristics comparable to noncancer patients following definitive radiotherapy for early glottic cancer. Patients should be advised to quit smoking and avoid vocal cord stripping as these factors are associated with worse voice quality after radiotherapy.[115] Severe complications defined as laryngectomy or permanent tracheostomy occur in only 1% of early glottic cancer patients treated with definitive radiotherapy.[113]

Reducing dose to the larynx improves speech and quality of life. Dornfeld et al. reviewed twenty-seven eligible cancer-free patients treated with IMRT who completed pretreatment and 1 year posttreatment diet and speech-related quality-of-life surveys. All dosimetric data were evaluated with patient quality-of-life scores. The authors observed a steep decline in speech-related quality-of-life score when the aryepiglottic folds, pre-epiglottic space, false cords, and lateral pharyngeal walls at the level of the vocal cords received a dose above 66 Gy.[42] In a review of 66 patients with head and neck cancers without laryngeal involvement, Sanguineti et al. observed a significant correlation between dose and volume of the larynx irradiated and grade 2 or higher edema. The larynx was defined as the soft tissue within the external cartilaginous framework as seen in Figure 27.12. Using the toxicity criteria defined by RTOG, grade 2 edema is defined as diffuse asymptomatic edema of the larynx.[116] Multivariate analysis found that the risk of grade 2 or higher laryngeal edema was correlated with the mean laryngeal dose, neck stage, and V_{50} of the larynx. For each 1% of laryngeal volume that received more than 50 Gy, there was a 3% increase in the rate of grade 2 or higher edema using 2 Gy/fraction. The lowest risk was found when the mean laryngeal dose was <43.5 Gy and the V_{50} was <27% (Fig. 27.13).[117] Rancati et al. found that both the Lyman and the Logit NTCP models fit their clinical data well for predicting RTOG grade 2 and 3 subacute/late laryngeal edema. A clear volume effect was found, consistent with a parallel architecture of the larynx. An equivalent

uniform dose <30 to 35 Gy was associated with a ≤10% risk of grade 2 and 3 laryngeal edema.[118]

Laryngeal edema can be persistent for many months. This requires close follow-up, as persistent or recurrent tumor may mask itself as radiation-related edema. Patients with laryngeal edema that worsens over time may require serial imaging and eventually a biopsy. Dexamethasone can be used to reduce radiation-induced edema. This can be combined with broad spectrum antibiotics if infection is suspected.

Less than 1% of patients will develop cartilage necrosis secondary to radiotherapy. Chondronecrosis often presents as pain, worsening voice quality, and edema, and can mimic recurrent tumor. Serial imaging and biopsy should be considered. Once necrosis has been established, a functioning larynx can be salvaged with hyperbaric oxygen.[119,120]

THYROID

Radiation-induced hypothyroidism can be centrally mediated through damage to the hypothalamic-pituitary axis or by damage to the thyroid gland itself. The incidence of radiation-induced hypothyroidism ranges from 14% to 67% in various reported series.[121,122] The wide range in incidence is in part due to heterogeneity in radiation dose and different follow-up

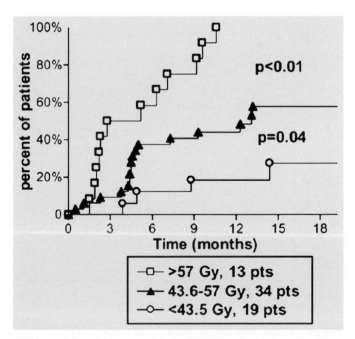

Figure 27.13. Mean dose to the larynx and percentage of patients with grade 2 or higher larynx edema. (Reprinted from Sanguineti et al. Dosimetric predictors of laryngeal edema. *Int J Radiat Oncol Biol Phys.* 2007;68:741–749, with permission.)

periods in each published series. Many series also included patients who also had surgical intervention. In addition, the definition of hypothyroidism varies from institution to institution with different threshold levels of thyroid stimulating hormone (TSH) and/or free T4.

Clinical manifestations of hypothyroidism are attributed to either the slowing of metabolic processes or the accumulation of matrix glycosaminoglycans in tissues. This can lead to depression, cold intolerance, weight gain, dry skin, hair loss, and fatigue. Physical findings include coarse hair, enlargement of the tongue, and dry skin. Thyroid function should be monitored in all patients who have received radiotherapy to the neck and/or skull base. Measuring serum TSH and free T4 will differentiate patients with central versus primary hypothyroidism. Primary hypothyroidism is caused by damage to the thyroid gland resulting in low serum free T4 with high serum TSH. Patients can also have subclinical hypothyroidism where there is high serum TSH with normal free T4. Secondary hypothyroidism is caused by damage to the pituitary-hypothalamic axis resulting in low serum free T4 and TSH.

In the absence of clinical symptoms, serum TSH and T4 levels may be checked every 6 months for the first 2 years after treatment and then annually as long as the levels are within normal limits. The time course for radiation-induced hypothyroidism is highly variable with a median time of 1.5 to 2 years in many series.[121-123] Patients will need lifelong testing as the incidence of hypothyroidism continues to increase with time. In a review of 147 patients at Queen Mary Hospital in Hong Kong who underwent laryngectomy and preoperative or postoperative radiotherapy for laryngeal carcinoma, the rate of hypothyroidism increased from 20% at 3 years to 93% at 10 years post therapy (Fig. 27.14).[124] With a median follow-up of 4.2 years, Tell et al. found that patients who also had surgery involving the thyroid gland in addition to radiotherapy had an increase in the incidence of hypothyroidism from 11%

to 41%. Similar to the Queen Mary series, patients receiving radiotherapy with or without surgery had a gradually increasing incidence of hypothyroidism with time from 7% at 1 year to 27% at 10 years after treatment. Of note, only 34 out of 308 patients in Tell's series had surgery involving the thyroid gland, which may explain the lower incidence of hypothyroidism compared to the Queen Mary series.[123]

Combined modality therapy with surgery and radiotherapy appears to result in a higher incidence of hypothyroidism. In a study of head and neck cancer patients by Cetinayak et al. with follow-up ranging from 25 to 44 months depending on the subgroup, 3% of patients had thyroid dysfunction postoperatively prior to radiotherapy. Following postoperative radiotherapy, the incidence increased to 12%. No patient who received definitive radiotherapy developed hypothyroidism during the follow-up period.[125] The incidence of hypothyroidism may vary based on the extent of thyroid gland removed prior to radiotherapy. With partial thyroidectomy for benign conditions, patients have a risk of hypothyroidism ranging from 18% to 35%.[126-129] Among patients with a portion of their thyroid gland removed, having a small thyroid remnant and higher thyroperoxidase antibody serum levels is associated with a higher incidence of hypothyroidism.[129] As previously mentioned, as high as 93% of patients who undergo total laryngectomy and radiotherapy may develop hypothyroidism 10 years after treatment.[124] The mean time to onset of hypothyroidism after laryngectomy and radiotherapy is earlier than after definitive radiotherapy alone. Onset is seen at 6 months with nearly half of the patients having hypothyroidism within 3 years following treatment. Factors associated with increased rates include (a) total laryngectomy, (b) extensive neck dissection, (c) dose to the remaining thyroid gland, and 4) presence of thyroiditis in the surgical specimen.[130]

There is suggestion of a dose-response relationship with the pituitary-hypothalamic axis and the thyroid gland. Bhandare et al. reported a 16% increase in the rate of primary hypothyroidism at 5 years when the dose to the thyroid gland increased beyond 45 Gy (Fig. 27.15). The authors also reported that the total dose to the thyroid gland was the only predictor for hypothyroidism on multivariate analysis.[131] The same authors did

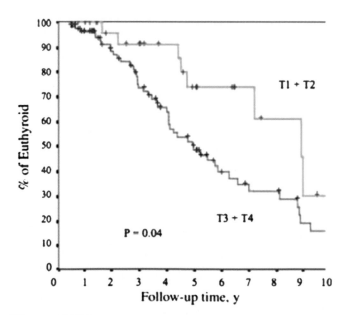

Figure 27.14. Posttherapy follow-up for T1-4 larynx carcinoma. Probability of developing hypothyroidism from the time of surgery. (Reprinted from Ho et al. Thyroid dysfunction in laryngectomees: 10 year after treatment. *Int J Radiat Oncol Biol Phys.* 2008;30:336–340, with permission.)

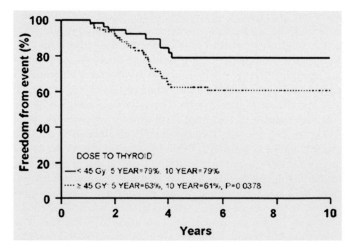

Figure 27.15. Estimate of freedom from central hypothyroidism based on dose <45 Gy and ≥45 Gy. (Reprinted from Bhandare et al. Primary and central hypothyroidism after radiotherapy for head and neck tumors. *Int J Radiat Oncol Biol Phys.* 2007;68(4):1131–1139, with permission.)

not find the total dose to affect the pituitary-hypothalamic axis on multivariate analysis. On the contrary, researchers from the proton facility at Massachusetts General Hospital found a dose-response relationship with patients treated with proton beam radiotherapy to the skull base. The 5- and 10-year rate of central hypothyroidism was 30% and 63% with no patients developing hypothyroidism if they received a maximum dose (D_{max}) to the entire pituitary gland <50 GyE. A limitation of this study is that only 12 of the 95 patients evaluated for central hypothyroidism received a dose <50 GyE.[132] Authors at St. Jude's hospital reported that hypothyroidism rates increased from 11% to 44% when the dose to the hypothalamic-pituitary axis increased above 42 Gy in children treated with craniospinal axis radiotherapy followed by boost radiotherapy for embryonal brain tumors.[133]

With modern radiotherapy techniques, physicians may be able to lower the dose to the thyroid gland compared to more traditional methods. A study by Vanderbilt University reported a higher dose to the thyroid gland with an IMRT plan that had no dose constraints on the dose to the thyroid gland compared to 3D conformal radiotherapy. This effect is reversed when dose constraints are used for the thyroid gland with reduced dose to the gland achievable with an IMRT plan.[134]

Once a patient is diagnosed with hypothyroidism, the free T4 and TSH will assist in determining central versus primary hypothyroidism. Patients suspected of central hypothyroidism present with low free T4 with low to normal levels of TSH as the hypothalamus-pituitary cannot compensate for the low thyroid hormone level. These patients should be approached with caution as patients with radiation-induced central hypopituitarism are also predisposed for other endocrinopathy. Referral to an endocrinologist may be warranted as supplementing T4 can lead to acute adrenal crisis due to adrenal insufficiency. Pituitary-adrenal function needs to be tested prior to initiating supplements usually with a Cortrosyn stimulation test. Patients with central hypothyroidism require T4 supplementation and are monitored clinically and with serum T4 levels.

Patients with primary hypothyroidism will present with high serum TSH levels with either normal to low serum free T4 levels. Patients with subclinical hypothyroidism should be treated to prevent progression to overt hypothyroidism. Radiation-induced hypothyroidism is usually a permanent condition that will require lifelong supplementation. It is recommended that patients be referred to either a primary care provider or an endocrinologist when hypothyroidism is discovered as multiple factors can affect serum T4 levels including diet and medications. In addition, patients will require periodic monitoring based on ongoing changes in thyroid function and with changes in their medications and general health.

AUDITORY SYSTEM

Toxicities to the auditory system can be broken down into effects on the external, middle, and inner ear. The external ear consists of the auricle and external auditory canal. Radiotherapy complications include acute and chronic otitis externa as well as canal stenosis. Symptoms of otitis externa include pain, pruritus, otorrhea, erythema, edema, and scaling. Patients who receive chemotherapy and high-dose radiotherapy to the external ear have an increased risk of acute and chronic otitis externa. Canal stenosis and atrophy are more dependent on fraction size.[135]

The middle ear space is an air-filled compartment containing the ossicles and is in continuity with the mastoid air cells. Radiotherapy to these structures can cause otitis media, mastoiditis, fibrosis, perforation of the tympanic membrane, and chorda tympani dysfunction. Higher dose to the mastoid and middle ear structures increases the incidence of these complications.[135] Otitis media develops as a result of mucosal vasodilation and eustachian tube dysfunction and can lead to conductive hearing loss. Analysis of 40 nasopharyngeal cancers patients in Shanghai, China, found a dose relationship between dose to the eustachian tube isthmus and middle ear cavity and the development of otitis media with effusion (Fig. 27.16). Patients underwent pure tone and impedance audiometry tests before and after radiotherapy. Investigators found that audiometry results worsened significantly with dose over 52 Gy to the eustachian tube isthmus and 46 Gy to the middle ear cavity.[136] Patients with these complications should be referred to a specialist otolaryngologist for management. Treatment options include observation, myringotomy with aspiration, or myringotomy with ventilation tube placement.

The inner ear comprises the cochlea and vestibular organs (Fig. 27.17). Damage to these structures can cause sensorineural hearing loss (SNHL), tinnitus, and vertigo. Vertigo results from high doses to the vestibular labyrinth causing labyrinthitis. These effects are increased with the addition of chemotherapy.

Radiation-induced hearing loss includes sensorineural, conductive, and mixed hearing loss (a combination of conductive and SNHL).[137] Conductive hearing loss results from middle ear fluid, tympanic membrane abnormalities, and problems with the ossicular chain.[138] SNHL results from damage to the cochlea or auditory nerve. The incidence increases with age

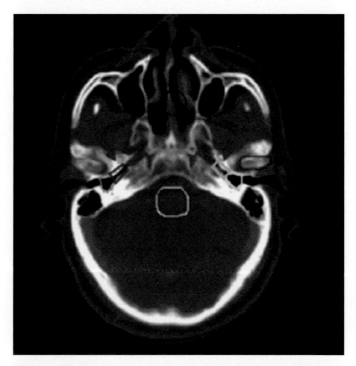

Figure 27.16. Contour of the middle ear cavity and isthmus of the Eustachian tube (*arrow*). (Reprinted from Wang et al. Analysis of anatomical factors controlling the morbidity of radiation-induced otitis media with effusion. *Radiother Oncol.* 2007;85:463–468, with permission.)

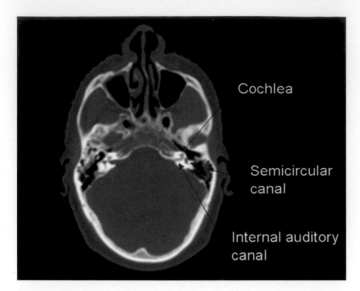

Figure 27.17. Treatment planning CT scan (bone window) illustrating location of cochlea, semicircular canal, and internal auditory canal.

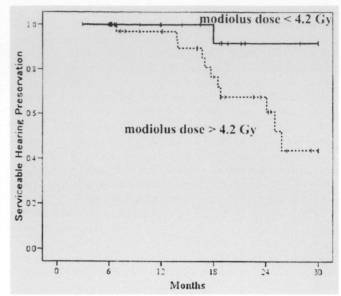

Figure 27.18. Maintenance of serviceable hearing and dose to the middle of the cochlea with single fraction gamma knife radiosurgery in patients <60 years old with an acoustic neuroma. (Reprinted from Kano et al. Predictors of hearing preservation after stereotactic radiosurgery for acoustic neuroma. *J Neurosurg.* 2009;111:863–873, with permission.)

and loud noise exposure. Mixed hearing loss can be caused by a combination of radiation damage to the middle ear structures either directly or by chronic processes such as fluid accumulation and damage to the nerve or cochlea.

In radiotherapy patients, the incidence of SNHL increases with increasing dose to the inner ear, combined chemotherapy with cisplatin, preexisting hearing loss, and advanced age of the patient.[139–141] In a University of Florida series, 37% of patients who received above 60.5 Gy to the cochlea had clinically overt hearing loss compared with 3% at doses below 60.5 Gy.[135] This dose constraint appears be generous as Van der Putten et al. observed asymmetric hearing loss in parotid cancer patients when doses to the cochlea and eustachian tube exceeded 50 Gy and Lee et al. observed increased hearing deficits in nasopharyngeal cancer patients when the cochlea dose exceeded 50 Gy.[142,143] The average latency for persistent SNHL was 1.8 years in this series. In fractionated radiotherapy series of children with gliomas, the incidence of SNHL increased significantly when the cochlea received >40 to 45 Gy compared to doses <30 Gy.[144] Calculated single dose thresholds for the cochlea and hearing preservation appear to be around 4 to 5.33 Gy. Massager and colleagues reported on acoustic neuroma patients who had stable or improved hearing after gamma knife radiosurgery with a median dose of 3.7 Gy and worsened hearing with 5.33 Gy to the cochlea.[145] Authors at the University of Pittsburgh recommended 4.2 Gy or less to the cochlea as serviceable hearing dropped significantly above this dose (Fig. 27.18).[146]

Cisplatin, an alkylating agent, and radiotherapy cause various forms of damage to the cochlea. These include atrophy of the stria vascularis, diminished spiral ganglion, and loss of inner and outer hair cells.[147,148] Thus, patients who undergo concurrent cisplatin and radiotherapy have synergistic effects on the hearing apparatus with more pronounced SNHL. Amifostine has been suggested to protect against ototoxicity in children with medulloblastoma who are treated with craniospinal radiotherapy and cisplatin. Grade 3 ototoxicity was decreased from 37% to 14.5% in a St. Jude study of 97 patients when amifostine was given twice daily during cisplatin infusion suggesting

a protective affect from the ototoxic effects of cisplatinum.[149] In another hypothesis generating study, Zurr and colleagues conducted a prospective phase III study on the affects of intra-arterial (IA) cisplatin compared to intravenous (IV) cisplatin concomitant with radiotherapy in patients with head and neck cancer. Patients who received IA cisplatin had approximately 10% less hearing loss at speech perception frequencies compared to the IV group. Of note, the median radiotherapy dose to the inner ear was 16.3 Gy in the IV chemoradiation group versus 10.8 Gy ($p < 0.05$) in the IA group suggesting the possibility that radiotherapy dose plays an important role as well.[150] Chan et al. reported that patients with nasopharyngeal cancer treated with either radiotherapy or chemoradiotherapy with cisplatin would have <15% risk of SNHL (≥15 dB loss) if the mean dose to the cochlea was reduced to <47 Gy. Authors used audiometric testing pretherapy and posttherapy at 6-month intervals and evaluated the effects of cisplatin dose and radiotherapy dose on the probability of SNHL (Fig. 27.19).[151] Another prospective study by investigators at the University of Utah reported dramatic affects of adding cisplatin to radiotherapy patients. There were 62 patients studied with pretreatment and posttreatment audiograms. Patients who received radiotherapy alone had no significant hearing loss when the cochlea dose was <40 Gy. This rose to +38.4 and +18.5 dB hearing loss when 100 and 40 mg/m² of cisplatin were added to radiotherapy, respectively. Their model predicts the threshold for hearing loss when patients receive cisplatin and radiotherapy to be 10 Gy.[152] In the event of total hearing loss, cochlear implantation in patients who have received radiotherapy is feasible as reported by Low et al.[153]

With use of IMRT or proton radiotherapy, the risk of acute and chronic adverse radiation affects on the auditory system can be reduced. By creating an avoidance structure that encompasses the external, middle, and inner ear, one can lower the dose and reduce the risk of sensorineural and/or conductive hearing loss.[154–157]

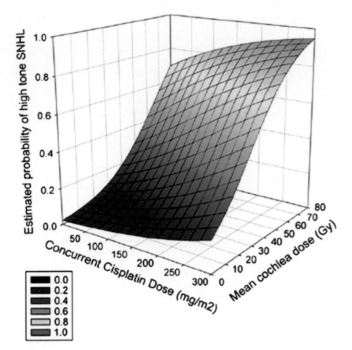

Figure 27.19. Relationship between probability of SNHL, concurrent cisplatin dose, and mean cochlea dose. (Reprinted from Chan et al. Sensorineural hearing loss after nasopharyngeal carcinoma: longitudinal analysis. *Int J Radiat Oncol Biol Phys.* 2009;73(5):1335–1342, with permission.)

CONCLUSION

Radiotherapy to the head and neck region is both challenging and rewarding. It is challenging due to the variety of normal organs and tissues in this region with differing degrees of radiation sensitivity all of which are interrelated, integrated, and coordinated to provide complex functions important to life and quality of life. The risk for severe acute toxicity and late complications with loss of function is high. However, the rewards are long-term survival with good function and meaningful quality of life, which can be achieved in many patients using patient immobilization devices, current imaging modalities, and treatment planning systems; meticulous attention to detail when defining and contouring GTV, CTV, PTV, and OAR (which requires a strong foundation in anatomy); strict treatment QA; and current treatment delivery systems that include image guidance and adaptive therapy.

REFERENCES

1. Elting LS, Cooksley CD, Chambers MS, et al. Risk, outcomes, and costs of radiation-induced oral mucositis among patients with head-and-neck malignancies. *Int J Radiat Oncol Biol Phys.* 2007;68(4):1110–1120.
2. Mirza N, Machtay M, Devine PA, et al. Gustatory impairment in patients undergoing head and neck irradiation. *Laryngoscope.* 2008;118(1):24–31.
3. Yamashita H, Nakagawa K, Tago M, et al. Taste dysfunction in patients receiving radiotherapy. *Head Neck.* 2006;28(6):508–516.
4. Yamashita H, Nakagawa K, Nakamura N, et al. Relation between acute and late irradiation impairment of four basic tastes and irradiated tongue volume in patients with head-and-neck cancer. *Int J Radiat Oncol Biol Phys.* 2006;66(5):1422–149.
5. Fernando IN, Patel T, Billingham L, et al. The effect of head and neck irradiation on taste dysfunction: a prospective study. *Clin Oncol (R Coll Radiol).* 1995;7(3):173–178.
6. Braam PM, Roesink JM, Moerland MA, et al. Long-term parotid gland function after radiotherapy. *Int J Radiat Oncol Biol Phys.* 2005;62(3):659–664.
7. Blanco AI, Chao KS, El Naqa I, et al. Dose-volume modeling of salivary function in patients with head-and-neck cancer receiving radiotherapy. *Int J Radiat Oncol Biol Phys.* 2005;62(4):1055–1069.

8. Li Y, Taylor JM, Ten Haken RK, et al. The impact of dose on parotid salivary recovery in head and neck cancer patients treated with radiation therapy. *Int J Radiat Oncol Biol Phys.* 2007;67(3):660–669.
9. Murdoch-Kinch CA, Kim HM, Vineberg KA, et al. Dose-effect relationships for the submandibular salivary glands and implications for their sparing by intensity modulated radiotherapy. *Int J Radiat Oncol Biol Phys.* 2008;72(2):373–382.
10. Jellema AP, Slotman BJ, Doornaert P, et al. Impact of radiation-induced xerostomia on quality of life after primary radiotherapy among patients with head and neck cancer. *Int J Radiat Oncol Biol Phys.* 2007;69(3):751–760.
11. Meirovitz A, Murdoch-Kinch CA, Schipper M, et al. Grading xerostomia by physicians or by patients after intensity-modulated radiotherapy of head-and-neck cancer. *Int J Radiat Oncol Biol Phys.* 2006;66(2):445–453.
12. Braam PM, Terhaard CH, Roesink JM, et al. Intensity-modulated radiotherapy significantly reduces xerostomia compared with conventional radiotherapy. *Int J Radiat Oncol Biol Phys.* 2006;66(4):975–980.
13. Pow EH, Kwong DL, McMillan AS, et al. Xerostomia and quality of life after intensity-modulated radiotherapy vs. conventional radiotherapy for early-stage nasopharyngeal carcinoma: initial report on a randomized controlled clinical trial. *Int J Radiat Oncol Biol Phys.* 2006;66(4):981–991.
14. Daly ME, Lieskovsky Y, Pawlicki T, et al. Evaluation of patterns of failure and subjective salivary function in patients treated with intensity modulated radiotherapy for head and neck squamous cell carcinoma. *Head Neck.* 2007;29(3):211–220.
15. Liu WS, Kuo HC, Lin JC, et al. Assessment of salivary function change in nasopharyngeal carcinoma treated by parotid-sparing radiotherapy. *Cancer J.* 2006;12(6):494–500.
16. Graff P, Lapeyre M, Desandes E, et al. Impact of intensity-modulated radiotherapy on health-related quality of life for head and neck cancer patients: matched-pair comparison with conventional radiotherapy. *Int J Radiat Oncol Biol Phys.* 2007;67(5):1309–1317.
17. McMillan AS, Pow EH, Kwong DL, et al. Preservation of quality of life after intensity-modulated radiotherapy for early-stage nasopharyngeal carcinoma: results of a prospective longitudinal study. *Head Neck.* 2006;28(8):712–722.
18. Portaluri M, Fucilli FI, Castagna R, et al. Three-dimensional conformal radiotherapy for locally advanced (Stage II and worse) head-and-neck cancer: dosimetric and clinical evaluation. *Int J Radiat Oncol Biol Phys.* 2006;66(4):1036–1043.
19. Antonadou D, Pepelassi M, Synodinou M, et al. Prophylactic use of amifostine to prevent radiochemotherapy-induced mucositis and xerostomia in head-and-neck cancer. *Int J Radiat Oncol Biol Phys.* 2002;52(3):739–747.
20. Jellema AP, Slotman BJ, Muller MJ, et al. Radiotherapy alone, versus radiotherapy with amifostine 3 times weekly, versus radiotherapy with amifostine 5 times weekly: a prospective randomized study in squamous cell head and neck cancer. *Cancer.* 2006;107(3):544–553.
21. Brizel DM, Wasserman TH, Henke M, et al. Phase III randomized trial of amifostine as a radioprotector in head and neck cancer. *J Clin Oncol.* 2000;18(19):3339–3345.
22. Buntzel J, Kuttner K, Frohlich D, et al. Selective cytoprotection with amifostine in concurrent radiochemotherapy for head and neck cancer. *Ann Oncol.* 1998;9(5):505–509.
23. Sasse AD, Clark LG, Sasse EC, et al. Amifostine reduces side effects and improves complete response rate during radiotherapy: results of a meta-analysis. *Int J Radiat Oncol Biol Phys.* 2006;64(3):784–791.
24. Wasserman TH, Brizel DM, Henke M, et al. Influence of intravenous amifostine on xerostomia, tumor control, and survival after radiotherapy for head-and- neck cancer: 2-year follow-up of a prospective, randomized, phase III trial. *Int J Radiat Oncol Biol Phys.* 2005;63(4):985–990.
25. Munter MW, Hoffner S, Hof H, et al. Changes in salivary gland function after radiotherapy of head and neck tumors measured by quantitative pertechnetate scintigraphy: comparison of intensity-modulated radiotherapy and conventional radiation therapy with and without Amifostine. *Int J Radiat Oncol Biol Phys.* 2007;67(3):651–659.
26. Buentzel J, Micke O, Adamietz IA, et al. Intravenous amifostine during chemoradiotherapy for head-and-neck cancer: a randomized placebo-controlled phase III study. *Int J Radiat Oncol Biol Phys.* 2006;64(3):684–691.
27. Anné PR, Machtay M, Rosenthal DI, et al. A phase II trial of subcutaneous amifostine and radiation therapy in patients with head-and-neck cancer. *Int J Radiat Oncol Biol Phys.* 2007;67(2):445–452.
28. Hamlar DD, Schuller DE, Gahbauer RA, et al. Determination of the efficacy of topical oral pilocarpine for postirradiation xerostomia in patients with head and neck carcinoma. *Laryngoscope.* 1996;106(8):972–976.
29. Zimmerman RP, Mark RJ, Tran LM, et al. Concomitant pilocarpine during head and neck irradiation is associated with decreased posttreatment xerostomia. *Int J Radiat Oncol Biol Phys.* 1997;37(3):571–575.
30. Valdez IH, Wolff A, Atkinson JC, et al. Use of pilocarpine during head and neck radiation therapy to reduce xerostomia and salivary dysfunction. *Cancer.* 1993;71(5):1848–1851.
31. Haddad P, Karimi M. A randomized, double-blind, placebo-controlled trial of concomitant pilocarpine with head and neck irradiation for prevention of radiation-induced xerostomia. *Radiother Oncol.* 2002;64(1):29–32.
32. Warde P, O'Sullivan B, Aslanidis J, et al. A phase III placebo-controlled trial of oral pilocarpine in patients undergoing radiotherapy for head-and-neck cancer. *Int J Radiat Oncol Biol Phys.* 2002;54(1):9–13.
33. Scarantino C, LeVeque F, Swann RS, et al. Effect of pilocarpine during radiation therapy: results of RTOG 97–09, a phase III randomized study in head and neck cancer patients. *J Support Oncol.* 2006;4(5):252–258.
34. Duke RL, Campbell BH, Indresano AT, et al. Dental status and quality of life in long-term head and neck cancer survivors. *Laryngoscope.* 2005;115(4):678–683.
35. Kaste SC, Goodman P, Leisenring W, et al. Impact of radiation and chemotherapy on risk of dental abnormalities. A report from the Childhood Cancer Survivor Study. *Cancer.* 2009;115:5817–5827.
36. Murray CG, Herson J, Daly TE, et al. Radiation necrosis of the mandible: a 10 year study. Part I. Factors influencing the onset of necrosis. *Int J Radiat Oncol Biol Phys.* 1980;6(5): 543–548.

37. Meraw SJ, Reeve CM. Dental considerations and treatment of the oncology patient receiving radiation therapy. *J Am Dent Assoc.* 1998;129(2):201–205.
38. Wahl MJ. Osteoradionecrosis prevention myths. *Int J Radiat Oncol Biol Phys.* 2006;64(3): 661–669.
39. Marx RE, Johnson RP, Kline SN. Prevention of osteoradionecrosis: a randomized prospective clinical trial of hyperbaric oxygen versus penicillin. *J Am Dent Assoc.* 1985;111(1):49–54.
40. Goldsmith T. Videofluoroscopic evaluation of oropharyngeal swallowing. In: CH, Som PM, eds. *Head and Neck Imaging.* Mosby, 2003:1727–1753.
41. Yao M, Karnell LH, Funk GF, et al. Health-related quality-of-life outcomes following IMRT versus conventional radiotherapy for oropharyngeal squamous cell carcinoma. *Int J Radiat Oncol Biol Phys.* 2007;69(5):1354–1360.
42. Dornfeld K, Simmons JR, Karnell L, et al. Radiation doses to structures within and adjacent to the larynx are correlated with long-term diet- and speech-related quality of life. *Int J Radiat Oncol Biol Phys.* 2007;68(3):750–757.
43. Goguen LA, Posner MR, Norris CM, et al. Dysphagia after sequential chemoradiation therapy for advanced head and neck cancer. *Otolaryngol Head Neck Surg.* 2006;134(6):916–922.
44. Terrell JE, Ronis DL, Fowler KE, et al. Clinical predictors of quality of life in patients with head and neck cancer. *Arch Otolaryngol Head Neck Surg.* 2004;130(4):401–408.
45. Eisbruch A, Lyden T, Bradford CR, et al. Objective assessment of swallowing dysfunction and aspiration after radiation concurrent with chemotherapy for head-and-neck cancer. *Int J Radiat Oncol Biol Phys.* 2002;53(1):23–28.
46. Kotz T, Costello R, Li Y, et al. Swallowing dysfunction after chemoradiation for advanced squamous cell carcinoma of the head and neck. *Head Neck.* 2004;26(4):365–372.
47. Stenson KM, MacCracken E, List M, et al. Swallowing function in patients with head and neck cancer prior to treatment. *Arch Otolaryngol Head Neck Surg.* 2000;126(3):371–377.
48. Langerman A, Maccracken E, Kasza K, et al. Aspiration in chemoradiated patients with head and neck cancer. *Arch Otolaryngol Head Neck Surg* 2007;133(12):1289–1295.
49. Carroll WR, Locher JL, Canon CL, et al. Pretreatment swallowing exercises improve swallow function after chemoradiation. *Laryngoscope.* 2008;118(1):39–43.
50. Kulbersh BD, Rosenthal EL, McGrew BM, et al. Pretreatment, preoperative swallowing exercises may improve dysphagia quality of life. *Laryngoscope.* 2006;116(6):883–886.
51. Smith JE, Suh JD, Erman A, et al. Risk factors predicting aspiration after free flap reconstruction of oral cavity and oropharyngeal defects. *Arch Otolaryngol Head Neck Surg.* 2008;134(11):1205–1208.
52. Eisbruch A, Schwartz M, Rasch C, et al. Dysphagia and aspiration after chemoradiotherapy for head-and-neck cancer: which anatomic structures are affected and can they be spared by IMRT? *Int J Radiat Oncol Biol Phys.* 2004;60(5):1425–1439.
53. Feng FY, Kim HM, Lyden TH, et al. Intensity-modulated radiotherapy of head and neck cancer aiming to reduce dysphagia: early dose-effect relationships for the swallowing structures. *Int J Radiat Oncol Biol Phys.* 2007;68(5):1289–1298.
54. Teguh DN, Levendag PC, Noever I, et al. Treatment techniques and site considerations regarding dysphagia-related quality of life in cancer of the oropharynx and nasopharynx. *Int J Radiat Oncol Biol Phys.* 2008;72(4):1119–1127.
55. Caglar HB, Tishler RB, Othus M, et al. Dose to larynx predicts for swallowing complications after intensity-modulated radiotherapy. *Int J Radiat Oncol Biol Phys.* 2008;72(4): 1110–1118.
56. Fua TF, Corry J, Milner AD, et al. Intensity-modulated radiotherapy for nasopharyngeal carcinoma: clinical correlation of dose to the pharyngo-esophageal axis and dysphagia. *Int J Radiat Oncol Biol Phys.* 2007;67(4):976–981.
57. Caudell JJ, Schaner PE, Desmond RA, et al. Dosimetric factors associated with long-term dysphagia after definitive radiotherapy for squamous cell carcinoma of the head and neck. *Int J Radiat Oncol Biol Phys.* 2010;76(2):403–409.
58. Forastiere AA, Goepfert H, Maor M, et al. Concurrent chemotherapy and radiotherapy for organ preservation in advanced laryngeal cancer. *N Engl J Med.* 2003;349(22):2091–2098.
59. Denis F, Garaud P, Bardet E, et al. Late toxicity results of the GORTEC 94-01 randomized trial comparing radiotherapy with concomitant radiochemotherapy for advanced-stage oropharynx carcinoma: comparison of LENT/SOMA, RTOG/EORTC, and NCI-CTC scoring systems. *Int J Radiat Oncol Biol Phys.* 2003;55(1):93–98.
60. Jaghagen EL, Bodin I, Isberg A. Pharyngeal swallowing dysfunction following treatment for oral and pharyngeal cancer—association with diminished intraoral sensation and discrimination ability. *Head Neck.* 2008;30(10):1344–1351.
61. Logemann JA, Pauloski BR, Rademaker AW, et al. Swallowing disorders in the first year after radiation and chemoradiation. *Head Neck.* 2008;30(2):148–158.
62. Pauloski BR, Rademaker AW, Logemann JA, et al. Relationship between swallow motility disorders on videofluorography and oral intake in patients treated for head and neck cancer with radiotherapy with or without chemotherapy. *Head Neck.* 2006;28(12): 1069–1076.
63. Salama JK, Stenson KM, List MA, et al. Characteristics associated with swallowing changes after concurrent chemotherapy and radiotherapy in patients with head and neck cancer. *Arch Otolaryngol Head Neck Surg.* 2008;134(10):1060–1065.
64. Lee WT, Akst LM, Adelstein DJ, et al. Risk factors for hypopharyngeal/upper esophageal stricture formation after concurrent chemoradiation. *Head Neck.* 2006;28(9):808–812.
65. Lee NY, O'Meara W, Chan K, et al. Concurrent chemotherapy and intensity-modulated radiotherapy for locoregionally advanced laryngeal and hypopharyngeal cancers. *Int J Radiat Oncol Biol Phys.*, 2007;69(2):459–468.
66. Lee NY, de Arruda FF, Puri DR, et al. A comparison of intensity-modulated radiation therapy and concomitant boost radiotherapy in the setting of concurrent chemotherapy for locally advanced oropharyngeal carcinoma. *Int J Radiat Oncol Biol Phys.* 2006;66(4): 966–974.
67. Chen AM, Li B., Jennelle RLS, et al. Late esophageal toxicity after radiation therapy for head and neck cancer. *Head Neck.* 2010;32:178–183
68. Dijkstra PU, Sterken MW, Pater R, et al. Exercise therapy for trismus in head and neck cancer. *Oral Oncol.* 2007;43(4):389–394.
69. Dijkstra PU, Huisman PM, Roodenburg JL, Criteria for trismus in head and neck oncology. *Int J Oral Maxillofac Surg.* 2006;35(4):337–342.
70. Sciubba JJ, Goldenberg D. Oral complications of radiotherapy. *Lancet Oncol.* 2006;7(2): 175–183.
71. Wang CJ, Huang EY, Hsu HC, et al. The degree and time-course assessment of radiation-induced trismus occurring after radiotherapy for nasopharyngeal cancer. *Laryngoscope.* 2005;115(8):1458–1460.
72. Teguh DN, Levendag PC, Voet P, et al. Trismus in patients with oropharyngeal cancer: relationship with dose in structures of mastication apparatus. *Head Neck.* 2008;30(5): 622–630.
73. Hsiung CY, Huang EY, Ting HM, et al. Intensity-modulated radiotherapy for nasopharyngeal carcinoma: the reduction of radiation-induced trismus. *Br J Radiol.* 2008;81(970): 809–814.
74. Delanian S, Balla-Mekias S, Lefaix JL. Striking regression of chronic radiotherapy damage in a clinical trial of combined pentoxifylline and tocopherol. *J Clin Oncol.* 1999;17(10): 3283–3290.
75. Lefaix JL, Delanian S, Vozenin MC, et al. Striking regression of subcutaneous fibrosis induced by high doses of gamma rays using a combination of pentoxifylline and alpha-tocopherol: an experimental study. *Int J Radiat Oncol Biol Phys.* 1999;43(4):839–847.
76. Chiao TB, Lee AJ. Role of pentoxifylline and vitamin E in attenuation of radiation-induced fibrosis. *Ann Pharmacother.* 2005;39(3):516–522.
77. Chua DT, Lo C, Yuen J, et al. A pilot study of pentoxifylline in the treatment of radiation-induced trismus. *Am J Clin Oncol.* 2001;24(4):366–369.
78. Sonis ST, Elting LS, Keefe D. et al. Perspectives on cancer therapy-induced mucosal injury: pathogenesis, measurement, epidemiology, and consequences for patients. *Cancer.* 2004;100(9 suppl):1995–2025.
79. Vera-Llonch M, Oster G, Hagiwara M, et al. Oral mucositis in patients undergoing radiation treatment for head and neck carcinoma. *Cancer.* 2006;106(2):329–336.
80. Withers HR, Peters LJ, Taylor JM, et al. Local control of carcinoma of the tonsil by radiation therapy: an analysis of patterns of fractionation in nine institutions. *Int J Radiat Oncol Biol Phys.* 1995;33(3):549–562.
81. Overgaard J, Hansen HS, Specht L, et al. Five compared with six fractions per week of conventional radiotherapy of squamous-cell carcinoma of head and neck: DAHANCA 6 and 7 randomised controlled trial. *Lancet.* 2003;362(9388):933–940.
82. Dreizen S, Bodey GP, Valdivieso M. Chemotherapy-associated oral infections in adults with solid tumors. *Oral Surg Oral Med Oral Pathol.* 1983;55(2):113–120.
83. Dahiya MC, Redding SW, Dahiya RS, et al. Oropharyngeal candidiasis caused by non-albicans yeast in patients receiving external beam radiotherapy for head-and-neck cancer. *Int J Radiat Oncol Biol Phys.* 2003;57(1):79–83.
84. Stokman MA, Spijkervet FK, Burlage FR, et al. Oral mucositis and selective elimination of oral flora in head and neck cancer patients receiving radiotherapy: a double-blind randomised clinical trial. *Br J Cancer.* 2003;88(7):1012–1016.
85. El-Sayed S, Nabid A, Shelley W, et al. Prophylaxis of radiation-associated mucositis in conventionally treated patients with head and neck cancer: a double-blind, phase III, randomized, controlled trial evaluating the clinical efficacy of an antimicrobial lozenge using a validated mucositis scoring system. *J Clin Oncol.* 2002;20(19):3956–3963.
86. Dodd MJ, Miaskowski C, Greenspan D, et al. Radiation-induced mucositis: a randomized clinical trial of micronized sucralfate versus salt & soda mouthwashes. *Cancer Invest.* 2003;21(1):21–33.
87. Foote RL, Loprinzi CL, Frank AR, et al. Randomized trial of a chlorhexidine mouthwash for alleviation of radiation-induced mucositis. *J Clin Oncol.* 1994;12(12):2630–2633.
88. Okuno SH, Foote RL, Loprinzi CL, et al. A randomized trial of a nonabsorbable antibiotic lozenge given to alleviate radiation-induced mucositis. *Cancer.* 1997;79(11):2193–2199.
89. Janjan NA, Weissman DE, Pahule A. Improved pain management with daily nursing intervention during radiation therapy for head and neck carcinoma. *Int J Radiat Oncol Biol Phys.* 1992;23(3):647–652.
90. Cerchietti LC, Navigante AH, Bonomi MR, et al. Effect of topical morphine for mucositis-associated pain following concomitant chemoradiotherapy for head and neck carcinoma. *Cancer.* 2002;95(10):2230–2236.
91. Ehrnrooth E, Grau C, Zachariae R, et al. Randomized trial of opioids versus tricyclic antidepressants for radiation-induced mucositis pain in head and neck cancer. *Acta Oncol.* 2001;40(6):745–750.
92. Berger A, Henderson M, Nadoolman W, et al. Oral capsaicin provides temporary relief for oral mucositis pain secondary to chemotherapy/radiation therapy. *J Pain Symptom Manage.* 1995;10(3):243–248.
93. Hensley ML, Hagerty KL, Kewalramani T, et al. American Society of Clinical Oncology 2008 clinical practice guideline update: use of chemotherapy and radiation therapy protectants. *J Clin Oncol.* 2009;27(1):127–145.
94. Bensadoun RJ, Franquin JC, Ciais G, et al. Low-energy He/Ne laser in the prevention of radiation-induced mucositis. A multicenter phase III randomized study in patients with head and neck cancer. *Support Care Cancer.* 1999;7(4):244–252.
95. Brizel DM, Murphy BA, Rosenthal DI, et al. Phase II study of palifermin and concurrent chemoradiation in head and neck squamous cell carcinoma. *J Clin Oncol.* 2008;26(15): 2489–2496.
96. Epstein JB, Silverman S Jr, Paggiarino DA, et al. Benzydamine HCl for prophylaxis of radiation-induced oral mucositis: results from a multicenter, randomized, double-blind, placebo-controlled clinical trial. *Cancer.* 2001;92(4):875–885.
97. Cerchietti LC, Navigante AH, Lutteral MA, et al. Double-blinded, placebo-controlled trial on intravenous L-alanyl-L-glutamine in the incidence of oral mucositis following chemoradiotherapy in patients with head-and-neck cancer. *Int J Radiat Oncol Biol Phys.* 2006;65(5):1330–1337.
98. Ertekin MV, Koc M, Karslioglu I, et al. Zinc sulfate in the prevention of radiation-induced oropharyngeal mucositis: a prospective, placebo-controlled, randomized study. *Int J Radiat Oncol Biol Phys.* 2004;58(1):167–174.
99. Ferreira PR, Fleck JF, Diehl A, et al. Protective effect of alpha-tocopherol in head and neck cancer radiation-induced mucositis: a double-blind randomized trial. *Head Neck.* 2004;26(4):313–321.

100. Nicolatou O, Sotiropoulou-Lontou A, Skarlatos J, et al. A pilot study of the effect of granulocyte-macrophage colony-stimulating factor on oral mucositis in head and neck cancer patients during X-radiation therapy: a preliminary report. *Int J Radiat Oncol Biol Phys.* 1998;42(3):551–556.

101. Rovirosa A, Ferre J, Biete A. Granulocyte macrophage-colony-stimulating factor mouth-washes heal oral ulcers during head and neck radiotherapy. *Int J Radiat Oncol Biol Phys.* 1998;41(4):747–754.

102. Makkonen TA, Minn H, Jekunen A, et al. Granulocyte macrophage-colony stimulating factor (GM-CSF) and sucralfate in prevention of radiation-induced mucositis: a prospective randomized study. *Int J Radiat Oncol Biol Phys.* 2000;46(3):525–534.

103. Sprinzl GM, Galvan O, de Vries A, et al. Local application of granulocyte-macrophage colony stimulating factor (GM-CSF) for the treatment of oral mucositis. *Eur J Cancer.* 2001;37(16):2003–2009.

104. Ryu JK, Swann S, LeVeque F, et al. The impact of concurrent granulocyte macrophage-colony stimulating factor on radiation-induced mucositis in head and neck cancer patients: a double-blind placebo-controlled prospective phase III study by Radiation Therapy Oncology Group 9901. *Int J Radiat Oncol Biol Phys.* 2007;67(3):643–650.

105. Goyal M, Shukla P, Gupta D, et al. Oral mucositis in morning vs. evening irradiated patients: a randomised prospective study. *Int J Radiat Biol.* 2009;85(6):504–509.

106. Kaanders JH, Fleming TJ, Ang KK, et al. Devices valuable in head and neck radiotherapy. *Int J Radiat Oncol Biol Phys.* 1992;23(3):639–645.

107. Sanguineti G, Endres EJ, Gunn BG, et al. Is there a "mucosa-sparing" benefit of IMRT for head-and-neck cancer? *Int J Radiat Oncol Biol Phys.* 2006;66(3):931–938.

108. Induction chemotherapy plus radiation compared with surgery plus radiation in patients with advanced laryngeal cancer. The Department of Veterans Affairs Laryngeal Cancer Study Group. *N Engl J Med.* 1991;324(24):1685–1690.

109. Soo KC, Tan EH, Wee J, et al. Surgery and adjuvant radiotherapy vs concurrent chemo-radiotherapy in stage III/IV nonmetastatic squamous cell head and neck cancer: a randomised comparison. *Br J Cancer.* 2005. 93(3):279–86.

110. Carrara-de Angelis E, Feher O, Barros AP, et al. Voice and swallowing in patients enrolled in a larynx preservation trial. *Arch Otolaryngol Head Neck Surg.* 2003;129(7):733–738.

111. Terrell JE, Fisher SG, Wolf GT. Long-term quality of life after treatment of laryngeal cancer. The Veterans Affairs Laryngeal Cancer Study Group. *Arch Otolaryngol Head Neck Surg.* 1998;124(9):964–971.

112. Rosier JF, Gregoire V, Counoy H, et al. Comparison of external radiotherapy, laser micro-surgery and partial laryngectomy for the treatment of T1N0M0 glottic carcinomas: a retrospective evaluation. *Radiother Oncol.* 1998;48(2):175–183.

113. Mendenhall WM, Amdur RJ, Morris CG, et al. T1-T2N0 squamous cell carcinoma of the glottic larynx treated with radiation therapy. *J Clin Oncol.* 2001;19(20):4029–4036.

114. Yamazaki H, Nishiyama K, Tanaka E, et al. Radiotherapy for early glottic carcinoma (T1N0M0): results of prospective randomized study of radiation fraction size and overall treatment time. *Int J Radiat Oncol Biol Phys.* 2006;64(1):77–82.

115. Verdonck-de Leeuw IM, Keus RB, Hilgers FJ, et al. Consequences of voice impairment in daily life for patients following radiotherapy for early glottic cancer: voice quality, vocal function, and vocal performance. *Int J Radiat Oncol Biol Phys.* 1999;44(5):1071–1078.

116. Cox JD, Stetz J, Pajak TF, Toxicity criteria of the Radiation Therapy Oncology Group (RTOG) and the European Organization for Research and Treatment of Cancer (EORTC). *Int J Radiat Oncol Biol Phys.* 1995;31(5):1341–1346.

117. Sanguineti G, Adapala P, Endres EJ, et al. Dosimetric predictors of laryngeal edema. *Int J Radiat Oncol Biol Phys.* 2007;68(3):741–749.

118. Rancati T, Fiorino C, Sanguineti G. NTCP modeling of subacute/late laryngeal edema scored by fiberoptic examination. *Int J Radiat Oncol Biol Phys.* 2009;75(3):915–923.

119. London SD, Park SS, Gampper TJ, et al. Hyperbaric oxygen for the management of radionecrosis of bone and cartilage. *Laryngoscope.* 1998;108(9):1291–1296.

120. Ferguson BJ, Hudson WR, Farmer JC Jr. Hyperbaric oxygen therapy for laryngeal radionecrosis. *Ann Otol Rhinol Laryngol.* 1987;96(1 pt 1):1–6.

121. Colevas AD, Read R, Thornhill J, et al. Hypothyroidism incidence after multimodality treatment for stage III and IV squamous cell carcinomas of the head and neck. *Int J Radiat Oncol Biol Phys.* 2001;51(3):599–604.

122. Mercado G, Adelstein DJ, Saxton JP, et al. Hypothyroidism: a frequent event after radiotherapy and after radiotherapy with chemotherapy for patients with head and neck carcinoma. *Cancer.* 2001;92(11):2892–2897.

123. Tell R, Lundell G, Nilsson B, et al. Long-term incidence of hypothyroidism after radiotherapy in patients with head-and-neck cancer. *Int J Radiat Oncol Biol Phys.* 2004;60(2):395–400.

124. Ho AC, Ho WK, Lam PK, et al. Thyroid dysfunction in laryngectomees-10 years after treatment. *Head Neck.* 2008;30(3):336–340.

125. Cetinayak O, Akman F, Kentli S, et al. Assessment of treatment-related thyroid dysfunction in patients with head and neck cancer. *Tumori.* 2008;94(1):19–23.

126. McHenry CR, Slusarczyk SJ. Hypothyroidism following hemithyroidectomy: incidence, risk factors, and management. *Surgery.* 2000;128(6):994–998.

127. Piper HG, Bugis SP, Wilkins GE, et al. Detecting and defining hypothyroidism after hemithyroidectomy. *Am J Surg.* 2005;189(5):587–591; discussion 591.

128. Miller FR, Paulson D, Prihoda TJ, et al. Risk factors for the development of hypothyroidism after hemithyroidectomy. *Arch Otolaryngol Head Neck Surg.* 2006;132(1):36–38.

129. De Carlucci D Jr, Tavares MR, Obara MT, et al. Thyroid function after unilateral total lobectomy: risk factors for postoperative hypothyroidism. *Arch Otolaryngol Head Neck Surg.* 2008;134(10):1076–1079.

130. Alkan S, Baylancicek S, Ciftcic M, et al. Thyroid dysfunction after combined therapy for laryngeal cancer: a prospective study. *Otolaryngol Head Neck Surg.* 2008;139(6):787–791.

131. Bhandare N, Kennedy L, Malyapa RS, et al. Primary and central hypothyroidism after radiotherapy for head-and-neck tumors. *Int J Radiat Oncol Biol Phys.* 2007. 68(4):1131–1139.

132. Pai HH, Thornton A, Katznelson L, et al. Hypothalamic/pituitary function following high-dose conformal radiotherapy to the base of skull: demonstration of a dose-effect relationship using dose-volume histogram analysis. *Int J Radiat Oncol Biol Phys.* 2001;49(4):1079–1092.

133. Laughton SJ, Merchant TE, Sklar CA, et al. Endocrine outcomes for children with embryonal brain tumors after risk-adapted craniospinal and conformal primary-site irradiation and high-dose chemotherapy with stem-cell rescue on the SJMB-96 trial. *J Clin Oncol.* 2008;26(7):1112–1118.

134. Diaz R, Jaboin JJ, Morales-Paliza M, et al. Hypothyroidism as a consequence of intensity-modulated radiotherapy with concurrent taxane-based chemotherapy for locally advanced head and neck cancer. *Int J Radiat Oncol Biol Phys.* 2010;77(2):468–476.

135. Bhandare N, Antonelli PJ, Morris CG, et al. Ototoxicity after radiotherapy for head and neck tumors. *Int J Radiat Oncol Biol Phys.* 2007;67(2):469–479.

136. Wang SZ, Wang WF, Zhang HY, et al. Analysis of anatomical factors controlling the morbidity of radiation-induced otitis media with effusion. *Radiother Oncol.* 2007;85(3):463–468.

137. Bennett M, Kaylie D, Warren F, et al. Chronic ear surgery in irradiated temporal bones. *Laryngoscope.* 2007;117(7):1240–1244.

138. Gyorkey J, Pollock FJ. Radiation necrosis of the ossicles. *AMA Arch Otolaryngol.* 1960;71:793–796.

139. Zuur CL, Simis YJ, Lansdaal PE, et al. Risk factors of ototoxicity after cisplatin-based chemo-irradiation in patients with locally advanced head-and-neck cancer: a multivariate analysis. *Int J Radiat Oncol Biol Phys.* 2007;68(5):1320–1325.

140. Zuur CL, Simis YJ, Lamers EA, et al. Risk factors for hearing loss in patients treated with intensity-modulated radiotherapy for head-and-neck tumors. *Int J Radiat Oncol Biol Phys.* 2009;74(2):490–496.

141. Low WK, Toh ST, Wee J, et al. Sensorineural hearing loss after radiotherapy and chemoradiotherapy: a single, blinded, randomized study. *J Clin Oncol.* 2006;24(12):1904–1909.

142. Van der Putten L, de Bree R, Plukker JT, et al. Permanent unilateral hearing loss after radiotherapy for parotid gland tumors. *Head Neck.* 2006;28(10):902–908.

143. Lee AW, Ng WT, Hung WM, et al. Major late toxicities after conformal radiotherapy for nasopharyngeal carcinoma-patient- and treatment-related risk factors. *Int J Radiat Oncol Biol Phys.* 2009;73(4):1121–1128.

144. Hua C, Bass JK, Khan R, et al. Hearing loss after radiotherapy for pediatric brain tumors: effect of cochlear dose. *Int J Radiat Oncol Biol Phys.* 2008;72(3):892–899.

145. Massager N, Nissim O, Delbrouck C, et al. Irradiation of cochlear structures during vestibular schwannoma radiosurgery and associated hearing outcome. *J Neurosurg.* 2007;107:733–739.

146. Kano H, Kondziolka D, Khan A, et al. Predictors of hearing preservation after stereotactic radiosurgery for acoustic neuroma. *J Neurosurg.* 2009;111(4):863–873.

147. Hoistad DL, Ondrey FG, Mutlu C, et al. Histopathology of human temporal bone after cis-platinum, radiation, or both. *Otolaryngol Head Neck Surg.* 1998;118(6):825–832.

148. Asenov DR, Kaga K, Tsuzuku T. Changes in the audiograms of a nasopharyngeal cancer patient during the course of treatment: a temporal bone histopathological study. *Acta Otolaryngol.* 2007;127(10):1105–1110.

149. Fouladi M, Chintagumpala M, Ashley D, et al. Amifostine protects against cisplatin-induced ototoxicity in children with average-risk medulloblastoma. *J Clin Oncol.* 2008;26(22):3749–3755.

150. Zuur CL, Simis YJ, Lansdaal PE, et al. Ototoxicity in a randomized phase III trial of intra-arterial compared with intravenous cisplatin chemoradiation in patients with locally advanced head and neck cancer. *J Clin Oncol.* 2007;25(24):3759–3765.

151. Chan SH, Ng WT, Kam KL, et al. Sensorineural hearing loss after treatment of nasopharyngeal carcinoma: a longitudinal analysis. *Int J Radiat Oncol Biol Phys.* 2009;73(5):1335–1342.

152. Hitchcock YJ, Tward JD, Szabo A, et al. Relative contributions of radiation and cisplatin-based chemotherapy to sensorineural hearing loss in head-and-neck cancer patients. *Int J Radiat Oncol Biol Phys.* 2009;73(3):779–788.

153. Low WK, Gopal K, Goh LK, et al. Cochlear implantation in postirradiated ears: outcomes and challenges. *Laryngoscope.* 2006;116(7):1258–1262.

154. Kozak KR, Adams J, Krejcarek SJ, et al. A dosimetric comparison of proton and intensity-modulated photon radiotherapy for pediatric parameningeal rhabdomyosarcomas. *Int J Radiat Oncol Biol Phys.* 2009;74(1):179–186.

155. Lee CT, Bilton SD, Famiglietti RM et al. Treatment planning with protons for pediatric retinoblastoma, medulloblastoma, and pelvic sarcoma: how do protons compare with other conformal techniques? *Int J Radiat Oncol Biol Phys.* 2005;63(2):362–372.

156. St. Clair WH, Adams JA, Bues M, et al. Advantage of protons compared to conventional x-ray or IMRT in the treatment of a pediatric patient with medulloblastoma. *Int J Radiat Oncol Biol Phys.* 2004;58(3):727–734.

157. MacDonald SM, Safai S, Trofimov A, et al. Proton Radiotherapy for childhood ependymoma: initial clinical outcomes and dose comparisons. *Int J Radiat Oncol Biol Phys.* 2008;71(4):979–986.

Daniel Gomez
Kenneth E. Rosenzweig

Lung

INTRODUCTION

Radiation therapy (RT) is one of the major treatment modalities in the treatment of lung cancer and other thoracic malignancies along with surgery and chemotherapy. RT is used in all therapeutic situations, including definitive, adjuvant, and palliative treatments. Radiation injury to the lung may have severe consequences and its avoidance is one of the principal determinants of radiation dose and fractionation.

The largest environmental exposure of RT is radon, specifically decay products from the chemically inert gas radon-222, which decays from uranium-238 and can diffuse through the soil and into the air. In fact, this isotope accounts for approximately 50% of all nonmedical exposure to radiation.[1] While in an open space the risk is relatively low, in confined areas like mines or homes the exposure can accumulate to measurable, clinically significant levels. There have been several studies published regarding the correlation of radon exposure with the development of lung cancer, many of which were meta-analyses due to the large number of cases required to achieve the necessary statistical power required to demonstrate this correlation. In one such representative study, the authors pooled 13 case-control studies assessing the relationship between residential radon and the incidence of lung cancer. The study examined 7,148 cases of lung cancer and 14,208 controls in nine European countries. Each study measured the radon gas concentration in the household air over a median of 5.34 years in becquerels per cubic meter (Bq/m^3). The authors found that the relative risk of lung cancer increased by 8.4% per 100 Bq/m^3 increase in radon levels. The relationship was linear in nature with no threshold, consistent with a stochastic effect.[1]

It is also notable that synergism exists between radon exposure and smoking in the development of lung cancer. Several studies have shown that even when accounting for smoking, the excess relative risks of radon exposure remain the same.[2] Statistically, this means that the risk of developing lung cancer with a lifetime history of smoking and radon exposure would be much greater than that in a never-smoker with the same radon exposure.[3]

THERAPEUTIC ROLE OF RADIATION FOR THORACIC MALIGNANCIES

RT is delivered to the lungs for a variety of cancers including non–small cell lung cancer (NSCLC), small cell lung cancer, lymphoma, esophageal cancer, breast cancer, thymoma, and

various pediatric malignancies. The dose of RT used varies widely. Lymphoma treatment will use doses ranging from 2,500 to 4,000 cGy. The typical breast cancer dose is 4,000 to 5,000 cGy and only a small portion of lung deep to the breast needs to be irradiated. Small cell lung cancer is typically irradiated in doses of 4,500 cGy delivered in 150-cGy fractions twice a day or 6,000 cGy in daily fraction. Locally advanced NSCLC receives 6,000 to 7,400 cGy. Early-stage NSCLC previously received similar doses as locally advanced disease, albeit in smaller volumes. Recently, there has been increasing use of stereotactic body radiotherapy with doses of 4,800 to 6,000 cGy delivered in three to four fractions.[4]

Chemotherapy is typically used in conjunction with RT for the definitive treatment of locally advanced lung cancers, lymphomas, breast cancers, and small cell lung cancers as well as all palliative situations. Chemotherapy can be used either sequentially or concurrently with RT. Various agents are used with different levels of expected pulmonary toxicity.

DEFINITION AND DIAGNOSIS OF RADIATION-INDUCED LUNG DISEASE

ACUTE/SUBACUTE TOXICITY

In the acute/subacute setting, radiation-induced lung disease (RILD) presents in the form of radiation pneumonitis (RP), a disease similar in clinical presentation to bacterial pneumonia. Symptoms generally arise approximately 2 weeks after the completion of treatment and include cough, dyspnea, chest pain, malaise, and occasionally fever. On physical examination, crackles/rales can often be appreciated on auscultation, and, depending on whether or not a pleural effusion is present, there may be dullness to percussion or decreased breath sounds at the base of the lung. There are no commonly used laboratory studies for the purposes of diagnosis, and no laboratory studies are unique to RP, though patients can have an elevated white blood cell count and lactate dehydrogenase level. In addition, various biomarkers are being tested for use in the prediction and diagnosis of RP, as is discussed in detail below.

A chest x-ray is the preferred initial imaging study for diagnosis, though, particularly in the early phases, this may not demonstrate any abnormalities. A computed tomography study is much more sensitive in delineating radiographic characteristics. The general progression of imaging findings is that of perivascular haziness followed by alveolar filling densities, primarily within the radiation portal. There may be a small pleural effusion present. While various nuclear imaging studies have been used in small studies, including single photon emission computed tomography imaging, none are in widespread use at this time.

RP is usually treated with prednisone, at least 60 mg/d for 2 weeks, then with a gradual taper over the next 3 to 12 weeks. It is notable that the prophylactic administration of glucocorticoids or antibiotics has not been shown to be beneficial in reducing the incidence in RP.[5,6]

CHRONIC TOXICITY

Late RILD is usually in the form of radiation-induced fibrosis (RIF). Characteristics of this disease can be chronic dyspnea, which can be debilitating in nature, as well as with the associated late complications of cor pulmonale and even respiratory failure. However, the severity of these symptoms is largely dependent on the amount of lung tissue involved, as small amounts of fibrotic tissue may be asymptomatic. Historically, RIF has been thought to be irreversible. However, a recent study demonstrated efficacy of Pentoxifylline in reducing long-term symptoms. Specifically, the authors studied the effect of Pentoxifylline and alpha-tocopherol in 55 patients with RIF after undergoing RT for breast cancer. It was found that the combination was continuously effective and resulted in exponential decreases in the fibrotic surface area. The mean time to the effect was 24 months and was shorter if the radiation had been administered within 6 years. There was also noted to be approximately a 50% decrease in symptom severity.[7] Therefore, this agent holds future promise in reducing the effects of this serious and potentially fatal condition.

CHANGES IN PULMONARY FUNCTION TESTS

The nature of the changes in pulmonary function tests (PFTs) is variable after thoracic RT. Indeed, although both forced expiratory volume in one second (FEV1), a measure of bronchial obstruction, and the diffusing capacity of the lung for carbon monoxide (DLCO), a measure of the efficiency of gas exchange from the alveoli into the blood stream, tend to decrease after thoracic radiation, in some patients these values increase due to a reduction in the size of the tumor. One study evaluated the change in 82 patients with inoperable NSCLC with involved field doses ranging from 60.8 to 94.5 Gy. The authors found that at 3 to 4 months after RT, FEV1 values decreased by 6% and DLCO values decreased by 14%. However, 38% and 21% of patients had an improvement in FEV1 and DLCO, respectively. Furthermore, 62% of patients with an improvement in DLCO were found to have a correlative improvement in FEV1, suggesting a common factor to these changes.[8]

In another study at Duke University, 13 patients were enrolled in a prospective trial to determine radiation-related changes in PFTs. The median dose was 71.4 Gy, and only four patients received chemotherapy. The authors found that at 6 months, all PFT values, including FEV1, forced vital capacity (FVC), and DLCO, had declined (89%, 89%, and 92% of baseline, respectively). However, at 1 year, the FEV1, FVC, and DLCO values were 100%, 105%, and 90% of baseline, respectively. After 12 months, the yearly decline in median of these same three values was 7%, 9.5%, and 3.5%, respectively (Fig. 28.1). In addition, 10/13 patients (77%) developed

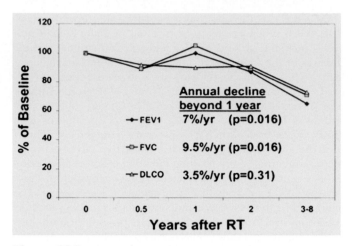

Figure 28.1. Changes in PFTs after high-dose thoracic RT. (From Miller KL, et al. Long-term changes in pulmonary function tests after definitive radiotherapy for lung cancer. *Int J Radiat Oncol Biol Phys.* 2003;56(3):611–615.)

respiratory symptoms that were concluded to be unrelated to cancer at time points between 6 weeks and 21 months. These symptoms included cough alone in 2/13 patients and 8/13 patients with dyspnea, which in 7/8 patients was progressive in nature, and one patient developed Grade 3 dyspnea requiring oxygen and steroids.[9] In a third study from MD Anderson Cancer Center, 100 patients with NSCLC from five protocols between 1992 and 2000 were evaluated with pre- RTA, and post-RT PFTs, and found that values for the FEV1/FVC, total lung capacity, and DLCO had decreased to 93%, 69%, and 83% of their baseline values after radiation treatment, respectively, and that FEV1/FVC and DLCO were reduced more in patients receiving concurrent chemotherapy.[10] Therefore, it can be concluded that as a result of RT to the lungs, while some patients will experience a transient improvement in PFTs due to reduction in tumor size, over the long term most patients will experience a decline in these values, with possible associated symptoms. Furthermore, diffusing capacity/DLCO is the most likely functional parameter to be affected.

KEY MOLECULES IN THE DEVELOPMENT OF RILD

Early histological studies on the effect of radiation on large animals demonstrated that the capillary endothelium appeared to be the initial site of post–irradiation pulmonary damage. Capillary luminar dilatation and congestion were some of the first changes to be observed within the first 2 weeks postirradiation. These changes led to an increase in vascular permeability and production of interstitial edema.[11] Irreversible fibrosis becomes histologically evident 36 weeks after whole-lung radiation in mice.[12] Further molecular biologic work uncovered autocrine, paracrine, and endocrine mechanisms that persist after radiation injury to the lung and can be the basis of the clinical pathologic expression of pulmonary fibrosis.[13]

Currently, lung radiation damage is believed to result from a combination of the direct effects of radiation, the inflammatory process, and abnormal wound healing.[14] The biological response of radiation is mediated by several mechanisms, including transforming growth factor-β (TGF-β), reactive oxygen and nitrogen species, cytokines, and the renin-angiotensin system.[15]

TGF-β is classified both as a cytokine and a growth factor. The TGF-β system seems to be involved in many human processes including wound healing and scar formation,[16] fibrotic diseases in the kidney and other organs,[17] immunodeficiency, arteriosclerosis, rheumatoid arthritis, and scleroderma.[15] TGF-β exists in three isoforms (TGF-β1–3). The biological activity of TGF-β is constrained by its production as a latent complex consisting of TBFβ1 associated with a latency-associated peptide (LAP). It is activated when it is dissociated from the LAP. Therefore, there is a large pool of inactive TGF-β that can be activated after a triggering event. Ionizing radiation is one of a few exogenous agents known to cause latent TGF-β1 activation in situ.[18] Active TGF-β binds to pairs of transmembrane receptors.[19] The activation of the TGF-β receptors initiates a signaling pathway that promotes terminal differentiation of progenitor fibroblasts to functional fibrocytes.[20] This fibroblast proliferation leads to increased extracellular matrix and collagen deposition and subsequently tumor remodeling.

Irradiation of the cytoplasm also stimulates signaling pathways that can influence on nuclear processes.[21] Ionizing radiation creates reactive oxygen species (ROS) in the cell. The low relative levels of ROS are amplified through interaction with reactive nitrogen species (RNS). This disturbance of the ROS/RNS system can drive the formation of superoxide dismutase, which in turn has an important role in the molecular pathology of fibrosis.[22]

The renin-angiotensin system is a complex hormonal system in which renin and angiotensin are released in the circulation. Their product, Angiotensin I is activated by the angiotensin-converting enzyme (ACE) to release the biologically active Angiotensin II.[23] ACE inhibitors have been shown to prevent the development of pulmonary hypertension in chronically hypoxic rats.[24] It appears that the activation of angiotensin receptors is involved pathogenesis of radiation injury.

ANATOMY

The external anatomy of the lung is dominated by fissures and a cardiac notch on each lung. On both the left and the right lungs, the oblique fissure extends from the surface of the lung to the hilum and divides the lung into upper and lower lobes, which are connected only by the lobar bronchi and vessels. On the right lung, a horizontal fissure passes from the anterior margin into the oblique fissure to separate the wedge-shaped middle lobe from the upper lobe. The visceral pleura covering the surface of the lung extends inward to line the depths of the fissures. The trachea divides into a left and a right main stem bronchi at the carina. The right main stem bronchus (approximately 4.5 cm long) gives off a right upper lobe bronchus and continues as the bronchus intermedius that separates into middle and lower lobe bronchi. The left main stem bronchus gives off three branches, but the upper and middle ones are fused before they separate into the upper lobe and lingular lobe. The other branch is the lower lobe bronchus. Each lobar bronchus in turn gives off segmental bronchi totaling ten segments on each side of the lung.

The trachea and proximal airways are lined with pseudostratified ciliated columnar epithelial cells with admixed mucus-producing goblet cells, as well as Clara, intermediate, and brush cells.[25] Below the layer of the epithelium is a layer of reserve epithelial cells. The functional subunit of the lung is the alveolar/capillary complex. The alveoli are lined with type I pneumocytes. They form a complete, thin lining of the alveoli.

Type II pneumocytes (cuboidal cells) reside in the alveolar lining and produce surfactant, which maintains a low level of surface tension in the air sacs. The alveolar lining cells are in close contact with their alveolar wall blood capillaries. Therefore, the air space within the alveoli is in close proximity to the bloodstream and any thickening of this distance can impair gas exchange.

PHYSIOLOGIC AND RADIOBIOLOGIC EFFECTS OF INJURY

After thoracic irradiation, there are two waves of increased vascular permeability. In one study in rats, after large single fractions of whole thorax irradiation, there was increased permeability at day 1, which normalized at day 4. The second wave of increased permeability occurred between 14 and 38 days after RT.[26] Other studies have shown abnormalities in plasminogen activator, angiotensin-converting enzyme, prostacyclin production, and surfactant production after exposure to large doses of single-fraction radiation.[25]

The morphologic changes in mice have been described in experimental animal models as three consecutive stages: acute, intermediate, and late. The higher the dose of the radiation, the more likely the progression to late stage.[27] Other studies have shown that irradiated rat lungs repair in a time- and dose-related manner after relatively low doses of radiation.[14]

Several investigators in the past have provided an overview on the sequence of events that leads to pulmonary injury after exposure to ionizing radiation. An excellent summary was published by Gross[28] and has since been revised based on recent data. The physiologic damage can be summarized as follows. Incident x- or γ-rays excite electrons, which then produce ion pairs and free radicals. These free radicals damage both DNA and macromolecules. Specifically in the lung, the macromolecules that are affected occur in the capillary endothelial cells, type I/type II pneumocytes, macrophages, and stromal fibroblasts. The classical cellular theory of RP is that in the "early" phase, there is loss of type I pneumocytes that line the alveoli, resulting in a sloughed epithelium, as well as the type II pneumocytes, which are the less-differentiated precursors to type I cells and secrete surfactant. When exposed to radiation, type II pneumocytes release surfactants into the alveoli, which can then persist for days to weeks.[29] On a microscopic level, there is increased capillary permeability and swelling of the basement membrane, which can then lead to vascular obstruction and interstitial edema. This increased vascular permeability can also facilitate the systemic release of surfactants through the blood stream.[30] These changes can be seen with radiation doses of >10 to 20 Gy.[31]

In the intermediate or "subacute" phase, the following microscopic changes can be seen: protein leakage, thickening of the alveolar septa, and changes in type II pneumocytes or macrophages. It is in these beginning phases that patients generally experience symptoms of RP, characterized by cough, dyspnea, and malaise.

In the "late" phase of radiation damage, there is a decrease in the number of multiple pulmonary cell types, including capillaries and pneumocytes (both types I and II). At the same time, there is an increase in collagen deposition that occurs, which can vary by the species of animal.[32] It is in this late time period that patients experience the fibrotic changes characteristic of late pulmonary damage, which are irreversible.

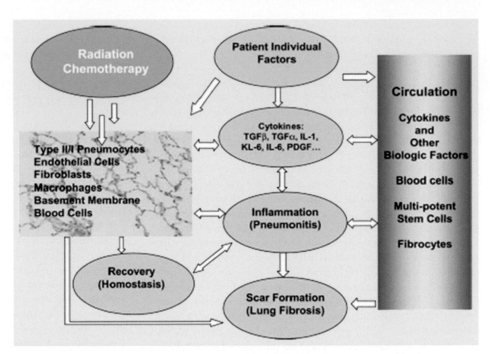

Figure 28.2. Molecular and cellular mechanisms of radiation-related pulmonary injury. (From Kong FM, et al. Non-small cell lung cancer therapy-related pulmonary toxicity: an update on radiation pneumonitis and fibrosis. *Semin Oncol.* 2005;32 (2 suppl 3):S42–S54.)

From these basic tenets, this hypothesis has been expanded due to the vast knowledge of molecular mechanisms that have been elucidated over the past 15 years. Indeed, the interactions that take place as a result of radiation are quite complex, as is demonstrated in Figure 28.2. A wide number of molecules circulate, such as fibroblasts, fibrocytes, and even blood and bone marrow cells, which create a self-perpetuating cycle that accentuates injury and impedes repair.[33] The molecules are produced in the region of treatment and either bind to cells of the same type (autocrine response), cells within the same tissue (paracrine response), or cells in distant tissues/organs (endocrine response).[34]

Some of the key molecular agents that play a role in RILD have been introduced above. Several investigators have attempted to elucidate the role of specific markers in this process, and the research in this area continues to evolve. Here, we will provide an overview of some of the research being performed to further characterize this very complex process.

TRANSFORMING GROWTH FACTOR-β

Chen et al.[35] performed a detailed assay of several serum markers in 24 patients who underwent radiation to the thorax and had follow-up of at least 12 months, thirteen of which had symptomatic pneumonitis. The authors found that both IL-1α and IL-6 levels were significantly higher before, during, and after radiation for those patients that had pneumonitis, while TGF-β1, MCP-1, and bFGF varied during the time period but did not correlate with symptoms.[35] In contrast, Anscher et al.[36] examined the correlation of plasma levels of TGF-β1 with the development of RP, and found that failure to normalize after treatment was associated with a higher risk of this toxicity. Supporting the latter study, Vujaskovic et al.[37] performed a pilot study of 27 patients with stage III NSCLC and found that patients who were diagnosed with RP had persistently elevated TGF-β1 levels throughout treatment, while patients without RP did not. As studies regarding the exact role of TGF-β in the development of RP have been contradictory, some authors have

proposed that there are two contrasting mechanisms in regard to this cytokine. In fact, TGF-β may be produced by both tumor cells and normal tissue, with the former causing a decrease in levels during treatment and the latter increasing. It may therefore be that this cytokine is predictive of toxicity only when the balance favors release by normal tissue.[38]

INTERLEUKINS

Interleukins are released by macrophages, pneumocytes, lymphocytes, and fibroblasts, and can be detected during an acute inflammatory phase. As noted above, IL-1 and IL-6 were found to be correlated with RP in the study by Chen et al.[35] Another study examined the relationship of IL-6 and IL-10 levels with the time course of RT. The authors found an inverse relationship of the levels of these two molecules, particularly within the first 2 weeks of treatment, with IL-6 levels remaining high throughout radiation treatment and IL-10 levels remaining low during this time period.[39] And in another study, IL-8 levels were found to vary according to whether or not a patient developed lung injury. Interestingly, IL-1 and IL-6 did not differ according to this endpoint.[40]

KL-6

KL-6 is expressed primarily on type II pneumocytes and bronchiolar epithelial cells, and is released when these cells are damaged.[34] Goto et al.[41] examined the role of KL-6 in this process and concluded that in patients with severe RP, there was a "consistent tendency" for these markers to increase after the diagnosis. In addition, Hara et al.[42] studied the correlation of KL-6 levels with RP in single-fraction stereotactic body radiation, and found that the magnitude of the increase of this level 2 months after treatment was predictive of RP, and that all patients who developed this toxicity were found to have at least a 50% (1.5-fold) increase in KL-6 levels. Finally, Matsuno et al.[43] assessed KL-6 levels at various time points from the beginning to the end of radiation, and found that beginning at 40 Gy, KL-6 levels were increased relative to the initial levels, and that levels of >1,000 U/mL were correlated with diffuse RP. Clearly, KL-6 plays some role in the acute-phase response.

SURFACTANT PROTEINS

As noted above, type II pneumocytes release surfactants, which can then be disseminated in the circulation due to increased vascular permeability. It therefore follows logically that molecules associated with surfactant may be of utility in predicting radiation-induced lung toxicity. Four surfactant proteins have been identified, SP-A, SP-B, SP-C, and SP-D.[44] Monitoring these proteins in serum has been found to be associated with pulmonary fibrosis, interstitial lung disease associated with collagen vascular disease, and acute respiratory distress syndrome.[45] Of the four proteins, SP-A and SP-D have been studied the most as predictive markers in RILD. In the above-cited study by Matsuno et al., which also examined the role of KL-6, the authors also studied the role of SP-D as a predictive molecule. The authors did not find a statistical difference between SP-D levels before treatment and at various dose levels, such that it did not provide utility in predicting the development of RP.[43] However, Sasaki et al.[46] examined 86 patients who underwent thoracic RT (lung, breast, or esophageal sites) at doses from 30 to 76 Gy, and monitored the SP-A and SP-D levels for 1 year after treatment, or until the development of RILD. The authors found that serum levels of SP-D were higher in the 19 patients who experienced SP-D compared to those who did not. Furthermore, the authors found that SP-D was more sensitive and specific in predicting RP than SP-A.[46] In addition, Sasaki et al.[46] measured SP-A and SP-D levels in 25 patients with lung tumors who underwent RT. Both proteins had a higher concentration in patients who experienced RP, and the authors concluded that these proteins may have diagnostic value in the detection of RP.[47]

ADHESION MOLECULES

In order to facilitate the inflammatory process that is characteristic of lung toxicity, particularly in the acute phase, adhesion molecules act to promote leukocyte accumulation in the treatment field. The most well-studied adhesion molecule in this regard is ICAM-1, which is present in vascular endothelial cells, epithelial cells, and lymphocytes.[34] While adhesion molecules have been found to be increased in the general malignant setting,[48] Kawana et al.[49] found that in rat models, ICAM-1 was significantly increased starting at 1 week after irradiation, but not at 8 weeks after radiation treatment. Similarly, Hallahan and Virudachalam[50] found that ICAM-1 expression increased 24 hours after radiation in mouse models, and that the dose required for increased expression was 2 Gy, then increasing in a dose-dependent manner. Therefore, while it is unclear how predictive ICAM-1 expression could be in the development of clinical symptoms, due to the high likelihood of increased levels in the background of malignancy, it does appear to play a prominent role in the development of the inflammatory process.

In summary, much progress has been made in elucidating the multifactorial mechanism of RP on the molecular level, though there is still a great deal that is unknown as to the role of specific cytokines and how the various pathways interact. The potential utility of further discovery in this field cannot be overstated, with the goal being individualized monitoring and

subsequent advances in prevention and treatment. The advent of techniques that assay a wide array of biomarkers has and will continue to be the driving force behind this process.

CLINICAL PREDICTORS OF RADIATION INJURY TO THE LUNG

Several studies have examined patient characteristics that may influence the development of RP. One factor that has been relatively consistent among studies is that of chemotherapy, particularly in the concurrent setting.[51–53] Other factors, such as age, tumor location, and KPS, have been inconsistent in their predictive value. For instance, in the earlier-cited study by Gopal et al.,[10] the authors found that concurrent chemoradiation was associated with a significantly lower post-RT TLC than radiation alone, 92% versus 107% of baseline, respectively. In addition, patient age of at least 60 years, N2, or higher nodal status, tumor volume of at least 100 cm^3, central tumor location, and the use of at least six treatment fields were also associated with a significantly lower post-RT DLCO. In contrast, other studies have not shown a difference in age, chemotherapy, or tumor location.[51,54,55] Table 28.1, taken from Hernando et al.[55] and Mehta et al.,[56] demonstrates the disparity between different studies in this regard.

PULMONARY FUNCTION TESTS AS PREDICTORS OF RILD

In studies regarding the predictive value of preradiation PFTs in predicting long-term function and the development of RILD, most investigators have found some relationship between poor initial function and RILD. Marks et al.[57] examined 100 patients receiving partial-lung irradiation, a model based on the pre-RT DLCO and the normal tissue complication probability (NTCP, defined below) was strongly predictive of the development of RT-induced symptoms. In another study by Robnett et al.,[6] in patients receiving definitive chemoradiation for lung cancer, pretreatment FEV1 was predictive of the development of RP. In particular, no patient suffering severe RP had a pretreatment FEV1 > 2.0 L. Inoue found that a low PaO$_2$ (<80 torr) prior to RT was predictive of severe RP.[58] Although the data have not been as comprehensive as those for dose-volume parameters, it does appear that pulmonary dysfunction prior to radiation exacerbates those processes that lead to both acute and chronic RILD.

DOSIMETRIC PREDICTORS OF RADIATION INJURY TO THE LUNG

Dose-Volume Histogram Parameters

Defining dose-volume histograms (DVH) parameters that have predictive value in determining RILD has been an area of active study for many years and has evolved with the development of more conformal techniques. The following definitions are useful in this discussion.

VX—Volume of total lung (including both right and left lungs) receiving at least X Gy. For instance, V_{20} is the volume of total lung receiving at least 20 Gy.

DX—Minimum dose to X% of volume of both lungs. For example, D35 is the minimum dose to the hottest 35% of the lungs.

| TABLE 28.1 | | Clinical Factors that may Influence the Rate of Symptomatic Radiation Pneumonitis with Non-Small-Cell Lung Cancer | | |

Author	No.	Increased Risk	No Change in Risk	Decreased Risk
Brooks et al. (1986)(26)	80	Chemotherapy	Age	
Schaake-Koning et al. (1992)(27)	331		Chemotherapy	
Jeremic et al. (1996)(28)	131		Chemotherapy	
Lee et al. (1996)(29)	79	Chemotherapy		
By hardt et al. (1998)(30)	461	Concurrent chemotherapy		
Monson et al. (1998)(31)	83	Smoking	Chemotherapy	Surgery
Yamada et al. (1998)(32)	60	Tumor location Concurrent chemotherapy		
Robert et al. (1999)(19)	43	Chemotherapy		
Quon et al. (2000)(33)	608		Age	
Robnett et al. (2000)(34)	148	Women Low KPS	Chemotherapy timing Tumor site	
Hernado et al. (2001)(35)	201		Age Tumor location	Smoking
Rancati et al. (2003)(36)	84		Age Chemotherapy	Surgery
Claude et al (2004)(37)	96	Age	Gender KPS Smoking Surgery Chemotherapy	

KPS, Karnofsky performance status.

Source: Adapted from Hernando et al. Radiation-induced pulmonary toxicity: a dose-volume histogram analysis in 201 patients with lung cancer. *Int J Radiat Oncol Biol Phys.* 2001;51(3):650–659.

Mean lung dose (MLD)—Mean dose to the total lung (including both right and left lungs).

NTCP—Probability of complication to the normal tissue (in this case, the lung), given certain dose-volume parameters. The significance of the NTCP will be defined further below.

The first step in defining relevant DVH parameters is to determine whether or not a threshold dose exists. In other words, is there a dose, or dose-volume combination, after which the incidence of complications rises sharply? Three recent studies demonstrate this principle. First, Gopal et al.[59] examined 26 patients who received thoracic RT for lung cancer, all treated with 3D-based planning, eleven of whom also received the radioprotector amifostine. The authors used DVH data to estimate the local dose-response relationship for DLCO and found that there was a pronounced decrease in DLCO when the local dose exceeded 13 Gy. Notably, this dose threshold increased to 36 Gy in the presence of amifostine. Furthermore, the study found that grade 2 or higher pulmonary symptoms were associated with a DLCO loss of at least 30%.[59]

In a similar study examining the risk of RP based on dose-volume combinations, Willner et al.[60] asked the question of what dose-volume combination is more important in terms of RP: "a little (dose) to a lot or a lot to a little?" The two authors display the figure (Fig. 28.3), highlighting this important distinction. Both DVHs have similar MLDs, but different high- and low-dose regions.

To answer this question, the authors analyzed DVH data from 49 patients treated with 3D-CRT to the thorax (48 with chemotherapy), 18 of which developed RP. Using a detailed DVH analysis, during which the authors defined low (≤10 Gy), moderate (<10–40 Gy), and high doses to the lungs as both one unit and as separate organs, as well as assessing the effect

of V_{10} to V_{40} and MLD, the study found that the risk of RP increased from 13% to 60% with increasing levels of the high dose region. This sharp correlation was not found at low doses. As Figure 28.4 shows, using logistic regression there was increasing steepness with higher doses and a better correlation with RP at higher radiation doses. Therefore, using these data, we

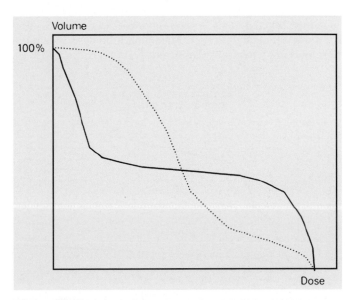

Figure 28.3. Difference between a DVH with a "lot to a little" versus "a little to a lot." (From Willner J, et al. A little to a lot or a lot to a little? An analysis of pneumonitis risk from DVH parameters of the lung in patients with lung cancer treated with 3-D conformal radiotherapy. *Strahlenther Onkol.* 2003;179(8):548–556.)

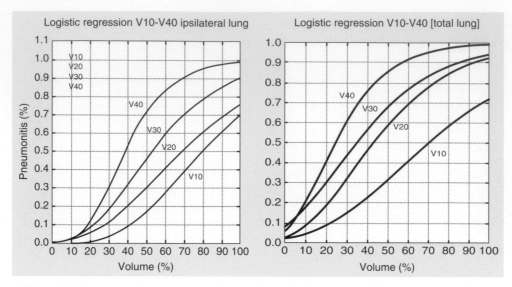

Figure 28.4. Dose-volume relationships in predicting RP from 10 to 40 Gy. (From Willner J, et al. A little to a lot or a lot to a little? An analysis of pneumonitis risk from DVH parameters of the lung in patients with lung cancer treated with 3-D conformal radiotherapy. *Strahlenther Onkol.* 2003;179(8):548–556.)

could extrapolate that doses of at least 20 Gy (V_{20} or higher) should be used to assess the risk of RP.[60]

Indeed, the V_{20} parameter is commonly used to predict rates of RP, as 20 Gy has been estimated to be a threshold dose at which lung tissue is no longer functional. In a now widely cited study, Graham et al.[61] examined the predictive value of V_{20} in RP. The authors found that the V_{20} stratified patients into four main groups for the development of pneumonitis, as demonstrated in Figure 28.5. With the incidence rising sharply after V_{20} values of 40% (Table 28.2).[61]

Schallenkamp et al.[62] reviewed 92 consecutive cases of patients treated with definitive thoracic RT. They evaluated DVHs using total lung dose and found that MLD, V_{10}, V_{13}, V_{15}, V_{20} and Veff were all significantly correlated with RP. However, when the gross tumor was subtracted from the total lung volume and heterogeneity corrections were used, only V_{10} and V_{13} retined their significance. Maximum lung dose (as a point dose) was not statistically significant.

There is some data to suggest that lower lobe of the lung is more susceptible to pneumonitis than other regions. This is perhaps due to the larger density of target cells in the lower lung. Yorke et al.,[63] found that there is an increased correlation between dosimetric predictors of RP in tumors located in the lower lobes as opposed to the upper lobes. In a recent paper, Bradley et al.[64] devised a nomogram to predict the incidence of RP based on the Radiation Therapy Oncology Group (RTOG) trial 93-11, as well as institutional data. The authors found that the most predictive parameter using the RTOG 93-11 database was a single-parameter model, the D15. Combining institutional and RTOG databases, a two-parameter model was most predictive, the two parameters being MLD and superior-to-inferior gross tumor volume position.[64] The nomogram is depicted in Figure 28.6 below.

THE NORMAL TISSUE COMPLICATION PROBABILITY MODEL

Radiation-induced lung injury is related to the dose of radiation delivered as well as the volume of lung irradiated. Numerous models have been established to estimate and predict RP. All models are based on dose and volume constraints.

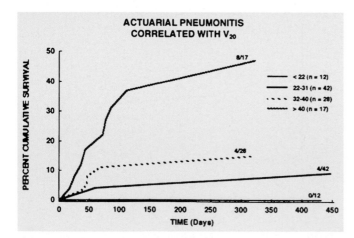

Figure 28.5. Incidences of RP given V_{20}. (From Graham MV, Purdy JA, Emami B, et al. Clinical dose-volume histogram analysis for pneumonitis after 3D treatment for non-small cell lung cancer (NSCLC). *Int J Radiat Oncol Biol Phys.* 1999;45(2):323–329, with permission.)

TABLE 28.2	Correlation Between V_{20} and Severity of Pneumonitis	
V_{20} (%)	Grade 2 (%)	Grades 3–5 (%)
<22	0	0
22–31	8	8
32–40	13	5 (1 fatal)
>40	19	23 (3 fatal)

Source: Graham MV, Purdy JA, Emami B, et al. Clinical dose-volume histogram analysis for pneumonitis after 3D treatment for non-small cell lung cancer (NSCLC). *Int J Radiat Oncol Biol Phys.* 1999;45(2):323–329, with permission.

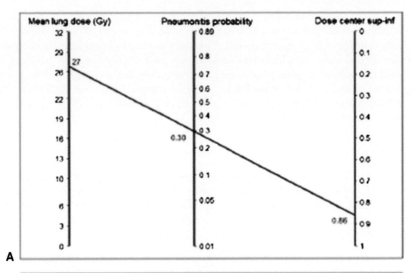

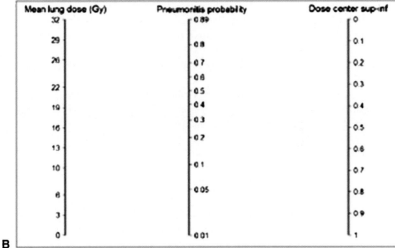

Figure 28.6. Nomogram to predict RP based on MLD and superior-inferior position of tumor. (From Bradley JD, et al. A nomogram to predict radiation pneumonitis, derived from a combined analysis of RTOG 9311 and institutional data. *Int J Radiat Oncol Biol Phys.* 2007;69(4):985–992.)

One of the earliest attempts to estimate the probability of lung complications was from Burman et al.[65] at Memorial Sloan-Kettering Cancer Center (MSKCC). They attempted to provide a quantitative method of estimating risk based on clinical data of specific doses and irradiated volumes of lung. The clinical data were provided by the landmark paper from Emami,[66] which provided the TD5 and TD50 for 1/3, 2/3 and whole-lung irradiation. Burman et al. utilized Lyman's model of interpolating clinical data to represent an NTCP. The model incorporated three quantities: complication probability, dose, and partial volume. A complication probability is subsequently generated as a means to compare treatment plans.

J.T. Lyman first introduced the concept of NTCP in a 1985 publication from the Lawrence Berkeley Laboratory. In this landmark study, Lyman outlined the concept of this parameter using the kidney. Cumulative DVHs were depicted for several possible treatment plans (2-field vs. 3-field vs. 4-field, etc.). From these histograms and previously published $TD_{50/5}$ values, defined as the probability that a dose will result in a 50% complication probability in 5 years, the probability of complication to a particular organ was defined in an equation relating the number of standard deviations between the mean $TD_{50/5}$ at that volume of tissue and the dose-volume combination that was present in the individual histogram. Or, put another way, the method combined what had been previously published

regarding the complication rates of different structures based on the volume irradiated and mathematically related these values to the individual patient's DVH.[67]

The NTCP model has been utilized in at least two Phase I protocols of dose escalation in NSCLC at the University of Michigan and at MSKCC.[68,69] At MSKCC, a fatal complication in an early dose escalation level compelled the use of the NTCP to help gauge risk in future patients. Initially, an NTCP value of 0.20 was utilized as a threshold. When this was determined to be safe, it was raised to 0.25 for the remainder of the protocol. At the University of Michigan, the NTCP model was used to generate a series of iso-complication plots that specified the dose of volume of uniformly irradiated ipsilateral normal lung expected to result in the same probability of grade 2 or higher RP. Using 2.1-Gy fractions, they were able to escalate small tumors to 102.9 Gy, intermediate-sized tumors to 75.6 to 84 Gy, and large tumors to 65.1 Gy.

Investigators at MDACC recently attempted to improve on the Lyman NTCP model by incorporating time-to-toxicity data and clinical risk factors in order to better predict rates of RP. The investigators reviewed the records of 576 patients with NSCLC and a history of RT. More specifically, this model does not measure the probability of *observing* a complication, as does the Lyman model, but the probability that a complication *would eventually occur* if the patient survived and underwent adequate follow-up. With patient smoking status taken into account as well, the revised model, termed the "generalized" Lyman model, provided NTCP estimates that were up to 27% different from the original model. The authors concluded that the inclusion of nondosimetric risk factors and time-to-event data can markedly affect outcome predictions made using the more binary approach in the original Lyman model.[70] The clinical significance of these revisions, as would be demonstrated in patient trials, is yet to be determined.

BREAST CANCER

Speirer et al. reported no cases of symptomatic RP in 118 patients treated with post–mastectomy electron beam radiotherapy. The NTCP in these patients was zero.[71] Pierce et al.[72] from the University of Michigan reported superior dosimetric calculations with standard tangents as opposed to partially wide tangents, mixed photon/electron or large tangent ("hockey stick") fields.

Recently, investigators have evaluated the use of accelerated partial-breast irradiation (APBI) as an alternative to whole-breast irradiation. The advantages of APBI include a shorter treatment time and a lower volume of irradiated breast. When APBI is delivered via 3D-CRT, there is a potential risk of RP. Recht et al.[73] reported four cases of pneumonitis out of 198 patients treated with APBI, all of whom received photons alone as opposed to mixed photons/electron or protons. The rate of pneumonitis was significantly higher in patients if the ipsilateral lung volume was too high. They recommended using mixed photons/electrons if necessary to keep the ipsilateral lung dose below the following constraints: ILV 20 Gy: 3%, ILV 10 Gy: 10%, ILV 5 Gy: 20%.

LYMPHOMA

Although the doses used to treat lymphoma tend to be low, the additional exposure to potentially toxic chemotherapy still leaves patients at risk for lung injury. Bleomycin especially has been associated with pulmonary toxicity. One study demonstrated that patients who received mantle or mediastinal radiation in addition to bleomycin had larger decreases in their PFTs.[74] Total body irradiation (TBI) as a component of allogeneic bone marrow transplantation is a frequently used in the treatment of leukemias and lymphomas. Studies have shown an 11% incidence of pneumonitis with a TBI dose of 12 Gy in six fractions. This decreases to 2.3% with the use of lung shielding.[75]

USE OF AMIFOSTINE

Amifostine (WR-2721) is a thiophosphate that was initially developed as a radioprotectant against nuclear fallout. (see Chapter 5.) It works through its active metabolite, a free thiol, which is thought to provide an alternative target for reactive species that would otherwise target DNA. Clinically, amifostine has been studied as a chemoprotectant from the nephrotoxic effects of cisplatin. It has been studied as a radioprotectant in multiple organ sites, especially the salivary gland and the esophagus. In lung cancer, the use of amifostine was the subject of RTOG Protocol 98-01, which failed to show a significant decrease in esophagus in patients treated with an aggressive regimen of concurrent chemoradiation. A separate study from the MD Anderson Cancer Center randomized 62 patients with inoperable NSCLC. Both arms received 69.6 Gy in 1.2-Gy bid fractions with concurrent cisplatin and etoposide. The experimental arm received 500 mg intravenous 20 to 30 minutes before treatment the first 2 days of each week. The treatments arms demonstrated similar median survival (19–20 months) and the amifostine arm showed a significant decrease in esophagitis and RP (16% vs. 0%, $p = 0.020$). There was no statistically significant difference in late clinical or radiographic pulmonary effects.[76]

Two studies from Greece[77,78] also showed a significant decrease in the rate of RP both in the setting of RT alone and chemoradiation.

Despite these positive results, amifostine is not commonly used clinically due to a variety of reasons. Clinically, it is difficult to administer with hypotension being a major side effect. In addition, the conflicting data of its ability to minimize esophagitis have dampened the enthusiasm of using it in thoracic malignancies.

REFERENCES

1. Darby S, Hill D, Auvinen A, et al. Radon in homes and risk of lung cancer: collaborative analysis of individual data from 13 European case-control studies. *BMJ.* 2005;330(7485):223.
2. Lubin JH, Steindorf K. Cigarette use and the estimation of lung cancer attributable to radon in the United States. *Radiat Res.* 1995;141(1):79–85.
3. Bochicchio F. The radon issue: considerations on regulatory approaches and exposure evaluations on the basis of recent epidemiological results. *Appl Radiat Isot.* 2008;66(11):6.
4. Onishi H, Araki T, Shirato H, et al. Stereotactic hypofractionated high-dose irradiation for stage I nonsmall cell lung carcinoma: clinical outcomes in 245 subjects in a Japanese multiinstitutional study. *Cancer.* 2004;101(7):1623–1631.
5. Kwok E, Chan CK. Corticosteroids and azathioprine do not prevent radiation-induced lung injury. *Can Respir J.* 1998;5(3):211–214.
6. Robnett TJ, Machtay M, Vines EF, et al. Factors predicting severe radiation pneumonitis in patients receiving definitive chemoradiation for lung cancer. *Int J Radiat Oncol Biol Phys.* 2000;48(1):89–94.
7. Delanian S, Porcher R, Rudant J, et al. Kinetics of response to long-term treatment combining pentoxifylline and tocopherol in patients with superficial radiation-induced fibrosis. *J Clin Oncol.* 2005;23(34):8570–8579.
8. De Jaeger K, Seppenwoolde Y, Boersma LJ, et al. Pulmonary function following high-dose radiotherapy of non-small-cell lung cancer. *Int J Radiat Oncol Biol Phys.* 2003;55(5):1331–1340.
9. Miller KL, Zhou SM, Barrier RC, Jr, et al. Long-term changes in pulmonary function tests after definitive radiotherapy for lung cancer. *Int J Radiat Oncol Biol Phys.* 2003;56(3):611–615.
10. Gopal R, Starkschall G, Tucker SL, et al. Effects of radiotherapy and chemotherapy on lung function in patients with non-small-cell lung cancer. *Int J Radiat Oncol Biol Phys.* 2003;56(1):114–120.
11. Moosavi H, McDonald S, Rubin P, et al. Early radiation dose-response in lung: an ultrastructural study. *Int J Radiat Oncol Biol Phys.* 1977;2(9-10):921–931.
12. Travis EL. The sequence of histological changes in mouse lungs after single doses of x-rays. *Int J Radiat Oncol Biol Phys.* 1980;6(3):345–347.
13. Rubin P, Finkelstein J, Shapiro D. Molecular biology mechanisms in the radiation induction of pulmonary injury syndromes: interrelationship between the alveolar macrophage and the septal fibroblast. *Int J Radiat Oncol Biol Phys.* 1992;24(1):93–101.
14. Ghosh SN, Wu Q, Mader M, et al. Vascular injury after whole thoracic x-ray irradiation in the rat. *Int J Radiat Oncol Biol Phys.* 2009;74(1):192–199.
15. Bentzen SM. Preventing or reducing late side effects of radiation therapy: radiobiology meets molecular pathology. *Nat Rev Cancer.* 2006;6(9):702–713.
16. Ferguson MW, Duncan J, Bond J, et al. Prophylactic administration of avotermin for improvement of skin scarring: three double-blind, placebo-controlled, phase I/II studies. *Lancet.* 2009;373(9671):1264–1274.
17. Schnaper HW, Jandeska S, Runyan CE, et al. TGF-beta signal transduction in chronic kidney disease. *Front Biosci.* 2009;14:2448–2465.
18. Ewan KB, Henshall-Powell RL, Ravani SA, et al. Transforming growth factor-beta1 mediates cellular response to DNA damage in situ. *Cancer Res.* 2002;62(20):5627–5631.
19. Wrana JL, Attisano L, Wieser R, et al. Mechanism of activation of the TGF-beta receptor. *Nature.* 1994;370(6488):341–347.
20. Herskind C, Rodemann HP. Spontaneous and radiation-induced differentiationof fibroblasts. *Exp Gerontol.* 2000;35(6-7):747–755.
21. Mikkelsen RB, Wardman P. Biological chemistry of reactive oxygen and nitrogen and radiation-induced signal transduction mechanisms. *Oncogene.* 2003;22(37):5734–5754.
22. Kinnula VL, Crapo JD. Superoxide dismutases in the lung and human lung diseases. *Am J Respir Crit Care Med.* 2003;167(12):1600–1619.
23. Robbins ME, Diz DI. Pathogenic role of the renin-angiotensin system in modulating radiation-induced late effects. *Int J Radiat Oncol Biol Phys.* 2006;64(1):6–12.
24. Zakheim RM, Mattioli L, Molteni A, et al. Prevention of pulmonary vascular changes of chronic alveolar hypoxia by inhibition of angiotensin I-converting enzyme in the rat. *Lab Invest.* 1975;33(1):57–61.
25. Fajardo L, Berthrong M, Anderson R. Respiratory tract. *Radiation Pathology.* New York, NY: Oxford University Press; 2001.

26. Evans ML, Graham MM, Mahler PA, et al. Changes in vascular permeability following thorax irradiation in the rat. *Radiat Res.* 1986;107(2):262–271.

27. Travis EL, Harley RA, Fenn JO, et al. Pathologic changes in the lung following single and multi-fraction irradiation. *Int J Radiat Oncol Biol Phys.* 1977;2(5-6):475–490.

28. Gross NJ. The pathogenesis of radiation-induced lung damage. *Lung.* 1981;159(3):115–125.

29. Rubin P, Finkelstein JN, Siemann DW, et al. Predictive biochemical assays for late radiation effects. *Int J Radiat Oncol Biol Phys.* 1986;12(4):469–476.

30. Rubin P, McDonald S, Maasilta P, et al. Serum markers for prediction of pulmonary radiation syndromes. Part I: Surfactant apoprotein. *Int J Radiat Oncol Biol Phys.* 1989;17(3):553–558.

31. Morgan GW, Breit SN. Radiation and the lung: a reevaluation of the mechanisms mediating pulmonary injury. *Int J Radiat Oncol Biol Phys.* 1995;31(2):361–369.

32. Down JD, Steel GG. The expression of early and late damage after thoracic irradiation: a comparison between CBA and C57Bl mice. *Radiat Res.* 1983;96(3):603–610.

33. Kong FM, Ten Haken R, Eisbruch A, et al. Non-small cell lung cancer therapy-related pulmonary toxicity: an update on radiation pneumonitis and fibrosis. *Semin Oncol.* 2005;32(2 Suppl 3):S42–S54.

34. Provatopoulou X, Athanasiou E, Gounaris A. Predictive markers of radiation pneumonitis. *Anticancer Res.* 2008;28(4C):2421–2432.

35. Chen Y, Williams J, Ding I, et al. Radiation pneumonitis and early circulatory cytokine markers. *Semin Radiat Oncol.* 2002;12(1 Suppl 1):26–33.

36. Anscher MS, Kong FM, Marks LB, et al. Changes in plasma transforming growth factor beta during radiotherapy and the risk of symptomatic radiation-induced pneumonitis. *Int J Radiat Oncol Biol Phys.* 1997;37(2):253–258.

37. Vujaskovic Z, Groen HJ. TGF-beta, radiation-induced pulmonary injury and lung cancer. *Int J Radiat Biol.* 2000;76(4):511–516.

38. Novakova-Jiresova A, Van Gameren MM, Coppes RP, et al. Transforming growth factor-beta plasma dynamics and post-irradiation lung injury in lung cancer patients. *Radiother Oncol.* 2004;71(2):183–189.

39. Arpin D, Perol D, Blay JY, et al. Early variations of circulating interleukin-6 and interleukin-10 levels during thoracic radiotherapy are predictive for radiation pneumonitis. *J Clin Oncol.* 2005;23(34):8748–8756.

40. Hart JP, Broadwater G, Rabbani Z, et al. Cytokine profiling for prediction of symptomatic radiation-induced lung injury. *Int J Radiat Oncol Biol Phys.* 2005;63(5):1448–1454.

41. Goto K, Kodama T, Sekine I, et al. Serum levels of KL-6 are useful biomarkers for severe radiation pneumonitis. *Lung Cancer.* 2001;34(1):141–148.

42. Hara R, Itami J, Komiyama T, et al. Serum levels of KL-6 for predicting the occurrence of radiation pneumonitis after stereotactic radiotherapy for lung tumors. *Chest.* 2004;125(1):340–344.

43. Matsuno Y, Satoh H, Ishikawa H, et al. Simultaneous measurements of KL-6 and SP-D in patients undergoing thoracic radiotherapy. *Med Oncol.* 2006;23(1):75–82.

44. Kuroki Y, Voelker DR. Pulmonary surfactant proteins. *J Biol Chem.* 1994;269(42):25943–25946.

45. Takahashi H, Sano H, Chiba H, et al. Pulmonary surfactant proteins A and D: innate immune functions and biomarkers for lung diseases. *Curr Pharm Des.* 2006;12(5):589–598.

46. Sasaki R, Soejima T, Matsumoto A, et al. Clinical significance of serum pulmonary surfactant proteins a and d for the early detection of radiation pneumonitis. *Int J Radiat Oncol Biol Phys.* 2001;50(2):301–307.

47. Takahashi H, Imai Y, Fujishima T, et al. Diagnostic significance of surfactant proteins A and D in sera from patients with radiation pneumonitis. *Eur Respir J.* 2001;17(3):481–487.

48. Tsujisaki M, Imai K, Hirata H, et al. Detection of circulating intercellular adhesion molecule-1 antigen in malignant diseases. *Clin Exp Immunol.* 1991;85(1):3–8.

49. Kawana A, Shioya S, Katoh H, et al. Expression of intercellular adhesion molecule-1 and lymphocyte function-associated antigen-1 on alveolar macrophages in the acute stage of radiation-induced lung injury in rats. *Radiat Res.* 1997;147(4):431–436.

50. Hallahan DE, Virudachalam S. Ionizing radiation mediates expression of cell adhesion molecules in distinct histological patterns within the lung. *Cancer Res.* 1997;57(11):2096–2099.

51. Brooks BJ, Jr, Seifter EJ, Walsh TE, et al. Pulmonary toxicity with combined modality therapy for limited stage small-cell lung cancer. *J Clin Oncol.* 1986;4(2):200–209.

52. Byhardt RW, Scott C, Sause WT, et al. Response, toxicity, failure patterns, and survival in five Radiation Therapy Oncology Group (RTOG) trials of sequential and/or concurrent chemotherapy and radiotherapy for locally advanced non-small-cell carcinoma of the lung. *Int J Radiat Oncol Biol Phys.* 1998;42(3):469–478.

53. Monson JM, Stark P, Reilly JJ, et al. Clinical radiation pneumonitis and radiographic changes after thoracic radiation therapy for lung carcinoma. *Cancer.* 1998;82(5):842–850.

54. Schaake-Koning C, van den Bogaert W, Dalesio O, et al. Effects of concomitant cisplatin and radiotherapy on inoperable non-small-cell lung cancer. *N Engl J Med.* 1992;326(8):524–530.

55. Hernando ML, Marks LB, Bentel GC, et al. Radiation-induced pulmonary toxicity: a dose-volume histogram analysis in 201 patients with lung cancer. *Int J Radiat Oncol Biol Phys.* 2001;51(3):650–659.

56. Mehta V. Radiation pneumonitis and pulmonary fibrosis in non-small-cell lung cancer: pulmonary function, prediction, and prevention. *Int J Radiat Oncol Biol Phys.* 2005;63(1):5–24.

57. Marks LB, Munley MT, Bentel GC, et al. Physical and biological predictors of changes in whole-lung function following thoracic irradiation. *Int J Radiat Oncol Biol Phys.* 1997;39(3):563–570.

58. Inoue A, Kunitoh H, Sekine I, et al. Radiation pneumonitis in lung cancer patients: a retrospective study of risk factors and the long-term prognosis. *Int J Radiat Oncol Biol Phys.* 2001;49(3):649–655.

59. Gopal R, Tucker SL, Komaki R, et al. The relationship between local dose and loss of function for irradiated lung. *Int J Radiat Oncol Biol Phys.* 2003;56(1):106–113.

60. Willner J, Jost A, Baier K, et al. A little to a lot or a lot to a little? An analysis of pneumonitis risk from dose-volume histogram parameters of the lung in patients with lung cancer treated with 3-D conformal radiotherapy. *Strahlenther Onkol.* 2003;179(8):548–556.

61. Graham MV, Purdy JA, Emami B, et al. Clinical dose-volume histogram analysis for pneumonitis after 3D treatment for non-small cell lung cancer (NSCLC). *Int J Radiat Oncol Biol Phys.* 1999;45(2):323–329.

62. Schallenkamp JM, Miller RC, Brinkmann DH, et al. Incidence of radiation pneumonitis after thoracic irradiation: Dose-volume correlates. *Int J Radiat Oncol Biol Phys.* 2007;67(2):410–416.

63. Yorke ED, Jackson A, Rosenzweig KE, et al. Dose-volume factors contributing to the incidence of radiation pneumonitis in non-small-cell lung cancer patients treated with three-dimensional conformal radiation therapy. *Int J Radiat Oncol Biol Phys.* 2002;54(2):329–339.

64. Bradley JD, Hope A, El Naqa I, et al. A nomogram to predict radiation pneumonitis, derived from a combined analysis of RTOG 9311 and institutional data. *Int J Radiat Oncol Biol Phys.* 2007;69(4):985–992.

65. Burman C, Kutcher GJ, Emami B, et al. Fitting of normal tissue tolerance data to an analytic function. *Int J Radiat Oncol Biol Phys.* 1991;21(1):123–135.

66. Emami B, Lyman J, Brown A, et al. Tolerance of normal tissue to therapeutic irradiation. *Int J Radiat Oncol Biol Phys.* 1991;21(1):109–122.

67. Lyman JT. Complication probability as assessed from dose-volume histograms. *Radiat Res Suppl.* 1985;8:S13–S19.

68. Hayman JA, Martel MK, Ten Haken RK, et al. Dose escalation in non-small-cell lung cancer using three-dimensional conformal radiation therapy: update of a phase I trial. *J Clin Oncol.* 2001;19(1):127–136.

69. Rosenzweig KE, Fox JL, Yorke E, et al. Results of a phase I dose-escalation study using three-dimensional conformal radiotherapy in the treatment of inoperable nonsmall cell lung carcinoma. *Cancer.* 2005;103(10):2118–2127.

70. Tucker SL, Liu HH, Liao Z, et al. Analysis of radiation pneumonitis risk using a generalized Lyman model. *Int J Radiat Oncol Biol Phys.* 2008;72(2):568–574.

71. Spierer MM, Hong LX, Wagman RT, et al. Postmastectomy CT-based electron beam radiotherapy: dosimetry, efficacy, and toxicity in 118 patients. *Int J Radiat Oncol Biol Phys.* 2004;60(4):1182–1189.

72. Pierce LJ, Butler JB, Martel MK, et al. Postmastectomy radiotherapy of the chest wall: dosimetric comparison of common techniques. *Int J Radiat Oncol Biol Phys.* 2002;52(5):1220–1230.

73. Recht A, Ancukiewicz M, Alm El-Din MA, et al. Lung dose-volume parameters and the risk of pneumonitis for patients treated with accelerated partial-breast irradiation using three-dimensional conformal radiotherapy. *J Clin Oncol.* 2009;27(24):3887–3893.

74. Hirsch A, Vander Els N, Straus DJ, et al. Effect of ABVD chemotherapy with and without mantle or mediastinal irradiation on pulmonary function and symptoms in early-stage Hodgkin's disease. *J Clin Oncol.* 1996;14(4):1297–1305.

75. Sampath S, Schultheiss TE, Wong J. Dose response and factors related to interstitial pneumonitis after bone marrow transplant. *Int J Radiat Oncol Biol Phys.* 2005;63(3):876–884.

76. Komaki R, Lee JS, Milas L, et al. Effects of amifostine on acute toxicity from concurrent chemotherapy and radiotherapy for inoperable non-small-cell lung cancer: report of a randomized comparative trial. *Int J Radiat Oncol Biol Phys.* 2004;58(5):1369–1377.

77. Antonadou D, Coliarakis N, Synodinou M, et al. Randomized phase III trial of radiation treatment +/– amifostine in patients with advanced-stage lung cancer. *Int J Radiat Oncol Biol Phys.* 2001;51(4):915–922.

78. Antonadou D, Throuvalas N, Petridis A, et al. Effect of amifostine on toxicities associated with radiochemotherapy in patients with locally advanced non-small-cell lung cancer. *Int J Radiat Oncol Biol Phys.* 2003;57(2):402–408.

Heart

Philippe Giraud, Mehdi Henni,
Michael Yassa, Jean-Marc Cosset

INTRODUCTION

The anatomical position of the heart, and the relative radiosensitivity of its structural components, make it a critical organ at risk when irradiating the thorax or the mediastinum. Radiation treatments for lymphomas, pulmonary tumors, and esophageal or breast cancer expose the heart to varying, nonnegligible doses of radiation, causing potentially lethal side effects. It has long been recognized that ionizing radiation and its sequelae represent the second most prevalent cause of death, after progression of disease, in cancer patients who have undergone mediastinal irradiation.[1,2]

Up until the 1960s, the heart was often considered a radioresistant organ. With the improvement in long-term survival of patients treated for Hodgkin disease and other lymphomas, radiation-related cardiac toxicities became evident.[1,3] However, because of the diversity of side effects and symptoms, the numerous confounding risk factors for cardiac disease (chemotherapy, hypercholesterolemia, tobacco use, etc.) and the difficulties in properly evaluating patients for cardiotoxicity, no definitive consensus has been reached on the true incidence of cardiac complications after radiation therapy. A review of the literature on the subject of cardiac toxicity from radiation treatments is further complicated by the fact that modern publications are based on patients who were treated 10 to 20 years ago, using older and less precise techniques, unrepresentative of today's practice. Technological advances, such as three-dimensional (3D) imaging, conformal radiotherapy, intensity-modulated radiation, and respiratory gating, should help to reduce the cardiac side effects of radiation therapy. Furthermore, the use of *de-escalated* doses in some pathology, notably Hodgkin disease, will have a positive impact on reducing, and maybe eliminating, cardiac side effects.[4]

The clinical pictures of cardiac complications are several. Early-onset cardiac toxicity is most often seen in the form of acute pericarditis, while late complications can range from chronic constrictive pericarditis and myocarditis, to coronary disease, valvulopathy or conduction deficits.

In the following chapter, we recall different anatomical subcomponents of the heart and explain the impact of ionizing radiation on each of these. Early- and late-appearing complications associated with radiation therapy, and methods aimed at reducing them, will be described. Finally, the role of

chemotherapy, especially anthracyclines, and its impact on the heart when used in adjunct with radiation will be reviewed.

ANATOMY AND PATHOLOGICAL CONCEPTS

EMBRYOLOGY

Although the anatomy of the heart may appear less complicated than some other vital organs, the heart plays a crucial role in life even as early as the third week of gestation.[5] The heart is indispensable to all stages of fetal development. By the ninth week of gestation, its genesis is almost complete. Postnatally, the heart will continue to develop mostly due to hyperplasia and hypertrophy of myocardial cells. At 6 months, the maximum number of these myocardial cells is reached. All subsequent modification of the heart muscle is due to either cellular hypertrophy or scarring fibrosis resulting from a pathological insult.[6]

ANATOMY

The heart is a four-chamber structure. Each pair of chambers (one atrium and one ventricle) acts as the right and left heart. The wall of these chambers will rhythmically contract, propulsing oxygenated or deoxygenated blood through either the systemic circulation or the pulmonary circulation, respectively. This cardiac wall is made up of three layers: endocardium, myocardium, and pericardium. The endocardium is the layer that lines the inside of the chambers, as well as the cardiac valves. It comprises an endothelium resting on conjunctive tissue. The myocardium is the muscular layer of the heart and is variable in size. It is made of striated muscular fiber unable to regenerate if damaged. The pericardium consists of a single layer of mesenchymal cells resting on a fine conjunctiva, forming an almost inextensible envelope.[5]

The heart has a fragile system of arterial vascularization with little area of overlap. Conversely, it is rich in capillaries, located mostly in the myocardium, and these act as an ideal target for ionizing radiation. It is these capillaries that will be damaged when irradiated causing adjacent epithelial cell damage. Indeed, late radiation toxicity is essentially a result of endothelial cell destruction inducing smooth muscle cell migration into surrounding blood vessel walls and causing lumen narrowing.[7]

In order to get a harmonious and progressive contractile wave through the muscles lining the cardiac chambers, the heart relies on a specialized neural network called the *nodal tissue*. An electric stimulus, usually originating from the nodal sinus and progressing through the AV node and down the Purkinje fibers, will conduct the contractile signal to help "push" blood in the correct direction.

PATHOPHYSIOLOGY OF IONIZING RADIATION EFFECTS ON THE HEART

The mechanism in which ionizing radiation damages the heart is poorly understood. It is probably a result of a chain reaction that starts with microvascular injury, which induces ischemia in the cardiac tissue and eventually leads to fibrosis.[3,8–11]

The pericardium is the most commonly affected heart tissue. Damage is manifested by a fibrotic thickening whose exact pathogenesis is unknown. Late ischemic damage is probably a result of microangiopathy[12]; however, other mechanisms might also play a role. These may include the persistence of an inflammatory exudate at the pericardial surface that sets off a cascade of biochemical reactions from the inhibition of tissue plasminogen activator to the production of collagen.[13] This is most often associated with an effusion rich in protein that may be quite significant in volume. Its insidious onset rarely causes tamponade.[3,10,11] With time, fibrosis may evolve to a chronic pericarditis, which remains fortunately rare.[12,14]

The myocardium, although less often affected than the pericardium, can develop more serious complications. The left ventricle is more commonly affected than the right because of its anterior position.[15,16] Radiation induces the deposition of fibrotic plaques in the myocardium that may become necrotic. These plaques usually arise in areas downstream of pathologically damaged coronary arteries.[9] Much like other radiation injury, damage to the myocardium is more a result of small capillary endothelial cell death rather than a direct insult to postmitotic myocytes.[14] This initiates intravascular thrombosis and microrupture of arterioles and capillaries, leading to a disruption of the vascular network in the myocardium. This, with time, will lead to hypoxia, progressing to ischemia, and eventually leading to myocardial fibrosis.[17]

The endocardium is affected much like the myocardium and develops fibrotic plaques when exposed to ionizing radiation. Rarely symptomatic, these lesions are a consequence of hypoxia and ischemia from damage to the arterial supply.[12,15]

Coronary artery involvement is often characterized by endoluminal fibromuscular hyperplasia, aggravating the risk of atherosclerosis.[18] The preexistence of coronary disease is most probably an important cofactor to subsequent radiation injury. However, the direct impact of radiation on endothelial cell cannot be ignored. The damaging effect is, as for other target tissue in the heart, a result of a thrombotic phenomenon and ischemia in downstream tissue leading to architectural (valvulopathy) and functional disruption (conduction anomalies).[3,10,19]

SYMPTOMATOLOGY

It is important to remember that symptomatic cardiac toxicity from ionizing radiation is often a late-occurring event and that most affected patients will have subclinical, asymptomatic cardiac dysfunction.[11,14] Table 29.1 shows main characteristics of cardiac toxicities induced by radiation therapy.

Cardiac complications are most often observed in patients treated for Hodgkin lymphoma and breast cancer: two upper body cancers with usually good prognosis and potentially long survival after treatment.

For Hodgkin disease, mantle irradiation was for a long time the standard technique (Fig. 29.1). More recent data suggests that low-dose, involved field radiation and chemotherapy are similar in efficacy compared to larger volume, high dose radiation. For breast cancer, dose to the heart is increased when treating the left breast. Furthermore, cardiac dose varies with the anatomical configuration of the breast, its location on the thoracic wall, and with the radiation technique used. Figure 29.2 shows the dose distribution when irradiating a left breast by the technique of tangential fields and an internal mammary field.

EARLY COMPLICATIONS

During the course of radiation treatments, cardiac symptoms are usually the result of pericardial disease (Table 29.1). This is an infrequent nonmalignant inflammation that rarely requires

TABLE 29.1	**Main Characteristics of Cardiac Toxicities from Radiation Therapy**					
	Time of Onset	*Symptoms*	*Pathogenesis*	*Dose Range (Gy)*	*Incidence*[a]	*Mortality*
Acute pericarditis	During or soon after RT	Fever, chest pain	Inflammatory?	>35	5%	Self resolving
Chronic pericarditis	1–2 years	Asymptomatic	Microangiopathy	35–40	1% 10%	1%
Myocarditis	Usually follows chronic pericarditis	Often asymptomatic, decreased EF	Microvascular damage	35–40	30%–50%[b]	<1%
Coronary artery disease	>5 years	Asymptomatic, nonspecific	Microvascular damage	>30	5%–10%	2.5%
Valvulopathy	>5 ans	Valvular dysfunction	Late fibrosis	30–40	15%–30%	
Conduction anomalies	>5 ans	Asymptomatic	Late fibrosis	30–40	NR	NR

[a]Mean incidence based on different publications.
[b]Autopsy series.
NR, not reported.

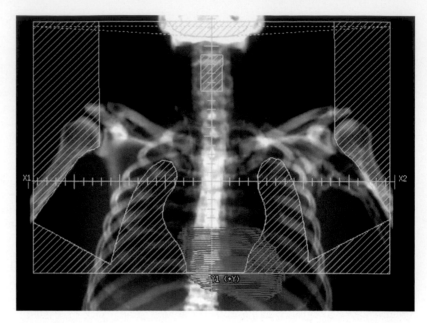

Figure 29.1. Anterior portal of a supradiaphragmatic radiation treatment for Hodgkin disease. Lung, heart, buccal, and laryngeal shields can be seen.

cessation of treatment. Incidence is higher when the volume of irradiated heart is more important.[20] Most often, the pericardial effusion is small and asymptomatic. Rarely, symptoms develop resembling that of an infectious pericarditis with fever and chest pain. On exam, a friction rub may be noted on auscultation and classic electrocardiogram changes of diffuse ST elevation and PR depression may be present. The episode usually resolves spontaneously within a few weeks. These symptoms are in no way a precursor of chronic constrictive pericarditis[14]; however, true acute constrictive pericarditis may still arise months, and up to 2 years, after radiotherapy.[20,21]

LATE COMPLICATIONS

Chronic Constrictive Pericarditis

Chronic pericarditis is a late-occurring complication of radiation therapy, arising months to years after treatment (Table 29.1). The incidence is 1% to 5% in breast and lung cancer patients,[21] but slightly higher with lymphoma (5%–10%).[22] These data are from older series looking at patients treated with obsolete techniques and often evaluated by subjective nonstandardized methods. In reality, the true incidence of chronic pericarditis depends largely on the physician's ability to recognize

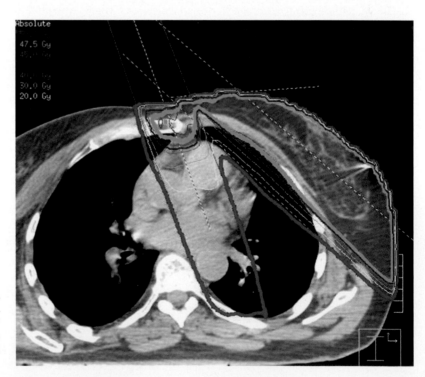

Figure 29.2. Radiation dose distribution for a treatment of a left breast by tangential fields and the internal mammary chain by direct anterior mixed electron/photon field. Isodoses are color coded, as per reference on the figure. The heart receives a dose between 1 and 40 Gy.

the subtle signs that may arise insidiously and to order the appropriate diagnostic test.[14] In a series of 2,232 Hodgkin lymphoma patients treated at Stanford University, the mortality rate from pericarditis was 0.7%.[23]

As for acute pericarditis, the symptoms of chronic pericarditis are nonspecific.[11] Often asymptomatic, it can be diagnosed by pulmonary radiograph, electrocardiogram, or cardiac echography. Catheterization by Swan-Ganz may be needed to confirm the diagnosis.[20] The majority of chronic pericarditis will also regress spontaneously, with no long-term adverse complication. However, some patients will develop a late constrictive pericarditis with rapidly progressing cardiac effusion that may result in tamponade requiring drainage or a pericardial window.[3,11,18] Other than this rare form of presentation, treatment is usually medical, with surgery reserved for life-threatening cases or highly exudative form of pericarditis.[20]

Dose per fraction and total dose constitute the main factors responsible for developing chronic pericarditis. As for the acute form, the risk is greater when a larger proportion of heart is irradiated.[13] Regarding total dose, the risk of pericarditis is present at 35 Gy, but increases significantly above 40 Gy. In fact, this threshold dose of 40 Gy has become a maximal limit of acceptable dose to the heart.[11,14,21] In the literature, the frequency of chronic pericarditis reported varies greatly, from 4% to 96%, but is probably more accurately estimated to be between 2% and 7% for mediastinal doses ranging from 35 to 40 Gy.[22]

Myocarditis

Generally, myocarditis arises in patients who already have chronic pericarditis with significant diastolic cardiac insufficiency (Table 29.1). Myocarditis often becomes evident when cardiac symptoms and signs persist despite treatment for pericarditis.[11]

The incidence of radiation-induced myocarditis is difficult to determine; it is probably low with modern-day techniques but increases when radiation is associated with chemotherapy, particularly anthracyclines.[14] In the latter case, myocarditis may be seen outside the context of a preexisting pericarditis.[11] Autopsy series have found myocardial fibrosis in 50% of patients irradiated at a young age.[15] Ventricular hypokinesia occurs

less frequently, being reported in 5% to 25% of cases.[24] Also, numerous publications on the long-term follow-up of patients with Hodgkin disease who underwent radiation therapy have shown decreased left ventricular ejection fraction in 30% to 50%.[22] The interpretation of all these data is subject to potential bias, such as the radiation technique used, the method of calculation of dose to the heart, and the retrospective nature of the data collection. It seems, from modern series, that patients treated with newer techniques have normal cardiac function and maintain this through long-term follow-up.[4]

The pathophysiology of this damage is microcirculation damage by ionizing radiation, with a resulting chronic diffuse ischemia of the myocardium. For most authors, biopsy is rarely indicated because of the poor correlation of the histological information and the functional outcome.[4]

The treatment of radiation-induced myocarditis is nonspecific and pertains more to medical treatment to correct the anomalies caused by cardiac insufficiency.[21]

Coronary Disease

Coronary complications from radiation occur less frequently than pericardial injury. The true incidence is probably underestimated because coronary disease is often asymptomatic (Table 29.1). However, coronary disease may lead to nonspecific secondary cardiac disease, which is in itself symptomatic, such as myocardiopathy, valvulopathy, and conduction anomalies.[19] Rutqvist et al.[25] found that the relative mortality rate for coronary artery disease was 3.2 in patients irradiated for left breast cancer. Cosset et al.[26] observed a 4% significant increase in the 10-year cumulative incidence of coronary disease in patients undergoing mediastinal radiation. The mortality from myocardial infarction was 2.5% in the Stanford series of young patients with Hodgkin disease, with a relative risk of 4 (Fig. 29.3).[27] These statistics have all been confirmed in numerous other studies.[11,28,29] As for cardiomyopathies, most studies reported a higher, and more severe, risk in patients irradiated at a young age.[11,14,22] In the report by Gustavsson et al.,[30] the relative risk of myocardial infarction in young patients undergoing irradiation was 41.5.[30] The risk of coronary artery disease is associated to total dose of radiation. Although the risk is relatively

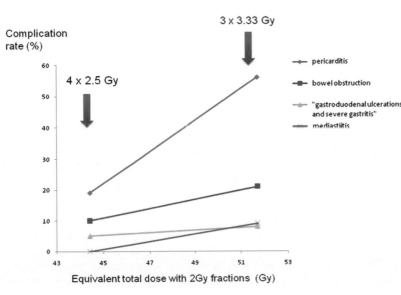

Figure 29.3. Complication rate of radiation treatment of Hodgkin disease as function of the equivalent total dose with 2-Gy fractions. (Modified from original figure published by Cosset JM, Henry-Amar M, Girinsky T, et al. Late toxicity of radiotherapy in Hodgkin's disease: the role of fraction size. *Acta Oncol.* 1988;27:123–130.)

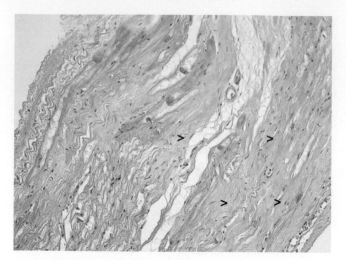

Figure 29.4. Interstitial fibrosis (*arrowheads*) of the myocardium and myocyte alterations in a patient treated by radiotherapy for Hodgkin disease (HES stain; obj ×10).

low for doses below 30 Gy, it is estimated at 37% if dose is above 40 Gy.[14,25,31] The subcarinal block, placed after 30 Gy to block the heart in the traditional 2D technique for patients with Hodgkin disease undergoing radiation therapy, does not properly shield the coronary ostia; thus, the risk of coronary artery disease is not significantly reduced.[14,27]

Coronary complications from radiation usually appear 5 to 6 years after treatment, which is longer than other cardiac complications. Proximal coronary artery involvement is frequent and often limited to only one main coronary artery.[13] This differs from the other etiologies of coronary disease. Screening is therefore possible in this group of patients, and angioplasty may remain a sufficient treatment to restore adequate blood perfusion to the myocardium.[15,32] If not, treatment of radiation-induced coronary artery disease is the same as for the classical form of the disease found in the normal population.[20] Figure 29.4 shows interstitial fibrosis (arrowheads) of the myocardium and myocyte alterations in a patient treated by radiotherapy for Hodgkin disease.

Other risk factors for cardiac disease, such as hypercholesterolemia or tobacco use, seem to accentuate coronary lesions, making the interpretation of the literature difficult.[11,14] Glanzman et al.,[22] in a report on patients who had undergone mediastinal irradiation, showed an excess mortality rate of 5% in patients with risk factors for cardiovascular disease, compared to no mortality increase for patients with no risk factors.

Valvulopathies

To prove a relation between ionizing radiation and a valvulopathy is difficult (Table 29.1). The most probable mechanism of valvulopathy is a perivalvular myocardial fibrosis that leads to a secondary dysfunction.[14] This indirect damage is difficult to analyze in the literature because the pre-existent cardiac function of patients is rarely documented and diagnostic procedures vary greatly.[22,30] With modern and more sophisticated diagnostic methods, the rate of valvulopathy is thought to be quite high and averages between 15% and 30%. The cumulative incidence at 20 and 25 years is reported to be 45% and 60%, respectively.[22,30] Valvular dysfunction is usually present as mitral or

aortic insufficiency.[10] Total dose is an important risk factor. Doses below 30 Gy do not seem to induce valvular damage; however, with doses of 31 to 40 Gy, the incidence of valvulopathy increases sharply to 12%.[22] Death from valvular disease in patients who have undergone mediastinal irradiation can reach 0.3%.[23]

Conduction Abnormalities

As for valvulopathies, it is difficult to demonstrate a direct relationship between ionizing radiation and conduction abnormalities. It is supposed that the disruption in the conduction pathways is a result of postradiation ischemia and fibrosis in the heart (Table 29.1). The conduction abnormalities are usually asymptomatic and diagnosed only on routine electrocardiogram. The typical pattern is an abnormal repolarization phase in the precordial leads.[33,34] However, more serious involvement, such as disruption of the atrioventricular or interventricular system, has been described from 1 to 23 years after radiation (on average, 13 years).[35]

At moderate doses (30 Gy) delivered with a conventional fractionation scheme (2 Gy per fraction), the risk of symptomatic conduction abnormalities is very low.[14] Lindahl et al.[36] observed repolarization anomalies in 35% of women who underwent radiation therapy for breast cancer and who received doses to the heart of more than 20 Gy.

SCREENING AND TREATMENT

It is mostly the long-term follow-up of patients treated for Hodgkin disease, which has forged our knowledge on cardiac toxicity from radiation therapy.[1,22,23,26,28,29,31,35,37-42] These patients, on average, received a significant dose of radiation to about 60% of the cardiac volume and 6.6% to 29% subsequently developed cardiac toxicity.[11] The relative risk of death from cardiac complications is between 2.2 and 7.2 in patients with Hodgkin disease who underwent mediastinal irradiation. Conversely, women treated for breast cancer receive less radiation to the heart, and so treatment tolerance and incidence of cardiac complications are lower.[25,36,43]

There is no specific treatment for radiation-induced cardiac complications[11,14,20]; prevention remains the best option. The effect of radiation on the heart is largely dependent on three factors: the volume, the total dose, and the dose per fraction of heart irradiated.[11,14] Reduction of these parameters has a positive impact and diminishes the potential cardiac toxicity associated with a radiation treatment plan.

The dose per fraction, in itself, is a nonnegligible factor. Cosset et al.[1,26] demonstrated that the cumulative incidence of pericarditis 5 years after treatment was 5% for a dose per fraction of 2 Gy and 7.5% for fractions of 3.3 Gy for an equal total dose.. The relative risk doubled when dose per fraction is equal or higher than 3 Gy compared to lower doses per fraction. However, a correlation between dose per fraction and myocardial infarction was not seen in this study.[1]

The volume of heart irradiated is probably the most important risk factor for cardiac toxicity from radiation. With a greater volume irradiated, there is an increased risk of heart complications. If the entire pericardium is irradiated, the incidence of acute and chronic complications is nearly 20%. This falls to 7% if only the left ventricle is shielded.[15] Three-dimensional conformal radiotherapy and intensity-modulated radiotherapy are now commonly used to decrease the volume of heart receiving radiation. Also, respiratory gating may present another solution

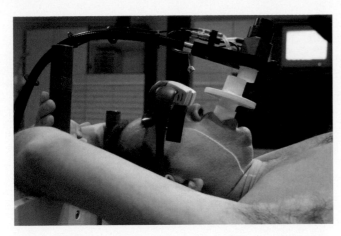

Figure 29.5. System for respiratory gating SDX (Dyn'R) by voluntary breath holding used at the *European Georges Pompidou Hospital*, with apparatus for visual feedback by video-glasses.

(Fig. 29.5). This technique allows the radiation to be administered cyclically during a precise phase of the respiratory cycle—usually a phase in which the heart is further from the radiation fields.[4, 44]

Total radiation dose is also a crucial factor determining cardiac toxicity. Studies of mantle irradiation for Hodgkin disease have shown that the cumulative incidence of pericarditis at 5 years increases with total dose to the heart.[1] Using similar fractionation, pericarditis incidence is 4% with a total dose of 36 Gy, and more than 10% for doses above 41 Gy. The relative risk was >3 for doses above 41 Gy.[1] Technically, for breast cancer patients undergoing internal mammary chain irradiation, dose to the heart, and cardiac complications, can be reduced using a mixed photon/electron technique.[43]

An essential and often overlooked factor is the decision to actually give a radiation treatment and the justification of the dose chosen. This is seen in the historical evolution of the treatment of Hodgkin disease where a de-escalation of radiation dose became the standard.[14,20] For early disease, dose has decreased dramatically, and radiation treatment is even omitted in some pediatric cases. In breast cancer, the indication and definition of target volumes is often rediscussed, particularly the regional nodal irradiation of the internal mammary chain.

Age of the patient also plays a crucial in the development of chronic cardiac toxicity. Patients irradiated before the age of 20 at doses above 35 Gy have a relative risk of death from myocardial infarction of 44. Relative risk of death from other cardiac causes is also high at 22.[27]

Treatment of cardiac complications is not specific to the cause. After failure of medical treatment, pericardiocentesis is usually the procedure of choice for reducing pericardial effusion or chronic pericarditis. Only when this fails is a pericardectomy proposed.[11,14,20,45] For coronary disease, correction and prevention of behavioral risk factors are essential.[22]

ASSOCIATION OF RADIATION THERAPY AND CHEMOTHERAPY

There are numerous cytotoxic medications causing potential cardiac toxicity. It is evident that combining these drugs with radiation therapy increases the likelihood of complications.[16,46–48] The typical example is the association of ionizing radiation with anthracyclines, notably doxorubicin.[46,47] The result is a diffuse fibrosis, physiologically different from the damage caused by radiation alone but with a similar symptomatology. The mechanism of action resulting in this damage is poorly understood. Chemotherapy does not directly impact endothelial cells, but rather causes myofibrillary damage that leads to myocyte degeneration. This damage is irreversible and eventually leads to myocardial fibrosis. When irradiation follows anthracycline treatment, it can aggravate cardiomyopathy by causing further damage to small blood vessels. Damage is therefore not synergistic but additive. When administration of anthracyclines follows irradiation, a phenomenon known as *radiation recall* may arise even months after the last radiation treatment. This will lead to an inflammatory response with endothelial damage similar to an early radiation injury.[46]

Cardiac complications may arise when radiation is administered to the mediastinum before, concurrently or after the use of anthracyclines; even with chemotherapy doses below the threshold thought safe (<450 mg/m²).[47] Of course, other existing factors are known to increase the risk of toxicity, such as age and preexisting cardiac disease. Doses of 20 to 30 Gy, when associated with anthracyclines, increase by a factor of 2 the risk of pericardial thickening seen with the use of chemotherapy alone.[14] A higher incidence of valvular damage, which is usually asymptomatic, is also observed with combination treatment with radiation therapy and anthracycline use.[11,49]

CONCLUSION

Although thoracic irradiation has indisputable benefits, it may also result in potentially severe complications. The risk of cardiac toxicity is increased in patients with preexisting heart disease and those undergoing radiation treatments at a young age. The association with chemotherapy, notably anthracyclines, also increases the risk of developing adverse events. In light of the term studies of patients treated for Hodgkin disease, much work has been done to develop techniques to decrease the risk to the heart. Various advances, such as proper delineation of radiation volumes, improved targeting of these volumes, modification of dose per fraction and radiation dose de-escalation, have all decreased the incidence and severity of cardiac complications. Initial results on cardiac toxicity in modern practice are promising; however, because the latency period for development of chronic complications is long, prudence and proper follow-up is still recommended.

SUMMARY

Irradiation of the heart may result in numerous complications, of which the most common is pericardial effusion. Thoracic and mediastinal irradiation of lymphoma, Hodgkin disease, and lung and breast cancer can result in adverse effects to every structural component of the heart. Potential injury includes acute and late pericarditis, cardiomyopathy, valvular disease, and conduction abnormalities. The pathophysiology of these various syndromes is probably similar, starting with microvascular injury and leading to subsequent myocardial ischemia, all causing late fibrous scars. Acute pericarditis is often asymptomatic and can resolve spontaneously. Late pericarditis affects approximately 5% of patients when the radiation dose to the heart exceeds 40 Gy with conventional fractionation. At this dose, the mortality rate is below 1%. Cardiomyopathy is rare and often asymptomatic. Coronary artery disease was for a long time unrecognized but is now diagnosed in 5% to 10% of patients. It is more likely to occur if the patient was young at the time of radiation treatment (<21 years), and the risk is further increased when other cardiovascular risk factors are present. Coronary artery disease may lead to myocardial infarction, valvular abnormalities, and cardiac rhythm changes. Conduction anomalies are seen in 5% of patients who have undergone radiation therapy to the thorax, valvular defects occur in 20% with resulting mortality in 0.5%. Radiation-induced heart injury seems to be related to total dose (>30 Gy), fraction size, and the volume of tissue irradiated. Because cardiac complications appear months to years following incidental irradiation of the heart, appropriate screening and long-term cardiac follow-up of these patients is essential.

REFERENCES

1. Cosset JM, Henry-Amar M, Pellae-Cosset B, et al. Pericarditis and myocardial infarction after Hodgkin's disease therapy. *Int J Radiat Oncol Biol Phys.* 1991;21:447–449.
2. Jones JM, Ribeiro GG. Mortality patterns over 34 years of breast cancer patients in a clinical trial of post-operative radiotherapy. *Clin Radiol.* 1989;40:204–208.
3. Cohn KE, Stewart JR, Fajardo LF, et al. Heart disease following radiation. *Medicine.* 1967;46:281–298.
4. Remouchamps VM, Vicini FA, Sharpe MB, et al. Significant reductions in heart and lung doses using deep inspiration breath hold with active breathing control and intensity-modulated radiation therapy for patients treated with locoregional breast irradiation. *Int J Radiat Oncol Biol Phys.* 2003;55(2):392–406.
5. Clark EB. Growth morphogenesis and function: the dynamics of heart development. In: Moller JH, Neal WA, Lock JE, eds. *Fetal, Neonatal, and Infant Heart Disease.* New York, NY: Appleton-Century-Crofts; 1990.
6. Fishman NH. Models of congenital heart disease in fetal lambs. *Circulation.* 1978;58:354–364.
7. Truesdell S, Schwartz C, Constine L, et al. Cardiovascular effects of cancer therapy. In: Schwartz C, Hobbie W, Constine L, et al., eds. *Survivors Of Childhood Cancers: Assessment and Management.* St. Louis, MO: Mosby Yearbook; 1994:159–176.
8. Archambeau J, Inès A, Fajardo LF. Response of swine skin microvasculature to acute single exposures of x-rays: quantification of endothelial changes. *Radiat Res.* 1984;98:37–51.
9. Fajardo LF, Stewart JR. Pathogenesis of radiation-induced myocardial fibrosis. *Lab Invest.* 1973;29:244–257.
10. Stewart JR, Cohn KE, Fajardo LF, et al. Radiation-induced heart disease. *Radiology.* 1967;89:302–310.
11. Stewart JR, Fajardo LF, Gillette SM, et al. Radiation injury to the heart. *Int J Radiat Oncol Biol Phys.* 1995;5:1205–1211.
12. Fajardo LF, Stewart JR, Cohn KE. Morphology of radiation-induced heart disease. *Arch Pathol.* 1968;86:512–519.
13. Ferrari E, Lagrange JL, Taillan B, et al. Complications cardiaques de la radiothérapie. *Ann Med Int.* 1993;1:23–27.
14. Girinski T, Cosset JM. Les effets tardifs pulmonaires et cardiaques induits par les radiations ionisantes seules ou associées à la chimiothérapie. *Cancer Radiother.* 1997;1:735–743.
15. Brosius FC, Waller BF, Roberts WC. Radiation heart disease. Analysis of 16 young (aged 15 to 33 years) necropsy patients who received over 3,500 rads to the heart. *Am J Med.* 1981;70:519–530.
16. Catane R, Schwade JG, Turrisi AT, et al. Pulmonary toxicity after radiation and bleomycin: a review. *Int J Radiat Oncol Biol Phys.* 1979;5:1513–1518.
17. Gillette EL, McChesney SL, Hoopes PJ. Isoeffect curves for radiation-induced cardiomyopathy in the dog. *Int J Radiat Oncol Biol Phys.* 1985;11:2091–2097.
18. Corn BW, Trock BJ, Goodman RL. Irradiation-related ischemic heart disease. *J Clin Oncol.* 1990;8:741–750.
19. Fajardo LF. Radiation-induced coronary artery disease. *Chest.* 1977;71:563–577.
20. Chappuis MA, Kaeser P, Enrico JF, et al. Péricardites et autres atteintes cardiaques, consequences tardives de la radiothérapie. *Rev Med Suisse Normande.* 1996;116:429–439.
21. Bourhis J. Les complications cardiaques de la radiothérapie. In: Bourhis J, Habrand JL, Mornex F, eds. *Secondary Effects and Complications of Radiotherapy.* Paris: Upjohn-France; 1995;81–85.
22. Glanzman C, Huguenin P, Lutolf UM, et al. Cardiac lesions after mediastinal irradiation for Hodgkin's disease. *Radiother Oncol.* 1994;30:43–54.
23. Hancock SL, Hoppe RT. Long-term complications of treatment and causes of mortality after Hodgkin's disease. *Sem Radiat Oncol.* 1996;6:225–242.
24. Morgan GM, Freeman AP, McLean RG, et al. Late cardiac, thyroid, and pulmonary sequelae of mantle radiotherapy for Hodgkin's disease. *Int J Radiat Oncol Biol Phys.* 1985;11:1925–1931.
25. Rutqvist LE, Lax I, Fornander T, et al. Cardiovascular mortality in a randomized trial of adjuvant radiation therapy versus surgery alone in primary breast cancer. *Int J Radiat Oncol Biol Phys.* 1992;22:887–896.
26. Cosset JM, Henry-Amar M, Girinsky T, et al. Late toxicity of radiotherapy in Hodgkin's disease: the role of fraction size. *Acta Oncol.* 1988;27:123–130.
27. Hancock SL, Donaldson SS. Radiation-related cardiac disease: risks after treatment of Hodgkin's disease during childhood and adolescence. *Proceedings of Second International Conference on the Long-term Complications Treatment of Children and Adolescents for Cancer,* Buffalo, NY, June 12–14, 1992.
28. Henry-Amar M, Hayat M, Meerwaldt J, et al. Causes of death after therapy for Hodgkin's disease entered on EORTC protocols. *Int J Radiat Oncol Biol Phys.* 1992;79:389–391.
29. Boivin JF, Hutchison GB, Lubin JH, et al. Coronary artery disease mortality in patients treated for Hodgkin's disease. *Cancer.* 1992;69:1241–1247.
30. Gustavsson A, Eskilsson J, Landberg T, et al. Late cardiac effects after mantle field radiotherapy in patients with Hodgkin's disease. *Ann Oncol.* 1990;1:355–363.
31. Hancock SL, Tucker MA, Hoppe RT. Factors affecting late mortality from heart disease after treatment of Hodgkin's disease. *JAMA.* 1993;16:1949–1955.
32. Om A, Ellahham S, Vetrovec GW. Radiation-induced coronary artery disease. *Am Heart J.* 1992;6:1598–1601.
33. Ebagosti A, Gueunoun M, Favre R, et al. Bloc auriculo-ventriculaire, complication de la radiothérapie du médiastin. *Arch Mal Cœur.* 1989;82:935–939.
34. Orzan F, Brusca A, Gaita F, et al. Associated cardiac lesions in patients with radiation-induced complete heart block. *Int J Cardiol.* 1993;39:151–156.
35. Putterman C, Polliack A. Late cardiovascular and pulmonary complications of therapy in Hodgkin's disease: report of three unusual case with a review of relevant literature. *Leuk Lymphoma.* 1992;7:109–115.
36. Lindahl J, Strender LE, Larsson LE, et al. Electrocardiographic changes after radiation therapy for carcinoma of the breast. *Acta Radiol Oncol.* 1983;22:433–440.
37. Appelfeld MM, Cole JF, Pollock SH, et al. The late appearance of chronic pericardial disease in patients treated by radiotherapy for Hodgkin's disease. *Ann Int Med.* 1981;94:338–341.
38. Coltart RS, Thom CH, Roberts JT, et al. Severe constrictive pericarditis after single 16 MeV anterior mantle irradiation for Hodgkin's disease. *Lancet.* 1985;3:488, 489.
39. Cosset JM, Henry-Amar M, Dietrich PY, et al. Les tumeurs solides secondaires après irradiation pour maladie de Hodgkin: l'expérience de l'Institut Gustave-Roussy. *Bull Cancer.* 1992;79:387, 388.
40. Hancock SL, Donaldson SS, Hoppe RT. Cardiac disease following treatment of Hodgkin's disease in children and adolescents. *J Clin Oncol.* 1993;7:1208–1215.
41. Tarbell NJ, Thompson L, Mauch P. Thoracic irradiation in Hodgkin's disease: disease control and long-term complications. *Int J Radiat Oncol Biol Phys.* 1990;18:275–281.
42. Adams MJ, Hardenbergh PH, Constine LS, et al. Radiation-associated cardiovascular disease. *Crit Rev Oncol Hematol.* 2003;45:55–75.
43. Pierce SM, Recht A, Lingos TI, et al. Long-term radiation complications following conservative surgery (CS) and radiation therapy (RT) in patients with early stage breast cancer. *Int J Radiat Oncol Biol Phys.* 1992;23:915–923.
44. Giraud PH, Reboul F, Clippe S, et al. La radiothérapie asservie à la respiration: techniques actuelles et bénéfices attendus. *Cancer Radiother.* (sous presse).
45. Nataf P, Cacoub P, Dorent R, et al. Results of subtotal pericardiectomy for constrictive pericarditis. *Eur J Cardio-thorac Surg.* 1993;7:252–256.
46. Billingham ME, Bristow MR, Glatstein E, et al. Adriamycin cardiotoxicity: endomyocardial biopsy evidence of enhancement of irradiation. *Am J Surg Pathol.* 1977;1:17–23.
47. Bristow MR. Anthracycline cardiotoxicity. In: Bristow MR, eds. *Drug-induced Heart Disease.* Amsterdam: Elsevier/North Holland; 1980:191–215.
48. Chan PYM, Kagan AR, Byfield JE, et al. Pulmonary complications of combined chemotherapy and radiotherapy in lung cancer. *Front Radiat Ther Oncol.* 1979;13:136–144.
49. Carlson RG, Mayfield WR, Normann S, et al. Radiation-associated valvular disease. *Chest.* 1991;99:538–545.

Kenneth D. Westover
Theodore S. Hong

Liver

INTRODUCTION

Radiation to the liver is a common occurrence in the modern management of gastrointestinal cancers. Radiation in the curative setting, particularly for gastric and pancreaticobiliary cancers, can result in significant doses of radiation to liver. Furthermore, as nonsurgical ablative therapies for liver tumors, such as stereotactic body radiation therapy (SBRT), become increasingly studied, there has been renewed interest in understanding the nature of radiation-induced liver damage.

CLINICAL PRESENTATION

Liver radiation was first reported in the 1920s, but radiation-induced liver disease (RILD) was not well characterized until the 1960s.[1,2] RILD typically occurs 4 to 8 weeks after radiation exposure but can happen as early as 2 weeks and as late as 7 months after completion of treatment. Clinical manifestations are similar to those seen with Budd-Chiari syndrome or suprahepatic vein obstruction seen following high-dose chemotherapy. Classically, patients present with ascites, fatigue, rapid weight gain, increased abdominal girth, and right upper quadrant discomfort. A moderate transaminitis is also seen with little or no increase in bilirubin levels. A 3- to 10-fold increase in the alkaline phosphatase level is also characteristic.[3] The elevation of the alkaline phosphatase is typically more dramatic than the transaminases.

At the tissue level venoocclusion is observed, characterized by severe congestion in the central portion of the parenchymal lobules. On gross pathology, hyperemia is apparent. Silver and aniline blue staining reveal reticulin and collagen deposition within the lumen of the afferent sinusoids. Within 6 months of injury, however, little congestion is seen and the liver ultrastructure is largely restored, although not entirely normal.[4] Transforming growth factor beta (TGF-β) is thought to mediate this process by stimulating migration of fibroblasts that proliferate and deposit collagen in areas of injury. This is similar to observations for other processes that lead to fibrosis of the liver including chronic hepatitis and cirrhosis.[5]

Aside from supportive measures, there are no established interventions for RILD. Anticoagulants, diuretics, and steroids have been suggested, but support for these is limited.[6,7] Although occasionally fatal, most patients recover from RILD in about 2 months.

HISTORICAL MODELS FOR TOXICITY

Predictors of RILD were first proposed based on data from trials in the 1970s and 1980s studying palliative whole liver irradiation for metastases. In an early study, 1,800 cGy delivered in 225 cGy fractions was shown to be safe in all patients treated, but 2,800 cGy in 350 cGy fractions was associated with RILD in 8 out of 25 patients.[8,9] In a later study by the RTOG, various dosing schemes were tested in 109 patients. Patients with solitary metastases received 3,040 cGy in 18 fractions or 3,000 cGy in 15 fractions followed by an optional 2,000 cGy boost in 10 fractions. Patients with multiple metastases received 3,000 cGy in 15 fractions; 2,560 cGy in 16 fractions; 2,000 cGy in 10 fractions; or 2,100 cGy in 7 fractions. In all dosing schemes, no RILD was observed.[10]

The upper limit of total liver dose was later established in a trial comparing total liver doses of 2,700 cGy versus 3,000 cGy versus 3,300 cGy using fractions of 150 cGy twice daily. Five of fifty-one patients on the 3,300 cGy arm developed biochemical RILD prompting early closure of the protocol.[11] In 1986 Austin-Seymour et al.[12] observed RILD in 1 out of 11 patients after treatment with charged particles for biliary cancer leading him to suggest that liver doses in excess of 3,500 cGy should be limited to 30% of the liver with 1,800 cGy delivered to the entire liver.

The tolerance for partial liver irradiation is substantially higher with safe delivery of up to 5,500 cGy to portions of the liver reported as early as 1965.[1] Later estimates given by Emami were based primarily on expert consensus, taking into account retrospective reports of 27 patients with suspected or proven RILD. For a fractionation scheme of 180 to 200 cGy/d, the TD 5/5 or 5% probability of RILD at 5 years for one third, two thirds, and whole liver irradiation was 5,000; 3,500; and 3,000 cGy, respectively. The TD 50/5 or 50% probability of RILD at 5 years for one third, two thirds, and whole liver irradiation was estimated at 5,500; 4,500; and 4,000 cGy, respectively.[13]

THE UNIVERSITY OF MICHIGAN MODEL

These estimates were further refined by studies from the University of Michigan based on prospective data from a group of about 200 patients who received liver irradiation for various hepatic malignancies. Some patients received concurrent hepatic arterial chemotherapy. Three-dimensional treatment planning allowed for construction of dose-volume histograms that were correlated with clinical complications. A DVH reduction scheme developed by Kutcher and Burman[14] allowed for direct comparison of DVH/toxicity data between patients. In total, 19 patients developed RILD. All these patients received whole liver radiation with a mean dose of 3,700 cGy.[15]

Using the data, a normal tissue complication probability (NTCP) model was developed. This model assumes a sigmoidal relationship between the dose of uniform radiation given to a volume of liver and the probability of toxicity. Three parameters were utilized including the TD_{50}, or whole-organ dose associated with a 50% probability of toxicity, "m" which defines the steepness of the dose response at TD_{50}, and "n" which takes into account the effect of volume on a scale of 0 to 1.

Fitting the data to clinical data sets has confirmed a number of prior observations about liver irradiation. For example, the n factor is generally high emphasizing the importance of the volume.[15] However, other important observations have emerged including differences in TD_{50} between subgroups. In one study, patients with hepatobiliary cancer had a TD_{50} of 3,980 cGy, whereas for patients with liver metastases, it was 4,580 cGy, suggesting a higher tolerance in patients with liver metastases compared to primary hepatobiliary malignancy. Further extrapolation using these models gave a final estimate of tolerance for one third or two thirds uniform partial liver irradiation at 10,000 and 5,400 cGy, respectively, for patients with liver metastases and 9,300 and 4,700 cGy for primary liver cancer based on a 150-cGy twice-daily fractionation schedule.[14,16]

Damage injury models have also been developed that include biological data. These models assume a parallel functional organ architecture such that the organ continues to function until a critical fraction of the organ becomes incapacitated. This idea is well validated for liver from the surgical literature where it has been observed that sparing 20% of liver at the time of partial hepatectomy rarely leads to liver failure.[17] Again, using the cohort from the University of Michigan, Jackson developed a damage injury model for liver that showed the TD_{50} to be 4,160 cGy for a group of patients with various hepatic malignancies.[18]

TOLERANCE WITH HYPOFRACTIONATION

Recent advances in imaging and radiation delivery have made it possible to give high doses of radiation to relatively small areas of disease within the body. SBRT utilizes multiple nonopposing beams that converge on a target to deliver high doses of radiation with little dose to surrounding tissues. Interest in treating liver lesions in this manner emerged from observations from surgical series involving colorectal patients who had oligometastatic disease to liver where it was shown that a long-term survival benefit could be obtained from partial hepatectomy provided that the primary disease was also controlled.[19] Trials are now underway to evaluate whether the same benefits might be achievable using SBRT for liver metastases.

Two recent liver SBRT trials included medically inoperable patients with solitary liver metastases showed encouraging local control rates of 71% to 92% at 2 years for all subjects with nearly complete control of tumors <2 cm at 2 years, although the survival of these patients was generally poor because of other competing factors.[20,21] Notably, one of the trials was designed to dose escalate in a personalized fashion based on the probability of developing RILD using the NTCP model mentioned above. In this trial, 68 patients consisting of 40 metastatic colorectal, 12 metastatic breast, and 16 other liver metastases were divided into three cohorts and treated with SBRT plans designed to give a 5%, 10%, or 20% risk of RILD according to the Lyman-Kutcher-Burman model. A correction for dose fractionation was based on an assumption of $\alpha/\beta =$ 2.5 Gy. Thirteen, thirty five, and twenty patients were treated in the low-, medium-, and high-risk strata. The median prescription dose was 41.4 Gy in six fractions with a range of 27.8 to 60 Gy. Liver was the dose-limiting structure in 48 patients. The median tumor volume was 75.2 mL, but also included large tumors up to 3,090 mL.

Surprisingly, no serious clinical or hepatic toxicities were observed even in the highest dose arm. Tai et al.[22] attempted to create a new expression of normalized total dose to convert NTCP data between different fractionation schemes. Data from four institutions with fraction sizes ranging from 150 to 600 cGy were analyzed and fitted. A new set of Lyman parameters were established that potentially better fit hypo fractionated regimens. As an example, regimens of 8.8 Gy times four fractions and a single fraction of 19.7 Gy had a classically predicted risk of 100%. However, with the new proposed parameters, risk of RILD for these to schedules was 6.6% and 7.8%, respectively, consistent with the observations of the Lee trial.[22]

Some have suggested that these observations argue for alternative biological explanations for results obtained by hypofractionation. One line of evidence points to the importance of immune responses in mediating some antitumor effects after radiation therapy, particularly hypofractionated therapy.[23,24] Indeed, several new studies focus on promoting antitumor immune responses using various agents including Iplilmumab.[25]

POTENTIATION OF TOXICITY

Additional factors appear to potentiate the effects of radiation in liver. The addition of chemotherapy to radiation in particular has increased hepatic toxicity in selected patients. Individual patients treated with lymphoma regimens such as ProMACE-MOPP and CHOP developed RILD after only 2,250 and 2,500 cGy, respectively to the whole liver.[26] Breast cancer radiation after doxorubicin has been associated with increased RILD in several patients.[27] Increased toxicity after vincristine has also been reported.[28]

Patients with cirrhosis and hepatocellular carcinoma also appear to have lower tolerances to liver radiation.[29] In one Japanese study of patients with hepatocellular carcinoma, RILD was not seen in 75 patients treated with proton-based radiation therapy.[30] However, in another study, 12 out of 68 patients with hepatocellular carcinoma (HCC) treated with 3D conformal radiation therapy developed RILD. Patients who developed RILD had a higher mean hepatic dose (2,504 cGy vs. 1,965 cGy, $p = 0.02$). When fitted to the NTCP model, the volume effect was found to be smaller for patients with HCC than with other hepatic malignancies.[31] Other studies have found an association with Hepatitis B infection and Child-Pugh B liver cirrhosis with development of RILD after radiation therapy.[32] Consequently, an unfavorable Child-Pugh score is occasionally used as an exclusion criteria for SBRT to liver.[33]

IMAGING

Characteristic radiological patterns after radiation exposure allow for some level of discrimination between benign radiation-induced changes and disease progression. Indeed, scattered reports suggest that 1 to 2 months after radiation exposure, high-dose regions will often show a low density (Fig. 30.1). This is most often seen at doses above 4,500 cGy, independent of signs or symptoms of RILD.[26,34]

Changes in the setting of stereotactic body radiosurgery were characterized in detail in a group of 36 German patients who received a single fraction of SBRT to the liver. Spiral CT scans were preformed before and 1 month after treatment with additional follow-up scanning every 3 to 5 months for a median of 8 months after treatment. The median radiation dose was 22 Gy. On noncontrast imaging, 74% of the studies showed a sharply demarcated hypodense area corresponding to the high-dose region at a median of 1.8 months. The change was correlated with a threshold dose of 13.7 Gy. On contrast imaging, three distinct, but interactive changes were observed. Type I reactions showed hypodensity in the portal venous phase and isodensity in the late phase. Type II reactions showed hypodensity in the portal venous phase and hyperdensity in the late phase. Type III reactions showed isodensity or hyperdensity in the portal venous phase and hyperdensity in the late phase. Type I and II

reactions were seen earlier and showed a lower threshold dose than type III reactions. Shifting from one reaction to another was also seen during follow-up.[35] There were no reports of RILD in these patients.

Recent efforts have focused on developing radiographic technologies to predict RILD. One promising approach used portal venous perfusion as measured by enhanced computer tomography. In a small study of ten patients treated with hepatic radiation, it was shown that on average each 100 cGy reduced venous perfusion by 1.2%.[36] Another approach used indocyanine green retention in liver in patients with HCC to predict development of RILD. No statistically significant correlation could be made, but other factors such as Child-Pugh score were observed.[37] With further development of these, or similar technologies it may be possible to monitor for RILD in real time while dose escalating with radiation therapy.

MANAGEMENT OF RILD

As mentioned previously, there are few data to support the use of a number of interventions for RILD. However, data from other causes of venoocclusive disease such as hematopoietic stem cell transplant, where more subjects are available for study, are likely applicable.[38] In general, ascites should be managed with sodium restriction, diuretics, and paracentesis. In extreme cases, ventilatory support may be required if mechanical respiratory failure develops. Anticoagulants and fibrinolytics such as heparin and tPA have been used, but response rates are generally low at approximately 30% with severe bleeding in about 25% of treated patients.[39,40] Defibrotide, a polydeoxyribonucleic acid with profibrinolytic and antithrombotic properties, has been used with some success.[41,42] As a last resort where medical therapy has failed, transjugular intrahepatic portosystemic shunts have also been used although this is controversial.[43,44]

Hepatocyte transplantation for hepatic injury after radiation is an area of active investigation and may provide new therapeutic options in the future. In one study, rats treated with partial hepatectomy, radiation, and then hepatocyte transplant showed a decrease in the incidence of RILD and improved survival compared to nontransplanted rats.[45–47] Advances in cryopreservation have made this approach a potentially viable alternative to whole liver transplantation which could be done with little lead time with autologous tissue.[48]

CONCLUSION

Development of RILD is dose dependent and influenced by a number of factors such as the volume of liver treated, general health of the liver at the time of irradiation, prior or concurrent chemotherapy, type of pathologic disease, and infection. Toxicity models are useful for predicting the baseline risk for developing RILD for a given patient and for comparing different subgroups for fractionated therapy. In general, a V30 (volume receiving at least 30 Gy) of 30% is a conservative constraint for upper abdominal radiation. However, these models do not appear to hold when applied to hypofractionated treatment and new models will need to be developed for such regimens. While radiographic changes after radiation are typical, there are no well-characterized radiographic signs of RILD, although promising technologies are under development (Table 30.1).

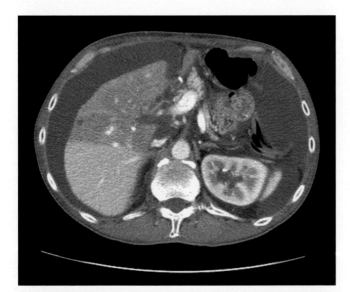

Figure 30.1. Hepatic changes after radiation therapy. Irradiated liver typically appears hypodense on CT. Note the sharp demarcation in the anterior aspect of the liver. Ascites is apparent in this patient with gastric cancer who developed RILD after six cycles of perioperative EOX (epirubicin, oxaliplatin, capecitabine) chemotherapy followed by chemoradiotherapy to the gastric bed that received 4,500 cGy. The mean dose to liver was <1,500 cGy and the V30 < 18%. Transaminases were slightly elevated, but alkaline phosphatase was markedly elevated.

TABLE 30.1		Summary of RILD According to Radiation Dose						
					5% Risk of RILD			
Total Patients	Cases of RILD	Fractionation	Model	Whole Liver	2/3 Liver	1/3 Liver	Reference
11	1	2–3 Gy daily	None	NA	NA	35 Gy	12
407	27	2 Gy daily[a]	None	30 Gy	35 Gy	50 Gy	13
407	27	2 Gy daily[a]	Lyman	30 Gy	34 Gy	43 Gy	49
79	9	1.5 Gy bid	Lyman	35 Gy	45 Gy	72 Gy	50
93	9	1.5 Gy bid	Damage	35 Gy	52 Gy	—	18
183	19	1.5 Gy bid	Lyman	31 Gy	47 Gy	90 Gy	16
183	19	1.5 Gy bid	Damage	32 Gy	43 Gy	99 Gy	16
183	19	1.5 Gy bid	Mean dose	31 Gy	—	—	16
LIVER METASTASES							
28	8	3.5 Gy daily	None	28 Gy	—	—	8
51	5	1.5 Gy bid	None	33 Gy	—	—	11
98	5	1.5 Gy bid	Lyman	37 Gy	54 Gy	107 Gy	15
PRIMARY LIVER CANCER							
105	14	1.5 Gy bid	Lyman	32 Gy	47 Gy	93 Gy	15

[a]Equivalent dose.

REFERENCES

1. Ingold JA, Reed GB, Kaplan HS, et al. Radiation hepatitis. Am J Roentgenol. 1965;93: 200–208.
2. Reed GB Jr, Cox AJ Jr. The human liver after radiation injury. A form of veno-occlusive disease. Am J Pathol. 1966;48:597–611.
3. Tefft M, Mitus A, Das L, et al. Irradiation of the liver in children: review of experience in the acute and chronic phases, and in the intact normal and partially resected. Am J Roentgenol. 1970;108:365–385.
4. Lewin K, Millis RR. Human radiation hepatitis. A morphologic study with emphasis on the late changes. Arch Pathol. 1973;96:21–26.
5. Castilla A, Prieto J, Fausto N. Transforming growth factors beta 1 and alpha in chronic liver disease. Effects of interferon alfa therapy. N Engl J Med. 1991;324:933–940.
6. Kinzie J, Studer RK, Perez B, et al. Noncytokinetic radiation injury: anticoagulants as radio-protective agents in experimental radiation hepatitis. Science. 1972;175:1481–1483.
7. Lightdale CJ, Wasser J, Coleman M, et al. Anticoagulation and high dose liver radiation: a preliminary report. Cancer. 1979;43:174–181.
8. Wharton JT, Delclos L, Gallager S, et al. Radiation hepatitis induced by abdominal irradiation with the cobalt 60 moving strip technique. Am J Roentgenol. 1973;117:73–80.
9. Perez CA, Korba A, Zivnuska F, et al. 60Co moving strip technique in the management of carcinoma of the ovary: analysis of tumor control and morbidity. Int J Radiat Oncol Biol Phys. 1978;4:379–388.
10. Borgelt BB, Gelber R, Brady LW, et al. The palliation of hepatic metastases: results of the Radiation Therapy Oncology Group pilot study. Int J Radiat Oncol Biol Phys. 1981;7: 587–591.
11. Russell AH, Clyde C, Wasserman TH, et al. Accelerated hyperfractionated hepatic irradiation in the management of patients with liver metastases: results of the RTOG dose escalating protocol. Int J Radiat Oncol Biol Phys. 1993;27:117–123.
12. Austin-Seymour MM, Chen GT, Castro JR, et al. Dose volume histogram analysis of liver radiation tolerance. Int J Radiat Oncol Biol Phys. 1986;12:31–35.
13. Emami B, Lyman J, Brown A, et al. Tolerance of normal tissue to therapeutic irradiation. Int J Radiat Oncol Biol Phys. 1991;21:109–122.
14. Kutcher GJ, Burman C. Calculation of complication probability factors for non-uniform normal tissue irradiation: the effective volume method. Int J Radiat Oncol Biol Phys. 1989;16:1623–1630.
15. Dawson LA, Normolle D, Balter JM, et al. Analysis of radiation-induced liver disease using the Lyman NTCP model. Int J Radiat Oncol Biol Phys. 2002;53:810–821.
16. Dawson LA, Ten Haken RK, Lawrence TS. Partial irradiation of the liver. Semin Radiat Oncol. 2001;11:240–246.
17. Penna C, Nordlinger B. Colorectal metastasis (liver and lung). Surg Clin North Am. 2002;82:1075–1090, x–xi.
18. Jackson A, Ten Haken RK, Robertson JM, et al. Analysis of clinical complication data for radiation hepatitis using a parallel architecture model. Int J Radiat Oncol Biol Phys. 1995;31:883–891.
19. Aloia TA, Vauthey JN, Loyer EM, et al. Solitary colorectal liver metastasis: resection determines outcome. Arch Surg. 2006;141:460–466; discussion 466–467.
20. Rusthoven KE, Kavanagh BD, Cardenes H, et al. Multi-institutional phase I/II trial of stereotactic body radiation therapy for liver metastases. Am J Clin Oncol. 2009;27:1572–1578.
21. Lee MT, Kim JJ, Dinniwell R, et al. Phase I study of individualized stereotactic body radiotherapy of liver metastases. Am J Clin Oncol. 2009;27:1585–1591.
22. Tai A, Erickson B, Li XA. Extrapolation of normal tissue complication probability for different fractionations in liver irradiation. Int J Radiat Oncol Biol Phys. 2009;74:283–289.
23. Lee Y, Auh SL, Wang Y, et al. Therapeutic effects of ablative radiation on local tumor require CD8+ T cells: changing strategies for cancer treatment. Blood. 2009;114:589–595.
24. Nakanishi M, Chuma M, Hige S, et al. Abscopal effect on hepatocellular carcinoma. Am J Gastroenterol. 2008;103:1320–1321.
25. Wolchok JD, Neyns B, Linette G, et al. Ipilimumab monotherapy in patients with pretreated advanced melanoma: a randomised, double-blind, multicentre, phase 2, dose-ranging study. Lancet Oncol. 2009;11:155–164.
26. Lawrence TS, Robertson JM, Anscher MS, et al. Hepatic toxicity resulting from cancer treatment. Int J Radiat Oncol Biol Phys. 1995;31:1237–1248.
27. Khozouz RF, Huq SZ, Perry MC. Radiation-induced liver disease. J Clin Oncol. 2008;26: 4844–4845.
28. Hansen MM, Ranek L, Walbom S, et al. Fatal hepatitis following irradiation and vincristine. Acta Med Scand. 1982;212:171–174.
29. Xu ZY, Liang SX, Zhu J, et al. Prediction of radiation-induced liver disease by Lyman normal-tissue complication probability model in three-dimensional conformal radiation therapy for primary liver carcinoma. Int J Radiat Oncol Biol Phys. 2006;65:189–195.
30. Tsuji H, Okumura T, Maruhashi A, et al. Dose-volume histogram analysis of patients with hepatocellular carcinoma regarding changes in liver function after proton therapy. Nippon Igaku Hoshasen Gakkai Zasshi. 1995;55:322–328.
31. Cheng JC, Wu JK, Huang CM, et al. Radiation-induced liver disease after radiotherapy for hepatocellular carcinoma: clinical manifestation and dosimetric description. Radiother Oncol. 2002;63:41–45.
32. Cheng JC, Wu JK, Lee PC, et al. Biologic susceptibility of hepatocellular carcinoma patients treated with radiotherapy to radiation-induced liver disease. Int J Radiat Oncol Biol Phys. 2004;60:1502–1509.
33. Tse RV, Hawkins M, Lockwood G, et al. Phase I study of individualized stereotactic body radiotherapy for hepatocellular carcinoma and intrahepatic cholangiocarcinoma. J Clin Oncol. 2008;26:657–664.
34. Yamasaki SA, Marn CS, Francis IR, et al. High-dose localized radiation therapy for treatment of hepatic malignant tumors: CT findings and their relation to radiation hepatitis. Am J Roentgenol. 1995;165:79–84.
35. Herfarth KK, Hof H, Bahner ML, et al. Assessment of focal liver reaction by multiphasic CT after stereotactic single-dose radiotherapy of liver tumors. Int J Radiat Oncol Biol Phys. 2003;57:444–451.
36. Cao Y, Platt JF, Francis IR, et al. The prediction of radiation-induced liver dysfunction using a local dose and regional venous perfusion model. Med Phys. 2007;34:604–612.
37. Lee IJ, Seong J, Shim SJ, et al. Radiotherapeutic parameters predictive of liver complications induced by liver tumor radiotherapy. Int J Radiat Oncol Biol Phys. 2009;73:154–158.
38. Senzolo M, Germani G, Cholongitas E, et al. Veno occlusive disease: update on clinical management. World J Gastroenterol. 2007;13:3918–3924.
39. Leahey AM, Bunin NJ. Recombinant human tissue plasminogen activator for the treatment of severe hepatic veno-occlusive disease in pediatric bone marrow transplant patients. Bone Marrow Transplant. 1996;17:1101–1104.
40. Bearman SI, Lee JL, Baron AE, et al. Treatment of hepatic venoocclusive disease with recombinant human tissue plasminogen activator and heparin in 42 marrow transplant patients. Blood. 1997;89:1501–1506.
41. Chopra R, Eaton JD, Grassi A, et al. Defibrotide for the treatment of hepatic venoocclusive disease: results of the European compassionate-use study. Br J Haematol. 2000;111: 1122–1129.

42. Richardson PG, Elias AD, Krishnan A, et al. Treatment of severe veno-occlusive disease with defibrotide: compassionate use results in response without significant toxicity in a high-risk population. *Blood.* 1998;92:737–744.

43. Senzolo M, Cholongitas E, Patch D, et al. TIPS for veno-occlusive disease: is the contraindication real? *Hepatology.* 2005;42:240–241; author reply 241.

44. Fried MW, Connaghan DG, Sharma S, et al. Transjugular intrahepatic portosystemic shunt for the management of severe venoocclusive disease following bone marrow transplantation. *Hepatology.* 1996;24:588–591.

45. Guha C, Parashar B, Deb NJ, et al. Normal hepatocytes correct serum bilirubin after repopulation of Gunn rat liver subjected to irradiation/partial resection. *Hepatology.* 2002;36:354–362.

46. Guha C, Sharma A, Gupta S, et al. Amelioration of radiation-induced liver damage in partially hepatectomized rats by hepatocyte transplantation. *Cancer Res.* 1999;59: 5871–5874.

47. Fox IJ, Chowdhury JR. Hepatocyte transplantation. *Am J Transplant* 2004;4(suppl 6): 7–13.

48. Jamal HZ, Weglarz TC, Sandgren EP. Cryopreserved mouse hepatocytes retain regenerative capacity in vivo. *Gastroenterology.* 2000;118:390–394.

49. Burman C, Kutcher GJ, Emami B, et al. Fitting of normal tissue tolerance data to an analytic function. *Int J Radiat Oncol Biol Phys.* 1991;21:123–135.

50. Lawrence TS, Ten Haken RK, Kessler ML, et al. The use of 3-D dose volume analysis to predict radiation hepatitis. *Int J Radiat Oncol Biol Phys.*1992;23:781–788.

Colleen A. Lawton
Eric P. Cohen
John E. Moulder

Kidney and Adrenal Gland

GROSS ANATOMY

The kidneys are bean-shaped, fist-sized, paired internal organs that are below the diaphragm in the retroperitoneal space (Fig. 31.1). The two kidneys are opposite each other, on each side of the lumbar spine, from the L1 to L3 level, the left usually a centimeter cephalad to the right. Their usual length in a healthy adult is 11 cm, with a range of 10 to 12.5 cm. Their width is half that, and their thickness half again in measurement. Kidneys are bigger in men than in women, and are bigger in taller than in shorter people. The kidney size declines with age. Kidneys are enveloped in a thin connective fascia, called *Gerota capsule*, which is in turn surrounded by the perinephric fat.

Internally, the relations of the kidneys differ on the right and on the left.[1] On the right, the liver abuts the lateral and anterior aspect, the colon abuts the lower pole, and the second portion of the duodenum abuts the medial aspect. On the left, the spleen and stomach are in relation to the anterior-superior aspect, the pancreas is anterior to the midportion, and the jejunum abuts the lower part of the left kidney. Posteriorly, the diaphragm covers the upper aspect of both kidneys, and the quadratus lumborum muscles cover most of the middle and lower aspects. The tops of both kidneys are subtended by the adrenal glands.

Anteriorly, the surface projection of the kidneys is that they are approximately bisected by the transpyloric plane, a line midway between the lower edge of the sternum and umbilicus. Posteriorly, the renal hila are at the level of L2, each about 5 cm from the sagittal midplane of the body. The kidneys move with position and with respiration, being a few centimeters lower in the standing position, and also a few centimeters lower in deep inspiration.

Kidneys are fully formed at birth, after which there is no formation of additional nephrons. About 1 out of 1,000 persons is born with a single kidney. Other infrequent abnormalities include so-called horseshoe kidneys, which are fused right and left kidneys that did not complete their migration out of the pelvis during development. Rarer still are ectopic kidneys, which are not in their usual position and also have abnormalities of form and structure.

RENAL PERFUSION

Renal perfusion is by renal arteries that directly come off the aorta, one to each kidney. At the renal hilum, at their junction with the renal parenchyma, these split into intrarenal branches that further subdivide to interlobar, then arcuate arteries. These subdivide into interlobular arteries that perfuse the glomeruli, which are the filtering elements of the kidneys. The glomeruli are located in the cortex of the kidney, which is the outer portion of the kidney; in healthy individuals it is about 1 cm in thickness. Glomeruli are up to 250 μm in diameter, so just at the limit of visibility to the human eye. There are about one million glomeruli in each kidney. The glomerular capillary network extends from the afferent to the efferent arteriole, the latter then subdividing into cortical capillaries that eventually coalesce into interlobular, arcuate, and interlobar veins. The renal veins then rejoin the systemic circulation, specifically the inferior vena cava. Because the abdominal aorta lies to the left of the vertebral column and the inferior vena cava lies to its right, the right renal artery is longer than is the left, and the left renal vein is longer than is the right.

HISTOLOGICAL ANATOMY

Kidneys have a cortex, which is the outer portion that contains the filtering glomeruli; and a medulla, the inner portion that contains the collecting tubules that drain to the urinary pelvis and ureters. Human kidney medulla is divided into more than a dozen triangular papillae, or pyramids, the tips of which are molded to urinary calyces, that themselves coalesce to the single urinary pelvis and ureter. Embryologically, the ureters and collecting systems of the kidneys derive from the ureteric bud, an endodermal derivative; whereas the glomeruli and cortical tubules derive from the metanephric cap, which derives from mesenchyme.

The functional unit of the kidneys is the nephron. A single nephron begins at a glomerulus and then continues in the proximal tubule. The loop of Henle follows and then a short distal tubule that continues into the collecting duct. The latter begin in the cortex and course toward the renal hilum through the renal medulla and then the papillae. They combine with other collecting ducts on their path to the papillary tips. The total length of a nephron is 50 to 55 mm; the length of a proximal tubule is 10 to 20 mm, a loop of Henle is 10 to 20 mm long, a distal tubule is 5 mm long, and a collecting duct is about 20 mm long.[2] These lengths are shorter at birth and reach adult length by the end of puberty.

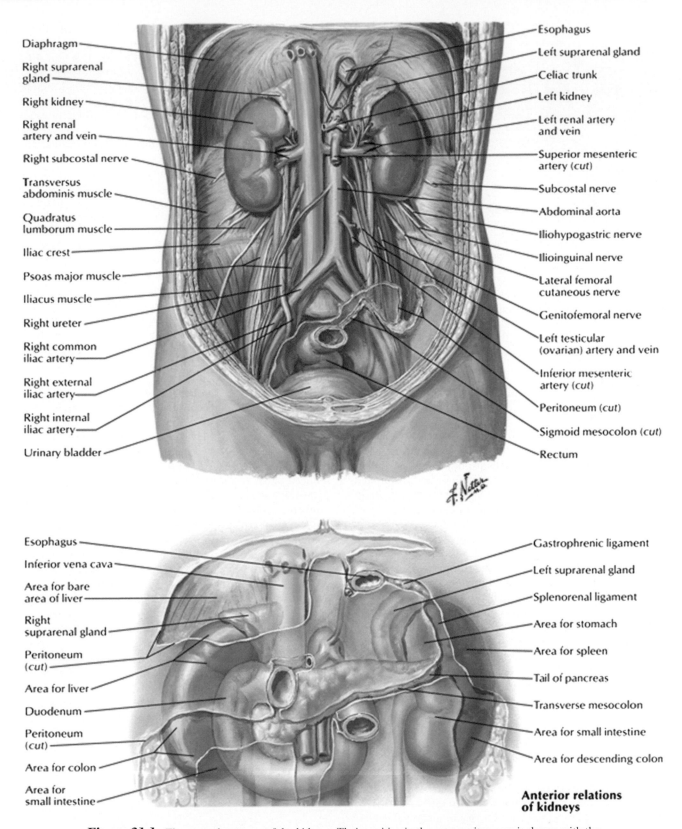

Figure 31.1. The normal anatomy of the kidneys. Their position in the retroperitoneum is shown, with the landmarks and adjacent structures as described in the text. (Netter medical illustration, used with permission of Elsevier; all rights reserved.)

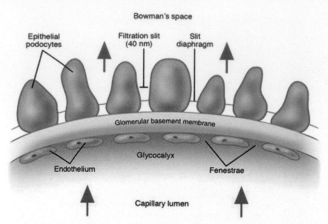

Figure 31.2. A diagram of the glomerular capillary wall, made of a fenestrated endothelium, a basement membrane, and epithelial foot processes. The foot processes form filtration slits spanned by slit diaphragms. Also shown is the endothelial cell coat, or glycocalyx. Some approximate dimensions are: minimum diameter of fenestra, 30 nm; glomerular basement membrane thickness, 200 to 400 nm; width of filtration slit, 40 nm. (Reprinted from Deen WM. What determines glomerular capillary permeability? *J Clin Invest.* 2004;114:1412–1414, with permission.)

HISTOLOGY

CELLULAR HISTOLOGY

A glomerulus is a tuft of filtering cells that are perfused by high-pressure capillaries. Each glomerulus is perfused from a single afferent arteriole that divides into numerous capillaries. These are lined by a fenestrated endothelium that is adjoined by the glomerular basement membrane[3] (Fig. 31.2). The outer aspect of the glomerular basement membrane is covered by interdigitating epithelial cells, the podocytes. Centrally, the capillary tufts are held together by the mesangial cells. Combined, these form the surface for glomerular filtration.

The proximal tubules are lined by cuboidal epithelial cells that are rich in mitochondria, which enable energy for transport. On the luminal side, there is a brush border that enhances the transport surface area. The loop of Henle is lined by a thinner epithelium that lies in close apposition to the medullary circulation of the vasa recta that descend from the efferent arterioles of the deep cortical glomeruli, into the medullary pyramids and reascend from them. The distal tubule is composed of a cuboidal epithelium that has no brush border. Before it joins the collecting duct, the distal tubule of a given nephron passes adjacent to its "parent" glomerulus and afferent arteriole, forming the juxtaglomerular apparatus. Collecting duct epithelium is of two main types, light and dark cells; the latter are less abundant, but richer in mitochondria.

The renal blood vessels have the usual endothelial lining, which becomes fenestrated at the glomerular capillaries. At 40 nm in width, these capillary fenestrae are too small to allow passage of blood cells, yet offer no barrier to macromolecules. The role of the fenestrae remains incompletely understood.

FUNCTIONAL HISTOLOGY

The functions of the kidney can be understood by its anatomy and histology. The renal arterial blood flow, to both kidneys combined, is 1 L/min (i.e., one fifth of the resting cardiac output). This is the highest blood flow rate in the body (per gram of tissue). At the glomeruli, the plasma water and constituent electrolytes are freely filtered, at a rate of over 100 mL/min in healthy adults (i.e., approximately 150 L/d). In healthy adults, the intact glomerular basement membrane ensures that cells and large molecular weight constituents of the blood are not lost by filtration. Glomerular filtration of the plasma water ensures a rapid filtering of the blood, and an indirect filtering of the extracellular and intracellular spaces. This is enabled by the high intracapillary pressure of glomeruli, which, at about 50 mm Hg, is much higher than the 15 mm Hg of normal tissue capillaries. The fine tuning of glomerular filtration pressure is in part enabled by the juxtaglomerular apparatus, which senses urinary electrolytes in the distal nephron and adapts the afferent arteriolar tone, in a feedback mode, to adjust the glomerular filtration. The filtrate is then processed by the tubules. In healthy adults, close to 99% of the filtered salt and water are reabsorbed (in particular, by the proximal tubule). Other constituent electrolytes (e.g., phosphorous and uric acid) are reabsorbed by the proximal tubule, but in a lesser fraction, thus allowing their removal by the urine. Urinary acidification is enabled by the reclamation of filtered bicarbonate, by intrarenal ammoniagenesis, and by the energy-dependent hydrogen ion secretion by the dark cells of the collecting ducts. The conservation of water is finely adapted to changing requirements by establishment of an osmotic gradient by the loops of Henle and their adjoining vasa recta, under the control of vasopressin.

Any injury to kidneys can thus impact glomerular filtration, salt and water balance, acid-base balance, water metabolism, and the homeostasis of other compounds such as phosphorus and uric acid. Importantly, the overall filtering function of kidneys may be reduced either by direct glomerular injury or by tubular injury. Agents that damage the renal tubules may cause reduced glomerular filtration because of altered tubuloglomerular feedback via the juxtaglomerular apparatus, or because of scarring that permanently impedes the tubular egress of glomerular filtrate.

The kidney cortex and medulla are further distinguished by their different tissue oxygen tensions. The cortex, with its blood flow of 4 L/min/g of tissue, has a tissue pO_2 of approximately 50 mm Hg, while the medulla, with a blood flow rate of <2 mL/min/g of tissue, has a tissue pO_2 of 10 to 20 mm Hg.[4] This may explain renal susceptibility to acute injury from hypoperfusion or radiocontrast. However, the medullary oxygen tension is not low enough to render it resistant to radiation injury; and in radiation nephropathy there is both medullary and cortical tissue injury.

Finally, the different cell types of the kidney have different proliferation rates. Thus, when expressed as a percentage of cells labeled with proliferating cell nuclear antigen, the proximal tubular epithelium has a labeling index of 0.22, whereas the glomerular endothelium has a labeling index of 0.42.[5] It is possible that this plays a role in radiation injury, rendering glomerular endothelium more apt to show injury (and to show it earlier) than the tubular epithelium.

IMAGING

ANATOMICAL IMAGING

The traditional method for imaging the kidney was the intravenous pyelogram (IVP), also referred to as an *excretory urography.* Given the current options of ultrasound, computed tomography (CT), and magnetic resonance (MR), all of which provide better images of the kidney, IVP has essentially been replaced.

Standard contrast-enhanced multidetector CT, or helical CT, provides excellent imaging of the kidney and the ureters. Cystic or solid tumors are easily seen with this technology. The CT urogram, which allows for the best imaging of the renal parenchyma, is done as follows. First a noncontrast CT is done of the kidneys and bladder to look for calcifications or stones. Next intravenous contrast is injected, and CT scanning at this point allows for imaging of the "corticomedullary phase" where the renal cortex enhances before the renal medulla. By 4 minutes following contrasting injection, the renal parenchyma is uniformly enhanced (the "nephrogram phase"), after which the contrast is in the collecting system and ureter. 3D images can be reformatted, mimicking an IVP, but with better resolution.[6]

It is reasonable to avoid use of potential nephrotoxins of any kind at time of renal irradiation. Intravenous radiocontrast may cause acute renal failure[7-10] and that could complicate the course of a subject undergoing radiation therapy. For patients who cannot have iodinated contrast, or if the CT is equivocal, MR is appropriate. Multiphase MR with intravenous gadolinium contrast produces renal images similar to contrast-enhanced multidetector CT.[6]

Ultrasound is a simple test often used to detect hydronephrosis and/or show overall kidney size. Color ultrasound can be used to detect venous involvement of renal tumors.[6]

FUNCTIONAL IMAGING

To get a sense of the function of the kidneys in preparation for surgical, medical, or radiation intervention, functional renal imaging can be of help. There are three methods to assess renal function: functional imaging, renography, and the quantification of renal function.[11] Functional renal imaging is done with ^{99}Tc-labeled agent. This provides anatomic, functional, and collecting system patency information.[11,12] Renography is the production of a renogram, which is a time-versus-activity graph that shows the uptake and excretion of a radiopharmaceutical (usually ^{99}Tc based) by the kidneys.[11,12] By graphing both kidneys, one can see differences (if any) in functionality. Quantification of renal function is a direct measure of the glomerular filtration rate (GFR), which can be useful because up to one half of renal function can be lost before serum creatinine levels become abnormal.[11,12] However, the result of ^{99}Tc-based tests for the GFR may have the same imprecisions as creatinine-based estimates, and these radiopharmaceutical tests are more expensive.

EFFECTS OF RENAL IRRADIATION IN HUMANS

The effects of radiation on the kidney have been studied fairly well in animal models (see "Renal Injury After Radiation Accidents or Radiological Terrorism"), but have not been systematically studied in the human. In a review article published in 1972, only 151 cases of radiation therapy renal toxicity had been reported.[13] Yet the effects of radiation on the kidney can, and have been, life threatening.[14,15]

Since the kidney is a paired organ, radiation to both kidneys will produce changes that are different than radiation to only one kidney. But even radiation to one kidney and its ipsilateral renal artery can produce renal artery stenosis with resulting increased renin secretion.[16,17] This has most often been seen in infants and children, and can be addressed surgically.[17]

Renal radiation injury can appear in the first few months following renal exposure; or it can manifest itself as late or chronic radiation nephropathy, which can occur years after the exposure, and which may not necessarily follow from an acute renal event.[18]

Most of the data regarding radiation renal toxicity relate to bilateral fractionated renal irradiation. Yet there are data from Willett et al.[19] suggesting that with fractionated radiation, a dose of 26 to 30 Gy will eliminate renal function in an irradiated kidney, even when the opposite kidney is spared and functional. With bilateral fractionated renal irradiation, multiple studies suggest that doses above 25 Gy will likely result in elimination of useful renal function.[20] Data from Emami et al.[21] suggest a dose for causing a 5% chance of dysfunction at 5 years (TD 5/5) for total bilateral renal radiation of 23 Gy, and a dose for causing a 50% chance of dysfunction at 5 years (TD 50/5) of 28 Gy.

To elucidate the effects of fractionated versus single-fraction irradiation of the kidney, one needs to look at the hematopoietic stem cell transplant (HSCT) literature, where single fractions of total body irradiation (TBI) have been used as well as fractionated regimens. Although these data are clouded by the use of nephrotoxic drugs in the peri-HSCT period, it still represents the best data to address the fractionation issue. Data from Sweden[22] directly address single-fraction tolerance in a group of patients who survived >6 months following an autologous HSCT. Their conditioning regimen included 7.5-Gy single-fraction TBI along with a myriad of chemotherapies. Twelve of seventy-two patients developed renal dysfunction, and the single most important risk factor for its development was radiation in the preparative regimen. The authors[22] suggest that the use of a fractionated regimen and/or a lower dose rate might reduce the incidence of renal injury. Data from two other institutions would suggest that these authors are correct, as both Lawton et al.[23] and Miralbell et al.[24] show that patients who received fractionated TBI where the renal dose was limited to approximately 10 Gy had a low incidence of renal toxicity. Thus the higher, yet fractionated, total dose of 10 Gy produced less renal toxicity than 7.5 Gy in a single fraction.

RENAL INJURY AFTER RADIATION ACCIDENTS OR RADIOLOGICAL TERRORISM

Most of the concern about radiation accidents and radiological terrorism has focused on acute injuries to the hematopoietic system and gastrointestinal tract, as well as on late stochastic effects such as cancer. However, other normal tissue injuries might also occur, including acute and chronic renal failure.[25-27] For example, Fliedner et al.[28] reported that "very severe" renal injury (acute and chronic) occurred in 13 of 45 radiation accident victims who received doses high enough to cause severe hematological injury, and Maekawa[29] reported that two victims of the Tokaimura criticality accident developed renal failure as part of multiple organ system failure.

EFFECTS OF RENAL IRRADIATION IN ANIMALS

RENAL TOLERANCE TO SINGLE-FRACTION IRRADIATION

Bilateral renal irradiation can produce renal injury in animals at relatively low doses. Specifying a unique renal tolerance dose is impossible as the value depends on species, age, and duration of follow-up. The single-fraction 50% lethal dose (LD_{50}) after 10 months of follow-up ranges from under 10 Gy in rats[30] to over 15 Gy in mice.[31] In the rat, radiation-induced renal failure occurs as early as 8 months after single doses as low as 9 Gy, and renal dysfunction (e.g., azotemia) is observed by 7 months after single doses as low as 7 Gy.[30] In the pig, renal dysfunction has been demonstrated 3 months after a single dose of 7.8 Gy[32]; and in dogs, renal dysfunction has been shown at 6 months after a single dose of 10 Gy.[33] Mice appear as the outliers, with single doses of 12 Gy and above being required to produce significant renal injury in less than about 9 months.[31,34-36]

When animals are exposed to TBI and hematopoietic death is prevented by HSCT, radiation nephropathy is a common late event. In the rat, radiation nephropathy is actually the dominant cause of chronic morbidity in pathogen-free rats given TBI plus HSCT.[30,37] Histopathological evidence of radiation nephropathy has also been observed in Rhesus monkeys 6 to 8 years after HSCT when the TBI dose was 7.2 to 8.5 Gy at 0.2 Gy/min.[38]

Dose-response curves for radiation-induced renal dysfunction are steep. For example, in rats the incidence of radiation-induced renal failure after 8 months of follow-up goes from 5% at 8.7 Gy to 88% at 9.5 Gy.[30] Similar steep dose-response curves are seen for end-points such as azotemia,[30,34,39] GFR,[32] creatinine clearance,[40] proteinuria,[40] and hypertension.[40]

EFFECTS OF FOLLOW-UP TIME, ANIMAL AGE, AND IRRADIATION VOLUME

The effects of follow-up time on the renal tolerance dose are significant, as the single-fraction LD_{50} for a 2 month-old rat drops from 11.5 Gy after 3 months of follow-up to <9.5 Gy after 9 months.[30] The effect of age-at-irradiation can also be significant, with tolerance doses for rats[41] and dogs[42] increasing by as much as 50% between perinatal and adult animals, while the tolerance dose in pigs decreases with age.[43] The effects of partial volume irradiation on renal tolerance are poorly known.

FRACTIONATION, RADIATION DOSE RATE, AND RENAL TOLERANCE

For radiation given in fractionated schedules, renal tolerance in animals is strongly influenced by fraction size[30,36,39,44]; and when the dose is highly fractionated, animals can survive for many months after doses as high as 30 Gy.[36,39,44,45] If the fractionation effect is expressed using a linear-quadratic model,[46] the consensus value for the α/β ratio is in the 1.5 to 2.5 Gy range; but values as low as 0.9 Gy and as high as 3.5 Gy are compatible with some studies.[46,47]

Renal tolerance in animals is affected relatively little by overall duration of treatment, provided that interfraction intervals are sufficiently long (>4 hours) to allow repair of sublethal damage.[44,48,49] As a result of the lack of dependence of renal tolerance on the duration of treatment, animal models indicate that the kidney has very little tolerance for reirradiation.[49-51]

Renal tolerance in animals can also be affected by the interfraction interval and the radiation dose rate. The half-life of repair of sublethal renal damage in rodents is 0.6 to 2.1 hours,[39,45,52,53] with some evidence that repair is faster for lower doses per fraction.[45,53] These repair rates indicate that interfraction intervals of 4 hours, as used in some clinical protocols, may only be barely adequate to ensure complete repair of sublethal damage between fractions. Renal tolerance increases substantially when dose rates as low as 2 to 5 Gy/h[54,55] are used. Insufficient data exist to specify at what dose-rate tolerance increases, but based on repair half-life, it could occur at dose rates as high as 10 Gy/h.

PROGRESSION OF RADIATION-INDUCED RENAL INJURY

Robbins and Bonsib[47] have reviewed the pathophysiology of radiation nephropathy in animal models in detail. The pattern is generally the same in all species, although the rate of progression is variable. The progression of radiation-induced renal damage has been best characterized in rat models (Fig. 31.3).

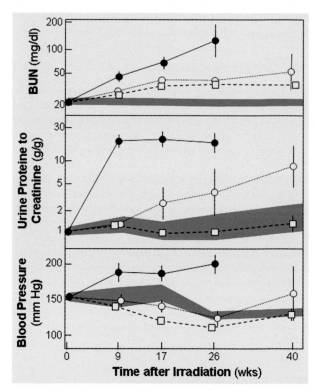

Figure 31.3. Progression of renal dysfunction in rats after irradiation. Data are shown for animals receiving irradiation alone (●); animals receiving irradiation plus therapy with an ACE inhibitor, captopril (○); and animals receiving irradiation plus therapy with an ARB, L-158,809 (□). Data for age-matched normal animals are shown as a gray area. Irradiation was given as 17-Gy TBI (in six fractions over 3 days) with an HSCT to prevent hematological toxicity. Drug therapy was begun 9 days prior to irradiation and was continued for the duration of the study. (Adapted from Moulder JE, Fish BL, Cohen EP, et al. Angiotensin II receptor antagonists in the prevention of radiation nephropathy. *Radiat Res.* 1996;146:106–110 with permission.)

After a dose of radiation sufficient to cause eventual renal failure, changes in glomerular permeability can be detected in the rat within 1 hour.[35] Overt proteinuria does not appear until at least 5 weeks later,[35,40,56] and this proteinuria is followed first by azotemia[40,56] and decreased creatinine clearance,[40] and then by hypertension.[40,56] Anemia develops along with the azotemia, but at a level disproportionate to the azotemia.[32,57] Azotemia becomes progressively worse over several months and can eventually lead to renal failure.[30,56] Serum renin activity, blood levels of angiotensin *II* (A*II*), renal A*II*, and A*II* receptor binding remain normal, at least until animals become severely azotemic and hypertensive.[56,58] Histopathological changes are first observed when azotemia reaches about double its normal value.[59]

MITIGATION AND TREATMENT OF EXPERIMENTAL RADIATION NEPHROPATHY

Antagonism of the renin-angiotensin system (RAS) has been shown to be highly effective for the mitigation and treatment of experimental radiation nephropathy.[37,58,60–63]. Established radiation nephropathy in the rat can be effectively *treated* with angiotensin-converting enzyme (ACE) inhibitors or with A*II* receptor blockers (ARBs).[58,64] Both ACE inhibitors[37,60–62] and ARBs[37,62,63] are also effective in reducing the incidence of radiation-induced renal failure when used after irradiation, but before there is physiological evidence of injury (Fig. 31.3) (i.e., in a *mitigation* regimen[65]). A delay in the start of treatment until weeks after irradiation does not decrease the efficacy of RAS antagonism,[62] and substantial preservation of renal function can be sustained in animals if therapy is stopped after several months.[62] Other types of antihypertensive drugs have not been shown to prevent radiation-induced renal injury in animals[61,66]; and no therapeutic approach assessed to date has been as effective as RAS antagonism for mitigation or treatment of experimental radiation nephropathy.[67] In fact, the only other pharmacologic approach with confirmed mitigation or treatment efficacy has been the use of anti-inflammatory agents.[60,68] We assessed pirfenidone (a phenyl-pyridone antifibrotic), thiaproline (1,3-thiazolidine-4-carboxylic acid, an inhibitor of collagen deposition), and all-trans retinoic acid (ATRA, an antithrombotic agent) for treatment of experimental radiation nephropathy; the first two agents had no efficacy, and ATRA exacerbated radiation nephropathy.[69] For mitigation of experimental radiation nephropathy, we have assessed spironolactone (an aldosterone inhibitor), genistein (a soy isoflavone), deferiprone (an iron chelator), apocynin (a substituted catechol that is a partial inhibitor of NADPH oxidase), and pravastatin; none of these agents were effective mitigators (Moulder JE, Cohen EP, Fish BL, unpublished data).

An obvious explanation for the efficacy of RAS antagonism would be that radiation leads to RAS activation and that such activation is detrimental; but there is no substantial evidence that the RAS is activated by irradiation.[32,58] The efficacy of RAS suppression in the absence of evidence for RAS activation is not unique to radiation injury,[70] and the lack of evidence for radiation-induced activation of the RAS has led to the hypothesis that even the normal activity of the RAS contributes to injury after irradiation.[56,58] A wide range of mechanisms have been proposed for the efficacy of RAS suppression in radiation nephropathy, including: unopposed stimulation of the A*II* type-2 receptor[71]; suppression of radiation-induced proliferation[72]; prevention of radiation-induced production of transforming growth factor (TGF)-β[73]; and suppression of chronic oxidative stress.[74,75] So far, none of these mechanisms has substantial support.[67]

PATHOGENESIS OF RADIATION NEPHROPATHY IN ANIMALS

All of the major features of clinical radiation nephropathy, including its characteristic glomerular lesions and mesangiolysis, are seen in mice, rats, dogs, pigs, and nonhuman primates (see review by Robbins and Bonsib[47]). However, neither the physiological nor the pathological studies in animals have resolved the issue of what the target cell(s) are for radiation nephropathy or what the pathophysiological mechanism(s) are. Arguments have been made that the target cells are parenchymal and that they are vascular; and arguments have been made that the target site is glomerular and that it is tubular.[47] There are data from animal studies to both support and oppose all of these arguments. The fact that postirradiation suppression of the RAS decreases the severity of radiation nephropathy[58,66] argues against a pathogenic mechanism based on simple mitotic cell death but does not itself directly point toward a mechanism.

HUMAN DATA

CLINICAL PRESENTATION

Radiation injury to kidneys was suspected a mere decade after the discovery of x-rays.[76] By 1927, radiation nephropathy was clinically delineated[77]; and by the early 1950s, its occurrence was quantified in terms of the doses required to cause it, and the frequency at which it occurred. Specifically, about 20% of subjects receiving more than 2,300 R (approximately 21.5 Gy) fractionated irradiation that included all of the kidneys developed radiation nephropathy.[14]

The typical presentation of radiation nephropathy is of decreased kidney function, proteinuria, hypertension, and disproportionally severe anemia occurring many months after sufficient radiation to the kidneys. There is elevation of the serum creatinine and BUN. There is fluid retention and edema. Hypertension is always present. The anemia is worse than would be expected for the degree of azotemia (decreased kidney function); and in some cases there are features of intravascular hemolysis and microangiopathic anemia.[78]

In his classic descriptions, Luxton[79] identified four variants of radiation nephritis: acute, chronic, and hypertensive forms, benign and malignant. These could occur at 6 months to 5 years after irradiation. The hypertensive forms were variants of the acute and chronic forms. The word *nephropathy* is now preferred to the word *nephritis*, since there is little inflammation in radiation nephropathy (see Refs. 80, 81 and see Fig. 31.4). The variant forms of radiation nephropathy may be more similar than different. In its modern forms, occurring after TBI-based HSCT or as a complication of radioisotope therapies, radiation nephropathy presents in a way similar to that of Luxton "acute radiation nephritis."

In the past 30 years, although classical radiation nephropathy has been uncommon, modern congeners have occurred after TBI and also after radioisotope therapies. In the case of TBI, this has been in subjects undergoing TBI in preparation for HSCT.[82]

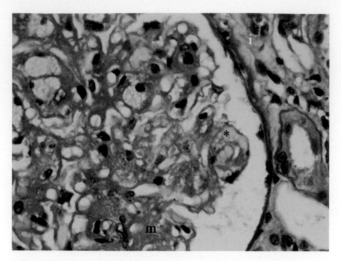

Figure 31.4. Light photomicrograph of a kidney biopsy in a recent case of BMT nephropathy (stained with periodic acid Schiff and viewed at 1,000×). There is mesangiolysis and increased mesangial matrix (m). There is interstitial expansion with edema and fibrosis (i). There is subendothelial widening with amorphous material (*), which narrows the glomerular capillary of the tuft. (Photomicrograph provided by Dr Louis Novoa-Takara, Department of Pathology, Medical College of Wisconsin.)

The actuarial occurrence rate of radiation nephropathy in these subjects can reach 20%.[82] The TBI doses that can cause radiation nephropathy are 10 Gy in a single fraction and 14 Gy in nine equal fractions (see further discussion later in this chapter). In those cases occurring after TBI, which we have called "BMT nephropathy,"[83] the average time of occurrence is 8 months after TBI. Thus, this congener of radiation nephropathy is different from the acute renal failure that can occur within thirty days after HSCT.[27,84] That form of acute renal failure is largely due to sepsis and use of nephrotoxic antibiotics. BMT nephropathy is also different from cyclosporine or tacrolimus toxicity, because these drug toxicities should improve with stopping the drug. In addition, BMT nephropathy has occurred in subjects who never were treated with cyclosporine or tacrolimus.[85]

Radiation nephropathy after radioisotope therapies may occur when the isotope has sufficient dose and energy to cause cellular injury, and when the pharmacokinetics of the carrier is such that kidneys are irradiated. Thus, ^{90}Y isotopes carried by immunoglobulins (e.g., ibritumomab tiuxetan) are not filtered by the glomeruli or secreted by the renal tubules because the immunoglobulin has a molecular weight of 150,000 or more, and thus kidneys will not receive high radiation doses. On the other hand, dota-D-phe(1)-tyr(3)-octreotide, which is labeled with the same β-emitting ^{90}Y, will be filtered by the glomeruli because the octreotide carrier has a molecular weight of 1,019 Da. It will pass through the filtration barrier, and it will then be taken up by the tubular cells that will thus be irradiated.[166]Ho attached to a phosphonate carrier has also caused radiation nephropathy.[86] The renal doses delivered by these isotopes are not known precisely, but have been estimated to be 7 to 20 Gy.[87–90]

UNILATERAL RADIATION NEPHROPATHY

Exposure of one kidney to sufficient irradiation may cause radiation nephropathy in that kidney.[19,91] The scarring kidney may secrete excess renin, thereby causing increased levels of AII and hypertension. The hypertension may be severe, and may by itself damage the opposite kidney, leading to loss of its function. Uninephrectomy of the irradiated kidney may relieve the hypertension.[92]

RADIATION-INDUCED RENOVASCULAR DISEASE

Radiation has been associated with worsening of atherosclerotic vascular disease.[93] Thus, renal arterial disease could result from either TBI or local kidney irradiation that included the renal artery(ies) in its field. Renal artery stenosis with hypertension and azotemia has been reported after local kidney irradiation.[94] Hypertension in unilateral renal artery stenosis could result from reduced renal blood flow causing renin and AII release, while the rise in BUN and serum creatinine would depend on the reduced renal blood flow on the side of the arterial stenosis and the hypertensive injury of the opposite kidney. Even worse hypertension and renal failure could occur with bilateral renal artery stenosis.

TESTING OF FUNCTION AND DEFINITION OF TOXICITY

The clinical expression of radiation nephropathy does not occur until months after irradiation. There are no known early biomarkers to predict the future development of radiation nephropathy. There is little or no information on age, sex, or ethnic sensitivity to radiation nephropathy, although a greater loss in kidney function after TBI/HSCT was associated with the ACE genotype in one study.[95] It is possible that a family history of kidney disease is associated with a risk of radiation nephropathy, but this has not been studied in detail.

As with any kidney disease, with loss of glomerular function there is a rise in serum creatinine and BUN. Subjects will have concomitant high blood pressure, in keeping with their degree of azotemia.[82] Classical descriptions of radiation nephropathy often included the development of malignant hypertension, which is very high blood pressure with hypertensive retinopathy. The retinopathy that may be seen after TBI/HSCT could also be a direct effect of TBI itself.[96]

In BMT nephropathy, the rate of decline of the kidney function may be rapid, at rates up to ten times faster than in other kidney diseases.[83] Thus, a patient with BMT nephropathy may evolve to complete kidney failure within 6 months of diagnosis. This evolution of kidney function can be graphed, as 100/serum creatinine versus time (Fig. 31.5).[97] or by using calculated values of the GFR, also graphed as a function of time. The graphing function of some electronic medical records can be very helpful to show this evolution, which is often biphasic, with a rapid decline in GFR followed by a slower one (Fig. 31.5).

Proteinuria in radiation nephropathy is on average about 2 g/d, which is at the lower limit of the "nephrotic" range. Higher values of proteinuria may suggest other kidney disease, such as membranous nephropathy associated with graft versus host disease.

Some BMT nephropathy cases have had hyperchloremic metabolic acidosis, along with hyperkalemia. Of these, a few have had low serum levels of aldosterone, perhaps in turn due to low levels of renin, and not due to adrenal insufficiency, per se.

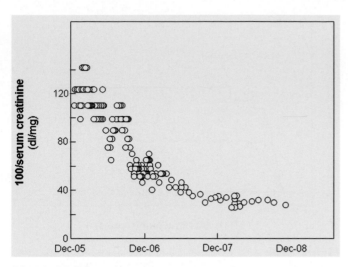

Figure 31.5. The evolution of kidney function in a recent case of BMT nephropathy. The kidney function, as estimated GFR, is graphed as the reciprocal of the serum creatinine, in mg/dL, ×100. This subject underwent TBI-based HSCT in December 2005 and had rapid loss of kidney function subsequently. There has been some stabilization of the kidney function over the past year, in association with referral to Nephrology Clinic and the use of the ACE inhibitor, captopril. This is the same subject whose biopsy photomicrograph is shown in Figure 31.4.

In subjects with BMT nephropathy, we have reported a transient rise in serum levels of lactate dehydrogenase, and a simultaneous thrombocytopenia, which tend to be more marked in those with more severe clinical presentations.[83] In the most severe forms of BMT nephropathy, the clinical presentation is reminiscent of hemolytic uremic syndrome (HUS) or thrombotic thrombocytopenic purpura (TTP). The pathogenesis of these severe forms may be the result of endothelial injury, with consequent platelet adherence to the injured endothelium and generation of a microangiopathic hemolytic anemia.

An additional hematologic aspect to radiation nephropathy, and also for its BMT nephropathy congener, is that the degree of anemia is more severe than would be expected for the degree of azotemia.[78] Red blood cell hemolysis and also low levels of erythropoietin may be the reason for this.

IMAGING

Renal imaging by ultrasound or nuclear medicine scanning has a limited role in radiation nephropathy. More involved studies, such as arteriography, would only be used after less invasive studies. CT scanning and MR scanning do not have an important role in imaging of radiation nephropathy.

Ultrasound may show findings suggestive of renal vascular disease, which could include asymmetry of kidney size, the smaller kidney possibly having an arterial stenosis. A unilateral cortical thinning (i.e., renal atrophy or even simple cyst formation) could also suggest ipsilateral renal artery stenosis.[98] More commonly, in established radiation nephropathy without renovascular disease, parenchymal scarring would be evident on ultrasound scans by increased echogenicity and loss of corticomedullary differentiation. Ultrasound also shows urinary tract obstruction well, because of the hypodense and distended collecting system that results from obstruction. The latter will not occur with uncomplicated radiation nephropathy, but

could result from retroperitoneal disease (e.g., cancerous infiltration that can be in the differential diagnosis in some cases).

Nuclear medicine scans may suggest chronic parenchymal disease by reduced or slowed parenchymal uptake of the tracer. The flow part of the nuclear medicine study may show asymmetry of flow, which could point to renovascular disease. Urinary obstruction would be suggested by a slowed excretion of the tracer.

In cases where one would suspect renovascular disease, renal arteriography would be indicated, but this is uncommon.

HISTOLOGY

In a subject at risk for radiation nephropathy, there are many other potential causes for kidney disease. These can include the effects of chemotherapy (e.g., kidney damage from cis-platinum or ifosfamide), side effects of immunodeficiency (e.g., interstitial nephritis from polyoma virus), and the effects of graft versus host disease.[99] Kidney biopsy may be useful to differentiate these causes and guide treatment. In BMT nephropathy, mesangiolysis is always present, there is limited tubulointerstitial inflammation, and there is substantial subendothelial expansion by low density material that seems mostly to be plasma proteins (Fig. 31.4) Inflammation is not prominent, which is why the word *nephropathy* is preferable to the word *nephritis*. Immune-type deposits are usually not prominent, but in some cases there may be deposition of C3, which may point to a role for the complement system in the pathogenesis. The light microscopic appearance of classical radiation nephropathy is similar to that of BMT nephropathy, as is the radiation nephropathy occurring after radioisotope therapies.[88]

DOSE, TIME, AND VOLUME RECOMMENDATIONS

RENAL RADIATION TOLERANCE

Earlier in this chapter we discussed data that suggest that the TD 5/5 for bilateral radiation of the kidneys is approximately 23 Gy, and that the TD 50/5 is approximately 28 Gy.[21,100] The initial work to identify these doses, which are based on fractionated radiation, comes from the treatment of patients with testicular and ovarian cancers.[14,15] Those data consisted of the 2-year results on 93 patients treated for testicular cancer with doses of 2,000 to 3,250 R (approximately 18.5–30 Gy). Of 55 patients treated with 2,500 to 3,250 R (approximately 23–30 Gy) in 3 to 6 weeks, 40% showed evidence of renal damage, as exhibited by proteinuria and either elevated BUN or hypertension or both.[14] The authors carefully evaluated the different radiation delivery methods and determined a central kidney dose, an average dose to the upper one third of the kidneys, and an average dose to the lower one third of the kidneys. They concluded that a dose of 2,300 R (approximately 21.5 Gy) delivered to the whole of both kidneys can cause hypertension and renal failure, and that it is best to protect one third of the entirety of both kidneys to minimize the risk of renal failure.[14]

More recently, Flentje et al.[101] analyzed a group of 142 patients with seminoma treated to the periaortic region with rotational techniques that produced significant renal radiation exposure. This group of patients had a median follow up of 8.2 years.

Their data supported a TD 50/5 of 28 Gy and a TD 5/5 of 23 Gy for fractionated bilateral whole-kidney radiation; this corresponds to practice guidelines used today.

TOLERANCE FOR PARTIAL VOLUME EXPOSURES

Tolerance doses for partial renal volume irradiation are more difficult to assess. Data from treatment of upper abdominal malignancies[19,102] support the data reported by Emami et al.[21] in that the TD 5/5 for treatment of one third of the total renal volume is approximately 50 Gy, and for treatment of two thirds of the total renal volume is approximately 30 Gy. Partial organ TD 50/5 is not known with any certainty.

RENAL TOLERANCE AFTER TBI USED FOR HSCT

There are extensive data on renal radiation toxicity in the HSCT literature that suggest a much lower dose threshold for renal radiation injury than the 23 Gy TD 5/5 Gy[21,100] found for fractionated local renal irradiation. By the 1980s, there were reports of renal toxicity in children undergoing HSCT with TBI as part of the conditioning regimen.[103–105] The first large series of pediatric HSCT patients reporting renal toxicity related to TBI was by Tarbell et al.[105] In that report, 29 patients who had undergone HSCT for acute lymphocytic leukemia or Stage IV neuroblastoma were alive and in remission 3 months after HSCT; 11 of these patients had developed renal dysfunction (a syndrome now called *BMT nephropathy*[83,106]). All patients had received TBI as part of the conditioning regimen. TBI ranged from one fraction of 8.5 Gy, to 12 or 13 Gy in six fractions, and 14 Gy in eight fractions; clearly all of these doses are well below the 23 to 28 Gy tolerance previously established. Other authors reported similar findings in the adult HSCT population. Lawton et al.[107] found a cumulative 20% incidence of renal dysfunction at 1 year in 103 adult patients who were conditioned with approximately 14-Gy TBI in nine fractions over 3 days. This again supports the concern that the tolerance of the kidneys to radiation is lowered when radiation is associated with chemotherapy, antibiotics, and antifungal agents.

Extensive work has been done to try to sort out the cause of the decrease in radiation tolerance in HSCT.[7,108–113] Certainly the drugs given in the peri-TBI period could play a role; these range from cytotoxic agents to nephrotoxins such as antifungal agents and aminoglycoside antibiotics. Issues related to the delivery of the TBI also appear to play a role. Miralbell et al.[7] suggested that both total dose and dose per fraction were important. Lawton et al.,[112] through the use of renal shielding to lower the total dose to the kidneys, suggested that total dose was the key factor (Fig. 31.6). Cheng et al.[108] supported the position that dose rate was a key factor. Kal et al.[113] looked at the concept of biologically effective dose (BED[46,114]) using a/b of 2.5 Gy and a repair half-time of 2 h. After synthesizing the HSCT literature on late renal dysfunction, their analysis supports a tolerance BED for bilateral kidney radiation of approximately 16 Gy and suggests renal shielding for patients receiving a BED >16 Gy to the kidneys. A BED of 16 Gy corresponds to approximately 10 Gy in six fractions or approximately 11 Gy in nine fractions (assuming a dose rate >5 cGy/min).[113]

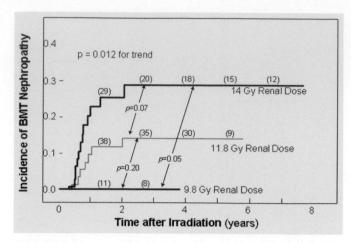

Figure 31.6. Actuarial incidence of BMT nephropathy after TBI-based HSCT as a function of renal dose. The number of patients at risk is shown in parentheses. Based on the Cox proportional hazard model, there is a significant trend ($p = 0.012$) for decreasing renal dose and the decreasing incidence of BMT nephropathy. (Adapted from Lawton CA, Barber-Derus SW, Murray KJ, et al. Influence of renal shielding on the incidence of late renal dysfunction associated with T-lymphocyte deplete bone marrow transplantation in adult patients. *Int J Radiat Oncol Biol Phys.* 1992;23:681–686, with permission.)

STRATEGIES FOR AVOIDING TOXICITY

If the determinants of normal tissue radiation injury were better known, be they genetic or environmental, there could be reliable and complete prevention or mitigation of radiation nephropathy. However, at present only the radiation dose and schedule are proven normal tissue injury modifiers, and dose reduction may diminish radiation's therapeutic benefit.

SHIELDING

The best method to avoid radiation toxicity to the kidneys is to avoid irradiating the kidneys altogether. However, there are situations, such as treatment of upper abdominal malignancies,[19] where this is not always possible. Current 3D and intensity modulated radiotherapy (IMRT) radiation techniques allow the treating radiation oncologist to spare most or at least some of one or both kidneys in some such cases.[115] In such cases, it is important to avoid kidney irradiation above the TD 5/5 doses previously discussed.[21]

The other situation where the treatment of the kidneys is difficult to avoid is in TBI for HSCT. Data from both the pediatric[105] and adult[107] HSCT populations with TBI as part of the conditioning regimen have shown significant renal toxicity if no measures are taken to shield/protect the kidneys. When TBI is delivered, and the doses to the kidneys are lowered, there is a significant decrease in the incidence of renal toxicity.[7,112] Lawton et al.[23] described the use of selective renal shielding to successfully decrease the risk of late renal toxicity in TBI patients. Their use of a posterior partial transmission renal shield, which results in a total dose to the kidneys of <10 Gy (Fig. 31.6), showed a decrease in the incidence of late renal toxicity which other authors have supported.[7,112]

LOWERING THE DOSE RATE

Lowering of the TBI dose rate (<10 cGy/min) in adults to decrease renal toxicity has been suggested by at least one group performing a comprehensive review of the dosimetric aspects of TBI,[108] but these authors did not see a dose-rate effect for TBI-induced renal damage in the pediatric population. Furthermore, decreasing the dose rate to <10 cGy/min lengthens the treatment delivery time significantly, which could be problematic for these medically frail patients.

PHARMACOLOGIC APPROACHES

Radioprotective agents such as amifostine could in theory prevent radiation nephropathy[116]; but when given at the time of irradiation, their use could also protect the cancerous tissues, making them inappropriate.

Experimental studies of the use of ACE inhibitors to mitigate radiation nephropathy showed that these drugs could be started at 3 weeks after irradiation and still exert a substantial long-term benefit.[117] There was by that time clear clinical evidence that the ACE inhibitor captopril could successfully slow the progression of diabetic nephropathy.[118] We thus conducted a randomized, placebo-controlled clinical trial to mitigate chronic renal failure in subjects undergoing TBI-based HSCT. That study shows that there is a favorable trend for captopril to reduce the occurrence of chronic renal failure and to reduce the incidence of the BMT nephropathy syndrome after HSCT.[119] During the time of this study, 74 subjects who were eligible for this study did not participate, either because of refusal or involvement in competing studies. They were thus a parallel cohort, providing an internal control group. Five of this group developed the BMT nephropathy syndrome or HUS. Their survival free of BMT nephropathy and their overall survival were the same as those of the placebo group in the study cohort. Thus, an additional analysis was done, combining the 74 nonstudy subjects with the placebo group. We then compared the study subjects on captopril to all subjects who did not take captopril. This showed a favorable trend for captopril to reduce the occurrence of BMT nephropathy ($p = 0.07$), and a significant ($p = 0.03$) benefit of captopril to improve patient survival in subjects undergoing TBI-based HSCT (Fig. 31.7).

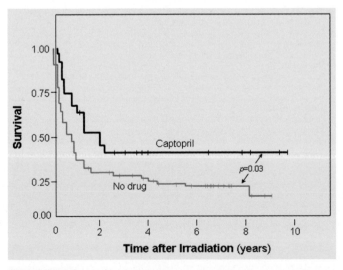

Figure 31.7. Actuarial patient survival in a clinical trial using the ACE inhibitor, captopril, to mitigate chronic renal failure in subjects undergoing TBI-based HSCT. Patients taking captopril in a randomized, placebo-controlled trial[119] are compared to patients not taking the drug (the latter group includes both the placebo group from the randomized trial and subjects who were eligible for this study but did not participate).

Chronic renal failure after HSCT is now widely recognized.[120] The occurrence of end-stage renal disease after HSCT is many-fold increased over its expected occurrence in an age-matched population.[121] When end-stage renal disease occurs, and there is the need for long-term dialysis, survival is poor. Further study of captopril or other A*II* antagonism after HSCT is thus justified. It is possible that studies in laboratory animals may point to other agents that can mitigate radiation nephropathy, in which case those agents merit testing in humans. Yet other drugs may be beneficial to mitigate chronic renal failure occurring after HSCT that is not preceded by TBI.

TREATMENT OF INJURY

Radiation nephropathy or its congeners, such as BMT nephropathy, may be treated as one would any form of kidney disease. Thus, for high blood pressure, there are many effective antihypertensive drugs, and for anemia, one can use parenteral erythropoietin. In our 20-year experience at the Froedtert Hospital and Medical College of Wisconsin, this "generic" approach has slowed, even arrested, the progression of renal failure in many cases of BMT nephropathy. Indeed, it is well established that hypertension aggravates most forms of kidney disease, and, conversely, that good control of the blood pressure slows down the progression of kidney diseases.[122]

ACE inhibitors and ARBs are very effective in the treatment of radiation nephropathy in laboratory rats.[58,64] We have shown the clear therapeutic benefit of ARBs in a case of radiation nephropathy occurring in a subject with a kidney transplant.[123] In addition, ACE inhibitors are the preferred agents for slowing the progression of most causes of chronic renal failure.[124] We thus recommend the use of ACE inhibitors or ARBs for treatment of established radiation nephropathy.

In cases of BMT nephropathy in which there is an associated HUS and thrombocytopenia, plasmapheresis has been used. That may attenuate the hematologic syndrome, but it does not help to relieve the renal failure.[125] In classical TTP, plasmapheresis is beneficial; but in those cases, the pathogenesis of the disease is based on blood-borne proteins, rather than a primary endothelial abnormality.

Despite appropriate treatment, radiation nephropathy may evolve to complete renal failure and the need for dialysis or kidney transplant (i.e., end-stage renal disease).[126,127] We have shown that survival on dialysis in such cases is poor.[127] Kidney transplantation may be possible. In cases where the marrow donor has remained healthy and is willing to donate a kidney to the recipient now ill with radiation nephropathy, it may be possible to avoid immunosuppression after the kidney transplant.[126] Use of a deceased-donor kidney remains possible; but in the recipient who has undergone previous HSCT, we recommend halving the immunosuppression because the recipient's bone marrow may not be fully functional.

ADRENALS

Although the adrenal glands are immediately adjacent to the kidneys (Fig. 31.1), they have different embryological origins,[6] and they are not radiosensitive.[128] Indeed, adrenal failure is not a known complication of TBI-based bone marrow transplantation,[129] whereas other endocrine insufficiency is well described after TBI, including gonadal and thyroid failures.[129,130]

Secondary adrenal insufficiency could occur after pituitary irradiation that destroys the pituitary gland.[131,132] It could also occur after prolonged use of high-dose corticosteroids that would suppress the endogenous corticosteroid production by the adrenal glands.

In limited studies of the pituitary-adrenal axis after 10 Gy TBI in rats with head shielding, we have found normal adrenal cell synthesis of corticosterone, and normal blood levels of corticosterone and its controller, adrenocorticotrophic hormone (ACTH). In these same studies, we have found an exaggerated pituitary ACTH response to corticotrophin-releasing hormone, at eight days after irradiation. Thus, transient pituitary-adrenal dysfunction after TBI may occur.

Adrenal injury has not been described after radioimmunotherapy. But given a specific combination of ligand and isotope, uptake in adrenal cortex or medulla could occur, thus causing direct adrenal insufficiency.

REFERENCES

1. The urinary organs. In: Williams PL, Warwick R, Dyson M, et al., eds. *Gray's Anatomy.* London: Churchill Livingstone; 1989:1397–1415.
2. Anatomy. In: Allen AC, ed. *The Kidney: Medical and Surgical Diseases.* New York, NY: Grune & Stratton; 1962:19–63.
3. Deen WM. What determines glomerular capillary permeability? *J Clin Invest.* 2004;114: 1412–1414.
4. Brezis M, Rosen S. Hypoxia of the renal medulla—its implications for disease. *N Engl J Med.* 1995;332:647–655.
5. Nadasdy T, Laszik Z, Blick KE, et al. Proliferative activity of intrinsic cell populations in the normal human kidney. *J Am Soc Nephrol.* 1994;4:2032–2039.
6. Brandt WE. Adrenal glands and kidney. In: Brandt WE, Helms CA, eds. *Fundamentals of Diagnostic Radiology.* Philadelphia, PA: Lippincott Williams & Wilkins; 2007:867–886.
7. Miralbell R, Sancho G, Bieri S, et al. Renal insufficiency in patients with hematologic malignancies undergoing total body irradiation and bone marrow transplantation: a prospective assessment. *Int J Radiat Oncol Biol Phys.* 2004;58:809–816.
8. Golman K, Almen T. Contrast media-induced nephrotoxicity. Survey and present state. *Invest Radiol.* 1985;20(suppl):S92–S97.
9. Tepel M, van der Giet M, Schwarzfeld C, et al. Prevention of radiographic-contrast-agent-induced reductions in renal function by acetylcysteine. *N Engl J Med.* 2000;343:180–184.
10. Bakris GL, Lass N, Gaber AO, et al. Radiocontrast medium-induced declines in renal function: a role for oxygen free radicals. *Am J Physiol.* 1990;258:F115–F120.
11. Genitourinary system and adrenal glands. In: Mettler FA, Guiberteau MM, eds. *Essentials of Nuclear Medicine Imaging.* Philadelphia, PA: Saunders Elsevier; 2006:293–324.
12. Ziessman HA, O'Malley JP, Thrall JT. *Nuclear Medicine: The Requisites.* Philadelphia, PA: Elsevier Mosby; 2006.
13. Maier JG. Effects of radiation on kidney, bladder, and prostate. *Front Rad Ther Oncol.* 1972;6:196–227.
14. Kunkler PB, Farr RF, Luxton RW. The limit of renal tolerance to X rays: an investigation into renal damage occurring following the treatment of tumours of the testis by abdominal baths. *Br J Radiol.* 1952;25:190–201.
15. Luxton RW. Radiation nephritis: a long-term study of 54 patients. *Lancet.* 1961;2: 1221–1224.
16. Crummy WE, Hellman S, Stansel HC, et al. Renal hypertension secondary to unilateral radiation damage relieved by nephrectomy. *Radiology.* 1965;84:108–111.
17. McGill CW, Holder TM, Smith TH, et al. Postradiation renovascular hypertension. *J Pediatr Surg.* 1979;14:831–833.
18. Turesson I. The progression rate of late radiation effects in normal tissue and its impact on dose-response relationships. *Radiother Oncol.* 1989;15:217–226.
19. Willett CG, Tepper JE, Orlow EL, et al. Renal complications secondary to radiation treatment of upper abdominal malignancies. *Int J Radiat Oncol Biol Phys.* 1986;12:1601–1604.
20. Cassady JR. Clinical radiation nephropathy. *Int J Radiat Oncol Biol Phys.* 1995;31:1249–1256.
21. Emami B, Lyman J, Brown A, et al. Tolerance of normal tissue to therapeutic irradiation. *Int J Radiat Oncol Biol Phys.* 1991;21:109–122.
22. Lönnerholm G, Carlson K, Bratteby LE, et al. Renal function after autologous bone marrow transplantation. *Bone Marrow Transplant.* 1991;8:129–134.
23. Lawton CA, Cohen EP, Murray KJ, et al. Long-term results of selective renal shielding in patients undergoing total body irradiation in preparation for bone marrow transplantation. *Bone Marrow Transplant.* 1997;12:1069–1074.
24. Miralbell R, Bieri S, Mermillod B, et al. Renal toxicity after allogeneic bone marrow transplantation: the combined effects of total-body irradiation and graft-versus-host disease. *J Clin Oncol.* 1996;14:579–585.
25. Moulder JE. Multiorgan problems associated with total and partial body irradiation. In: Ricks RC, Berger ME, O'Hara FM, eds. *The Medical Basis for Radiation-Accident Preparedness: The Clinical Care of Victims.* Boca Raton, FL: Parthenon Publishing Group; 2002:175–189.
26. Coleman CN, Blakely WF, Fike JR, et al. Molecular and cellular biology of moderate-dose (1–10 Gy) radiation and potential mechanisms of radiation protection: Report of a workshop at Bethesda, Maryland, December 17–18, 2001. *Radiat Res.* 2003;159:812–834.
27. Moulder JE, Cohen EP. Radiation-induced multi-organ involvement and failure: the contribution of radiation effects on the renal system. *Br J Radiol.* 2005;27(suppl):82–88.
28. Fliedner TM, Dörr HD, Meineke V. Multi-organ involvement as a pathogenetic principle of the radiation syndromes: a study involving 110 case histories documented in SEARCH and classified as the bases of haematopoietic indicators of effect. *Br J Radiol.* 2005;27(suppl):1–8.
29. Maekawa K. Overview of medical care for highly exposed victims in the Tokaimura accident. In: Ricks RC, Berger ME, O'Hara FM, eds. *The Medical Basis for Radiation-Accident Preparedness: The Clinical Care of Victims.* Boca Raton, FL: Parthenon Publishing Group; 2002:313–318.
30. Moulder JE, Fish BL. Late toxicity of total body irradiation with bone marrow transplantation in a rat model. *Int J Radiat Oncol Biol Phys.* 1989;16:1501–1509.
31. Williams MV, Denekamp J. Sequential functional testing of radiation-induced renal damage in the mouse. *Radiat Res.* 1983;94:305–317.
32. Robbins MEC, Campling D, Rezvani M, et al. Radiation nephropathy in mature pigs following the irradiation of both kidneys. *Int J Radiat Biol.* 1989;56:83–98.
33. Prescott DM, Hoopes PJ, Thrall DE. Modification of radiation damage in the canine kidney by hyperthermia: a histologic and functional study. *Radiat Res.* 1990;124:317–325.
34. Liao ZX, Travis EL. Unilateral nephrectomy 24 hours after bilateral kidney irradiation reduces damage to the function and structure of the remaining kidney. *Radiat Res.* 1994;139:290–299.
35. Sharma M, Sharma R, Ge XL, et al. Early detection of radiation-induced glomerular injury by albumin permeability assay. *Radiat Res.* 2001;155:474–480.
36. Williams MV, Denekamp J. Radiation induced renal damage in mice: influence of fraction size. *Int J Radiat Oncol Biol Phys.* 1984;10:885–893.
37. Moulder JE, Fish BL, Cohen EP, et al. Angiotensin II receptor antagonists in the prevention of radiation nephropathy. *Radiat Res.* 1996;146:106–110.
38. van Kleef EM, Zurcher C, Oussoren YG, et al. Long-term effects of total body irradiation on the kidney of Rhesus monkeys. *Int J Radiat Biol.* 2000;76:641–648.
39. van Rongen E, Kuijpers WC, Madhuizen HT. Fractionation effects and repair kinetics in rat kidney. *Int J Radiat Oncol Biol Phys.* 1990;18:1093–1106.
40. Cohen EP, Moulder JE, Fish BL, et al. Prophylaxis of experimental bone marrow transplant nephropathy. *J Lab Clin Med.* 1994;124:371–380.
41. Moulder JE, Fish BL. Age-dependence of radiation nephropathy in the rat. *Radiat Res.* 1997;147:349–353.
42. Phemister RD, Thomassen RW, Norridin RW, et al. Renal failure in perinatally irradiated beagles. *Radiat Res.* 1973;55:399–410.
43. Robbins MEC, Campling D, Rezvani M, et al. The effect of age and the proportion of renal tissue irradiated on the apparent radiosensitivity of the pig kidney. *Int J Radiat Biol.* 1989;59:99–106.
44. Hopewell JW, Berry RJ. Radiation tolerance of the pig kidney: a model for determining overall time and fraction factors for preserving renal function. *Int J Radiat Oncol Biol Phys.* 1975;1:61–68.
45. Moulder JE, Fish BL. Rate of repair of sublethal radiation injury in the rat kidney. In: Paliwal BR, Fowler JF, Herbert DE, et al., eds. *Prediction of Response in Radiation Therapy.* New York, NY: American Institute of Physics; 1989:131–143.
46. Fowler JF. The linear-quadratic formula and progress in fractionated radiotherapy. *Br J Radiol.* 1989;62:679–694.
47. Robbins MEC, Bonsib SM. Radiation nephropathy: a review. *Scanning Microsc.* 1995;9: 535–560.
48. Williams MV, Denekamp J. Radiation induced renal damage in mice: influence of overall treatment time. *Radiother Oncol.* 1984;1:355–367.
49. Rockwell S, Moulder JE. Biological factors of importance in split-course radiotherapy. In: Paliwal BR, Herbert DE, Orton CG, eds. *Optimization of Cancer Radiotherapy.* New York, NY: American Institute of Physics; 1985:171–182.
50. Robbins ME, Bywaters T, Rezvani M, et al. Residual radiation-induced damage to the kidney of the pig as assayed by retreatment. *Int J Radiat Biol.* 1991;60:917–928.
51. Stewart FA, Oussoren Y, van Tinteren H, et al. Loss of reirradiation tolerance in the kidney with increasing time after single or fractionated partial tolerance doses. *Int J Radiat Biol.* 1994;66:169–179.
52. Joiner MC, Rojas A, Johns H. Renal damage in the mouse: repair kinetics at 2 and 7 Gy per fraction. *Radiat Res.* 1993;134:355–363.
53. Rojas A, Joiner MC. The influence of dose per fraction on repair kinetics. *Radiother Oncol.* 1989;14:329–336.
54. Moulder JE, Fish BL, Wilson JF. Tumor and normal tissue tolerance for fractionated low-dose-rate radiotherapy. *Int J Radiat Oncol Biol Phys.* 1990;19:341–348.
55. Safwat A, Nielsen OS, El-Bakky HA, et al. Renal damage after total body irradiation in a mouse model for bone marrow transplantation: effect of radiation dose rate. *Radiother Oncol.* 1995;34:203–209.
56. Cohen EP, Fish BL, Moulder JE. The renin-angiotensin system in experimental radiation nephropathy. *J Lab Clin Med.* 2002;139:251–257.
57. Down JD, Berman AJ, Warhol M, et al. Late tissue-specific toxicity of total body irradiation and busulfan in a murine bone marrow transplant model. *Int J Radiat Oncol Biol Phys.* 1989;17:109–116.
58. Cohen EP, Joines MM, Moulder JE. Prevention and treatment of radiation injuries—the role of the renin-angiotensin system. In: Rubin P, Constine LS, Mark LB, et al., eds. *Late Effects of Cancer Treatment on Normal Tissues.* Heidelberg: Springer-Verlag; 2008:69–76.
59. Cohen EP, Molteni A, Hill P, et al. Captopril preserves function and ultrastructure in experimental radiation nephropathy. *Lab Invest.* 1996;75:349–360.
60. Geraci JP, Sun MC, Mariano MS. Amelioration of radiation nephropathy in rats by postirradiation treatment with dexamethasone and/or captopril. *Radiat Res.* 1995;143: 58–68.

61. Juncos LI, Carrasco Dueñas S, Cornejo JC, et al. Long-term enalapril and hydrochlorothiazide in radiation nephritis. *Nephron.* 1993;64:249–255.

62. Moulder JE, Fish BL, Cohen EP. Brief pharmacologic intervention in experimental radiation nephropathy. *Radiat Res.* 1998;150:535–541.

63. Oikawa T, Freeman M, Lo W, et al. Modulation of plasminogen activator inhibitor-1 *in vivo:* a new mechanism for the anti-fibrotic effect of renin-angiotensin inhibition. *Kidney Int.* 1997;51:164–172.

64. Moulder JE, Fish BL, Cohen EP. Radiation nephropathy is treatable with an angiotensin converting enzyme inhibitor or an angiotensin II type-1 (AT₁) receptor antagonist. *Radiother Oncol.* 1998;46:307–315.

65. Stone HB, Moulder JE, Coleman CN, et al. Models for evaluating agents intended for the prophylaxis, mitigation and treatment of radiation injuries. Report of an NCI workshop, December 3–4, 2003. *Radiat Res.* 2004;162:711–728.

66. Moulder JE, Robbins MEC, Cohen EP, et al. Pharmacologic modification of radiation-induced late normal tissue injury. *Cancer Treat Res.* 1998;93:129–151.

67. Moulder JE, Cohen EP. Future strategies for mitigation and treatment of chronic radiation-induced normal tissue injury. *Semin Radiat Oncol.* 2007;17:141–148.

68. Verheij M, Stewart FA, Oussoren Y, et al. Amelioration of radiation nephropathy by acetyl-salicylic acid. *Int J Radiat Biol.* 1995;67:587–596.

69. Moulder JE, Fish BL, Regner KR, et al. Retinoic acid exacerbates radiation nephropathy. *Radiat Res.* 2002;157:199–203.

70. Rosenberg ME, Smith LJ, Correa-Rotter R, et al. The paradox of the renin-angiotensin system in chronic renal disease. *Kidney Int.* 1994;45:403–410.

71. Cohen EP, Fish BL, Sharma M, et al. The role of the angiotensin II type-2 receptor in radiation nephropathy. *Trans Res.* 2007;150:106–115.

72. Moulder JE, Fish BL, Regner KR, et al. Angiotensin II blockade reduces radiation-induced proliferation in experimental radiation nephropathy. *Radiat Res.* 2002;157:393–401.

73. Datta PK, Moulder JE, Fish BL, et al. TGF-ß1 production in radiation nephropathy: role of angiotensin II. *Int J Radiat Biol.* 1999;75:473–479.

74. Robbins ME, Diz DI. Pathogenic role of the renin-angiotensin system in modulating radiation-induced late effects. *Int J Radiat Oncol Biol Phys.* 2006;64:6–12.

75. Zhao W, Diz DI, Robbins ME. Oxidative damage pathways in relation to normal tissue injury. *Br J Radiol.* 2007;80 S23–S31.

76. Edsall DL. The attitude of the clinician in regard to exposing patients to the x-ray. *J Am Med Assoc.* 1906;47:1425–1429.

77. Domagk G. Röntgenstrahlenschädigungen der niere beim menschen [Radiation damage of the human kidney]. *Med Klinik (Berlin).* 1927;23:345–347.

78. Cohen EP, Lawton CA, Moulder JE. Bone marrow transplant nephropathy: radiation nephritis revisited. *Nephron.* 1995;70:217–222.

79. Luxton RW. Radiation nephritis. *Quart J Med.* 1953;22:215–242.

80. Zuelzer WW, Palmer HD, Newton WA. Unusual glomerulonephritis in young children probably radiation nephritis. *Am J Pathol.* 1950;26:1019–1039.

81. Rubenstone AI, Fitch LB. Radiation nephritis. A clinicopathologic study. *Am J Med.* 1962;33:545–554.

82. Cohen EP. Radiation nephropathy after bone marrow transplantation. *Kidney Int.* 2000;58:903–918.

83. Cohen EP, Lawton CA, Moulder JE, et al. Clinical course of late-onset bone marrow transplant nephropathy. *Nephron.* 1993;64:626–635.

84. Cohen EP. Acute renal failure after bone marrow transplantation. In: Molitoris B, Finn W, eds. *Acute Renal Failure.* Philadelphia, PA: WB Saunders; 2001:344–348.

85. Chappell ME, Keeling DM, Prentice HG, et al. Haemolytic uraemic syndrome after bone marrow transplantation: an adverse effect of total body irradiation. *Bone Marrow Transplant.* 1988;3:339–347.

86. Giralt S, Bensinger W, Goodman M, et al. ¹⁶⁶Ho-DOTMP plus melphalan followed by peripheral blood stem cell transplantation in patients with multiple myeloma: results of two phase 1/2 trials. *Blood.* 2003;102:2684–2691.

87. O'Donoghue J. Relevance of external beam dose-response relationships to kidney toxicity associated with radionuclide therapy. *Cancer Biother Radiopharm.* 2004;19:378–387.

88. Moll S, Nickeleit V, Mueller-Brand J, et al. A new cause of renal thrombotic microangiopathy: yttrium 90-DOTATOC internal radiotherapy. *Am J Kid Dis.* 2001;37:847–851.

89. Lambert B, Cybulla M, Weiner SM, et al. Renal toxicity after radionuclide therapy. *Radiat Res.* 2004;161:607–611.

90. Wessels BW, Konijnenberg MW, Dale RG, et al. MIRD Pamphlet No. 20: the effect of model assumptions on kidney dosimetry and response-implications for radionuclide therapy. *J Nuc Med.* 2008;49:1884–1899.

91. Thompson PL, Mackey IR, Robson GSM, et al. Late radiation nephritis after gastric x-irradiation for peptic ulcer. *Quart J Med.* 1971;40:145–157.

92. Dean A, Abels J. Study by newer renal function tests of an unusual case of hypertension following irradiation of one kidney and the relief of the patient by nephrectomy. *J Urol.* 1944;52:497–501.

93. Akasheh M, Priyanath A, Pello N, et al. Accelerated atherosclerosis in a patient with post-BMT nephropathy. *Bone Marrow Transplant.* 1999;23:199.

94. Staab GE, Tegtmeyer CJ, Constable WC. Radiation-induced renovascular hypertension. *Am J Roentgenol.* 1976;126:634–637.

95. Juckett MB, Cohen EP, Keever-Taylor CA, et al. Loss of renal function following bone marrow transplantation: an analysis of angiotensin converting enzyme D/I polymorphism and other clinical risk factors. *Bone Marrow Transplant.* 2001;27:451–456.

96. Bernauer W, Gratwohl A, Keller A, et al. Microvasculopathy in the ocular fundus after bone marrow transplantation. *Ann Int Med.* 1991;115:925–930.

97. Cohen EP, Lemann J. The role of the laboratory in evaluation of kidney function. *Clin Chem.* 1991;37:785–796.

98. Cohen EP, Elliott WC Jr. The role of ischemia in acquired cystic kidney disease. *Am J Kid Dis.* 1990;15:55–60.

99. Troxell ML, Pilapil M, Miklos DB, et al. Renal pathology in hematopoietic cell transplantation recipients. *Mod Pathol.* 2008;21:396–406.

100. Milano MT, Constine LS, Okunieff P. Normal tissue tolerance dose metrics for radiation therapy of major organs. *Sem Rad Onc.* 2007;17:131–140.

101. Flentje M, Hensley F, Gademann G, et al. Renal tolerance to nonhomogenous irradiation: comparison of observed effects to predictions of normal tissue complication probability from different biophysical models. *Int J Radiat Oncol Biol Phys.* 1993;27:25–30.

102. Kim TH, Somerville PJ, Freeman CR. Unilateral radiation nephropathy—the long-term significance. *Int J Radiat Oncol Biol Phys.* 1984;10:2053–2059.

103. Kamil ES, Latta H, Johnston WH, et al. Radiation nephritis following bone marrow transplantation. *Kidney Int.* 1978;14:713.

104. Bergstein J, Andreoli SP, Provisor AJ, et al. Radiation nephritis following total-body irradiation and cyclophosphamide in preparation for bone marrow transplantation. *Transplantation.* 1986;41:63–66.

105. Tarbell NJ, Guinan EC, Niemeyer C, et al. Late onset of renal dysfunction in survivors of bone marrow transplantation. *Int J Radiat Oncol Biol Phys.* 1988;15:99–104.

106. Moulder JE, Fish BL, Cohen EP. Treatment of radiation nephropathy with ACE inhibitors. *Int J Radiat Oncol Biol Phys.* 1993;27:93–99.

107. Lawton CA, Cohen EP, Barber-Derus SW, et al. Late renal dysfunction in adult survivors of bone marrow transplantation. *Cancer.* 1991;67:2795–2800.

108. Cheng JC, Schultheiss TE, Wong JY. Impact of drug therapy, radiation dose, and dose rate on renal toxicity following bone marrow transplantation. *Int J Radiat Oncol Biol Phys.* 2008;71:1436–1443.

109. Delgado J, Cooper N, Thomson K, et al. The importance of age, fludarabine, and total body irradiation in the incidence and severity of chronic renal failure after allogeneic hematopoietic cell transplantation. *Biol Blood Marrow Transplant.* 2006;12:75–83.

110. Lawton CA, Fish BL, Moulder JE. Effect of nephrotoxic drugs in the development of radiation nephropathy after bone marrow transplantation. *Int J Radiat Oncol Biol Phys.* 1994;28:883–889.

111. Van Why SK, Friedman AL, Wei LJ, et al. Renal insufficiency after bone marrow transplantation in children. *Bone Marrow Transplant.* 1991;7:383–388.

112. Lawton CA, Barber-Derus SW, Murray KJ, et al. Influence of renal shielding on the incidence of late renal dysfunction associated with T-lymphocyte deplete bone marrow transplantation in adult patients. *Int J Radiat Oncol Biol Phys.* 1992;23:681–686.

113. Kal HB, van Kempen-Harteveld ML. Renal dysfunction after total body irradiation: dose-effect relationship. *Int J Radiat Oncol Biol Phys.* 2006;65:1228–1232.

114. Barendsen GW. Dose fractionation, dose rate and iso-effect relationships for normal tissue responses. *Int J Radiat Oncol Biol Phys.* 1982;8:1981–1997.

115. Abrams RA, Choo J. Pancreatic cancer. In: Gunderson LL, Tepper JE, eds. *Clinical Radiation Oncology.* Philadelphia, PA: Saunders; 2006:1061–1082.

116. Kaldir M, Cosar-Alas R, Cermik TF, et al. Amifostine use in radiation-induced kidney damage. *Strahlen Onkol.* 2008;184:370–375.

117. Moulder JE, Fish BL, Cohen EP. Noncontinuous use of angiotensin converting enzyme inhibitors in the treatment of experimental bone marrow transplant nephropathy. *Bone Marrow Transplant.* 1997;19:729–736.

118. Lewis EJ, Hunsicker LG, Bain RP, et al. The effect of angiotensin-converting-enzyme inhibition on diabetic nephropathy. *N Engl J Med.* 1993;329:1456–1462.

119. Cohen EP, Irving AA, Drobyski WR, et al. Captopril to mitigate chronic renal failure after hematopoietic stem cell transplantation: a randomized controlled trial. *Int J Radiat Oncol Biol Phys.* 2008;70:1546–1551.

120. Weiss AS, Sandmaier BM, Storer B, et al. Chronic kidney disease following non-myeloablative hematopoietic cell transplantation. *Am J Transplant.* 2006;6:89–94.

121. Cohen EP, Drobysjki WR, Moulder JE. Significant increase in end-stage renal disease after hematopoietic stem cell transplantation. *Bone Marrow Transplant.* 2007;39:571–572.

122. Sarnak MJ, Greene T, Wang X, et al. The effect of a lower target blood pressure on the progression of kidney disease: long-term follow-up of the modification of diet in renal disease study. *Ann Int Med.* 2005;142:342–351.

123. Cohen EP, Hussain S, Moulder JE. Successful treatment of radiation nephropathy with angiotensin II blockade. *Int J Radiat Oncol Biol Phys.* 2003;55:190–193.

124. Jafar TH, Stark PC, Schmid CH, et al. Progression of chronic kidney disease: the role of blood pressure control, proteinuria, and angiotensin-converting enzyme inhibition: a patient-level meta-analysis. *Ann Int Med.* 2003;139:244–252.

125. Sarode R, McFarland JG, Flomenberg N, et al. Therapeutic plasma exchange does not appear to be effective in the management of thrombotic thrombocytopenic purpura/hemolytic uremic syndrome following bone marrow transplantation. *Bone Marrow Transplant.* 1995;16:271–275.

126. Butcher JA, Hariharan S, Adams MB, et al. Renal transplantation for end-stage renal disease following bone marrow transplantation: a report of six cases, with and without immunosuppression. *Clin Transplant.* 1999;13:330–335.

127. Cohen EP, Piering WF, Kabler-Babbitt C, et al. End-stage renal disease (ESRD) after bone marrow transplantation: poor survival compared to other causes of ESRD. *Nephron.* 1998;79:408–412.

128. Rubin P, Casarett GW. The adrenal glands. In: *Clinical Radiation Pathology.* Philadelphia, PA: WB Saunders Co.; 1968:740–749.

129. Kauppila M, Koskinen P, Irjala K, et al. Long-term effects of allogeneic bone marrow transplantation (BMT) on pituitary, gonad, thyroid and adrenal function in adults. *Bone Marrow Transplant.* 1998;22:331–337.

130. Boulad F, Sands S, Sklar C. Late complications after bone marrow transplantation in children and adolescents. *Curr Probl Pediatr.* 1998;28:277–297.

131. Sanders JE, Pritchard S, Mahoney P, et al. Growth and development following marrow transplantation for leukemia. *Blood.* 1986;68:1129–1135.

132. Littley MD, Shalet SM, Beardwell CG, et al. Hypopituitarism following external radiotherapy for pituitary tumours in adults. *Quart J Med.* 1989;70:145–160.

Josephine Kang
Anthony L. Zietman

Urinary Function

BACKGROUND

Much of what is known about tolerance of the lower urinary tract to radiation comes from experience treating pelvic malignancies with radiation. Effects of radiation on the bladder and urethra have been documented following treatment of various pelvic malignancies such as bladder, prostate, gynecologic, and anorectal cancers. Dose and degree of exposure vary with the site and method of treatment, ranging from bladder cancer, where a substantial portion of the bladder is deliberately targeted with external beam radiation, to prostate cancer, where both prostate and prostatic urethra are targeted and adjacent bladder tissue is incidentally exposed. There can be homogeneous or heterogeneous distribution of radiation dose depending on whether radiation is delivered as external beam therapy, brachytherapy (BT) or a combination of the two. Furthermore, radiation is often combined with chemotherapy, which can result in heightened sensitivity of normal tissue to radiation. Over the past decade, dose escalation studies in prostate cancer have shed light on the effects of higher radiation doses on the lower urinary tract. Toxicity can be divided into acute and long-term effects. In this chapter, we discuss the pathogenesis and clinical manifestation of lower urinary tract toxicity after exposure to radiation.

THE LOWER URINARY TRACT: ANATOMY

The lower urinary tract consists of the bladder, which serves to store urine, and the urethra, which acts as a drainage tube for urine to exit the body. Storage and emptying of the bladder are regulated by the internal and external urethral sphincters. Successful micturition results from appropriate interaction between the bladder muscle and supporting neurovascular structures. The muscular bladder wall contracts, internal and external sphincters are relaxed, and urine is expulsed through the urethra.

BLADDER

The normal bladder is a hollow, highly compliant organ that can comfortably hold approximately 500 mL of urine when full. When empty, it lies as a pyramid-shaped viscus within the pelvic cavity between the pubis and rectum in the male, and between the pubis and uterus in the female. As it fills with urine, it rises above the pelvis minor toward the abdomen and becomes more rounded in shape.

The bladder can be divided into two main parts: the body, where urine is collected and stored, and the neck, which traverses the urogenital diaphragm to connect with the urethra (Fig. 32.1). Superiorly, the body of the bladder is covered with peritoneum. The apex of the bladder body ends as a fibrous cord, a derivative of the urachus called the *median umbilical ligament*. This extends from the apex to the umbilicus between the transversalis fascia and the peritoneum. Posteriorly, the base of the bladder body lies adjacent to the rectum, and in males, it is separated from the rectum by the vas deferens, seminal vesicles, and ureters, which travel superolaterally to the seminal vesicles before entering the bladder (Fig. 32.2A). In females, the bladder base is separated from the rectum by the uterus and vagina (Fig. 32.2B). The ureters enter the bladder wall inferomedially on opposite sides at an oblique angle. The two ureteric orifices and the internal urethral orifice at the neck of the bladder form the three points of the bladder trigone.

The inferior and lateral surfaces of the bladder body are adjacent to the pubic bone, levator ani muscles, and obturator internus muscles, and have surrounding retropubic and perivesicular fat and connective tissue. Inferiorly, the body of the bladder transitions into the bladder neck, which is 2 to 3 cm long, funnel shaped, and connects to the urethra. As the bladder fills, the bladder body rises from the pelvic cavity toward the abdomen, while the neck of the bladder remains held in place by the puboprostatic ligament in males, and the pubovesical ligaments in females.

The bladder mucosa, or urothelium, is lined with three to seven layers of transitional cells (Fig. 32.3). These cells can be subdivided into three basic layers: basal, intermediate, and superficial, which are connected by tight junctions. The urothelium is coated with a layer of glycosaminoglycans, which act as a protective coating separating urine from underlying bladder wall.[1] Together, the urothelium and glycosaminoglycan layer act as a permeability barrier, allowing for urine to be stored in the bladder without transfer of urine electrolytes and other permeable molecules. It appears smooth when the bladder is distended and contracts into numerous folds when the bladder is empty. Underneath the urothelium lies the basement membrane and lamina propria, which is composed of sparse smooth

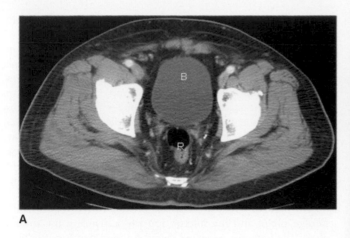

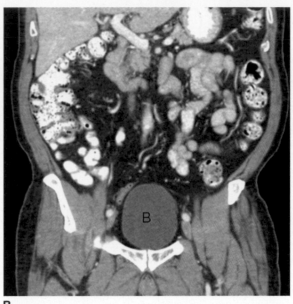

A

B

Figure 32.1. Normal bladder anatomy (CT) **A**: Axial CT image demonstrating anatomic relationship of a distended bladder (B) to rectum (R) posteriorly, and femoral heads laterally. **B**: Coronal CT image demonstrates relationship of distended bladder (B) to pubic symphysis inferiorly and pelvic bones laterally.

muscle fibers and loose connective tissue. Beneath this lies the detrusor muscle layer, which is composed of smooth muscle fibers arranged in various directions, converging at the bladder neck to form an outer longitudinal layer, a middle circular layer, and an inner longitudinal layer (Fig. 32.4). The inner and outer layers of the detrusor muscle extend down toward the urethra in both men and women. The middle layer ends at the bladder neck.

The bladder receives efferent innervation from the autonomic nervous system. Parasympathetic fibers arise from spinal cord levels S3-4, and reach the bladder via the sacral and pelvic nerves. Sympathetic innervation of the bladder arises from spinal cord levels T11-L2, and controls the trigonal region of the bladder, along with seminal vesicles and ampulla of the vas in men. Afferent sensation of stretch and bladder wall distention arising from the bladder body and the bladder neck/trigone are carried via the pelvic nerve and sympathetic pathways to the T11-L2 level, respectively.

URETHRA

The bladder neck connects to the urethra, which serves to drain urine from the body. Except during micturition, the urethra is a virtual space. It consists of a mucosa and two smooth muscle layers. The inner longitudinal layer is a direct continuation of the inner detrusor muscle layer and is most developed anteriorly. The middle circular layer is a direct continuation of the outer detrusor muscle layer, and is present throughout the entire length of the female urethra, and the posterior urethra in the male, serving as an involuntary sphincter. The external sphincter is innervated by the pudendal nerve and allows for voluntary release of urine. The external sphincter is composed of circularly oriented striated muscle and lies between the superior and inferior layers of the urogenital diaphragm in both males and females (Fig. 32.2).

In males, the urethra is approximately 17 to 18 cm long and can be divided anatomically into three main parts: the prostatic

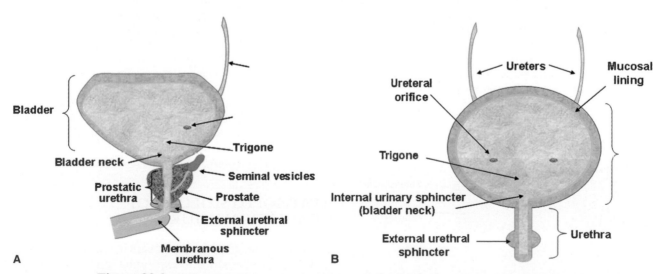

A

B

Figure 32.2. **A**: Male bladder anatomy (sagittal view). **B**: Female bladder anatomy (coronal view).

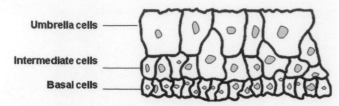

Figure 32.3. Urinary bladder epithelium. Transitional epithelium is composed of three distinct cell layers. Basal cell layers are 5 to 10 μm in diameter and germinal in nature. Intermediate cells are 20 μm in diameter. The diameter of superficial umbrella cells is dependent on the degree of bladder stretch, ranging from 50 to 120 μm across. Umbrella cells are joined together by tight junctions.

urethra, the membranous urethra, and the penile urethra. The prostatic urethra, approximately 3 to 4 cm in length, runs through the prostate gland and is lined with transitional epithelium. The ejaculatory ducts and several prostatic ducts open into the prostatic urethra to deliver sperm and ejaculatory fluids. The membranous urethra is only 1 to 2 cm in length and lined with pseudostratified columnar epithelium. It runs from the prostate apex to the bulb of the penis, traversing through the external urethral sphincter and the urogenital diaphragm. The bulbourethral glands open on the lateral surfaces of the membranous and penile urethra. The penile urethra is approximately 15 cm in length, and is lined with pseudostratified epithelium proximally, and nonkeratinized stratified squamous epithelium distally.

In females, the urethra is approximately 3 to 4 cm long, and extends from the bladder neck to the urethral orifice that lies between the clitoris and vaginal opening. The proximal one third of the urethra is lined with transitional epithelium, and the distal two thirds is lined with squamous epithelium. The paraurethral glands and ducts (Skene glands) surround the urethra. The middle third of the female urethra traverses the urogenital diaphragm, where the striated muscles of the external sphincter and pelvic floor contribute to the voluntary sphincteric control (Fig. 32.2B).

MICTURITION

Urinary continence is regulated by the internal and external urinary sphincters. The internal sphincter is composed of smooth muscle derived from the outermost layer of the destrusor muscle and can stand intravesical pressures of 30 to 40 mm without opening.[2] Involuntary continence is maintained by sympathetic innervation from T11-L2, which innervates the smooth muscles of the internal urinary sphincter and bladder trigone. At rest, the internal sphincter is increased in tone. Inhibition of the internal sphincter and motor control of the detrusor

muscles arise from the gray matter of the spinal cord at the level of S2-3.

The external sphincter is composed of striated muscles, and is further supported by striated muscles of the pelvic floor, especially the levator ani. It is innervated via the pudendal nerves, which arise from spinal cord levels S2 and 3. During voluntary contraction, the external urethral sphincter and levator ani muscles compress the urethra circumferentially and also elongate it by pulling it cephalad. The contribution of the external sphincter to normal resting urethral pressure is unclear, but it is clear that the external sphincter plays an important role in preventing stress incontinence. Intravesical pressures >70 to 100 mm are required to open the external sphincter forcefully.[2]

The cycle of micturition can be divided into two phases, the storage phase and the micturition phase. During the storage phase, the detrusor muscle is relaxed and expands as the bladder fills with urine. Bladder pressure remains low, due to the high compliance of the bladder wall. The bladder neck remains contracted, generating resistance to prevent involuntary leakage. Sympathetic innervation to the internal urinary sphincter maintains continence.

The conscious urge to urinate begins once the bladder fills with 150 to 200 mL of urine. Voluntary voiding begins when neurons in the pontine micturition center fire, causing excitation of sacral preganglionic neurons and relaxation of the external urinary sphincter. This causes contraction of the detrusor muscles, with sharp rise in intravesical pressure. The bladder neck and urethral muscles relax, allowing the detrusor contractions to result in expulsion of nearly all the urine, with approximately 5 to 10 postvoid residual volume. The perineal muscles and external sphincter can be contracted during micturition to prevent urine from passing down the urethra. Average urine flow rate in males is 20 to 25 mL/s, and in females is 25 to 30 mL/s.

AGE EFFECTS

Aging is associated with deterioration of detrusor muscle function, bladder wall fibrosis with resultant loss of functional capacity, and heightened sensitivity to neurotransmitters such as norepinephrine.[3] Urodynamic studies demonstrated increased postvoid residual volume and decreased peak flow rates in the elderly. However, maximum detrusor pressure does not correlate with age, which suggests that detrusor contraction velocity, rather than contraction strength, diminishes with age.[4,5]

In females, age-related changes from hormonal fluctuations and vaginal deliveries result in weakening of the pelvic floor muscles and stress incontinence.

In males, hyperplasia of prostatic stromal and epithelial cells occurs with age. An estimated 50% of men have histologic evidence of benign prostatic hyperplasia (BPH) by age 50 years and >75% by age 80 years.[6] BPH and compression of the prostatic urethra cause lower urinary tract symptoms such as urinary hesitancy, weak stream, overflow incontinence, increased frequency, and sensation of incomplete emptying.

PATHOPHYSIOLOGY OF RADIATION INJURY

Studies of radiation-induced bladder injury in animal models have been essential in expanding our knowledge on the pathophysiology of radiation injury. Various techniques, including

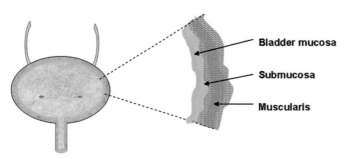

Figure 32.4. Layers of the bladder wall.

measurement of urinary frequency, bladder compliance, cystometry and histologic examination of irradiated bladder tissue, have been utilized to determine radiation-induced changes that can occur in the bladder wall and their effects on bladder function.[7-15] Studies in mice demonstrate the murine bladder has a triphasic response to radiation. The early, or acute phase, starts during radiation exposure and resolves several weeks after radiation is complete. This is followed by a latent period, which is time dependent on the amount of dose received. Finally, there is a progressive, irreversible late phase, where reduction in bladder storage capacity leads to symptoms of urgency and increased frequency. It is hypothesized that the human bladder also responds to radiation in a triphasic pattern. In humans, the late phase can occur up to 10 years after initial radiation exposure.[16,17] The pathophysiology behind the early and late effects of radiation on the bladder has not been fully delineated, but what we have learned from animal studies is summarized below.

BLADDER EPITHELIUM

The urothelium acts as a protective barrier that allows urine to be stored for long periods of time while maintaining initial composition. Viewed in cross section, the urothelium is composed of three main layers: basal, intermediate, and superficial (Fig. 32.3). When the urothelial barrier is disrupted, movement of urinary constituents into underlying lamina propria and bladder muscle can occur, resulting in irritative bladder symptoms such as frequency, urgency, and dysuria.

Under normal conditions, the urothelium undergoes proliferation at a low rate.[7,9,18] In mice, the rate of turnover has been estimated to range anywhere from 6 weeks to a year.[9] Basal cells divide to form intermediate cells, and intermediate cells fuse to form the superficial cells.[8,19]

Histologically, urothelial cells exhibit signs of damage such as nuclear irregularity, cellular edema, and increase in lysosomal and autophagic vacuoles, 3 months after radiation. At 6 to 12 months after radiation exposure, loss of normal cell differentiation and changes in cellular proliferation pattern can be noted (Fig. 32.5).[8,20,21]

Studies suggest that the urothelium becomes depleted in cells after exposure to radiation. This depletion is evident within weeks and requires months for recovery to occur, depending on the dose.[22-25] A single dose of 20 Gy delivered to the murine bladder results in significantly decreased number of superficial urothelial cells during the acute phase (days 0–31) and late recovery phase (days 90, 120).[24] Using measurement of urinary frequency and cystometry in murine bladders, Stewart et al. demonstrated that the early, acute phase of radiation-induced damage occurs 1 to 3 weeks after irradiation, and manifests as a dose-dependent increase in urinary frequency. Late bladder damage manifests approximately 6 months after radiation and inversely correlates to dose of radiation. Late damage is persistent, irreversible, and is associated with focal hyperplasia, fibrosis, ulceration, epithelial denudation, and pathologic changes such as nuclear irregularity, cellular edema, and increase in autophagic vacuoles,[10] predominantly noted in intermediate and basal urothelial cells. These changes manifest by 3 months after radiation.[7] Increased bladder wall thickness, collagen deposition, and changes in collagen composition in the irradiated murine bladder have been noted in quantitative immunohistochemical studies, but do not correlate with bladder function or late radiation sequelae. Denudation and hyperproliferative reactions in the urothelium, however, were inversely correlated with bladder capacity and are believed to be involved in the pathogenesis of radiation-induced late effects.[15]

Additional studies have demonstrated that radiation disrupts the protective glycosaminoglycan layer and decreases the density of uroplakin-III.[24] In humans, the uroplakins form polygonal-shaped plaques that occupy 70% to 90% of the apical surface area,[26] and it is hypothesized that these proteins maintain integrity of the urothelial barrier to urine.

In summary, exposure to radiation results in disruption of the normal glycosaminoglycan layer and decrease in urothelial proliferation, with resultant interruption of tight junctions and surface uroplakins. This increases exposure of underlying tissue to urine and its caustic solutes, contributing to irritative voiding symptoms that are encountered with radiation. It is hypothesized that these changes contribute to acute radiation-induced toxicity. Furthermore, when radiation is administered in conjunction with chemotherapeutic agents

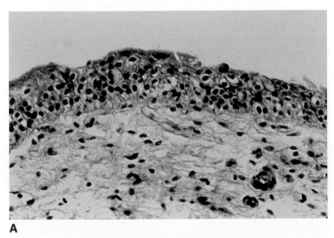 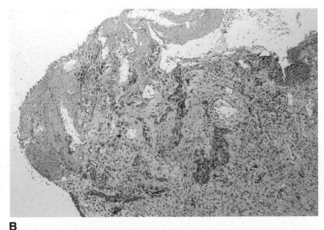

A   **B**

Figure 32.5. Histology of normal bladder versus irradiated bladder. **A:** Normal bladder mucosa, showing organized lamina propria. **B:** Example of radiation cystitis with epithelial proliferation and reactive changes in the lamina propria. (Images courtesy of Dr. Robert H. Young, Department of Pathology, Massachusetts General Hospital.)

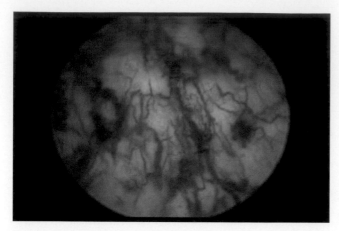

Figure 32.6. Bladder mucosa telangiectasia.

such as cyclophosphamide, there can be synergistic effects that lead to greater severity in both early and late radiation effects, compared to radiation alone.[27] Over time, radiation exposure leads to denudation and focal hyperproliferation of the urothelium, along with loss of normal cell differentiation. However, the contribution of such changes to manifestation of late radiation-induced toxicity is unclear. Finally, animal studies suggest increased risk of secondary malignancies, arising from the urothelium after exposure to radiation.[21]

VASCULATURE

The time course and extent of radiation-induced damage to the bladder vasculature has also been studied in animal models. Approximately 3 months after radiation, edema of the vascular endothelium can be noted. By 6 to 12 months, endothelial cell proliferation, perivascular fibrosis, and vascular occlusion occur and can be seen years after radiation exposure. In severe cases, focal bladder ischemia can result,[20] leading to fibrosis of the bladder wall.

The alteration of balance between endothelial cell growth and small vessel maturation is hypothesized to cause development of telangiectasia (Fig. 32.6). These thin-walled, tortuous,

abnormally dilated vessels manifest as a late dose-dependent response to radiation.[28] Bladder wall telangiectasias are prone to rupture and bleed, resulting in microscopic or frank hematuria. In severe cases, excessive bleeding requires surgical intervention.

SMOOTH MUSCLE

The three smooth muscle layers of the bladder wall contribute to compliance and elasticity. Acute response to radiation is associated with a dose-dependent decrease in bladder capacity that manifests as soon as 2 weeks after radiation exposure[29,30] and resolves within several weeks. Pathologic changes include cellular edema, inflammation, and cell death, which may contribute to early changes in bladder function.

The late response to radiation is mostly irreversible and manifests as loss of bladder compliance and capacity, after a latent period ranging from 35 to 401 days in animal studies.[31] Loss of smooth muscle, infiltration of fibroblasts, and increase in collagen deposition, along with microvascular occlusion, are hypothesized to contribute to loss of appropriate bladder function and resulting contracture (Fig. 32.7).

NEURAL TISSUE

The extent of radiation-induced injury to the richly innervated bladder wall has not been well studied. However, animal experiments suggest that early changes in bladder function after exposure to radiation are largely attributable to smooth muscle edema and loss of the endothelial barrier, rather than nerve function.[7,8,21] Radiation-induced injury may lead to stimulation of sensory nerves that transmit sensation of fullness and pain, which can result in lower urinary tract symptoms. Clinically, a significant number of patients undergoing radiation to the bladder or surrounding structures have undergone prior surgical procedures such as radical prostatectomy or hysterectomy, which may result in injury to bladder wall innervation. Thus it is unclear whether radiation in the adjuvant setting contributes to exacerbation of underlying mechanical nerve damage.

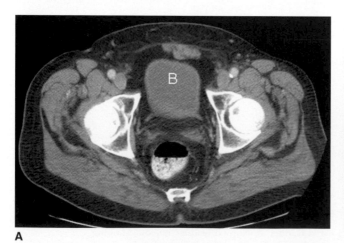
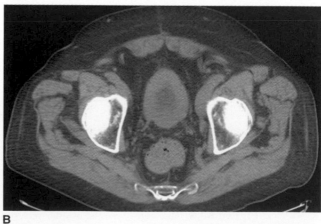

A   B

Figure 32.7. Normal versus contracted bladder. **A**: CT scan of normal bladder (B). **B**: CT scan of contracted bladder (B) after radiation therapy, with reduced capacity to store urine.

TABLE 32.1	RTOG Acute Radiation Morbidity Scoring Criteria			
0	*1*	*2*	*3*	*4*
No change	Frequency of urination or nocturia twice pretreatment habit/ dysuria, urgency not requiring medication	Frequency of urination or nocturia that is less frequent than every hour. Dysuria, urgency, bladder spasm requiring local anesthetic	Frequency with urgency and nocturia hourly or more frequently/dysuria, pelvis pain or bladder spasm requiring regular, frequent narcotic/gross hematuria with/without clot passage	Hematuria requiring transfusion/acute bladder obstruction not secondary to clot passage, ulceration or necrosis

CLINICAL MANIFESTATION OF RADIATION INJURY

The clinical manifestation of radiation to the lower urinary tract can be categorized into acute and late reactions. Acute reactions occur during and up to 3 months after radiation exposure. Most acute symptoms subside within several weeks of standard radiation therapy. Late reactions occur at least 3 months after radiation exposure.

ACUTE TOXICITY

Acute radiation-induced symptoms can be irritative or obstructive, and depend on gender, region of exposure, and dose. Radiation-induced inflammation, edema, and loss of urothelial integrity are thought to be the underlying events that contribute to acute symptoms. Irritative symptoms include increased urinary frequency, dysuria, urgency, and nocturia. Obstructive symptoms include weak stream, incomplete voiding, hesitancy, and in rare cases, complete obstruction with overflow incontinence. It is difficult to distinguish between the side effects of radiation to the prostate and radiation to the bladder, as both can manifest similarly. The reported incidence of acute toxicity varies from 23% to 80% in patients treated with radiation to the pelvis for various malignancies.[32–39] Such wide range in incidence rates reflects the heterogeneity in treatment techniques, dose, and treatment fields for different malignancies and also reflects the inherent difficulty in collecting such subjective data.

The Radiation Therapy Oncology Group (RTOG) has published scoring criteria for a qualitative assessment of the degree of acute radiation morbidity[40] (Table 32.1). Acute toxicity is scored from days 1 through 90. Symptoms related to radiation exposure must be distinguished from underlying disease. Grade I criteria are defined as frequency of urination or nocturia that is twice pretreatment habit, or dysuria, or urgency, not requiring medication. Grade II criteria include urinary frequency or nocturia that is less frequent than every hour, or dysuria, urgency, bladder spasms requiring pharmacologic intervention. Grade III criteria are defined as frequency and nocturia that is hourly or greater, or gross hematuria, or dysuria, pelvic pain, or bladder spasm requiring regular, frequent doses of narcotics. Grade IV criteria include hematuria that requires transfusion or acute bladder obstruction that is not secondary to clots, ulceration, or necrosis.

LATE TOXICITY

Late effects of radiation arise from epithelial and microvascular alterations, nerve damage, fibrosis, and changes in bladder physiology. Clinical manifestation ranges from decreased bladder capacity, to ureteral strictures, to secondary malignancies. In contrast to acute toxicity, late toxicity tends to be chronic and irreversible.

Depending on site and dose of radiation, late toxicity can involve the entire bladder, a portion of bladder mucosa, or the urethra. Fibrotic constriction of the bladder occurs months to years after radiation, with collagen deposition and replacement of smooth muscle tissue with fibroblasts. If bladder contracture is severe, there will be incontinence, pronounced frequency, and sensation of incomplete emptying. Such changes in bladder function are reflected in cystometric studies as reduced capacity and loss of compliance (Fig. 32.8). Chronic urethritis and

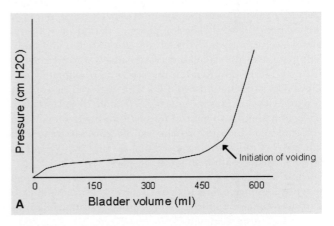

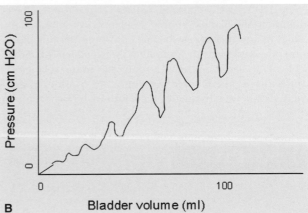

Figure 32.8. Cystometrogram of the normal versus contracted bladder. **A:** Normal, compliant bladder displays minimal increase in pressure (<15 cm H_2O) as it fills to capacity, until voiding is initiated. **B:** Fibrotic or contracted bladder will display unstable contractions and increased pressure as it fills to decreased capacity (approximately 100 cc).

urethral strictures are additional complications that can occur. For example, the rate of urethral stricture after EBRT for prostate cancer is estimated to be 2% to 5% in patients without prior Tranurethral Resection of the Prostate, external Beam Radiation Therapy (TURP), and 6% to 16% with TURP prior to radiation treatment.[41,42] Hematuria can occur as a result of chronic cystitis and/or telangiectasia. This situation is commonly compounded in the elderly by the use of Coumadin. Hemorrhagic cystitis, a rare and potentially severe long-term side effect of radiation, is very uncommon with recent technologic advances in radiation therapy, that allow safe delivery of high doses of radiation to tumor while sparing adjacent bladder tissue.

It is important to distinguish side effects of radiation from effects of underlying disease and the natural aging process, as well as effects of pelvic surgery and chemotherapy. Patients with increased frequency, incontinence, hematuria, or dysuria may be presenting with late effects of bladder contracture and fibrosis, but it is important to rule out urinary tract infection, neuromuscular dysfunction from other comorbid conditions such as diabetes, or obstructive symptoms of BPH in males. It is also important to rule out secondary malignancies such as transitional cell carcinoma or recurrence of primary tumor.

In general, time to onset of late toxicity typically occurs 2 to 3 years after treatment, with a median time of approximately 13 to 20 months.[33,34,43–48] The latency of several months before the onset of late clinical symptoms in patients parallels the time of onset in mouse models, where a dose-dependent decrement of bladder capacity and increment in urinary frequency occurs after a latent phase.[7,11] The long latency period prior to onset of late lower urinary tract toxicity was illustrated in one study of 1,784 patients with stage IB cervical cancer, who were treated with external beam radiation therapy of approximately 45 Gy followed by tandem and ovoid BT. The actuarial risk of hematuria at 5, 10, and 20 years was 6%, 7%, and 10%, respectively. Regression analysis to control for confounding factors was not performed. A study of prostate cancer patients treated with high doses of radiation suggested that as many as 50% will have had one episode of hematuria by 15 years.[49]

These studies, along with several other case reports, suggest the true incidence of late toxicity to the lower urinary tract may be underestimated in most patients, since symptoms can manifest decades after treatment.[50–52]

The RTOG has published criteria to grade late effects of radiation to the bladder, noting that late effects of radiation on normal tissues increase with time, and long periods of observation are necessary to accurately assess effects of radiation (Table 32.2). Slight epithelial atrophy and minor telangiectasia manifesting as microscopic hematuria are considered grade I toxicity. Moderate frequency, generalized telangiectasia, and intermittent macroscopic hematuria are criteria for grade II late toxicity. Severe frequency and dysuria, frequent hematuria, severe telangiectasia, and reduction in bladder capacity to <150 mL are criteria for grade III late toxicity. Necrosis, bladder contraction to <100 mL capacity, and severe hemorrhagic cystitis are criteria for grade IV toxicity.

SECONDARY MALIGNANCIES

In addition, secondary malignancies develop many years after radiation, as long as 10 years for ovarian cancer[53] and 20 years for cervical cancer.[54] Secondary bladder malignancies after radiation therapy are typically high-grade, transitional cell carcinomas with poor prognosis.[55]

An increased risk of secondary bladder malignancy after radiation exposure from the Chernobyl nuclear reactor meltdown and the Japanese atomic bomb has been documented, and reflects a long latency period between exposure to radiation and development of secondary malignancy.[56,57] The Japanese atomic bomb survivor cohort is a well-defined cohort of approximately 86,000 individuals, with majority (73%) exposed to doses <50 mSv, followed since 1950 to determine cause of death and cancer incidence (Hall). A total of 222 bladder cancers were documented to occur between 1950 and 1977. For the first 12 to 15 years after exposure, incidence was not significantly different from that of nonexposed individuals. For the next 15 to 30 year follow-up period and >30 year follow-up period, there is doubling of relative risk that is independent of age group. Based on these data, the United Nations released a report in 2000 stating there is a significant correlation between radiation exposure and bladder cancer risk.[58–60]

Retrospective series analyzing risk of secondary malignancy after treatment for various pelvic malignancies illustrate increased risk. Analysis of secondary malignancy risk after external beam radiation therapy for prostate cancer using Surveillance, Epidemiology, and End Results data also demonstrate an increased risk of secondary bladder cancer with an odds ratio of 1.63 with a 95% confidence interval of 1.44 to 1.84.[61] Analysis of secondary bladder malignancies after radiation treatment in 2,674 patients with cervical cancer demonstrates an incidence rate of 57.6 times that of the general female population.[54] Case-controlled series in 251 women treated with either radiation or surgery alone for ovarian cancer suggest a nearly twofold increased risk in secondary bladder malignancy for patients treated with radiation.[53]

These studies underscore the importance of long-term follow-up for patients treated with pelvic radiation, as long-term toxicity can manifest decades after initial treatment, as bladder fibrosis, contractures, hematuria, and secondary malignancies.

TABLE 32.2		RTOG/EORTC Late Radiation Morbidity Scoring Scheme		
0	1	2	3	4
None	Slight epithelial atrophy; minor telangiectasia (microscopic hematuria)	Moderate frequency; generalized telangiectasia; intermittent macroscopic hematuria	Severe frequency and dysuria; severe telangiectasia; frequent hematuria; reduction in bladder capacity (<150 cc)	Necrosis/contracted bladder (capacity <100 cc)

SCORING SYSTEMS

Several validated scoring systems have been proposed to rate bladder toxicity. Acute and late toxicity can be assessed in a variety of ways: symptomatically, radiographically, cystoscopically, cystometrically, and histologically. The RTOG-LENT/SOMA criteria[40] is one scoring system that has been presented in an attempt to standardize subjective and objective data. The American Urological Association's Symptom Score consists of seven questions related to voiding symptoms, and each question is scored from 0 to 5. Scores of 0 to 7, 8 to 19, and 20 to 35 signify mild, moderate, and severe symptoms, respectively. In addition, there is a quality of life score; this questionnaire is utilized to assess symptoms of BPH in males but can also tract acute effects of radiation during treatment. There are several additional patient-assessment scales, including the Clark and Talcott scales and the Expanded Prostate Cancer Index Composite (EPIC), being integrated into current clinical trials.[62] The Common Toxicity Criteria/Adverse Events reporting version 3 has been utilized by the RTOG gynecologic group as of 2007 and includes bladder spasms, cystitis, fistula, urinary incontinence, leak (including anastomotic, but without development of a fistula), obstruction, perforation, prolapse of stoma, renal failure, stricture/stenosis, urinary frequency/urgency, urinary retention, urine color change, and "other" under gynecologic criteria, but fails to distinguish between acute or long-term effects.

MANAGEMENT OF ACUTE AND LATE TOXICITY

As described above, acute radiation-induced symptoms, such as frequency, hematuria, and/or dysuria, are secondary to irritation and inflammation of the urothelium and bladder smooth muscle. Such symptoms typically resolve within several weeks of completion of radiation and can be managed conservatively. Alpha-blockers, such as terazosin, doxazosin, tamsulosin, and alfuzosin, are commonly prescribed to relieve irritative and obstructive side effects by relaxing the prostatic smooth muscle and promoting complete emptying of the bladder. Terazosin and doxazosin are nonselective α-blockers and are associated with side effects of dizziness and hypotension. Tamsulosin and alfuzosin are selective α-blockers that have fewer side effects. Phenazopyridine hydrochloride can be used as an analgesic on the bladder mucosa for patients with significant dysuria. Select patients with irritative symptoms may also benefit from non-steroidal anti-inflammatory drugs.

Individuals with increased urinary urgency may benefit from anticholinergics such as tolterodine, or antisposmodics such as oxybutynin. However, such agents should be used with caution since they can exacerbate existing obstructive symptoms or precipitate acute retention.

Long-term complications from radiation arise from bladder wall fibrosis, decreased capacity and compliance, and telangiectasia formation. Side effects related to decreased compliance and contracture are chronic and for the most part, irreversible. Symptomatic relief may be derived from usage of α-blockers or anticholinergics and antispasmodics. Hematuria is managed according to severity. Microscopic hematuria may occur from telangiectasia in the bladder mucosa and can be managed conservatively. Sometimes cystoscopic fulguration will be required. In extreme cases, formalin instillation may be required to stop the bleeding though this treatment in its turn can cause a fibrotic, contracted bladder. It is important to rule out a secondary bladder malignancy, and cystoscopic evaluation is necessary, particularly in patients with long onset from initial radiation therapy.

Hemorrhagic cystitis is an uncommon late side effect of radiation. Management options include intravesical formalin therapy, selective embolization of hypogastric arteries, or hyperbaric oxygen therapy. Bladder reconstruction or cystectomy is reserved for severe cases.

RADIATION TOLERANCE OF THE LOWER URINARY TRACT

Emami et al.[63] pooled data from a number of studies utilizing radiation to treat pelvic malignancies, and reported the bladder TD 5/5 (5% severe late toxicity at 5 years) is 65 Gy for irradiation of a contracted whole bladder, versus 80 Gy for irradiation of two thirds of the bladder. TD 50/5 was estimated to be 80 Gy. This study did not utilize 3D imaging and it is argued that with advances in radiation technique, the actual TD 5/5 to the bladder may be higher.

A similar study done by Marks et al. estimated bladder toxicity based on literature reviews of prostate, bladder, and cervical cancers.[41] Incidence of grades 3 to 4 toxicity and dose-volume relationships after external beam radiation therapy and BT were estimated (Table 32.3) Marks et al. estimated a clinical complication rate of approximately 5% to 10% with a whole bladder dose of 50 Gy, and higher complication rates with doses

TABLE 32.3		Risk of Grade ≥3 Bladder Complications Following RT for Bladder Cancer				
Reference	*Patients*	*Total Bladder Dose (Gy)*	*Fraction Size (Gy)*	*Total Equivalent Bladder Dose[a]*	*Risk Grade ≥3 (%)*
Shipley et al.[64]	55	66	1.8	64.3	11
Quilty et al.[36,37]	24	50	2.5	53.1	8
Duncan and Quilty[43]	889	55–57.5	2.75–2.88	60.2–63.8	17
Yu et al.[66]	309	63	2	63	2
Corcoran et al.[85]	34	63	2.4	69.3	12
Marcial et al.[86]	96	55–60	2–2.75	60–65	2
Scholten et al.[67]	123	36	6	54	0
Mameghan et al.[87]	330	45–65	1.8–2.5	43.9–69	2

[a]Total equivalent dose at 2 Gy was calculated assuming α/β ratio of 6.

of 50 to 65 Gy. Thus, whole bladder irradiation to >50 Gy in 2-Gy fractions was associated with significant risk of bladder dysfunction.

Exposure of approximately one third to half of the bladder volume to a dose of 50 to 65 Gy resulted in approximately 5% to 10% complication rates. Irradiation of smaller portions of the bladder (<20%) to higher doses of 65 to 75 Gy resulted in late toxicity in approximately 5% to 10% of patients. Partial bladder volume irradiation to doses >75 to 80 Gy was hypothesized, therefore, to carry >10% risk of serious injury. The urethral tolerance dose was estimated to be greater than approximately 60 to 70 Gy, with strictures resulting in approximately 0% to 5% of patients. These data are based on older studies and may overestimate the risk of bladder injury with current radiation techniques.

Based on these results, Marks distinguished a difference between "global" injury of the whole bladder and "focal" injury of a small portion of the bladder. Treatment of bladder cancer, for example, typically results in "global" injury to the whole bladder, and manifests as symptoms of urinary frequency, urgency, decreased bladder capacity, and cystitis.[33,36,43,64–66] Treatment of gynecologic malignancies, with intracavitary implant placement, or treatment of prostate cancer with high dose boost, is more often associated with "focal" injury and manifests with bleeding, ulceration, stone formation, and fistulas. By delineating between global and focal injury, Marks et al. proposed there should be two separate dose-response curves for essentially two different mechanisms of bladder injury.

Studies suggest that larger fraction size or accelerated fractionation may increase risk of lower urinary tract complications.[36,67,68]

Data on the radiation tolerance of the bladder are difficult to interpret due to inherent challenges in defining the bladder volume, which is in constant flux. Despite attempts to standardize bladder volume by having patients treated with empty or full bladders, there is still widespread variability from day to day.[69–76] Such variability results from differing amounts of postvoid residual after emptying the bladder, combined with movement from respiration and secondary effects of bowel filling. One study assessed motion of the empty bladder in bladder cancer patients, by utilizing weekly CT scans,[76] and found that a minimum 2-cm margin was required in order to cover the entire bladder and account for daily variation in size and location. Another study assessed motion of the full bladder on dose volume histogram (DVH) calculations in prostate cancer patients, who received four CT scans over the course of treatment at 2-week intervals.[74] Study size was small; however, the authors noted a trend toward decreased total bladder volume over time, of approximately 4%/week, with the conclusion that DVH calculations based on initial CT scans are not reliable, and underscore the challenges that exist in accurately calculating dose distribution and predicting toxicity.

In conclusion, it is challenging to accurately determine bladder tolerance for the range of techniques, doses, and fractionation schemes encountered in external beam treatments for pelvic malignancies. Dose distribution varies markedly between cancers; thus, it becomes difficult to extrapolate data between different cancers. With this in mind, we briefly discuss various bladder tolerance parameters with regard to three major disease subsets: prostate, bladder, and gynecologic malignancy.

QUALITY OF LIFE

The incidence and severity of lower urinary tract dysfunction after radiation has been documented in numerous studies, underscoring the direct physical sequelae of therapy. However, patient-centered measures to document quality of life are equally important and reflect the true impact of radiation,

Quality-of-life data from patients treated for various pelvic malignancies have shown relatively few long-term effects of radiation on bladder function, with low incidence of distressful symptoms. One study from Massachusetts General Hospital followed long-term survivors with invasive bladder cancer who were treated with TURB, chemotherapy, and bladder radiation to 64 to 65 Gy.[77] Patients underwent urodynamic testing and a quality-of-life questionnaire was completed at a median follow-up time of 6.3 years. Urodynamic studies demonstrated normal bladder parameters in 75% of patients. Twenty-two percent of patients had reduced bladder compliance, which is a recognized late complication of radiation; of this group, only a third reported distress due to symptoms. Two out of twelve women had bladder hypersensitivity, involuntary detrusor contractions, and incontinence. Overall, 19% of patients had issues with continence, with 11% requiring pads (all female). However, only half of the patients with continence problems described their symptoms as distressful. Less common were issues with flow (5%) and urgency (16%). This low level of symptom-induced distress parallels results of questionnaires from Italian and Swedish studies, where >74% of patients report good urinary function after bladder radiation.[78–80]

Another study focused on patients treated with either radiation, surgery, hormones, or active surveillance for early-stage prostate cancer.[81] A cross-sectional survey of patients treated 12 to 24 months prior, and was compared to a reference group. As expected, patients who had undergone radiation to the prostate had a statistically significant increase in urinary obstructive or irritative symptoms, and reported significantly worse quality of life with respect to urinary control.

A study by Miller et al. evaluated 709 patients with prostate cancer who had undergone external beam radiation, BT, or radical prostatectomy, with evaluation at median follow-up of 2.6 and 6.2 years.[82] Patients were compared to an age-matched control group. A prostate-cancer specific (EPIC) questionnaire was utilized to detect differences in urinary irritative symptoms (hematuria, weak stream, frequency, dysuria) and incontinence (leakage, dribbling, use of pads). There was a significant difference in extent of urinary symptoms in patients treated with external beam radiation and BT compared to control. When compared to initial follow-up assessment, the BT cohort reported reduction in moderate to severe urinary symptoms, from 23% to 16%, which was statistically significant. These results are consistent with other studies that demonstrate urinary symptoms after BT manifest predominantly within the first 2 years, and improve gradually thereafter. There was no significant difference in urinary irritative symptoms between initial and second assessment in the cohort that received external beam radiation, although a trend toward improvement was noted. However, there was significantly increased incidence of urinary incontinence, but these results are difficult to interpret since the cohort included patients who received salvage surgery after radiation for local recurrences.

For men treated with prostate BT, long-term issues were described in a series characterizing patient-reported quality of life among 72 patients, at a median follow-up of 5 years after implant placement.[83] Forty percent of BT patients reported some degree of urinary. In contrast, a separate study looked at patients post-BT with median follow-up of 64 months, with EPIC incontinence summary scores, and found no difference in long-term urinary control.[84]

REFERENCES

1. Parsons CL, Boychuk D, Jones S, et al. Bladder surface glycosaminoglycans: an epithelial permeability barrier. *J Urol.* 1990;143(1):139–142.
2. Kleeman FJ. The physiology of the internal urinary sphincter. *J Urol.* 1970;104(4):549–554.
3. Siroky MB. The aging bladder. *Rev Urol.* 2004;6(suppl 1):S3–S7.
4. Madersbacher S, Pycha A, Schatzl G, et al. The aging lower urinary tract: a comparative urodynamic study of men and women. *Urology.* 1998;51(2):206–212.
5. Malone-Lee J, Wahedna I. Characterisation of detrusor contractile function in relation to old age. *Br J Urol.* 1993;72(6):873–880.
6. Guess HA, Arrighi HM, Metter EJ, et al. Cumulative prevalence of prostatism matches the autopsy prevalence of benign prostatic hyperplasia. *Prostate.* 1990;17(3):241–246.
7. Stewart FA. The proliferative and functional response of mouse bladder to treatment with radiation and cyclophosphamide. *Radiother Oncol.* 1985;4(4):353–362.
8. Stewart FA. Mechanism of bladder damage and repair after treatment with radiation and cytostatic drugs. *Br J Cancer Suppl.* 1986;7:280–291.
9. Stewart FA, Denekamp J, Hirst DG. Proliferation kinetics of the mouse bladder after irradiation. *Cell Tissue Kinet.* 1980;13(1):75–89.
10. Stewart FA, Lundbeck F, Oussoren Y, et al. Acute and late radiation damage in mouse bladder: a comparison of urination frequency and cystometry. *Int J Radiat Oncol Biol Phys.* 1991;21(5):1211–1219.
11. Stewart FA, Michael BD, Denekamp J. Late radiation damage in the mouse bladder as measured by increased urination frequency. *Radiat Res.* 1978;75(3):649–659.
12. Stewart FA, Oussoren Y, Luts A. Long-term recovery and reirradiation tolerance of mouse bladder. *Int J Radiat Oncol Biol Phys.* 1990;18(6):1399–1406.
13. Stewart FA, Randhawa VS, Michael BD. Multifraction irradiation of mouse bladders. *Radiother Oncol.* 1984;2(2):131–140.
14. Stewart FA, Randhawa VS, Michael BD, et al. Repair during fractionated irradiation of the mouse bladder. *Br J Radiol.* 1981;54(645):799–804.
15. Kraft M, Oussoren Y, Stewart FA, et al. Radiation-induced changes in transforming growth factor beta and collagen expression in the murine bladder wall and its correlation with bladder function. *Radiat Res.* 1996;146(6):619–627.
16. Farquharson DI, Shingleton HM, Soong SJ, et al. The adverse effects of cervical cancer treatment on bladder function. *Gynecol Oncol.* 1987;27(1):15–23.
17. Perez CA, Lee HK, Georgiou A, et al. Technical factors affecting morbidity in definitive irradiation for localized carcinoma of the prostate. *Int J Radiat Oncol Biol Phys.* 1994;28(4):811–819.
18. Farsund T. Cell kinetics of mouse urinary bladder epithelium. I. Circadian and age variations in cell proliferation and nuclear DNA content. *Virchows Arch B Cell Pathol.* 1975;18(1):35–49.
19. Martin BF. Cell replacement and differentiation in transitional epithelium: a histological and autoradiographic study of the guinea-pig bladder and ureter. *J Anat.* 1972;112(pt 3):433–455.
20. Antonakopoulos GN, Hicks RM, Berry RJ. The subcellular basis of damage to the human urinary bladder induced by irradiation. *J Pathol.* 1984;143(2):103–116.
21. Antonakopoulos GN, Hicks RM, Hamilton E, et al. Early and late morphological changes (including carcinoma of the urothelium) induced by irradiation of the rat urinary bladder. *Br J Cancer.* 1982;46(3):403–416.
22. Reitan JB. Some long-term cell kinetic effects of ionizing radiation on mouse bladder urothelium. *Cell Tissue Kinet.* 1986;19(5):511–517.
23. Reitan JB, Feren K. Scanning electron microscopy of the irradiated mouse bladder urothelium. *Scan Electron Microsc.* 1986;2(pt 2):773–780.
24. Jaal J, Dorr W. Radiation-induced damage to mouse urothelial barrier. *Radiother Oncol.* 2006;80(2):250–256.
25. Schreiber H, Oehlert W, Kugler K. Regeneration and proliferation kinetics of normal and x-irradiated transitional epithelium in the rat. *Virchows Arch B Cell Pathol.* 1969;4(1):30–44.
26. Lewis SA. Everything you wanted to know about the bladder epithelium but were afraid to ask. *Am J Physiol Renal Physiol.* 2000;278(6):F867–F874.
27. Edrees G, Luts A, Stewart F. Bladder damage in mice after combined treatment with cyclophosphamide and X-rays: the influence of timing and sequence. *Radiother Oncol.* 1988;11(4):349–360.
28. Turesson I. Characteristics of dose-response relationships for late radiation effects: an analysis of skin telangiectasia and of head and neck morbidity. *Radiother Oncol.* 1991;20(3):149–158.
29. Lundbeck F, Djurhuus JC, Vaeth M. Bladder filling in mice: an experimental in vivo model to evaluate the reservoir function of the urinary bladder in a long time study. *J Urol.* 1989;141(5):1245–1249.
30. Lundbeck F, Ulso N, Overgaard J. Cystometric evaluation of early and late irradiation damage to the mouse urinary bladder. *Radiother Oncol.* 1989;15(4):383–392.
31. Bentzen SM, Lundbeck F, Christensen LL, et al. Fractionation sensitivity and latency of late radiation injury to the mouse urinary bladder. *Radiother Oncol.* 1992;25(4):301–307.
32. Amdur RJ, Parsons JT, Fitzgerald LT, et al. Adenocarcinoma of the prostate treated with external-beam radiation therapy: 5-year minimum follow-up. *Radiother Oncol.* 1990;18(3):235–246.
33. Duncan W, Williams JR, Kerr GR, et al. An analysis of the radiation related morbidity observed in a randomized trial of neutron therapy for bladder cancer. *Int J Radiat Oncol Biol Phys.* 1986;12(12):2085–2092.
34. Pilepich MV, Krall JM, Sause WT, et al. Correlation of radiotherapeutic parameters and treatment related morbidity in carcinoma of the prostate–analysis of RTOG study 75-06. *Int J Radiat Oncol Biol Phys.* 1987;13(3):351–357.
35. Pilepich MV. Radiation Therapy Oncology Group studies in carcinoma of the prostate. *NCI Monogr.* 1988;7:61–65.
36. Quilty PM, Duncan W, Kerr GR. Results of a randomised study to evaluate influence of dose on morbidity in radiotherapy for bladder cancer. *Clin Radiol.* 1985;36(6):615–618.
37. Quilty PM, Duncan W. Primary radical radiotherapy for T3 transitional cell cancer of the bladder: an analysis of survival and control. *Int J Radiat Oncol Biol Phys.* 1986;12(6):853–860.
38. Sack H, Nosbuesch H, Stuetzer H. Radiotherapy of prostate carcinoma: results of treatment and complications. *Radiother Oncol.* 1987;10(1):7–15.
39. Sakurai M, Saijo N, Shinkai T, et al. The protective effect of 2-mercapto-ethane sulfonate (MESNA) on hemorrhagic cystitis induced by high-dose ifosfamide treatment tested by a randomized crossover trial. *Jpn J Clin Oncol.* 1986;16(2):153–156.
40. Cox JD, Stetz J, Pajak TF. Toxicity criteria of the Radiation Therapy Oncology Group (RTOG) and the European Organization for Research and Treatment of Cancer (EORTC). *Int J Radiat Oncol Biol Phys.* 1995;31(5):1341–1346.
41. Marks LB, Carroll PR, Dugan TC, et al. The response of the urinary bladder, urethra, and ureter to radiation and chemotherapy. *Int J Radiat Oncol Biol Phys.* 1995;31(5):1257–1280.
42. Sandhu AS, Zelefsky MJ, Lee HJ, et al. Long-term urinary toxicity after 3-dimensional conformal radiotherapy for prostate cancer in patients with prior history of transurethral resection. *Int J Radiat Oncol Biol Phys.* 2000;48(3):643–647.
43. Duncan W, Quilty PM. The results of a series of 963 patients with transitional cell carcinoma of the urinary bladder primarily treated by radical megavoltage X-ray therapy. *Radiother Oncol.* 1986;7(4):299–310.
44. Green N, Treible D, Wallack H. Prostate cancer: post-irradiation incontinence. *J Urol.* 1990;144(2 pt 1):307–309.
45. Greskovich FJ, Zagars GK, Sherman NE, et al. Complications following external beam radiation therapy for prostate cancer: an analysis of patients treated with and without staging pelvic lymphadenectomy. *J Urol.* 1991;146(3):798–802.
46. Lawton CA, Won M, Pilepich MV, et al. Long-term treatment sequelae following external beam irradiation for adenocarcinoma of the prostate: analysis of RTOG studies 7506 and 7706. *Int J Radiat Oncol Biol Phys.* 1991;21(4):935–939.
47. Pilepich MV, Perez CA, Walz BJ, et al. Complications of definitive radiotherapy for carcinoma of the prostate. *Int J Radiat Oncol Biol Phys.* 1981;7(10):1341–1348.
48. Perez CA, Breaux S, Bedwinek JM, et al. Radiation therapy alone in the treatment of carcinoma of the uterine cervix. II. Analysis of complications. *Cancer.* 1984;54(2):235–246.
49. Gardner BG, Zietman AL, Shipley WU, et al. Late normal tissue sequelae in the second decade after high dose radiation therapy with combined photons and conformal protons for locally advanced prostate cancer. *J Urol.* 2002;167(1):123–126.
50. Eifel PJ, Levenback C, Wharton JT, et al. Time course and incidence of late complications in patients treated with radiation therapy for FIGO stage IB carcinoma of the uterine cervix. *Int J Radiat Oncol Biol Phys.* 1995;32(5):1289–1300.
51. Zoubek J, McGuire EJ, Noll F, et al. The late occurrence of urinary tract damage in patients successfully treated by radiotherapy for cervical carcinoma. *J Urol.* 1989;141(6):1347–1349.
52. Kottmeier HL. Complications following radiation therapy in carcinoma of the cervix and their treatment. *Am J Obstet Gynecol.* 1964;88:854–866.
53. Kaldor JM, Day NE, Kittelmann B, et al. Bladder tumours following chemotherapy and radiotherapy for ovarian cancer: a case-control study. *Int J Cancer.* 1995;63(1):1–6.
54. Duncan RE, Bennett DW, Evans AT, et al. Radiation-induced bladder tumors. *J Urol.* 1977;118(1 pt 1):43–45.
55. Quilty PM, Kerr GR. Bladder cancer following low or high dose pelvic irradiation. *Clin Radiol.* 1987;38(6):583–585.
56. Romanenko A, Morimura K, Wei M, et al. DNA damage repair in bladder urothelium after the Chernobyl accident in Ukraine. *J Urol.* 2002;168(3):973–977.
57. Hall P. Radiation-associated urinary bladder cancer. *Scand J Urol Nephrol Suppl.* 2008;42(218):85–88.
58. Pierce DA, Shimizu Y, Preston DL, et al. Studies of the mortality of atomic bomb survivors. Report 12, Part I. Cancer: 1950–1990. *Radiat Res.* 1996;146(1):1–27.
59. Ron E, Preston DL, Mabuchi K, et al. Cancer incidence in atomic bomb survivors. Part IV: Comparison of cancer incidence and mortality. *Radiat Res.* 1994;137(2 suppl):S98–S112.
60. Thompson DE, Mabuchi K, Ron E, et al. Cancer incidence in atomic bomb survivors. Part II: solid tumors, 1958–1987. *Radiat Res.* 1994;137(2 suppl):S17–S67.
61. Moon K, Stukenborg GJ, Keim J, et al. Cancer incidence after localized therapy for prostate cancer. *Cancer.* 2006;107(5):991–998.
62. Clark JA, Talcott JA. Symptom indexes to assess outcomes of treatment for early prostate cancer. *Med Care.* 2001;39(10):1118–1130.
63. Emami B, Lyman J, Brown A, et al. Tolerance of normal tissue to therapeutic irradiation. *Int J Radiat Oncol Biol Phys.* 1991;21(1):109–122.
64. Shipley WU, Rose MA, Perrone TL, et al. Full-dose irradiation for patients with invasive bladder carcinoma: clinical and histological factors prognostic of improved survival. *J Urol.* 1985;134(4):679–683.
65. Shipley WU, Prout GR Jr, Coachman NM, et al. Radiation therapy for localized prostate carcinoma: experience at the Massachusetts General Hospital (1973–1981). *NCI Monogr.* 1988;64(7):67–73.

66. Yu WS, Sagerman RH, Chung CT, et al. Bladder carcinoma: experience with radical and preoperative radiotherapy in 421 patients. *Cancer.* 1985;56(6):1293–1299.

67. Scholten AN, Leer JW, Collins CD, et al. Hypofractionated radiotherapy for invasive bladder cancer. *Radiother Oncol.* 1997;43(2):163–169.

68. Moonen L, van der Voet H, Horenblas S, et al. A feasibility study of accelerated fractionation in radiotherapy of carcinoma of the urinary bladder. *Int J Radiat Oncol Biol Phys.* 1997;37(3):537–542.

69. Hellebust TP, Dale E, Skjonsberg A, et al. Inter fraction variations in rectum and bladder volumes and dose distributions during high dose rate brachytherapy treatment of the uterine cervix investigated by repetitive CT-examinations. *Radiother Oncol.* 2001;60(3):273–280.

70. Holloway CL, Macklin E, Cormack RA, et al. Should the organs at risk be contoured in vaginal cuff brachytherapy? An analysis of within-patient variance brachytherapy. *Int J Radiat Oncol Biol Phys.* 2008;1(1):11.

71. Jhingran A, Sam M, Salehpour M, et al. A pilot study to evaluate consistency of bladder filling and vaginal movement in patients receiving pelvic IMRT. In: *Proceedings of the 87th Annual Meeting of the American Radium Society,* Barcelona, Spain, 2005.

72. Turner SL, Swindell R, Bowl N, et al. Bladder movement during radiation therapy for bladder cancer: implications for treatment planning. *Int J Radiat Oncol Biol Phys.* 1997;39(2):355–360.

73. Muren LP, Smaaland R, Dahl O. Organ motion, set-up variation and treatment margins in radical radiotherapy of urinary bladder cancer. *Radiother Oncol.* 2003;69(3):291–304.

74. Lebesque JV, Bruce AM, Kroes AP, et al. Variation in volumes, dose-volume histograms, and estimated normal tissue complication probabilities of rectum and bladder during conformal radiotherapy of T3 prostate cancer. *Int J Radiat Oncol Biol Phys.* 1995;33(5):1109–1119.

75. Roeske JC, Forman JD, Mesina CF, et al. Evaluation of changes in the size and location of the prostate, seminal vesicles, bladder, and rectum during a course of external beam radiation therapy. *Int J Radiat Oncol Biol Phys.* 1995;33(5):1321–1329.

76. Roof K MD, Sarkar S, Zietman A, et al. A 3-D CT based analysis of inter-fraction bladder motion during radiotherapeutic treatment of bladder cancer. *Int J Radiat Oncol Biol Phys.* 2000.

77. Zietman AL, Sacco D, Skowronski U, et al. Organ conservation in invasive bladder cancer by transurethral resection, chemotherapy and radiation: results of a urodynamic and quality of life study on long-term survivors. *J Urol.* 2003;170(5):1772–1776.

78. Henningsohn L, Wijkstrom H, Dickman PW, et al. Distressful symptoms after radical radiotherapy for urinary bladder cancer. *Radiother Oncol.* 2002;62(2):215–225.

79. Caffo O, Fellin G, Graffer U, et al. Assessment of quality of life after radical radiotherapy for prostate cancer. *Br J Urol.* 1996;78(4):557–563.

80. Caffo O, Fellin G, Graffer U, et al. Assessment of quality of life after cystectomy or conservative therapy for patients with infiltrating bladder carcinoma: a survey by a self-administered questionnaire. *Cancer.* 1996;78(5):1089–1097.

81. Talcott JA, Manola J, Clark JA, et al. Time course and predictors of symptoms after primary prostate cancer therapy. *J Clin Oncol.* 2003;21(21):3979–3986.

82. Miller DC, Sanda MG, Dunn RL, et al. Long-term outcomes among localized prostate cancer survivors: health-related quality-of-life changes after radical prostatectomy, external radiation, and brachytherapy. *J Clin Oncol.* 2005;23(12):2772–2780.

83. Talcott JA, Clark JA, Stark PC, et al. Long-term treatment related complications of brachytherapy for early prostate cancer: a survey of patients previously treated. *J Urol.* 2001;166(2):494–499.

84. Merrick GS, Wallner KE, Butler WM. Minimizing prostate brachytherapy-related morbidity. *Urology.* 2003;62(5):786–792.

85. Corcoran MO, Thomas DM, Lim A, et al. Invasive bladder cancer treated by radical external radiotherapy. *Br J Urol.* 1985;57(1):40–42.

86. Marcial VA, Thomas DM, Lim A, et al. A Radiation Therapy Oncology Group Study. Split-course radiotherapy of carcinoma of the urinary bladder stages C and D1. *Am J Clin Oncol.* 1985;8(3):185–199.

87. Mameghan H, Fisher RJ, Watt WH, et al. The management of invasive transitional cell carcinoma of the bladder. Results of definitive and preoperative radiation therapy in 390 patients treated at the Prince of Wales Hospital, Sydney, Australia. *Cancer.* 1992;69(11):2771–2778.

Sexual Function

BACKGROUND

The untoward effects of radiation on sexual function have been documented in patients after treatment of pelvic malignancies. In males, the primary manifestation of sexual dysfunction after radiation exposure is failure to achieve erection. However, other detrimental impacts of radiation have been reported, including lack of ejaculation, decreased sexual desire, decreased orgasm and decreased sexual satisfaction.[1–3]

Erectile dysfunction incidence has been reported to range from 38% up to 84% after radiation treatment.[4,5] According to prospective studies, 36% to 59% and 24% to 50% of patients experience erectile dysfunction after external beam radiotherapy and brachytherapy, respectively.[6–10] The reported prevalence of sexual dysfunction after radiation varies widely due to disparity in mode of data collection, differences in length of follow-up, and patient selection.

The distal internal pudendal arteries and their terminal branches, the common penile, dorsal and cavernosal arteries, are closely situated to the prostate. Thus, critical vascular structures that support penile erection are exposed to radiation during treatment for prostate cancer, as well as other pelvic malignancies such as anal, rectal, and bladder cancer.

PHYSIOLOGY OF MALE SEXUAL FUNCTION

PENILE STRUCTURE, VASCULATURE, INNERVATION

The adult male penis ranges from 8.85 to 10.7 cm in length in its flaccid, unstretched state. When erect, the penile length ranges from 12.89 to 15.5 cm.[11] The penis is composed of two functional compartments: the paired corpora cavernosa and the corpus spongiosum (Fig. 33.1). The corpora cavernosa is composed of smooth muscle fibers with a parenchyma of endothelial cell-lined sinuses, helicine arteries, and nerve terminals. The corpus spongiosum surrounds the urethra. The site of divergence between the corpora cavernosa and spongiosum is referred to as the *penile bulb*.

The penis is richly innervated by somatic and autonomic nerve fibers, which are both parasympathetic and sympathetic. The major efferent parasympathetic pathway originates at the level of S2-4 and travels along the pelvic nerve, passing inferiorly and laterally to the prostate, entering the corporeal body along the cavernous artery at the crura of the corpora as preganglionic nerve fibers. Acetylcholine is believed to be the neurotransmitter released from the preganglionic parasympathetic neurons. Postganglionic fibers terminate either on the vascular smooth muscle of the corporeal arterioles or on the nonvascular smooth muscle of the trabecular tissue that surrounds the corporeal lacunae. Parasympathetic innervation is responsible for causing vasodilation of the corporeal bodies during erection, which results in several-fold increase in blood flow, expanding the sinusoidal spaces to lengthen and enlarge the penis. This causes compression of the subtunical venular plexus against the tunica albuginea, reducing outflow of the blood to a minimum. Concomitant smooth muscle relaxation is mediated by nitric oxide, which is produced by the sinusoidal endothelial cells.

Sympathetic innervation maintains the penis in the flaccid state and mediates detumescence after orgasm is achieved. When flaccid, inflow of blood through the constricted helicine arteries is minimal, and the subtunical venular plexus has free outflow. Sympathetic innervation also controls ejaculation. Penile sensation is mediated by branches of the pudendal nerves.

SEXUAL RESPONSE

The male sexual response cycle can be functionally divided into a defined sequence of libido/sexual desire, erection, ejaculation, orgasm, and detumescence. Thus, sexual dysfunction can occur at multiple levels. Sexual libido/desire is multifactorial. Testosterone, psychosocial factors, and dopaminergic receptor activation are all thought to contribute to sex-seeking behavior.[12,13] Erection is achieved when parasympathetic innervation causes penile vasodilation and culminates in ejaculation and orgasm. In order to achieve adequate penile erection, it is necessary to have cavernous nerves that facilitate nitric oxide supply and resulting smooth muscle relaxation; adequate arterial inflow through the internal pudendal and accessory pudendal arteries; and erectile tissue that can function appropriately to mediate veno-occlusion, trapping blood in the penis to maintain erection. Ejaculation is controlled by sympathetic innervation through a spinal cord reflex arc. It is possible for orgasm to occur without preceding erection and ejaculation; or conversely, ejaculation can occur in the absence of organism. In the final phase of detumescence, the arterioles vasoconstrict and blood is diverted away from the cavernous sinuses, allowing venous drainage to occur through initial 10-fold increase in blood outflow until pretumescence level is reached. This is mediated through local penile alpha-adrenergic receptor activation.[13]

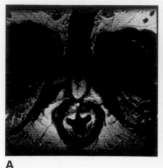
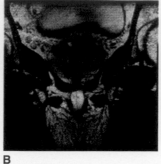
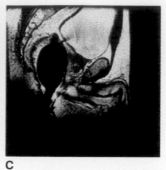

A   **B**   **C**

Figure 33.1. Endorectal magnetic resonance images of the male pelvis in (**A**) axial, (**B**) coronal, and (**C**) sagittal planes. Bulb of penis is outlined in red in each image. (From Fisch BM, et al. Dose of radiation received by the bulb of the penis correlates with risk of impotence after three-dimensional conformal radiotherapy for prostate cancer. *Urology.* 2001;57(5):955–959 with permission.)

RADIATION INJURY

Although the impact of radiation exposure on sexual function is well established, the etiology and pathophysiology is less established and is multifactorial. In males, arterial damage and vascular changes have been implicated as a main cause of erectile dysfunction after radiation, resulting in arterial occlusion and resultant cavernosal artery insufficiency; however, exposure of the neurovascular bundle to high radiation doses and structural alterations in penile corporal smooth muscle have also been implicated. We will now discuss what is known about the etiology and pathophysiology of radiation-induced sexual dysfunction.

ETIOLOGY

In 1984, a study by Goldstein et al. examined fifteen patients, prior to and after pelvic radiation treatment, with nocturnal penile tumescence testing, bulbocavernous reflex latency, perineal electromyography, penile Doppler ultrasonography, and endocrine screening of the hypothalamic-pituitary-gonadal axis in an effort to identify the etiology of postradiation sexual dysfunction.[14] All fifteen patients were measured 14 months after radiation and noted worsening in erectile function. Penile Doppler evaluation revealed abnormalities in all fifteen patients after radiation treatment, with decreased blood flow in the cavernosal arterial system. In addition, two patients underwent selective pudendal arteriography and were diagnosed with occlusive vascular disease in the distal internal pudendal and penile arteries, within the pelvic radiation field. Therefore, this study suggested a vasculogenic etiology for postradiation erectile dysfunction.

In contrast, a smaller study by Mittal et al.[15] examined six patients, before and 6 to 9 months after radiation for prostate cancer, and found no changes in penile blood flow. Penile brachial index and penile flow index were measured. However, this study was limited by small number of patients and evaluation of erectile function only 6 to 9 months after treatment, which may be an insufficient length of time to truly capture the changes in penile vasculature after radiation. In addition, penile brachial index has now been supplanted by more modern techniques of penile vasculature evaluation utilizing Doppler ultrasonography or cavernosography.

In 1998, Zelefsky and Eid[16] evaluated ninety eight patients with treatment-induced erectile dysfunction after radical prostatectomy, external beam radiation or brachytherapy for prostate cancer. Mean dose of radiation to the prostate was 70.2 Gy.

Duplex ultrasonography was utilized, before and after intracorporal prostaglandin injections, to establish the degree of penile blood flow, and categorize the etiology of impotence into arteriogenic, cavernosal, mixed arteriogenic/cavernosal, or neurogenic. Results revealed the predominant etiology of erectile dysfunction in patients after radiation treatment to be arteriogenic in nature, with 63% of impotent patients after radiation diagnosed with arteriogenic dysfunction, in contrast to 32% of patients after radical prostatectomy. On the other hand, of patients who had undergone radical prostatectomy, predominant cause of erectile dysfunction was cavernosal, followed by arteriogenic and neurogenic. Thus this study, similar to that of Goldstein et al., suggests radiation results in sexual dysfunction through disruption of the arteriolar system supplying the penile corporal muscles.

Similar results were noted in a study by Mulhall et al.[17] Sixteen males with erectile dysfunction after external beam radiation for prostate cancer (mean dose: 72 Gy) were evaluated at a mean duration of 11 months posttreatment, with dynamic infusion cavernosometry/cavernosography. There was 100% incidence of cavernosal artery insufficiency and 90% incidence of corporovenoocclusive dysfunction, suggesting significant alteration in erectile hemodynamics of both arterial and venous etiology.

A study by Wiedermann et al.[18] demonstrated decreased intracoronary smooth muscle response to nitroglycerin after exposure to high-dose irradiation. Carrier et al.[19] demonstrated a dose-dependent reduction in nitric oxide synthase containing nerve fibers in the rat penis after radiation, implying decrease in nitric oxide–mediated smooth muscle relaxation may also contribute to erectile dysfunction after pelvic radiation.

The etiology of erectile dysfunction after brachytherapy has also been studied, with conflicting data. Some studies suggest radiation dose to the neurovascular bundle may be correlated to erectile dysfunction,[20] while others suggest no correlation.[21]

PATHOPHYSIOLOGY

The acute phase of radiation damage occurs weeks to months after radiation exposure, and results from microvessel damage. Chronic damage occurs months to years after therapy and is presumed to result from endarteritis obliterans. Assessment of postradiation sexual dysfunction should ideally be conducted after an appropriate duration of time has elapsed and should take baseline function and comorbidities into account.

At low doses of radiation, well below 12 Gy, endothelial cells exhibit morphologic changes, including cellular retraction and disruption of capillary structure.[22,23] In general, doses >20 Gy are required to sustain injury to larger arterial vessels. To put this in perspective, patients treated with radiation for prostate cancer typically receive in excess of 80 Gy, well above doses required for large vessel damage. A study by van der Wielen et al.[24] assessed changes in the penile arteries of the rat after fractionated irradiation to the prostate, and demonstrated marked changes in the arteries of the corpora cavernosa, 9 weeks postradiation, with loss of smooth muscle cells, thickening of the intima and small vessel occlusions.

FACTORS CONTRIBUTING TO TOXICITY

Radiation field size and target extent are also hypothesized to contribute to extension of vascular injury and therefore correspond to sexual dysfunction. Smaller fields may allow for collateralization outside of the targeted area, establishing blood flow to circumvent deleterious effects of arterial occlusion.[23]

Several studies demonstrate a dose- and target-dependent effect of radiation on erectile dysfunction. Roach et al. reviewed 158 patients after external beam radiation therapy for prostate cancer. At 5 year follow-up, patients with median penile dose of 52.5 Gy or higher had the greatest risk of erectile dysfunction, which was statistically significant.[25] Dose of radiation to the penile bulb may also impact the prevalence of radiation-induced sexual effects. A study by Fisch et al.[26] demonstrated dose of radiation to the penile bulb correlated with risk of impotence after external beam radiation treatment for prostate cancer. Patients who received 70 Gy or more to 70% of the bulb of the penis were at significantly higher risk of having erectile dysfunction, compared to those who received <40 Gy (Fig. 33.2).

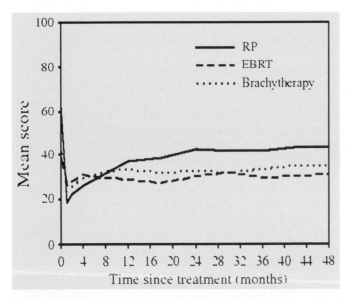

Figure 33.2. Longitudinal mean scores for sexual function, measured using the University of California-Los Angeles Prostate Cancer Index. Higher scores reflect better sexual function. Sample size was as follows: 0 months ($n = 475$), 1 months ($n = 400$), 2 months ($n = 420$ months), 4 months ($n = 412$), 8 months ($n = 402$), 12 months ($n = 392$), 18 months ($n = 385$), 24 months ($n = 357$), 30 months ($n = 341$), 36 months ($n = 329$), 42 months ($n = 303$), and 48 months ($n = 290$). RP, radical prostatectomy; EBRT, external beam radiation therapy. (Adapted from Gore JL, et al. Survivorship beyond convalescence: 48-month quality-of-life outcomes after treatment for localized prostate cancer. *J Natl Cancer Inst.* 2009;101(12): 888–892 with permission.)

In contrast, a study by van der Wielen et al. did not show any correlation between radiation-associated erectile dysfunction at 2 years, and radiation dose to the crura or penile bulb. Ninety-six patients were analyzed, and dose-volume parameters to the proximal corpora cavernosa, the superior-most 1-cm segment of the crura, and the penile bulb were calculated.[27]

Treatment modality has been shown to impact preservation of potency. Namiki et al.[28] compared the sequelae of radiation treatment for prostate cancer in patients treated with conformal 3D radiation treatment versus those who received intensity-modulated radiotherapy. UCLA prostate cancer index and Medical Outcomes Study 36 Item Healthy Survey was used to quantitate the effect of radiation on sexual function. At 18-month follow-up, the intensity modulated radiotherapy (IMRT) group had better sexual function compared to the 3D conformal radiation group. At 5-year follow-up, the difference was sustained, with sexual function substantially decreased compared to baseline in the patients treated with 3D conformal radiation, whereas patients treated with IMRT had a nonstatistically significant decrease in sexual function.

TREATMENT OPTIONS FOR RADIATION-INDUCED SEXUAL DYSFUNCTION

Several options are available to successfully treat sexual dysfunction after radiation therapy. Phosphodiesterase-5 inhibitors (sildenafil [Viagra], tadalafil [Cialis], vardanafil [Levitra]) have been showed to significantly improve erectile dysfunction. Side effects, most commonly headaches, flushing or dyspepsia, are mild or moderate in nature. A randomized controlled trial by Incrocci et al.[29,30] studied patients with erectile dysfunction after external beam radiation treatment for prostate cancer. Patients received either sildenafil or placebo and data were collected using the Internal Index of Erectile Function (IIEF) questionnaire,[31] which assesses five domains of sexual function: erectile function, orgasmic function, sexual desire, intercourse satisfaction, and overall satisfaction. For almost all items, sildenafil caused a significant increase in scores compared with baseline. Ninety percent of patients needed 100-mg sildenafil for success. At 2-year follow-up, 24% of patients were still using sildenafil. Sixty percent stopped due to lack of efficacy, 24% stopped due to costs, and 16% due to other side effects. Only 8% required alternative treatments for erectile dysfunction, such as intracavernosal injections or vacuum devices.

Tadalafil is a newer phosphodiesterase-5 inhibitor that has a longer duration of action, up to 36 hours. A randomized, double-blind study by Incrocci et al.[32] compared tadalafil to placebo and showed a significant difference between tadalafil and placebo in all items of the IIEF questionnaire. The 20-mg dose was well tolerated with mild-to-moderate side effects, none of which led to drug discontinuation. Common side effects of headache and dyspepsia decreased over time.

In patients who fail to respond to sildenafil, a trial of tadalafil or verdenafil may prove efficacious. Second-line treatment strategies include intracavernosal injections with alprostadil and penile implants, which have been used with success in patients after radiation therapy.[33] Vacuum erection devices are another option for patients who are refractory to oral therapy, or may be used in combination with medication.

QUALITY OF LIFE

Quality-of-life outcomes in patients who have undergone radiation for pelvic malignancies have been documented using various patient-centered questionnaires, and specifically address the impact of radiation on sexual function. One study from Massachusetts General Hospital reported quality-of-life outcomes in 409 patients, 36 months after treatment for prostate cancer with radical prostatectomy, external beam radiation therapy, or brachytherapy, and stratified patients based on pretreatment function.[34] Sexual function was measured using the validated Prostate Cancer Symptom Indices and patients were stratified according to their baseline sexual function as normal, intermediate, or poor. Outcomes were reported as improved, preserved, or worsened. This produced distinct 36-month outcomes. For external beam radiation treatment, 74% and 72% of patients with baseline normal and intermediate sexual function, respectively, reported diminished function. In comparison, 54% and 62% of patients with baseline normal and intermediate sexual function, respectively, reported treatment related dysfunction after brachytherapy, suggesting brachytherapy patients have higher preservation of sexual function in comparison to patients who receive external beam radiation. In contrast, patients with baseline poor sexual function experienced minimal increase in preexisting dysfunction after radiation treatment.

Gore et al.[35] analyzed quality-of-life outcomes in patients treated for prostate cancer and published 48-month outcomes. Sexual dysfunction was quantitated using the UCLA Prostate Cancer Index, with higher score reflecting better function. Sexual dysfunction was common in patients regardless of radiation treatment modality. Progressive decline in sexual function was noted in patients treated with external beam radiation, but a trend toward slight improvement in sexual function was observed in patients treated with brachytherapy.

Sanda et al.[36] characterized quality of life after treatment for prostate cancer utilizing the Expanded Prostate-Cancer Index Composite (EPIC-26) and Service Satisfaction Scale for Cancer Care, collected from patients before treatment and up to 24 months afterward. The questionnaire specifically addressed poor erections, difficulty with orgasm, quality and reliability of erections, sexual function, and overall problems with sexuality. Older age, large prostate size, and higher pretreatment PSA score were found to correlate with worse sexual function after treatment. Sexual quality of life was also reported by the patients' partners. 22% of those in the external beam radiation group and 13% of those in the brachytherapy group reported distress related to the patient's erectile dysfunction.

FEMALE SEXUAL FUNCTION

BACKGROUND

Much of what is known about the effects of radiation on female sexual function has been gleaned from decades of treating pelvic malignancies with radiation in various treatment modalities, including external beam radiation and low and high dose-rate brachytherapy. Radiation can have a variety of sequelae on female sexual function, including vaginal fibrosis, shortening, decreased libido, and reduced lubrication. The frequency of such side effects varies widely, ranging from 4% to 100% incidence of vaginal shortening, 55% vaginal stenosis, and 17% to 58% percent vaginal dryness in women after treatment with radiation and/or surgery.[37–42] It is difficult to distinguish some of these sequelae from effects of surgical manipulation.

PHYSIOLOGY OF FEMALE SEXUAL FUNCTION

The female sexual response cycle has been characterized by Masters and Johnson to occur in four phases[43]: excitement, plateau, orgasmic, and resolution, and is mediated by the parasympathetic and sympathetic nervous system. During sexual arousal, there is increased blood flow to the clitoral cavernosal and labial arteries, resulting in increased tumescence and engorgement of the glans clitoris and labia minora. Unlike the penis, the clitoris and vestibular bulbs lack the subalbugineal layer between the erectile tissue and tunica albuginea layer. In males, this layer is composed of a venous plexus that becomes compressed against the tunica albuginea, resulting in penile rigidity due to reduced venous outflow.

The vaginal wall also becomes engorged, with increased capillary pressure, causing increased transudation of fluid through the endothelium. This results in lubrication of the vaginal wall.[44] Additional lubrication is provided by secretion from the Bartholin glands. The vagina also lengthens and dilates during sexual arousal as a result of relaxation of the vaginal wall smooth muscle.

ETIOLOGY OF RADIATION INJURY

The etiology of female sexual dysfunction after radiation is multifactorial and complicated, resulting from a combination of vascular, neurogenic, hormonal, muscular as well as psychogenic causes. As female patients with pelvic malignancies are often treated with surgery in addition to radiation, it can be more difficult to ascertain whether sexual sequelae are due predominantly to surgery, radiation, or hormonal changes from both.

Vascular injury from radiation is a known complication and, as discussed above, is dose dependent and phasic in nature, with acute and chronic manifestations. Microscopic changes include infiltration of inflammatory cells and alterations of microvasculature (Fig. 33.3).

Vascular insufficiency of the iliohypogastric and pudendal arterial beds has been demonstrated to result in diminished genital blood flow, causing failure to achieve vaginal and clitoral engorgement, as well as vaginal wall and clitoral smooth muscle fibrosis. Ultimately, such vascular injury results in vaginal dryness, dyspareunia, and difficulty achieving physiologic arousal, as well as vaginal stenosis and scarring.[45]

The effect of radiation on neurogenic sexual dysfunction is less well characterized. Hormonal effects, resulting from premature ovarian failure or surgically induced menopause, leads to decreased estrogen, vaginal dryness, and lack of sexual arousal, which contribute to the radiation-induced sexual dysfunction.

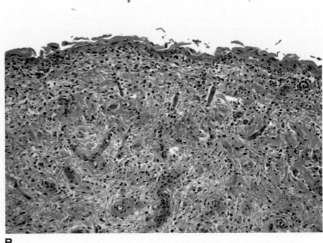

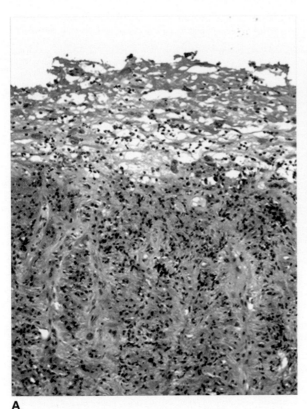

Figure 33.3. Postradiation changes in the vagina. **A:** Denuded vaginal mucosa status post radiation treatment with acute inflammatory and atypical stromal cells in an edematous submucosa. (Courtesy of Dr Michelle Hirsch, BWH.). **B:** Vaginal mucosa status post radiation treatment with a fibrotic submucosa that contains chronic inflammatory cells and dilated blood vessels.

TREATMENT

Vaginal dilation is commonly used to prevent vaginal stenosis after pelvic radiation therapy. Women with decreased estrogen secondary to oophorectomy can have vaginal atrophy and resultant dyspareunia; vaginal lubricants can be utilized to facilitate intercourse, or low-dose estrogen may also be beneficial, either in the form of a vaginal ring or suppository. A small study utilizing a clitoral vacuum device in thirteen women treated with radiotherapy for cervical cancer demonstrated improvement in sexual function.[46]

QUALITY-OF-LIFE OUTCOMES

Jensen et al.[47] reviewed incidence of sexual dysfunction in women treated with radiation for cervical cancer. 119 patients were assessed with a validated questionnaire at the termination of radiation, and at select time points up to 24 months afterward. Compared to an age-matched control group, 85% reported little or no sexual interest; 35% reported moderate-to-severe lack of lubrication, 55% reported some degree of dyspareunia, and 30% reported overall dissatisfaction with sexual life. 50% of women reported reduction in vaginal dimension. Thus, despite cure from disease, women continued to experience persistent sexual dysfunction up to 2 years after radiation.

Bergmark et al.[48] developed a questionnaire to assess treatment-related changes in sexual function in women treated for cervical cancer, which assessed symptoms of sexual dysfunction, including reduced sexual interest, altered responses to sexual arousal, vaginal shortness, vaginal inelasticity, frequency of intercourse and orgasm, and orgasmic pleasure, as well as dyspareunia. Of the 256 women who completed the questionnaire, 93 were treated with surgery alone, 22 were treated with radiotherapy alone, and 136 were treated with a combination of surgery and radiation. Radiation was intracavitary, external, or a combination of both. The women were compared to a control group. The difference in frequency of orgasmic frequency and pleasure was small, suggesting little to no effect of radiation. Vaginal changes included dyspareunia, genital swelling and lack of vaginal lubrication, and reduction in perceived vaginal length and elasticity during intercourse. When compared to women treated with surgery alone, the addition of intracavitary or external radiotherapy or both, or instead of surgery, had little effect on the risk of reduced vaginal lubrication, genital swelling, vaginal shortness, or inelasticity, suggesting a substantial component of sexual dysfunction arises from surgical treatment of cervical cancer, not radiation itself.

REFERENCES

1. Beckendorf V, Hay M, Rozan R, et al. Changes in sexual function after radiotherapy treatment of prostate cancer. *Br J Urol.* 1996;77(1):118–123.
2. Helgason AR, Fredrikson M, Adolfsson J, et al. Decreased sexual capacity after external radiation therapy for prostate cancer impairs quality of life. *Int J Radiat Oncol Biol Phys.* 1995;32(1):33–39.
3. Joly F, Brune D, Couette JE, et al. Health-related quality of life and sequelae in patients treated with brachytherapy and external beam irradiation for localized prostate cancer. *Ann Oncol.* 1998;9(7):751–757.
4. Incrocci L, Slob AK, Levendag PC. Sexual (dys)function after radiotherapy for prostate cancer: a review. *Int J Radiat Oncol Biol Phys.* 2002;52(3):681–693.
5. van der Wielen GJ, van Putten WL, Incrocci L. Sexual function after three-dimensional conformal radiotherapy for prostate cancer: results from a dose-escalation trial. *Int J Radiat Oncol Biol Phys.* 2007;68(2):479–484.
6. Merrick GS, Wallner KE, Butler WM, et al. Erectile function after prostate brachytherapy. *Int J Radiat Oncol Biol Phys.* 2005;62(2):437–447.

7. Potters L, Torre T, Ashley R, et al. Potency after permanent prostate brachytherapy for localized prostate cancer. *Int J Radiat Oncol Biol Phys.* 2001;50(5):1235–1242.
8. Stone NN, Stock RG. Long-term urinary, sexual, and rectal morbidity in patients treated with iodine-125 prostate brachytherapy followed up for a minimum of 5 years. *Urology.* 2007;69(2):338–342.
9. Turner SL, Swindell R, Bowl N, et al. Bladder movement during radiation therapy for bladder cancer: implications for treatment planning. *Int J Radiat Oncol Biol Phys.* Sep 1 1997;39(2):355–360.
10. Sandhu AS, Zelefsky MJ, Lee HJ, et al. Long-term urinary toxicity after 3-dimensional conformal radiotherapy for prostate cancer in patients with prior history of transurethral resection. *Int J Radiat Oncol Biol Phys.* Oct 1 2000;48(3):643–647.
11. Wessells H, Lue TF, McAninch JW. Penile length in the flaccid and erect states: guidelines for penile augmentation. *J Urol.* 1996;156(3):995–997.
12. Brown WA, Monti PM, Corriveau DP. Serum testosterone and sexual activity and interest in men. *Arch Sex Behav.* 1978;7(2):97–103.
13. Kandeel FR, Koussa VK, Swerdloff RS. Male sexual function and its disorders: physiology, pathophysiology, clinical investigation, and treatment. *Endocr Rev.* 2001;22(3):342–388.
14. Goldstein I, Feldman MI, Deckers PJ, et al. Radiation-associated impotence. A clinical study of its mechanism. *JAMA.* 1984;251(7):903–910.
15. Mittal B. A study of penile circulation before and after radiation in patients with prostate cancer and its effect on impotence. *Int J Radiat Oncol Biol Phys.* 1985;11(6):1121–1125.
16. Zelefsky MJ, Eid JF. Elucidating the etiology of erectile dysfunction after definitive therapy for prostatic cancer. *Int J Radiat Oncol Biol Phys.* 1998;40(1):129–133.
17. Mulhall J, Ahmed A, Parker M, et al. The hemodynamics of erectile dysfunction following external beam radiation for prostate cancer. *J Sex Med.* 2005;2(3):432–437.
18. Wiedermann JG, Leavy JA, Amols H, et al. Effects of high-dose intracoronary irradiation on vasomotor function and smooth muscle histopathology. *Am J Physiol.* 1994;267(1 pt 2):H125–H132.
19. Carrier S, Hricak H, Lee SS, et al. Radiation-induced decrease in nitric oxide synthase—containing nerves in the rat penis. *Radiology.* 1995;195(1):95–99.
20. DiBiase SJ, Wallner K, Tralins K, et al. Brachytherapy radiation doses to the neurovascular bundles. *Int J Radiat Oncol Biol Phys.* 2000;46(5):1301–1307.
21. Merrick GS, Butler WM, Dorsey AT, et al. A comparison of radiation dose to the neurovascular bundles in men with and without prostate brachytherapy-induced erectile dysfunction. *Int J Radiat Oncol Biol Phys.* 2000;48(4):1069–1074.
22. Fajardo LF, Berthrong M. Vascular lesions following radiation. *Pathol Annu.* 1988;23(pt 1):297–330.
23. Himmel PD, Hassett JM. Radiation-induced chronic arterial injury. *Semin Surg Oncol.* 1986;2(4):225–247.
24. van der Wielen GJ, Vermeij M, de Jong BW, et al. Changes in the penile arteries of the rat after fractionated irradiation of the prostate: a pilot study. *J Sex Med.* 2009;6(7):1908–1913.
25. Roach M, Winter K, Michalski JM, et al. Penile bulb dose and impotence after three-dimensional conformal radiotherapy for prostate cancer on RTOG 9406: findings from a prospective, multi-institutional, phase I/II dose-escalation study. *Int J Radiat Oncol Biol Phys.* 2004;60(5):1351–1356.
26. Fisch BM, Pickett B, Weinberg V, et al. Dose of radiation received by the bulb of the penis correlates with risk of impotence after three-dimensional conformal radiotherapy for prostate cancer. *Urology.* 2001;57(5):955–959.
27. van der Wielen GJ, Hoogeman MS, Dohle GR, et al. Dose-volume parameters of the corpora cavernosa do not correlate with erectile dysfunction after external beam radiotherapy for prostate cancer: results from a dose-escalation trial. *Int J Radiat Oncol Biol Phys.* 2008;71(3):795–800.
28. Namiki S, Ishidoya S, Ito A, et al. Five-year follow-up of health-related quality of life after intensity-modulated radiation therapy for prostate cancer. *Jpn J Clin Oncol.* 2009;39(11):732–738.
29. Incrocci L, Koper PC, Hop WC, et al. Sildenafil citrate (Viagra) and erectile dysfunction following external beam radiotherapy for prostate cancer: a randomized, double-blind, placebo-controlled, cross-over study. *Int J Radiat Oncol Biol Phys.* 2001;51(5):1190–1195.
30. Incrocci L, Hop WC, Slob AK. Efficacy of sildenafil in an open-label study as a continuation of a double-blind study in the treatment of erectile dysfunction after radiotherapy for prostate cancer. *Urology.* 2003;62(1):116–120.
31. Rosen RC, Riley A, Wagner G, et al. The international index of erectile function (IIEF): a multidimensional scale for assessment of erectile dysfunction. *Urology.* 1997;49(6):822–830.
32. Incrocci L, Slob AK, Hop WC. Tadalafil (Cialis) and erectile dysfunction after radiotherapy for prostate cancer: an open-label extension of a blinded trial. *Urology.* 2007;70(6):1190–1193.
33. Pierce LJ, Shimizu Y, Preston DL, et al. Studies of the mortality of atomic bomb survivors. Report 12, Part I. Cancer: 1950-1990. *Radiat Res.* 1996;146(1):1–27.
34. Chen RC, Clark JA, Talcott JA. Individualizing quality-of-life outcomes reporting: how localized prostate cancer treatments affect patients with different levels of baseline urinary, bowel, and sexual function. *J Clin Oncol.* 2009;27(24):3916–3922.
35. Gore JL, Kwan L, Lee SP, et al. Survivorship beyond convalescence: 48-month quality-of-life outcomes after treatment for localized prostate cancer. *J Natl Cancer Inst* 2009;101(12):888–892.
36. Sanda MG, Dunn RL, Michalski J, et al. Quality of life and satisfaction with outcome among prostate-cancer survivors. *N Engl J Med.* 2008;358(12):1250–1261.
37. Abitbol MM, Davenport JH. Sexual dysfunction after therapy for cervical carcinoma. *Am J Obstet Gynecol.* 1974;119(2):181–189.
38. Bertelsen K. Sexual dysfunction after treatment of cervical cancer. *Dan Med Bull.* 1983;30(suppl 2):31–34.
39. Flay LD, Matthews JH. The effects of radiotherapy and surgery on the sexual function of women treated for cervical cancer. *Int J Radiat Oncol Biol Phys.* 1995;31(2):399–404.
40. Schover LR, Fife M, Gershenson DM. Sexual dysfunction and treatment for early stage cervical cancer. *Cancer.* 1989;63(1):204–212.
41. Vasicka A, Popovich NR, Brausch CC. Postradiation course of patients with cervical carcinoma; a clinical study of psychic, sexual, and physical well-being of sixteen patients. *Obstet Gynecol.* 1958;11(4):403–414.
42. Nunns D, Williamson K, Swaney L, et al. The morbidity of surgery and adjuvant radiotherapy in the management of endometrial carcinoma. *Int J Gynecol Cancer.* 2000;10(3):233–238.
43. Masters WH, Johnson VE. *Human Sexual Response.* Boston, MA: Little Brown & Co.; 1966.
44. Levin RJ. The physiology of sexual function in women. *Clin Obstet Gynaecol.* 1980;7(2):213–252.
45. Goldstein I, Berman JR. Vasculogenic female sexual dysfunction: vaginal engorgement and clitoral erectile insufficiency syndromes. *Int J Impot Res.* 1998;10(suppl 2):S84–S90; discussion S98–S101.
46. Schroder M, Mell LK, Hurteau JA, et al. Clitoral therapy device for treatment of sexual dysfunction in irradiated cervical cancer patients. *Int J Radiat Oncol Biol Phys.* 2005;61(4):1078–1086.
47. Jensen PT, Groenvold M, Klee MC, et al. Longitudinal study of sexual function and vaginal changes after radiotherapy for cervical cancer. *Int J Radiat Oncol Biol Phys.* 2003;56(4):937–949.
48. Bergmark K, Avall-Lundqvist E, Dickman PW, et al. Vaginal changes and sexuality in women with a history of cervical cancer. *N Engl J Med.* 1999. 340(18):1383–1389.

Testes

ANATOMY OF THE TESTES

The testes are suspended within the scrotum by the spermatic cord[1] (Fig. 34.1). The spermatic cord is composed of the vas deferens, testicular vessels, and spermatic fascia.[2] The average testis is $4 \times 3 \times 2.5$ cm in diameter.[3] The epididymis is attached to the posterolateral surface of the testis and the vas deferens lies on the medial aspect. The superficial fascia of the abdominal wall is replaced within the scrotal wall by smooth muscle called *dartos muscle*.[1]

Three layers cover the testes from the outside and include the tunica vaginalis, tunica albuginea, and tunica vasculosa.[4] The testis is covered anteriorly and laterally by the tunica vaginalis[3], which is the lower end of the peritoneal processus vaginalis.[4] The tunica albuginea is a dense fascial covering overlying the testis, which then forms a dense fibrous mediastinum that connects the lobules within the testis.[3] The tunica vaginalis covers this layer, except at the posterior aspect of the testis, where vessels and nerves enter.[4] The tunica vasculosa contains blood vessels and delicate loose connective tissue, which extends over the tunica albuginea and covers the septa and all the testicular lobules.[4]

The connective tissue protruding from the tunica albuginea into the interior of the testis is the mediastinum of testis.[5] Incomplete septa radiate from the mediastinum to attach to the inner surface of the tunica albuginea to form 200 to 300 lobules[2] with frequent intercommunication between the lobules.[6]

Each lobule contains one or more convoluted seminiferous tubules.[2] These tubules are enmeshed in connective tissue rich in blood and lymphatic vessels, nerves, and interstitial cells of Leydig which occupy much of the space between the seminiferous tubules.[6]

The walls of the seminiferous tubules are lined by primitive germ cells and Sertoli cells.[7] Seminiferous tubules produce spermatozoa, whereas interstitial cells secrete testicular androgens.[6] Seminiferous tubules enter the fibrous tissue of the mediastinum testis, forming the anastomosing tubes of the rete testis. At the upper pole of the mediastinum, 12 to 20 ductules (ductuli efferentes) perforate the tunica albuginea to pass from the testis to the epididymis.[4]

Spermatozoa are produced through a process of spermatogenesis that includes cell division through mitosis and meiosis and the final differentiation of spermatozoids, which is called *spermiogenesis*.[6]

Tight junctions between adjacent Sertoli cells near the basal layer form a blood-testis barrier that prevents many large molecules from passing from the interstitial tissue and the part of the tubule near the basal lamina to the lumen.[7] Sertoli cells do not divide during the reproductive period and are resistant to adverse conditions such as infection, malnutrition, and radiation and have a much better survival rate after these insults than the spermatogenic cells.[6]

Sertoli cells also have several other functions:

(a) They support, protect, and regulate nutrition of the developing spermatozoa.[6]
(b) They secrete a fluid into the seminiferous tubules that is used for sperm transport.[6]
(c) Sertoli cells have several additional functions.[7] They contain the enzyme responsible for conversion of androgens to estrogens, and they can produce estrogens. They also secrete androgen-binding protein that helps maintain the supply of androgen in the tubular fluid. Sertoli cells also produce inhibin, which in turn inhibits follicle-stimulating hormone (FSH) secretion in the pituitary.[6]

Müllerian inhibiting substance (also called *Müllerian regression factor*) is also secreted by Sertoli cells and causes regression of the Müllerian ducts in the male fetus by apoptosis.[7]

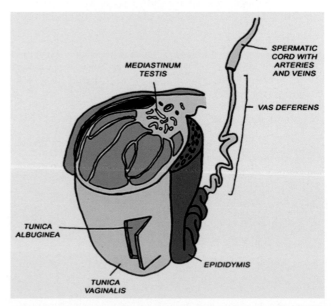

Figure 34.1. Testicular anatomy. (Courtesy of Ahmed Fahim.)

The interstitial tissue of the testis is an important site of production of androgens. The connective tissue between the seminiferous tubules consists of various cell types, including fibroblasts, undifferentiated connective cells, mast cells, and macrophages. During puberty, Leydig, cells of the testis become apparent, and have the characteristics of steroid-secreting cells.[6]

THE BLOOD AND LYMPHATIC SUPPLY OF THE TESTIS

The blood supply of the testes is from the aorta through the testicular artery branch.[1] Venous blood drains through the pampiniform plexus, which surround the testicular artery and form the testicular veins.[2] The right testicular vein drains into the inferior vena cava and the left into the left renal vein.[1]

The lymphatic drainage of the wall of the scrotum and the layers surrounding the testes is into superficial nodes, while the lymphatic drainage of the testes is to the para-aortic nodes.[1]

FUNCTIONAL AND STRUCTURAL UNITS IMPORTANT IN RADIATION DAMAGE

The testis is made up of germ cells and interstitial or Leydig cells, in a connective tissue stroma (Fig. 34.2). The germ cells within the testis are sensitive to radiation damage and include stem cells, spermatogonia, spermatocytes, and spermatids. The various types of germ cells are significantly different in their susceptibility to radiation-induced apoptosis.[8,9] These differences are important since apoptosis is the main mechanism of death of testicular germ cells after exposure to ionizing radiation.[10]

Leydig cells are more resistant to radiation damage. Hence, the lower chance of decreases in testosterone with low radiation doses. Luteinizing hormone (LH) and FSH are pituitary hormones that regulate testicular function. LH secretion is under negative feedback control by gonadal steroids. FSH secretion is under negative feedback control of both the gonadal steroids and the peptide hormone inhibin produced by the Sertoli cells. Leydig cells are stimulated by LH to produce testosterone. LH stimulates the transfer of cholesterol in

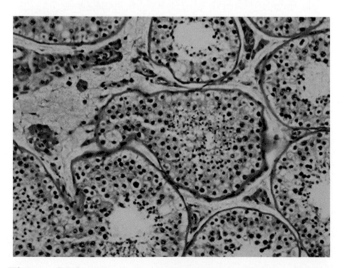

Figure 34.2. H&E of the normal testicle. (Courtesy of Merce Jorda.)

the mitochondria,[11] leading to the first step in conversion of cholesterol to testosterone. The resulting testosterone then has an inhibitory effect on LH production. Conversely, LH production is expected to increase with lowering of testosterone levels. Testosterone inhibits LH production by decreasing gonadotrophin release hormone in the hypothalamus and subsequent inhibition of the pituitary gland hormone secretion.[12,13]

EFFECTS OF FRACTIONATED AND SINGLE DOSE RADIATION ON STRUCTURE

ANIMAL DATA

Liu et al. studied apoptosis in mouse male germ cells after whole-body radiation doses of up to 200 mGy. They found that doses ranging from 25 to 200 mGy induced p53 protein expression leading to significant increases in apoptosis in both spermatogonia and spermatocytes, with a maximal effect at 75 mGy. However, if 75 mGy were given before high-dose radiation, this would lead to the induction of a significant adaptive response that decreased cell death after the high-dose irradiation.[14]

Henriksen et al. examined irradiated rat testes at 8 hours or more after 3 Gy of radiation and showed that spermatogonia at stages II to VI of seminiferous tubules were the most sensitive germ cells to radiation-induced apoptosis.[15]

Andrieu et al.[16] studied the early protective effects of amifostine against radiation-induced damage in the rat testis. The four study groups were as follows: group A control, group B 200 mg/kg amifostine, group C radiation alone (6 Gy), and group D amifostine given 15 to 30 minutes before 6 Gy testicular irradiation. The size of the testicles decreased in the treatment groups. The decrease in width after irradiation was found to be significantly less in the amifostine plus radiation group. A significant reduction of testis weight relative to body weight was seen in the irradiated testes, but not in the amifostine plus irradiation group. Primary spermatocyte numbers were significantly higher in the amifostine plus radiation group when compared with radiation alone group. Pretreatment with amifostine reduced the decrease of primary spermatocyte counts by a factor of 1.28. Furthermore, electron microscopic analysis showed normal testicular ultrastructure with the addition of amifostine prior to irradiation, though there was significant damage evident in the radiation alone group.

Mazonakis et al.[17] used three humanoid phantoms representing patients of 5, 10, and 15 years of age to measure the scattered dose to the testes using a 6- or 18-MVp linear accelerator with multileaf collimation (MLC). The radiation fields were those commonly used for treatment of various pediatric tumors such as central nervous system tumors, acute leukemia, neuroblastoma, Hodgkin disease, Wilms tumor, and sarcoma. Testicular dose measurements were performed using thermoluminescent dosimeters.

They found that the scattered dose to testes was between 0.4 and 145 cGy for a tumor dose ranging from 12 to 55 Gy. The value depended on the patient's size and the particular type of treatment. Furthermore, they found that the use of conventional blocks for field shaping increased the gonadal dose up to a factor of 2 compared to that measured using MLC. Abdominal irradiation with18-MVp instead of 6-MVp x-rays reduced the gonadal dose by a factor in excess of 1.3.

Testicular dose from radiotherapy was lower than that required to induce permanent gonadal damage. The above scattered dose reductions are also consistent with those reported by Stern.[18]

HUMAN DATA

Before delving into the details of the radiation effects on the testicle, it is important to note some physiologic effects of testosterone and the effect of age to help in interpreting the available literature on the radiation effects in humans. Testosterone deficiency has been associated with reduced lean body mass and muscle mass, increased fat content, reduced sexual function, decrease in bone mineral density and increased osteoporosis, increase in fatigue, depression, and reduced intellectual activity, among other effects.[19–21] In addition, there is a strong association between low levels of testosterone and development of the metabolic syndrome such as obesity and abdominal fat distribution, diabetes, and hypertension.[22–24] Furthermore, some authors report an age-related physiological decrease in serum testosterone levels with increasing age.[25,26] The decrease in testosterone levels was calculated to be about 0.4%/yr from the age of 40 years based on population-based studies. An age-related increase in sex hormone binding globulin, leading to a decrease in the biologically active unbound testosterone, has also been reported.[26]

LEYDIG CELL DYSFUNCTION

Leydig cell dysfunction after radiation therapy can be defined as the elevation of LH levels in the presence of reduced or normal testosterone levels.[27–30] In general, radiation-induced Leydig cell dysfunction occurs after testicular doses of >20 Gy.[27,31] Therefore, most male survivors of childhood cancer will produce normal amounts of testosterone and develop normal secondary sexual characteristics.

GERM CELL DAMAGE

Testicular spermatogenesis is very sensitive to radiation therapy.[32,33] Even testicular doses as low as 10 cGy can cause morphological and quantitative changes to spermatogonia.[34,35] Permanent infertility appears after fractionated doses of 2 Gy.[34,36] A single dose of 3.5 to 6 Gy to the testicles may result in long-term or permanently reduced spermatogenesis or azospermia.[32,33] Fractionated radiation can cause more damage than single fractions due to the long cell cycle of stem cells (>2 weeks) coupled with the decrease in radiation sensitivity as the cells progress through spermatogenesis and mature. Kutzner and Loos reported on their study using thermoluminescence dosimetry in patients who received head-neck, mantle, or abdominal radiation with cobalt-60 or linear accelerator treatment units. Critical levels for the gonads were only reached in patients receiving abdominal irradiation. Testicular doses of up to 2 Gy were reached in these patients due to a scattered dose of approximately 5% of the 40 Gy prescribed tumor dose. This was found to lead to possible permanent azoospermia.[37]

GENETIC EFFECTS

The frequency of congenital abnormalities in the offspring of childhood cancer survivors has been estimated through epidemiologic studies.[38–42] This method of risk assessment is difficult because of the long latency period between parental irradiation and occurrence of a birth defect. Moreover, uncertainties might exist due to the difficulty to distinguish background from radiation-induced genetic disorders. Mazonakis et al.[43] estimated risk based on the accurate determination of gonadal dose and the use of the appropriate risk factor proposed by the ICRP.[44] This method can provide direct estimates of the risk for hereditary effects. The estimated risk values associated with pediatric radiotherapy should be regarded as low taking into account that the incidence of serious birth defects in human population ascribed to background radiation is 6%.[45]

RADIATION EFFECTS ON THE TESTICLE IN CANCER TREATMENT

Testicular Effects of Bone Marrow Transplantation

Adolescents and adults receiving chemotherapy as part of the conditioning regimen for bone marrow transplantation (BMT) can have testicular dysfunction following BMT[46] with or without total body irradiation (TBI).[47] Children undergoing transplants have spontaneous pubertal development and completion of puberty although they may still have a lower testicular volume due to germinal epithelial damage.[47] This was confirmed by Ogilvy-Stuart et al.[48] who reported normal puberty and testosterone levels in all boys who underwent BMT with TBI at a young age.

Intensive treatment before BMT may have a direct effect on the Leydig cell function. However, it is likely that this effect may be due in part to the reduced testicular volume and the resulting testicular structural changes that affect Leydig cell function.[46] It is important to note that the conditioning regimen before BMT will frequently produce infertility, especially if it includes TBI, and the disturbance of the gonadal function is permanent.

Ishiguro et al.[49] studied 30 patients who had undergone allogeneic BMT during childhood or adolescence for both benign and malignant diagnoses. Patients underwent various conditioning regimens that generally included chemotherapy (most commonly cyclophosphamide) and were divided into three groups for the purpose of the study depending on whether they received chemotherapy alone (five patients) or radiation (with or without gonadal shielding—9 and 16 patients, respectively). Six to twelve Gy of TBI in three to six fractions, or 3 to 10 Gy of thoracoabdominal irradiation with gonadal shield in one to five fractions was given. Testicular growth and function were evaluated by serial measurements of testicular volume, basal LH, basal FSH, and testosterone levels and by gonadotropin-releasing hormone provocative test.

Gonadal shielding was helpful since lower testicular volume was seen at last evaluation in the radiation group without gonadal shield compared to those who had shielding ($p < 0.005$).[49] Furthermore, patients without testicular shielding showed a smaller median testicular volume in adult (median: 7 mL) compared to patients with testicular shield (median: 15 mL) or with chemotherapy alone (median: 12 mL) as part of the preparative regimen. Furthermore, testicular volume showed a tendency to stop at 10 mL in those without gonadal shield seen on serial measurement. With regard to fertility, only one patient fathered a child after reaching spontaneous puberty.

Of note is that, only 20% to 30% of patients with testicular shield or chemotherapy alone experienced raised peak FSH levels, yet 90% of patients without testicular shield had raised peak FSH levels indicating germinal epithelium damage.[49] Other studies confirmed these findings, with two thirds of patients treated with radiation having raised serum levels of FSH indicative of permanent germinal epithelium damage.[50,51]

Although gonadal shielding was effective in protecting testicular growth, damage of testicular germinal epithelium is seen in these patients, as well as partial Leydig cell dysfunction and loss of fertility. It is important to note that the contribution of chemotherapy to the dysfunction could not be separated and accurately assessed in this series.

Normalization of FSH was found to occur in patients with time in some series[52,53] but not in others. This may be dependent on the differences in cumulative doses of chemotherapy and exposure to alkylating agents before BMT.

Most patients experienced elevated peak LH levels with normal serum testosterone and diminished testosterone/ LH ratio in patients without testicular shield compared with patients with testicular shield or chemotherapy only.[49] Although spontaneous puberty occurred in all patients, all except four had an elevated LH and normal testosterone levels.

Long-term data regarding long-term recovery of testicular function after a median follow-up of 20 years were reported by Sanders et al. They followed 463 men treated with 10, 12, or 14 to 15.5 Gy TBI. After median follow-up of over 20 years, 81 (18%) of these men had testicular recovery (i.e., normal LH, FSH, and testosterone levels with evidence of sperm production). However, only five men (1%) fathered children. Furthermore, this rate was even lower in those who received 12 Gy or more (2 of 392 or 0.5%).

Anserini et al.[54] reported similar results following treatment with TBI (9.9 or 13.2 Gy) and cyclophosphamide. Azoospermia was found in 41 of 48 men (85%), with oligospermia in the remaining seven patients. It is important to note that the prevalent use of alkylating agents in the conditioning regimens of some of these protocols may add to testicular toxicity, and thus it becomes difficult to determine the relative contributions of each treatment modality to testicular dysfunction.

RADIOIODINE RADIATION AND TESTICULAR FUNCTION

Krassas and Pontikides[55] reported on the effect of iodine-131 therapy on gonadal function in the context of treatment of differentiated thyroid carcinoma. A major concern for male patients is the risk of azoospermia and permanent infertility due to damage of spermatogonia. For patients treated with a single ablation dose, testicular function recovered within months and the risk of infertility was diminished. Gonadal damage may be cumulative in those requiring multiple administrations. Long-term storage of semen should be addressed prior to therapy in young male patients, especially in those with metastatic or pelvic disease as well as in patients likely to be given cumulative doses >14 GBq of iodine-131. However, male patients should be counseled on sperm banking even when lower doses are planned.

EFFECT OF LOCALIZED EXTERNAL BEAM RADIATION ON TESTICULAR FUNCTION

CRANIAL RADIATION

Tamminga et al.[56] studied the accumulation of DNA damage in the shielded testes tissue to investigate whether paternal cranial irradiation can affect the germline. They reported that localized paternal cranial irradiation results in a significant accumulation of unrepaired DNA lesions in sperm cells and could lead to a profound epigenetic dysregulation in the unexposed progeny if conceived a week after paternal exposure.

Testicular function was studied in long-term survivors of acute lymphoblastic leukemia treated with identical chemotherapy regimens on two consecutive Children Cancer Study.[57] Patients also received either 18 or 24 Gy to one of the following fields: craniospinal plus 12 Gy abdominal RT including the gonads (group 1); craniospinal (group 2); or cranial (group 3). Their last evaluation took place a median of 5 years after discontinuing therapy. Raised levels of FSH and/ or reduced testicular volume were significantly associated with field treated; 55% of group 1, 17% of group 2, and 0% of group 3 were abnormal ($p = 0.002$). On the other hand, plasma concentrations of LH and testosterone, and pubertal development, were unaffected in the majority of subjects regardless of RT field.

RECTAL CANCER RADIATION

Radiation for treatment of pelvic tumors such as rectal and prostate cancers can potentially deliver radiation dose to the testes. Clinical data have shown that the testes receive from 3% to 17% of the administered radiation dose given for rectal cancer.[58-60]

Dueland et al.[60] studied the effect of radiation therapy (46–50 Gy) on the sex hormone levels in 25 male rectal cancer patients (mean age: 65 years), receiving pelvic radiation therapy. Serum testosterone, FSH, and LH were determined before start of treatment, at the 10th and 25th fractions, and 4 to 6 weeks after completion of radiotherapy. Five weeks of radiation therapy (46–50 Gy) resulted in a 100% increase in serum FSH, a 70% increase in LH, and a 25% reduction in testosterone levels. After treatment, 35% of the patients had serum testosterone levels below the lower limit of reference. The mean radiation dose to the testicles was 8.4 Gy. A reduction in testosterone values was observed after a mean dose of 3.3 Gy. Radiation therapy for rectal cancer resulted in a significant increase in serum FSH and LH and a significant decrease in testosterone levels, indicating that sex hormone production is sensitive to radiation exposure in patients with a mean age of 65 years. It is not clear, however, whether the effect of radiation therapy on hormone levels is permanent or only temporary.

However, longer follow-up after radiation was seen in the study by Bruheim et al.[61]. They studied patients with rectal cancer found on the Norwegian tumor registry from 1993 to 2003, using the surgical patients as control. Serum FSH was three times higher in the radiotherapy group than in the control surgery alone group ($p < 0.001$), and serum LH was 1.7 times higher ($p < 0.001$). In the radiotherapy group, 27% of patients had testosterone levels below the reference range compared to 10% of the nonirradiated patients ($p < 0.001$). Irradiated patients also had lower serum testosterone and lower calculated free testosterone than control subjects. Total testosterone, calculated free testosterone, and gonadotropins were related to the distance from the bony pelvic structures to the caudal field edge. One caveat to the study is that they used the distance from a bony landmark as the surrogate for testicle position and that they had older patients in the radiation group. Furthermore, recovery of endocrine function has been described following scattered radiation dose to the testes.[62]

RADIATION FOR PROSTATE CANCER

The testicular effects of radiation therapy after treatment of localized prostate cancer have been investigated. In one study, a dose of 66 to 70 Gy (with a testicular dose of about 2 Gy) resulted in a small, yet significant (9%) decrease in serum testosterone levels 3 months after treatment.[63] Thus, radiation treatment of prostate cancer may affect Leydig cell function in men of about 70 years of age.

Furthermore, Daniell et al.[64] found similar results in the postprostatectomy setting. They compared serum levels of hormones taken 3 to 8 years after primary treatment for localized prostate carcinoma in 33 men who had external beam radiation versus in 55 men who had radical prostatectomy. In irradiated men, total testosterone levels averaged 27.3% less, free testosterone levels 31.6% less, dihydrotestosterone levels 33.4% less, LH levels 52.7% greater, and FSH levels 100% greater than those values in men who had prostatectomy. The differences in gonadotropin levels of LH and FSH were greater in men older than 70 years of age.

However, other studies have shown different results. For example, although significant decreases in testosterone levels were seen 1 week and 3 months after treatment, the level returned to baseline 12 months after treatment.[30] Furthermore, other studies did not show any significant decrease in testosterone levels after radiation therapy with testicular doses of 2.5 to 6 Gy.[29,65] The effect of prostate cancer radiation on gonadotropins was more consistent among studies, showing significant increase in plasma LH and FSH levels,[29,30,65] which was persistent 1 to 2 years after radiation.[65,29]

RADIATION FOR SEMINOMA

Effect on Sperm Count

Patients with seminoma commonly present with impaired spermatogenesis. One out of two patients will have abnormal semen analyses including low sperm counts at baseline even before any treatment is initiated.[66,67] This renders subsequent assessments of the effect of treatment on fertility more difficult.

Patients with seminoma who received radiation after orchiectomy were found to have reduction in sperm count 1 year after the radiation when they received a testicular dose of 0.32 Gy, while a lower dose of 0.09 Gy did not have a significant effect on sperm count.[68] However, in other series, aspermia was not seen at doses of <0.5 Gy. It was found to occur in over 70% of patients who received >0.65 Gy to the remaining testicle with subsequent recovery after 30 to 80 weeks from the radiation.[69] Furthermore, Gordon et al.[67] reported on testicular function of men with seminoma who were treated with orchiectomy and radiotherapy on the SWOG 8711 protocol. Patients receiving a testicular dose below 0.79 Gy, had a drop in sperm count to

a nadir at about 6 months, followed by recovery by 12 months with a longer delay seen following higher doses.

Treating a para-aortic field instead of the classic "dog-leg" field, which includes the ipsilateral internal iliac nodes, can decrease the testicular dose from a median dose of 0.32 to 0.09 Gy[68] with patients receiving para-aortic treatment showing no reduction in sperm count, while patients receiving "dog-leg" radiotherapy showing a 50% reduction in sperm count at 1 year.

Effect on Gonadotropins and Testosterone

Hormone production in these younger patients was more resistant to radiation as evidenced by normal serum testosterone levels in these patients who had orchiectomy for seminoma and were then treated with 20 Gy for carcinoma in situ in the remaining testicle. The serum testosterone levels were stable, suggesting that male sex hormone production is relatively resistant to irradiation in younger patients.[27]

Changes in gonadotropins can be seen in some patients and treatment field factors as well as shielding may help prevent these effects. Treating a para-aortic field instead of the classic "dog-leg" field decreases testicular dose,[68] so patients treated using para-aortic fields do not have significant changes in endocrine profile. On the other hand, patients receiving "dog-leg" radiotherapy had an elevation of serum FSH levels for up to 3 years. No change in serum testosterone was seen, however.

The Role of Chemotherapy in Toxicity

Chemotherapeutic agents may affect spermatogenesis independent of radiation (Table 34.1). Akylating agents (cyclophosphamide, procarbazine, nitrogen mustard, and others) are especially effective in inducing germ cell damage with up to an 85% chance of azoospermia (Table 34.2).[70-73] Furthermore, cyclophosphamide damage is dose dependent. Patients are likely to retain fertility at doses of <4 g/m², while loss of fertility is likely at doses above 9 g/m².[70,72-74]

In summary, radiotherapy-induced damage to the testis varies by radiation dose, proximity of the radiation field border to the testis, fractionation scheme, chemotherapy use, and testicular shielding. Within the testes, germ cells are more sensitive to radiation than Leydig cells. Thus, germ cells can be damaged with doses even <1 Gy, whereas 20 to 30 Gy are generally required for Leydig cell damage. Permanent azoospermia results from doses of >3 to 4 Gy. The potential for a return of spermatogenesis in the intermediate dose range of 1 to 3 Gy is variable.

Effect of Scattered Radiation

Kinsella et al.[75] studied 17 patients who received low-dose scattered irradiation during treatment of Hodgkin disease and found the following testicular dose effects.

Doses of <0.2 Gy had no significant effect on FSH levels or sperm counts.

Doses between 0.2 and 0.7 Gy caused a transient dose-dependent increase in FSH and reduction in sperm concentration, with a return to normal values within 12 to 24 months.

Higher doses between 1.2 and 3 Gy[76,77] in 14 to 26 fractions given during inverted Y-inguinal field irradiation for Hodgkin

TABLE 34.1	Fertility in Adult Men Following Chemotherapy for Treatment of Different Malignancies
Diagnosis and Treatment	*Fertility Posttreatment*
Hodgkin disease	
MOPP	Azoospermia in >90%
COPP	Azoospermia in >90%
ABVD	Temporary azoospermia with normal sperm count in all at 18 months
Non-Hodgkin lymphoma	
CHOP	Permanent azoospermia in ~30%
VACOP-B	Normospermia in >95%
VEEP	Normospermia in >95%
Bone marrow transplant for a variety of malignancies	
Cyclophosphamide alone	FSH raised in 40%
High-dose melphalan	FSH raised in >95%
BEAM	FSH raised in >95%
Testicular cancer	
Cisplatin/carboplatin	Normospermia in 50% at 2 y based therapy and 80% at 5 y

ABVD, doxorubicin hydrochloride, bleomycin, vinblastine, and dacarbazine; BEAM, carmustine, etoposide, Ara-C, and melphalan; CHOP, cyclophosphamide, doxorubicin, vincristine, and prednisolone; COPP, cyclophosphamide, vincristine, procarbazine, and prednisolone; FSH, follicle-stimulating hormone; MOPP, mustine, vincristine, procarbazine, and prednisolone; VACOP-B, vinblastine, doxorubicin, prednisolone, vincristine, cyclophosphamide, and bleomycin; VEEP, vincristine, etoposide, epirubicin, and prednisolone. Adapted from Meistrich ML, Vassilopoulou-Sellin R, Lipshultz LI. Gonadal dysfunction. In: DeVita VT, Hellman S, Rosenberg SA, eds. *Cancer: Principles and Practice of Oncology.* 7th ed. New York, NY: Lippincott Williams & Wilkins; 2005:2560–2574.

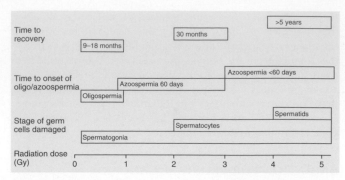

Figure 34.3. Radiation effects on the testicle and their duration following various radiation doses. From Howell SJ, Shalet SM. Spermatogenesis after cancer treatment: damage and recovery. *J Natl Cancer Monogr Inst.* 2005;34:12–17, with permission.

EFFECTS OF SINGLE DOSE RADIATION

The effect of single dose radiation on the testis has been addressed in detail by Rowley et al.[33] and discussed in detail by Howell and Shalet[78] (Fig. 34.3). They describe that the more immature cells are more radiosensitive. Spermatogonia showed morphological and quantitative changes at doses as low as 0.1 Gy. Spermatocytes show damage at doses of 2 to 3 Gy, with reduction in spermatid numbers. Damage to spermatids occurs at doses of 4 to 6 Gy with significant decrease in the number of spermatozoa.

The decline in sperm count following damage to more immature cells, with doses of up to 3 Gy, occurred over 60 to 70 days, with doses above 0.8 Gy resulting in azoospermia and doses below 0.8 Gy giving rise to oligospermia. A much faster fall in sperm counts occurred following doses of 4 Gy and above because of damage to spermatids.

Recovery of spermatogenesis takes place from surviving stem cells (type A spermatogonia) and is dependent on the dose of radiation. Complete recovery, as indicated by a return to preirradiation sperm counts and germinal cell numbers, takes place within 9 to 18 months following radiation with 1 Gy or less, 30 months for 2 to 3 Gy, and 5 years or more for doses of 4 Gy and above. It is important to note here that others consider 3 to 4 Gy a threshold for permanent azoospermia. Radiation doses exceeding 6 Gy resulted in permanent azoospermia.

STRATEGIES FOR AVOIDING TOXICITY

THE ROLE OF CRYOPRESERVATION PRIOR TO RADIATION OF TREATMENT OF TESTICULAR CANCER

Paul and Gilbert[79] evaluated semen quality including count, motility, and morphology in postorchiectomy patients before and after radiation treatment for stage I testicular seminoma. This study included 14 patients with unilateral testicular seminoma and a normal contralateral testicle seen between April 1997 and July 2003. The study confirmed that semen abnormalities were common before radiation treatment in patients with testicular carcinoma, since abnormal semen analyses were present in 11 of the 14 study patients (79%) prior to initiating radiation. Interestingly, two of these patients (14%) demonstrated an improvement in their semen analyses after receiving radiation. Of the nine patients (65%) who demonstrated worsening of their

disease led to more severe and possibly permanent effects. All patients were azoospermic following treatment, and recovery was not seen in patients receiving doses of 1.4 to 2.6 Gy after 17 to 43 months' follow-up.

A return of fertility in the two patients with testicular radiation doses of 1.2 Gy, indicating that this may represent a threshold for permanent testicular damage.

TABLE 34.2		Fertility in Men Following Radiation	
Effector Cell	*Dose*	*Clinical Effect*	*Time to Recovery*
Spermatogonia	≥0.1 Gy	Oligospermia[a]	9–18 mo
Spermatocytes	≥2 Gy	Azoospermia after 60 d	30 mo
Spermatids	≥4 Gy	Azoospermia < 60 d	5 y[b]

[a]Azoospermia may occur with doses >0.75 Gy.
[b]Doses >4 to 6 Gy may lead to permanent azoospermia.
Based on data from Howell SJ, Shalet SM. Spermatogenesis after cancer treatment: damage and recovery. *J Natl Cancer Monogr Inst.* 2005;34:12–17.

semen analyses after radiation, seven (50%) had preradiation abnormalities that worsened after therapy, one of which later returned to its preradiation baseline. The authors concluded that cryopreservation prior to radiation therapy would be beneficial in patients with testicular seminoma.

THE ROLE OF TESTICULAR SHIELDING AND RADIATION FIELD ON DOSE

Testicular shielding can affect testicular dose. The type of shielding used is important as demonstrated by Mazonakis et al.[80] who compared the use of a conventional 8-cm-thick lead block with the use of a commercially available round testicular shield. They found that the round shield reduced the gonadal dose by >66% compared with a <41% reduction with the conventional shield. Others have shown that shielding can reduce the dose received by the remaining testis from "dog-leg" fields to between 1% and 2% of the prescription dose.[68]

The distance from the testicles is another important factor that may be modified. Specifically, the level of the lower field border is one of the important factors influencing the dose to the testicles during pelvic radiotherapy.[59,81] The reduction of radiation field size in seminoma patients, that is, treating a para-aortic field instead of the classic "dog-leg" field, can decrease the testicular dose from a median dose of 0.32 to 0.09 Gy.[68]

Attempts at using antioxidants failed to prevent testicular damage. Hoyes et al.[82] investigated the ability of dietary vitamin C (ascorbic acid) to mitigate radiation-induced damage to the testis using testicular weight and sperm counts as biological endpoints. Their results suggest that vitamin C does no abrogate the effects of radiation in this setting.

DETECTION AND TREATMENT OF INJURY

Testing of testicular function includes testing for sperm count and morphology, tests to determine testosterone levels in the serum as well as LH and FSH levels and the ratio of testosterone to LH, and testosterone levels.

Leydig Cell Dysfunction

The most common presenting symptom of Leydig cell dysfunction is decreased libido in adults. Hormone replacement therapies are available, although care should be taken to avoid their use in hormone sensitive tumors such as prostate cancer. In patients at risk for osteoporosis in the presence of lowered testosterone, bone densitometry can aid in early detection and management.

In children, delayed puberty may occur. Tanner staging and testicular exam to assess for atrophy should be included as part of their routine physical exams. LH and testosterone levels should be drawn at age 13 and subsequent follow-up referral to an endocrinologist made if needed.

Germ Cell Damage

No treatments are available at this time to treat radiation damage to germ cells after radiation is delivered. Prevention and possible sperm banking before treatment are the best methods to mitigate the subsequent challenges facing these individuals. For patients with temporary azoopermia, recommendations to avoid conception for 12 months to allow the new generation of spermatogonia to complete their cycle into spermatozoa to avoid fertilization with sperm that may have radiation-induced genetic defects.

REFERENCES

1. Khatri VP, Asensio JA, eds. *Operative Surgery Manual.* Philadelphia, PA: Elsevier Science; 2003.
2. Brooks JD. Anatomy of the lower urinary tract and male genitalia. In: Wein AJ, Kavoussi LR, Novick AC, Partin AW, Peters CA, eds. *Campbell-Walsh Urology.* 9th ed. Philadelphia, PA: Saunders-Elsevier; 2007.
3. Olumi AF, Richie JP. Urologic surgery-spermatic cord, epididymis, and testes. In: Townsend CM, Beauchamp RD, Mark Evers BM, Mattox KL, eds. *Sabiston Textbook of Surgery: The Biological Basis of Modern Surgical Practice.* 18th ed. Philadelphia, PA: Saunders Elsevier; 2007.
4. Bannister LH, Dyson M. Reproductive system. In: Williams PL, ed. *Gray's Anatomy: The Anatomical Basis of Medicine and Surgery.* 38th ed. Philadelphia, PA: Harcourt Brace and Company; 1999.
5. Feneis H, Dauber W. *Pocket Atlas of Human Anatomy.* 5th ed. Thieme: Stuttgard; 2007.
6. Abrahamsohn PA. The male reproductive system. In: Junqueira LC, Carneiro J, eds. *Basic Histology: Text & Atlas.* 11th ed. Philadelphia, PA: McGraw-Hill; 2005.
7. Ganong WF. Endocrinology, metabolism, & reproductive function. the gonads: development & function of the reproductive system. In: Ganong WF, ed. *Review of Medical Physiology.* 22nd ed. Philadelphia, PA: The McGraw-Hill Companies, Inc.; 2005.
8. Hasegawa M, Wilson G, Russell LD, et al. Radiation- induced cell death in the mouse testis: relationship to apoptosis. *Radiat Res.* 1997;147:457–467.
9. Hasegawa M, Zhang Y, Niibe H, et al. Resistance of differentiating spermatogonia to radiation-induced apoptosis and loss in p53-deficient mice. *Radiat Res.* 1998;149:263–270.
10. Sapp WJ, Philpott DE, Williams CS, et al. Comparative study of spermatogonial survival after x-ray exposure, high LET (HZE) irradiation or spaceflight. *Adv Space Res.* 1992;12:179–189.
11. Amory JK, Bremner WJ. Endocrine regulation of testicular function in men: implications for contraceptive development. *Mol Cell Endocrinol.* 2001;182:175–179.
12. Matsumoto AM, Bremner WJ. Modulation of pulsatile gonadotropin secretion by testosterone in men. *J Clin Endocrinol Metab.* 1984;58:609–614.
13. Sheckter A, Matsumoto AM, Bremner WJ. Testosterone administration inhibits gonadotropin secretion by an effect of the human pituitary. *J Clin Endocriol Metab.* 1989;68:397–401.
14. Liu G, Gong P, Zhao H, et al. Effect of low-level radiation on the death of male germ cells. *Radiat Res.* 2006;165:379–389.
15. Henriksen K, Kulmala J, Toppari J, et al. Stage-specific apoptosis in the rat seminiferous epithelium: quantification of irradiation effects. *J Androl.* 1996;17:394–402.
16. Andrieu MN, Kurtman C, Hicsonmez A, et al. In vivo study to evaluate the protective effects of amifostine on radiation-induced damage of testis tissue. *Oncology.* 2005;69:44–51.
17. Mazonakis M, Zacharopoulou F, Kachris S, et al. Radiotherapy for common pediatric malignancies a phantom study. *Strahlenther Onkol.* 2007;183:332–337.
18. Stern RL. Peripheral dose from a linear accelerator equipped with multileaf collimation. *Med Phys.* 1999;26:559–563.
19. Kim YC. Testosterone supplementation in the aging male. *Int J Impot Res.* 1999;11:343–352.
20. Morley JE, Kaiser FE, Sih R, et al. Testosterone and frailty. *Clin Geriatr Med.* 1997;13:685–695.
21. Sternbach H. Age-associated testosterone decline in men: clinical issues for psychiatry. *Am J Psychiatry.* 1998;155:1310–1318.
22. Svartberg J, Jenssen T, Sundsfjord J, et al. The Tromsø Study. The associations of endogenous testosterone and sex hormone-binding globulin with glycosylated hemoglobin levels, in community dwelling men. *Diabetes Metab.* 2004;30:29–34.
23. Svartberg J, von Mülen D, Sundsfjord J, et al. The Tromsø study. Waist circumference and testosterone levels in community dwelling men. *Eur J Epidemiol.* 2004;19:657–663.
24. Svartberg J, von Mülen D, Schirmer H, et al. The Tromsø Study. Association of endogenous testosterone with blood pressure and left ventricular mass in men. *Eur J Endocrinol.* 2004;150:65–71.
25. Bremner WJ, Vitiello MV, Prinz PN. Loss of circadian rhythmicity in blood testosterone levels with aging in normal men. *J Clin Endocrinol Metab.* 1983;56:1278–1281.
26. Nankin HR, Calkins JH. Decreased bioavailable testosterone in aging normal and impotent men. *J Clin Endocrinol Metab.* 1986;63:1418–1420.
27. Giwercman A, von-der-Maase H, Berthelsen JG, et al. Localized irradiation of testes with carcinoma in situ: effects on Leydig cell function and eradication of malignant germ cells in 20 patients. *J Clin Endocrinol Metab.* 1991;73:596–603.
28. Nader S, Schultz PN, Cundiff JH, et al. Endocrine profiles of patients with testicular tumors treated with radiotherapy. *Int J Radiat Oncol Biol Phys.* 1983;9:1723–1726.
29. Seal US, the Veteran Administration Uro-Oncology Research Group. FSH and LH elevation after radiation for treatment of cancer of the prostate. *Invest Urol.* 1979;16:278–280.
30. Tomic R, Bergman B, Damber JE, et al. Effects of external radiation therapy for cancer of the prostate on the serum concentrations of testosterone, follicle-stimulating hormone, luteinizing hormone and prolactin. *J Urol.* 1983;130:287–289.
31. Sklar C. Reproductive physiology and treatment-related loss of sex hormone production. *Med Pediatr Oncol.* 1999;33:2–8.
32. Heller CG, Wootton P, Rowley MJ, et al. Action of radiation on human spermatogenesis. *Excerpta Med Int Congr Ser.* 1966;112:408–410.
33. Rowley MJ, Leach DR, Warner GA, et al. Effect of graded doses of ionizing radiation on the human testis. *Radiat Res.* 1974;59:665–678.
34. Howell S, Shalet S. Gonadal damage from chemotherapy and radiotherapy. *Endocrinol Metab Clin North Am.* 1998;27:927–943.
35. Waring AB, Wallace WHB. Subfertility following treatment for childhood cancer. *Hosp Med.* 2000;61:550–557.
36. Ash P. The influence of radiation on fertility in man. *Br J Radiol.* 1980;53:271–278.
37. Kutzner J, Loos R. Determination of gonald dose in radiotherapy with thermoluminescent dosimetry. *Klin Padiatr.* 1987;199(3):239–242.

38. Boice JD, Tawn EJ, Winter JF, et al. Genetic effects of radiotherapy for childhood cancer. *Health Phys.* 2003;85:65–80.

39. Byrne J, Rasmussen SA, Steinhorn SC, et al. Genetic disease in offspring of long-term survivors of childhood and adolescent cancer. *Am J Hum Genet.* 1998;62:45–52.

40. Green DM, Fiorello A, Zevon MA, et al. Birth defects and childhood cancer in offspring of survivors of childhood cancer. *Arch Pediatr Adolesc Med.* 1997;151:379–383.

41. Hermann T, Thiede G, Trott KR, et al. Offsprings of preconceptially irradiated patients. Final report of a longitudinal study 1976–1994 and recommendations for patient's advisory. *Strahlenther Onkol.* 2004;180:21–30.

42. Kenney LB, Nicholson HS, Brasseux C, et al. Birth defects in offspring of adult survivors of childhood acute lymphoblastic leukaemia: a CCG/NIH report. *Cancer.* 1996;78:169–176.

43. Mazonakis M, Zacharopoulou F, Kachris S, et al. Radiotherapy for common pediatric malignancies a phantom study. *Strahlenther Onkol.* 2007;183:332–337.

44. ICRP, International Commission on Radiological Protection. Publication 60. *Recommendations of the International Commission on Radiological Protection.* Oxford: Pergamon Press; 1991.

45. Hall EJ, ed. *Radiobiology for the Radiologist.* 5th ed. Philadelphia, PA: Lippincott Williams & Wilkins; 2000.

46. Howell SJ, Shalet SM. Testicular function following chemotherapy. *Hum Reprod Update.* 2001;7:363–369.

47. Bakker B, Massa GG, Oostdijk W, et al. Pubertal development and growth after total-body irradiation and bone marrow transplantation for haematological malignancies. *Eur J Pediatr.* 2000;159:31–37.

47. Bakker B, Massa GG, Oostdijk W, et al. Pubertal development and growth after total-body irradiation and bone marrow transplantation for haematological malignancies. *Eur J Pediatr.* 2000;159:31–37.

48. Ogilvy-Stuart AL, Clark DJ, Wallace WH, et al. Endocrine deficit after fractionated total body irradiation. *Arch Dis Child.* 1992;67:1107–1110.

49. Ishiguro H, Yasuda Y, Tomita Y et al. Gonadal shielding to irradiation is effective in protecting testicular growth and function in long-term survivors of bone marrow transplantation during childhood or adolescence. *Bone Marrow Transplant.* 2007;39:483–490.

50. Shalet SM. Effect of irradiation treatment on gonadal function in men treated for germ cell cancer. *Eur Urol.* 1993;23:148–151.

51. Sklar CA, Robison LL, Nesbit ME, et al. Effects of radiation on testicular function in long-term survivors of childhood acute lymphoblastic leukemia: a report from the Children Cancer Study Group. *J Clin Oncol.* 1990;8:1981–1987.

52. Sanders JE, The Seattle Marrow Transplant Team. The impact of marrow transplant preparative regimens on subsequent growth and development. *Semin Hematol.* 1991;28:244–249.

53. Sklar CA, Kim TH, Ramsay NK. Testicular function following bone marrow transplantation performed during or after puberty. *Cancer.* 1984;53:1498–1501.

54. Anserini P, Chiodi S, Spinelli S, et al. Semen analysis following allogeneic bone marrow transplantation. Additional data for evidence-based counselling. *Bone Marrow Transplant.* 2002;30:447–451.

55. Krassas GE, Pontikides N Gonadal effect of radiation from I-131 in male patients with thyroid carcinoma. *Arch Androl.* 2005;51(3):171–175.

56. Tamminga J, Koturbash I, Baker M, et al. Paternal cranial irradiation induces distant bystander DNA damage in the germline and leads to epigenetic alterations in the offspring *Cell Cycle.* 2008;7(9):1238–1245.

57. Sklar CA, Robison LL, Nesbit ME, et al. Effects of radiation on testicular function in long-term survivors of childhood acute lymphoblastic leukemia: a report from the Children's Cancer Study Group. *J Clin Oncol.* 1990;8(12):1981–1987.

58. Piroth MD, Hensley F, Wannenmacher M, et al. Male gonadal dose in adjuvant 3-D-pelvic irradiation after anterior resection of rectal cancer: influence to fertility. *Strahlenther Onkol.* 2003;179:754–759.

59. Hermann RM, Henkel K, Christiansen H, et al. Testicular dose and hormonal changes after radiotherapy of rectal cancer. *Radiother Oncol.* 2005;75:83–88.

60. Dueland S, Guren MG, Olsen DR, et al. Radiation therapy induced changes in male sex hormone levels in rectal cancer patients. *Radiother Oncol.* 2003;68:249–253.

61. Bruheim K, Svartberg J, Carlsen E. Radiotherapy for rectal cancer is associated with reduced serum testosterone and increased FSH and LH. *Int J Radiat Oncol Biol Phys.* 2008;70(3):722–727.

62. Shapiro E, Kinsella TJ, Makuch RW, et al. Effects of fractionated irradiation of endocrine aspects of testicular function. *J Clin Oncol.* 1985;3:1232–1239.

63. Zagars GK, Pollack A. Serum testosterone levels after external beam radiation for clinically localized prostate cancer. *Int J Radiat Oncol.* 1997;39(1):85–89.

64. Daniell HW, Clark JC, Pereira SE, et al. Hypogonadism following prostate-bed radiation therapy for prostate cancer. *Cancer.* 2001;91(10):1889–1895.

65. Grigsby PW, Perez CA. The effects of external beam radiotherapy on endocrine function in patients with carcinoma of the prostate. *J Urol.* 1986;135:726–727.

66. Petersen PM, Skakkebaek NE, Vistisen K, et al. Semen quality and reproductive hormones before orchiectomy in men with testicular cancer. *J Clin Oncol.* 1999;17:941–947.

67. Gordon W Jr, Siegmund K, Stanisic TH, et al. Southwest Oncology Group. A study of reproductive function in patients with seminoma treated with radiotherapy and orchidectomy: (SWOG-8711). *Int J Radiat Oncol Biol Phys.* 1997;38:83–94.

68. Jacobsen KD, Olsen DR, Fossa K, et al. External beam abdominal radiotherapy in patients with seminoma stage I: field type, testicular dose, and spermatogenesis. *Int J Radiat Oncol Biol Phys.* 1997;38:95–102.

69. Hahn EW, Feingold SM, Simpson L, et al. Recovery from aspermia induced by low-dose radiation in seminoma patients. *Cancer.* 1982;50:337–340.

70. Krueser ED, Felsenberg D, Behles C. Long-term gonadal dysfunction and its impact on bone mineralization in patients following COPP/ABVD chemotherapy for Hodgkin's disease. *Ann Oncol.* 1992;3(suppl 4):105–110.

71. Kulkarni S, Sastry P, Saikia T, et al. Gonadal function following ABVD therapy for Hodgkin's disease. *Am J Clin Oncol.* 1997;20:354–357.

72. Relander T, Cavallin-StahlE, Garwicz S. Gonadal and sexual function in men treated for childhood cancer. *Med Pediatr Oncol.* 2000;35:52–63.

73. Schultheiss TE, Kun LE, Ang KK, et al. Radiation response of the central nervous system. *Int J Radiat Oncol Biol Phys.* 1995;31:1093–1112.

74. Hill M, Milan S, Cunningham D, et al. Evaluation of the efficacy of the VEEP regimen in adult Hodgkin's disease with assessment of gonadal and cardiac toxicity. *J Clin Oncol.* 1995;13:387–395.

75. Kinsella TJ, Trivette G, Rowland J, et al. Long-term follow-up of testicular function following radiation therapy for early-stage Hodgkin's disease. *J Clin Oncol.* 1989;7:718–724.

76. Centola GM, Keller JW, Henzler M, et al. Effect of low-dose testicular irradiation on sperm count and fertility in patients with testicular seminoma. *J Androl.* 1994;15:608–613.

77. Speiser B, Rubin P, Casarett G. Aspermia following lower truncal irradiation in Hodgkin's disease. *Cancer.* 1973;32:692–698.

78. Howell SJ, Shalet SM. Spermatogenesis after cancer treatment: damage and recovery. *J Natl Cancer Monogr Inst.* 2005;34:12–17.

79. Paul EM, Gilbert BR. Cryopreservation prior to radiation therapy in testis cancer patients: is it necessary? *Fertil Steril.* P-48 abstract pS153.

80. Mazonakis M, Damilakis J, Varveris H, et al. Radiation dose to testes and risk of infertility from radiotherapy for rectal cancer. *Oncol Rep.* 2006;15:729–733.

81. Amies CJ, Mameghan H, Rose A, et al. Testicular doses in definitive radiation therapy for localized prostate cancer. *Int J Radiat Oncol Biol Phys.* 1995;32:839–846.

82. Hoyes KP, Morris ID, Sharmat HL, et al. Effect of dietary vitamin C on radiation induced damage to the testis. *J. Radiol Prot.* 1995;15(2):143–150.

Christopher J. Anker
David K. Gaffney

Ovary

INTRODUCTION

Over the past few decades, the number of cancer survivors has significantly increased, including those diagnosed as children and young adults.[1] Approximately 8% of female cancers occur before age 40.[2] Ovaries are the most radiosensitive portion of the female reproductive tract, putting patients at risk for infertility and menopause-related complications at a young age.[3] In a report from the Childhood Cancer Survivor Study (CCSS), 2,819 survivors of childhood cancer over 18 years old were compared with a control group of 1,065 female siblings of participants.[4] The cumulative incidence of premature ovarian failure (POF) in the survivor group was 8% compared to 0.9% in the siblings. Medical professionals need to have the ability to identify those at risk for ovarian damage and prevent its occurrence if possible.

DESCRIPTION OF GROSS ANATOMY, LOCATION, AND IMAGING OF NORMAL STRUCTURE

GROSS ANATOMY

For premenopausal women for whom therapeutic radiation is planned, it is essential to ascertain whether the ovaries are in the radiation field. The ovaries are ovoid structures whose size depends on a woman's age, hormonal status, and menstrual cycle stage.[5] Typical dimensions of an adult ovary are 2.5- to 5-cm long, 1.5- to 3-cm wide, and 1- to 2-cm thick.[6,7] Normalcy of size is best assessed by measuring volume,[7] calculated assuming an ellipsoid shape (0.523 × length × width × thickness). The normal mean volume measured via ultrasonography in a large patient series was 3 cc (95% confidence interval [CI], 0.2–9.1 cc) before menarche, 9.8 cc (95% CI, 2.5–21.9 cc) in menstruating women, and 5.8 cc (95% CI, 1.2–14.1 cc) in postmenopausal women.[8]

Three anchoring structures are connected to the ovary: the suspensory ligament (Fig. 35.1), the utero-ovarian ligament (Fig. 35.1), and the mesovarium (Fig. 35.2).[6,9] The broad ligament of the uterus is a double layer of peritoneum (mesentery) that extends from the sides of the uterus to the lateral walls and floor of the pelvis (Fig. 35.2). The mesovarium is the part of the broad ligament by which the ovary is suspended, which anchors the ovary to the posterior surface of the broad ligament.

The utero-ovarian ligament, which anchors the ovary to the uterus, lies posterior-superiorly between the layers of the broad ligament (Fig. 35.1). Laterally, the broad ligament drapes superiorly over the ovarian vessels (artery and vein) as the suspensory ligament of the ovary, anchoring the ovary to the pelvic sidewall. The round ligament lies antero-inferiorly between the layers of the broad ligament, and it courses through the inguinal canal functioning to maintain anteversion of the uterus (Fig. 35.3).[9]

In nulliparous women, the ovary is usually found near the lateral pelvic sidewall in the ovarian fossa,[10] a shallow peritoneal depression also known as the *fossa of Waldeyer*.[11] This area is delineated by the ureter and internal iliac artery posteriorly,

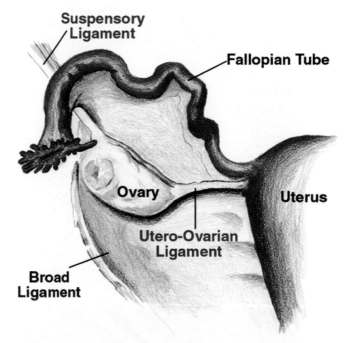

Figure 35.1. Posterior view shows the broad ligament and ovarian attachments with the fallopian tube separated from the ovary. The suspensory ligament extends from the superolateral part of the broad ligament to the pelvic sidewall. The medially located utero-ovarian ligament is enclosed between the two peritoneal layers of the broad ligament. (Reprinted from Saksouk FA, Johnson SC. Recognition of the ovaries and ovarian origin of pelvic masses with CT. *Radiographics.* 2004;24(suppl 1):S133–S146, with permission.)

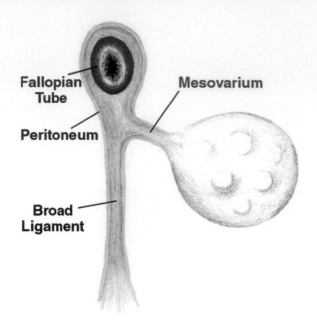

Figure 35.2. Sagittal view shows the mesovarium anchoring the ovary to the posterosuperior aspect of the broad ligament. The mesovarium is the primary route of transit for blood vessels entering and exiting the ovarian hilum. (Reprinted from Saksouk FA, Johnson SC. Recognition of the ovaries and ovarian origin of pelvic masses with CT. *Radiographics.* 2004;24(suppl 1):S133–S146, with permission.)

by the external iliac vein superiorly, and by the obliterated umbilical artery anteriorly (Figs. 35.3 and 35.4).[5] During the first pregnancy, the enlarging uterus and stretched broad ligament pull the ovaries into the abdomen. Following delivery, the broad ligament may remain elongated causing increased ovarian mobility. As a result, the ovaries often do not return to their initial position in the pelvis.[10]

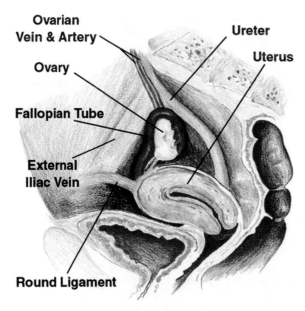

Figure 35.3. Ovarian fossa at the posterolateral pelvic sidewall. The fossa is bounded posteriorly by the ureter and superiorly by the external iliac vein. The ovary is draped by the fallopian tube, which arches over much of the ovarian surface. (Reprinted from Saksouk FA, Johnson SC. Recognition of the ovaries and ovarian origin of pelvic masses with CT. *Radiographics.* 2004;24(suppl 1):S133–S146, with permission.)

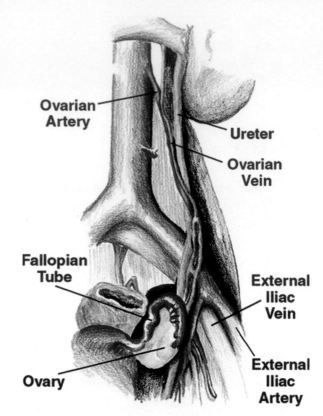

Figure 35.4. Illustration shows the ovarian artery and vein without the overlying peritoneum and suspensory ligament. The vessels are medial to the ureter in the upper abdomen, cross obliquely anterior to the ureter in the middle to lower lumbar region, and are lateral to the ureter in the lower abdomen and pelvis. (Reprinted from Saksouk FA, Johnson SC. Recognition of the ovaries and ovarian origin of pelvic masses with CT. *Radiographics.* 2004;24(suppl 1):S133–S146, with permission.)

Ovarian location is influenced by uterine and ovarian size, urinary bladder filling, rectosigmoid colon distension, and coexisting pelvic masses. Because the mesovarium anchors the ovary to the posterior layer of the broad ligament, the normal ovary is located in the posterior pelvic compartment. This area is above the uterine fundus but not between the uterus and bladder or in the anterior cul-de-sac (Fig. 35.3).[7] Potential ovarian locations include the posterior cul-de-sac, the adnexal regions beside the uterus, and posterior or superior to the uterine fundus. When the uterus is retroverted, one or both ovaries could be ventral and lateral to the uterus.[12]

IMAGING OF NORMAL STRUCTURE

As the diagnosis of cancer often involves a computed tomography (CT) scan, it is essential to know how to locate an ovary on this imaging modality. The ovarian vein is often easily identified on CT. The left ovarian vein drains into the left renal vein, and the right drains into the inferior vena cava below the level of the renal vessels (Fig. 35.5A).[5,6] The ovarian artery is smaller and less consistently identifiable with CT than the vein. The vessels may be followed caudally along the anterior surface of the psoas muscle to the true pelvis and to the suspensory ligament of the ovary (Fig. 35.5B). The suspensory ligament leads to the ovary and

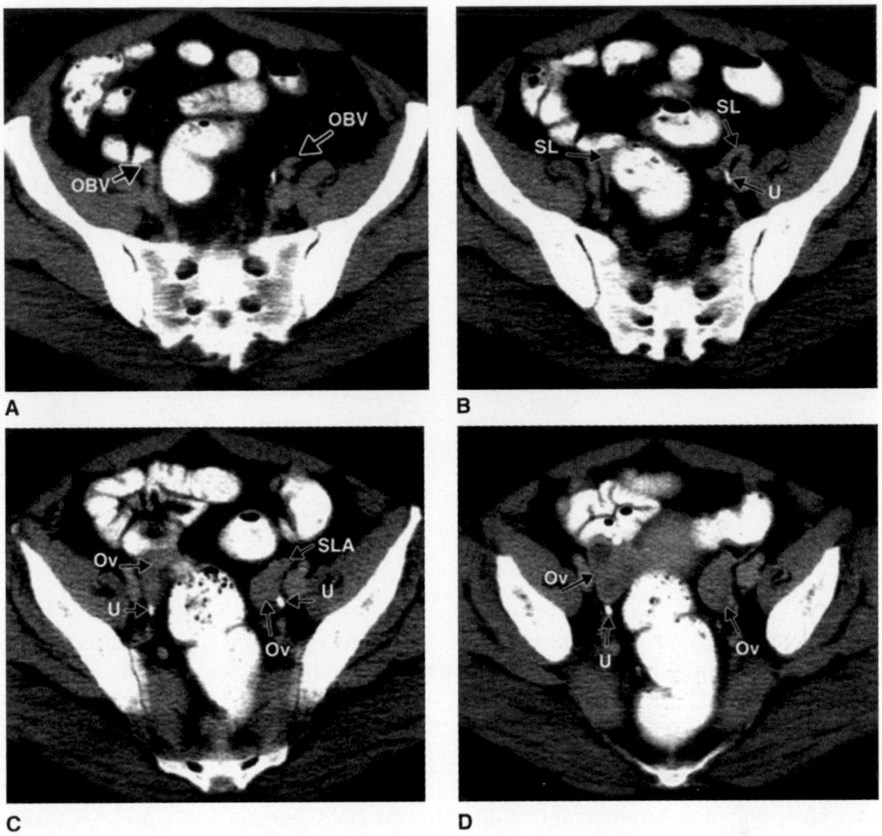

Figure 35.5. CT features of normal ovaries. **A**: CT scan shows ovarian blood vessels (OBVs) coursing in the upper pelvis lateral to the ureters. **B**: CT scan shows that the OBVs are continuous with the suspensory ligaments (SL), which are visualized near the external iliac vessels. The left suspensory ligament is seen as a narrow soft-tissue band that demonstrates subtle widening as it approaches the ovary. **C**: CT scan shows that the suspensory ligaments lead to the ovaries, which are typically located in the ovarian fossa and bounded by the ureters and external iliac veins. **D**: CT scan shows that the ovaries have a characteristic morphologic appearance, with distinct cystic follicles seen in the right ovary. SLA, ovarian attachment of the left suspensory ligament; Ov, ovaries; U: ureter. (Reprinted from Saksouk FA, Johnson SC. Recognition of the ovaries and ovarian origin of pelvic masses with CT. *Radiographics.* 2004;24(suppl 1): S133–S146, with permission.)

is a reliable anatomic landmark for localization.[13] It may be seen on CT in continuity with the ovarian vessels as a short and narrow fan-shaped soft tissue band (Fig. 35.5C). At its ovarian attachment, it may be noted as a linear band slightly thicker than the ovarian vein leading into it. When visualized axially on CT imaging, it usually extends along the direction of the external or common iliac vessels. This structure is more commonly identifiable than the other ovarian ligamentous attachments.[13]

Ovaries have a distinct morphologic appearance that varies with a patient's age and hormonal status.[14] In women of child-bearing age, the majority of normal ovaries are identifiable. They often contain visible cystic follicles or physiologic cysts, which are seen as characteristic fluid-attenuating areas. Postmenopausal ovaries are small and often not recognizable.

If locating the ovaries is challenging on CT, alternate imaging modalities such as ultrasound or MRI may be useful.[7,8,15] Furthermore, MRI/CT fusion for radiation treatment planning may help for particularly difficult cases.[15]

DESCRIPTION OF HISTOLOGICAL ANATOMY OF STRUCTURE, INCLUDING FUNCTIONAL UNITS IMPORTANT IN RADIATION DAMAGE

NEUROENDOCRINE CONTROL OF REPRODUCTIVE CYCLE

Normal reproductive function in women involves a cyclical process of follicle development, ovulation, corpus luteum development, and luteal regression. This system is controlled through the interdependent functioning of the hypothalamus, pituitary, and

ovary (Fig. 35.6).[16] Gonadotropin-releasing hormone (GnRH) from the hypothalamus initiates follicle-stimulating hormone (FSH) and luteinizing hormone (LH) production by the pituitary. FSH stimulates follicle formation and development of ova. LH is required for the synthesis of androgens from theca cells within the developing follicle, and FSH controls aromatization of these androgen precursors in the granulosa cells. The follicle secretes increasing titers of estradiol (E_2) and inhibin A and B. This positively feeds back to the hypothalamic-hypophyseal axis producing an LH surge, which in turn causes ovulation.[16]

The remaining follicle cells transform into a corpus luteum, which secretes E_2, progesterone, and inhibin A. This stimulates development of the uterine lining. Progesterone inhibits FSH secretion and thus development of other ova, as well as uterine contractions. If fertilization fails to occur, the corpus luteum disintegrates. Progesterone titers decrease, and FSH stimulates development of additional ova.[16]

FUNCTIONAL HISTOLOGY

The follicle, the functional unit within the ovary, consists of the sex-steroid-producing cells (i.e., granulosa and thecal cells) and the germ cells that eventually become ova.[17] The connective tissue of the ovarian cortex is where ovarian follicles are located.[3] There are a fixed number of follicles, and as an embryo approximately 7 million germ cells are in ovarian rudiment. This decreases to 1 to 2 million by birth, and 300,000 by puberty. Menopause occurs when this number drops to 1,000 to 2,000. During a woman's lifespan, approximately 400 eventually mature and ovulate. The remaining follicles undergo atresia, and follicular decline accelerates in the decade preceding menopause.[16,17] Since the process of involution may begin at

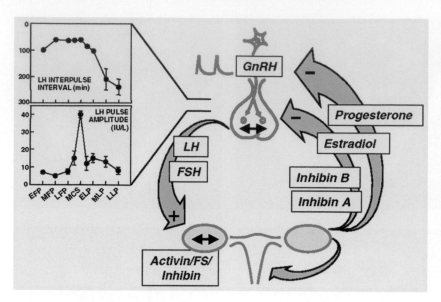

Figure 35.6. The reproductive system operates in a classic endocrine feedback mode as follows: stimulation of LH and FSH secretion from the pituitary by the pulsatile release of GnRH; stimulation of ovarian secretion of E_2, progesterone, and the inhibins by FSH and LH; and negative feedback of ovarian steroids and inhibins on the hypothalamus and pituitary. The horizontal arrows within the pituitary and ovary indicate the autocrine and paracrine actions of the activin/follistatin/inhibin system. The inset documents the dynamic changes in the interpulse interval and amplitude of LH across the early (EFP), mid-(MFP), and late (LFP) follicular phases, midcycle surge (MCS) and early (ELP), mid-(MLP), and late (LLP) luteal phases of the menstrual cycle. (Reprinted from Hall JE. Neuroendocrine physiology of the early and late menopause. *Endocrinol Metab Clin North Am.* 2004;33:637–659, with permission.)

any stage of follicular development, the normal ovary contains both degenerating ova and follicles in various sizes and stages of development.[18]

OVARIAN PATHOLOGY FOLLOWING RADIATION

Ovarian follicles are remarkably vulnerable to DNA damage from ionizing radiation.[19] Following radiation, the most consistent and clear histological change is atrophy of the ovarian cortex.[3] There is demise of primordial follicles and absence of mature follicles, as well as a loss of normal cortical stromal cells. Although this atrophy occurs in essentially all patients uniformly throughout the cortex with external beam radiation, atrophy following brachytherapy ranges from mild to severe and only occurs in approximately one half of the cases. Ovaries become smaller and collagen seems to be the sole component of the cortex.[3] At the cellular level, the follicles die an interphase death via apoptosis, like lymphocytes.[19–21] Oocytes show the rapid onset of pyknosis, chromosome condensation, nuclear envelope disruption, and cytoplasmic vacuolization. This results in ovarian atrophy and reduced follicle stores. Both mature and maturing follicles are equally damaged. There is essentially no latent period, and sterilization of damaged follicles is immediate. This limits the sublethal damage repair typically achieved with fractionation of radiation therapy.[22]

DATA FOR FRACTIONATED AND SINGLE DOSE EFFECTS ON STRUCTURE

ANIMAL DATA

Animal data show that oocyte radiosensitivity varies widely according to the stage of the follicle/oocyte and the species.[23,24] Most of the data come from older literature where units of roentgen (R) were used. For radiation protection purposes, an exposure of 1 R approximately results in an absorbed dose of 0.01 Gy. The oocytes of rats and mice are highly sensitive to radiation. These rodents frequently have one or two litters when subjected to substerilizing doses of radiation, resulting from eggs that were in the process of follicular maturation at the time of exposure. When these follicles have all been used, the animal becomes sterile, since the small primordial oocytes are highly sensitive and would have been destroyed.[24] For example, the exposure of young mice to 25 R (0.25 Gy) whole-body irradiation had little effect on the number of offspring born within 3 months of treatment, but the *total* reproductive capacity (number of litters and litter size) was reduced by 50%.[25] LD_{50} (Lethal Dose, 50%) is the dose required to destroy 50% of oocytes. The LD_{50} for mouse oocytes has been estimated to be only 15 R (0.15 Gy),[26] compared to 1 Gy for the rat.[27] The histological changes involved in rat follicular destruction during the acute clinical period are shown in Figure 35.7.[18] In regard to dose escalation toxicity, Ingram[28] exposed adult rats to varying single fraction radiation doses of 31, 78, 315, and 630 R. At a mean follow-up of 288 days, the number of surviving oocytes was reduced to 83%, 51%, 4%, and 1%, respectively.

Some morphological and physiological characteristics of the female guinea pig make it a more accurate model for human females, including similar ovarian structure and density, a long estrous cycle with follicle secretion, and a long gestation period with folliculogenesis starting in utero.[29,30] Two distinct types of immature oocytes are contained in the ovaries of guinea pigs: an oocyte of the true diplotene type with a large nucleus, similar to resting oocytes in the ovaries of humans, monkeys, cows, and pigs, and another with a contracted nucleus.[31] The LD_{50} of the large oocytes was found to be around 4 Gy based on histological analysis.[31] Comparatively little is known regarding oocyte radiosensitivity for primates. As in other species, germ cell survival depends on dose and stage of oogenesis. Doses above 20 Gy are adequate to eliminate all growing follicles, while doses of 70 to 120 Gy are required to kill all primordial oocytes.[32]

HUMAN DATA

In women, it has been well accepted for decades that the radiation dose required for complete and permanent sterility is related to the age at the time of radiation, or more precisely how many oocytes remain.[3,15,18,33] Dose tolerance variability in the literature reflects how chemotherapy and age play large roles in toxicity. Because of the frequency of female genital tract cancer as well as cancer in the vicinity of the ovaries, considerable information has been gathered regarding ovarian radiosensitivity.

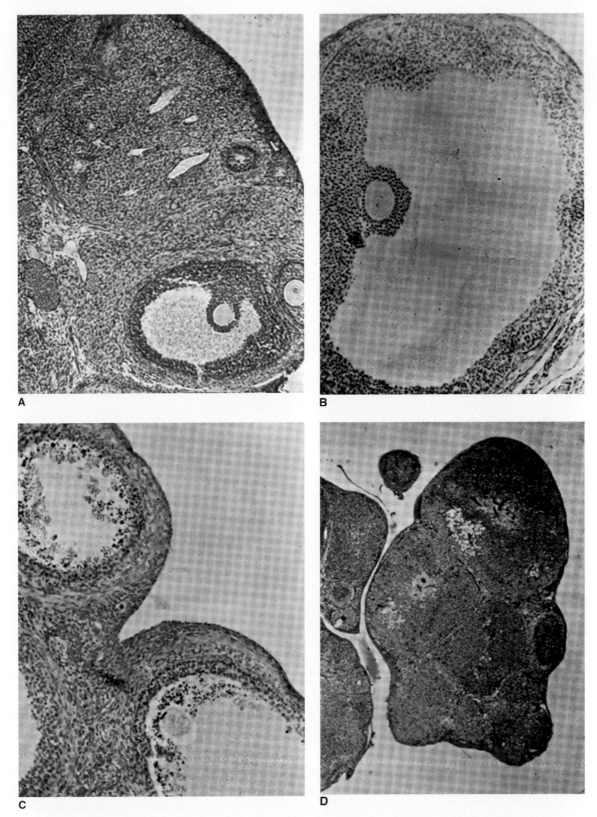

Figure 35.7. A: Normal rat ovary. Normal follicles in various stages of development and sizes (approximately ×100) **B**: Normal mature ovarian follicle of rat. Note the fluid-filled cavity surrounded by a wall of stratified granulosa cells and the oocyte embedded in the hillock of granulosa cells (approximately ×200). **C**: Rat ovary 1 day after a single x-ray dose of 750 R. Note the numerical reduction of granulosa cells, disorganization of the granulosa cell wall of the follicles, and degeneration and necrosis of the remaining cells in these follicles of intermediate size (approximately ×100). **D**: Rat ovary 25 days after a single x-ray dose of 750 R. Note the disappearance of developing follicles, remains of follicles damaged or destroyed and fatty metamorphosis of corpora lutea (approximately ×25). (From Rubin P, Casarett G. The female genital tract. In: *Clinical Radiation Pathology.* Vol I. Philadelphia, PA: W.B. Saunders Company; 1968:396–423.)

External Beam Radiation Therapy

In order to cause POF, both ovaries need to be damaged by radiation. Wallace et al.[34] studied 38 patients who received whole abdominal radiation (20–30 Gy) during early childhood. Twenty-seven failed to undergo or complete pubertal development (pubertal failure). Premature menopause (median age, 23.5 years) occurred in a further 10, including 4 patients who had documented conceptions (dose range, 20–26.5 Gy). However, there were no live births, and all miscarriages occurred in the second trimester. For 15 patients who received flank irradiation (dose range, 20–30 Gy), thereby sparing or near sparing the contralateral ovary, ovarian function (median age at last assessment, 15.2 years) was normal in all but one in whom pubertal failure occurred.

In the past, low dose radiation was actually used to "stimulate" the ovary by causing superovulation. One such regimen involved three weekly treatments, in which a total dose of 0.65 Gy was delivered to each ovary while 0.90 Gy was delivered to the pituitary.[35] In a series of 644 women radiated with this method, 351 (55%) were able to conceive. No evidence of excess genetic abnormalities was noted in the children and grandchildren of these women. Despite the utility and safety of this procedure, it has been replaced with more modern fertility treatments that do not harbor such concerns of oocyte mutations. Also, it is recognized that any radiation dose is damaging and results in the loss of ovarian follicles. Glucksman noted that doses as low as 170 R caused temporary sterility in women for 12 to 36 months, although the age range to expect this effect is not specified. Despite recovery of function, premature menopause is likely, due to the loss of oocytes.[36]

Ovarian ablation using radiation was a procedure once popular in the treatment of various benign conditions as well as metastatic breast cancer. This technique was used to avoid hospitalization, anesthesia, and the discomfort of oophorectomy. Doll and Smith[37] reported on the radiation treatment of "metropathia hemorrhagica" in 2,068 women, 99% of whom were over 35 years old. Doses of 625 to 1,050 R in two to four fractions caused cessation of menses in 97% of women, with the rest requiring one to two additional fractions to achieve permanent amenorrhea. Above 40 years old, doses >600 to 650 R have been found to consistently cause permanent sterility.[38–42]

The likelihood of ovarian failure at younger ages varies. Although Peck et al.[42] found that all patients under 40 were sterilized by a dose of 625 R, other studies clearly show much higher doses may be required for younger patients. Mills et al. evaluated 188 acute lymphoblastic leukemia (ALL) survivors who were premenarchal at diagnosis, at a time when they were at least 18 years old, at least 2 years out from diagnosis, while they were alive and in remission. Their siblings served as controls. For craniospinal irradiation (CSI) doses <24 Gy, no delay in menarche was noted. However, those who received 24 Gy CSI with or without abdominal radiation had significantly later menarche than the control subjects, with a hazard ratio (HR) of 0.5 (95% CI: 0.3–0.7 [$p = 0.0002$]). Sixty-seven percent of this group had an elevated FSH.[43] Jacox[41] reported on one 21-year-old patient who delivered a normal child despite receiving 640 R and being amenorrheic for 2 years. Lushbaugh and Casarett[44] reported doses above 20 Gy given over 5 to 6 weeks are required to induce complete failure in the majority of pediatric patients. In other series, conceptions have even occurred for women under 20 who have received up to 30 Gy.[36, 45–47]

Effect of Fractionation

Ovarian recovery has some dependency on fractionation of radiation, as most notably reported by Sanders et al. when evaluating patients who received various regimens of total body irradiation (TBI). For those under 25 years of age, increased recovery was noted for the 12-Gy fractionated TBI group (7 of 29 patients, 24%) compared to the 10-Gy single dose group (2 of 36 patients, 6%). However, at fractionated doses above 15 Gy ovarian failure was seen in all cases, and above age 25 no ovarian recovery occurred regardless of dose and fractionation.[48] Of note, since oocytes die via apoptosis, the effect of fractionation on survival is diminished compared to cells eliminated via a mitotic death.[22]

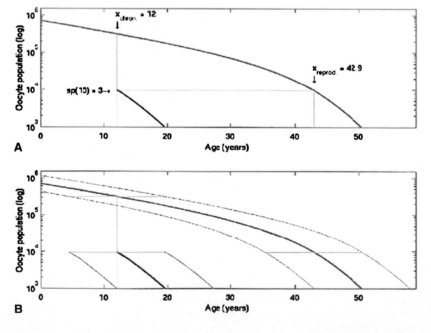

Figure 35.8. **A:** An example of the method for predicting ovarian failure after treatment. The chronologic age, x_{chron}, is 12 years, and the dose, z, is 10 Gy. The average oocyte population at x_{chron} is 312,000. The surviving percentage after 10 Gy is $\log_{10}g$ (10) = 3.01%, corresponding to a population after treatment of 9,600. This new population is the average population at age 42.9 years, the reproductive age, x_{reprod}, after treatment. The average 42.9-year-old patient is expected to have ovarian failure in 7.5 years, at age 50.4 years. Hence, the 12-year-old patient is expected to experience ovarian failure in 7.5 years, at age 19.5 years. **B:** The same example, with confidence intervals included. Average untreated menopause occurs at 50.4 years ± (1.96 × 3.9) years. Average menopause after treatment is the predicted age of menopause (19.5 years) ± (1.96 × 3.9) years. (From Wallace WH, Thomson AB, Saran F, et al. Predicting age of ovarian failure after radiation to a field that includes the ovaries. *Int J Radiat Oncol Biol Phys.* 2005;62:738–744.)

Dose Toxicity Model and Recommendations

Wallace et al.[15] have mathematically correlated the issue of age and radiosensitivity. They determined that the change in rate of follicle decline likely represents an instantaneous rate of temporal change based on the remaining pool, best represented by the Faddy and Gosden model. This model was solved based on data involving ovarian failure following TBI, including the finding that the surviving fraction for TBI patients receiving 14.4 Gy is 0.66%. The graphical solution to this model is represented by Figure 35.8A. Also based on these data, the surviving percentage function, $g(z)$, for a given dose (z) was determined to be $g(z) = 10^{(2-0.15z)}$, which decreases exponentially from 100% at zero dosage ($z = 0$). If one solves $g(z) = 50$ for z, then $z = LD_{50} = 1.99$ Gy.

From the solution to the Faddy-Gosden equation and the surviving percentage function, the authors developed a straightforward method to determine the age of menopause expected for women of any age (x_{chron}, years) receiving a given dose (z, Gy). Ovarian failure occurs at an average age of 50.4 years.[49] Assuming a patient has an average number of oocytes, the population before radiation will be $y(x_{chron})$, which may be determined from the curve in Figure 35.8A. After treatment, the surviving fraction is $g(z)/100$. Therefore, the oocyte number following radiation is the product of $y(x_{chron})$ and $g(z)/100$. This new posttreatment oocyte population corresponds to their reproductive age, x_{reprod}, which normally occurs at an age between x_{chron} and 50.4 years. The remaining reproductive life span of the patient may thus be calculated as $50.4-x_{reprod}$. Furthermore, a patient's age of ovarian failure may be predicted as $x_{chron} + (50.4-x_{reprod})$ years. Wallace et al. provided an example calculation for a patient with $x_{chron} = 12$ years receiving a dose $z = 10$ Gy, shown in Figure 35.8A. This calculation with 95% CI is depicted in Figure 35.8B. For quick reference, Wallace et al.[15] performed a range of calculations to develop a table depicting the expected age of menopause for women age 0 to 30 receiving doses from 3 to 12 Gy (Table 35.1).

The authors also calculated the effective dose of radiation that would result in immediate and permanent sterilization in 97.5% of patients. The results were 20.3 Gy at birth, 18.4 Gy at 10 years, 16.5 Gy at 20 years, and 14.3 Gy at 30 years. The average sterilizing dose at which 50% of patients will develop immediate ovarian failure was calculated to be 18.9 Gy at

TABLE 35.1	Predicted Age at Ovarian Failure with 95% Confidence Limits for Ages at Treatment from 0 to 30 Years and for Doses 3, 6, 9, and 12 Gy											
	3 Gy			*6 Gy*			*9 Gy*			*12 Gy*		
Age	Low	Mean	High	Low	Mean	High	Low	Mean	High	Low	Mean	High
0	31.2	35.1	39	18.7	22.6	26.5	9.8	13.7	17.6	4	7.9	11.8
1	31.3	35.2	39.1	19	22.9	26.8	10.4	14.3	18.2	4.8	8.7	12.6
2	31.5	35.4	39.3	19.3	23.2	27.1	10.9	14.8	18.7	5.5	9.4	13.3
3	31.6	35.5	39.4	19.7	23.6	27.5	11.5	15.4	19.3	6.2	10.1	14
4	31.7	35.6	39.5	20.1	24	27.9	12.1	16	19.9	6.9	10.8	14.7
5	31.9	35.8	39.7	20.5	24.4	28.3	12.7	16.6	20.5	7.7	11.6	15.5
6	32.1	36.0	39.9	20.9	24.8	28.7	13.3	17.2	21.1	8.4	12.3	16.2
7	32.2	36.1	40	21.3	25.2	29.1	13.9	17.8	21.7	9.1	13.0	16.9
8	32.4	36.3	40.2	21.7	25.6	29.5	14.6	18.5	22.4	9.9	13.8	17.7
9	32.6	36.5	40.4	22.1	26	29.9	15.2	19.1	23.0	10.6	14.5	18.4
10	32.8	36.7	40.6	22.6	26.5	30.4	15.8	17.7	23.6	11.4	15.3	19.2
11	33	36.9	40.8	23	26.9	30.8	16.5	20.4	24.3	12.1	16.0	19.9
12	33.2	37.1	41	23.5	27.4	31.3	17.1	21.0	24.9	12.9	16.8	20.7
13	33.4	37.3	41.2	23.9	27.8	31.7	17.8	21.7	25.6	13.6	17.5	21.4
14	33.6	37.5	41.4	24.4	28.3	32.2	18.5	22.4	26.3	14.4	18.3	22.2
15	33.9	37.8	41.7	24.9	28.8	32.7	19.1	23.0	26.9	15.1	19.0	22.9
16	34.1	38.0	41.9	25.4	29.3	33.2	19.8	23.9	27.6	15.9	19.8	23.7
17	34.3	38.2	42.1	25.9	29.8	33.7	20.5	24.4	28.3	17.0	20.5	24.4
18	34.6	38.5	42.4	26.4	30.3	34.2	21.2	25.1	29.0	18.0	21.3	25.2
19	34.9	38.8	42.7	27.0	30.9	34.8	21.8	25.7	29.6	19.0	22.0	25.9
20	35.1	39	42.9	27.5	31.4	35.3	22.5	26.4	30.3	20.0	22.8	26.7
21	35.4	39.3	43.2	28.0	31.9	35.5	23.2	27.1	31.0	21.0	23.5	27.4
22	35.7	39.6	43.5	28.6	32.5	36.4	23.9	27.8	31.7	22.0	24.3	28.2
23	36	39.9	43.8	29.1	33.0	36.9	24.6	28.5	32.4	23.0	25.0	28.9
24	36.3	40.2	44.1	29.7	33.6	37.5	25.3	29.2	33.1	24.0	25.7	29.6
25	36.7	40.6	44.5	30.3	34.2	38.1	25.9	29.8	33.7	25.0	26.5	30.4
26	37	40.9	44.8	30.8	34.7	38.6	26.6	30.5	34.4	26.0	27.2	31.1
27	37.3	41.2	45.1	31.4	35.5	39.2	27.3	31.2	35.1	27.0	27.9	31.8
28	37.7	41.6	45.5	32.0	35.9	37.8	28.0	31.9	35.8	28.0	28.7	32.6
29	38	41.9	45.8	32.5	36.4	40.3	29.0	32.6	36.5	29.0	29.4	33.3
30	38.3	42.2	46.1	33.1	37	40.9	30.0	33.2	37.1	30.0	30.1	34.0

Source: From Wallace WH, Thomson AB, Saran F, et al. Predicting age of ovarian failure after radiation to a field that includes the ovaries. *Int J Radiat Oncol Biol Phys*. 2005;62:738–744. Permission pending.

birth, 16.9 Gy at 10 years, 14.9 Gy at 20 years, and 12.1 Gy at 30 years.[15] However, the dose to the ovaries should be kept well below these doses as any dose may be damaging. Although a dose of 6 Gy has historically been described as the dose that causes sterilization for women over 40,[38–42] as described previously, younger women may achieve pregnancy despite higher doses.[36,41,45–47] However, based on the results of Wallace et al. (Table 35.1), even an ovarian dose of 6 Gy for 10- and 20-year-old patients could cause menopause at an average age of 26.5 and 31.4 years, respectively. This outcome would likely be undesirable for most women, as recent trends reveal it is becoming increasingly common for women in their late 30s to early 40s to attempt pregnancy for the first time.[50] Therefore, attempts should be made to limit the ovarian dose as much as reasonably possible.

Radionucleotide Therapy

Radiation given in the form of radionucleotide therapy may have a noticeable, although temporary, effect on female fertility. Radioactive [131]Iodine (RAI) is the most common radionucleotide administered, and its damaging effects are the result of beta particle emission. Bal et al.[51] evaluated 1,282 women treated with RAI, 692 (54%) of whom were premenopausal between the ages of 18 and 45. The goal was to assess female fertility and genetic risk to offspring. For a prescription dose range of 25 to 150 mCi, ovarian absorbed dose was 0.035 to 0.06 Gy (mean, 0.12 Gy ± 0.11). Forty women had 50 pregnancies, with 3 spontaneous abortions and 44 babies with normal birth weight and developmental milestones. The authors concluded that female fertility is not affected by high dose RAI treatment, and there is no apparent genetic risk to offspring.

The topic of ^{131}I toxicity was thoroughly examined by Sawka et al.,[52] who reviewed data from 16 studies of 3,023 women and adolescents with differentiated thyroid cancer (DTC). They found that changes in menstrual timing or flow following RAI treatment for DTC may occur in approximately 12% to 31% of women. Temporary interruption of menses may be present in 8% to 27% of women, starting 1 to 6 months or cycles after administration of therapeutic RAI and continuing between 1 and 10 months or cycles. Transient elevations of serum gonadotrophins (FSH and LH) have been noted with these episodes of temporary oligomenorrhoea, indicating a temporary decline in ovarian function. Overall, these menstrual and hormone abnormalities have been noted to end within a year from receiving RAI. Women in their mid-30s or older are at higher risk of experiencing these effects compared to younger women. Menopause may occur slightly earlier for women treated with RAI (mean or median age in the late 40s) versus women who did not receive this therapy (mean or median age in the early 50s). In general, RAI treatment for DTC was not associated with an increased long-term risk of infertility, induced abortions, miscarriage, stillbirths, 1-year neonatal mortality, or congenital defects, especially when compared with controls.[52]

CHEMOTHERAPY

In patients being treated for various cancers, on multivariate analysis the use of chemotherapy has been predictive of POF along with radiation dosage and age.[53] Chemotherapy

TABLE 35.2	Cytotoxic Agents According to Degree of Gonadotoxicity

High risk
  Cyclophosphamide
  Cholarambucil
  Melphalan
  Busulfan
  Nitrogen mustard
  Procarbazine
Intermediate risk
  Cisplatin
  Adriamycin
Low/no risk
  Methotrexate
  5-Fluorouracil
  Vincristine
  Bleomycin
  Actinomycin D

Source: Reprinted from Sonmezer M, Oktay K. Fertility preservation in female patients. *Hum Reprod Update*. 2004;10(3):251–266, with permission.

damages the steroid-producing cells of the ovary (granulosa and theca cells) more than oocytes, as most anticancer drugs have a greater effect on dividing cells. Typically, the ovaries of women who have received chemotherapy have a normal to mildly decreased number of primordial follicles, and a greater decrease in the number of larger maturing follicles.[54,55] Clinically, many postmenarchal women are amenorrheic during chemotherapy, often having elevated gonadotropin levels, but menstrual function and fertility return months to years after chemotherapy administration has ended.[56–58]

The likelihood of ovarian toxicity is age, drug, and dose dependent. As with radiation, younger women are less often affected than older women, likely because they have more oocytes in reserve.[59] The main offending agents are alkylators, although many other agents have been found to cause toxicity.[60] The effect of various chemotherapy agents on ovarian function varies widely, some having no effect and others producing permanent hypogonadism (Table 35.2).[60]

The toxicity of chemotherapy regimens is more easily assessed than for single agents, as patients are most often treated with multiple drugs. For example, ABVD (adriamycin, bleomycin, vinblastine, and dacarbazine) is significantly less likely to cause amenorrhea than MOPP (mechlorethamine, vincristine, procarbazine, and prednisone).[61] However, there have been reports of normal pregnancies and deliveries in patients who underwent autologous bone marrow transplantation involving high dose cyclophosphamide even after receiving MOPP.[56] Amenorrhea, not menopause, is the endpoint most frequently evaluated in various series involving chemotherapy. Serum gonadotropin and E_2 concentrations are much less often evaluated, and when recorded women with normal ovarian function and those with hypogonadism often have overlapping values.[62]

Chemotherapy does not appear to cause increased risk of congenital abnormalities[63] and children appear to develop normally.[64] Although an elevated risk of spontaneous abortion has been noted,[65] chemotherapy does not appear to cause increased risk of miscarriage, fetal demise, or low birth weight according to the available data.[66]

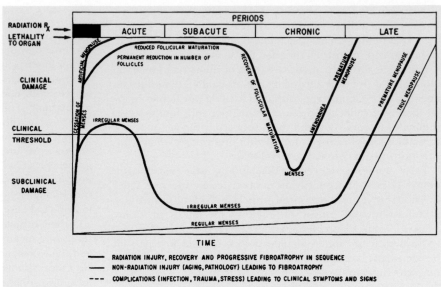

Figure 35.9. The ovary is a radiosensitive organ requiring only modest doses for complete ablation. The cessation of menses after irradiation may not occur at the first menstrual period but may require a few cycles (*upper line*). Temporary cessation or sterilization can result with a few hundred roentgens or rads; despite recovery, a premature menopause is most likely to occur (*lower line*). The loss of granulosa cells as well as the primary oocytes leads to the parallel changes of depression of endocrine levels (estrogens) and of reproductive capacity. (Reprinted from Rubin P, Casarett G. The female genital tract. In: *Clinical Radiation Pathology.* Vol I. Philadelphia, PA: W.B. Saunders Company; 1968:396–423, with pernmission.)

TESTING OF FUNCTION FOLLOWING IRRADIATION & DEFINITION OF TOXICITY (ACUTE, SUBACUTE, AND LATE EFFECTS)

ACUTE

Within 4 to 8 weeks after radiation exposure, serum E2 levels decline. Serum levels of FSH and LH rise progressively.[19] Temporary amenorrhea results from the depletion of maturing follicles, while permanent amenorrhea results from destruction of primordial follicles.[67]

SUBACUTE

Women whose ovaries were irradiated with very small doses causing at most only brief amenorrhea or sterility may show complete recovery even after 6 to 18 months, although the number of primordial follicles will be decreased (Fig. 35.9).[18] Larger doses (e.g., 170 R, or 1.7 Gy) may cause a reduction or absence of mature or developing follicles, associated with continued temporary amenorrhea or sterility. At high enough doses, permanent sterility will occur with the ovary having complete or near complete absence of normal follicles. Some follicles will be in the process of gradual atrophy, in association with the beginning of secondary involutional changes in secondary genitalia and the symptoms of menopause.[18]

LATE EFFECTS

Premature Ovarian Failure

Larger doses (1.7–2.5 Gy or more for younger women) may cause significant but temporary amenorrhea or sterility, with recommencement of ovulation not occurring for years.[18] Pathologically, ovaries have a sizable reduction of primordial follicles, and followed longitudinally these ovaries have marked premature involution. Doses high enough to cause permanent sterility may cause total or near total absence of primordial follicles, with involution of the remaining follicles, and degenera-

tion and decrease of the corpora lutea and interstitial gland cells. This occurs concurrently with vascular sclerosis and replacement fibrosis.[3,18] Even ovaries that have recovered partly or almost entirely will show evidence of residual damage.[18]

A major toxicity of concern resulting from radiation is POF with its resulting loss of reproductive potential. POF is defined as cessation of menstruation (hypergonadotrophic amenorrhea) before the age of 40 years, and it occurs in up to 0.9% of women in the general population.[16] The end of ovarian function results in a remarkable decrease in ovarian steroid and inhibin production. The ultimate result is the freeing of the hypothalamus and pituitary gland from ovarian negative feedback, and gonadotropin levels rise (Fig. 35.10).[16] Ovarian failure may also be defined as failure to undergo or complete pubertal development, as LH and FSH may remain normal in a prepubertal child. Therefore, it may be necessary to wait until a patient is 10- to 12 years old before detecting these abnormalities is possible. Primary amenorrhea is defined as the lack of spontaneous onset of menstrual function (a) by

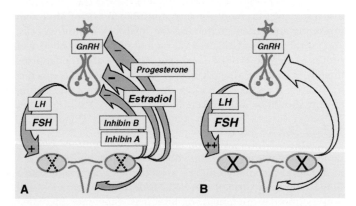

Figure 35.10. During the menopausal transition (A), the decrease in ovarian feedback is characterized by lower levels of inhibin B, inhibin A, and progesterone, whereas E$_2$ levels are normal or elevated. After menopause (B), FSH and LH levels increase dramatically, reflecting stimulation by GnRH in the absence of ovarian restraint. (Reprinted from Hall JE. Neuroendocrine physiology of the early and late menopause. *Endocrinol Metab Clin North Am.* 2004;33:637–659, with permission).

14 years of age in the absence of development of secondary sexual characteristics or (b) by 16 years of age with secondary sexual development.[68] Secondary amenorrhea is cessation of spontaneous menstrual function for >6 months. Menopause is defined as the permanent cessation of menstrual function, although it is not officially recognized until after 12 months of amenorrhea.[69] Coinciding symptoms include hot flashes, vaginal dryness, headaches, dizziness, sweating, and numbness or tingling of fingers.[70] Of additional concern is the fact that any premature loss of estrogen production predisposes women for osteoporosis and coronary artery disease.

Early studies produced understanding that cessation of menses does not necessarily mean absence of endocrine activity. Diczfalusy et al.[39] measured urinary excretion of estrone, estradiol-17β, and estriol in 96-hour specimens of urine collected from 17 premenopausal cancer patients. This was performed at five different time points: (a) the first part of the menstrual cycle (follicular phase), (b) the second part of the cycle (luteal phase), (c) 2 months following ovarian irradiation, (d) 4 months following ovarian irradiation, and (e) 7 months following radiation, after an oophorectomy that was performed at 5 months post radiation. Of the three evaluated hormones, the decrease in estriol was most marked at 90%, whereas estrone and E_2 only decreased by 50%. The drop in the ratio of estriol to estrone and E_2 was significantly higher for radiated patients versus those undergoing bilateral oophorectomy ($p = 0.001$), indicating that surgical castration did not diminish the excretion of estrogen more than irradiation. Neither procedure fully eliminates estrogen production, as adrenals continue to produce estrogen.

The precursor to ovarian failure is decreased ovarian reserve, defined by a poor ovarian response to stimulation.[16] This suggests a decreased number of oocytes. Even if a woman has normal ovulatory cycles, FSH levels that are elevated early in the menstrual cycle may indicate diminished ovarian reserve. Serum FSH levels are usually under 10 mIU/mL in most assays on day 3 of the menstrual cycle. FSH levels more than 15 mIU/mL on day 3 suggest a reduced ovarian reserve and a decreased chance of pregnancy, with an extremely low probability at levels above 20 mIU/mL. Serum E_2 levels above 80 pg/mL indicate abnormal folliculogenesis.[71] Other tests of ovarian reserve include: the clomiphene citrate challenge test;[72] the GnRH agonist test;[73] measurements of serum inhibin B[74] or of Mullerian inhibiting substance[75] reflecting the health of granulosa cells; and antral follicle assessment via vaginal ultrasound. Abnormal results of these tests portend a pregnancy probability of approximately 5%, although each has its own sensitivity and specificity. If a test is abnormal, a more aggressive approach to testing fertility should be undertaken.[66]

Second Malignancy

Benign ovarian tumors occur with a remarkably high frequency in sublethally irradiated mice.[76] Most female mice exposed to a single total body dose of 87 to 350 R developed granulosa-cell tumors, tubular adenomas, or luteomas. Incidence increased with time from exposure, with potentially all animals affected after 17 months. However, similar effects have not been observed for human ovaries. In a review of 2,068 women who received 350 to 720 R to the ovaries for menorrhagia, there were no excess cases of ovarian cancer observed after mean of 19 years.[37]

Genetic Effect of Radiation on Offspring

There is concern regarding radiation-induced genetic abnormalities that could potentially produce birth defects and cancer in offspring (e.g., germ-line mutations and chromosomal aberrations). Theoretically, since radiation-induced mutagenesis is a stochastic effect, any radiation dose involves a risk of causing a mutation.[22] Following substantial doses of radiation which do not cause sterility, there is a residual increase in genic or chromosomal abnormalities in oocytes. Although high doses of radiation in experimental animals have caused a range of disorders in their progeny,[23] multiple large studies involving humans have not found any increased risk of genetic disease. The most significant human cohort evaluated in regard to the genetic effects of ionizing radiation involves the survivors of the atomic bombings and their offspring. The initial survivors exposed to radiation received a mean dose of approximately 0.2 Gy, and this group and their descendants have been followed since the late 1940s. No excess abnormalities have been noted for various outcomes including: stillbirth, mortality, malformations, chromosome aberrations, DNA studies, protein electrophoresis, weight, and sex ratio.[77, 78] Little[79] performed a thorough review of studies involving the Chernobyl accident, and found no consistent evidence of a harmful effect on congenital abnormalities or other pregnancy outcome measures. The UNSCEAR (United Nations Scientific Committee on Effects of Atomic Radiation) report also studied various other groups exposed to radiation, including patients receiving radiation treatments, populations living in areas with elevated background radiation, the population in Hungary exposed to Chernobyl radionuclides (e.g., ^{131}I), and radiologic technicians. The investigators found little risk of hereditary damage in all these groups exposed to moderately low levels of ionizing radiation.[77] A case control study was performed using computerized record linkage to ascertain the incidence of cancer in parents of children born with an anomaly versus a matched sample of children's parents without abnormalities. Over 170,000 parents were analyzed, and the cancer incidence was similar between groups with no association found between congenital abnormalities and cancer treatment method (including radiation therapy and chemotherapy with alkylating agents).[80] Multiple large studies comparing cancer survivors and case-control sibling matches have found no increased incidence of genetic disease in offspring.[81-83] Furthermore, various investigators have not found any excess cases of stillbirths, low birth weight, congenital malformations, abnormal karyotypes, or cancer in the offspring of women treated for Hodgkin lymphoma.[84,85]

In contrast to these reassuring studies, Green et al.[86] reported on a series of pregnancy outcomes that included 427 pregnancies sustained 20 weeks or more after treatment for Wilms tumor. The authors found a trend toward an increased risk of congenital anomalies in previously radiated women ($p = 0.054$). No influence of radiation dose was found on the likelihood of abnormalities. Despite being the largest follow-up series of Wilms tumor patients, the sample size of this series is small. The patient number is particularly limited compared to the previously discussed substantial series involving parental radiation exposure or therapy, all of which did not find an increased risk of congenital anomalies. In addition, anomalies noted such as cleft palate and lip found in 3 patients could have been hereditary in nature. Ventricular septal defects, which occurred in 3 children, are the most common congenital defect and may have been spontaneous in nature rather than due to radiation.[86,87]

Pregnancy Outcomes Following Pelvic Radiation

Although genetic abnormalities are not seen in offspring, some genetic effects may be deduced from observations of increased incidence of spontaneous abortion. Alternatively, radiation effects on the uterus could be attributed to undesirable pregnancy outcomes. Hawkins[88] studied female survivors given abdominal or gonadal irradiation versus controls. There were increased miscarriages for first pregnancies (19% vs. 8%) and all pregnancies (17% vs. 9%), as well as an increased incidence low birth weight. However, consistent with larger scale studies, there was no effect on the sex ratio and no increase in serious congenital abnormalities. The authors concluded that there was no association of radiation with potentially mutagenic harm to germ cells.

Pregnancy outcomes have been studied in over 300 children borne from Wilms tumor survivors.[86] Adverse neonatal outcomes including low birth weight (<2,500 g) and preterm birth occurred more frequently for irradiated survivors. Higher radiation doses correlated with increased risk. Since pregnancies conceived with male survivors did not have these abnormalities, it is thought unlikely that radiation-induced genetic oocyte mutations were the cause. Mulvihill et al.[89,90] found an increase in low birth weight and spontaneous abortions, especially if conception occurred <1 year after radiation. Thus, the authors suggested this could represent defects in factors (e.g., uterine or hormonal) that normally maintain gestations. Therefore, it is recommended for patients to delay pregnancy for 1 year following radiation. Uterine dysfunction following prepubertal irradiation has been noted with TBI doses as low as 14.4 Gy,

indicating children of this age are particularly sensitive to uterine radiation.[91] Critchley and Wallace[92] evaluated patients who received TBI and or flank radiation as children. Despite estrogen replacement, uteruses were only 40% of normal adult size. If pregnancy was achieved, there was still a risk of early pregnancy loss, premature labor, and low birth weight due to impaired uterine growth and blood flow.

In summary, pelvic irradiation appears to be correlated with complications such as miscarriage, preterm labor and delivery, low birth weight, and placenta accreata. Genetic damage to oocytes cannot explain these findings. One possible mechanism is that radiation causes small arteriolar damage leading to decreased fetoplacental blood flow, thus impairing fetal growth.[88] Preterm labor and delivery could result from decreased uterine elasticity and volume from myometrial changes related to radiation.[92] Placenta accreata or percreta may be the result of radiation damage to the endometrium, causing disorders of placental attachment.[93,94]

STRATEGIES FOR AVOIDING TOXICITY

INTRODUCTION

Potential options to avoid ovarian toxicity vary widely between patients depending on the risk of ovarian involvement with cancer, the types of cancer treatment, patient age, the time available before the start of treatment, the estrogen sensitivity of the tumor, and partner availability for fertilization.[60] Figure 35.11 provides an algorithm as to how to approach fertility preservation strategies.

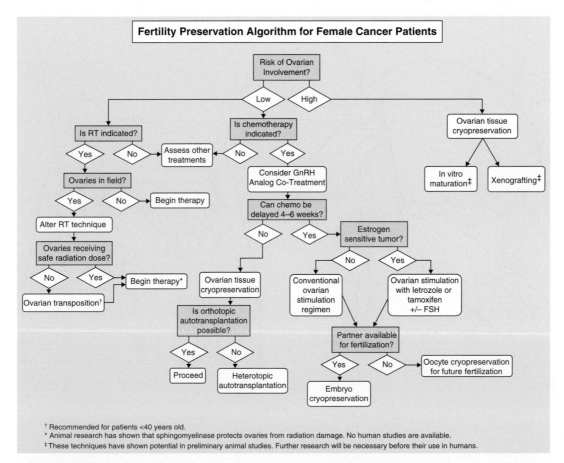

† Recommended for patients <40 years old.
* Animal research has shown that sphingomyelinase protects ovaries from radiation damage. No human studies are available.
‡ These techniques have shown potential in preliminary animal studies. Further research will be necessary before their use in humans.

Figure 35.11. Fertility preservation algorithm for the female cancer patient. Options differ based on the risk of ovarian involvement with cancer, the treatment modalities used, patient age, time available before the start of treatment, the estrogen sensitivity of the tumor, and partner availability for fertilization.

RADIATION TECHNIQUE

It is always appropriate to choose a radiation beam orientation that minimizes ovarian dose. For example, attention to the beam angle may limit ovarian dose for patients undergoing cranio-spinal radiation (CSI). Harden et al.[95] evaluated eight females with medulloblastoma, all of whom had a pelvic MRI in the treatment position to localize the ovaries before treatment planning. Doses ranged from 23.4 Gy in 13 fractions to 35 Gy in 19 fractions. Plans were compared using conventional spinal fields (one or two fields used depending on patient height) versus a half beam block at the inferior border to achieve a nondivergent edge (two fields used in each case). They found that with a non-

divergent beam inferiorly, the mean ovarian dose was reduced by a median value of 2.45 Gy (range, 0.6–19.5 Gy). The median percent dose reduction was 66.8% (range, 2.6–84.6%). This modified technique doubled the number of patients receiving <4 Gy to a single ovary from three to six, and three patients received <1.5 Gy. In conclusion, they recommend using a half beam block at the inferior spinal border to decrease dose.

Peripheral dose from head leakage as well as collimator and patient scatter must be taken into consideration, as their contribution to ovarian dose may be significant.[96] Increased head leakage occurs with intensity-modulated radiation therapy (IMRT) compared with three-dimensional conformal radiation therapy (3DCRT) due to the additional monitor units required for

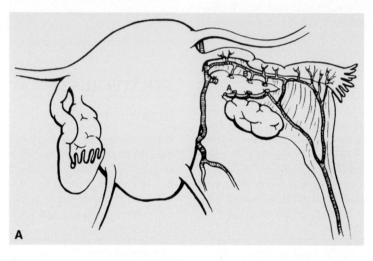

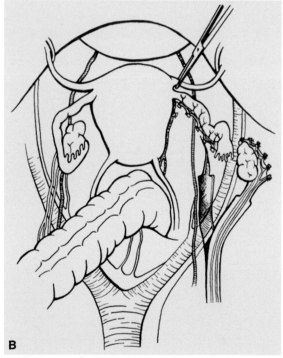

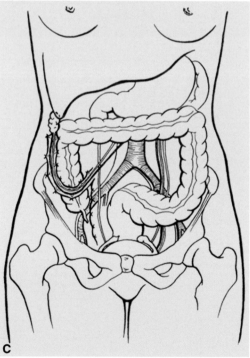

Figure 35.12. **A**: The peritoneum of the mesovarium is opened and the utero-ovarian ligament and the utero-ovarian artery (A) are divided. The marginal tubal artery (B) can be visualized. **B**: The ovary is completely disconnected from the fallopian tube and it is moved dividing the peritoneum on both sides above the ovarian funiculus. **C**: Position of the right ovary when transposed into the paracolic gutter. The left ovary will also be transposed into the paracolic gutter, at the same height. (Reprinted from Gaetini A, De Simone M, Urgesi A, et al. Lateral high abdominal ovariopexy: an original surgical technique for protection of the ovaries during curative radiotherapy for Hodgkin's disease. *J Surg Oncol.* 1988;39:22–28, with permission.)

treatment delivery.[97] For distant targets such as the breast and central nervous system, ovarian dose is increased although the absolute dose may be very small.[98] However, ovaries outside the field edge but within the range of internal scatter may receive a lower peripheral dose using IMRT. This is due to reduced internal scatter from smaller effective field sizes with IMRT dynamic multi–leaf collimators, which outweighs the effect of lower head leakage from 3DCRT.[99] The method and frequency of patient positioning verification may affect ovarian dose as well, especially with the increasing popularity of image-guided radiation therapy (IGRT) techniques such as cone beam CT.[100]

OVARIAN TRANSPOSITION (OOPHOROPEXY)

If it is not possible to sufficiently limit the ovarian dose by altering radiation treatment technique, it may be appropriate to displace the ovary from the radiation portals. The procedures used to accomplish this are ovarian transposition or oophoropexy.

Details of Surgical Procedure

For transposition of the ovary via laparotomy, the peritoneum of the mesovarium is opened, exposing the utero-ovarian ligament and the utero-ovarian artery (Fig. 35.12A).[101] These structures are divided in succession, and then the remaining mesovarium between the ovaries and fallopian tubes is incised (Fig. 35.12B). Next, the peritoneum along the infundibulopelvic ligament is incised up to the level of the aortic bifurcation[102] or paracolic gutter.[103] The ovary, now vascularized only by ovarian vessels, is mobilized with the vessels ideally at least 3 cm from the border of the radiation field (Fig. 35.12C).[101] Ovaries are most commonly

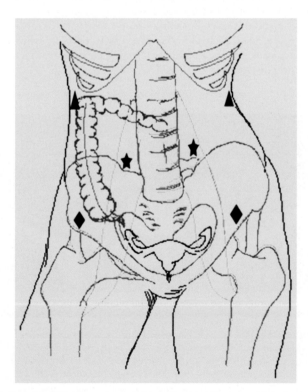

Figure 35.13. Schematic drawing shows common locations for ovarian transposition: laterally within pelvis, in lower paracolic gutters (◆), anterior to psoas muscles (★), and in intra-abdominal paracolic gutters (▲). Reprinted with permission from the American Journal of Roentgenology. (From Sella T, Mironov S, Hricak H. Imaging of transposed ovaries in patients with cervical carcinoma. *Am J Roentgenol.* 2005;184:1602–1610.)

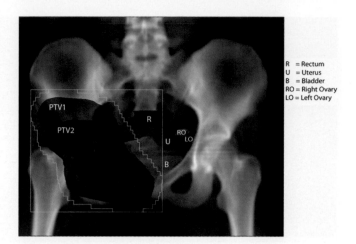

Figure 35.14. The AP radiation portal for a 16-year-old girl status post resection of a right hip Ewing sarcoma. The right (*orange*) and the left (*light green*) ovaries were mobilized to the left pelvic sidewall, both in continuity with their fallopian tubes. The ovaries would have been at the field edge without this procedure, but are now well outside the field edge (*yellow*) surrounding PTV1 and PTV2.

positioned laterally to the intra-abdominal or lower paracolic gutters, close to the lateral aspect of the colon near the iliac fossa level, or to the posterior intraperitoneal space in the upper pelvis, lateral or anterolateral to the psoas muscle (Fig. 35.13).[104] The radiation oncologist should communicate the borders of the treatment field to the surgeon, so they may determine the optimal location for ovarian transposition as a team. Metallic clips should be attached to the borders of the ovaries so that radiation oncologists may identify each ovary's new position.[105] It has been found that transposed ovaries can potentially migrate back to their original position, so transposition is best done immediately preceding radiation therapy using nonabsorbable sutures.[105,106]

A laparoscopic transposition method is now preferred, as it is less invasive and radiation need not be delayed while awaiting laparotomy incision healing.[107] Radiation may begin within 1 to 2 days following laparoscopy. Additional benefits are lower rates of complications,[103] better cosmesis, and lower cost.[103,108]

In some instances, the ovaries may not need to be moved very far to be out of the treatment field. In this situation, the ovary may be moved in continuity with the fallopian tube, and potentially no ligaments need to be divided. This arrangement may facilitate later attempts at pregnancy, although pregnancy is still possible with ovarian transplantation far from the fallopian tube.[109] Figure 35.14 shows the anterior-posterior (AP) radiation portal for a 16-year-old girl in need of adjuvant radiation following resection of a right hip Ewing sarcoma. Thirty-six Gray was prescribed to the lower-risk planning target volume (PTV1), with 45 Gy prescribed to the higher-risk area (PTV2). Her right ovary (orange) was mobilized to the left pelvic sidewall in continuity with its fallopian tube, and the left ovary (light green) was moved slightly superiorly above the iliac vessels. This procedure placed the ovaries out of the radiation field, resulting in the delivery of only a small scatter dose ranging from 0.50 to 0.84 Gy (Fig. 35.15) Oophoropexy may be performed medially as well, during which the ovaries are placed in the midline of the true pelvis and sutured to the surface of the uterus.[110] In this technique, central shielding is required to further protect the ovaries.

Stillman et al.[62] evaluated prognostic factors for ovarian failure in a cohort of patients ages 1 to 17 years old. Of 25 patients with both ovaries in-field (mean dose: 32 Gy; range: 12–50),

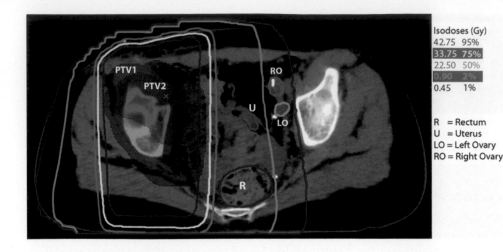

Figure 35.15. Only a small scatter dose ranging from 1.1% (0.50 Gy) to 1.9% (0.84 Gy) of the prescription dose (45 Gy to PTV2 with 36 Gy to PTV1) is reaching the ovaries. Assistance in ovarian identification is provided by the radio-opaque clips attached during transposition.

there was 68% ovarian failure. For 35 patients with at least one in-field ovary (mean dose: 2.9 Gy; range: 0.9–10), there was 14% failure. For 34 patients with both ovaries outside the treatment field (mean dose: 0.54 Gy, range: 0.05–1.5), there were no failures. Therefore, it is recommended to surgically move both ovaries out of the radiation field, as damaging even one ovary increases the chance of POF.

Indications

There is no age at which ovarian transposition is contraindicated, and it is appropriate to discuss this procedure with all premenopausal women. However, it is generally not recommended for those over 40 years old, as women in this age group have an intrinsically reduced fertilization potential and therefore a higher risk for ovarian failure despite transposition.[108] However,

for women under 40 this procedure has been associated with preservation of ovarian function in 88.6% of cases.[109] Transposition is not recommended for cancers for which there is a high risk of ovarian metastases (Table 35.3).[60] In one report, 2 out of 107 patients developed ovarian metastases following transposition for Stage IB cervical cancer. Therefore, the authors advised against transposition for tumors >3 cm in diameter because of increased risk of metastases.[111]

Identifying Surgically Transposed Ovaries

The CT identification of surgically transposed arteries is aided by identifying surgical clips marking their location,[112] recognizing characteristic morphologic features of ovaries such as physiologic cysts, and tracking ovarian blood vessels (OBVs) toward the ovaries (Fig. 35.16).[6,113] Ovarian vessels in lateral transposition typically deviate laterally near the iliac fossa rather than coursing inferiorly into the pelvis.

TABLE 35.3	The Risk of Ovarian Metastasis According to Cancer Types

Cancers with low risk of ovarian involvement
  Wilms tumor
  Ewing sarcoma
  Breast cancer
    Stages I–III
    Infiltrative ductal histological subtype
  Non-Hodgkin lymphoma
  Hodgkin lymphoma
  Nongenital rhabdomyosarcoma
  Osteogenic sarcoma
  Squamous cell carcinoma of the cervix
Cancers with moderate risk of ovarian involvement
  Adenocarcinoma/adenosquamous carcinoma of the cervix
  Colon cancer
  Breast cancer
    Stage IV
    Infiltrative lobular histological subtype
Cancers with high risk of ovarian involvement
  Leukemia
  Neuroblastoma
  Burkitt lymphoma

Source: Reprinted from Sonmezer M, Oktay K. Fertility preservation in female patients. *Hum Reprod Update.* 2004;10(3):251–266, with permission.

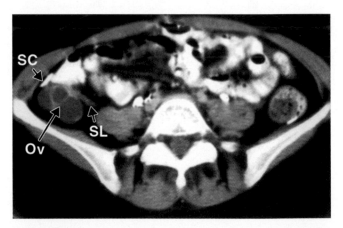

Figure 35.16. Surgically transposed ovary in a young patient with cervical cancer. CT scan shows the right ovary (Ov) positioned close to the colon at the level of the iliac fossa; the ovary is characterized by its multiple physiologic cysts. The laterally placed surgical clip (SC) is a marker for the ovary. In cases of lateral transposition, the OBVs typically course laterally near the iliac fossa and lead to the suspensory ligament (SL), which is seen joining the ovary. (Reprinted from Saksouk FA, Johnson SC. Recognition of the ovaries and ovarian origin of pelvic masses with CT. *Radiographics.* 2004;24(suppl 1):S133–S146, with permission.)

Outcomes with Lateral Versus Medial Transposition

The planned radiation field guides the proper location to fix transposed ovaries.[109] Lateral transposition has always been the procedure of choice for various carcinomas including cervical cancer, although medial transposition was initially performed for Hodgkin lymphoma. Hadar et al.[114] evaluated the postoperative CT scans of 16 patients following ovarian transposition. A gynecological oncologist performed lateral transposition on seven patients with cervical cancer, and nine patients with Hodgkin lymphoma had medial transposition. The location of each ovary was depicted on diagrams of the respective radiation fields. For those receiving lateral transposition, all 13 ovaries were easily identified, and 11 of the 13 ovaries (for 6 of 7 patients) were outside the radiation field (Fig. 35.17). The single patient with in-field ovaries received 4.5 Gy and developed POF. For the medially transposed group, only 13 of 18 ovaries were easily identified despite the fact that metallic clips were placed on each ovary (Fig. 35.18). Three of the 13 identified ovaries were completely outside the field ($p = 0.005$), but they still received 3 Gy. The authors concluded that lateral transposition is preferable to medial for patients with lymphoma requiring pelvic radiation. Even given proper placement of the ovary, scatter and transmission through central ovarian shielding can result in delivery of 8% to 15% of the prescription dose to the ovaries.[105,110] Clough et al.[108] demonstrated that it is possible to mobilize an ovary well out of an inverted-Y Hodgkin lymphoma radiation field via lateral transposition (Fig. 35.19).

Gaetini et al.[101] evaluated 6 patients with Hodgkin lymphoma, for whom lateral high ovarian transposition (LHAO) was performed before pelvic radiation. Doses were also calculated assuming the ovaries were either in their normal position

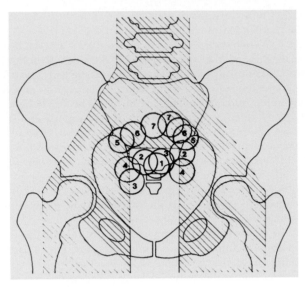

Figure 35.18. Schematic representation of the female pelvis. The transposed ovaries (medial ovarian transposition) are depicted according to their position on the computed tomography scan. Each number represents a single patient. The shaded area represents the radiation field. (Reprinted from Wiley-Liss, Inc., a subsidiary of John Wiley & Sons, Inc. Hadar H, Loven D, Herskovitz P, et al. An evaluation of lateral and medial transposition of the ovaries out of radiation fields. *Cancer.* 1994;74:774–779, with permission. Copyright 1994 American Cancer Society.)

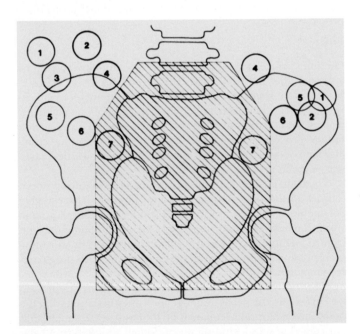

Figure 35.17. Schematic representation of the female pelvis. The transposed ovaries (lateral ovarian transposition) are depicted according to their position on the computed tomography scan. Each number represents a single patient. The shaded area represents the radiation field. (Reprinted from Wiley-Liss, Inc., a subsidiary of John Wiley & Sons, Inc. Hadar H, Loven D, Herskovitz P, et al. An evaluation of lateral and medial transposition of the ovaries out of radiation fields. *Cancer.* 1994;74:774–779, with permission. Copyright 1994 American Cancer Society.)

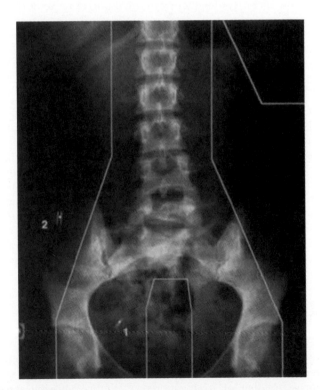

Figure 35.19. Laparoscopic transposition of the right ovary before inverted Y radiotherapy for Hodgkin's disease. The irradiation field is outlined with a white line. Two metal clips have been applied on the transposed ovary (2), whereas one clip marks the original position of the ovary before transposition (1). (From Clough KB, Goffinet F, Labib A, et al. Laparoscopic unilateral ovarian transposition prior to irradiation: prospective study of 20 cases. *Cancer.* 1996;77(2):2638–2645.)

or if they were transposed medially. They found that for a total nodal irradiation dose of 36 Gy, the ovaries would have received 35.3 ± 0.90 Gy in their natural position and 5.3 ± 2.2 Gy if placed medially. Instead, they were exposed to 3.2 ± 0.75 Gy following LHAO, significantly less dose than if placed medially ($p < 0.01$). All patients but one had continued normal menses and hormone values, and one patient gave birth to a healthy baby. Howard[115] performed a compilation of 10 case reports and small series comparing medial and lateral transposition. Ovarian failure occurred in 50% of patients with a medial transposition, but only 14% of patients with a lateral procedure. They concluded that superior outcomes are achieved with lateral transposition. In addition, lateral oophoropexy significantly decreases toxicity for patients receiving CSI as the ovaries may be moved out of the spinal field.[116]

In the case of brachytherapy, lateral transposition is an effective method for minimizing radiation exposure. For 14 patients receiving brachytherapy alone, Clough et al.[108] were consistently able to limit the ovarian dose, as calculated by computerized dosimetry, to under 3.3% (2.2 Gy) of a prescription dose of 65 Gy. The only two cases of menopause reported for patients receiving brachytherapy alone involved women over 40 years old. Haie-Meder et al.[53] did not report any instances of ovarian failure for 23 patients under 40 receiving brachytherapy alone to 60 Gy, with a median dose of 2.2 ± 1.30 Gy (3.7% dose).

Although pregnancies have been achieved following lateral ovarian transposition (LOT),[101,102] when ovaries are moved to an abdominal location a second procedure may be necessary to allow for spontaneous pregnancy.[109] Furthermore, if in vitro fertilization (IVF) is subsequently needed, oocyte retrieval could be more challenging. Therefore, candidates for ovarian transposition should be selected considering all the variables that affect its success.

Complications

The most common complication from ovarian transposition is the development of ovarian cysts, with an incidence ranging from 0% to 23%.[103,117–119] Some older series involving a laparotomy reported incidences of painful cysts ranging as high as 21% to 23%.[117,119] However, a recent report of 28 patients undergoing serial CT scans following laparoscopic transposition revealed cysts in only 2 patients, and although removed they were asymptomatic.[103] Ovarian cysts may be suppressed with oral contraceptives or GNRH-α with surgery reserved for patients refractory to medical treatment.[117] Chronic ovarian pain, vascular injury to ovaries, and infarction of the fallopian tubes are rare but have been reported as well.[102,105,118,119]

CRYOPRESERVATION

Embryo

Cryopreservation of embryos is an established technique after IVF. Implantation potential of frozen-thawed embryos approaches that of fresh embryos.[120] Embryo survival rates range from 35% to 90%, implantation rates from 8% to 30%, and cumulative pregnancy rates can exceed 60%.[60] However, there are a few potential drawbacks to this procedure. For one, the patient either needs a male partner or a donor sperm for oocyte fertilization.[60] Delays in initiating cancer therapy might be unacceptable, as treatment may be scheduled to begin before the 2 to 3 weeks required for ovulation induction and retrieval.[121] Even if time is available, the potential harm of supraphysiological E_2 levels must be considered for estrogen-sensitive tumors.[50] Agents involved in the treatment of anovulatory infertility include selective estrogen receptor modulators (e.g., tamoxifen) and aromatase inhibitors (e.g., letrozole).[122] A regimen of letrozole and FSH has been found to result in lower E_2 levels and higher oocyte recovery than tamoxifen with FSH or tamoxifen alone, making it a particularly appealing option for estrogen-sensitive tumors.[122,123] In addition, this treatment does not appear to increase the risk of cancer recurrence.[124]

Oocyte

Oocyte cryopreservation is an investigational procedure for women without a partner who decide against a sperm donor for IVF. As this process requires ovarian stimulation for the maturation of the oocyte, the potential pitfalls of delaying cancer treatment and stimulating estrogen-sensitive tumors remain. This process is less successful than IVF due to the fragility of the meiotic spindle and the formation of ice crystals,[125] although improved success may be obtained with the fast-freeze process of vitrification.[126] A recent meta-analysis of the vitrification process found that the modern mean fertilization rate, live-birth rate per injected oocyte, and live-birth rate per oocyte transfer were 75.4%, 4.6%, and 39%, respectively.[126] Of note, there is a theoretical concern of increased karyotypic abnormalities due to potential damage to the oocyte metaphase spindle during cryopreservation. However, these deleterious effects have not yet been observed.[127–129] The Practice Committee of the American Society for Reproductive Medicine recommends offering this procedure to women given informed consent in an institutional-review-board (IRB)-approved investigational protocol.[130]

Ovary

Ovarian tissue cryopreservation is another investigational approach that holds promise. Unlike embryo or oocyte cryopreservation, there is no need for ovarian stimulation with its resulting delay in cancer treatment.[60] In addition, no partner is needed, and the reimplanted ovarian tissue could produce hormones. Primordial follicles are much more resistant to cryoinjury than oocytes due to their slower metabolic rates, decreased size, and absent zona pellucida.[50]

The main challenge in this process involves maturing stored follicles to the necessary stage for fertilization. Three potential methods to accomplish this include autotransplantation (orthotopically or heterotopically), xenotransplantation, and in vitro maturation.[121] Autotransplantation currently shows the most potential, with return of ovarian function and pregnancy seen in animal studies and a few human cases.[131–134] Orthotopic ovarian transplantation involves placing thawed slices of ovarian cortex into the pelvis under general anesthesia, allowing the possibility of natural pregnancy. Heterotopic transplantation is performed in sites including the abdomen and forearm,[135] and has advantages of not requiring general anesthesia and more easily monitored follicle development. This procedure may be preferable over ovarian transposition when the likelihood of success is low and/or the chance of developing ovarian cancer or metastases is high.[135] In either case, it is highly recommended that the patient not delay childbearing as the functionality of the transplanted tissue is between 9 months and 3 years.[136]

Consideration must be given to the possible future risk of developing ovarian cancer, particularly for women with BRCA mutations, and the theoretical concern of reimplantation of metastatic cells from the primary tumor.[60] Malignancies at intermediate risk of ovarian involvement are cervical, colon, and advanced breast cancer, and tumors at higher risk are neuroblastoma, Burkitt lymphoma, and leukemias (Table 35.3).[60] Histological and molecular analysis should be used to rule out ovarian micrometastases.[137] For patients with a high risk of ovarian metastases, xenotransplantation to immunodeficient mice has the potential to eliminate the risk of cancer transmission and relapse, as cancer cells are not able to penetrate the zona pellucida. Mature human follicles have been grown in ovarian tissue xenotransplanted to mice[138] and oocytes have been retrieved successfully.[139] Although bovine oocytes have been fertilized using this method, subsequent embryonic development has not been successful.[140] In addition, this process remains experimental in part due to concerns of transmission of zoonoses to humans.[50] Isolating primordial follicles from cryopreserved ovarian tissue for the purpose of in vitro maturation has been partially successful in mice, but has not yet been investigated in humans.[141]

SYSTEMIC PROPHYLACTIC TREATMENT

The use of a GnRH analogue as a cotreatment during cancer therapy is based on the postulated role of gonadal suppression.[60] Some success in primordial follicle preservation has been found both in Rhesus monkeys and humans receiving chemotherapy.[142-144] Despite fairly preliminary data, many patients, such as those with breast cancer and Hodgkin lymphoma, are receiving this treatment during chemotherapy.[121] However, no protective effect from a GnRH analogue has been noted for Rhesus monkeys against radiation-induced ovarian injury.[145]

A potentially promising radioprotective agent has been studied by Morita et al.[20,21] They demonstrated that the sphingomyelin pathway regulates oocyte apoptosis, and that sphingosine-1-phosphate (SIP) is an apoptotic inhibitor. In vivo treatment entirely prevented radiation induced oocyte loss and preserved fertility in mice,[20] without propagating genomic damage in offspring.[146] Although this has not yet been tested in humans, the future utility of this agent is promising.

OVARIAN GERMLINE STEM CELL TRANSPLANTATION

Traditional dogma has been that female mammals are born with all the oocytes they will ever have. However, recent studies have provided evidence of a female germline stem cell (FGSC) population capable of replenishing the ovarian follicular pool. Zou et al.[147] have established neonatal and adult FGSC lines, which are chromosomally normal and have high telomerase activity. These FGSCs were infected with green fluorescent protein (GFP) virus and then transplanted into ovaries sterilized by chemotherapy. Control ovaries did not show any immature oocytes or follicles following sterilization, but transplanted cells underwent oogenesis and recipient mice produced progeny with the GFP transgene.

Additional work will be needed to determine the effect FGSCs have on the postnatal ovarian follicle pool. It is possible the potential of these cells is only realized after culture in vitro.

Their activity may be suppressed in vivo, as without intervention they currently fail to sustain ovarian function during the lifespan of a normal female mouse. It should be considered that age- or treatment-related ovarian failure may result from impairment in somatic cell support of FGSC activity.[148] Furthermore, research is needed to determine if a similar population of FGSCs exists in human ovaries. Promising findings include the discovery of stem-like cells with germline characteristics in the ovarian surface epithelium of postmenopausal women.[149,150] With future research, someday stem cell-based regenerative medicine may be an option to control the timing of ovarian failure.

TREATMENT OF INJURY

PREMATURE OVARIAN FAILURE

Once POF has occurred, it is irreversible. Therefore, with POF comes menopause and its associated symptoms and risks. For women who do not have hormonally sensitive cancer, consideration should be given to prescribing them hormone replacement therapy (HRT).[151] Verschuuren et al.[151] found that HRT often was not offered to menopausal patients treated for Hodgkin lymphoma and urged caretakers to consider this therapy. Of course, the benefits in quality of life must be balanced with the risks, such as increasing the chance of developing breast cancer. However, women who develop treatment-related POF have a reduced risk of breast cancer. Also, there exists no evidence that women who develop treatment-related POF have an increased risk of breast cancer when compared with women who remain premenopausal after this treatment.[151]

UTERINE INJURY

Hormone replacement may be beneficial for women treated previously with pelvic radiation, in an attempt to ameliorate reduced uterine volume and blood flow. In a series of patients who received TBI, blood flow was significantly improved following three cycles of physiologic hormone replacement although it was still subnormal.[152] To monitor for potential uterine complications from pelvic radiation, placental attachment can be evaluated with sonography in the late second and third trimesters.[153] Fetal growth may be monitored via serial sonograms every 4 to 6 weeks in the late second and third trimesters. Unfortunately, no reliable method exists for prediction and prevention of preterm labor and delivery.[154]

CONCLUSIONS

TIME, DOSE, AND VOLUME RECOMMENDATIONS

The best model available to predict toxicity of the ovary has been described by Wallace et al. (Fig. 35.8 and Table 35.1). The average dose at which 50% of patients will develop immediate ovarian failure was calculated to be 18.9 Gy at birth, 16.9 Gy at 10 years old, 14.9 Gy at 20 years old, and 12.1 Gy at 30 years old.[15] However, merely preventing immediate sterilization is inadequate, as much lower ovarian doses may still preclude any chance of pregnancy. Therefore, the expected age of menopause for a given dose should be determined from Figure 35.8 or Table 35.1, and this information should be relayed to the patient in the context of weighing all risks and benefits of radiation treatment.

Although the authors recognized the limitation of this model in regard to the potentially sparing effect of fractionation, the fact that oocytes die via apoptosis likely limits interfraction sublethal damage repair.[22] This model is therefore reasonable to apply to various fractionation regimens. The effect of partially radiating a single ovary is unknown, although it is noted that radiation to both ovaries is typically required to produce ovarian failure. Whenever possible, sparing both ovaries should be performed to decrease the subsequent risk of POF.[62] In addition, it is important to remember ovaries have some degree of mobility in the pelvis, especially following pregnancy.[10] Therefore, ovaries close to the field edge are at risk to receive a significantly different dose than that predicted at the time of simulation.[15]

RECOMMENDATIONS TO PRESERVE FERTILITY

For patients who lose and later regain ovarian function following high dose radiotherapy or chemotherapy, it is recognized that the number of follicles in reserve is reduced. Therefore, it is strongly recommended that child bearing is not delayed more than necessary. It is recommended to attempt conceiving a few years after a disease-free interval, but not <6 to 12 months due to possible toxicity from treatment to developing oocytes.[89,90,155]

Predicting the likelihood and age of POF is facilitated by the model developed by Wallace et al.,[15] which should be helpful when counseling patients about family planning. Although the toxicity of chemotherapy is well documented, the likelihood of infertility is less easily predicted than with radiation and pregnancies have been documented despite high dose therapy with alkylators. Therefore, for women with a history of ovary-toxic chemotherapy about to undergo pelvic radiation, it may be reasonable to offer ovarian transposition/oophoropexy to those who wish to conceive or delay menopause. There are other options for preserving fertility that should be considered (Fig. 35.11).[60] These complex decisions are aided by inclusion of the appropriate specialists, including medical, radiation, and gynecologic oncologists, as well as fertility specialists.

REFERENCES

1. Jemal A, Siegel R, Ward E, et al. Cancer statistics, 2008. *CA Cancer J Clin.* 2008;58:71–96.
2. *Surveillance, Epidemiology, and End Results.* http://seer.cancer.gov. Accessed April 1, 2008.
3. Fajardo L. *Pathology of Radiation Injury.* 1st ed. New York, NY: Masson Publishing; 1982.
4. Sklar CA, Mertens AC, Mitby P, et al. Premature menopause in survivors of childhood cancer: a report from the childhood cancer survivor study. *J Natl Cancer Inst.* 2006;98:890–896.
5. Gardner E, Gray D, O'Rahilly R, eds. Female genital organs. In: *Anatomy: A Regional Study of Human Structure.* 3rd ed. Philadelphia, PA: Saunders; 1969.
6. Saksouk FA, Johnson SC. Recognition of the ovaries and ovarian origin of pelvic masses with CT. *Radiographics.* 2004;24(suppl 1):S133–S146.
7. Waldroup L, Liu J. Sonographic Anatomy of the Female Pelvis. In: *Diagnostic Medical Sonography: Obstetrics and Gynecology.* Philadelphia, PA: Lippincott Williams & Wilkins; 1991.
8. Cohen HL, Tice HM, Mandel FS. Ovarian volumes measured by US: bigger than we think. *Radiology.* 1990;177:189–192.
9. Moore K, Dalley A, eds. Pelvis and perineum. In: *Clinically Oriented Anatomy.* 4th ed. Philadelphia, PA: Lippincott Williams & Wilkins; 1999.
10. Thorek P. Pelvic viscera in the female. In: *Anatomy in Surgery.* 3rd ed. New York, NY: Springer-Verlag; 1985.
11. Bloom M, Van Dongen L. The Ovaries. In: *Clinical Gynaecology: Integration of Structure and Function.* Philadelphia, PA: Lippincott; 1972.
12. Doherty M. *Clinical Anatomy of the Pelvis.* 2nd ed. Philadelphia, PA: Saunders; 2000.
13. Bazot M, Deligne L, Boudghene F, et al. Correlation between computed tomography and gross anatomy of the suspensory ligament of the ovary. *Surg Radiol Anat.* 1999;21:341–346.
14. Langer JE, Jacobs JE. High-resolution computed tomography of the female pelvis: spectrum of normal appearances. *Semin Roentgenol.* 1996;31:267–278.
15. Wallace WH, Thomson AB, Saran F, et al. Predicting age of ovarian failure after radiation to a field that includes the ovaries. *Int J Radiat Oncol Biol Phys.* 2005;62:738–744.
16. Hall JE. Neuroendocrine physiology of the early and late menopause. *Endocrinol Metab Clin North Am.* 2004;33:637–659.
17. Sklar C. Reproductive physiology and treatment-related loss of sex hormone production. *Med Pediatr Oncol.* 1999;33:2–8.
18. Rubin P, Casarett G. The female genital tract. In: *Clinical Radiation Pathology.* Vol I. Philadelphia, PA: W.B. Saunders Company; 1968:396–423.
19. Mandl AM. A quantitative study of the sensitivity of oocytes to x-irradiation. *Proc R Soc Lond B Biol Sci.* 1959;150:53–71.
20. Morita Y, Perez GI, Paris F, et al. Oocyte apoptosis is suppressed by disruption of the acid sphingomyelinase gene or by sphingosine-1-phosphate therapy. *Nat Med.* 2000;6:1109–1114.
21. Morita Y, Tilly JL. Oocyte apoptosis: like sand through an hourglass. *Dev Biol.* 1999;213:1–17.
22. Hall E, Giaccia A. *Radiobiology for the Radiologist.* 5th ed. Philadelphia, PA: Lippincott Williams & Wilkins; 2005.
23. Adriaens I, Smitz J, Jacquet P. The current knowledge on radiosensitivity of ovarian follicle development stages. *Hum Reprod Update.* 2009.
24. Baker TG. Comparative aspects of the effects of radiation during oogenesis. *Mutat Res.* 1971;11:9–22.
25. Peters H, Levy E. Effect of irradiation in infancy on the fertility of female mice. *Radiat Res.* 1963;18:421–428.
26. Mandl AM. The radiosensitivity of germ cells. *Biol Rev Camb Philos Soc.* 1964;39:288–371.
27. Mole RH, Papworth DG. The sensitivity of rat oocytes to x-rays. *Int J Radiat Biol Relat Stud Phys Chem Med.* 1966;10:609–615.
28. Ingram DL. Fertility and oocyte numbers after x-irradiation of the ovary. *J Endocrinol.* 1958;17:81–90.
29. Bookhout CG. The development of the guinea pig ovary from sexual differentiation to maturity. *J Morphol.* 1945;77:233–265.
30. Deansely R. Follicle formation in guinea-pigs and rabbits. A comparative study with notes on the rete ovarii. *J Reprod Fertil.* 1975;45:371–374.
31. Jacquet P, Vankerkom J, Lambiet-Collier M. The female guinea pig, a useful model for the genetic hazard of radiation in man; preliminary results on germ cell radiosensitivity in foetal, neonatal and adult animals. *Int J Radiat Biol.* 1994;65:357–367.
32. Baker TG. The sensitivity of oocytes in post-natal rhesus monkeys to x-irradiation. *J Reprod Fertil.* 1966;12:183–192.
33. Wallace WH, Thomson AB, Kelsey TW. The radiosensitivity of the human oocyte. *Hum Reprod.* 2003;18:117–121.
34. Wallace WH, Shalet SM, Crowne EC, et al. Ovarian failure following abdominal irradiation in childhood: natural history and prognosis. *Clin Oncol (R Coll Radiol).* 1989;1:75–79.
35. Kaplan I. Genetic effects in children and grandchildren, of women treated for infertility and sterility by roentgen therapy; report of a study of thirty-three years. *Radiology.* 1959;72:518–521, passim.
36. Glucksmann A. The Effects of Radiation on Reproductive Organs. *Br J Radiol.* 1947;1(suppl):101–109.
37. Doll R, Smith PG. The long-term effects of x irradiation in patients treated for metropathia haemorrhagica. *Br J Radiol.* 1968;41:362–368.
38. Ash P. The influence of radiation on fertility in man. *Br J Radiol.* 1980;53:271–278.
39. Diczfalusy E, Notter G, Edsmyr F, et al. Estrogen excretion in breast cancer patients before and after ovarian irradiation and oophorectomy. *J Clin Endocrinol Metab.* 1959;19:1230–1244.
40. Dunlap C. The effect of roentgen rays and exposure to radium on fertility. *Hum Fertil.* 1947;12:33.
41. Jacox H. Recovery following human ovarian irradiation. *Radiology.* 1939;32:538–545.
42. Peck W, McGreer J, Kretzschman N, et al. Castration of the female by irradiation: the results in 334 patients. *Radiology.* 1940;34:176–186.
43. Mills JL, Fears TR, Robison LL, et al. Menarche in a cohort of 188 long-term survivors of acute lymphoblastic leukemia. *J Pediatr.* 1997;131:598–602.
44. Lushbaugh CC, Casarett GW. The effects of gonadal irradiation in clinical radiation therapy: a review. *Cancer.* 1976;37:1111–1125.
45. Gans B, Bahary C, Levie B. Ovarian regeneration and pregnancy following massive radiotherapy for dysgerminoma. Report of a case. *Obstet Gynecol.* 1963;22:596–600.
46. Green DM, Yakar D, Brecher ML, et al. Ovarian function in adolescent women following successful treatment for non-Hodgkin's lymphoma. *Am J Pediatr Hematol Oncol.* 1983;5:27–31.
47. Horning SJ, Hoppe RT, Kaplan HS, et al. Female reproductive potential after treatment for Hodgkin's disease. *New Engl J Med.* 1981;304:1377–1382.
48. Sanders JE, Buckner CD, Amos D, et al. Ovarian function following marrow transplantation for aplastic anemia or leukemia. *J Clin Oncol.* 1988;6:813–818.
49. Treloar AE. Menstrual cyclicity and the pre-menopause. *Maturitas.* 1981;3:249–264.
50. Seli E, Tangir J. Fertility preservation options for female patients with malignancies. *Curr Opin Obstet Gynecol.* 2005;17:299–308.
51. Bal C, Kumar A, Tripathi M, et al. High-dose radioiodine treatment for differentiated thyroid carcinoma is not associated with change in female fertility or any genetic risk to the offspring. *Int J Radiat Oncol Biol Phys.* 2005;63:449–455.
52. Sawka AM, Lea J, Alshehri B, et al. A systematic review of the gonadal effects of therapeutic radioactive iodine in male thyroid cancer survivors. *Clin Endocrinol (Oxf).* 2008;68:610–617.
53. Haie-Meder C, Mlika-Cabanne N, Michel G, et al. Radiotherapy after ovarian transposition: ovarian function and fertility preservation. *Int J Radiat Oncol Biol Phys.* 1993;25:419–424.
54. Nicosia SV, Matus-Ridley M, Meadows AT. Gonadal effects of cancer therapy in girls. *Cancer.* 1985;55:2364–2372.
55. Warne GL, Fairley KF, Hobbs JB, et al. Cyclophosphamide-induced ovarian failure. *New Engl J Med.* 1973;289:1159–1162.
56. Hershlag A, Schuster MW. Return of fertility after autologous stem cell transplantation. *Fertil Steril.* 2002;77:419–421.

57. Bakri YN, Pedersen P, Nassar M. Normal pregnancy after curative multiagent chemotherapy for choriocarcinoma with brain metastases. *Acta Obstet Gynecol Scand.* 1991;70:611–613.
58. Siris ES, Leventhal BG, Vaitukaitis JL. Effects of childhood leukemia and chemotherapy on puberty and reproductive function in girls. *New Engl J Med.* 1976;294:1143–1146.
59. Koyama H, Wada T, Nishizawa Y, et al. Cyclophosphamide-induced ovarian failure and its therapeutic significance in patients with breast cancer. *Cancer.* 1977;39:1403–1409.
60. Sonmezer M, Oktay K. Fertility preservation in female patients. *Hum Reprod Update.* 2004;10(3):251–266.
61. Santoro A, Bonadonna G, Valagussa P, et al. Long-term results of combined chemotherapy–radiotherapy approach in Hodgkin's disease: superiority of ABVD plus radiotherapy versus MOPP plus radiotherapy. *J Clin Oncol.* 1987;5:27–37.
62. Stillman RJ, Schinfeld JS, Schiff I, et al. Ovarian failure in long-term survivors of childhood malignancy. *Am J Obstet Gynecol.* 1981;139:62–66.
63. Li FP, Fine W, Jaffe N, et al. Offspring of patients treated for cancer in childhood. *J Natl Cancer Inst.* 1979;62:1193–1197.
64. Blatt J, Mulvihill JJ, Ziegler JL, et al. Pregnancy outcome following cancer chemotherapy. *Am J Med.* 1980;69:828–832.
65. Holmes GE, Holmes FF. Pregnancy outcome of patients treated for Hodgkin's disease: a controlled study. *Cancer.* 1978;41:1317–1322.
66. Green DM, Whitton JA, Stovall M, et al. Pregnancy outcome of female survivors of childhood cancer: a report from the Childhood Cancer Survivor Study. *Am J Obstet Gynecol.* 2002;187:1070–1080.
67. Falcone T, Attaran M, Bedaiwy MA, et al. Ovarian function preservation in the cancer patient. *Fertil Steril.* 2004;81:243–257.
68. Speroff L, Glass RH, Kase N. *Clinical Gynecologic Endocrinology and Infertility.* 2nd ed. Baltimore, MD: Williams & Wilkins Co.; 1978.
69. Soules MR, Sherman S, Parrott E, et al. Executive summary: stages of Reproductive Aging Workshop (STRAW). *Climacteric.* 2001;4:267–272.
70. National Institutes of Health State-of-the-Science Conference statement: management of menopause-related symptoms. *Ann Intern Med.* 2005;142:1003–1013.
71. Scott RT, Opsahl MS, Leonardi MR, et al. Life table analysis of pregnancy rates in a general infertility population relative to ovarian reserve and patient age. *Hum Reprod.* 1995;10:1706–1710.
72. Navot D, Rosenwaks Z, Margalioth EJ. Prognostic assessment of female fecundity. *Lancet.* 1987;2:645–647.
73. Galtier-Dereure F, De Bouard V, Picto MC, et al. Ovarian reserve test with the gonadotrophin-releasing hormone agonist buserelin: correlation with in-vitro fertilization outcome. *Hum Reprod.* 1996;11:1393–1398.
74. Seifer DB, Scott RT, Jr, Bergh PA, et al. Women with declining ovarian reserve may demonstrate a decrease in day 3 serum inhibin B before a rise in day 3 follicle-stimulating hormone. *Fertil Steril.* 1999;72:63–65.
75. van Rooij IA, Broekmans FJ, te Velde ER, et al. Serum anti-mullerian hormone levels: a novel measure of ovarian reserve. *Hum Reprod.* 2002;17:3065–3071.
76. Errera M, Forssberg A. *Mechanisms in Radiobiology.* New York, NY: Academic Press; 1960.
77. UNSCEAR 2000 published. United Nations Scientific Committee on the Effects of Atomic Radiation. *Health Phys.* 2001;80:291.
78. Yamada M, Sasaki H, Mimori Y, et al. Prevalence and risks of dementia in the Japanese population: RERF's adult health study Hiroshima subjects. Radiation Effects Research Foundation. *J Am Geriatr Soc.* 1999;47:189–195.
79. Little J. The Chernobyl accident, congenital anomalies and other reproductive outcomes. *Paediatr Perinat Epidemiol.* 1993;7:121–151.
80. Dodds L, Marrett LD, Tomkins DJ, et al. Case-control study of congenital anomalies in children of cancer patients. *Br Med J.* 1993;307:164–168.
81. Meistrich ML, Byrne J. Genetic disease in offspring of long-term survivors of childhood and adolescent cancer treated with potentially mutagenic therapies. *Am J Hum Genet.* 2002;70:1069–1071.
82. Byrne J, Rasmussen SA, Steinhorn SC, et al. Genetic disease in offspring of long-term survivors of childhood and adolescent cancer. *Am J Hum Genet.* 1998;62:45–52.
83. Boice JD Jr, Tawn EJ, Winther JF, et al. Genetic effects of radiotherapy for childhood cancer. *Health Phys.* 2003;85:65–80.
84. Aisner J, Wiernik PH, Pearl P. Pregnancy outcome in patients treated for Hodgkin's disease. *J Clin Oncol.* 1993;11:507–512.
85. Swerdlow AJ, Jacobs PA, Marks A, et al. Fertility, reproductive outcomes, and health of offspring, of patients treated for Hodgkin's disease: an investigation including chromosome examinations. *Br J Cancer.* 1996;74:291–296.
86. Green DM, Peabody EM, Nan B, et al. Pregnancy outcome after treatment for Wilms tumor: a report from the National Wilms Tumor Study Group. *J Clin Oncol.* 2002;20:2506–2513.
87. Marshall FF. Pregnancy outcome after treatment for Wilms tumor: a report from the National Wilms Tumor Study Group. *J Urol.* 2003;170:695–696.
88. Hawkins MM. Is there evidence of a therapy-related increase in germ cell mutation among childhood cancer survivors? *J Natl Cancer Inst.* 1991;83:1643–1650.
89. Mulvihill JJ, McKeen EA, Rosner F, et al. Pregnancy outcome in cancer patients. Experience in a large cooperative group. *Cancer.* 1987;60:1143–1150.
90. Mulvihill JJ, Myers MH, Connelly RR, et al. Cancer in offspring of long-term survivors of childhood and adolescent cancer. *Lancet.* 1987;2:813–817.
91. Bath LE, Critchley HO, Chambers SE, et al. Ovarian and uterine characteristics after total body irradiation in childhood and adolescence: response to sex steroid replacement. *Br J Obstet Gynaecol.* 1999;106:1265–1272.
92. Critchley HO, Wallace WH. Impact of cancer treatment on uterine function. *J Natl Cancer Inst Monogr.* 2005;(34):64–68.
93. Norwitz ER, Stern HM, Grier H, et al. Placenta percreta and uterine rupture associated with prior whole body radiation therapy. *Obstet Gynecol.* 2001;98:929–931.
94. Pridjian G, Rich NE, Montag AG. Pregnancy hemoperitoneum and placenta percreta in a patient with previous pelvic irradiation and ovarian failure. *Am J Obstet Gynecol.* 1990;162:1205–1206.
95. Harden SV, Twyman N, Lomas DJ, et al. A method for reducing ovarian doses in whole neuro-axis irradiation for medulloblastoma. *Radiother Oncol.* 2003;69:183–188.
96. Stovall M, Blackwell CR, Cundiff J, et al. Fetal dose from radiotherapy with photon beams: report of AAPM Radiation Therapy Committee Task Group No. 36. *Med Phys.* 1995;22:63–82.
97. Followill D, Geis P, Boyer A. Estimates of whole-body dose equivalent produced by beam intensity modulated conformal therapy. *Int J Radiat Oncol Biol Phys.* 1997;38:667–672.
98. Klein EE, Maserang B, Wood R, et al. Peripheral doses from pediatric IMRT. *Med Phys.* 2006;33:2525–2531.
99. Mansur DB, Klein EE, Maserang BP. Measured peripheral dose in pediatric radiation therapy: a comparison of intensity-modulated and conformal techniques. *Radiother Oncol.* 2007;82:179–184.
100. Walter C, Boda-Heggemann J, Wertz H, et al. Phantom and in-vivo measurements of dose exposure by image-guided radiotherapy (IGRT): MV portal images vs. kV portal images vs. cone-beam CT. *Radiother Oncol.* 2007;85:418–423.
101. Gaetini A, De Simone M, Urgesi A, et al. Lateral high abdominal ovariopexy: an original surgical technique for protection of the ovaries during curative radiotherapy for Hodgkin's disease. *J Surg Oncol.* 1988;39:22–28.
102. Morice P, Castaigne D, Haie-Meder C, et al. Laparoscopic ovarian transposition for pelvic malignancies: indications and functional outcomes. *Fertil Steril.* 1998;70:956–960.
103. Pahisa J, Martinez-Roman S, Martinez-Zamora MA, et al. Laparoscopic ovarian transposition in patients with early cervical cancer. *Int J Gynecol Cancer.* 2008;18:584–589.
104. Sella T, Mironov S, Hricak H. Imaging of transposed ovaries in patients with cervical carcinoma. *Am J Roentgenol.* 2005;184:1602–1610.
105. Williams RS, Littell RD, Mendenhall NP. Laparoscopic oophoropexy and ovarian function in the treatment of Hodgkin disease. *Cancer.* 1999;86:2138–2142.
106. Treissman MJ, Miller D, McComb PF. Laparoscopic lateral ovarian transposition. *Fertil Steril.* 1996;65:1229–1231.
107. Williams RS, Mendenhall N. Laparoscopic oophoropexy for preservation of ovarian function before pelvic node irradiation. *Obstet Gynecol.* 1992;80:541–543.
108. Clough KB, Goffinet F, Labib A, et al. Laparoscopic unilateral ovarian transposition prior to irradiation: prospective study of 20 cases. *Cancer.* 1996;77(2):2638–2645.
109. Bisharah M, Tulandi T. Laparoscopic preservation of ovarian function: an underused procedure. *Am J Obstet Gynecol.* 2003;188:367–370.
110. Ray GR, Trueblood HW, Enright LP, et al. Oophoropexy: a means of preserving ovarian function following pelvic megavoltage radiotherapy for Hodgkin's disease. *Radiology.* 1970;96:175–180.
111. Morice P, Haie-Meder C, Pautier P, et al. Ovarian metastasis on transposed ovary in patients treated for squamous cell carcinoma of the uterine cervix: report of two cases and surgical implications. *Gynecol Oncol.* 2001;83:605–607.
112. Chambers SK, Chambers JT, Kier R, et al. Sequelae of lateral ovarian transposition in irradiated cervical cancer patients. *Int J Radiat Oncol Biol Phys.* 1991;20:1305–1308.
113. Bashist B, Friedman WN, Killackey MA. Surgical transposition of the ovary: radiologic appearance. *Radiology.* 1989;173:857–860.
114. Hadar H, Loven D, Herskovitz P, et al. An evaluation of lateral and medial transposition of the ovaries out of radiation fields. *Cancer.* 1994;74:774–779.
115. Howard FM. Laparoscopic lateral ovarian transposition before radiation treatment of Hodgkin disease. *J Am Assoc Gynecol Laparosc.* 1997;4:601–604.
116. Kuohung W, Ram K, Cheng DM, et al. Laparoscopic oophoropexy prior to radiation for pediatric brain tumor and subsequent ovarian function. *Hum Reprod.* 2008;23:117–121.
117. Morice P, Juncker L, Rey A, et al. Ovarian transposition for patients with cervical carcinoma treated by radiosurgical combination. *Fertil Steril.* 2000;74:743–748.
118. Gabriel DA, Bernard SA, Lambert J, et al. Oophoropexy and the management of Hodgkin's disease. A reevaluation of the risks and benefits. *Arch Surg.* 1986;121:1083–1085.
119. Anderson B, LaPolla J, Turner D, et al. Ovarian transposition in cervical cancer. *Gynecol Oncol.* 1993;49:206–214.
120. Veeck LL, Bodine R, Clarke RN, et al. High pregnancy rates can be achieved after freezing and thawing human blastocysts. *Fertil Steril.* 2004;82:1418–1427.
121. Marhhom E, Cohen I. Fertility preservation options for women with malignancies. *Obstet Gynecol Surv.* 2007;62:58–72.
122. Oktay K, Buyuk E, Libertella N, et al. Fertility preservation in breast cancer patients: a prospective controlled comparison of ovarian stimulation with tamoxifen and letrozole for embryo cryopreservation. *J Clin Oncol.* 2005;23:4347–4353.
123. Oktay K. Further evidence on the safety and success of ovarian stimulation with letrozole and tamoxifen in breast cancer patients undergoing in vitro fertilization to cryopreserve their embryos for fertility preservation. *J Clin Oncol.* 2005;23:3858–3859.
124. Azim AA, Costantini-Ferrando M, Oktay K. Safety of fertility preservation by ovarian stimulation with letrozole and gonadotropins in patients with breast cancer: a prospective controlled study. *J Clin Oncol.* 2008;26:2630–2635.
125. Shaw JM, Oranratnachai A, Trounson AO. Fundamental cryobiology of mammalian oocytes and ovarian tissue. *Theriogenology.* 2000;53:59–72.
126. Oktay K, Cil AP, Bang H. Efficiency of oocyte cryopreservation: a meta-analysis. *Fertil Steril.* 2006;86:70–80.
127. Chian RC, Gilbert L, Huang JY, et al. Live birth after vitrification of in vitro matured human oocytes. *Fertil Steril.* 2009;91:372–376.
128. Chian RC, Huang JY, Gilbert L, et al. Obstetric outcomes following vitrification of in vitro and in vivo matured oocytes. *Fertil Steril.* 2008.
129. Soderstrom-Anttila V, Salokorpi T, Pihlaja M, et al. Obstetric and perinatal outcome and preliminary results of development of children born after in vitro maturation of oocytes. *Hum Reprod.* 2006;21:1508–1513.
130. Ovarian tissue and oocyte cryopreservation. *Fertil Steril.* 2004;82:993–998.
131. Gosden RG, Baird DT, Wade JC, et al. Restoration of fertility to oophorectomized sheep by ovarian autografts stored at −196°C. *Hum Reprod.* 1994;9:597–603.
132. Silber SJ, Lenahan KM, Levine DJ, et al. Ovarian transplantation between monozygotic twins discordant for premature ovarian failure. *New Engl J Med.* 2005;353:58–63.

133. Donnez J, Dolmans MM, Demylle D, et al. Restoration of ovarian function after orthotopic (intraovarian and periovarian) transplantation of cryopreserved ovarian tissue in a woman treated by bone marrow transplantation for sickle cell anaemia: case report. *Hum Reprod.* 2006;21:183–188.

134. Donnez J, Dolmans MM, Demylle D, et al. Livebirth after orthotopic transplantation of cryopreserved ovarian tissue. *Lancet.* 2004;364:1405–1410.

135. Oktay K, Buyuk E, Rosenwaks Z, et al. A technique for transplantation of ovarian cortical strips to the forearm. *Fertil Steril.* 2003;80:193–198.

136. Oktay K, Economos K, Kan M, et al. Endocrine function and oocyte retrieval after autologous transplantation of ovarian cortical strips to the forearm. *JAMA.* 2001;286:1490–1493.

137. Oktay KH, Yih M. Preliminary experience with orthotopic and heterotopic transplantation of ovarian cortical strips. *Semin Reprod Med.* 2002;20:63–74.

138. Oktay K, Newton H, Mullan J, et al. Development of human primordial follicles to antral stages in SCID/hpg mice stimulated with follicle stimulating hormone. *Hum Reprod.* 1998;13:1133–1138.

139. Revel A. Human oocyte retrieval from nude mice transplanted with human ovarian cortex [abstract]. *Hum Reprod.* 2000;15 (Abstract Book 1).

140. Senbon S, Ishii K, Fukumi Y, et al. Fertilization and development of bovine oocytes grown in female SCID mice. *Zygote.* 2005;13:309–315.

141. Revel A, Koler M, Simon A, et al. Oocyte collection during cryopreservation of the ovarian cortex. *Fertil Steril.* 2003;79:1237–1239.

142. Ataya K, Rao LV, Lawrence E, et al. Luteinizing hormone-releasing hormone agonist inhibits cyclophosphamide-induced ovarian follicular depletion in rhesus monkeys. *Biol Reprod.* 1995;52:365–372.

143. Recchia F, Sica G, De Filippis S, et al. Goserelin as ovarian protection in the adjuvant treatment of premenopausal breast cancer: a phase II pilot study. *Anticancer Drugs.* 2002;13:417–424.

144. Recchia F, Saggio G, Amiconi G, et al. Gonadotropin-releasing hormone analogues added to adjuvant chemotherapy protect ovarian function and improve clinical outcomes in young women with early breast carcinoma. *Cancer.* 2006;106:514–523.

145. Ataya K, Pydyn E, Ramahi-Ataya A, et al. Is radiation-induced ovarian failure in rhesus monkeys preventable by luteinizing hormone-releasing hormone agonists?: preliminary observations. *J Clin Endocrinol Metab.* 1995;80:790–795.

146. Paris F, Perez GI, Fuks Z, et al. Sphingosine 1-phosphate preserves fertility in irradiated female mice without propagating genomic damage in offspring. *Nat Med.* 2002;8:901–902.

147. Zou K, Yuan Z, Yang Z, et al. Production of offspring from a germline stem cell line derived from neonatal ovaries. *Nat Cell Biol.* 2009;11:631–636.

148. Tilly JL, Telfer EE. Purification of germline stem cells from adult mammalian ovaries: a step closer towards control of the female biological clock? *Mol Hum Reprod.* 2009;15:393–398.

149. Virant-Klun I, Rozman P, Cvjeticanin B, et al. Parthenogenetic embryo-like structures in the human ovarian surface epithelium cell culture in postmenopausal women with no naturally present follicles and oocytes. *Stem Cells Dev.* 2008;76:843–856.

150. Virant-Klun I, Zech N, Rozman P, et al. Putative stem cells with an embryonic character isolated from the ovarian surface epithelium of women with no naturally present follicles and oocytes. *Differentiation.* 2008;76:843–856.

151. Verschuuren SI, Schaap JJ, Veer MB, et al. Optimal treatment of premature ovarian failure after treatment for Hodgkin's lymphoma is often withheld. *Acta Obstet Gynecol Scand.* 2006;85:997–1002.

152. Holm K, Nysom K, Brocks V, et al. Ultrasound B-mode changes in the uterus and ovaries and Doppler changes in the uterus after total body irradiation and allogeneic bone marrow transplantation in childhood. *Bone Marrow Transplant.* 1999;23:259–263.

153. Palacios Jaraquemada JM, Bruno CH. Accuracy of ultrasonography and magnetic resonance imaging in the diagnosis of placenta accreta. *Obstet Gynecol.* 2007;109:203.

154. Harkness UF, Mari G. Diagnosis and management of intrauterine growth restriction. *Clin Perinatol.* 2004;31:743–764, vi.

155. Meirow D, Nugent D. The effects of radiotherapy and chemotherapy on female reproduction. *Hum Reprod Update.* 2001;7:535–543.

CHAPTER
36

Victor J. Gonzalez
David K. Gaffney

Vagina

INTRODUCTION

Gynecologic malignancies are common cancers in women, with an estimated 50,000 cases of endometrial, cervical, and vaginal cancer diagnosed in the United States in 2008.[1] Given the proximity of the genital tract organs to adjacent critical structures, surgery is often of limited benefit in bulky and locally advanced disease, and radiation therapy plays a central role in the management of these cases. In the treatment of endometrial and cervical cancer, the proximal vagina is subjected to high doses of radiation. While the vagina proper is less frequently involved with malignant disease, the usual treatment of disease in this location is radiation therapy. A thorough understanding of the factors influencing radiation injury is therefore necessary for the successful radiotherapeutic management of intrapelvic neoplasms in women.

ANATOMY

The vagina is a fibromuscular tube extending from the vaginal vestibule, or introitus, to the uterine cervix. The average vaginal length is 7.5 cm in adults. Anatomically, the vagina is typically divided into three distinct sections based on vascular supply. The superior and middle third of the vagina are supplied by the uterine and vaginal branches of the internal iliac arteries, while the distal vagina is supplied by the middle rectal and internal pudendal arteries. The distal location of these branches at the terminus of the internal iliac artery may inhibit revascularization following microvascular injury and therefore may contribute to the increased radiosensitivity of the distal vagina relative to the proximal organ. The proximal vagina forms fornices with the cervix, which projects into the apical lumen of the tube. The anterior vaginal wall is shorter than the posterior vaginal wall, which extends superiorly beyond the cervical os (Fig. 36.1).

The anatomic borders of the vagina are not typically well defined on radiographic studies. Visualization of the introitus can be facilitated by placement of a radio-opaque marker or BB at the time of imaging. Visualization of the superior extent of the vagina can be achieved by insertion of a radio-opaque rod or iodine-infused tampon in the vagina at the time of imaging[2] (Fig. 36.2). Some authors favor the use of iodine instilled into the vagina over rigid intravaginal rods at the time of radiotherapy planning due to less anatomic distortion[3,4] (Fig. 36.3). In relationship to the bony pelvis, the vaginal apex typically ranges from 2 to 3.5 cm above the pubic symphysis on AP radiographs.[5] This relationship is highly variable and should be corroborated on CT scan when defining radiation field borders.

Histology

The vagina shares the general characteristics of the hollow viscera. A stratified layer of postmitotic cells overlies a proliferative layer of basal cells with underlying supportive layers of connective tissue and muscle. These are divided into mucosa, submucosa, muscularis propria, and adventitia. The vaginal mucosa is composed of a stratified squamous epithelium, which is of variable thickness. The thickness of this layer is dependent on age and hormonal status; decreasing thickness is associated with advanced age and hypoestrogenic states. Beneath the stratified, postmitotic layer lies a vegetative basal cell layer. Unlike the epithelium of the cervix, the normal vaginal epithelium is typically devoid of mucus-producing glands. Secretions are produced by cervical mucus and accessory glands located near the introitus.

The mucosal and submucosal layers contain a rich network of anastamosing lymphatics and blood vessels. These lymphatics are fairly superficial. One pathologic study found 95% of the vaginal lymphatic ducts within 3 mm depth from the vaginal surface, with no lymphatics beyond 4 mm depth.[6] This depth is pertinent when choosing prescription depth for adjuvant vaginal cuff irradiation following hysterectomy for cervical or endometrial cancer as these paracervical vaginal lymphatics may potentially harbor micrometastatic disease.

The muscularis layer is composed of smooth muscle fibers arranged in two layers with the inner layer arranged circularly and the thicker outer layer arranged longitudinally. The radial-most extent of the vagina is defined by a thin adventitia. Once tumor penetrates beyond the adventitia, there are no physical barriers to the tumor spread. MRI provides excellent soft tissue visualization and can help identify extension of vaginal tumor into paravaginal fat and adjacent organs.[7]

RADIATION EFFECTS

Acute Radiation Injury

PATHOLOGIC CHANGES. Acute radiation changes seen within the vaginal mucosa are not unique to the vagina and essentially parallel the sequence of radiation injury seen within oral mucosa. Cells within the rapidly proliferating basal layer are markedly sensitive to conventional doses of radiation.

Figure 36.1. Normal vaginal anatomy on cadaver and MRI. *Upper panels:* Upper left image depicts normal anatomy at the level of the midvagina, and upper right image depicts axial T2-weighted fast SE image at the same level. The urethral sphincter, vaginal muscularis, and rectal muscularis show low signal intensity and the vaginal venous plexus shows high signal intensity. Pr, puborectal muscle; R, rectum; US, urethral sphincter; V, vaginal muscularis; VP, vaginal venous plexus. *Lower panels:* Lower right panel depicts sagittal T2-weighted MR image. Arrows show the collapsed vaginal walls. The superior extent of the anterior vaginal wall ends at the level of the cervix, while the superior extent of the posterior vaginal wall extends above the cervical os. Lower left panel depicts coronal T2-weighted MR image. Pr, puborectal sling; V, vagina; PD, pelvic diaphragm. (Reprinted from Siegelman ES, Outwater EK, Banner MP. et al. High-resolution MR imaging of the vagina. *Radiographics.* 1997;17:1183–1203, with permission. Anatomic section reprinted from "The Visible Human Project" obtained on the Internet from the National Library of Medicine, permission pending. Normal vaginal anatomy on cadaver and MRI.)

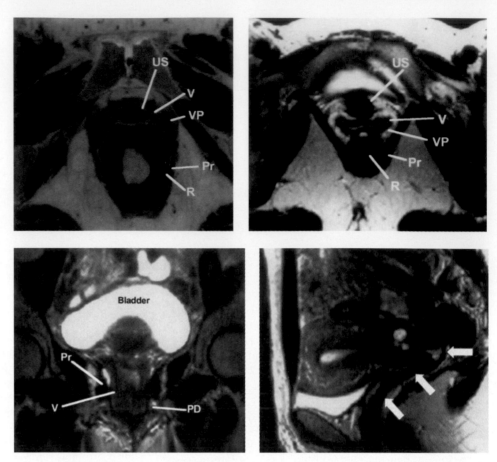

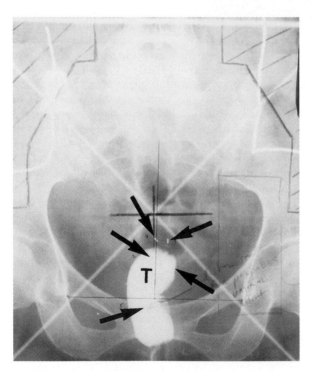

Figure 36.2. Simulation radiograph of patient before definitive radiation for cervical cancer. A vaginal contrast tampon (T) and five seeds outline the contour of the cervix and the vagina. (Reprinted from Weidner GJ, Mayr NA, Saw CB, et al. Radiation field simulation of gynecologic malignancies: localization of the cervix and vagina with a flexible vaginal localizer contrast tampon. *Radiology.* 1999;211(3):876–881, with permission.)

Superficial ulceration occurs when the rate of epithelial sloughing exceeds the rate of replacement by mitotic basal cells. Microscopically, this is seen as epithelial thinning. The acute period is characterized by vascular congestion, submucosal hemorrhage, and migration of lymphocytes and granulocytes into the squamous epithelium.[8] Acute histologic changes also include hyalinization and collagenization of connective tissues within the submucosa, thickening of vascular walls with possible luminal obliteration, hyalinization and fibrosis of the muscularis, and development of a dense inflammatory infiltrate[8–10] (Fig. 36.4).

Acute cytologic changes are seen in Pap smears shortly after initiation of radiation treatment. These include cytoplasmic vacuolation, anisocytosis, and balloon degeneration[11] (Fig. 36.5). These changes exhibit an orderly progression with changes in basal cell shape visible as early as day 1 following radium treatment. Anisocytosis of basal cells becomes marked by 10 days posttreatment. Multinucleated cells may be seen in the precornified layer. A prominent leukocytic infiltrate is typically seen by day 20. Maximum cellular changes appear 10 to 12 days after completion of fractionated radiation.

Early data suggested that the percentage of cells showing characteristic radiation changes had prognostic significance in cervical cancer. Much attention was dedicated to this "sensitization response" or "radiation response" of normal vaginal epithelium.[12] In addition to having predictive value, the degree of radiation changes in normal epithelium was also found to correlate with the incidence of severe complications. Although early studies failed to find a clear correlation between radium dose and complications, these studies did not calculate

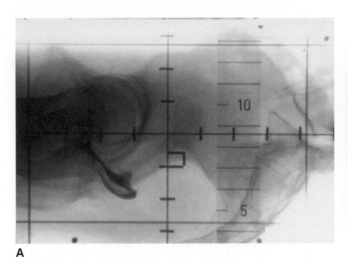

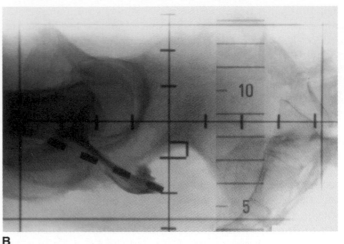

A   **B**

Figure 36.3. The upper panel depicts a lateral film of a cervical carcinoma patient with contrast in the vagina. The lower panel depicts a lateral film of the same patient with contrast and rod in the vagina. The rod creates superior displacement of the vaginal apex. (Reprinted from Wiggenraad RG, Coerkamp EG, Tamminga RI, et al. Contrast vaginography is more accurate than the radiopaque rod for localization of the vagina. *Int J Radiat Oncol Biol Phys.* 2000;48(5):1439–1442, with permission.)

vaginal surface dose (VSD), which is dependent on technical factors at the time of implant (ovoid size, applicator geometry, etc.). It is therefore possible that the aforementioned radiation response is more representative of mucosal dose than of intrinsic radiosensitivity.

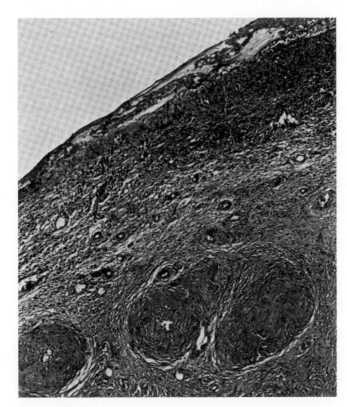

Figure 36.4. Ulceration of the cervicovaginal mucosa following radiotherapy. The epithelium is absent and a fibrinous layer covers a surface of granulation tissue and collagen. Marked arteriolar narrowing is present. (Reprinted from Fajardo LF. *Pathology of Radiation Injury.* New York: Masson Publishing; 1982:110, with permission [pending].)

CLINICAL CHANGES. Clinically, depletion of mitotic basal cells is seen as ulceration when the rate of epithelial sloughing exceeds the rate of replacement. Immediately following low dose rate (LDR) brachytherapy, ulceration with overlying fibropurulent exudate may be seen in areas that were in contact with the source.[8] This is believed to result from a combination of both acute radiation injury and direct pressure from the applicator. Clinical symptoms usually peak 1 to 2 weeks out from completion of treatment. The time course for the development of acute changes with brachytherapy alone is similar following LDR or high dose rate (HDR) treatment.

Despite the frequent observation of vaginal ulceration at the end of treatment, these injuries are typically well tolerated and often asymptomatic. Unlike the oral mucosa and the vulva, the

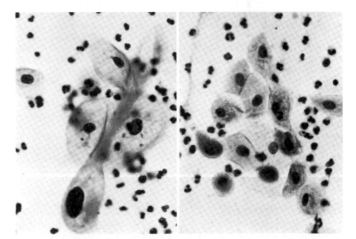

Figure 36.5. Acute cytologic changes in cervical smears following radiotherapy. Size of both cytoplasm and nuclei is markedly increased. Cytoplasmic vacuolization and bizarre morphology are also present. (Reprinted from Rubin P, Casaret GW. *Clinical Radiation Pathology.* Philadelphia, PA: WB Saunders and Company; 1968:415, permission pending.)

vagina proper is relatively insensate.[9] Thus, significant vaginal pain during treatment is atypical and should be investigated. Caffo et al. reported the results of a daily quality-of-life questionnaire filled out by 25 patients undergoing adjuvant external beam radiation with or without LDR brachytherapy for endometrial and cervical cancer. There was a trend toward increased vaginal discomfort at the end of the treatment course, which did not reach statistical significance.[13] Davidson et al. reported on quality of life during radiation therapy for cervical cancer in 89 patients. The vaginal and sexual dysfunction subsections of the LENT-SOMA scale were used. The only statistically significant difference between pretreatment and posttreatment scores was seen with a worsening of day 70 vaginal toxicity scores. There was, however, significant heterogeneity in responses, with many patients reporting symptomatic improvement over baseline after treatment. The authors attribute these results to the fact that their population included patients with locally advanced disease who may have had palliation of symptoms.[14]

Ulcerations are prone to serous discharge. Decreased mucus production in the setting of mucosal injury further predisposes to development of infection. Superficial vault ulceration typically resolves in 3 to 6 months,[15] but may progress to long-term necrosis.

The clinical diagnosis of necrosis implies full thickness ulceration and loss of basal cell layer with resultant delayed healing. This inclusion of "delayed healing" poses a diagnostic dilemma in the acute setting. While histologically identical to ulceration, the term *necrosis* is often used by clinicians to describe persistent ulceration after an interval of time. Given this ambiguity, historical data include a broad range for incidence of acute necrosis following vaginal irradiation. Ulceration is not uncommon during the course of vaginal irradiation but may be of limited clinical relevance. Many authors retrospectively defined vaginal cuff ulceration as necrosis if it persisted 3 months posttreatment. Hintz et al. defined necrosis as a "clinically apparent area of de-epithelialized mucosa occurring or still present 6 weeks after cessation of all radiation."[16] In this sense, necrosis is a consequential late effect that results from depletion of the mitotically active basal cell layer within the vaginal epithelium.

In patients undergoing hysterectomy 1 month following concurrent chemoradiation for cervical cancer, gross alterations seen at time of surgery include vaginal and cervical ulceration, severe narrowing of the vaginal stump, obliteration of the vaginal fornices, and adhesions between the cervix and vaginal walls.[17]

Late Radiation Injury

PATHOLOGIC CHANGES. Following radiation, histologic and cytologic changes are common and may persist indefinitely. Abitbol et al. reported on 17 patients who had vaginal biopsies performed more than 1 year after external beam radiation therapy (EBRT) and LDR intracavitary radium for early-stage cervical cancer.[10] These biopsies consistently demonstrated marked mucosal atrophy with epithelial thinning; often with complete loss of the overlying stratified squamous layer leaving only a residual basal cell layer. Hyalinization and collagenization of the connective tissues within the submucosa may also frequently be observed. The prominent leukocytic infiltrate seen acutely may persist. Fibrosis of the muscular layer may be evident. Vascular changes are seen including fibrosis of vessel walls, intimal proliferation, and a resultant decrease in

luminal diameter.[8–10] These vaso-occlusive changes are felt to compromise blood delivery to the injured tissues. The resultant tissue hypoxia may lead to persistent ulceration and fistula formation to adjacent viscera.[10] By 2 years postradiation, there has typically been complete or near complete re-epithelialization of the mucosa as well as resolution of inflammatory changes,[18] but other histologic changes may persist indefinitely.

The frequency of cytologic abnormalities seen on postradiation therapy Pap smears decreases with time. Whereas up to 100% smears will show some abnormalities within the first 6 months postradiation, these changes gradually diminish.[11] Still, some studies have suggested that most patients will show characteristic changes in vaginal cytology for up to 10 years posttreatment.[19] In the surveillance setting, it is important to distinguish postradiation atypia from new or recurrent malignancy. It is therefore important for clinicians to relay a history of radiotherapy to the examining cytopathologist.

Detection of glandular cells in posthysterectomy smears poses a diagnostic dilemma when smears are performed for surveillance of adenocarcinoma. Yavuz et al. reviewed 508 posthysterectomy vaginal smears, 183 of whom had received adjuvant radiation therapy. Benign glandular cells were identified in 17 patients, all of whom had prior radiation. The authors concluded that radiation can induce metaplasia which may be misinterpreted as recurrent adenocarcinoma.[20]

Gross changes in the vagina following radiotherapy include mucosal pallor, telangiectasia, adhesions, vaginal stenosis, and vaginal shortening.[10] Fine adhesions, termed *synechiae*, develop between adjacent areas of denuded epithelium. These may form within weeks of completion of radiation. Synechiae are initially easy to break; however, with time they become more fibrous and resilient. Clinically, adhesions and stenosis may make vaginal exam difficult or impossible and impede disease surveillance. In addition, these side effects can significantly affect sexual function.

CLINICAL CHANGES

Vaginal Stenosis and Shortening. Stenosis and shortening are the most frequent late consequences of vaginal irradiation. These changes are secondary to circumferential fibrosis as well as the development of intraluminal adhesions. The typical time course for the initial development of clinically apparent vaginal stenosis is 3 to 6 months but may occur at later times. The incidence of vaginal stenosis following radiation therapy for nonovarian gynecologic malignancy is highly variable among series but has been reported as high as 88%.[21] It is important to recognize the heterogeneity in reporting methods among different series. Whereas some studies report stenosis and shortening only based on patient report, others have used more rigorous methods including colpometry and measurement of vaginal length.

Multiple studies have specifically reported on vaginal stenosis and shortening following radiation. Brand et al. published a retrospective review of prospectively gathered data on vaginal stenosis following whole pelvic radiation with or without intracavitary brachytherapy in 188 patients with cervical cancer. Stenosis was documented in 38% of patients with a median time to onset of symptoms of 7.5 months (range: 26 days–>5 years).[22] A retrospective study of 97 patients treated for early-stage cervical cancer with surgery, radiotherapy, or both and who were disease free more than 1 year from completion of treatment indicated significant narrowing on pelvic exam (admitting only one finger) or obliteration of greater than two thirds of the vagina in 71% of patients who received radiotherapy compared to 17% in those treated with surgery alone.[10] Hartman et al. published a retrospective review of 221 patients treated with RT for cervical cancer. Patients received 3,000 cGy EBRT followed by 6,000 cGy of LDR brachytherapy to point A. Some degree of vaginal stenosis was noted in 88% of patients and 38% had stenosis causing occlusion of greater than one third of the vagina. These are among the highest reported rates of vaginal stenosis. Potential causes for this high incidence include the use of older techniques without calculation of VSDs, the combination of external beam irradiation and brachytherapy, and the lack of posttreatment counseling regarding mechanical dilatation.[21].

Eifel et al. published a retrospective review of 1,784 patients treated with radiation therapy at MDACC for stage 1B cervical cancer. The majority of patients received combination external beam and LDR brachytherapy. The risk of severe vaginal shortening (>50% length) was significantly higher for patients treated after age 50 (5% at 10 years vs. 1%).[23] This study also documented a steady increase in the incidence late vaginal stenosis with new cases reported up to 15 years post-treatment. In contrast, Sorbe and Smeds using colpometry following vaginal cuff HDR brachytherapy documented no additional cases of shortening after 36 months.[24]

Bruner et al. prospectively measured vaginal length in 90 patients who had undergone external beam and intracavitary radiotherapy for cervical or endometrial cancer. Patients treated for cervical cancer had vaginal shortening ranging from 0.6 to 1.5 cm shorter than those with endometrial cancer. The authors attribute this difference to the higher VSDs in the cervical cancer group.[25]

Acute shortening of the vagina occurring during the course of radiation treatment has been documented.[5] Katz et al. measured vaginal length in patients receiving intravaginal brachytherapy with or without external beam radiation. Measurements were performed at the time of first and second brachytherapy insertions. They reported an average 5 mm shortening in vaginal length in patients receiving external beam radiation, but no significant shortening in those receiving brachytherapy alone.[5] In a Swedish series of 404 women treated with vaginal cuff HDR alone, Sorbe and Smeds showed that on average, 88% of total vaginal length reduction occurred within the first 12 months following treatment with stabilization after 36 months.[24]

Vaginal Necrosis. Vaginal necrosis develops from acute injury following the depletion of a critical level of progenitor basal cell.[26] For this reason, it is considered to be a consequential late effect. The incidence of necrosis is dependent on total dose, fractionation, location, and technique. Eifel et al. reported on 1,784 patients treated with definitive external beam and LDR intracavitary brachytherapy for early-stage cervical cancer. Limiting total VSD to 140 Gy, they documented a 6% incidence of necrosis. Among patients with necrosis, 90% of cases developed within 15 months of completion of treatment and 2% of patients had necrosis for >3 months. Among 65 cases of necrosis, three experienced progression to fistulas.[23]

The risk of vaginal necrosis following a given dose of radiation varies significantly based on anatomic location. In a retrospective review of 16 patients with vaginal cancer treated with a combination of EBRT and LDR (including interstitial and

intracavitary), Hintz et al. documented five cases of ulcerations. All occurred on the posterior vaginal wall and four occurred in the distal one third of the vaginal canal.[16] Likewise, toxicity studies of vaginal intracavitary brachytherapy for carcinoma in situ have consistently shown an increased incidence of ulceration and fistula development when the distal vagina is included in the treatment volume.[27] Several hypotheses have been proposed to account for the increased radiation sensitivity of the distal vagina. It is felt that differences in blood supply between the proximal and distal vagina may in part account for this dichotomy. Additionally, the proximity of the distal vagina and introitus to the anus predisposes the vagina to fecal contamination. Superinfection with enteric bacteria may prevent re-epithelialization following radiation injury and promote necrosis.[16] Regardless of the mechanism, retrospective studies of patients treated for vaginal cancer have consistently shown increased sensitivity of the distal vagina to ionizing radiation in comparison to the proximal vagina.

Rectovaginal/Vesicovaginal Fistula. Rectovaginal and vesicovaginal fistulas are among the most devastating potential complications of radiation therapy for gynecologic malignancies. Rectovaginal fistula development is often preceded by pelvic pain and nonhealing rectal ulceration. Symptoms include rectal bleeding, and passage of vaginal flatus or stool.[28] The most common symptom of vesicovaginal fistula development is passage of watery discharge per the vagina. Radiographically, vesicovaginal fistula may be suggested by the presence of air in the bladder in the absence of instrumentation. Diagnosis is usually made on vaginoscopy or cystoscopy, but dynamic contrast-enhanced CT or contrast MRI can be helpful in making the diagnosis[29] (Fig. 36.6). Typically, fistula formation occurs within the first 2 years after completion of radiotherapy.[28] Vaginal necrosis and rectal or bladder invasion by tumor are the main risk factors for the development of fistulas.[30,31] In a review of 193 patients treated for vaginal cancer at MDACC, Frank et al. reported two vesicovaginal fistulas. Both cases occurred in patients with anterior wall tumors. Similarly, 73% of major rectal complications occurred in patients with posterior wall tumors.[32]

Several studies have shown a significant increase in fistula development with interstitial brachytherapy for cervical cancer over intracavitary brachytherapy. Aristizabal et al. reported a 22% incidence of severe complications (10/45) in patients who received interstitial brachytherapy compared to 7% (3/43) in patients who had intracavitary brachytherapy. Severe complications included four cases of rectovaginal and vesicovaginal fistulas in the interstitial group but no grade 3 or higher toxicity in the intracavitary group.[33]

While bowel or bladder invasion have been found in multiple radiation series to be major risk factors for fistula development, it is not clear whether this risk exists independent of treatment modality. Some authors argue that the high rate of fistula development following definitive doses of radiation in patients with invasion of adjacent organs should preclude the use of aggressive therapy in this setting. Others argue that many patients with locally advanced disease are still curable with aggressive treatment and are at risk of fistula development even without aggressive treatment. The decision to proceed with definitive treatment in the setting of locally advanced disease should include a thorough discussion of risks as well as likelihood of long-term disease control prior to initiation of therapy.

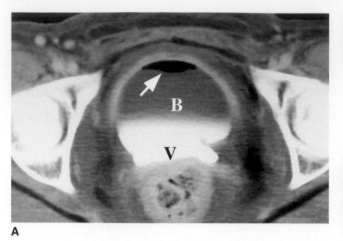

A

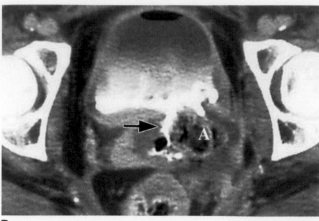

B

Figure 36.6. Vesicovaginal fistula seen on axial and sagittal imaging. **A:** Shows CT image, with excretion of intravenous contrast into the bladder (B), and extension of contrast material from the bladder into the vagina (V) due to fistula. Air in the bladder in the absence of catheterization (*arrow*) is also consistent with fistula. **B:** Shows a CT image of a patient with abscess of the rectovaginal pouch (A). Contrast material (*arrow*) is leaking from the bladder into the abscess cavity and into the vagina. As with the patient in *Panel A*, an air-fluid level is seen in the bladder. **C:** shows a sagittal MR image (fast spin-echo) of a patient with vesicovaginal fistula (*arrow*). The urine is hyperintense and delineates the fistula. (Reprinted from Yu NC, Raman SS, Patel M, et al. Fistulas of the genitourinary tract: a radiologic review. *Radiographics.* 2004;24(5):1331–1352, with permission.)

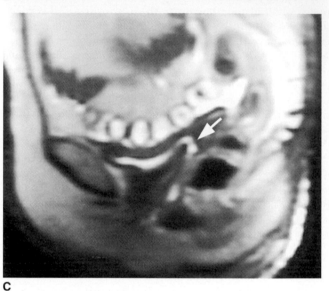

C

Sexual Dysfunction. Physician assessment of late radiotherapy vaginal morbidity has been shown to significantly underestimate patient-reported discomfort and sexual dysfunction. A 2008 study from Norway reported significant discordance between physician assessment and patient-reported vaginal morbidity with physicians reporting a 23% rate of grade 3 to 4 vaginal morbidity compared to a patient-reported 58% incidence of this level of morbidity.[34]

Sexual dysfunction following pelvic radiotherapy is often multifactorial. Symptoms that may directly impair sexual function include vaginal dryness, vaginal stenosis, and shortening. Vaginal dryness may be compounded by treatment-induced ovarian failure. These factors may result in dyspareunia and postcoital bleeding or may make sexual intercourse impossible. Bergmark et al. sent out sexual quality of life questionnaires to women in Sweden who had undergone treatment for cervical cancer and controls. Results were obtained for 256 women with a history of cervical cancer and 489 controls. There was an increase in patient-reported vaginal side effects with increased number of treatment modalities. Among patients who had received surgery, external beam radiation, and brachytherapy, 33% reported moderate or substantial decrease in vaginal length. The incidence of vaginal shortening was similar among patients who had received surgery alone or radiation alone

(19% and 22%, respectively). Likewise, decreased lubrication was greatest in among patients who had received both surgery and radiation. These changes correlated with a significant decrease in body image but did not correlate significantly with decreased sexual satisfaction.[35]

Grading of Radiation Injury

Grading of radiation injury may take into account acute and late structural and functional changes. Multiple grading schemes have been used in the past when analyzing radiation injury. Unfortunately, a lack of standardization makes it difficult to compare older reports. Several attempts at standardizing radiation injury to the vagina have been proposed. The most widely utilized grading systems include the Franco-Italian glossary,[36] RTOG/EORTC, NCI Common Toxicity Criteria (CTC) and the subjective, objective, management and analytic (SOMA) scale. Of these systems, the Franco-Italian glossary is the only one designed specifically for scoring complications from treatment of gynecologic cancers. The SOMA system is unique in that it quantifies subjective quality-of-life information including sexual dysfunction. While being the most comprehensive schema for grading vaginal injury, the SOMA scale is not routinely used outside of clinical trials (Table 36.1).

TABLE 36.1	Frequently Used Grading Systems for Vaginal Radiation Injury			
Endpoint	*Grade 1*	*Grade 2*	*Grade 3*	*Grade 4*
CTCAE v3				
Vaginal mucositis	Erythema of the mucosa, minimal symptoms	Patchy ulcerations; moderate symptoms or dyspareunia	Confluent ulcerations; bleeding with trauma; unable to tolerate vaginal exam, sexual intercourse or tampon placement	Tissue necrosis; significant spontaneous bleeding; life-threatening consequences
Vaginitis	Mild, intervention not indicated	Moderate, intervention indicated	Severe, not relieved with treatment; ulceration, but operative intervention not indicated	Ulceration and operative intervention indicated
Vaginal stenosis/ shortening	Vaginal narrowing and/or shortening not interfering with function	Vaginal narrowing and/or shortening interfering with function	Complete obliteration; not surgically correctable	—
Vaginal dryness	Mild	Interfering with sexual function; dyspareunia; intervention indicated	—	—
Fistula	Asymptomatic, radiographic findings only	Symptomatic, noninvasive intervention indicated	Symptomatic, interfering with ADL; invasive intervention indicated	Life-threatening consequences; operative intervention requiring partial or full organ resection; permanent urinary diversion
SOMA				
Subjective				
Dyspareunia, dryness, bleeding pain	Occasional	Intermittent	Persistent	Refractory
Objective				
Stenosis/length	>2/3 normal length	1/3 to 2/3 normal length	<1/3 normal length	Obliteration
Dryness	Asymptomatic	Symptomatic	Secondary dysfunction	
Ulceration/necrosis	Superficial, <1 cm^2	Superficial, >1 cm^2	Deep ulcer	Fistulae
Atrophy	Patchy	Confluent	Nonconfluent	Diffuse
Appearance	Telangiectasia without bleeding	Telangiectasia with gross bleeding		
Synechiae		Partial	Complete	
Bleeding		On contact	Intermittent	Persistent
Management				
Dyspareunia/pain	Occasional nonnarcotic	Regular nonnarcotic	Regular narcotic	Surgical intervention
Atrophy	Occasional hormone cream	Intermittent hormone cream	Regular hormone cream	
Bleeding	Iron therapy	Occasional transfusion	Frequent transfusion	
Stenosis	Occasional dilation	Intermittent dilation	Persistent dilation	
Dryness	Hormone replacement	Artificial lubrication		
Ulceration	Conservative	Debridement	Hyperbaric O$_2$	Graft, surgical repair
FRANCO-ITALIAN GLOSSARY				
Vaginitis	Acute symptoms of vulvovaginitis interrupting the treatment for more than 10% of the planned overall treatment time or lasting more than two weeks after the completion of treatment	Repeated infectious vaginitis		Death due to complication
Stenosis	Vaginal narrowing and/or shortening to 1/2 or <1/2 the original dimensions	Vaginal narrowing and/or shortening to more than 1/2 of the original dimensions	Complete vaginal stenosis	Death due to complication

(*continued*)

TABLE 36.1	Frequently Used Grading Systems for Vaginal Radiation Injury *(Continued)*			
Endpoint	*Grade 1*	*Grade 2*	*Grade 3*	*Grade 4*
Dyspareunia	Mild dyspareunia	Moderate dyspareunia	Severe dyspareunia	Death due to complication
Edema/telangiectasia	Asymptomatic vaginal or vulvar edema with or without telangiectasia.	Symptomatic vulvar edema and/or telangiectasia and/or fibrosis	Vulvar and/or vaginal and/or uterine necrosis requiring surgery.	Death due to complication
Perforation/tear	Uterine perforation or pyometra or hematometra not requiring surgery. Immediately repairable vaginal tear	Uterine perforation or pyometra requiring surgical laparotomy or drainage surgery	Posttreatement peritonitis or uterine perforation requiring major surgery	Death due to complication
Rectum			Rectovaginal fistula	
Bladder and urethra		Immediate or early postoperative vesicovaginal fistula with complete healing and normal function after treatment	Early or late vesicovaginal fistula with permanent anatomical and/or functional damage	
RTOG/EORTC				
Subcutaneous tissue	Slight induration (fibrosis) and loss of subcutaneous fat	Moderate fibrosis but asymptomatic; Slight field contracture; <10% linear reduction	Severe induration and loss of subcutaneous tissue; Field contracture > 10% linear measurement	Necrosis
Mucous membrane	Slight atrophy and dryness	Moderate atrophy and telangiectasia; Little mucous	Marked atrophy with complete dryness; Severe telangiectasia	Ulceration

DATA FOR RADIATION INJURY

Data for radiation injury to the vagina come from the treatment of several different intrapelvic diseases requiring a range of radiation doses and utilizing a variety of different treatment modalities. While this heterogeneity of treatments makes it difficult to generalize across disease sites, each one provides unique insights into specific aspects of radiation injury to the organ.

Animal Data

Animal data regarding radiation tolerance of the vagina are extremely limited. The reason for this paucity of animal data is unclear; however, several factors are probably responsible. Due to its proximity to the bowel and bladder, severe vaginal complications are typically not dose-limiting factors during radiation treatment. This may have reduced the need for an animal model for vaginal injury. Likewise, the vagina is easily accessible and biopsy studies assessing normal tissue response to radiation were conducted early in the history of cervical cancer treatment.

Human Data

PROXIMAL VAGINAL INJURY. The greatest volume of data for radiation injury to the proximal vagina comes from the treatment of cervical cancer. While endometrial cancer is more common, cervical cancer is more likely to involve the vagina and more often requires the treatment of gross disease

with higher radiation doses. The proximal vaginal mucosa is a frequent site of extension and varying degrees of the vagina are included in the treatment volume based on clinician judgment. Large prospective randomized trials also make it easier to compare toxicity between studies; however, most of these studies fail to document vaginal injury.

There are less data on high-grade vaginal injury associated with treatment of endometrial cancer. This is likely due to the predominant role of radiation as adjuvant treatment following surgery and, consequently, the use of lower radiation doses. Due to the frequency of adjuvant radiation for endometrial cancer, there are increased data on late low-grade injury (i.e., stenosis and shortening).

Brachytherapy Plus External Beam. When drawing conclusions from historic studies using brachytherapy, it is important to recognize the factors that may limit their applicability to modern radiation treatment. Given the proximity of tumor volumes to adjacent critical structures, the steep dose gradients generated during brachytherapy make it uniquely suited for the treatment of gynecologic malignancies. At the same time, this sharp dose drop off can result in extremely high doses to adjacent mucosa. Thus, when mucosal doses are not reported, it is difficult to compare vaginal toxicity between studies.

In addition to the difficulties of dose reporting, estimating vaginal radiation injury from studies using brachytherapy is further complicated by the variety of different treatment techniques. Cervical brachytherapy is routinely performed with an intracavitary applicator consisting of an intrauterine tandem and extrauterine colpostats or ring. Interstitial brachytherapy has been used for bulky cervical and endometrial cancer. Adjuvant vaginal cuff brachytherapy can be performed with ovoids alone or a vaginal cylinder. Lastly, comparison is further confounded by differences in dose rate that can significantly affect toxicity. Studies reporting vaginal injury following brachytherapy and external beam irradiation are summarized in Table 36.2. Most studies report <4% incidence of grade 3 or higher late vaginal toxicity utilizing therapeutic doses with a suggestion of increased radiosensitivity in the distal vagina. Using a combined VSD from external beam and LDR brachytherapy of <140 Gy, Eifel et al. demonstrated a 5-year actuarial incidence of grade 3 or higher vaginal toxicity of 2.3%.[23] Au et al. reviewed records of 274 patients treated with definitive radiation for FIGO I to IV cervical cancer between 1987 and 1997 at Mallinckrodt. The majority of patients (95%) were treated with EBRT and Fletcher-Suit tandem and ovoids LDR brachytherapy. LDR alone was used in the remaining 5%. External beam doses ranged from 20 to 40 Gy at 1.8/fraction, while LDR doses ranged from 48 to 64 Gy to point A in two fractions. This correlated to VSDs ranging from 56 to 300 Gy. Total surface doses of 150 Gy yielded a 3.6% incidence of grade 3 complications. Biologically equivalent dose (BED) was calculated for each regimen using the linear quadratic model with nominal $\alpha/\beta = 3$ and $\mu = 0.46$ and correlated with incidence of complications using logistic regression. With an external beam dose of 20 Gy, the calculated TD_5 for grade 3 complications using LDR was 238 Gy total mucosal dose.[22]

Rodrigus et al. published a retrospective review of 147 patients treated with definitive RT for cervical cancer in the Netherlands. Standardized treatment was administered giving 40 Gy to the whole pelvis AP:PA in 2 Gy/fraction. This was followed by two tandem and ovoid insertions delivering total doses of either 25 Gy to point A (54 cGy/h) or 20 Gy to point A (107 cGy/h).

Individualized dose optimization was not performed and VSDs or rectal doses were not reported. Using this approach, 12% of patients had moderate or higher vaginal symptoms. Eleven patients (7%) developed rectovaginal fistulas one patient (<1%) developed a vesicovaginal fistula.[37] This relatively high incidence of fistula development with conservative doses suggests that prescribing to point A without individualizing treatment may result in excessive VSDs.

Hamberger et al. reported on the MDACC experience treating 111 cervical cancer patients with EBRT and LDR between 1967 and 1974. All patients received between 40 and 60 Gy of external beam radiation to the pelvis followed by LDR intracavitary brachytherapy in the form of either tandem and ovoids or tandem and cylinder in cases of narrow vaginal vaults or extensive vaginal disease. Ten patients developed vaginal fistulas. Among these, 8/10 had received total surface doses of >9,000 cGy and all occurred in patients treated with vaginal cylinders. The increased incidence of vaginal injury with the use of cylinders as opposed to ovoids could be attributable to increased radiosensitivity of the distal vagina or the fact that patients treated with cylinders had more advanced stage disease.[38]

Nori et al. reported on 300 patients who received adjuvant radiation for early-stage endometrial cancer. Radiation consisted of external beam (40 Gy/20 fractions with four field technique) plus HDR intracavitary vaginal cuff brachytherapy (7 Gy × 3–5 mm depth). At a median follow-up of 12 years, the authors reported a 2.5% incidence of grade 1 to 2 vaginal stenosis and 0.7% incidence of vaginal necrosis with no cases of rectovaginal or vesicovaginal fistulas.[39]

Perez et al. published a retrospective review of 811 patients with endometrial or cervical cancer who underwent radiation alone at Mallinckrodt between 1959 and 1977. The authors reported nine cases of vesicovaginal fistulas, seven cases of rectovaginal fistulas, and eight cases of vaginal vault necrosis. A wide

TABLE 36.2	Studies Reporting Late Radiation Injury to the Proximal Vagina Using EBRT and Brachytherapy						
Author/Institution	*Design*	*N*	*Treatment*	*Mean VSD*	*Endpoint*	*Incidence*
Au[63]/Mallinkrodt	Retrospective review	274	95% EBRT 20–40 Gy/1.8 + T&O LDR 24–32 Gy to point A × 2	150–186 Gy	Grade 3 vaginal toxicity	3.6%
Rodrigus[37]/ Netherlands	Retrospective review	147	EBRT 40 Gy per 20 fx + T&O 25 Gy to point A × 2 at 54 cGy/h *or* T&O 20 Gy to point A × 2 at 107 cGy/h	Not reported	Fistula	8%
Hamberger[38]/ MDACC	Retrospective review	111	50 Gy EBRT + LDR		Fistula	7%[a]
		21	60 Gy EBRT + LDR		Fistula	19%
Perez[40]/Mallinkrodt	Retrospective review 1957–1977	811	EBRT + LDR	<80 Gy to point A	Grade 2 or higher	<5%
				>80 Gy to point A	Grade 2 or higher	10%–25%

[a]All occurrences were in patients with advanced disease.

BED, biologically equivalent dose; EBRT, external beam radiation therapy; ED, equivalent dose; fx, fraction; f/u, follow-up; Gy, gray; LDR, low dose rate; T&O, tandem and ovoid; VSD, vaginal surface dose.

range of doses was utilized along with a variety of techniques. They demonstrated <5% incidence of grade 2 or higher complications when doses of <8,000 cGy were utilized. Above 8,000 cGy, the incidence of grade 2 or higher toxicity increased to 10% to 25%. VSDs were not reported. Still, this study is notable because of the large number of patients and the relatively low rate of high-grade vaginal injury using simple techniques.[40]

Hintz et al. reported on a series of 16 patients treated with a variety of radiation techniques for vaginal cancer. They reported no cases of proximal vaginal necrosis requiring surgery when combined external beam and LDR brachytherapy mucosal doses up to 140 Gy were administered. In contrast, three patients had distal necrosis after receiving >98 Gy.[16] All cases of necrosis occurred in the posterior vaginal wall.

Brachytherapy Alone. Most of the data for exclusive brachytherapy to the proximal vagina come from the adjuvant setting. Alektiar et al. reported on 382 patients with intermediate-risk endometrial cancer treated postoperatively with vaginal cuff HDR at Memorial Sloan Kettering cancer center. Median dose was 21 Gy in three fractions prescribed to 5-mm depth. At 4 years median follow-up, there was one case of grade 3 or higher vaginal toxicity. This single case of vaginal necrosis occurred in a patient who had received 7 Gy × 3 prescribed to 5-mm depth for a VSD of 11.4 Gy/fraction[41] (BED$_3$ at 0.5 mm = 70).

Onsrud et al. illustrated the role of VSD on late vaginal toxicity. They reported on 217 patients who received adjuvant vaginal cuff HDR brachytherapy for stage I to II endometrial cancer. All patients received 5.5 Gy × 4 fractions prescribed to various depths. At VSDs of >40 Gy, there was a 40% incidence grade 1 to 2 late vaginal toxicity. In comparison, 12% with VSDs of <30 Gy had vaginal toxicity reported. The role of prescription depth selection is further discussed in the section on reducing toxicity.

Sorbe and Smeds reported the results of their experience in Sweden using cobalt-60 HDR vaginal cuff brachytherapy as adjuvant treatment for endometrial cancer. Data were prospectively gathered on 404 patients and included colpometric measurements using a vaginal obturator. Four different treatment fractionation schedules were used: 4.5 Gy × 6, 5 Gy × 6, 6 Gy × 5, and 9 Gy × 4. Doses were prescribed to 1 cm depth and α/β was calculated using a maximum likelihood method. Dose per fraction was the most important predictive factor for shortening. At 5 years, average vaginal length relative to baseline was 59% for the 4.5-Gy group, 50% for the 5-Gy group, 40% for the 6-Gy group, and 21% for the 9-Gy/fraction group[24] (Fig. 36.7).

Pearcey et al. performed a retrospective analysis of 1,800 patients who received adjuvant vaginal intracavitary HDR brachytherapy for low-to-intermediate risk endometrial cancer. Their analysis included published and unpublished results from 13 institutions. Patients were treated with a variety of fractionation schemes. The authors calculated late and early BED at the vaginal surface and at a depth of 5 mm. Significant late complications were reported in only 2 of 1,098 patients who received a BED of <100 Gy$_3$, in contrast to14% of patients (82/594) who received BED >100 Gy$_3$[42] Studies reporting vaginal injury following vaginal cuff HDR are summarized in Table 36.3. In general, severe late toxicity is low if a late BED of <100 Gy is maintained, though grade 1 to 2 fibrosis and vaginal shortening is relatively common (12%–37%) and is dose dependent.

Ebrt Alone. Given the proximity of the uterus to the rectum and urinary bladder, external beam radiation alone has not routinely been used to treat cervical and endometrial cancer.

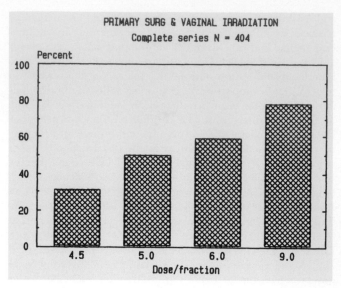

Figure 36.7. Percentage of vaginal shortening as a function of fraction size. Vaginal shortening is depicted as a percentage of the original vaginal length at the start of radiation therapy. Vaginal shortening increases as dose per fraction increases ($p < 0.0001$, linear regression analysis). (Reprinted from Sorbe BG, Smeds AC. Postoperative vaginal irradiation with high dose rate afterloading technique in endometrial carcinoma stage I. *Int J Radiat Oncol Biol Phys.* 1990;18(2):305–314, with permission [pending].)

Consequently, data on proximal vaginal injury following external beam radiation alone are relatively limited. Toxicity data are available for lower dose adjuvant irradiation for endometrial and cervical cancer. Keys et al. documented an increase in grade 3 and 4 toxicities in patients receiving adjuvant whole pelvic radiation following hysterectomy, but the report does not specifically address vaginal injury.[43]

Higher doses of external beam radiation have routinely been utilized for treatment of locally advanced cervical cancer in situations where brachytherapy is not possible. These situations may arise from technical limitations including vaginal stenosis and tumor bulk or poor patient functional status. A retrospective review from China reported late toxicity on 96 patients with stage IIb cervical cancer treated with external cobalt-60 irradiation. Patients received 60 Gy to the whole pelvis with a four-field technique followed by a 10-Gy boost using 2-Gy daily fractions. Four patients also received LDR brachytherapy. All patients had >5 years follow-up. Two patients developed rectovaginal fistulas for an overall 2.7% incidence of high-grade vaginal toxicity.[44]

Barraclough et al. reported their experience (1996–2004) in Manchester treating cervical cancer patients with definitive external beam radiation when brachytherapy could not be used. In their series, 44 patients were treated using 3D conformal techniques. All patients received between 54 and 70 Gy with two thirds receiving >60 Gy. For the initial 40 to 45 Gy, 2 to 2.25 Gy/fraction were delivered. For the boost portion, dose per fractions of up to 2.5 Gy were utilized. With a median follow-up of 2.3 years, grade 1 vaginal shortening (<1/2 original length) was reported in 18% of patients and grade 2 shortening (>1/2 original length) was reported in 4.5% of patients. One patient with bladder invasion by tumor developed a vesicovaginal fistula during treatment.[45]

There has been growing interest in utilizing hypofractionated external beam radiation as a replacement for brachytherapy.

TABLE 36.3			Studies Reporting Late Radiation Injury to the Proximal Vagina Using HDR					
	N	Design	Treatment	Mean VSD	2 Gy ED	BED (Late) $\alpha/\beta = 3$	Endpoint	Incidence
Noyes[100]	63	Phase II	Vaginal cuff 16.2 Gy × 2 = 32.4 Gy	32.4 Gy		207.4 Gy	Necrosis	0%
							Apical fibrosis	22%
							Stenosis	1.6%
Sorbe[24]	290	Phase III RCT	Vaginal cuff 2.5 Gy × 6 = 15 Gy	22.5 Gy	30.4 Gy		Vaginal shortening	Mean = 2.1 cm
			5 Gy × 6 = 30 Gy	45 Gy	94.5 Gy		Vaginal shortening	Mean = 0.3 cm[a]
Alektiar[41]	382	Retrospective review	Vaginal cuff Mean 7 Gy × 3 = 21 Gy	34.2 Gy		70 Gy at 0.5 cm	Necrosis	3%
Onsrud[68]	217	Phase III RCT	Vaginal cuff 5.5 Gy × 4 = 22 Gy	<30 Gy			Grade 1–2 fibrosis	12%
				30–40 Gy			Grade 1–2 fibrosis	26%
				>40 Gy			Grade 1–2 fibrosis	37%
Pearcey[42]	1,800	Retrospective review	Vaginal cuff		<60 Gy	<100 Gy	Severe late toxicity[b]	0.2% (2/1,098)
					>60 Gy	>100 Gy	Severe late toxicity[b]	14% (82/594)

[a]Statistically significant ($p < 0.05$).
[b]Pooled toxicity for all organs.
BED, biologically equivalent dose; ED, equivalent dose; f/u, follow-up; Gy, gray; VSD, vaginal surface dose.

Whereas bowel toxicity has previously been the major limiting factor to such an approach, improvements in imaging, treatment planning, and dose delivery make it feasible to safely deliver higher doses to the vagina with external beam treatment. Molla et al. reported their results treating 16 patients with endometrial and cervical cancer using definitive external beam radiation. All patients received pelvic radiotherapy to 45 to 50.4 Gy in 1.8 Gy/fraction followed by stereotactic boost to the vaginal vault with or without inclusion of the parametria. Postoperative treatment was delivered in 12 patients (2 × 7 Gy to the Plannin Target Volume (PTV) with a 4 to 7-day interval between fractions). In the four nonoperated patients, a dose of 4 Gy/fraction was given for five fractions at 2 to 3 days' interval. For each boost fraction, daily immobilization and alignment were performed using a vacuum body cast, IR guidance (ExacTrac, BrainLAB), and a rectal balloon. At a median follow-up of 12.6 months, the authors reported seven (44%) total cases of grade 1 sexual dysfunction using LENT-SOMA criteria and no grade two or higher toxicities. No rectovaginal or vesicovaginal fistulas were reported.[46] These early results are similar to other studies documenting sexual changes following whole pelvic irradiation to 50 Gy followed by 35-Gy intracavitary LDR boost.[47]

DISTAL VAGINAL INJURY. In contrast to cervical and endometrial cancer, vaginal cancer is rare. This, combined with its comparatively poor prognosis, limits the availability of long-term data. Despite a lack of standardized treatments, retrospective studies from the treatment of vaginal cancer are the few available sources of toxicity data following high radiation doses to the distal vagina. Studies reporting vaginal injury following radiation treatment of vaginal cancer are summarized in Table 36.5.

Lian et al. reported on 55 patients with vaginal cancer treated with a variety of radiation techniques. The highest doses were delivered in patients who received brachytherapy and external beam (70.9–72.6 Gy); the lowest doses were delivered in patients

who received intracavitary brachytherapy alone (43.5-Gy HDR, 60-Gy LDR). Techniques differed based on location of the tumor within the vagina, with interstitial brachytherapy used for tumors located in the anterior wall and in the lower two thirds of the vagina, and intracavitary brachytherapy used for tumors in the posterior wall and upper third of the vagina. Using SOMA criteria, 29 patients (53%) experienced grade 1 to 2 vaginal toxicity and 6 (10%) experienced grade 3 to 4 vaginal injury. Five percent of patients developed rectovaginal fistulas. Radiation dose of >70 Gy was found to correlate significantly with the incidence of vaginal toxicity. Location in the vagina did not correlate with incidence of toxicity using techniques adapted to location.[48]

In the retrospective toxicity analysis by Hintz et al.,[16] three patients were treated with intracavitary LDR brachytherapy alone up to 8,000 cGy with no necrosis or fistula. Total doses >9,800 cGy to the vaginal mucosa were associated with increased incidence of necrosis, and there were no cases of necrosis requiring surgery in patients receiving <9,800 cGy total vaginal mucosal dose.[16]

De Crevoisier et al. reported a retrospective analysis of 91 patients who underwent definitive radiotherapy for vaginal carcinoma. All patients received 45 to 50 Gy of external beam radiation to the pelvis using 1.8 to 2 Gy/fraction. Pelvic irradiation was followed by an intracavitary boost using customized acrylic multichannel intravaginal applicators. Thirty-nine patients received interstitial brachytherapy in addition to external beam and intracavitary brachytherapy. The minimum prescription dose to the Clinical Target Volume (CTV) was 60 Gy. With a median follow-up of 4.3 years, the authors reported 13 grade 2 or 3 vaginal toxicities (Franco-Italian glossary) with three documented fistulas. Overall, the incidence of severe late vaginal toxicity was 18%. Both involvement of multiple vaginal segments and FIGO stage were associated with vaginal stenosis. The addition of interstitial brachytherapy was not found to correlate with increased toxicity.[49]

Frank et al. reported the MDACC experience with definitive RT for vaginal cancer. In their series, 193 patients were treated between 1970 and 2000 with a variety of techniques. Ninety-five percent of patients received external beam radiation and the majority also received brachytherapy. For early-stage lesions, patients typically received 40 to 45 Gy external beam radiation followed by an LDR brachytherapy boost. The mean total dose to the vaginal surface (for superficial tumors) and tumor volume (for deeper lesions) was 85 Gy. The majority of patients with advanced lesions (66%) were treated with external beam radiation alone to a mean dose of 64 Gy. Patients with advanced disease who were treated with external beam and brachytherapy received a mean dose of 76 Gy. At a median follow-up of 11 years, seven patients (3%) had developed fistulas (5 GI, 2 vesicovaginal). The majority of severe rectal complications occurred in patients with tumors involving the posterior vaginal wall, while both vesicovaginal fistulas occurred with tumors involving the anterior wall. Both FIGO stage and smoking were significantly correlated with risk of late complications on univariate analysis.[32]

Mock et al. reported on 86 patients with vaginal cancer treated with HDR brachytherapy with or without external beam radiation. Seventy-three received intracavitary HDR with a vaginal cylinder prescribed to depth of 0.5 to 0.75 cm. Two to six insertions of 5 to 8 Gy each were performed. In patients receiving both EBRT and HDR, this yielded a mean VSD of 94 Gy (31–158 Gy) and a BED (early) of 182 Gy_{10} (55–351 Gy). Eight patients received interstitial brachytherapy. Using EORTC grading system, 13% had grade 1 and 3% of patients experienced grade 2 vaginal toxicity. There was an increased incidence in late vaginal complications with 11% of patients experiencing grade 1 to 2 toxicity and 4% experiencing grade 3 to 4 toxicity. There was a significantly greater incidence of severe toxicity in patients receiving combined external beam and brachytherapy compared to those receiving brachytherapy alone. However, this effect was not controlled for dose that was consistently higher for combined therapy.[50]

Ogino et al. reported on 20 patients with vaginal intraepithelial neoplasia treated with intracavitary HDR. Doses ranged from 15 to 30 Gy given in three to six fractions. Of the two patients treated to the entire vaginal length, one patient had moderate and one had severe vaginal toxicity. These patients had received four and five fractions of 5 Gy.[27]

Samant et al. reported on 12 patients with vaginal cancer treated with concurrent cisplatin-based chemoradiation. All patients received pelvic external beam radiation with a mean dose of 45 Gy in 25 fractions followed by brachytherapy. Ten patients received interstitial brachytherapy and two received intracavitary treatment. The median prescribed dose from brachytherapy was 30 Gy given in either one LDR or three HDR insertions. Two patients (17%) developed vesicovaginal fistulas. Both had received interstitial brachytherapy to 25 and 30 Gy. Four patients (33%) developed significant vaginal vault fibrosis.[51]

Barillot et al. reported a retrospective review of 642 patients with cervical cancer treated with radical RT at the Centre GF Leclerc France from 1970 to 1994. Patients were treated according to Fletcher tables and later ICRU guideline. Vaginal cylinders were used for patients with narrow vaults or extension of tumor into the distal third of the vagina. Use of brachytherapy to the entire vagina was strongly correlated with incidence of

G3-4 genital complications (OR = 9.3, p = 0.002 for G3-4 with use of vaginal cylinder).[52]

The results of studies reporting on vaginal radiation injury following treatment for vaginal cancer are summarized in Table 36.4. While the majority of patients experience low-grade late toxicity, the incidence of severe late toxicity is typically <4%.

DOSE RATE DATA

For a given degree of acute effect or tumor control, LDR brachytherapy preferentially spares late-responding normal tissues compared to HDR. Thus, to maintain equivalent tumor control and toxicity to traditional LDR while using HDR, increased normal tissue must be spared. In HDR, selective dwell times give more flexibility for modifying dose distribution and improving normal tissue avoidance. These geometric advantages are necessary to overcome the inherent radiobiologic disadvantage of HDR in terms of late tissue injury.

Clinical Data for Dose Rate

LDR. Low dose rateLDR brachytherapy is typically defined as <200 cGy/h. Traditionally in the treatment of cervical cancer, the dose rate at point A is 40 to 60 cGy/h. Prior to the widespread acceptance of HDR brachytherapy, multiple clinical studies compared outcomes with different LDRs. Lambin et al. reported the results of a randomized study comparing two LDRs for cervical cancer. Two hundred and four patients received 60-Gy brachytherapy using custom intrauterine and intravaginal applicators followed by hysterectomy. There was a statistically significant increase in all late complications with 73 cGy/h versus 38 cGy/h. There was a nonsignificant increase in the incidence of severe toxicity in 73 cGy/h arm with four vesicovaginal fistulas versus two in 38 cGy/h arm.[53]

Haie-Meder et al. reported the results of a randomized trial comparing two LDRs of intracavitary brachytherapy for preop cervical cancer. A total of 204 patients were randomized to receive 60 Gy (to point A) delivered at either 40 cGy/h versus 80 cGy/h via a custom intravaginal applicator. The authors demonstrated a statistically significant increase in complications in the higher dose-rate group. Four vesicovaginal fistulas were reported in the 80 cGy/h arm versus two in the 40 cGy/h arm. Dyspareunia was reported in 17 patients receiving 80 cGy/h versus seven patients in the 40 cGy/h arm. Ureterovaginal fistulas were reported in seven total patients.[54] The use of adjuvant surgery may have contributed to the relatively high incidence of ureterovaginal fistulas seen on this trial.

HDR. Fu and Phillips performed a literature review of all published English literature series comparing HDR and LDR. Within individual institutions, they found comparable rates of toxicity. However, they were unable to compare across institutions due to differences in techniques, fractionation, doses, and reporting.[55]

Akine et al. published their analysis of 300 patients treated for cervical cancer with EBRT and either intracavitary LDR or HDR brachytherapy. Pelvic dose from EBRT was 48 to 52 Gy. LDR treatment was given in one to two applications delivering 11 to 52 Gy to point A. HDR treatment was given in four fractions of 5 to 20 Gy. A dose-response equation was generated from the cases of radiation injury in the LDR group and

TABLE 36.4	Retrospective Studies Reporting Radiation Injury to the Vagina in Treatment of Vaginal Cancer						
Author/ Institution (y)	N	F/u (y)	EBRT Dose	Brachy Modality/ Dose	Endpoint	Incidence	Comments
de Crevoisier[49]/ Gustave-Roussy Institute	91	4.3	45–50 Gy 1.8–2 Gy/fx ± parametrial/ iliac boost to 60 Gy	IC LDR using ± IS in 39 patients/ total dose including EBRT = 60 Gy	Grade 2–3 vaginal stenosis Vaginal fistula	14% 3%	FIGO stage and involvement of multiple vaginal segments correlated with severe toxicity
Chyle[72]/MDACC (1953–1991)	301	12.9 mean (among 112 patients alive at f/u)	Stage dependent	Stage dependent/ mean total dose = 74.7 Gy, (10–154 Gy)	Serious ulceration/ necrosis Vaginal fistula	3% 4%	FIGO stage, tumor size, and staging LAD correlated with severe toxicity. No ulceration in patients receiving EBRT alone
Dixit[101]/India (1985–1989)	70	All >2 y	45–60 Gy 1.8–2 Gy/fx	33 cases—IC LDR with cylinder/20–25 Gy 5 mm depth (400 cGy/h) 12 cascs—IC LDR with tandem and cylinder/22.5 Gy to PtA (140–160 cGy/h)	Vaginal fistula	3%	No severe toxicity if dose <70 Gy total Young mean age (47 yo)
Frank[32]/MDACC (1970–2000)	193	11 median	Early stage 40–45 Gy Advanced mean 64 Gy (EBRT alone)	LDR boost/mean total tumor dose – 85 Gy LDR boost/mean total dose of 76 Gy	Vaginal fistula	3%	FIGO stage and smoking correlated with severe complications. 21% major complications for stages III–IVa
Lian[48]/University of Alberta (1986–2006)	30	4.2	EBRT alone 60.5 Gy EBRT + brachy 43.3–45 Gy external	 IS LDR = 27.6 Gy IC LDR = 28 Gy IC HDR = 25.5 Gy to surface	Any SOMA vaginal toxicity Any SOMA vaginal toxicity Any SOMA vaginal toxicity Any SOMA vaginal toxicity	47% (8/17) 78% (7/9) 83% (5/6) 85% (11/13)	10% fistula incidence, all cases occurring in EBRT + brachy group
Marcus[102]/ University of Florida (1964–1975)	22		Early stages I–II, EBRT 40–50 Gy Late stages II–IV, 37.5–60 Gy	IC LDR 40–70 Gy to vaginal surface IS LDR 15–50 Gy to target	Vaginal necrosis lasting >3 mo or requiring surgery	11%	No major complications at total doses of <9,000 rad
Mock[50]/Vienna (1986–1998)	28		EBRT + HDR				

fx, fraction; f/u, follow-up; IC, intracavitary; IS, interstitial; LAD, lymphadenectomy; LDR, low dose rate.

correlated to the incidence of toxicity in the HDR group (4%). From this, the authors concluded that the clinically equivalent dose for HDR is two-thirds the LDR dose. While the analysis is valid, it should be noted that only 1 of the 12 major events (a rectovaginal fistula) was due to vaginal injury.[56] Other retrospective studies have reported local control and late effects equivalent to LDR with HDR when HDR was given in three to five fractions and total dose reduced to 60% to 80% of traditional LDR doses. [55,57,58]

As discussed in the section on stenosis and fibrosis, Sorbe and Smeds demonstrated in a randomized study that increased dose per fraction was strongly correlated with vaginal shortening. The study that utilized prospectively gathered colpometry from 404 patients treated randomized to one of four HDR regimens. At 5 years, average vaginal length relative to baseline was 59% for the 4.5 Gy × 6 group, 50% for the 5 Gy × 6 group, 40% for the 6 Gy × 5 group, and 21% for the 9 Gy × 4 group[24] (Fig. 36.6).

Orton et al. published the results of a questionnaire sent to all known HDR facilities worldwide. Clinicians reported results on 17,067 patients. HDR doses of >7 Gy/fraction were associated with increased incidence of moderate and severe toxicity (11.2% vs. 7.6%).[59]

SPECIAL CONSIDERATIONS

Pediatric Treatment

Limited data for late vaginal radiation injury come from the treatment of pediatric vaginal rhabdomyosarcoma. The Institut Gustave Roussy reported their long-term results following brachytherapy for vulvar and vaginal rhabdomyosarcoma in 39 girls (mean age = 2.6 years). The series spanned from 1971 and 2005. Radiation therapy consisted of 60 to 65 Gy LDR endocavitary brachytherapy (or interstitial treatment for patients with vulvar involvement) following induction chemotherapy. Prior to 1991, this dose was prescribed to cover the initial, prechemotherapy target volume. After 1991, only the residual tumor following induction chemotherapy was included. This practice change corresponded with a 50% reduction in treatment volume. Consequently, the incidence of long-term vaginal and urethral stricture decreased from 75% to 21%.[60]

Reirradiation

There are limited data reporting vaginal injury following repeat irradiation. Beriwal reported on 18 patients who underwent HDR brachytherapy for recurrent or primary vaginal cancer. Five patients had received prior radiation. Seventeen patients received external beam radiation to a median dose of 45 Gy. All patients then had additional HDR brachytherapy either with an interstitial template[13] or with an intracavitary applicator. The interstitial dose was 18.75 Gy in five fractions given twice daily. At a median follow-up of 18 months, two patients had developed grade 3 or higher toxicity (rectovaginal fistula and chronic vaginal ulcer). Both patients had received prior radiation.[61]

A larger retrospective study from China reported 73 cases treated with reirradiation for recurrent vaginal malignancy following initial radiotherapy for cervical cancer. Patients treated before 1981 received intracavitary radium with 60 to 74 Gy prescribed to point A given in four weekly fractions. After 1981, patients were treated with cobalt-60 HDR twice-weekly 5 Gy × 10

total fractions for a total dose of 50 Gy. A vaginal mold was used for lesions in the middle or lower vagina with a dose of 30 to 40 Gy given in six fractions prescribed to a depth of 5 mm below the vaginal surface. The majority of severe toxicities were rectal, again demonstrating the increased radiosensitivity of bowel relative to the vagina. Still, 11% of patients developed rectovaginal fistulas and one patient developed a vesicovaginal fistula.[62]

FACTORS CONTRIBUTING TO INJURY

Patient-Related Factors Contributing to Toxicity

In general, hypertension, diabetes, and active collagen vascular disease are felt to increase risk of radiation-related toxicity.[63,64] These factors all correlate with vascular injury, which is believed to delay wound healing. The role of vascular insult in vaginal radiation injury is supported by histologic findings following radiation as well as by case reports of revascularization leading to resolution of previously nonhealing vaginal necrosis.[42]

Multiple studies have demonstrated an increased incidence of fistula development following treatment for vaginal cancer that has invaded the bladder or rectum. This incidence has been reported as high as 25% in some series.[30–32]

Data from MDACC have consistently shown increased risk of injury in smokers treated with radiation for gynecologic malignancies. Eifel showed an increased incidence in rectal, small bowel, and bladder complications in smokers treated with radiation for localized cervical cancer. Although vaginal injury was not specifically addressed, rectovaginal and vesicovaginal fistula development were coded as rectal and bladder complications, respectively. Likewise, a retrospective review of patients treated at MDACC for vaginal cancer showed a 25% 5-year risk of complications in current smokers versus a 5% risk in never smokers.[32] This correlation has also been demonstrated by other authors. Moore et al. reported on 23 patients with stage IVa cervical cancer and bladder extension. No correlation was shown between technique and fistula incidence, but there was a significantly higher incidence of fistula development among smokers (73% vs. 27%, $p = 0.03$).[31]

Age over 50 at the time of treatment has been correlated with increased risk of vaginal stenosis.[22] Presumably this is secondary to the loss of the protective effects of estrogen on the vaginal mucosa of postmenopausal women.

Radiation Factors Contributing to Toxicity

Due to the rapid dose fall-off with brachytherapy, multiple technical factors can dramatically affect VSD and dose rate. VSDs are therefore significantly higher than doses at point A. Au and Grigsby calculated mucosal surface dose from 274 patients treated with Fletcher Suit LDR. A rate of 65 cGy/h at point A yielded an average mucosal dose rate of 175 cGy/h (270% of point A).[65] The single common factor contributing to increased vaginal toxicity with radiation technique is increased surface dose.

TANDEM AND OVOID. Treatment with short source-surface distances results in significantly greater VSDs for the same dose at depth.[15,66] Comparing two different colpostat sizes delivering 70 Gy to point A, a 1-cm colpostat gives 350-Gy mucosal dose relative to 120 Gy using 2.5-cm diameter colpostats.[15] Using a tandem and ring HDR system prescribed to point

A, Bergmark documented a 44% change in VSD with source position changes of <1 mm.[67] In clinical practice, multiple studies have shown a strong correlation between decreased colpostat diameter and increased vaginal toxicity. Mini-colpostats have been associated with increased grade 3 to 4 GI and GU toxicity over standard Fletcher systems.[68] In addition to increasing ovoid size, vaginal injury can be minimized by judicious use of vaginal packing to reduce dose to uninvolved tissues. This can be done with gauze soaked in petroleum jelly or 40% iodine for visualization on radiographs.

VAGINAL CYLINDER. Short source to surface distances may contribute to vaginal injury when treating with vaginal cylinders. Increased cylinder diameter has been shown to improve VSD.[69] Clinically, vaginal complications following intracavitary HDR brachytherapy have been found to be higher in patients treated with cylinders of <2.5 cm in diameter.[70] It is therefore recommended that the largest comfortable diameter cylinder be used. If patient anatomy dictates the use of a small diameter cylinder, care should be taken not to exceed vaginal mucosal tolerance.

Prescription depth selection is a major determinant of surface dose and consequently vaginal injury. Onsrud et al. documented a significant decrease in the incidence of late vaginal complications following an institutional switch from a standardized 5-mm prescription depth to a customized depth. In their series, 217 patients underwent adjuvant intravaginal brachytherapy following hysterectomy for early-stage endometrial cancer. Prescription depth was individualized down to a minimum of 3 mm based on the physician's clinical estimate of mucosal thickness. Four fractions of 5.5 Gy were administered with HDR (0.5–1.4 Gy/min) using 2 to 4 cm diameter cylinders. In patients with 5-mm prescription depth, 34% experienced grade 1 to 2 vaginal reactions (Franco Italian glossary). In contrast, 18% of patients in the customized depth group (median depth) experienced grade 1 to 2 complications. As would be expected, there was also a strong correlation between the calculated VSD and the incidence of complications; 12% of patients experiencing grade 1 to 2 vaginal reactions following VSD of <30 Gy versus 37% of patients receiving >40 Gy to surface.[70]

Several authors have recommended optimization of HDR cylinder plans using calculation points at the cylinder apex in addition to the lateral walls. Both Nag and Li[69,71] have shown that optimization without calculation points placed along the curved end of the tandem can result in hot spots at the vaginal apex in excess of 150% of lateral wall dose.

Some authors have advocated for the use of multichannel cylinders for irradiation of vaginal tumors.[72] Such applicators give increased flexibility and allow for noncircumferential vaginal irradiation. When such an approach is used, it is imperative that VSDs be calculated due to the increased proximity of sources to the mucosa. Several authors have documented increased incidence of vaginal necrosis, fistula, and chronic ulceration with sources on the surface of an intravaginal obturator.[16,73]

INTERSTITIAL. Multiple retrospective studies have demonstrated an increased incidence of vaginal necrosis and fistula with the addition of interstitial brachytherapy to external beam radiation.[74] However, these studies did not control for increased dose used when combined modalities were administered. Toxicity following interstitial brachytherapy may be more a function of dose heterogeneity than of prescribed dose. Several authors have recommended using hotspot volume as a constraint in interstitial brachytherapy.[75,76] Erickson recommends that no more than 25% of the implant volume exceed 10% of the prescription dose.

VOLUME CONSIDERATIONS. Although partial volume tolerances have not been established for the vagina, studies have illustrated a general trend of increased toxicity with increased volume irradiated. Increased length of vagina irradiated has been correlated with increased stenosis and fistula development.[15,27,49,77]

Circumferential vaginal irradiation has been associated with an increased incidence of symptomatic fibrosis. Stryker et al.[78] reported increased incidence of grade 3 SOMA vaginal stenosis with the use of vaginal cylinder intracavitary boost versus noncircumferential interstitial boost. Authors have recommended limiting treatment to <75% of the vaginal circumference when possible.[79]

Other treatment Factors Contributing to Toxicity

CHEMOTHERAPY. Despite multiple randomized trials for cervical cancer looking at the use of concurrent chemoradiation, vaginal injury has not been routinely addressed. Greven et al. reported vaginal toxicity data on 44 patients treated with adjuvant cisplatin-based chemoradiation for high-risk endometrial cancer. Patients received 45-Gy EBRT to the pelvis followed by intracavitary brachytherapy (20 Gy LDR or 3 × 6 Gy HDR prescribed to the vaginal surface). They documented four cases of grade 1 acute vaginal toxicity,[80] nine grade 1, and five grade 2 late vaginal mucosal injury.[81] This incidence is compatible with other studies treating with similar radiation regimens without chemotherapy. Other authors have reported increased incidence of soft tissue necrosis and fistula development with concurrent chemoradiation for vaginal cancer, but the number of patients is limited.[82]

Samant et al. reported on 12 patients treated with concurrent cisplatin and radiation for primary vaginal cancer. The median external beam radiation dose was 45 Gy and the median intracavitary surface dose was 30 Gy. The authors reported two cases of rectovaginal fistula formation (both in patients treated with interstitial brachytherapy) and four cases of significant vaginal vault fibrosis at a median follow-up of 50 months.[51]

Dalrymple et al. reported their experience with concurrent 5-fluorouracil-based chemotherapy and radiation for early-stage primary vaginal cancer. External beam radiation and LDR intracavitary brachytherapy were administered to a median total dose of 63 Gy. They reported no case of vaginal fistula.[44]

Vaginal necrosis as a radiation recall reaction has been reported following administration of Idarubicin in a patient previously treated with radiation for vaginal cancer 3 years prior.[83]

Overall, chemotherapy has not been clearly demonstrated to increase the risk of vaginal radiation injury. However, few studies have specifically addressed late vaginal toxicity.

SURGERY. Multiple studies have shown an increased incidence in fistula formation in patients undergoing surgery in addition to pelvic radiation.[23,74,84-86] An early retrospective series from MDACC showed a fourfold increase in fistula development in patients who underwent hysterectomy following

TABLE 36.5	Known Risk Factors for Vaginal Radiation Injury
Risk Factor	*Endpoint*
Distal location	Necrosis
High cumulative surface dose	Fistula, stenosis, shortening, necrosis
Increased dose rate	Stenosis, shortening, necrosis
Age > 50	Stenosis
Circumferential irradiation	Stenosis
Reirradiation	Fistula, necrosis
Increased length	Stenosis, shortening
Bowel or bladder invasion	Fistula
Surgery	Fistula
Smoking	Fistula

radiation. Interestingly, the interval between surgery and fistula development was significantly greater in the patients who received radiation versus patients who developed fistulas following surgery alone (11.6 vs. 7.7 weeks, respectively).[84] A later series from MDACC of more than 1,700 patients treated for early-stage cervical cancer documented a 5.2% risk of fistula formation in patients who received pretreatment laparotomy versus 2.9% in those treated with RT alone. Similarly, the risk of fistula development in patients undergoing adjuvant hysterectomy was 5.3% versus 2.6% in the nonoperated group.[87] Bergmark et al. reported a significant increase in subjective vaginal changes in patients who had undergone surgery and radiation as opposed to patients treated with either as a single modality[35] (Table 36.5).

PREVENTION AND TREATMENT OF RADIATION INJURY

Acute Toxicity

Maintenance of hygiene, treatment of infection, and control of pain with oral or topical analgesics are the mainstays of management for acute vaginal radiation injury.[88] Candida is a frequent cause of vaginitis and clinicians should have a low threshold for starting treatment with topical antifungals. The confluent pattern of radiation mucositis should be distinguished from the more discretely marginated ulcerations of Herpes Simplex Virus. These are typically seen on the labia and may be aggravated by pelvic irradiation.[89] Topical analgesics such as lidocaine may help vaginitis. Oral pain medications may be required.

Reduction of trauma to a denuded epithelium in the form of abstinence from intercourse is typically recommended in symptomatic patients. While providing a treatment break may seem intuitive for patients having severe acute toxicity, extending duration of treatment has been associated with loss of local control in cervical cancer without any significant reduction in toxicity.[23,90,91]

Late Toxicity

PREVENTION. Given the correlation between acute vaginal toxicity and development of long-term necrosis and fistula, methods to limit acute vaginal injury may decrease the development of late injuries.

Mechanical vaginal dilation in the form of regular intercourse or the use of a rigid obturator is routinely recommended following vaginal radiation therapy.[92] There is nonrandomized data supporting the use of mechanical dilators for maintenance of vaginal patency. Pitkin documented that patients who remained sexually active are more likely to have normal vaginal caliber. Likewise, Sorbe and Smeds found that continued sexual activity was significantly associated with decreased vaginal shortening following intravaginal brachytherapy.[24]

Topical estrogen has been shown to reduce the incidence of late vaginal toxicity in a randomized controlled trial. Pitkin et al. performed a double-blinded placebo trial in which patients who had received radiation were randomized to 0.1% topical dienestrol intravaginally or placebo. These were applied nightly three times weekly for 6 to 9 months following radiation. Patients randomized to estrogen had a significantly lower incidence of stenosis and dyspareunia and showed less cytologic changes in vaginal epithelium on smears.[92] Topical mitomycin-c has also been reported to prevent postradiotherapy vaginal stenosis in two small series.[93,94]

While effective at decreasing incidence of vaginal symptoms, topical estrogens are systemically absorbed and may therefore be contraindicated from an oncologic perspective.[95] In patients with an intact uterus, unopposed estrogen therapy is generally not advised following radiation therapy in women with adenocarcinomas. In the setting of postradiotherapy cervical os stenosis, estrogen supplementation without progesterone may lead to endometrial proliferation with resultant hematocolpos.[89,96]

TREATMENT. Once fibrosis has ensued, it is not clear to what degree mechanical dilation can reverse stenosis and shortening. There have been case reports of development of rectovaginal fistulas in patients starting mechanical dilatation with a vaginal obturator following the onset of stenosis, but this appears to occur only rarely.[97] Regardless of its ability to reverse existing fibrosis, gentle dilation is recommended to prevent progression of stenosis. When conservative measures have failed, surgery should be considered for management of severe stenosis.

Conservative management of radiation necrosis includes local debridement, H_2O_2 douches, antibiotics, antifungals, estrogen. Biopsy of persistent ulceration is necessary to differentiate necrosis from recurrent tumor. However, multiple biopsies should be avoided as this practice has been anecdotally implicated in increased risk of fistula formation.[98] Hyperbaric oxygen has been reported to facilitate healing of persistent vaginal necrosis in at least two small series.[99,100] Fink et al. reported on 14 patients who underwent hyperbaric oxygen treatment for radiation injury following treatment for gynecologic cancers. Of the 14 patients, 5 had treatment for vaginal necrosis or vaginitis. All patients with vaginal ulceration experienced a >50% reduction in the size of their lesions.[100]

Radiation-induced vesicovaginal or rectovaginal fistulas can be challenging to manage. Nonsurgical interventions such as urinary diversion in the case of vesicovaginal fistula may be effective. However, fecal diversion for rectovaginal fistula without additional surgery has not been typically found to be effective.[101]

Successful management of sexual dysfunction requires an understanding of the underlying causes of the dysfunction. Oftentimes, patients avoid sexual intercourse following radiation out of concern for injury. Reassurance and encouragement may be all that is required in these situations. Despite the fact that sexual dysfunction can significantly impact subjective well-being, patients are often reluctant to report sexual difficulties following radiation because they feel they are not "serious enough." Routine inquiry should therefore be made regarding sexual function at time of posttreatment evaluation. Patients should be counseled regarding adequate lubrication and routine dilatation. Denton and Maher found level 2C evidence supporting the use of mechanical dilatation and level 2A evidence for the use of topical estrogen in the management of postradiotherapy sexual dysfunction.[18]

CONCLUSION

Despite the high radiation tolerance of the vagina relative to adjacent critical organs, brachytherapy can significantly increase VSDs and, consequently, the risk of severe late injury. The impact of potential loss of vaginal function should be considered when selecting fractionation regimens. Mucosal doses should never be assumed to be within tolerance without being implicitly calculated. Additionally, patients should be educated on appropriate measures for the prevention of stenosis following vaginal irradiation.

REFERENCES

1. American Cancer Society: Key Statistics. 2009. Available from: www.cancer.org.
2. Weidner GJ, Mayr NA, Saw CB, et al. Radiation field simulation of gynecologic malignancies: localization of the cervix and vagina with a flexible vaginal localizer contrast tampon. *Radiology.* 1999;211(3):876–881.
3. Kim CR, Eaton BA, Stevens KR Jr. Localization of the apex of the vagina: implications for radiation therapy planning. *Radiology.* 1999;212(1):155–158.
4. Wiggenraad RG, Coerkamp EG, Tamminga RJ, et al. Contrast vaginography is more accurate than the radiopaque rod for localization of the vagina. *Int J Radiat Oncol Biol Phys.* 2000;48(5):1439–1442.
5. Katz A, Njuguna E, Rakowsky E, et al. Early development of vaginal shortening during radiation therapy for endometrial or cervical cancer. *Int J Gynecol Cancer.* 2001;11(3):234–235.
6. Choo JJ, Scudiere J, Bitterman P, et al. Vaginal lymphatic channel location and its implication for intracavitary brachytherapy radiation treatment. *Brachytherapy.* 2005;4(3):236–240.
7. Siegelman ES, Outwater EK, Banner MP, et al. High-resolution MR imaging of the vagina. *Radiographics.* 1997;17(5):1183–1203.
8. Fajardo LF. *Pathology of Radiation Injury.* New York, NY: Masson Pub. USA; 1982.
9. Rubin P, Casarett GW. *Clinical Radiation Pathology [by] Philip Rubin [and] George W. Casarett.* Philadelphia, London: Saunders; 1968.
10. Abitbol MM, Davenport JH. The irradiated vagina. *Obstet Gynecol.* 1974;44(2):249–256.
11. Gupta S, Gupta YN, Sanyal B. Radiation changes in vaginal and cervical cytology in carcinoma of the cervix uteri. *J Surg Oncol.* 1982;19(2):71–73.
12. Graham RM. The effect of radiation on vaginal cells in cervical carcinoma; description of cellular changes. *Surg Gynecol Obstet.* 1947;84:153–183.
13. Caffo O, Amichetti M, Mussari S, et al. Physical side effects and quality of life during postoperative radiotherapy for uterine cancer: prospective evaluation by a diary card. *Gynecol Oncol.* 2003;88(3):270–276.
14. Davidson SE, Burns MP, Routledge JA, et al. The impact of radiotherapy for carcinoma of the cervix on sexual function assessed using the LENT SOMA scales. *Radiother Oncol.* 2003;68(3):241–247.
15. Fletcher GH. *Textbook of Radiotherapy.* 2nd ed. Philadelphia, PA: Lea & Febiger; 1973.
16. Hintz BL, Kagan AR, Chan P, et al. Radiation tolerance of the vaginal mucosa. *Int J Radiat Oncol Biol Phys.* 1980;6(6):711–716.
17. Zannoni GF, Vellone VG. Accuracy of Papanicolaou smears in cervical cancer patients treated with radiochemotherapy followed by radical surgery. *Am J Clin Pathol.* 2008;130(5):787–794.
18. Denton AS, Maher EJ. Interventions for the physical aspects of sexual dysfunction in women following pelvic radiotherapy. *Cochrane Database Syst Rev.* 2003;(1).CD003750.
19. Kaufman RH, Topek NH, Wall JA. Late irradiation changes in vaginal cytology. *Am J Obstet Gynecol.* 1961;81:859–866.
20. Yavuz E, Ozluk Y, Kucucuk S, et al. Radiation-induced benign glandular cells in posthysterectomy smears: a cytomorphologic and clinical analysis. *Int J Gynecol Cancer.* 2006;16(2):670–674.
21. Hartman P, Diddle AW. Vaginal stenosis following irradiation therapy for carcinoma of the cervix uteri. *Cancer.* 1972;30(2):426–429.
22. Brand AH, Bull CA, Cakir B. Vaginal stenosis in patients treated with radiotherapy for carcinoma of the cervix. *Int J Gynecol Cancer.* 2006;16(1):288–293.
23. Eifel PJ, Levenback C, Wharton JT, et al. Time course and incidence of late complications in patients treated with radiation therapy for FIGO stage IB carcinoma of the uterine cervix. *Int J Radiat Oncol Biol Phys.* 1995;32(5):1289–1300.
24. Sorbe BG, Smeds AC. Postoperative vaginal irradiation with high dose rate afterloading technique in endometrial carcinoma stage I. *Int J Radiat Oncol Biol Phys.* 1990;18(2):305–314.
25. Bruner DW, Lanciano R, Keegan M, et al. Vaginal stenosis and sexual function following intracavitary radiation for the treatment of cervical and endometrial carcinoma. *Int J Radiat Oncol Biol Phys.* 1993;27(4):825–830.
26. Meyer J. *Radiation Injury: Advances in Management and Prevention.* Basel; New York, NY: Karger; 1999.
27. Ogino I, Kitamura T, Okajima H, et al. High-dose-rate intracavitary brachytherapy in the management of cervical and vaginal intraepithelial neoplasia. *Int J Radiat Oncol Biol Phys.* 1998;40(4):881–887.
28. Saclarides TJ, Rectovaginal fistula. *Surg Clin North Am.* 2002;82(6):1261–1272.
29. Yu NC, Raman SS, Patel M, et al. Fistulas of the genitourinary tract: a radiologic review. *Radiographics.* 2004;24(5):1331–1352.
30. Chau PM, Fletcher GH, Rutledge FN, et al. Complications in high dose whole pelvis irradiation in female pelvic cancer. *Am J Roentgenol Radium Ther Nucl Med.* 1962;87:22–40.
31. Moore KN, Gold MA, McMeekin DS, et al. Vesicovaginal fistula formation in patients with stage IVA cervical carcinoma. *Gynecol Oncol.* 2007;106(3):498–501.
32. Frank SJ, Jhingran A, Levenback C, et al. Definitive radiation therapy for squamous cell carcinoma of the vagina. *Int J Radiat Oncol Biol Phys.* 2005;62(1):138–147.
33. Aristizabal SA, Woolfitt B, Valencia A, et al. Interstitial parametrial implants in carcinoma of the cervix stage II-B. *Int J Radiat Oncol Biol Phys.* 1987;13(3):445–450.
34. Vistad I, Cvancarova M, Fossa SD, et al. Postradiotherapy morbidity in long-term survivors after locally advanced cervical cancer: how well do physicians' assessments agree with those of their patients? *Int J Radiat Oncol Biol Phys.* 2008;71(5):1335–1342.
35. Bergmark K, Avall-Lundqvist E, Dickman PW, et al. Vaginal changes and sexuality in women with a history of cervical cancer. *N Engl J Med.* 1999;340(18):1383–1389.
36. Chassagne D, Sismondi P, Horiot JC, et al. A glossary for reporting complications of treatment in gynecological cancers. *Radiother Oncol.* 1993;26(3):195–202.
37. Rodrigus P, De Winter K, Leers WH, et al. Late radiotherapeutic morbidity in patients with carcinoma of the uterine cervix: the application of the French-Italian glossary. *Radiother Oncol.* 1996;40(2):153–157.
38. Hamberger AD, Unal A, Gershenson DM, et al. Analysis of the severe complications of irradiation of carcinoma of the cervix: whole pelvis irradiation and intracavitary radium. *Int J Radiat Oncol Biol Phys.* 1983;9(3):367–371.
39. Nori D, Merimsky O, Batata M, et al. Postoperative high dose-rate intravaginal brachytherapy combined with external irradiation for early stage endometrial cancer: a long-term follow-up. *Int J Radiat Oncol Biol Phys.* 1994;30(4):831–837.
40. Perez CA, Breaux S, Bedwinek JM, et al. Radiation therapy alone in the treatment of carcinoma of the uterine cervix. II. Analysis of complications. *Cancer.* 1984;54(2):235–246.
41. Alektiar KM, Venkatraman E, Chi DS, et al. Intravaginal brachytherapy alone for intermediate-risk endometrial cancer. *Int J Radiat Oncol Biol Phys.* 2005;62(1):111–117.
42. Pearcey RG, Petereit DG. Post-operative high dose rate brachytherapy in patients with low to intermediate risk endometrial cancer. *Radiother Oncol.* 2000;56(1):17–22.
43. Keys HM, Roberts JA, Brunetto VL, et al. A phase III trial of surgery with or without adjunctive external pelvic radiation therapy in intermediate risk endometrial adenocarcinoma: a Gynecologic Oncology Group study. *Gynecol Oncol.* 2004;92(3):744–751.
44. Lei ZZ, He FZ. External cobalt 60 irradiation alone for stage IIB carcinoma of the uterine cervix. *Int J Radiat Oncol Biol Phys.* 1989;16(2):339–341.
45. Barraclough LH, Swindell R, Livsey JE, et al. External beam boost for cancer of the cervix uteri when intracavitary therapy cannot be performed. *Int J Radiat Oncol Biol Phys.* 2008;71(3):772–778.
46. Molla M, Escude L, Nouet P, et al. Fractionated stereotactic radiotherapy boost for gynecologic tumors: an alternative to brachytherapy? *Int J Radiat Oncol Biol Phys.* 2005;62(1):118–124.
47. Jensen PT, Groenvold M, Klee MC, et al. Longitudinal study of sexual function and vaginal changes after radiotherapy for cervical cancer. *Int J Radiat Oncol Biol Phys.* 2003;56(4):937–949.
48. Lian J, Dundas G, Carlone M, et al. Twenty-year review of radiotherapy for vaginal cancer: An institutional experience. *Gynecol Oncol.* 2008;111(2):298–306.
49. de Crevoisier R, Sanfilippo N, Gerbaulet A, et al. Exclusive radiotherapy for primary squamous cell carcinoma of the vagina. *Radiother Oncol.* 2007;85(3):362–370.
50. Mock U, Kucera H, Fellner C, et al. High-dose-rate (HDR) brachytherapy with or without external beam radiotherapy in the treatment of primary vaginal carcinoma: long-term results and side effects. *Int J Radiat Oncol Biol Phys.* 2003;56(4):950–957.
51. Barillot I, Horiot JC, Maingon P, et al. Impact on treatment outcome and late effects of customized treatment planning in cervix carcinomas: baseline results to compare new strategies. *Int J Radiat Oncol Biol Phys.* 2000;48(1):189–200.
52. Nag S. *Principles and Practice of Brachytherapy.* Armonk, NY: Futura Pub.; 1997.
53. Lambin P, Gerbaulet A, Kramar A, et al. Phase III trial comparing two low dose rates in brachytherapy of cervix carcinoma: report at two years. *Int J Radiat Oncol Biol Phys.* 1993;25(3):405–412.
54. Haie-Meder C, Kramar A, Lambin P, et al. Analysis of complications in a prospective randomized trial comparing two brachytherapy low dose rates in cervical carcinoma. *Int J Radiat Oncol Biol Phys.* 1994;29(5):953–960.
55. Fu KK, Phillips TL. High-dose-rate versus low-dose-rate intracavitary brachytherapy for carcinoma of the cervix. *Int J Radiat Oncol Biol Phys.* 1990;19(3):791–796.
56. Akine Y, Tokita N, Ogino T, et al. Dose equivalence for high-dose-rate to low-dose-rate intracavitary irradiation in the treatment of cancer of the uterine cervix. *Int J Radiat Oncol Biol Phys.* 1990;19(6):1511–1514.
57. Orton CG, Seyedsadr M, Somnay A. Comparison of high and low dose rate remote afterloading for cervix cancer and the importance of fractionation. *Int J Radiat Oncol Biol Phys.* 1991;21(6):1425–1434.

58. Magne N, Oberlin O, Martelli H, et al. Vulval and vaginal rhabdomyosarcoma in children: update and reappraisal of institut gustave roussy brachytherapy experience. *Int J Radiat Oncol Biol Phys.* 2008;72(3):878–883.

59. Beriwal S, Heron DE, Mogus R, et al. High-dose rate brachytherapy (HDRB) for primary or recurrent cancer in the vagina. *Radiat Oncol.* 2008;3:7.

60. Xiang EW, Shu-mo C, Ya-qin D, et al. Treatment of late recurrent vaginal malignancy after initial radiotherapy for carcinoma of the cervix: an analysis of 73 cases. *Gynecol Oncol.* 1998;69(2):125–129.

61. Chon BH, Loeffler JS. The effect of nonmalignant systemic disease on tolerance to radiation therapy. *Oncologist.* 2002;7(2):136–143.

62. Hoffman KE, Horowitz NS, Russell AH. Healing of vulvo-vaginal radionecrosis following revascularization. *Gynecol Oncol.* 2007;106(1):262–264.

63. Au SP, Grigsby PW. The irradiation tolerance dose of the proximal vagina. *Radiother Oncol.* 2003;67(1):77–85.

64. Griffin NB. The gross radiation changes of the vagina. *South Med J.* 1968;61(10):1052–1056.

65. Berger D, Dimopoulos J, Georg P, et al. Uncertainties in assessment of the vaginal dose for intracavitary brachytherapy of cervical cancer using a tandem-ring applicator. *Int J Radiat Oncol Biol Phys.* 2007;67(5):1451–1459.

66. Paris KJ, Spanos WJ Jr, Day TG Jr, et al. Incidence of complications with mini vaginal culpostats in carcinoma of the uterine cervix. *Int J Radiat Oncol Biol Phys.* 1991;21(4):911–917.

67. Nag S, Erickson B, Parikh S, et al. The American Brachytherapy Society recommendations for high-dose-rate brachytherapy for carcinoma of the endometrium. *Int J Radiat Oncol Biol Phys.* 2000;48(3):779–790.

68. Onsrud M, Strickert T, Marthinsen AB. Late reactions after postoperative high-dose-rate intravaginal brachytherapy for endometrial cancer: a comparison of standardized and individualized target volumes. *Int J Radiat Oncol Biol Phys.* 2001;49(3):749–755.

69. Li S, Aref I, Walker E, et al. Effects of prescription depth, cylinder size, treatment length, tip space, and curved end on doses in high-dose-rate vaginal brachytherapy. *Int J Radiat Oncol Biol Phys.* 2007;67(4):1268–1277.

70. Demanes DJ, Rege S, Rodriquez RR, et al. The use and advantages of a multichannel vaginal cylinder in high-dose-rate brachytherapy. *Int J Radiat Oncol Biol Phys.* 1999;44(1):211–219.

71. Aristizabal SA, Surwit EA, Hevezi JM, et al. Treatment of advanced cancer of the cervix with transperineal interstitial irradiation. *Int J Radiat Oncol Biol Phys.* 1983;9(7):1013–1017.

72. Chyle V, Zagars GK, Wheeler JA, et al. Definitive radiotherapy for carcinoma of the vagina: outcome and prognostic factors. *Int J Radiat Oncol Biol Phys.* 1996;35(5):891–905.

73. Ampuero F, Doss LL, Khan M, et al. The Syed-Neblett interstitial template in locally advanced gynecological malignancies. *Int J Radiat Oncol Biol Phys.* 1983;9(12):1897–1903.

74. Erickson B, Gillin MT. Interstitial implantation of gynecologic malignancies. *J Surg Oncol.* 1997;66(4):285–295.

75. Tyree WC, Cardenes H, Randall M, et al. High-dose-rate brachytherapy for vaginal cancer: learning from treatment complications. *Int J Gynecol Cancer.* 2002;12(1):27–31.

76. Stryker JA. Radiotherapy for vaginal carcinoma: a 23-year review. *Br J Radiol.* 2000;73(875):1200–1205.

77. Hoskins WJ, Perez CA, Young RC. *Principles and Practice of Gynecologic Oncology.* 3rd ed. Philadelphia, PA: Lippincott Williams & Wilkins; 2000.

78. Greven K, Winter K, Underhill K, et al. Preliminary analysis of RTOG 9708: adjuvant postoperative radiotherapy combined with cisplatin/paclitaxel chemotherapy after surgery for patients with high-risk endometrial cancer. *Int J Radiat Oncol Biol Phys.* 2004;59(1):168–173.

79. Greven K, Winter K, Underhill K, et al. Final analysis of RTOG 9708: adjuvant postoperative irradiation combined with cisplatin/paclitaxel chemotherapy following surgery for patients with high-risk endometrial cancer. *Gynecol Oncol.* 2006;103(1):155–159.

80. Kavanagh BD, Bentel GC, Montana GS. Soft tissue complication rates after low dose rate brachytherapy using customized perineal templates. *Int J Radiat Oncol Biol Phys.* 1994;30(2):508.

81. Gabel C, Eifel PJ, Tornos C, et al. Radiation recall reaction to idarubicin resulting in vaginal necrosis. *Gynecol Oncol.* 1995;57(2):266–269.

82. Boronow RC, Rutledge F. Vesicovaginal fistula, radiation, and gynecologic cancer. *Am J Obstet Gynecol.* 1971;111(1):85–90.

83. Fine BA, Hempling RE, Piver MS, et al. Severe radiation morbidity in carcinoma of the cervix: impact of pretherapy surgical staging and previous surgery. *Int J Radiat Oncol Biol Phys.* 1995;31(4):717–723.

84. Rotman M, John MJ, Roussis K, et al. The intracavitary applicator in relation to complications of pelvic radiation—the Ernst system. *Int J Radiat Oncol Biol Phys.* 1978;4(11–12):951–956.

85. Bourne RG, Kearsley JH, Grove WD, et al. The relationship between early and late gastrointestinal complications of radiation therapy for carcinoma of the cervix. *Int J Radiat Oncol Biol Phys.* 1983;9(10):1445–1450.

86. Grigsby PW, Russell A, Bruner D, et al. Late injury of cancer therapy on the female reproductive tract. *Int J Radiat Oncol Biol Phys.* 1995;31(5):1281–1299.

87. Abeloff MD. *Abeloff's Clinical Oncology.* 4th ed. Philadelphia, PA: Churchill Livingstone/Elsevier; 2008.

88. Perez CA, Grigsby PW, Castro-Vita H, et al. Carcinoma of the uterine cervix. I. Impact of prolongation of overall treatment time and timing of brachytherapy on outcome of radiation therapy. *Int J Radiat Oncol Biol Phys.* 1995;32(5):1275–1288.

89. Perez CA, Grigsby PW, Castro-Vita H, et al. Carcinoma of the uterine cervix. II. Lack of impact of prolongation of overall treatment time on morbidity of radiation therapy. *Int J Radiat Oncol Biol Phys.* 1996;34(1):3–11.

90. Pitkin RM, Buchsbaum HJ, Lenz H. Estrogen and the irradiated vagina. *Obstet Gynecol.* 1975;46(2):243–245.

91. Sobotkowski J, Markowska J, Fijuth J, et al. Preliminary results of mitomycin C local application as post-treatment prevention of vaginal radiation-induced morbidity in women with cervical cancer. *Eur J Gynaecol Oncol.* 2006;27(4):356–358.

92. Betalli P, De Corti F, Minucci D, et al. Successful topical treatment with mitomycin-C in a female with post-brachytherapy vaginal stricture. *Pediatr Blood Cancer.* 2008;51(4):550–552.

93. Hintz BL, Kagan AR, Gilbert HA, et al. Systemic absorption of conjugated estrogenic cream by the irradiated vagina. *Gynecol Oncol.* 1981;12(1):75–82.

94. Vernooij CB, Kruitwagen RF, Rodrigus P, et al. Hematometra after radiotherapy for cervical carcinoma. *Gynecol Oncol.* 1997;67(3):325–327.

95. White ID, Faithfull S. Vaginal dilation associated with pelvic radiotherapy: a UK survey of current practice. *Int J Gynecol Cancer.* 2006;16(3):1140–1146.

96. Boronow RC. Management of radiation-induced vaginal fistulas. *Am J Obstet Gynecol.* 1971;110(1):1–8.

97. Williams JA Jr, Clarke D, Dennis WA, et al. The treatment of pelvic soft tissue radiation necrosis with hyperbaric oxygen. *Am J Obstet Gynecol.* 1992;167(2):412–415; discussion 415–416.

98. Fink D, Chetty N, Lehm JP, et al. Hyperbaric oxygen therapy for delayed radiation injuries in gynecological cancers. *Int J Gynecol Cancer.* 2006;16(2):638–642.

99. Piekarski JH, Jereczek-Fossa BA, Nejc D, et al. Does fecal diversion offer any chance for spontaneous closure of the radiation-induced rectovaginal fistula? *Int J Gynecol Cancer.* 2008;18(1):66–70.

100. Noyes WR, Bastin K, Edwards SA, et al. Postoperative vaginal cuff irradiation using high dose rate remote afterloading: A phase II clinical protocol. *Int J Radiat Oncolo Biol Phys* 1995;32(5):1439–1443.

101. Dixit S, Singhal S, Baboo HA. Squamous cell carcinoma of the vagina: A review of 70 cases. *Gynecol Oncol* 1993;48(1):80–87.

102. Marcus RB, Million RR, Daly JW. Carcinoma of the vagina. *Cancer* 1978;42(5):2507–2512.

Lisa Hazard
Bruce Minsky

Esophagus

ANATOMY

The esophagus is a tube-shaped organ that propels food from the pharynx to the stomach. The proximal extent of the esophagus is contiguous with the laryngopharynx and begins at the inferior edge of the cricoid cartilage, corresponding to approximately the level of the C6 vertebral body. The inferior pharyngeal constrictor muscles merge with the cricophayrngeus muscle, forming the upper esophageal sphincter. This sphincter is contracted at rest, preventing reflux of food into the pharynx. The sphincter consists of striated muscle that is under conscious control and can be relaxed to allow passage of food. Inferiorly, the esophagus passes through the esophageal hiatus of the diaphragm at about the level of the T10 vertebral body, thus exiting the thorax and entering the abdomen. The lower portion of the esophagus contains a 2 to 4 cm long segment of thickened muscle known as the *lower esophageal sphincter*. Like the upper esophageal sphincter, this sphincter is contracted at rest to prevent reflux of the contents of the stomach into the esophagus and can be relaxed to allow passage of food during swallowing. Unlike the upper esophageal sphincter, however, the lower esophageal sphincter contains smooth muscle and is not under conscious control. The esophagus is typically about 25 to 30 cm in length and 5 mm in thickness. When collapsed, the esophagus contains luminal folds, which allow for expansion of the esophageal diameter to accommodate a food bolus. Anatomy of the esophagus is depicted in Figure 37.1.

For purposes of contouring the esophagus on CT scan during radiation treatment planning, the superior level is at the bottom of the cricoid cartilage, and the inferior level is the gastroesophageal junction.[1,2] Others have described the superior extent as the thoracic inlet and the inferior extent as the diaphragm.[3]

HISTOLOGY

The esophagus is formed by four layers: the mucosa, submucosa, muscularis propria, and adventitia (Figs. 37.2 and 37.3). Starting from the innermost layer, the mucosa is formed by the nonkeratinized, stratified squamous epithelium, the lamina propria, and the muscularis mucosa. The superficial layer of the epithelium serves as a permeability barrier. The deep layer of the epithelium contains basal cells, which are capable of

replication and serve to regenerate the epithelium. A loose network of connective tissue, the lamina propria, underlies the epithelium. Beneath the lamina propria is the muscularis mucosae, a thin layer of smooth muscle. Next is a dense network of connective tissue, the submucosa, which contains a plexus of blood vessels and lymphatic channels as well as the neurons of Meissner plexus (which carries afferent sensory nerve impulses to the brainstem) and esophageal glands. These

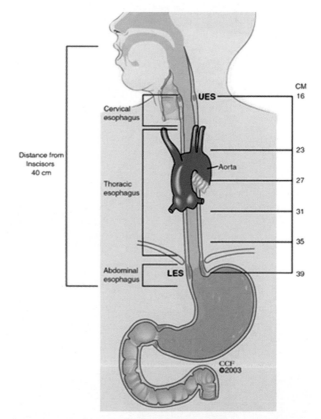

Figure 37.1. Schematic diagram of esophageal anatomy. UES, upper esophageal sphincter; LES, lower esophageal sphincter. (Reprinted from Vollweiler J, Vaiez M. The Esophagus: anatomy, physiology, and diseases. In: Cummings C, ed. *Otolaryngology: Head and Neck Surgery.* 4th ed. Philadelphia, PA: Mosby; 2005, with permission. Copyright Elsevier.)

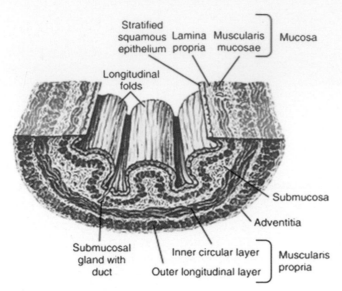

Figure 37.2. Histology of the esophagus. (Reprinted from Long J, Orlando R. Anatomy, histology, embryology, and developmental anomalies of the esophagus. In: Feldman MS, ed. *Sleisenger and Fordtran's Gastrointestinal and Liver Disease.* 8th ed. Philadelphia; 2009, with permission. Copyright Elsevier.)

glands secrete mucous, involved in lubrication, and factors involved in epithelial repair. The muscularia propria is the muscle layer underneath the submucosa. The upper portion of the esophagus contains striated muscles, the lower portion contains smooth muscle, and the midesophagus contains both. The inner muscle layer is circular, while the outer muscle layer is longitudinal. The myenteric or Auerbach nerve plexus is located between these two muscle layers and is responsible for peristalsis. The adventitia is the outermost connective tissue layer covering the esophagus; as a retroperitoneal organ the esophagus does not have a serosal layer.

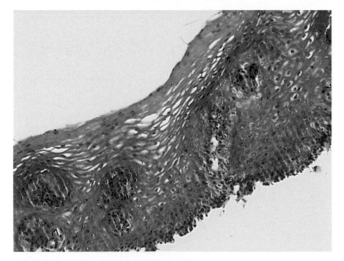

Figure 37.3. Micrograph of the esophageal epithelium. (Reprinted from Long J, Orlando R. Anatomy, histology, embryology, and developmental anomalies of the esophagus. In: Feldman MS, ed. *Sleisenger and Fordtran's Gastrointestinal and Liver Disease.* 8th ed. Philadelphia; 2009, with permission. Copyright Elsevier.)

SWALLOWING MECHANISM

As described above, the pharyngeal portion of the esophagus is under conscious control. With swallowing, the larynx elevates and the epiglottis seals the airway. The pharyngeal muscles contract and propel food through the upper esophageal sphincter. The upper esophageal sphincter, which is contracted at rest, relaxes in response to swallowing. The food bolus is then propelled through the esophagus via the primary peristaltic wave, which is a coordinated contraction of the smooth muscle beginning in the upper portion of the esophagus and proceeds distally. The smooth muscle of the esophagus is under involuntary control and is innervated by the vagus nerve. The lower esophageal sphincter relaxes and allows passage of food through the stomach. Secondary peristalsis, which is also coordinated, occurs in response to sensory receptors in the esophagus rather than swallowing. Residual food bolus can stimulate sensory receptors in the esophagus to initiate a secondary peristalsis at the level of the retained food, thus clearing residual food following primary peristalsis.

ACUTE PATHOLOGICAL CHANGES FOLLOWING IRRADIATION

The mucosal layer of the esophagus undergoes rapid renewal with high rates of cell turnover, and as such the mucosal layer of the esophagus is an acutely reacting tissue.[4] Acute radiation changes based on animal models include cytoplasmic vacuolization of and reduction/absence of mitoses in the basal layer of the mucosa as well as thinning of the epithelium.[5,6] Submucosal edema can also occur.[6,7] During recovery of the tissue following radiation, foci of proliferating basal cells form and regeneration of epithelium occurs. Regeneration of epithelium is typically complete, though thickening is common, with the epithelium often raised in multiple folds. Epithelial atrophy rather than thickening is occasionally seen.[7] The rapidity of regeneration of the basal cells correlates with survival in mouse studies.[6] In addition to epithelial destruction, endothelial damage can occur.

In a mouse model, Phillips and Ross[6] noted vacuolization, absence of mitoses, submucosal edema, and thinning of the squamous epithelium 3 days after a single large dose of radiation. They detected simultaneous areas of epithelial denudation and regeneration 1 to 2 weeks following radiation treatment, and complete epithelial regeneration 3 to 4 weeks following radiation treatment.[6] In a dog model, Engelstad et al.[8] described degenerative changes in the mucosa following high dose radiation, with entire loss of epithelium in some animals. Complete epithelial regeneration occurred in most animals.[8]

Human models demonstrate similar acute pathological changes to those described in animals. Mascarenhas et al.[5] performed endoscopy with biopsy in 38 lung carcinoma patients following a dose of 30 to 40 Gy standard fraction radiation therapy, and reported cytoplasmic vacuolization in 95% of patients, decreased basal mitotic activity in 86%, and atrophy in 55%. The decrease in basal cell mitotic activity observed in radiation esophagitis is distinct from peptic ulceration, in which basal hyperplasia typically occurs.[5] Human studies have shown complete epithelial regeneration 3 months to 2 years following completion of radiation therapy, though the epithelium may be thicker.[7] However, after high dose radiation, the epithelium may

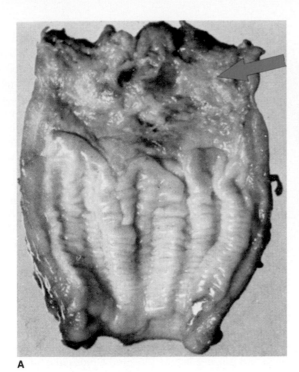

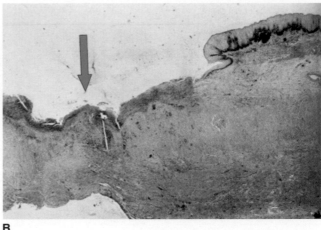

Figure 37.4. **A**: Surgical specimen with radiation necrosis (*arrow*) and complete epithelial denudation. **B**: Microscopic detail of surgical specimen in panel A, with loss of epithelium on the left side of the micrograph (*arrow*). (Reprinted from the Radiological Society of North America, with permission.[11])

not be able to regenerate. Seaman and Ackerman[11] described a patient who underwent partial esophagectomy 12 months postradiation due to dysphagia following 73-Gy radiation therapy in 48 days via 24-mega-electron volt (MeV) betatron machine. The surgical specimen showed thickened mucosa arranged in prominent longitudinal folds in some areas, with complete absence of mucosa and partial destruction of the muscle layer in an area corresponding to the high dose radiation field (Fig. 37.4).

In summary, acute radiation damage occurs primarily due to epithelial cell destruction. Surviving basal cells regenerate the epithelium. If insufficient numbers of basal cells survive, regeneration may not occur.

LATE PATHOLOGICAL CHANGES

While acute radiation damage occurs primarily in the epithelial layer, late radiation damage (occurring 3 months or longer following completion of radiation) largely results from changes in the deeper layers of the esophagus, most prominently the submucosal and muscular layers.[4,9] The lamina propria, which is the connective tissue layer that underlies the epithelium, and the submucosa, which is the connective tissue layer that underlies the muscularis mucosae, may show homogenization of collagen, small vessel telangiectasia, and atypical fibroblasts.[7,9–11] Fibrosis and thickening of the submucosal and muscular layers can occur.[7,9–11] In a dog model, Gillette et al.[12] analyzed esophageal specimens 2 years after receiving up to 72-Gy radiation, 1.5 Gy/fraction. Histologically, these specimens demonstrated a decrease in the percentage of the glandular tissue and an increase in the percentage of lamina propria and muscle tissue.[12] If the fibrosis is severe, luminal narrowing can result.[7] Luminal narrowing is largely due to thickening of the submucoal layer.[7,11] Infiltration of inflammatory cells in the muscular layer, and in particular surrounding the ganglion cells of

the mesenteric plexus, has been reported in opossum[13] and in humans.[9] Subacute and chronic ulceration can also rarely occur.[9] Endothelial cells can demonstrate hypertrophy and dysmorphic changes, and thickening and hyalinization of arterioles can occur, with intimal fibrosis.[7]

Seaman and Ackerman[11] reported pathologic changes at autopsy 9 months postradiation in a patient receiving 76 Gy in 36 days via 24-MeV betatron machine. This patient had radiological evidence of esophageal stricture prior to death. Microscopic examination of the esophagus showed marked thickening of the esophageal wall, predominantly due to thickening of the submucosa. The muscle layer showed cytoplasmic vacuolization with abnormal nuclei in regions of mild to moderate radiation damage and showed loss of nuclear detail

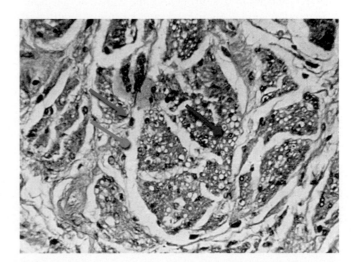

Figure 37.5. Esophageal muscle showing abnormal nuclei (*green arrow*), cytoplasmic vacuolization (*red diamond arrow*), and edema separating muscle bundles (*blue circle arrow*). (Reprinted from the Radiological Society of North America, with permission.[11])

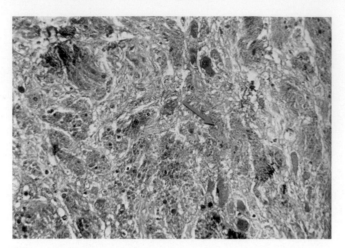

Figure 37.6. Radiation effect on muscle, demonstrating loss of nuclear detail and absence of cellular delineation (*arrow*). (Reprinted from the Radiological Society of North America, with permission.[11])

and absence of cellular delineation (termed *homogenization* by the authors) in areas of severe radiation damage. Seaman and Ackerman[11] noted minimal vascular changes, and concluded that late damage to the esophagus is primarily due to direct effects on the muscle and connective tissue layers rather than secondary ischemia due to vascular damage.[11] These findings are depicted in Figures 37.5 and 37.6. In summary, late radiation changes are marked by fibrosis and inflammation of the submucosal and muscular layers.

CLINICAL MANIFESTATIONS

ACUTE ESOPHAGITIS

Cause, Symptoms, and Time Course

Acute symptoms are related to primarily to mucosal damage, which manifests as esophagitis. Symptoms include dysphagia, odynophagia, and substernal burning pain. The severity of symptoms typically progresses throughout the course of radiation.

In a mouse model, Michalowski and Hornsey[14] reported that 100% of mice developed ulceration by day 7 following a single dose of 27 Gy, but by day 14 only 10% had ulceration and by day 21 none had ulceration. Phillips and Ross[6] noted decreased food intake and weight loss in mice 2 to 3 weeks following radiation treatment, which corresponded to histological changes of radiation esophagitis in the mucosa. Epithelial regeneration occurred in 3 to 4 weeks following radiation in survivors. In the absence of epithelial regeneration, death typically occurred 2 to 3 weeks after radiation, and was related to starvation and dehydration from mucosal damage rather than perforation.[6]

In humans, radiation esophagitis typically begins at weeks 2 to 3 during standard fraction radiation (1.8–2 Gy/d), and resolves within 4 weeks of completion of radiation therapy,[15] but can last for several months, particularly in patients who develop grade 3 or higher esophagitis. Hirota et al.[16] reported that patients with endoscopic grade 2 or less esophagitis recovered in a few weeks with conservative management and did not require repeat endoscopy. In three patients who developed grade 3 esophagitis by endoscopic criteria during radiation therapy and who underwent repeat endoscopy following

completion of radiation, two patients had resolution to grade 1 to 2 esophagitis on repeat endoscopy within 2 to 4 weeks following completion of radiation, but the third patient had persistent grade 3 esophagitis on endoscopy 3 months following completion of radiation therapy.[16] Seaman and Ackerman[11] noted that in 11 patients with mild radiation esophagitis symptoms resolved several weeks following completion of radiation, whereas four patients with moderately severe esophagitis had persistent symptoms 2 to 3 months following completion of therapy. Werner-Wasik et al.[17] evaluated four Radiation Therapy Oncology Group (RTOG) prospective studies utilizing concurrent chemoradiation in non–small cell lung cancer, and reported that esophagitis symptoms peaked within 1 month from the start of a 6-week course of radiation in 38% of patients, within 2 months in 49% of patients, and within 3 months in 3%. Therefore, symptoms peaked within about 2 weeks of finishing radiation in the vast majority of patients.

Radiographic Findings

Double contrast barium esophagogram demonstrates characteristic changes in acute radiation esophagitis. In single contrast barium esophagogram, findings may be absent or subtle. Seaman and Ackerman[11] in 1957 and Goldstein et al.[10] in 1975 did not consistently identify changes on single contrast esophagogram, though Seaman and Ackerman[11] noted fine serrations of the margin of the barium column in a minority of patients. Lamanna et al.[18] reported that esophagogram was normal in 80% of patients with symptoms of radiation esophagitis. On the other hand, Collazzo et al.[19] evaluated 13 patients with acute radiation esophagitis who underwent double-contrast barium (8 patients) or single contrast barium esophagogram (5 patients), and found that all patients had changes in the esophagogram; 37% of patients undergoing double contrast study had multiple small, discrete ulcers, 50% had a distinctive granular appearance of the mucosa, and 13% had both of these changes (Fig. 37.7). In the patients who underwent single contrast study, two had esophageal narrowing, one had narrowing and ulceration, and two had thickened esophageal folds. In reality, patients who develop symptoms of radiation esophagitis in the appropriate clinical setting will be treated symptomatically, and confirmation by esophagogram is of little utility. Double contrast esophagogram may be useful when the diagnosis of radiation esophagitis is in question.

Propulsion of food through the esophagus is often slowed during and immediately following thoracic radiation. In a study of 25 patients, Lamanna et al.[18] showed prolonged transit times on technetium transit scintigraphy in a majority of patients after 20 Gy, and in all but one patient after 45 Gy. Symptoms of dysphagia and weight loss, however, did not correspond to prolonged transit times.

Endoscopy can reveal characteristic changes including erythema, submucosal edema and endothelial proliferation, friability, and epithelial necrosis. None of these changes, however, are pathognomonic.[5,20] Hirota et al.[16] reported that 17% of 23 patients treated with mediastinal radiation therapy alone (median dose: 60 Gy) had endoscopic grade 2 esophagitis and none had grade 4, whereas 31% of 59 patients treated with chemotherapy concurrent with mediastinal radiation (median dose: 56 Gy) had endoscopic grade 2 esophagitis, and 27% had grade 4 (see Table 37.1 for definition of endoscopic grade). Mascarenhas showed signs of esophagitis in 17 of 38 lung cancer

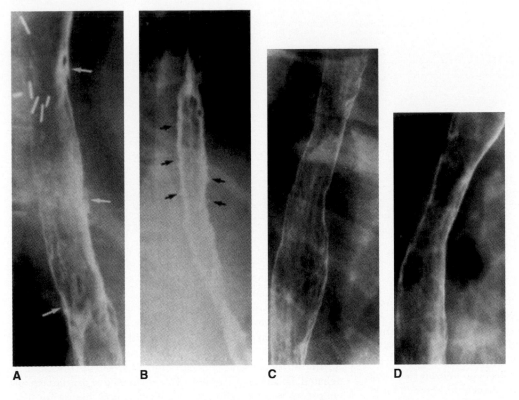

Figure 37.7. Acute radiation esophagitis findings on double contrast barium esophagogram. **A, B**: Multiple small ulcers (*arrows*) in patients suffering from acute radiation esophagitis. **C, D**: Granular appearance to the mucosa and esophageal narrowing in patients suffering from acute radiation esophagitis. (Reprinted from the American Roentgen Ray Society, with permission.[19])

patients (45%) who underwent planned endoscopy after 30 to 40 Gy. Of the 17 patients with signs of esophagitis, 9 (53%) had mild mucosal redness, 7 (41%) had redness and edema, and 1 (6%) had friability.[5] Slanina et al.[21] performed endoscopy before and after 40 to 44 Gy mantle field radiation therapy in Hodgkin Disease patients, and failed to identify pathologic findings in the mucosa of the esophagus. Minimal inflammation, erosions, and capillary ectasia were seen in the duodenal and gastric mucosa.[21] The reasons for these conflicting results compared to

the Mascarenhas study are not clear, though a study by Soffer et al.[22] reported that 44% of lung cancer patients have underlying esophagitis prior to initiation of radiation, perhaps due to lifestyle factors such as smoking or alcohol use. Therefore, higher rates of esophagitis may have been seen in the study of lung cancer patients by Mascarenhas et al.[5] compared to the Hodgkin disease by Slanina et al.[21] because of underlying pretreatment factors. Endoscopic changes related to acute and chronic radiation damage are depicted in Figure 37.8.

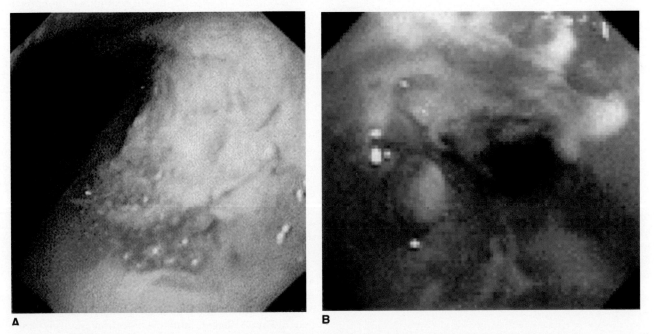

Figure 37.8. A: Endoscopic image of superficial ulceration related to acute radiation injury. **B**: Deep ulceration related to chronic radiation injury. (Reprinted from Elsevier, with permission.[78])

TABLE 37.1	**Definitions for Acute Radiation Esophagitis**		
Grade	CTCAE v.4.0	RTOG Criteria	Endoscopic Criteria
1	Asymptomatic; clinical or diagnostic observations only; intervention not indicated	Mild dyphagia or odynophagia, may require topical anesthetics/may require nonnarcotic analgesics/may require soft diet	Erythema
2	Symptomatic; altered eating/swallowing (e.g., altered dietary habits, oral supplements)	Moderate dysphagia or odynophagia/ may require narcotic analgesics/may require puree or liquid diet	Erosion/sloughing
3	Severely altered eating/swallowing (e.g., inadequate oral caloric or fluid intake); tube feeding; hospitalization indicated; TPN indicated	Severe dysphagia or odynophagia with dehydration or weight loss requiring NG tube feeding, IV fluids, or hyperalimentation	Ulcer, hemorrhage, stricture
4	Life-threatening consequences; urgent operative intervention indicated	Complete obstruction, perforation, or fistula	

CTCAE, Common terminology criteria for adverse events; RTOG, Radiation Therapy Oncology Group.

Scoring Systems

The National Cancer Institute's Common terminology criteria for adverse events (NCI-CTC) version 4.0 define esophageal toxicity gradation based primarily on clinical symptoms. These definitions are similar to those described by the RTOG in the past. Current RTOG protocols utilized NCI-CTC criteria. Endoscopic-based definitions have also been utilized (see Table 37.1). Hirota et al.[16] reported high correlation between endoscopic evaluation of esophagitis and RTOG grade (Spearman coefficient of 0.42, $p < 0.0001$). RTOG grade 3 score had predictive value for ulceration on endoscopy. This study did observe, however, that 7 of 16 patients with endoscopic grade 3 esophagitis had only clinical (RTOG) grade 0 and 1 esophagitis. Mascarenhas et al.[5] also reported good correlation between clinical symptoms of esophagitis and endoscopic findings. In this study, 38 patients undergoing split course radiation therapy for lung carcinoma underwent planned endoscopy after 30 to 40 Gy.[5] No patients had severe esophagitis symptoms at the time of endoscopy, while 18 had mild to moderate symptoms. Of 18 patients who reported symptoms of esophagitis, 12 (67%) had endoscopic findings of esophagitis. Of the 12 patients with clinical and endoscopic esophagitis, biopsy confirmed pathologic findings of esophagitis in 8 (67%). Biopsy findings were inconclusive in the remaining 4. Of 20 patients who did not report symptoms of dysphagia, 5 (25%) had endoscopic findings of esophagitis. Therefore, while correlation between endoscopic findings and symptoms of esophagitis is good, it is not perfect.

Werner-Wasik et al.[23] utilized esophagitis index for evaluation of acute esophageal toxicity. This index records esophageal toxicity score weekly during chemoradiation and at regular intervals following completion of radiation therapy. A graph of time versus grade is generated, and the area under the curve is calculated to determine the esophagitis index. This index incorporates not only maximum grade, but also the duration of symptoms, and is therefore more informative. However, it is a more labor intensive and cumbersome evaluation of toxicity compared to maximum grade. It has utility in research studies to more accurately define esophageal toxicity.

Concomitant Infection

Opportunistic infection secondary to breakdown of the protective mucosal barrier can mimic or worsen radiation esophagitis,

and should remain in the differential diagnosis under appropriate clinical circumstances. The most common opportunistic infection associated with thoracic radiation is candidiasis. Herpes and cytomegalovirus infections could also potentially mimic radiation esophagitis, and should remain in the differential diagnosis.[20]

The incidence and clinical significance of this infection is debated. Hirota et al.[16] noted a 16% incidence of candidiasis on endoscopy in 82 patients treated with radiation therapy for thoracic malignancies. The incidence of candidiasis did not differ between the 23 patients treated with radiation alone versus the 59 patients treated with chemoradiation. Soffer et al.[22] reported a 31% incidence of candidiasis on endoscopy in 26 patients undergoing thoracic radiation. Eight of nineteen patients (42%) with histologic evidence of esophagitis on biopsy had candidiasis, whereas none of seven patients with normal histologic biopsy had candidiasis, suggesting that radiation esophagitis predisposed to this opportunisitic infection. Interestingly, only one of the eight patients with candidiasis (13%) had a severe symptom of esophagitis, suggesting that the infection is not necessarily clinically significant.

Perez et al.[80] reviewed endoscopy records in 16 patients with esophagitis symptoms during or after thoracic radiation. All patients had endoscopic findings of esophagitis, and 6 of 16 patients (37.5%) had infectious esophagitis (candida in five cases and herpes simplex virus in one case). One of 16 patients (6%) had adenocarcinoma on biopsy. Therefore, a total of 7 of 16 patients (44%) had potential cause of esophagitis other than radiation (infection or malignancy). However, the area of esophagitis corresponded to the area of radiation exposure, even in those patients with infection, and none of the patients had oral signs or symptoms of candidiasis or herpes infection. Correlation with the radiation field suggests that radiation damage may have predisposed to infection, rather than infection occurring independent of radiation damage. This suggestion that radiation damage predisposes to opportunistic infection is consistent with the previously described trial by Hirota et al.[16]

It remains controversial whether treatment of candidial infection is warranted. Some authors recommend esophagosocopy in order to identify infection.[16,22] Others have advocated empiric treatment with antifungal therapy, while others suggest that radiation-related candidial infection is rarely symptomatic, and therefore treatment may not be necessary.[16] Given the expense and risks of endoscopy, its routine use during radiation is not warranted to identify infection. Endoscopy can be considered if symptoms do not resolve in the typical time frame (4–8 weeks) following completion of radiation therapy, or in an immunocompromised patient in whom infection is a significant concern.[24]

LATE

Dysmotility and Stricture

The most common late symptom from radiation-induced esophageal damage is dysphagia to solid foods from dysmotility and esophageal stricture.[25] Changes in motility and stricture occur due to muscular damage, submucosal fibrosis, and possibly nerve damage.[20]

Because of similarities in the opossum and human esophagus, opossum models have provided valuable information regarding the mechanism of action of esophageal late toxicity as well as dose dependence. Like humans, opossums have striated muscle in the upper third of the esophagus, smooth muscle in the lower one third and in the lower esophageal sphincter, and mixed types in the middle third. Northway et al.[13] evaluated manometry and esophagogram with swallowing in irradiated opossum and showed failure to complete the primary peristaltic wave at a single dose of 22.5 Gy. Tertiary contractions would then occur, resulting in trapping of barium. Unlike primary and secondary peristalsis seen in normal swallowing, tertiary contractions were uncoordinated and ineffective. A decrease in the relaxation of the lower esophageal sphincter was observed, without a decrease in resting lower esophageal sphincter pressure. Thus, propulsion of food into the stomach was impaired.

Human studies have also demonstrated failure of the primary peristaltic wave following radiation and failure of the lower of esophageal sphincter to relax. Goldstein et al.[10] evaluated 30 patients who developed persistent dysphagia following 45 to 60 Gy mediastinal radiation. Esophagogram showed failure to complete primary peristaltic wave, with disruption of the wave at the level of the irradiated esophagus. Repetitive nonperistaltic (tertiary) waves occurred distal to the point of disruption of the primary wave. The lower esophageal sphincter also failed to relax in several patients. Lepke et al.[26] reported abnormal peristalsis occurring 4 to 12 weeks following radiation based

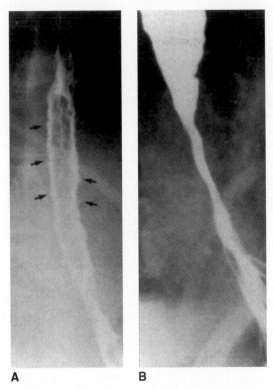

A   **B**

Figure 37.9. **A**: Acute radiation change with granular mucosa. **B**: Radiation-induced stricture 11 months following completion of radiation. (Reprinted from the American Roentgen Ray Society, with permission.[19])

on esophagogram. The esophagogram demonstrated smooth tapering at the level of stricture. Other authors have described the smooth tapering on esophagogram as a characteristic of radiation-induced stricture (Fig. 37.9).[20,27] Kaplinsky et al.[27] reported prolonged midesophagus retention with impaired, slow emptying into the stomach on esophageal dynamic scanning with Technetium dimethyl phosphonate in a patient with radiation-induced stricture. Endoscopy often does not reveal a mucosal abnormality as the cause of damage is submucosal and muscular, though mucosal friability and telangiectasia have

	Definitions for Acute Radiation Esophagitis Based on CTCAE (Common Terminology Criteria for Adverse Events) v.4.0 Criteria
TABLE 37.2	

Grade	Stenosis	Fistula	Ulceration	Perforation
1	Asymptomatic; clinical or diagnostic observations only; intervention not indicated	Asymptomatic; clinical or diagnostic observations only; intervention not indicated	Asymptomatic; clinical or diagnostic observations only; intervention not indicated	
2	Symptomatic; altered GI function;	Symptomatic; altered GI function (e.g., altered dietary habits, diarrhea, or GI fluid loss);	Symptomatic; altered GI function (e.g. altered dietary habits, vomiting, diarrhea)	Symptomatic; medical intervention indicated
3	Severely altered GI function; tube feeding; hospitalization indicated; elective operative intervention indicated	Severely altered GI function (e.g., bowel rest, altered dietary habits, diarrhea, or GI fluid loss); tube feeding; hospitalization indicated; TPN	Debilitating symptoms; severely altered GI function; TPN indicated; elective operative or endoscopic intervention indicated	Severe symptoms; elective operative intervention indicated
4	Life-threatening consequences; urgent operative intervention indicated	Life-threatening consequences; urgent intervention indicated	Life-threatening consequences; urgent operative intervention indicated	Life-threatening consequences; urgent operative intervention indicated

been reported.[20, 27] Median time to development of esophageal stricture is 6 months following completion of radiation, but has been reported as early as 3 to 4 months and as late as 16 years.[11,20,26–29]

Papazian et al.[9] reported formation of mucosal bridges across the lumen of the esophagus in a patient 3 years after 45-Gy mediastinal radiation therapy for treatment of Hodgkin disease. The bridges were visible on both endoscopy and CT scan, and consisted of normal overlying epithelium and chronic inflammation in the underlying lamina propria. Mucosal bridges have been described in inflammatory bowel disease and gastroesophageal reflux disease, and have been hypothesized to be a healing process of mucosal damage. Papazian et al.[9] hypothesize that the formation of the bridges occurred in this patient in part due to poor oral intake following radiation, such that food boluses could not prevent the formation of these bridges.

In summary, late radiation-induced dysphagia is marked by histological fibrosis and inflammation of the submucosal and muscular layers, smooth tapering at the level of stricture on esophagogram, and disordered motility on esophageal manometry with interruption of the primary peristaltic wave and esophageal spasm.[27] The NCI-CTC version 4.0 criteria for esophageal stenosis is described in Table 37.2. Studies reporting risks of late esophageal stricture are described in Table 37.3.

Ulceration, Fistula Formation, and Perforation

Esophageal ulceration related to radiation rather than persistent or recurrent cancer is uncommon.[9] In a study by Vanagunas et al.,[20] ulceration occurred in 10% of patients with abnormality on esophagogram. Tracheal-esophageal fistula is a rare but life-threatening complication.[10,11,20,30] The NCI-CTC version 4.0 criteria for these late esophageal toxicities is described in Table 37.2.

TABLE 37.3	Late Esophageal Toxicity						
Author	N	Dose (Gy)	Fx	Chemo	Late	Stricture	Fistula/Perforation
Prospective Data							
Ball[43]	23	60	Sfx	None		0%[a]	
	29	60	Afx	None		23%[a]	
	24	60	Sfx	CON		4%[a]	
	23	60	Afx	CON		0%[a]	
Saunders[58]	563	54	CHART	None		7%	
		60	Sfx	None		5%	
Cox[38] RTOG 83-11	641	60–74.4	Hfx	None	0%[b]		
	207	79.2	Hfx	None	1%		
Kramer[40] RTOG 73-03	136	50 preop	Sfx	None	0.8%		
	141	60 post-op	Sfx	None	6%		
Pooled Data from Prospective RTOG Studies							
Byhdart[54]	152	60	Sfx	IND	2%		
	109	60	Sfx	IND and CON	4%		
	200	69.6	Hfx	CON	8%		
Retrospective Data							
O'Rourke[29]	57	56–60	Sfx	59% ANY		58%	3.5%
DeRen[41]	869	50–79	Sfx	None			0.8%
Beatty[42]	152	60–70	Sfx	None		18%[c]	
Morichause-Beachant		<50			1.2%		
		>60			6%		
Bradley[46]	166	60–70	Sfx	22% IND, 25% CON		2%	0%
Takeda[74]	35	50–67	Sfx	9% IND and CON, 85% CON	3%	3%	0%
Singh[3]	207	60–74	Sfx	21% IND, 26% CON		6%[b]	0.5%
Rosenman[24]	48	60–74	Sfx			6%[d]	
Hishikawa[61]	17	55 EBRT + 17 HDR	Sfx	NS			12%
Seaman[11]	20	40–76	Sfx	None		25%[e]	10%[e]
Goldstein[10]	30	45–60	Sfx	None		17%	3%[f]

[a]Requiring dilation.
[b]Grade 3+
[c]Four of five patients undergoing autopsy had malignant stricture.
[d]Grade 2.
[e]Four of five patients with these toxicities received dose >65 Gy.
[f]Frank ulceration followed by trachea-esophageal stricture occurred in 1 of 30 patients at a dose of 58 Gy.

Afx, accelerated fractionation; ANY, Chemo given but sequence with radiation unknown; CHART, continuous hyperfractionated accelerated radiation therapy (54 Gy, 1.5 Gy/fraction, TID over 12 days); CON, concurrent chemotherapy; fx, fractionation; Gr, grade, Hfx, hyperfractionation; IND, induction chemotherapy, Sfx, standard fractionation, N, number, NR, not reported, RTOG, Radiation Therapy Oncology Group.

Studies reporting risks of late esophageal fistula and perforation are described in Table 37.3.

Radiation-Induced Esophageal Malignancy

Thoracic radiation is associated with a small but tangible risk of secondary malignancy in the esophagus, most commonly squamous cell carcinoma.[31] Less than 1% of esophageal malignancies are radiation induced.[32] By definition, radiation-induced malignancy occurs within the radiation field and occurs more than 5 years following radiation exposure.[33] In a literature review of radiation-induced esophageal malignancy, Micke et al.[31] identified 66 cases. The median dose of radiation was 40 Gy (range: 18.6–68 Gy), and the median time to secondary cancer in the esophagus was 15 years (range: 2–63 years).[31] Squamous cell carcinoma was by far the most likely histology, though small-cell carcinoma and adenocarcinoma were also reported. Ahsan et al.[34] reported a 5.42-fold increased risk of esophageal squamous cell carcinoma in breast cancer patients who received radiation compared with those who did not. Vanagunas et al.[20] report two patients developing secondary squamous cell carcinoma in the treated esophagus 16 and 24 years following radiation therapy. In both cases, the patients developed stricture 2 to 4 years prior to the development of cancer, and biopsies of the strictured esophagus revealed radiation damage with fibrovascular proliferation, suggesting that the malignancy tends to arise in areas of significant chronic radiation damage. While controversial, some authors have suggested a reduced latency period between development of secondary malignancy and higher radiation dose. Micke et al.[31] reported a non-statistically significant trend toward reduced latency time and higher dose in radiation-induced esophageal malignancy ($p = 0.07$).[31]

FACTORS INFLUENCING ACUTE ESOPHAGITIS

DOSE DEPENDENCE

Animal Data

In their work in the opossum model, Northway et al.[13] showed a decrease in the relaxation of the lower esophageal sphincter during swallowing at doses of 20 and 22.5 Gy, but not lower doses.[13] At a dose of 20 Gy, the response to balloon dilation returned to normal at 14 weeks following radiation, but at 22.5 Gy the animals did not regain a normal response. Animals consumed normal amounts of food after 15 Gy, 75% of normal after 20 Gy, and no food was consumed at 22.5 Gy. Phillips and Ross noted that a single dose of 20 Gy resulted in thinning of the epithelium and depletion of basal cells in mice, but that doses above 25 Gy there was complete obliteration of basal cells and epithelial denudation in more than half of the animals.[6] While these doses are difficult to extrapolate to humans, the findings suggest that (a) there is a dose response to radiation and (b) there is a sharp increase in persistent dysmotility after a certain tolerance dose.

Human Data on Acute Injury

Esophagitis typically occurs after approximately 20 to 30 Gy radiation therapy in standard fractionation, with a minimum dose of about 15 Gy required to result in symptoms.[4,25,35]

The occurrence of esophagitis is rare with doses <20 Gy in standard fractionation.[11] Most patients receiving doses >40 Gy will experience esophagitis. Seaman and Ackerman[11] reported that all of 20 patients receiving 40 to 76 Gy radiation therapy via 24-MEV betatron experienced some degree of esophagitis (mild in 55%, moderately severe in 20%, and severe in 25%). At doses of 60 Gy, Corder et al.[36] reported 82% incidence of esophagitis (any grade). In the acute setting, Lamanna et al.[18] showed prolonged transit times on technetium scintigraphy in a majority of patients after 20 Gy and in all but one patient after 45 Gy, suggesting dose response. Werner-Wasik et al.[37] evaluated esophagitis in four prospective RTOG non-small lung cancer cell trials using chemoradiation, and reported that higher tumor dose was associated with higher incidence of esophagitis. However, dose was not predictive of the severity esophagitis.[37] A separate single institution study by Werner-Wasik et al.[23] failed to show correlation between radiation dose and esophagitis in the dose range of 45 to 69.6 Gy. The RTOG 83-11 trial, which was a dose escalation study and utilized hyperfractionation (1.2 Gy BID to 60–79 Gy total), reported that the grade 3 or greater acute esophageal toxicity was 5% in 83 patients in the 60-Gy group, 9% in 127 patients in the 64.8-Gy group, 7% in 211 patients in the 74.4-Gy group, and 4% in the 207 patients on the 79.9-Gy group; differences between groups did not reach statistical significance.[38] In a phase I/II study of induction chemotherapy followed by standard fractionation radiation, Rosenman et al.[24] reported that 0 of 3 patients receiving 60 Gy developed grade 3 or 4 esophagitis, whereas 4 of 45 (9%) of patients receiving 66 to 74 Gy did. The only case of grade 4 esophagitis occurred in a patient receiving 74 Gy. Therefore, the majority of data demonstrate a dose response for the occurrence of acute esophagitis, though there is no dramatic dose dependence in the range of doses used for esophageal or lung malignancies. Table 37.4 summarizes acute toxicity in selected clinical trials.

Human Data on Late Injury

Seaman and Ackerman[11] first reported radiation tolerance dose of the esophagus in 1957 based on observations from 20 lung cancer patients treated with 24-MeV beam via a betatron machine to doses of 60 to 75 Gy. Of five patients with severe esophageal injury (permanent stricture requiring dilation or fistula), four (80%) had received 65 to 75 Gy over 35 to 50 days. Of four patients with moderate toxicity, three (75%) received >60 Gy over 30 to 40 days. The conclusion of the authors was that 60 Gy, given at a rate of about 10 Gy/wk, was "about the upper limit of tolerance." Philips and Margolis estimated a steep dose-response curve, and predicted that stricture and ulceration would increase from 5% to 50% between 63 and 66.5 Gy.[6] Morichau-Beauchant et al.[28] reported that complications rates were 1% to 2% for a dose <50 Gy versus 5% to 6% for doses >60 Gy in 6 weeks. In the radiation only arm of RTOG 85-01, 54 patients received a total dose of 64 Gy at 2 Gy/fraction. The incidence of grade 3 or higher late esophageal toxicity was 19%.[39] The RTOG reported late esophageal toxicity in 0.8% of head and neck cancer patients treated to 50 Gy preoperatively versus 6% of patients treated to 60 Gy postoperatively. Stricture rates were 1.2% for patients with lung cancer treated to 60 Gy in 6 weeks.[40] DeRen et al.[41] reported on 869 esophageal cancer patients treated to 50 to 79 Gy and noted a very low overall fistula rate (0.8%), but the authors did not provide information on dose in patients who developed fistula.[41]

TABLE 37.4   Acute Esophagitis

Author	Dose (Range)	Fx	Chemo	N	≥ Gr 3	Any Gr	Predictors[a]
Retrospective Data							
MacGuire[84]	78.8 (64.2–85.6)	64% Ahfx, 36% Sfx	47% IND, 7% CON	91	11%	70%	None
Takeda[74]	60 (50–67)	Sfx	9% IND AND CON, 86% CON	35	0%	71%	V_{35}
Singh[3]	70 (60–74)	Sfx	21% IND, 26% CON	207	5%	7%	CON, Max esoph dose >58 Gy
Kim[2]	60 (54–66)	Sfx	CON	74	20%	NR	CON Ch, $V_{60} > 30\%$
	60 (54–60)	Sfx	15% IND, 85% None	50	2%	NR	
Werner-Wasik[23]	59.9 (45–69.6)	Sfx	None	36	6%	61%	Hfx
		Sfx	IND	11	0%	82%	
		Sfx	CON	51	18%	92%	
		Hfx	CON	7	43%	100%	
Bradley[46]	70 (60–74)	Sfx	22% IND, 25% CON	166	5%	27%	A55, V_{60}, CON Ch
Pooled Data from Prospective RTOG Studies							
Byhardt[54]	60	Sfx	IND	152	1.3%	NR	Hfx-CON Ch
	60	Sfx	IND AND CON	209	6%	NR	
	69.6	Hfx	CON	200	34%	NR	
Werner-Wasik[17]	69.6	Hfx	None	560	7%	NR	CON Ch
	69.6	Hfx	CON	122	41%	NR	
Prospective Data							
Cox[38]	60–79.2	Hfx	None	848	6%	NR	None
Saunders[58]	54	CHART	None	563	19%	NR	CHART
	60	Sfx	None		3%	NR	
Ball[43]	60	Sfx	None	23	9%	79%	Afx
	60	Afx	None	29	35%	100%	
	60	Sfx	CON	24	29%	96%	
	60	Afx	CON	23	39%	95%	
Sause[56]	60	Sfx	IND	152	0%	NR	None
	60	Sfx	None	152	0%	NR	
	69.6	Hfx	None	154	1.3%	NR	
Curran[57]	60	Sfx	CON	200	23%/33%[b]	NR	CON Ch
	60	Hfx	IND	200	30%[c]	NR	
	69.6	Hfx	CON	193	42%/60%[b]	NR	
Furuse[55]	56	Sfx	CON	156	3%	64%	None
	56	Sfx	IND	158	2%	65%	

[a]Statistically significant predictors for acute esophagitis on multivariate analysis.
[b]Incidence in patients <70 years old/≥70 years old.
[c]Reported for all grade ≥3 non–hematologic toxicity, not strictly esophagitis.
A55, surface area of the esophagus receiving 55 Gy; Afx, accelerated fractionation; Ch, chemotherapy; CHART,= continuous hyperfractionated accelerated radiation therapy (54 Gy, 1.5 Gy/fraction, TID over 12 days); CON, concurrent chemotherapy; fx, fractionation; Gr, grade; Hfx, hyperfractionation; IND, induction chemotherapy; Sfx, standard fractionation; N, number; NR, not reported; RTOG, Radiation Therapy Oncology Group; V_{60}, volume of the esophagus receiving 60 Gy.

Beatty et al.[42] noted that although 27 of 152 (18%) of esophagus cancer patients in their study developed stricture attributed to radiation therapy, on post mortem examination four of five patients diagnosed with benign stricture had malignancy in the stricture site.[42] Although O'Rourke et al.[29] demonstrated a late complication rate of 30% in 80 esophagus cancer patients treated with 56 to 60 Gy radiation, another 28% of patients developed malignant stricture. Therefore, clinically diagnosed stricture may grossly overestimate the risk of radiation-related stricture formation and may be an early sign of tumor recurrence.

In summary, the risk of late radiation-induced stricture formation is about 1% following 50 Gy and 5% following 60 Gy. Rate of fistula formation is <1% following 70 Gy.

Table 37.3 summarizes selected clinical trials reporting last esophageal toxicity.

DOSE-VOLUME DEPENDENCE

Acute

The influence of the length of irradiated esophagus on the risk of toxicity remains debated. Michalowski and Hornsey[14] reported that the dose required to produce ulceration in 50% of mice was 24.5 Gy when half of the esophagus was irradiated, versus 22 Gy when the whole esophagus was irradiated. Clinical studies in humans have largely failed to validate that length of esophagus irradiated predicts for acute toxicity. However, more sophisticated analysis of three-dimensional (3D) data indicates that volume or area of treated esophagus does correlate with acute toxicity.

Much of the information related to esophageal toxicity and length of esophagus comes from lung cancer studies. Ball et al.[43] reported that length of treatment field of <14 cm, 14 to 15.9 cm, and >16 cm did not correlate with esophagitis in 100 patients. Choy et al.[44] also found no correlation between the grade of esophagitis and the length of the esophagus treated in either the boost or the primary field in 120 patients. Werner-Wasik prospectively evaluated 105 patients treated with radiation or chemoradiation, and did not find a correlation between the length of esophagus treated and the incidence or severity of esophagitis. In contrast, a study by Langer et al.[64] suggested increased esophagitis with >16 cm of esophagus irradiated compared to <16 cm, though formal statistical analysis was not performed. In this study of concurrent chemoradiation, five of six patients with <16 cm esophagus irradiated had grade 1 esophagitis, whereas eight of nine patients with >16 cm esophagus irradiated experienced grade 2 esophagitis.[45] Similarly, a phase I/II study using carboplatin and paclitaxel induction chemotherapy followed by 60 to 74 Gy standard fractionation radiation therapy by Rosenman et al.[24] identified a higher incidence of esophagitis in non–small cell lung cancer patients in whom >13.5 cm of the esophageal length received 40 Gy ($p = 0.05$) or 60 Gy ($p = 0.02$).

Length of irradiated esophagus may lack the sophistication required to reliably predict toxicity risk. The advent of 3D CT-based planning has allowed more precise collection and analysis of dose-volume distribution, and radiation oncologists continue to develop a more comprehensive understanding of the impact of the volume of irradiated tissue on toxicity. Singh et al.[3] analyzed predictors of esophagitis in non–small cell lung cancer patients treated with 3D conformal radiation therapy. Maximal esophageal point dose of 58 Gy or higher was associated with an increased incidence of grade 3 or higher radiation esophagitis on multivariate analysis.[3] Bradley et al.[46] analyzed this same group of patients, but limited the analysis to patients with detailed dose-volume data. They reported that the area of esophagus receiving +55 Gy, the volume of esophagus receiving ≥60 Gy, and the use of chemotherapy were each associated with a statistically significant increase in acute esophagitis risk. In a single institution retrospective series of lung cancer patients, Kim et al.[2] reported that the risk of acute esophagitis was increased when the volume of esophagus receiving >60 Gy exceeded 30%. Length of esophagus treated did not correlate with esophagitis in this study. In the chemoradiation arm of RTOG 85-01, esophagus cancer patients received 30 Gy to the whole esophagus followed by a cone-down of 20 Gy to the primary tumor plus 5-cm proximal and distal margins.[39] The fraction size was 2 Gy/d and 5-FU/cisplatin was delivered concurrently. In contrast, esophagus cancer patients enrolled in RTOG 0113 received 50.4 Gy to the primary tumor with 5-cm margins. The fraction size was 1.8 Gy/d and taxol/cisplatin ± 5-FU was delivered concurrently. The incidence of late grade 3+ toxicity was higher in RTOG 85-01 (21%) versus RTOG 0113 (8%–12%).[47]

The esophagus is a hollow tube, and dose to the hollow interior of the tube rather than the mucosal surface or the muscular wall of the esophagus is unlikely to be important. Therefore, it has been hypothesized that dose to a given surface area may be a superior predictor of toxicity compared to dose a given volume. Bradley et al. evaluated 3D data in 166 lung cancer patients, including dose-volume data and dose surface area data. Both the surface area receiving >55 Gy (A55) and the volume receiving 60 Gy (V_{60}) were predictive of acute esophagitis on multivariate analysis. The authors discuss the relative merits of evaluation of dose surface area rather than dose volume in a hollow tubular organ, but concede that their study demonstrated that both dose surface area and volume were predictive of esophagitis, and therefore the superiority of evaluation of surface area rather than volume in the clinical setting is unknown. In contrast, a study by Maguire et al.[48] analyzed dose-volume histogram (DVH) parameters in relation to esophageal toxicity in 91 lung cancer patients treated to a median of 78.8 Gy, and did not identify dose surface area or dose-volume parameters that were predictive of acute esophagitis.

Late

Emami et al.[81] estimated the TD 5/5 (tolerance dose at which there is 5% risk of complication at 5 years following radiation) for esophageal stricture or perforation to be 60 Gy if one third of the esophagus is irradiated, 58 Gy when two thirds is irradiated, and 55 Gy when the entire esophagus is irradiated. The TD 50/5 (tolerance does at which there is a 50% risk of complication at 5 years) was estimated to be 72 Gy for one third, 70 Gy for two thirds, and 68 Gy for the entire esophagus receiving radiation.

While the aforementioned study by Maguire et al.[48] did not identify DVH parameters predictive of acute esophageal toxicity, they did identify factors associated with late toxicity.[48] Specifically, the percentage of esophageal volume receiving >50 Gy is associated with late toxicity on multivariate analysis. Patients who received >50 Gy to >32% (median for all patients) of the esophageal volume had a significantly greater incidence of late toxicity. Overall, 13% of patients experienced late esophageal toxicity.

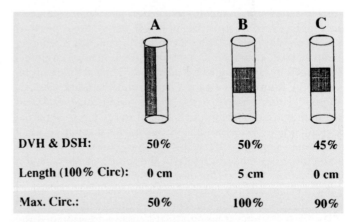

Figure 37.10. Radiation dose distribution (*shaded area*) in the esophagus in three hypothetical cases. Although DVH and dose surface histogram (DSH) are identical for cases A and B, only case B has 100% circumference of the esophagus treated. Therefore, it is hypothesized that epithelial regeneration will be able to occur sufficiently in case A but not case B, resulting in high likelihood of late stricture formation in case B. Case C treats 90% of the circumference of the esophagus, and therefore late toxicity has been hypothesized to be similar to case B. (Reprinted from Elsevier, with permission.[48])

While more sophisticated than 2D evaluation of esophageal length, DVH data have a severe limitation: they do not provide spatial information. The esophagus functions in series, such that destruction of the complete circumference of a small volume of esophagus could result in dysfunction of the entire organ. Therefore, if 50% of the volume of the esophagus is treated, but at no point is the entire circumference of the esophagus treated, then significant toxicity may not occur. On the other hand, if only 10% of the volume of the esophagus is treated, but the entire circumference of the esophagus is treated to high dose, it is possible that toxicity may occur. Figure 37.10 illustrates limitations of DVH in evaluation of the esophagus. Indeed, Maguire et al.[48] observed that patients who received >80 Gy to any portion of the entire organ circumference had increased risk of late (but not acute) toxicity on multivariate analysis. These findings suggest that efforts to spare full circumferential treatment of the esophagus could influence late toxicity.

Modern radiation therapy techniques such as intensity-modulated radiation therapy (IMRT) can generate exquisite dose distributions, with sharp dose fall off and sparing of organs at risk. While intriguing, a reduction in esophageal toxicity with IMRT has not been demonstrated in a clinical setting, and localization of the target and critical organs in the thorax remains a significant challenge due to respiration. Furthermore, the circumference of the esophagus may vary based on filling and edema, and patients undergoing radiation therapy may develop esophageal dysmotility and edema during the course of therapy, which could influence dose distributions. Finally, IMRT may deliver low dose radiation to a larger volume of normal tissue, which may have undesirable effects that are to date not well understood or quantified.

Stereotactic body radiotherapy (SBRT) is emerging as a tool to deliver high dose per fraction radiation therapy with high precision immobilization devices such as a stereotactic body frame and high-quality imaging such as daily pretreatment CT scans to verify positioning. Respiratory gating is also being investigated. Even with the aid of these precision immobilization and localization devices, set-up error and organ movement occur. Furthermore, as discussed above, the esophagus functions in series and complete destruction of a small volume of the esophagus could cause organ failure. Large doses per fraction, as employed in SBRT, are expected to allow less recovery of normal tissue compared to standard fractionation. Nonetheless, SBRT in targets adjacent to the esophagus holds promise for the future. As we gain a better understanding of dose-volume relationships to toxicity, and as sophisticated treatment and immobilization techniques allow us to reliably treat partial circumference of the esophagus, it may be possible to identify patients appropriate for SBRT. Poltinnikov et al. evaluated predictors of esophageal injury in the setting of reirradiation of non–small cell lung cancer patients using stereotactic body frame and median dose of 32 Gy, with median fraction size of 4 Gy. The authors divide the esophagus into "esophageal discs" (ED), each 1.5 mm in longitudinal length, and evaluated the percentage of esophageal circumference receiving prescription dose in each ED. The summation of all EDs represented the length of the esophagus within the radiation portal. This analysis included both length of esophagus treated and circumference of esophagus treated and is therefore more descriptive than a standard DVH. Overall, the length of the esophagus within the radiation portal did not correlate with risk of esophageal toxicity. However, none of the patients in this study had >9 cm esophagus in the radiation portal, so conclusions about esophageal length on toxicity risk are difficult to draw. An increased number of esophageal discs in which 50% of the volume of the disc received ≥50%, ≥80%, or ≥100% of the prescribed dose *was* associated with esophageal toxicity, suggesting circumference as well as length of esophagus treated contributes to toxicity.

In the currently open RTOG study 0613, which delivers 60 Gy in three fractions SBRT to stage I and II non–small cell lung cancer patients, normal tissue limitations included that any point in the esophagus should not receive more than 27 Gy total (9 Gy/fraction or 45% of the target dose).

PRETREATMENT DYSPHAGIA AND ESOPHAGITIS

Macquire et al. reported that preradiation dysphagia correlated with grade 3 acute esophagitis on multivariate analysis in a study of lung cancer patients. Another study by Soffer et al.[22] in which all patients underwent pretreatment EGD showed that 11 of 25 lung cancer patients (44%) had findings of esophagitis on EGD prior to initiation of radiation.[22] Lifestyle factors such as smoking that predispose to cancer may also predispose to esophageal inflammation and irritation and may contribute to the incidence of esophageal toxicity observed with thoracic radiation.

CHEMOTHERAPY AS A RADIOSENSITIZER

Chemotherapy acts as a radiation sensitizer and can therefore increase toxicity. The timing of chemotherapy in relation to radiation dramatically impacts the associated toxicity. Sherman et al.[49] evaluated adriamycin given 24 hours versus 7 days prior to total body radiation in mice. If low dose rate (LDR [5 cGy/h]) radiation was utilized, then the dose of radiation necessary to result in esophageal toxicity was dramatically reduced when adriamcyin was administered 24 hours prior to radiation, but not when the adriamycin was administered 7 days prior to radiation. If high dose rate (HDR [70 cGy/h]) radiation was utilized, then there was an increase in esophageal toxicity if adriamycin was given 24 hours *or* 7 days prior to radiation. In the absence of adriamycin, LDR reduced esophageal toxicity compared to HDR. In the presence of adriamycin 24 hours prior to radiation, the toxicity-sparing effects of lower dose rate were still observed, but these effects were less pronounced, suggesting chemotherapy prior to radiation reduces the benefits of LDR. Other studies have shown that radiation dose rate affects tolerance of the GI tract to radiation in experimental systems as well as in clinical studies.[50–53]

In human studies, the use of chemotherapy *prior* to radiation has not resulted in a clear increase in acute esophageal toxicity, but the use of chemotherapy *during* radiation therapy has.[2,3,17,46,54–57] In a combined analysis of five RTOG prospective lung cancer studies, Byhardt et al.[54] reported a 1.3% of severe (grade 3 or higher) acute esophagitis in patients undergoing induction chemotherapy followed by standard fractionation radiation therapy, 6% in patients undergoing induction chemotherapy followed by concurrent standard fractionation radiation therapy, and 34% in patients undergoing concurrent chemotherapy and hyperfractionated radiation therapy (69.6 Gy delivered 1.2 Gy BID).[54] Werner-Wasik et al.[17] reported that the addition of concurrent chemotherapy to hyperfractionated radiation therapy was associated with a 12-fold increase in

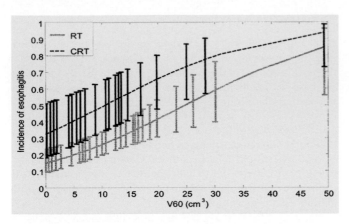

Figure 37.11. Rate of ≥ grade 1 acute esophagitis as a function of the volume of esophagus receiving ≥60 Gy (V_{60}). 95% confidence intervals are represented by error bars; $p < 0.0004$ RT versus CRT. RT, radiation therapy or sequential chemotherapy followed by radiation therapy; CRT, concurrent chemoradiation. (Reprinted from Elsevier, with permission.[46])

the risk of acute esophagitis. Bradley et al.[46] noted a near doubling in the incidence of acute esophagitis with the addition of chemotherapy (Fig. 37.11).

While the vast majority of trials have demonstrated increased toxicity with concurrent versus sequential chemotherapy and radiation therapy, a randomized study from Japan failed to identify an increase in esophagitis.[55] Although the incidence of late esophageal toxicity in the radiation alone versus chemoradiation arms of RTOG 8501 was similar (22% vs. 19%, respectively) since the doses of radiation were different (64 Gy vs. 50 Gy), these data do not help answer the question.[39]

Endoscopic as well as clinical findings of esophagitis are increasing with the use of concurrent chemotherapy. Hirota et al.[16] performed endoscopy in 82 patients with thoracic malignancy treated with radiation therapy. Endoscopy was performed either during or immediately following radiation therapy. Twenty-three of the patients underwent radiation alone, and 59 underwent cisplatin or carboplatinum-based chemoradiation. The use of chemotherapy concurrent with radiation was associated with a higher incidence of ulceration, hemorrhage or stricture on endoscopy, with 27% of chemoradiation patients having these findings versus 0% of radiation alone patients ($p < 0.004$). In terms of symptomatic (RTOG) esophagitis, 8.5% of chemoradiation patients experienced grade 3 toxicity versus none of the patients who received radiation alone. This difference did not reach statistical significance.

In their single institution review of 105 non–small cell lung cancer patients, Werner-Wasik et al.[23] note that concurrent chemotherapy not only increased the incidence of severe esophagitis but also increased the duration of time that patients suffered from esophagitis. Median duration of acute esophagitis was 14 days for patients treated with RT alone, 19 days for induction chemotherapy/standard RT, 29 days for concurrent chemotherapy/standard RT ($p = 0.0004$ compared to RT alone), and 87 days for concurrent chemotherapy/hyperfractionated RT group ($p = 0.002$ compared to RT alone).

In summary, concurrent but not sequential chemoradiation is associated with increased incidence and duration of esophagitis. Table 37.4 summarizes studies evaluating predictors of radiation esophagitis, including chemotherapy.

DOSE FRACTIONATION

Hyperfractionation

Pure hyperfractionation delivers the same total dose over the same time period, but delivers it in twice as many fractions. Therefore, the dose per fraction is smaller. The goal of hyperfractionation is to decrease late effects, as the incidence of late toxicity is highly dependent on dose per fraction. However, acute reacting tissues, which include most tumors, are also spared with smaller dose per fraction, albeit to a lesser extent than late reacting tissues. Therefore, in order to maintain tumor control, a higher total dose is often utilized, which has been referred to as *impure hyperfractionation*. Alternatively, rather than a higher dose, the dose can be delivered over a shorter overall time period, because acutely reacting tissues are sensitive to total time, and therefore tumor control can be maintained while using lower dose per fraction. This method has been referred to as *accelerated hyperfractionation*. Impure hyperfractionation or accelerated hyperfractionation can theoretically result in improved tumor control with equivalent late toxicity. However, acute toxicities may be more severe.

When chemotherapy is delivered concurrent with radiation therapy, the risk of severe esophagitis is increased with the use of hyperfractionation.[23,54] In the absence of concurrent chemotherapy, it is not clear that hyperfractionation increases acute esophagitis.[56] The RTOG 94-10 study randomized non–small cell lung cancer patients to concurrent vinblastine/cisplatin chemotherapy with daily radiation (60 Gy, 2 Gy/fraction) versus twice daily radiation (69.6 Gy, 1.2 Gy/fraction), and showed a higher incidence of grade 3 or higher esophagitis in the "impure" hyperfractionation arm. In a prospective randomized study by Turrisi et al.,[82] 417 small-cell lung cancer patients were randomized to daily radiation therapy (45 Gy, 1.8 Gy/fraction over 5 weeks) versus accelerated hyperfractionated radiation (45 Gy, 1.5 Gy BID over 3 weeks). Both arms received concurrent chemotherapy. The incidence of grade 3 or higher esophagitis was 27% in the BID groups versus 11% in the QD group ($p < 0.001$). Werner Wasik reported that hyperfractionated radiation (69.6 Gy, 1.2 Gy BID) with concurrent chemotherapy predicted for higher incidence of esophagitis as well as length of time spent suffering with esophagitis compared to standard fractionation with or without concurrent chemotherapy.[23] Hyperfractionation to a dose of 69.6 Gy in lung cancer is associated with 34% to 41% incidence of severe esophagitis if concurrent chemotherapy is given, and 1% to 7% if radiation alone is given, as summarized in Table 37.4.[17,23,54,56]

Pure accelerated radiation therapy delivers the same dose per fraction and total dose over a shorter time period, in an attempt to improve tumor control. However, acute toxicity is also expected to be more severe. Ball et al.[43] reported a four arm randomized trial in non–small cell lung cancer comparing standard fractionation (60 Gy in 30 fractions once daily) versus accelerated fractionation (60 Gy in 30 fractions twice daily).[43] On multivariate analysis, the incidence of grade 3 or higher esophagitis was increased from 9% to 35% with accelerated fractionation, and the duration of symptomatic esophagitis was significantly prolonged from 1.4 months with conventional fractionation to 3.2 months with hyperfractionation. Another randomized prospective trial compared continuous hyperfractionated accelerated radiation therapy (CHART), which delivers 1.5 Gy TID to 54 Gy total over 12 days, versus standard fractionation (60 Gy delivered daily over 30 fractions).

The rate of severe esophagitis was 19% with CHART versus 3% with standard fractionation.[58]

While acute toxicity was higher in the CHART arm of this study, late toxicity was mild and did not differ between the two arms. Similarly, RTOG 83-11, which used pure hyperfractionation, reported very little late toxicity, despite a high rate of acute toxicity. The hyperfractionation could perhaps account for low incidence of late effects. The reported late toxicities must be evaluated with caution, however, as median survival in these trials was short due to the poor prognosis of locally advanced non–small-cell lung cancer.

Table 37.5 summarizes esophagitis rates using various dose-fractionation schemes, lists acute and late biologically equivalent doses (BEDs) as well as total treatment time. As expected, the accelerated fractionation schedules, in which radiation was delivered over 3 weeks, had higher rates of esophagitis despite equivalent or lower acute BED based on linear quadratic model. This finding is due to the dependence of acute reacting tissue on total time. The impure hyperfractionation has lower acute BED compared to standard fractionation based on linear quadratic model. Despite the lower acute BED, there is a modest increase in esophagitis with hyperfractionation in the absence of chemotherapy, perhaps due to some degree of acceleration in time of delivery. In the presence of chemotherapy, there was a more dramatic increase in esophagitis compared to standard fractionation. This correlates with the previously described mouse model by Sherman et al.,[49] which suggested chemotherapy eliminates some of the toxicity-sparing effects of LDR radiation.

Hypofractionation

As predicted by radiobiological models, high dose per fraction has been associated with higher toxicity in animal and human studies. Phillips and Ross[6] observed that the lethal dose delivered to the thorax in 50% mice at 28 days was 57.45 Gy in ten fractions but was 26.82 Gy in a single fraction. These deaths were associated with epithelial denudation and starvation and dehydration, and were attributed to esophageal damage. In human studies, hypofractionation has been utilized most extensively in the setting of brachytherapy, and high doses per fraction have been associated with high rates of ulceration, perforation, fistula formation, stricture, and hemorrhage (see "Brachytherapy" section).

BRACHYTHERAPY

Brachytherapy delivers high dose to the esophageal mucosa and fibromuscular wall through endoscopic placement of a radioactive source in the esophagus. LDR and HDR brachytherapy have both been utilized alone or in combination with external beam radiation therapy (EBRT) in the setting of esophagus cancer. A high risk of acute and late toxicity is reported in some series, likely due to the use of high dose per fraction as well as high total dose (in particular when intraluminal brachytherapy is combined with EBRT). In addition, dose is often prescribed to a depth of 1 cm in order to deliver sufficient dose to tumor, with the result that the mucosal surface with receives significantly greater than prescription dose.[59,60]

As with EBRT, dose per fraction influences toxicity of brachytherapy. Hishikawa et al.[61] reported a 90% ulceration rate with 20-Gy single dose intraluminal brachytherapy. On the contrary, doses of 12 Gy in two fractions or 18 Gy in three fractions had lower rates of ulceration. Stricture formation occurred in 4 of 12 patients (33%) who survived 2 years. In a prospective trial, Homs et al.[60] delivered 12-Gy single dose intraluminal HDR brachytherapy and reported 12% major complication rate.

Several prospective trials have evaluated brachytherapy in addition to EBRT and generally have shown unacceptably high toxicity. A randomized trial of 50 patients conducted in India compared 55 Gy EBRT versus 35 Gy EBRT plus 12 Gy HDR. HDR was delivered in two fractions, 1 week apart. While local control rate was higher in the brachytherapy arm, late stricture formation was also higher (8% in the EBRT + brachytherapy arm vs. 4% in the EBRT arm).[62] Another trial from China randomized 200 patients to EBRT 70 Gy in 35 fractions, or EBRT 50 Gy in 25 fractions plus intermediate dose brachytherapy boost, either 19.6 Gy in 3 fractions or 26.16 Gy in 4 fractions. Perforation or hemorrhage was 12.6% in both arms.[63] Hishikawa et al.[61] reported 88% risk of ulceration and 12% risk of fistula formation with median dose of 55 Gy EBRT + 17 Gy HDR brachytherapy. When dose was decreased to 57 Gy EBRT + 12 Gy in 2 fractions HDR brachytherapy, ulceration rate was reduced to 50%, with no reports of fistula formation.[61] These trials did not utilize concurrent chemotherapy, which is now considered standard of care for definitive treatment of esophageal carcinoma, and which is expected to increase radiation related toxicity. RTOG 92-07 was a phase I/II study of external beam radiation (50 Gy) and concurrent 5-FU/cisplatin chemotherapy plus esophageal brachytherapy boost (15 Gy HDR

				≥ *Grade 3 Esophagitis,*	≥ *Grade 3 Esophagitis,*
Fractionation	*Acute BED*[a]	*Late BED*[a]	*Time (Wk)*	*No Chemo*	*Con Chemo*
69.6 Gy, 1.2 Gy/fx BID	51	97	5.8	7%[23]	34%[54]
60 Gy, 2 Gy/fx QD	61	100	6	1.3%[54]	6%–29%[23,43,54]
54 Gy, 1.5 Gy/fx TID	48	81	3	19%[58]	—
60 Gy, 2 Gy/fx BID	61	100	3	35%[43]	
45 Gy, 1.5 Gy/fx BID	53	72	3	—	27%[82]
45 Gy, 1.8 Gy/fx QD	53	72	5		11%[82]

TABLE 37.5 — **Esophagitis Rates Based on Fractionation**

[a]Assuming α/β ratio of 3 for late-responding tissue and 10 for early-responding tissue.
BED, biologically equivalent dose; fx, fraction.

delivered at 5 Gy/fraction or 20 Gy LDR at a dose rate of 0.5–1.0 Gy/h, both prescribed to a depth of 1 cm).[59] Esophageal fistula occurred in 12% of patients, and life-threatening toxicity occurred in 24%. Treatment-related death rate was 10%. Toxicity was considered unacceptable.

AGE

Age may also have an effect. The RTOG 94-10 trial reported that patients ≥70 years of age had 33% incidence of severe esophagitis compared to 23% in younger patients.[64] Other studies have not confirmed this finding.[2,46]

PROPHYLAXIS OF RADIATION TOXICITY

Radiation esophagitis has the potential to influence local control and survival if the severity of the toxicity results in treatment breaks. In the setting of head and neck squamous cell carcinoma, each day break in treatment is associated with approximately 1% loss in local control.[65] Treatment breaks have been associated with a decrease in overall survival in unresectable lung cancer.[66] Therefore, prophylaxis against esophagitis, which can require a treatment break, is desirable both for patient comfort and safety but also for tumor control.

CYCLOOXYGENASE INHIBITORS

Nonsteroidal anti-inflammatory agents (NSAIDs) block the synthesis of prostaglandins, which in turn trigger inflammation. Radiation has been shown to increase the synthesis of prostaglandins in gastrointestinal tissues.[22,67,68] Therefore, NSAIDs, primarily cyclooxygenase inhibitors, have been investigated for prevention of radiation induced esophagitis.

Cyclooxygenase inhibitors (including indomethacin and sodium meclofenamate) have reduced radiation-induced histologic damage in animal studies.[13,69,70] A mouse model showed reduction in weight loss and improvement in survival in addition to reduction in histologic changes with the addition of indomethacin to 28 to 30 Gy single fraction radiation therapy

to the esophagus, without protection of cancer cells.[69] These advantages were not noted at lower or higher radiation dose.

Despite promise in animal studies, these medications have not demonstrated sufficient efficacy in clinical trials to warrant routine use.[13,22,71,72] A failure to show clinical benefit in humans despite promising evidence in animal models may be due to differences in species, but could also be due to higher dose of drugs per kilogram utilized in animal models, or higher dose per fraction radiation in animal models. Finally, in mouse models, a narrow window of therapeutic benefit was identified, presumably due to a steep radiation dose-response to esophagitis.[69] Therefore, the radiation doses tested in human studies may be outside the therapeutic window.

AMIFOSTINE

Amifostine, a thiophosphate (Ethyol; MedImmune, Inc, Gaithersburg, MD), has been studied as a radioprotector. Its sulfhydryl (thiol) group can act as a free-radical scavenger and thus protect against oxygen-based free-radical generation by ionizing radiation. In addition, the sulfhydryl groups can donate a hydrogen atom to aid in repair of DNA damage. Amifostine is a prodrug that requires dephosphorylation by alkaline phosphatase, which is present in normal tissues. The active metabolite WR-1065 can then enter the cell. Amiofostine is taken up more quickly by normal tissues compared to tumor, and therefore tumor sparing is expected to be minimal if radiation is delivered promptly (within 30 minutes) following the administration of amifostine.[73]

In mouse models, amifostine administration increased the lethal dose in 50% of animals (LD_{50}) following thoracic radiation from 38 to 60 Gy, and protected against both acute and late esophageal damage.[74] The protection factor (dose of radiation required to produce a given lethality in the presence of the drug divided by the dose of radiation required to produce the same lethality in the absence of the drug) was approximately 1.5.

Human studies of amifostine on esophageal toxicity are summarized in Table 37.6. A statistically significant reduction in acute esophagatitis has been demonstrated in 3 randomized trials of NSCLC patients.[15,75,76] A fourth, larger trial by the RTOG failed to show a reduction in esophagitis.[77] However, swallowing dysfunction as measured by patient diaries was significantly

TABLE 37.6	Randomized Trials of Radiation With or Without Amifostine			
Author	*Dose*	*RT Dose*	*Amifostine*	*Gr 3/4 Esophagitis*
Antonadou[15] (*N* = 146)	340 mg/m² daily 15 min prior to RT	55–60 Gy QD	Yes	4%[a,b]
			No	42%[a,b]
Antonadou[75] (*N* = 68)	300 mg/m² daily 15–20 min prior to RT	55–60 Gy QD	Yes	39%
			No	84%
Komaki[76] (*N* = 60)	500 mg/m² IV two times per week	69.6 Gy BID	Yes	7%[a,c]
			No	31%[a,c]
Leong[83] (*N* = 60)	740 mg/m² IV weekly	60–66 Gy QD	Yes	43%[e]
			No	70%[e]
RTOG 98-01[25] (*N* = 243)	500 mg/m² IV four times per week	69.6 BID	Yes	30%[d]
			No	34%

[a]*p* < 0.05.
[b]Grade 2 or higher.
[c]Requiring morphine.
[d]Esophagitis by NCI-CTCAE criteria was not reduced, but swallowing function measured on patient diaries was lower with amifostine (*p* = 0.03).
[e]Grade 2 or 3 toxicity reported.
Gr, grade; IV= intravenous; NS, nonsignificant; RT, radiation therapy; wk, week. All studies used concurrent chemo except Antonadou 2001 study.

lower in the amifostine group. None of these trials showed a reduction in response rates of the cancer. About 5% of patients receiving amifostine will experience nausea and vomiting, and 7% to 22% will experience hypotension.[15,75] While results in terms of esophagitis have been encouraging, the therapeutic ratio is debated.

TREATMENT

RADIATION ESOPHAGITIS

After radiation esophagitis has developed, antacid medications including H2 blockers and proton-pump inhibitors are often utilized. The radiation damage is not caused by acid production.[20] However, acid production can worsen symptoms, particularly in patients with lower esophageal carcinoma in whom acid reflux into the treated esophagus may occur. Of interest, in the study by Mascarenhas et al.[5] in which patients underwent planned endoscopy after 30 to 40 Gy, 18 of 38 patients (47%) showed endoscopic signs of gastritis, which was confirmed by biopsy findings in 14 of 18 (78%). The stomach was not included in the radiation portal in these patients, and the authors postulate that hypersecretion of hydrochloric acid occurred in response to changes in the esophagus. These findings suggest a role for antacid therapy in radiation esophagitis, despite the fact that the esophagitis itself is not caused by acid hypersecretion.

Sucralfate has also been utilized, though its clinical utility is debated. Sucralfate is a basic aluminum salt used in the treatment of peptic ulcers and reflux esophagitis. Its mechanism is multifaceted. It is believed to reduce pepsin and bile acids and also to form a protective coating by binding of protein molecules, thus becoming viscous and adhesive. It is also thought to stimulate ulcer repair. Taal et al.[78] completed a pilot study in 10 patients with radiation esophagitis. Sucralfate was administered four times per day for 6 weeks. Only minor relief of pain was noted in four patients, and endoscopy after 6 weeks of treatment failed to show improvement. The same authors subsequently monitored the degree of coating of the esophagus using sucralfate labeled with technetium 99m in 26 esophagus cancer patients with endoscopically proven radiation esophagitis (11 acute, 15 chronic). Radiolabeled albumin was also administered as a control. Although 24 (92%) of patients were found to have radioactivity, only 8 (31%) of patients were found to have selective binding of sucralfate. The rest also demonstrated the presence of radiolabeled albumin in addition to sucralfate, suggesting non-specific binding, likely due to poor esophageal motility. Scans remained positive for radioactivity in only 15% of patients after 1 to 2 hours, suggesting the duration of adherence of sucralfate to the damaged esophagus is insufficient to provide symptomatic relief. The authors note that perhaps more frequent administration may be useful. The degree of binding was not related to depth of ulceration or to acute versus chronic damage. Sucralfate adheres to ulcer proteins in the presence of acid, and one hypothesis proposed by the authors is that a relative lack of acid in the esophagus impairs binding.[78] McGinnis et al.[71] completed a phase III randomized trial of placebo versus sucralfate in the treatment of radiation esophagitis, and sucralfate showed no advantage.[71]

Radiation esophagitis is essentially treated symptomatically. Healing is a matter of time. Until healing occurs, pain medications, soft or liquid diet, and topical anesthetics can be utilized. Triple mix (2% viscous lidocaine, diphenhydramine hydrochloride, and aluminum hydroxide-magnesium carbonate) is commonly utilized. If nutritional intake is severely limited, temporary placement of a feeding tube should be considered. A low-acid, bland diet has been advocated, with recommendations against coffee, hot beverages, spicy foods, citrus fruits and juices, tomato products, alcohol, and tobacco.[25]

RADIATION-INDUCED STRICTURE

The treatment of esophageal stricture is generally dilation, and repeated dilations are typically required. O'Rourke et al.[29] found that an average of 2.5 dilations were required to provide relief of dysphagia, and median time between dilations was 5 months.[29] Of 17 patients with radiation-induced esophageal stricture in this study, 70% were able to tolerate a full or soft diet. Though thickened, the esophageal wall may in fact be weaker in the area of stricture, and a concern of perforation exists.[20] However, this complication is infrequent.[29]

Dysphagia due to late radiation damage mimics esophageal spasm, and calcium channel blockers including nifedipine have anecdotally improved symptoms.[27,79]

FISTULA

Tracheoesophageal fistula is a life-threatening complication and treatment is difficult.[20] Esophageal stents to cover the fistula can be considered. However, migration of the stent is a concern. Percutaneous gastrostomy tube may be required for nutrition, with strict NPO status. Even in the absence of oral intake, aspiration of secretions is a major concern, and spit fistula (which diverts secretions through an ostomy in the neck) may be necessary.

CONCLUSION

Radiation injury to the esophagus is marked by epithelial damage with resultant esophagitis in the short term and submucosal and muscular fibrosis in the long term, with stricture and dysphagia the most common late injury. While esophagitis occurs to some degree in a majority of patients receiving more than 40-Gy standard fractionation radiation therapy, severe esophagitis occurs in a minority of patients, with risk of grade 3 or higher esophagitis of <2% at 60 Gy. Concurrent chemotherapy and altered fractionation together increase this risk to >30%. The risk of acute and late toxicity appears to be related to volume of esophagus treated, though data on dose-volume relationships remain poorly defined and are a topic of ongoing investigation. Amifostine is promising in the prevention of severe esophagitis, though the cost-benefit ratio of this treatment is not clear, and therefore its use is not routine.

REFERENCES

1. Bradley J, Movsas B. Radiation esophagitis: predictive factors and preventive strategies. *Semin Radiat Oncol.* 2004;14(4):280–286.
2. Kim TH, Cho KH, Pyo HR, et al. Dose-volumetric parameters of acute esophageal toxicity in patients with lung cancer treated with three-dimensional conformal radiotherapy. *Int J Radiat Oncol Biol Phys.* 2005;62(4):995–1002.
3. Singh AK, Lockett MA, Bradley JD. Predictors of radiation-induced esophageal toxicity in patients with non-small-cell lung cancer treated with three-dimensional conformal radiotherapy. *Int J Radiat Oncol Biol Phys.* 2003;55(2):337–341.
4. Coia LR, Myerson RJ, Tepper JE. Late effects of radiation therapy on the gastrointestinal tract. *Int J Radiat Oncol Biol Phys.* 1995;31(5):1213–1236.

5. Mascarenhas F, Silvestre ME, Sa da Costa M, et al. Acute secondary effects in the esophagus in patients undergoing radiotherapy for carcinoma of the lung. *Am J Clin Oncol.* 1989;12(1):34–40.

6. Phillips TL, Ross G. Time-dose relationships in the mouse esophagus. *Radiology.* 1974;113(2):435–440.

7. Berthrong M, Fajardo LF. Radiation injury in surgical pathology. Part II. Alimentary tract. *Am J Surg Pathol.* 1981;5(2):153–178.

8. Engelstad R. Uber die Wirhungen de Rontgenstrahlen auf Osophagus und Trachea. *Acta Radiol.* 1934;15:608–614.

9. Papazian A, Capron JP, Ducroix JP, et al. Mucosal bridges of the upper esophagus after radiotherapy for Hodgkin's disease. *Gastroenterology.* 1983;84(5 pt 1):1028–1031.

10. Goldstein HM, Rogers LF, Fletcher GH, et al. Radiological manifestations of radiation-induced injury to the normal upper gastrointestinal tract. *Radiology.* 1975;117(1):135–140.

11. Seaman WB, Ackerman LV. The effect of radiation on the esophagus; a clinical and histologic study of the effects produced by the betatron. *Radiology.* 1957;68(4):534–541.

12. Gillette SM, Poulson JM, Deschesne KM, et al. Response of the canine esophagus to irradiation. *Radiat Res.* 1998;150(3):365–368.

13. Northway MG, Libshitz HI, Osborne BM, et al. Radiation esophagitis in the opossum: radioprotection with indomethacin. *Gastroenterology.* 1980;78(5 pt 1):883–892.

14. Michalowski A, Hornsey S. Assays of damage to the alimentary canal. *Br J Cancer Suppl.* 1986;7:1–6.

15. Antonadou D, Coliarakis N, Synodinou M, et al. Randomized phase III trial of radiation treatment ± amifostine in patients with advanced-stage lung cancer. *Int J Radiat Oncol Biol Phys.* 2001;51(4):915–922.

16. Hirota S, Tsujino K, Endo M, et al. Dosimetric predictors of radiation esophagitis in patients treated for non-small-cell lung cancer with carboplatin/paclitaxel/radiotherapy. *Int J Radiat Oncol Biol Phys.* 2001;51(2):291–295.

17. Werner-Wasik M, Scott C, Graham ML, et al. Interfraction interval does not affect survival of patients with non-small cell lung cancer treated with chemotherapy and/or hyperfractionated radiotherapy: a multivariate analysis of 1076 RTOG patients. *Int J Radiat Oncol Biol Phys.* 1999;44(2):327–331.

18. LaManna MM, Parker JA, Wolodzko JG, et al. Radionuclide esophageal and intestinal transit scintigraphy in patients undergoing radiation therapy. *Radiat Med.* 1985;3(1):13–16.

19. Collazzo LA, Levine MS, Rubesin SE, et al. Acute radiation esophagitis: radiographic findings. *AJR Am J Roentgenol.* 1997;169(4):1067–1070.

20. Vanagunas A, Jacob P, Olinger E. Radiation-induced esophageal injury: a spectrum from esophagitis to cancer. *Am J Gastroenterol.* 1990;85(7):808–812.

21. Slanina J, Frohlich J, Oehlert W, et al. Endoscopic and biopsy findings in the esophageal, gastric and duodenal mucosa before and after radiotherapy for Hodgkin's disease. *Strahlentherapie.* 1985;161(4):216–220.

22. Soffer EE, Mitros F, Doornbos JF, et al. Morphology and pathology of radiation-induced esophagitis. Double-blind study of naproxen vs placebo for prevention of radiation injury. *Dig Dis Sci.* 1994;39(3):655–660.

23. Werner-Wasik M, Pequignot E, Leeper D, et al. Predictors of severe esophagitis include use of concurrent chemotherapy, but not the length of irradiated esophagus: a multivariate analysis of patients with lung cancer treated with nonoperative therapy. *Int J Radiat Oncol Biol Phys.* 2000;48(3):689–696.

24. Rosenman JG, Halle JS, Socinski MA, et al. High-dose conformal radiotherapy for treatment of stage IIIA/IIIB non-small-cell lung cancer: technical issues and results of a phase I/II trial. *Int J Radiat Oncol Biol Phys.* 2002;54(2):348–356.

25. Werner-Wasik M. Treatment-related esophagitis. *Semin Oncol.* 2005;32(2 suppl 3):S60–S66.

26. Lepke RA, Libshitz HI. Radiation-induced injury of the esophagus. *Radiology.* 1983;148(2):375–378.

27. Kaplinsky C, Kornreich L, Tiomny E, et al. Esophageal obstruction 14 years after treatment for Hodgkin's disease. *Cancer.* 1991;68(4):903–905.

28. Morichau-Beauchant M, Touchard G, Battandier D, et al. Chronic radiation-induced esophagitis after treatment of oropharyngolaryngeal cancer: a little-known anatomo-clinical entity. *Gastroenterol Clin Biol.* 1983;7(11):843–850.

29. O'Rourke IC, Tiver K, Bull C, et al. Swallowing performance after radiation therapy for carcinoma of the esophagus. *Cancer.* 1988;61(10):2022–2026.

30. Marks JE, Moran EM, Griem ML, et al. Extended mantle radiotherapy in Hodgkin's disease and malignant lymphoma. *Am J Roentgenol Radium Ther Nucl Med.* 1974;121(4):772–788.

31. Micke O, Schafer U, Glashorster M, et al. Radiation-induced esophageal carcinoma 30 years after mediastinal irradiation: case report and review of the literature. *Jpn J Clin Oncol.* 1999;29(3):164–170.

32. Marchese MJ, Liskow A, Chang CH. Radiation therapy associated cancer of the esophagus. *N Y State J Med.* 1986;86(3):152–153.

33. Black WC, III, Ackerman LV. Carcinoma of the Large Intestine as a Late Complication of Pelvic Radiotherapy. *Clin Radiol.* 1965;16:278–281.

34. Ahsan H, Neugut AI. Radiation therapy for breast cancer and increased risk for esophageal carcinoma. *Ann Intern Med.* 1998;128(2):114–117.

35. Cox JD, Byhardt RW, Wilson JF, et al. Complications of radiation therapy and factors in their prevention. *World J Surg.* 1986;10(2):171–188.

36. Corder MP, Tewfik HH, Clamon GH, et al. Radiotherapy plus razoxane for advanced limited extent carcinoma of the lung. *Cancer.* 1984;53(9):1852–1856.

37. Werner-Wasik M, Axelrod RS, Friedland DP, et al. Phase II: trial of twice weekly amifostine in patients with non-small cell lung cancer treated with chemoradiotherapy. *Semin Radiat Oncol.* 2002;12(1 suppl 1):34–39.

38. Cox JD, Azarnia N, Byhardt RW, et al. A randomized phase I/II trial of hyperfractionated radiation therapy with total doses of 60.0 Gy to 79.2 Gy: possible survival benefit with greater than or equal to 69.6 Gy in favorable patients with Radiation Therapy Oncology Group stage III non-small-cell lung carcinoma: report of Radiation Therapy Oncology Group 83–11. *J Clin Oncol.* 1990;8(9):1543–1555.

39. Cooper JS, Guo MD, Herskovic A, et al. Chemoradiotherapy of locally advanced esophageal cancer: long-term follow-up of a prospective randomized trial (RTOG 85–01). Radiation Therapy Oncology Group. *JAMA.* 1999;281(17):1623–1627.

40. Kramer S, Gelber RD, Snow JB, et al. Combined radiation therapy and surgery in the management of advanced head and neck cancer: final report of study 73-03 of the Radiation Therapy Oncology Group. *Head Neck Surg.* 1987;10(1):19–30.

41. DeRen S. Ten-year follow-up of esophageal cancer treated by radical radiation therapy: analysis of 869 patients. *Int J Radiat Oncol Biol Phys.* 1989;16:329–334.

42. Beatty JD, DeBoer G, Rider WD. Carcinoma of the esophagus: pretreatment assessment, correlation of radiation treatment parameters with survival, and identification and management of radiation treatment failure. *Cancer.* 1979;43(6):2254–2267.

43. Ball D, Bishop J, Smith J, et al. A phase III study of accelerated radiotherapy with and without carboplatin in nonsmall cell lung cancer: an interim toxicity analysis of the first 100 patients. *Int J Radiat Oncol Biol Phys.* 1995;31(2):267–272.

44. Choy H, LaPorte K, Knill-Selby E, et al. Esophagitis in combined modality therapy for locally advanced non-small cell lung cancer. *Semin Radiat Oncol.* 1999;9(2 suppl 1):90–96.

45. Langer CJ. Concurrent chemoradiation using paclitaxel and carboplatin in locally advanced non-small cell lung cancer. *Semin Radiat Oncol.* 1999;9(2 suppl 1):108–116.

46. Bradley J, Deasy JO, Bentzen S, et al. Dosimetric correlates for acute esophagitis in patients treated with radiotherapy for lung carcinoma. *Int J Radiat Oncol Biol Phys.* 2004;58(4):1106–1113.

47. Ajani JA, Winter K, Komaki R, et al. Phase II randomized trial of two nonoperative regimens of induction chemotherapy followed by chemoradiation in patients with localized carcinoma of the esophagus: RTOG 0113. *J Clin Oncol.* 2008;26(28):4551–4556.

48. Maguire PD, Sibley GS, Zhou SM, et al. Clinical and dosimetric predictors of radiation-induced esophageal toxicity. *Int J Radiat Oncol Biol Phys.* 1999;45(1):97–103.

49. Sherman DM, Carabell SC, Belli JA, et al. The effect of dose rate and adriamycin on the tolerance of thoracic radiation in mice. *Int J Radiat Oncol Biol Phys.* 1982;8(1):45–51.

50. Hornsey S, Alper T. Unexpected dose-rate effect in the killing of mice by radiation. *Nature.* 1966;210(5032):212–213.

51. Hornsey S, Vatistas S. Some Characteristics of the survival curve of crypt cells of the small intestine of the mouse deduced after whole body X irradiation. *Br J Radiol.* 1963;36:795–800.

52. Neal FE. Variation of acute mortality with dose-rate in mice exposed to single large doses of whole-body x-radiation. *Int J Radiat Biol.* 1960;2:295–300.

53. Cassady JR, Richter MP, Piro AJ, et al. Radiation-adriamycin interactions: preliminary clinical observations. *Cancer.* 1975;36(3):946–949.

54. Byhardt RW, Scott C, Sause WT, et al. Response, toxicity, failure patterns, and survival in five Radiation Therapy Oncology Group (RTOG) trials of sequential and/or concurrent chemotherapy and radiotherapy for locally advanced non-small-cell carcinoma of the lung. *Int J Radiat Oncol Biol Phys.* 1998;42(3):469–478.

55. Furuse K, Fukuoka M, Kawahara M, et al. Phase III study of concurrent versus sequential thoracic radiotherapy in combination with mitomycin, vindesine, and cisplatin in unresectable stage III non-small-cell lung cancer. *J Clin Oncol.* 1999;17(9):2692–2699.

56. Sause W, Kolesar P, Taylor SI, et al. Final results of phase III trial in regionally advanced unresectable non-small cell lung cancer: Radiation Therapy Oncology Group, Eastern Cooperative Oncology Group, and Southwest Oncology Group. *Chest.* 2000;117(2):358–364.

57. Curran W, Scott C, Langer C, et al. Phase III comparison of sequential vs concurrent chemoradiation for patients (pts) with unresected stage III non small cell lung cancer (NSCLC): initial report of radiation oncology group (RTOG) 9410. *Proc Am Soc Clin Oncol.* 2000;19:abstr 1891.

58. Saunders M, Dische S, Barrett A, et al. Continuous hyperfractionated accelerated radiotherapy (CHART) versus conventional radiotherapy in non-small-cell lung cancer: a randomised multicentre trial. CHART Steering Committee. *Lancet.* 1997;350(9072):161–165.

59. Gaspar LE, Winter K, Kocha WI, et al. A phase I/II study of external beam radiation, brachytherapy, and concurrent chemotherapy for patients with localized carcinoma of the esophagus (Radiation Therapy Oncology Group Study 9207): final report. *Cancer.* 2000;88(5):988–995.

60. Homs MY, Steyerberg EW, Eijkenboom WM, et al. Single-dose brachytherapy versus metal stent placement for the palliation of dysphagia from oesophageal cancer: multicentre randomised trial. *Lancet.* 2004;364(9444):1497–1504.

61. Hishikawa Y, Izumi M, Kurisu K, et al. Esophageal ulceration following high-dose-rate intraluminal brachytherapy for esophageal cancer. *Radiother Oncol.* 1993;28(3):252–254.

62. Sur RK, Singh DP, Sharma SC, et al. Radiation therapy of esophageal cancer: role of high dose rate brachytherapy. *Int J Radiat Oncol Biol Phys.* 1992;22(5):1043–1046.

63. Yin W. Brachytherapy of carcinoma of the esophagus in China, 1970–1974 and 1982–1984. In: Martinez A, Orton CG, Mould RF, eds. *Brachytherapy: HDR and LDR.* Columbia, MD: Nucletron Corp.; 1990:52–56.

64. Langer C, Hsu C, Curran W. Elderly patients (pts) with locally advanced non-small cell lung cancer (LA-NSCLC) benefit from combined modality therapy: secondary analysis of Radiation Therapy Oncology Group (RTOG) 94-10. *Proc Am Soc Clin Oncol.* 2002;21:299a (abstr 1193).

65. Hall E, Giaccia A. Time, dose, and fractionation in radiotherapy. In: Hall E, Giaccia A, eds. *Radiobiology for the Radiobiologist.* Philadelphia, PA: Lippincott Williams & Wilkins; 2006:388.

66. Cox JD, Pajak TF, Asbell S, et al. Interruptions of high-dose radiation therapy decrease long-term survival of favorable patients with unresectable non-small cell carcinoma of the lung: analysis of 1244 cases from 3 Radiation Therapy Oncology Group (RTOG) trials. *Int J Radiat Oncol Biol Phys.* 1993;27(3):493–498.

67. Gal D, Strickland DM, Lifshitz S, et al. Effect of radiation on prostaglandin production by human bowel in vitro. *Int J Radiat Oncol Biol Phys.* 1984;10(5):653–657.

68. Tanner NS, Stamford IF, Bennett A. Plasma prostaglandins in mucositis due to radiotherapy and chemotherapy for head and neck cancer. *Br J Cancer.* 1981;43(6):767–771.

69. Tochner Z, Barnes M, Mitchell JB, et al. Protection by indomethacin against acute radiation esophagitis. *Digestion.* 1990;47(2):81–87.

70. Ambrus JL, Ambrus CM, Lillie DB, et al. Effect of sodium meclofenamate on radiation-induced esophagitis and cystitis. *J Med.* 1984;15(2):81–92.

71. McGinnis WL, Loprinzi CL, Buskirk SJ, et al. Placebo-controlled trial of sucralfate for inhibiting radiation-induced esophagitis. *J Clin Oncol.* 1997;15(3):1239–1243.

72. Nicolopoulos N, Mantidis A, Stathopoulos E, et al. Prophylactic administration of indomethacin for irradiation esophagitis. *Radiother Oncol.* 1985;3(1):23–25.

73. Hall E, Giaccia A. Radioprotectors. In: Hall E, Giaccia A, eds. *Radiobiology for the Radiobiologist.* Philadelphia, PA: Lippincott Williams & Wilkins; 2006:131–132.

74. Takeda K, Nemoto K, Saito H, et al. Dosimetric correlations of acute esophagitis in lung cancer patients treated with radiotherapy. *Int J Radiat Oncol Biol Phys.* 2005;62(3):626–629.

75. Antonadou D, Throuvalas N, Petridis A, et al. Effect of amifostine on toxicities associated with radiochemotherapy in patients with locally advanced non-small-cell lung cancer. *Int J Radiat Oncol Biol Phys.* 2003;57(2):402–408.

76. Komaki R, Lee JS, Kaplan B, et al. Randomized phase III study of chemoradiation with or without amifostine for patients with favorable performance status inoperable stage II-III non-small cell lung cancer: preliminary results. *Semin Radiat Oncol.* 2002;12(1 suppl 1): 46–49.

77. Movsas B, Scott C, Langer C, et al. Phase III study of amifostine in patients with locally advanced non-small cell lung cancer receiving intensive chemoradiation: Radiation Therapy Oncology Group 98–01. *Proc Am Soc Clin Oncol.* 2003;22:636 (abst 2459).

78. Taal BG, Vales Olmos RA, Boot H, et al. Assessment of sucralfate coating by sequential scintigraphic imaging in radiation-induced esophageal lesions. *Gastrointest Endosc.* 1995;41(2):109–114.

79. Finkelstein E. Nifedipine for radiation oesophagitis. *Lancet.* 1986;1(8491):1205–1206.

80. Perez CA, Stanley K, Rubin P, et al. A prospective randomized study of various irradiation doses and fractionation schedules in the treatment of inoperable non-oat-cell carcinoma of the lung. Preliminary report by the Radiation Therapy Oncology Group. *Cancer.* 1980;45(11):2744–53.

81. Emami B, Lyman J, Brown A, et al. Tolerance of normal tissue to therapeutic irradiation. *Int J Radiat Oncol Biol Phys.* 1991;21(1):109–22.

82. Turrisi AT 3rd, Kim K, Blum R, et al. Twice-daily compared with once-daily thoracic radiotherapy in limited small-cell lung cancer treated concurrently with cisplatin and etoposide. *N Engl J Med.* 1999;340(4):265–71.

83. Leong SS, Tan EH, Fong KW, et al. Randomized double-blind trial of combined modality treatment with or without amifostine in unresectable stage III non-small-cell lung cancer. *J Clin Oncol.* 2003;21(9):1767–74.

84. MacGuire PD, Sibley GS, Zhou S-M, et al. Clinical and dosimetric predictors of radiation-induced esophageal toxicity. *Int J Radiat Oncol Biol Phys.* 45(1):97–103.

CHAPTER
38

Martin Hauer-Jensen, James W. Denham
Nils Hovdenak, K. Sree Kumar

Small Bowel and Colon

INTRODUCTION

Up to 70% of cancer patients may undergo radiation therapy at some point in the history of the disease, and radiation therapy plays a definitive role in 25% of cancer cures. Recent advances in treatment planning and dose delivery have made it possible to limit radiation to the tumor volume with greater precision. Nevertheless, with few exceptions, the radiation dose conforms to a target that is inherently uncertain. Therefore, normal tissue toxicity continues to be the single-most important obstacle to cancer cure and an important concern of radiation oncologists in their daily practice.

Normal tissue toxicity is a particularly critical consideration (a) in retreatment situations, (b) whenever treatment regimens with nonstandard time-dose-fractionation parameters are used, (c) in protocols with dose escalation, (d) whenever radiation is combined with other cytotoxic or biological therapies, (e) in patients with predisposing factors or comorbidities that make them particularly sensitive to radiation, as well as (f) in developing countries or other areas where sophisticated treatment planning and delivery technologies may not be widely available.

During radiation therapy of tumors in the abdomen or pelvis, the small bowel, colon, and rectum are important normal tissues at risk. While the mechanisms and pathophysiology of radiation injury in these organs have a lot in common, there are also important anatomical and physiological differences. These differences result in distinct clinical presentation of radiation toxicities and require different strategies for workup and therapy.

By definition, intestinal radiation toxicity is classified as acute (early) when it occurs during or within 3 months of radiation therapy, or delayed (chronic) when it occurs more than 3 months after radiation therapy. Early intestinal radiation toxicity affects patients' quality of life during and shortly after treatment. The symptoms are generally transient and cease after completion of radiation therapy. In some cases, however, early toxicity may be severe enough to require treatment interruption, deintensification of treatment, or other alterations of the original treatment plan. In these instances, the tumor control probability may be compromised. Delayed intestinal radiation injuries are highly important as a cancer survivorship issue. This is due to its often progressive nature, lack of

effective treatment options, and substantial long-term morbidity and mortality, thereby reducing the "uncomplicated cancer cure rate."

This chapter will discuss pertinent anatomical features of the small and large bowel, as well as the epidemiology, pathology, and clinical presentation of intestinal radiation injury. Principles of diagnostic workup and available treatment options in patients with suspected radiation induced bowel injury will also be presented, along with pharmacological approaches used to minimize bowel injury in the clinic. Finally, a section is included related to gastrointestinal (GI) injury in the setting of radiological/nuclear accidents or terrorist scenarios and ongoing efforts to develop effective medical countermeasures.

GROSS ANATOMICAL FEATURES OF THE SMALL AND LARGE INTESTINE

The average length of the small intestine is 5.5 to 6 m in the adult human. The small intestine comprises three segments, the duodenum, the jejunum, and the ileum. The duodenum extends from the pylorus to the ligament of Treitz and measures about 30 cm. There is no exact anatomical landmark indicating the transition between the jejunum and the ileum, but the ileum is somewhat paler in color, smaller in caliber, and exhibits more mesenteric fat than the jejunum. The length of the jejunum is about 2.5 m, while the ileum is slightly longer at about 3 m. While the duodenum is almost entirely fixed in the retroperitoneal position, the jejunum and ileum are located intraperitoneally and thus fully mobile when not tethered by intraperitoneal adhesions. The distal part of the ileum, however, is relatively fixed in its location in the lower right quadrant of the abdomen at its connection to the cecum.

The main functions of the small intestine are to digest and absorb nutrients, while propelling the intestinal contents in the aboral direction. Certain specialized functions take place in specific segments of the small intestine. For example, absorption of vitamin B_{12} and bile salts occurs mainly in the distal ileum.

The lower part of the digestive system, the colon, rectum, and anus, measures 1.5 to 1.8 m in total length. The colon consists

421

of the cecum and the ascending, transverse, descending, and sigmoid colon. The location of the ascending and descending colon is retroperitoneal, while the transverse and sigmoid colon are intraperitoneal. There is no clear anatomic demarcation of the transition between the sigmoid and rectum. By one convention, the transition is considered to be 16 cm from the anal verge, measured by rigid proctoscopy, but a generally agreed upon consensus has not been arrived at. The primary function of the colon is the absorption of water and electrolytes.

HISTOLOGY OF THE SMALL AND LARGE INTESTINE

The normal intestinal architecture is depicted in Figure 38.1. At a superficial inspection, the three sections of the small intestine are relatively similar, at the histological level. However, there are many important differences. For example, submucosal glands are found normally in the duodenum (so-called Brunner glands) but are only present in the other segments during pathological states. The villi of the jejunum are much, much longer than those of the ileum. Mucin-containing goblet cells become more abundant toward the distal small intestine. While there is lymphoid tissue throughout the small bowel, the so-called Peyer patches occur almost exclusively in the ileum. In contrast to the small bowel, the large bowel exhibits many straight mucus-secreting crypts, but no villi.

Except for the anal canal, which is covered by stratified squamous epithelium, the intestine is lined by a single layer columnar epithelium. The epithelial lining of the intestine covers an area roughly 200 times that of the surface of the skin and is the most rapidly renewing system in the body. Epithelial cells proliferate in the intestinal crypts, migrate toward the tip of the villi (or in the colon, onto the surface), from where they are eventually shed into the intestinal lumen.

The crypts of both small and large intestines are separated from each other by a loose connective tissue, the *lamina propria*, which contains many leukocytes and an abundance of capillaries. The *muscularis mucosae* is a thin layer of smooth muscle that forms the boundary between the intestinal mucosa and the *submucosa*, which is normally a thin layer of connective tissue. The *muscularis propria* is situated peripheral (away from the bowel lumen) to the submucosa. It consists of an inner circular layer and an outer longitudinal layer of smooth muscle. In the colon, the longitudinal muscle, rather than being a layer is concentrated into three distinct bands, the so-called *taenia coli*. The parts of the intestine that are located intraperitoneally are covered by the *visceral peritoneum*, a single layer of mesothelial cells. Under normal circumstances, the visceral peritoneum is separated from the longitudinal muscle only by an extremely thin layer of connective tissue.

The proliferation characteristics of the intestinal epithelium have been subject of considerable experimental work, mainly in rodents, and have been best studied in the small intestine. Figure 38.1B–D shows an example of the proliferative organization of the intestinal epithelium. The cell cycle time for the proliferating cells in the mouse small intestinal crypt is about 12 to 13 hours. Notably, the cell cycle time for the stem cells in the crypts is considerably longer, approximately 24 hours. The transit time for cells from the crypt base to the villus tip is about 6 to 8 days in the normal situation, and it takes 48 to 72 hours from when a cell enters the villus base until it is shed from the

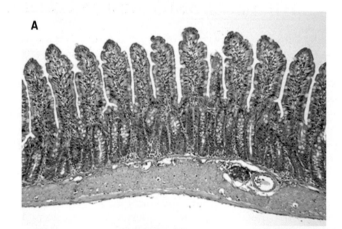

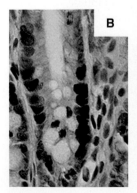
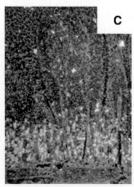
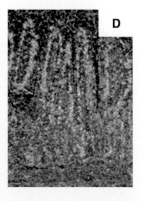

Figure 38.1. Normal small intestine and proliferation of intestinal epithelium. **A**: Normal small intestinal architecture (original magnification 2×). **B**: Intestinal crypt labeled with bromodeoxyuridine to demonstrate cells that are actively synthesizing DNA (original magnification 60×). **C**: Oblique dark field microscopic image of intestine 3 hours after injection of 3H-thymidine. The label (showing up as orange) has predominantly been taken up by crypt cells that actively synthesize DNA (original magnification 5×). **D**: Oblique dark field microscopic image of intestine 48 hours after injection of 3H-thymidine. The label has migrated upward and is now mostly outlining the villi (original magnification 5×).

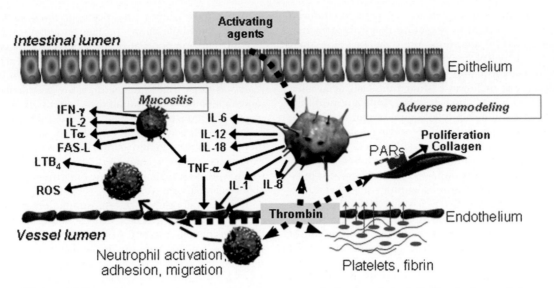

Figure 38.2. Involvement of the intestinal immune system and microvascular endothelium in the regulation of acute radiation mucositis and subsequent adverse tissue remodeling (intestinal fibrosis). When the mucosal barrier becomes disrupted, as after radiation exposure, bacterial products and other activating agents gain access to subepithelial intestinal tissue where they stimulate a variety of immune cells to produce cytokines and other proinflammatory and anti-inflammatory mediators. Moreover, radiation-induced endothelial dysfunction leads to endothelial dysfunction with loss of thromboresistance, resulting in thrombin formation, neutrophil recruitment and activation, and stimulation of mesenchymal cells.

villus tip.[1] In human intestine, the crypts are larger than in the mouse and they exhibit a lower fraction of cells in the S phase of the mitotic cycle, and the cell cycle time is about 30 hours, that is, about 2.5 times that in mouse intestine.[2]

Despite the attention that has been devoted to the epithelial lining of the intestine as the primary target for radiation injury, it is important to recognize that the intestine also contains a variety of other cell types, many of which exert a profound influence on the radiation response. For example, the microvascular endothelium, the intestinal immune system, and the enteric nervous system all participate in orchestrating and modulating the radiation response of the intestine. Some of these interactions are shown in Figure 38.2.

INCIDENCE AND PREVALENCE OF INTESTINAL RADIATION TOXICITY

INCIDENCE

An estimated 200,000 patients in the United States undergo radiation therapy of abdominal, pelvic, or retroperitoneal tumors each year and are thus at risk for developing early and delayed intestinal radiation toxicity. Symptoms of acute bowel toxicity occur in about 60% to 80% of these patients, and deintensification of treatment is estimated to be required in 5% to 15%, depending on treatment parameters, patient characteristics, and patient and physician threshold for what constitutes acceptable toxicity.

When estimating the incidence of delayed intestinal radiation injury, it is important to recognize that radiation therapy carries a continued, lifetime risk of late complications.[3] Therefore, incidence figures in the literature must be interpreted based on the duration and method of follow-up. Clinical studies published up to the mid-1990s generally reported an incidence of chronic symptoms after postoperative therapy of rectal cancer in the 30% to 40% range at 5 years, and late small-bowel obstruction requiring surgery in 5% to 15%.[4,5] Among women treated for cervical cancer, the reported incidence of serious delayed bowel toxicity at 20 years was 10% to 15%.[6] This is consistent with another study that showed chronic diarrhea in 13% after radiation therapy for gynecological cancer.[7] A study of patients who had undergone radiation therapy for prostate cancer, albeit with older techniques that would be considered outdated in developed countries today, revealed major bowel problems in 11% of the patients.[8] A large-scale trial comparing androgen deprivation and radiation to the prostate and seminal vesicles to 66 Gy with radiation alone in men with locally advanced prostate cancer found that the prevalence of National Cancer Institute's Common Toxicity Criteria for Adverse Events (CTCAE) grade 2 or greater delayed proctopathy was approximately 10%.[9] The increasing use of modern dose-sculpting radiation therapy, as well as the increased awareness of the risk and consequences of delayed bowel injury, may eventually lower the incidence of late complications.[10,11]

The incidence and severity of intestinal radiation toxicity depend on a number of therapy-related and patient-related factors.[12] Therapy-related factors include radiation dose, volume of bowel irradiated, time-dose-fractionation parameters, and concomitant chemotherapy or biotherapy. Previous abdominal surgery increases the risk of radiation-induced bowel injury because peritoneal adhesions lead to fixation of small-bowel loops in the radiation field.[13,14] Certain comorbidities, for example, inflammatory bowel disease,[15] diabetes,[16] vascular disorders,[17] and collagen vascular disease, particularly scleroderma[18,19] predispose patients to complications after radiation therapy. Tobacco smoking appears to be a strong independent predictor of major intestinal complications after pelvic radiation therapy.[20]

In considering the true incidence of radiation-induced bowel injury, it is important to recognize that only a fraction of patients seek medical attention. Many patients alter their dietary habits and accept restriction to their normal daily activities without expectation of successful intervention.[21] Subtle manifestations of bowel dysfunction, such as accelerated osteoporosis or anemia, may lead to significant morbidity even though their relationship to radiation treatment may not be obvious. Moreover, present toxicity scoring systems do not adequately consider specific symptoms although they may have major impact on patients' functional and psychosocial quality of life. For example, a patient who, after radiotherapy for prostate cancer, is required to be within 15 minutes of a toilet due to fecal urgency may not be classified as having sustained severe GI toxicity, but is nevertheless severely restricted in terms of professional and social function. For these and other reasons, most studies greatly underestimate the true incidence of delayed bowel toxicity. It is possible that modified toxicity scoring systems or scoring systems that specifically focus on GI side effects will be able to more accurately reflect the burden of delayed radiation enteropathy on patients.[22,23] Studies in which patients have been carefully examined show that chronic symptoms or signs of intestinal dysfunction are present in 60% to 90% of patients after abdominal radiotherapy.[24–26] After adjuvant radiation therapy of rectal cancer, more than 50% of patients develop persistent anorectal dysfunction with symptoms that include intermittent incontinence, bleeding, or fecal urgency.[27] Delayed injury of the rectum is also common after radiation therapy of cancer of the prostate and cervical cancer.[26,28]

PREVALENCE

The incidence of a disorder reflects the frequency with which a disorder occurs in a specific group of patients. In contrast, the prevalence reflects the total burden of the disorder on patients, their families, the health care system, and society. Nevertheless, there is a relative paucity of information about the prevalence of chronic radiation toxicities in the cancer survivor population.[29] The prevalence of bowel injury depends not only on the rate of occurrence, but also on several other factors: that is, (a) long-term survival rates (cancers that have favorable survival rates contribute more to the prevalence than cancers with poor prognosis), (b) relative incidence of specific cancers at various sites (common cancers contribute more than rare cancers), and (c) patient age (tumors that occur predominantly in younger patients contribute more [greater number of patient years at risk] than tumors that occur in older patients). Following prostatic and seminal vesicle irradiation, the actuarial probability of CTCAE grade 2 or greater delayed proctopathy at 5 years was three times greater than the prevalence rate at the same timepoint.[9] This finding draws attention to the possibility of grossly discrepant estimates when different methods of analysis are used. It is clear therefore that an understanding of the methodology used to derive injury rates is necessary if different experiences are to be compared. Moreover, it raises the issue of which type of estimate is most meaningful to the patient who is about to embark on treatment.

If the overall prevalence of postradiation toxicities could be estimated accurately, bowel toxicity would likely head the list by a considerable margin: According to the Surveillance, Epidemiology, and End Results Program of the National Cancer Institute, the number of cancer survivors in the United States exceeded 10 million in 2005 and increases by about 2% per year. Currently, more than 3% of the US population are cancer survivors and more than half are survivors of abdominal or pelvic cancers. A graphic representation of the dramatic increase in the number of cancer survivors (cancer prevalence) relative to the number of new cases (cancer incidence) and deaths (cancer mortality rate) is shown in Figure 38.3. Of note is that an estimated 60% are more than 5 years out from their diagnosis, a time when survivors after most solid tumor are considered "cured." If one assumes that half of these patients have undergone (or will undergo) radiation therapy and that 60% of them will develop some degree of intestinal dysfunction, a conservative estimate of the number of patients with postradiation intestinal dysfunction living in the United States is about 1.5 million. The paucity of useful information regarding the prevalence of chronic bowel toxicity is not surprising. Current toxicity scoring scales rely heavily on symptom reporting rather than on objectively measured signs. Moreover, many of the symptoms are nonspecific, so causal attribution can be problematic.[30] The impact of toxicity also depends to a large extent on how patients perceive and adapt to their symptoms. While accurate quantification of prevailing levels of dysfunction is difficult, there is clearly a need for new toxicity scoring methods based on objective, measurable criteria that more accurately reflect the impact of radiation therapy on long-term physical and psychosocial outcomes.[30]

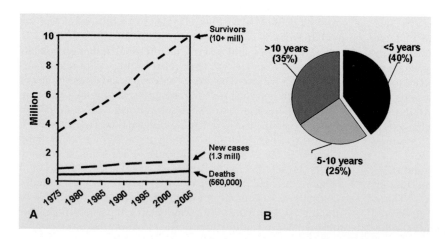

Figure 38.3. Cancer survivors in the US population. **A:** Increase in the number of cancer survivors (cancer prevalence) during the 30-year period 1975 to 2005. Note that in contrast to an exponential increase in the number of cancer survivors, there has been only modest change in the number of new cancer cases (cancer incidence) and deaths (cancer mortality rate). **B:** Time since initial cancer diagnosis in cancer survivors. Note that about 60% of cancer survivors are >5 years from the time of diagnosis and can thus be considered long-term cancer survivors.

PATHOLOGY AND PATHOPHYSIOLOGY OF RADIATION-INDUCED BOWEL INJURY

The pathology of intestinal radiation injury is only discussed briefly. For more comprehensive descriptions, the reader is referred to excellent reviews by Fajardo[31,32] and Carr.[33] An in-depth discussion of cellular and molecular mechanisms of intestinal radiation injury can be found in a review by Hauer-Jensen.[34] Examples of typical histological changes that may occur during radiation therapy for prostate cancer are depicted in Figure 38.4.

Radiation injuries to normal tissues arise from a combination of three different pathogenetic processes: (a) direct cellular cytocidal effects (clonogenic and apoptotic cell death), (b) direct cellular functional (noncytocidal) effects, and (c) indirect effects (reactive and downstream cellular or tissue phenomena).[35,36]

Early intestinal injury becomes manifest within days of the initial radiation exposure. It is primarily a result of cell death in the crypt epithelium, resulting in insufficient replacement of the villus epithelium, breakdown of the mucosal barrier, and mucosal inflammation. In addition, a number of adaptive responses occur, including accelerated, compensatory proliferation[37,38] during which crypt cell cycle times may be as short as 6 hours.[39] The power of compensatory proliferation is evident from the fact that, during pelvic radiation therapy, intestinal permeability and histological injury are maximal in the middle of the radiation course and actually improve toward the end, despite continued daily irradiation and increasing symptoms of bowel toxicity.[40,41]

The relative importance of mitotic (clonogenic) death versus apoptosis in the intestinal epithelium and their relationship to the intestinal radiation response are unclear. In fact, recent studies in genetically modified mice strongly suggest that intestinal crypt cell apoptosis does not play a major role in the intestinal radiation response.[42] The issue is further complicated by the fact that many preclinical studies have been performed with single doses of radiation, a situation that differs substantially from the fractionated radiation schedules used in clinically. Temporal shifts in the relative significance of clonogenic cell death, apoptosis, start time and intensity of compensatory proliferation, and cell migration during courses of fractionated irradiation are factors that further complicate extrapolation of animal experiments to the clinical situation.

An important characteristic of normal tissue injury during schedules of fractionated radiation therapy is that a series of insults is delivered—over a period of several weeks—to tissues that undergo a dynamic spectrum of injury, repair, inflammation, and compensatory responses. During a course of fractionated radiation therapy, cellular and molecular responses will be exacerbated, suppressed, or altered, and the "normal" tissue that is irradiated toward the end of a treatment course differs substantially from the normal tissue that was irradiated at the beginning.[36]

The pathogenesis of chronic radiation enteropathy is complex and involves changes in most compartments of the intestinal wall. Prominent structural features include atrophy of the mucosa, fibrosis of the intestinal wall, vascular sclerosis, and loss of mucin-producing goblet cells. Functional changes are dominated by malabsorption and dysmotility.[43,44] Adverse intestinal remodeling may lead to life-threatening complications, such as intestinal obstruction, perforation, or fistula formation.

Most of the varied manifestations of delayed injury are unrelated to active inflammation. Hence, when referring to the chronic forms of bowel and rectal injury, the terms *radiation enteropathy* and *radiation proctopathy* are generally preferred over the commonly used terms *radiation enteritis* and *radiation proctitis.*

In contrast to the traditional notion that acute and delayed tissue injury are unrelated, clinical studies,[9,30,45–48] preclinical time-dose-fractionation studies,[49–51] and animal studies using modifiers of acute injury[52,53] demonstrate that acute injury often contributes to development of chronic changes.[35,36]

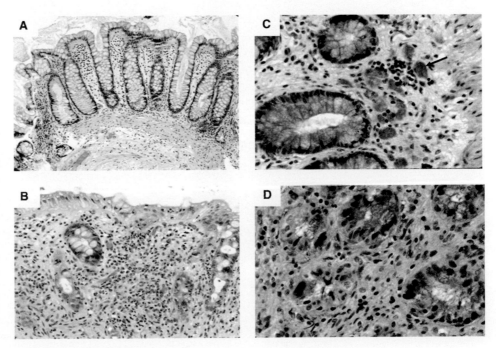

Figure 38.4. Endoscopic biopsies of rectal mucosa obtained from patients before and during radiation therapy of prostate cancer. **A**: Normal rectal mucosa before start of radiation therapy (original magnification 10×). **B**: Glandular atrophy and moderate mucosal inflammation 2 weeks into a course of radiation therapy (original magnification 20×). **C**: Para-aminosalicylic acid (PAS)-positive "mucophages" (*arrow*) 2 weeks into a course of radiation therapy (original magnification 40×). **D**: Mucosal inflammation and loss of PAS-positive goblet cells after 6 weeks' radiation therapy (original magnification 40×).

The clinical significance of these observations is that modifiers that ameliorate early toxicity may also reduce the incidence and severity of delayed radiation enteropathy, even if administration of the modifier may be discontinued shortly after radiation therapy.

CLINICAL PRESENTATION

RADIATION ENTEROPATHY

Nausea, abdominal pain, and diarrhea are main symptoms of early small-bowel toxicity. Fatigue is another symptom that may be quite prominent, albeit nonspecific. Nausea occurs relatively early during a typical course of radiation therapy, while diarrhea and abdominal pain usually arise 2 to 3 weeks into the course of radiation therapy. In most patients, the acute symptoms of bowel toxicity resolve within 2 to 4 weeks of completing treatment.

Symptoms of delayed bowel toxicity present after a latency period. The latency period is typically 6 months to 3 years after radiation therapy. In some patients, however, chronic bowel dysfunction develops in direct continuity with the acute symptoms. Conversely, latency periods of more than 30 years are not uncommon.

The main clinical features of delayed radiation injury of the small intestine are malabsorption and dysmotility. Patients often present with intermittent constipation and diarrhea and are not seldom metabolically deranged and malnourished. Progressive intestinal wall fibrosis may cause stricture formation, and localized areas of ischemic bowel necrosis may disrupt intestinal. In fact, a surprising number of patients with radiation enteropathy present

initially as surgical emergencies, with acute intestinal obstruction, fistulae, or bowel perforation. An example of a rather typical operative site from a patient admitted for radiation-induced small-bowel obstruction 30 years after radiation therapy of vaginal cancer with corresponding histopathology is shown in Figure 38.5. Massive bleeding is an infrequent manifestation of small-bowel radiation injury.[54] Polyvisceral necrosis is an exceedingly rare, but devastating complication.[55,56] It does not result from direct radiation injury to the GI tract, but rather from ischemic gangrene because of central vascular injury. There may be an increased risk of ischemic bowel complications when antiangiogenic therapies are used in conjunction with radiation therapy.[57]

The prognosis of patients with severe delayed small-bowel radiation injury is poor. Corrective surgery is associated with high postoperative morbidity and mortality, and some patients will require prolonged parenteral nutrition. Long term, the majority of patients have persistent or recurrent symptoms, and about 10% die as a direct result of radiation enteropathy.[58–64]

Symptoms and signs of delayed radiation injury of the colon differ to a certain extent from those of small-bowel injury. This reflects the primary role of the colon in water absorption and as fecal conduit rather than in uptake of nutrients. Patients with colonic injury typically suffer from intermittent diarrhea and constipation on the basis of fibrotic strictures or pseudo-obstruction (functional obstruction without anatomical stricture). These patients are not commonly metabolically deranged.

Compared to patients with small-bowel injury, the long-term prognosis of patients with colonic injury is somewhat more favorable, mainly because of less pronounced metabolic and nutritional derangement and because of the relative "expendability" of the colon.

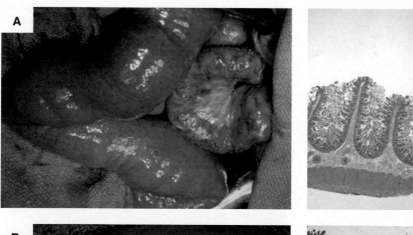
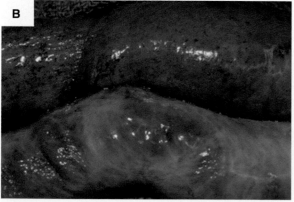
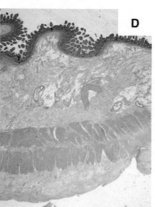

Figure 38.5. Operative site at laparotomy for radiation enteropathy with intestinal obstruction, and characteristic histopathologic changes. **A**: Severely contracted loop of small intestine with severe stenosis (right) next to a loop of proximal (normal) intestine. **B**: Intestinal loop exhibiting moderate chronic radiation injury with fibrin deposition and subserosal fibrosis. **C**: Histological appearance of normal intestine for comparison with the image in panel **D** (original magnification 2×). **D**: Histological appearance of resected small intestine from a woman with severe delayed radiation enteropathy. Note the very atrophic mucosa and severely fibrotic submucosa and subserosa (original magnification 2×, same as panel **C**).

RADIATION PROCTOPATHY

Acute radiation injury of the rectum is characterized by diarrhea, tenesmus (fecal urgency with crampy rectal pain), and bloody stools. Interestingly, even when virtually no small bowel is included in the radiation field during pelvic irradiation, symptoms from the upper abdomen are not uncommon, thus suggesting involvement of neurogenic mechanisms, cytokines, or other circulating factors.

Frequent or clustered bowel movements, anal discharge, rectal pain, urgency, tenesmus, incontinence, and hematochezia (rectal bleeding) are the main clinical features of delayed radiation injury of the rectum (radiation proctopathy). The clinical picture depends on what type of injury predominates in each patient. Bleeding may be the predominant symptom in patients with severe mucosal injury, rectal pain may predominate in patients with chronic rectal ulcers, whereas urgency may be the chief complaint in patients where fibrosis causes loss of anorectal compliance. In many cases, the patient is more socially disabled by the need to find a lavatory quickly, that is, by urgency and tenesmus, than by the episodic passage of blood in the bowel movements.[9,30,65] Attempts to characterize the various clinical presentations that can be included under the title *delayed radiation proctopathy* illustrate the complexity of the issue and the need to distinguish radiation induced symptoms and signs from those caused by preexisting morbidities.[30]

Delayed proctopathy often follows a remittent course, possibly due to exacerbation of symptoms associated with periodic breakdown of the mucosa. In many patients, hematochezia is at its worst 18 to 24 months after radiation therapy, but may then improve spontaneously. This is sometimes accompanied by visible reduction of the telangiectasia in affected mucosa.[66]

DIAGNOSTIC EVALUATION

RADIATION ENTEROPATHY

Acute intestinal radiation toxicity seldom poses diagnostic dilemmas because of the rather well-defined clinical picture and temporal relationship to radiation therapy. Therefore, diagnostic tests are seldom indicated. In contrast, the diagnosis and therapy of delayed radiation enteropathy is much less straightforward and can be quite challenging. This is due to the multifaceted nature of the disorder, variations among patients in terms of the dominant pathophysiological process(es), and the need to consider tumor recurrence as a differential diagnosis. In general, a pathophysiology-based approach is

TABLE 38.1	Pathophysiological Features and Clinical Presentation of Patients with Delayed Radiation Enteropathy
Pathophysiological Feature	*Clinical Sign or Symptom*
Mucosal dysfunction	Lactose intolerance
	Malabsorption
	Steatorrhea
	Weight loss
Stricture or stagnant loop syndrome	Abdominal pain, intestinal obstruction
Fistulae	Diarrhea
Postoperative changes	Bacterial overgrowth
	Short bowel
Intestinal dysmotility	Bloating
	Constipation
	Diarrhea
Abnormal bile acid recirculation	Cholerrheic diarrhea

clearly preferable to an empiric (trial-and-error) approach in the diagnosis of delayed radiation enteropathy.

The clinical manifestations of small-bowel radiation injury usually result from (a) mucosal dysfunction because of atrophy, reduced activity of brush border membrane enzymes, reduced mucosal blood flow, and/or impaired lymph drainage, and/or (b) intestinal dysmotility with bacterial overgrowth and digestive dysfunction because of stricture formation and neuromuscular dysfunction. The relative significance of these processes varies from patient to patient, and it is important to individualize the choice of diagnostic tests, as well as the therapeutic approach. Table 38.1 summarizes common pathophysiological features of delayed radiation enteropathy and their corresponding hallmark symptoms.

Diagnostic tests to consider in the work-up of patients with chronic-recurrent abdominal symptoms after radiation therapy must be individualized and may include imaging (e.g., computed tomography, ultrasonography, magnetic resonance imaging (MRI) (Fig. 38.6), enteroclysis, and/or fistulograms), measurement of intestinal transit, endoscopy, tests for malabsorption (e.g., fecal fat excretion, bile acid breath tests), tests for maldigestion (e.g., xylose breath test), motility studies, assessment of mucosal permeability, and histopathologic examination of mucosal biopsies. Capsule endoscopy is generally contraindicated because of the risk of impaction in intestinal strictures.

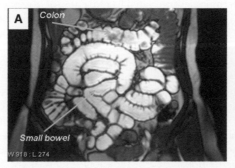

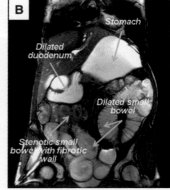

Figure 38.6. MRI of the small intestine used in the diagnosis of radiation enteropathy. **A:** Normal MRI exam (T2-weighted image). **B:** MRI exam of patient with radiation enteropathy (T2-weighted image). Note dilated loops of bowel and signs of bowel stenosis with intestinal wall thickening.

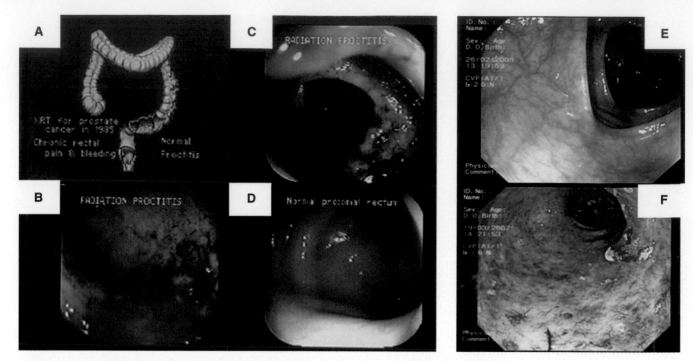

Figure 38.7. Endoscopic images from patients with radiation proctopathy. **A**: Diagram showing overview of rectum and normal proximal colon. **B,C**: Endoscopic view of rectal mucosa with severe chronic hemorrhagic changes. **D**: Endoscopic view of normal proximal rectum for comparison. **E**: Endoscopic view of normal colon. **F**: Endoscopic view of widespread telangiectasia of the rectal mucosa after radiation therapy.

The goal of the workup should be to make a diagnosis that is as precise as possible in terms of determining the underlying pathophysiology and the anatomic location and extent of pathology in each individual patient, and to provide a guide for treatment.

As mentioned above, the metabolic and nutritional impact of radiation injury in the colon is less than injury in the small bowel. Therefore, the purpose of diagnostic workup in patients with colonic radiation injury is mainly to clarify anatomical details, rule out malignancy by colonoscopy, and delineate strictures and fistulae by appropriate radiological imaging studies.

RADIATION PROCTOPATHY

As is the case for acute radiation enteropathy, the diagnosis of acute radiation proctopathy is usually straightforward, and there is little need for diagnostic studies.

More care is required in the diagnosis of delayed proctopathy. Preexisting and concurrent pathologies unrelated to radiation may be mistaken for delayed proctopathy and therefore not be managed appropriately.[30,67,68] Figure 38.7 shows characteristic endoscopic images from patients with delayed proctopathy after pelvic radiation therapy. Hematochezia is usually due to the development of friable rectal mucosa with telangiectatic vessels. In patients with hematochezia, it is important to always rule out neoplastic or nonneoplastic lesions proximal to the rectum by colonoscopy. This is true even when a firm diagnosis of chronic radiation proctopathy has been established by endoscopy and biopsies. Points of bowel fixation, decreased compliance, and strictures may be demonstrated by radiological contrast. As fibrosis is one of the hallmark features of chronicity, endorectal ultrasonography may be helpful. Anorectal function tests, which are usually normal or near-normal during the early postradiation period, frequently show abnormal results during the chronic phase.[69] Notably, such studies may provide valuable information in clinical trials where the focus is on anorectal radiation toxicity. On the other hand, anorectal function tests are less helpful in the everyday clinical decision-making process, and thus not indicated as part of the routine diagnostic workup of patients with radiation proctopathy.

RADIATION DOSE, VOLUME, AND TOLERANCE CONSIDERATIONS

Given the high prevalence of radiation-induced enteropathic and proctopathic morbidity in the community, it may seem surprising that the relationships between radiation dose, the volume irradiated, and these entities are not well defined. The most important reasons for this are the subjective nature of the scoring scales that are used to define the severity of radiation-induced morbidity, the difficulty in distinguishing radiation-induced morbidity from preexisting or concurrent gut pathologies or physiological variations, and the problem of knowing what volumes of gut have received particular doses of radiation. The commonly used CTC scales rely heavily on the accurate reporting of symptoms and therapeutic interventions. Descriptions of physical injury and radiation pathology play no role in symptom grading until surgical intervention becomes necessary. Moreover, the same scale is used to define the severity of acute and delayed proctopathic symptoms. If these issues were not significant enough, fecal urgency, which is a common and disabling manifestation of radiation-induced proctopathy, is not even captured on the scale.

Measurement of volume irradiated has improved considerably in the last 15 years as progressive improvements to the software of radiotherapy planning systems have taken place. Nowadays, dose-volume histograms are routinely generated for each patient receiving definitive radiotherapy. Unfortunately, the mobility and periodic distensions and contractions of virtually all parts of the gut make precise dose-volume relationships difficult to estimate. However, progress has been made and the relationship between the mucosal injuries that lead to delayed rectal bleeding and dose-volume histogram profiles generated prior to treatment is now better understood.[70-73] For example, it is now clear that radiation-induced rectal bleeding is significantly increased in men who have received 70 Gy or more to a quarter or more of their rectal volumes.[74] Efforts to define other dose volume histogram/symptom relationships are ongoing.

The concept of tolerance dose has been the subject of much discussion in recent years. It was developed long before efforts to assess the impact of radiation morbidity on the men and women who attempt to live with it. The Litwin questionnaire[75] was one of the first to successfully capture the "problem" and "distress" levels caused by dysfunctional rectal, urinary, and sexual symptoms in men treated for prostate cancer. A thorough exploration of the problems and distress caused by rectal symptoms prior to, during, and in the three years following prostatic irradiation has been provided recently.[30] This report, based on responses to a modification of the Litwin questionnaire, provides a good insight into the level of symptoms, and problems they cause, that men are able to tolerate.

THERAPY

ACUTE RADIATION ENTEROPATHY

The management of acute radiation toxicity of the small bowel and colon is symptomatic and therefore follows the general guidelines for treating similar symptoms in other situations. Hence, conventional antidiarrheal, antiemetic, spasmolytic, and defoaming agents are mainstays in the management of acute bowel toxicity. The somatostatin analog, octreotide, has been shown to ameliorate intestinal radiation toxicity in preclinical studies,[53,76] and a clinical trial has confirmed the superiority of octreotide over conventional antidiarrheals.[77] Therefore, patients with severe diarrhea who do not respond to first-line antidiarrheal medication should be considered candidates for treatment with octreotide or other somatostatin analogs. When emesis is a problem, a serotonin (5-hydroxytryptamine, 5-HT$_3$) receptor antagonist may be used to relieve symptoms. Prophylactic therapy may be considered in patients at high risk of radiation-induced emesis[78] and administration of steroids may be beneficial in addition.[79] Complications requiring surgical intervention (severe bleeding or perforation) are exceedingly rare in the acute setting.

DELAYED RADIATION ENTEROPATHY

Delayed radiation enteropathy, when uncomplicated by intestinal obstruction, perforation, or fistula formation, is usually managed nonoperatively. The diagnostic strategies and tests described above help distinguish radiation enteropathy from other conditions, rule out cancer recurrence, and identify pathophysiological processes in the individual patient that may be amenable to therapy. For example, a patient with a stricture

TABLE 38.2	Principles of Pathophysiology-directed Therapy of Delayed Radiation Enteropathy
Underlying Pathophysiology	*Therapeutic Options*
Nutritional deficits	Correction of specific deficits Caloric supplementation Low-fat diet Lactose-free diet Supplementary parenteral nutrition Elemental diet Total parenteral nutrition
Intestinal dysmotility	Loperamide Octreotide Prokinetic agents Dietary counseling
Bile acid malabsorption	Cholestyramine
Bacterial overgrowth	Antibiotics

in the distal ileum may be helped by elective surgical resection, but only if functional testing before and after a course of antimicrobial therapy rules out widespread mucosal dysfunction. In general, medical management of patients with delayed radiation enteropathy should be directed at the specific underlying abnormalities, depending on the outcome of diagnostic studies, as summarized in Table 38.2. A more comprehensive discussion of diagnosis and management principles and algorithms in chronic radiation enteropathy is beyond the scope of this review, but can be found elsewhere.[24,43,68,80,81]

While most patients with delayed radiation enteropathy can be managed conservatively, complications that require surgery are not infrequent. The main indications for surgical intervention include intestinal obstruction, perforation, and fistula formation, and more occasionally severe bleeding and malabsorption. Because of radiation-induced alterations in the intestine and mesentery and poor nutritional status, wound healing is usually delayed, and surgery carries a high risk of anastomotic dehiscence and iatrogenic fistulae. Several animal and clinical studies show that the risk of anastomotic dehiscence is reduced if at least one limb of the anastomosis is free of radiation injury.

As is the case for the medical management of patients with delayed radiation enteropathy, surgical management should be highly individualized. Surgical options include resection of involved intestinal segments, intestinal bypass procedures, enterostomy, or—in select patients—stricturoplasty.[82]

During surgery, dissection, including lysis of adhesions, should be kept to a minimum to preserve as much of the precarious intestinal blood supply as possible. It is also important to focus on conserving functional intestinal length. Early clinical studies often recommended enteric bypass procedures over surgical resection. However, it is now clear that resection is highly preferable to bypass, both in terms of short- and long-term outcome. For this reason, bypass procedures should only be performed when resection is not technically possible or as a temporary measure in unstable patients. Whether stapled or hand-sewn anastomoses are preferable remains unresolved. At any rate, caution is warranted in the use of conventional side-to-side staplers in situations where the intestine exhibits fibrotic thickening, as compression may cause staple line ischemia. Simple diverting procedures are generally an unsatisfactory alternative and should be reserved for highly unstable patients where the intent is to perform a more definitive procedure at a later date. The use of a temporary diverting enterostomy to protect an intestinal anastomosis, on the other hand, may reduce the risk of postoperative complications. While temporary enterostomies do require a second surgical procedure for closure, the second operation can usually be performed under more favorable circumstances, in the elective setting, and with the patient in a better nutritional state.

Patients with fistulae pose particularly challenging therapeutic problems. Fistulae that develop because of radiation injury almost never heal on conservative management, such as gut rest, low residue diets, or total parenteral nutrition. Hence, in patients with reasonable performance status, radiation-induced fistulae are a clear indication for surgery. Most patients are malnourished, and efforts to improve the patient's nutritional status preoperatively often fail because of radiation-induced intestinal dysfunction. Surgery in patients with radiation-induced fistulae is often extremely difficult, since the surrounding tissue frequently exhibits a combination of prominent inflammatory changes and severe radiation fibrosis. Details regarding surgical management of radiation-induced fistulae can be found in an excellent review by Durdey and Williams.[83]

ACUTE RADIATION PROCTOPATHY

As for radiation injury of the small bowel and colon, management of acute radiation proctopathy is symptomatic and follows the general treatment guidelines for similar symptoms in other situations. Topical lignocaine preparations may exert a soothing effect on anorectal irritation, and loperamide can be used to reduce tenesmus. Steroid-containing suppositories may be helpful when inflammatory symptoms are severe, although this treatment is only supported by weak evidence.

DELAYED RADIATION PROCTOPATHY

Denton et al.[84] have published a comprehensive review of strategies for treatment of delayed radiation proctopathy. Rectal bleeding is frequently the main symptom, but urgency and frequency can be even more difficult to control with medication and be even more disabling. When simple dietary alterations, including ingestion of increased amounts of dietary fiber, and agents such as loperamide are unhelpful, substantial changes in lifestyle may occur as the patient loses confidence in venturing too far from a lavatory.

First-line therapy for radiation proctopathy with bleeding is sucralfate enemas, which often have rapid and dramatic effect. Moreover, treatment with sucralfate enemas is the only evidence-based drug therapy (although with weak evidence) and has virtually no side effects. Sucralfate is an aluminum hydroxide complex of sulfated sucrose that provides a protective "film" by forming a complex with proteins in injured mucosa. It also increases local levels of fibroblast growth factors and mucosal prostaglandins. The effect of sucralfate enemas in the treatment of chronic radiation proctopathy is clearly superior to that of steroids and 5-aminosalicylic acid,[85] which have not been shown to be effective. It must be pointed out that the benefit of sucralfate in the chronic setting is in stark contrast to the lack of effect of this drug in the acute setting in most studies.[86–89]

A beneficial effect of short chain fatty acids (SCFAs) in the management of chronic radiation proctopathy has been described in several noncontrolled studies. SCFA are fatty acids with one to six carbons that have a trophic effect on the colonic mucosa. SCFA enemas appear to provide at least temporary benefit in some patients with hemorrhagic radiation proctopathy.[90,91] Butyric acid has interesting anti-inflammatory properties, including potent inhibition of nuclear factor κB (NF-κB) activation, and a shift in the Th1/Th2 cytokine balance toward a type 2 cytokine profile. While one randomized trial showed that butyrate enemas were highly effective in reducing symptoms and endoscopic signs of radiation proctitis,[92] another randomized study showed no benefit.[93] Compliance issues may be significant with the use of butyrate enemas because of the exceptionally offensive odor.

In patients with hemorrhagic proctitis refractory to sucralfate enemas, bleeding can often be controlled with local (endoscopic) interventions. Such approaches include topical formalin application[94–96] or coagulation using electrocautery,[97] laser therapy,[98–101] or argon plasma beam coagulation.[102–105] Argon lasers seem to be associated with less fibrosis and stricture formation than Nd:YAG lasers, and the argon plasma coagulator has the advantage that it can be applied tangentially, that is, to lesions that are difficult to treat with other methods.

In patients where sucralfate enemas and local therapies fail, or in patients with intractable pain because of rectal ulcers, hyperbaric oxygen (HBO) therapy may be considered.[106,107] Several uncontrolled studies suggest a benefit of HBO in patients with severe radiation proctopathy.[108] However, a proper "placebo"-controlled assessment of HBO has yet to be performed and, in fact, may never be performed because of the difficulties associated with conducting such a trial.

A number of other non–surgical therapies for radiation proctopathy have been suggested in anecdotal case reports or case series. For example, botulinum anatoxin injections were proposed as a treatment of painful radiation proctitis.[109] A small phase II study with oral supplement of antioxidant vitamins (vitamins C and E) suggested a benefit in some patients with radiation proctitis.[110] The merit of these therapies is difficult to assess.

Surgical management of radiation proctopathy is a an option for patients with persistent, transfusion-dependent bleeding that is refractory to the therapies discussed above, and in patients with large nonhealing ulcers, intractable pain, or complications such as stenosis or fistula formation. Such patients may be considered for restorative surgery, for example, by resection with coloanal anastomosis with or without a colonic J-pouch. These operations are technically challenging, but, in experienced hands, have a reasonable success rate. Restorative surgery is contraindicated in patients with grossly abnormal sphincter function. Proctectomy and/or diverting colostomy should only be considered as a last resort in patients where more conservative treatment options have failed, when reparative surgery is unsuccessful, or when it is contraindicated.

PRECLINICAL AND CLINICAL STRATEGIES TO PREVENT BOWEL INJURY AFTER RADIATION THERAPY

There have been major advances in our understanding of the complex pathogenetic mechanisms that have led to development of radiation-induced bowel injury during the last 20 to 30 years. As a result, there has been extensive preclinical and, albeit to a lesser extent, clinical evaluation of pharmacological compounds, biological response modifiers, nutritional supplements, and dietary interventions as strategies to prevent radiation enteropathy. Despite promising results with some of these interventions, very few are in general use in the clinic, as shown by several evidence-based clinical reviews.[79,111–114]

Prophylactic interventions aimed at ameliorating normal tissue radiation injury fall in two conceptually different categories. The first involves strategies that interfere with more or less radiation-specific mechanisms of injury, for example, antioxidants, free radical scavengers, and other cytoprotective agents. The second, fundamentally different approach is the modulation of various pathophysiological, cellular, or molecular tissue characteristics to increase radiation tolerance or enhance repair capacity.

ANTIOXIDANTS, FREE RADICAL SCAVENGERS, AND CYTOPROTECTIVE AGENTS

Cellular injury in response to low linear energy transfer radiation is largely mediated by reactive oxygen species. Therefore, antioxidants and free radical scavengers have been actively pursued as potential protective strategies.

Superoxide dismutase (SOD) has been the subject of particularly active investigation. Preclinical gene therapy studies show that magnesium superoxide dismutase (MnSOD) can ameliorate radiation toxicity in lung and esophagus.[115,116] There is also some suggestion that SOD, delivered locally, may be a radioprotector in the intestine.[117]

A French group reported that SOD, administered several months after irradiation, reversed fibrosis in irradiated skin.[118,119] However, a small pilot study with a low molecular weight SOD mimic found no evidence of reversal of fibrosis in the irradiated intestine (Hauer-Jensen, unpublished data, 1998). Moreover, in the clinical situation, reversal of fibrosis may be difficult to apply to the intestine, because many patients present with life-threatening complications that require urgent intervention, for example, intestinal obstruction, perforation, or fistulae.

The most thoroughly studied radioprotective agent is the aminothiol, amifostine (WR2721, ethyol), a free radical scavenger developed after the Second World War to protect troops on the nuclear battlefield. Amifostine reduces the incidence of early and delayed radiotherapeutic injury at several anatomical sites. However, the practicalities of administering the drug 30 minutes prior to each radiation exposure, high cost, side effects such as vomiting and hypotension, and lingering doubt as to the absence of tumor protection[120] have hampered widespread clinical use of amifostine. Amifostine protects both small and large intestine in preclinical studies,[121,122] and recent clinical studies also suggest that amifostine protects against GI radiation toxicity.[123,124] Interestingly, topically applied amifostine protects the small intestine of rats from injury after localized irradiation.[125] Moreover, clinical studies[126,127] suggest that intrarectal instillation of amifostine, 30 minutes prior to irradiation of the prostate protected against radiation proctitis. Larger-scale randomized trials using topical application of amifostine are clearly warranted-

In addition to its effects on blow flow, the phosphodiesterase inhibitor, pentoxifylline, has diverse biochemical and antioxidant properties. Pentoxifylline was initially suggested to have a beneficial effect in radiation necrosis of the skin[128] and, in combination with the antioxidant vitamin E, has been reported to reverse established fibrosis in chronic radiation skin damage.[129] Given prophylactically, pentoxifylline may reduce radiation injury in some organs,[130] although it does not appear to be effective in reducing injury after localized bowel irradiation.[131]

Prostaglandins or other modifiers of cyclooxygenase (COX) activity or components of the arachidonic acid cascade have been actively pursued as radioprotectors. The exact mechanisms by which these compounds confer cytoprotection are still not fully understood. Prostaglandin E2 (PGE2), enprostil (a PGE2 analog), and misoprostol (a PGE1 analog) protect against intestinal radiation toxicity in animal models.[132–135] In a small, but provocative, clinical study, misoprostol suppositories effectively reduced symptoms of acute radiation proctopathy in patients undergoing radiation therapy of prostate cancer.[136]

A number of other antioxidants, free radical scavengers, and cytoprotective compounds have been shown to modulate the intestinal radiation responses in animal models, but have not yet undergone systematic clinical investigation. Examples include the L-cysteine prodrug, ribose-cysteine, which stimulates glutathione biosynthesis[122,137]; tirizalad and other peroxidation inhibitors[138–140]; as well as vitamins A and E.[122,141,142]

CYTOKINES, GROWTH FACTORS, AND CHEMOKINES

Many preclinical studies have demonstrated that prophylactic or therapeutic modulation of cytokines or cytokine receptors can ameliorate intestinal radiation toxicity. However, clinical trials to assess cytokine modulation in terms of efficacy, toxicity, and differential protection have yet to be performed.

Among the interleukins (IL), preclinical evidence suggests a protective effect of IL-1,[143,144] IL-7,[145] and IL-11.[146–148] As discussed under "Post-Exposure Countermeasures against Intestinal Radiation Injury," local (intraluminal) application of IL-11 appears to be a promising approach by which systemic toxicity of this cytokine can be avoided and a protective effect on the bowel still be retained.[149]

Angiogenic growth factors, for example, acidic fibroblast growth factor (aFGF, FGF-1), basic fibroblast growth factor (bFGF, FGF-2), and vascular endothelial growth factor (VEGF), protect against acute small-bowel radiation toxicity in animal models.[150,151] While these cytokines may confer some protection, the use of angiogenic growth factors in cancer patients is highly problematic.

The keratinocyte growth factors, KGF-1 (FGF-7) and KGF-2 (FGF-10), have been subject of significant interest as radioprotectors, and KGF-1 ameliorates acute intestinal radiation toxicity in animal models.[152,153] Most of the beneficial effects of the KGFs are likely related to their epithelial growth-promoting activities. In contrast to aFGF and bFGF, which activate several FGF receptors, KGF activates mainly the receptor FGFR2IIIb on epithelial cells and therefore may have greater target-cell specificity.

Transforming growth factor beta 1 (TGFβ1) has been the subject of particularly intense investigation because of its fibrogenic properties. Numerous clinical and animal studies have provided strong correlative evidence supporting a role for TGFβ1 in radiation fibrosis in many organs, including the intestine. A preclinical study has demonstrated a direct mechanistic role for TGFβ1 in intestinal radiation fibrosis, as well as the potential for anti-TGFβ1 strategies to ameliorate delayed radiation enteropathy.[154] Substantial efforts are currently devoted to development of small molecule inhibitors of TGFβ and TGFβ signaling.[155]

Evidence from preclinical studies suggests that other cytokines may be considered as intestinal radiation response modifiers. Hence, stem cell factor (mast cell growth factor, c-Kit ligand), growth hormone (GH), insulinlike growth factor-1 (IGF-1), and certain chemokines (cytokines with the ability to induce directed migration of cells, such as inflammatory cells, to sites of tissue injury) also have the ability to protect the intestine against acute radiation injury.[156–160] The potential of these mediators as modifiers of the intestinal radiation response in the clinical situation is still unknown.

ENTEROTROPHIC STRATEGIES

There has been long-standing interest in the use of enterotrophic strategies (i.e., interventions that promote growth of the intestinal mucosa) to ameliorate intestinal radiation toxicity. The purpose of enterotrophic interventions is to increase the resistance of the intestinal mucosa to radiation injury and/or enhance its capacity for recovery after radiation exposure. Enterotrophic strategies with the potential to protect the intestine from radiation injury include cytokines (discussed in the previous section), GI peptide hormones, and various nutrients.

Elemental diets are enteroprotective in animal studies, but results from clinical trials are mixed.[161–165] There was substantial interest in elemental diets for intestinal radioprotection in the 1970s and 1980s, but this interest has now waned due to cost, logistics, compliance issues, and questions about the clinical benefit.

Several different nutrients, such as fiber, short-chain fatty acids, and the amino acids glutamine and arginine, enhance growth of the intestinal mucosa and ameliorate small-bowel radiation toxicity in preclinical and, in some cases, clinical studies. Of these, the semiessential amino acid, glutamine, has been subject to the most extensive studies. Glutamine supports mucosal structure and recovery and ameliorates intestinal radiation toxicity in some preclinical studies,[166,167] but not in others.[168,169] A large randomized trial showed that glutamine had no effect on acute intestinal toxicity in patients undergoing pelvic radiation therapy.[170]

Numerous GI peptide hormones have potent enterotrophic activities. This category includes, for example, GH, neurotensin, cholecystokinin, bombesin, and peptide YY. While these peptides have protective effects in various types of intestinal injury, they have not yet been subjected to systematic testing in radiation injury. The enterotrophic peptide hormone, glucagon-like peptide-2 (GLP-2) and synthetic analogs, are currently being investigated as an enteroprotective intervention. Preclinical results with GLP-2 in radiation enteropathy, albeit in a single dose radiation model, appear encouraging,[171,172] particularly when administration occurs before irradiation.

A common concern with enterotrophic strategies is that, while they may protect against adverse effects in the intestine, they may also enhance growth or metastatic potential of tumors, especially those of epithelial origin. A significant problem is that clinical studies that use radioprotection as the main endpoint are seldom adequately powered and of sufficient duration to rule out a clinically significant degree of tumor protection. It is essential that such studies be performed if this area of investigation is to be advanced.

ANTI-INFLAMMATORY STRATEGIES

Even though the common use of the term radiation *enteritis* implies an aspect of inflammation, the use of traditional anti-inflammatory drugs to ameliorate radiation enteropathy has been disappointing.

Acetylsalicylic acid (aspirin), an anti-inflammatory agent with antiplatelet properties, may be of some benefit in intestinal radiation toxicity,[173] whereas other nonsteroidal anti-inflammatories (NSAIDs) are clearly not protective.[174] Sulfasalazine may be moderately effective in reducing acute radiation-induced intestinal side effects.[175] In contrast, salicylic acid derivatives developed specifically for therapy of inflammatory bowel disease, while potent anti-inflammatory drugs, are not only ineffective, but may possibly even be harmful in the prophylaxis of acute intestinal radiation toxicity.[176–179] Given topically as enemas, these compounds also have no effect on chronic radiation proctitis.[180] The immunomodulator orazipone, on the other hand, did reduce intestinal radiation injury after localized irradiation in a rat model, although the exact mechanism by which this broad-based locally acting immunomodulator ameliorates radiation enteropathy remains to be elucidated.[181] It is possible that future agents, targeted to specific aspects of the inflammatory process, may prove more effective in modifying the intestinal radiation response.

MODULATION OF INTRALUMINAL CONTENTS

Modification of various intraluminal factors, notably bacteria, bile, and pancreatic secretions, has been explored for many years as strategies to ameliorate intestinal radiation injury.

Combined evidence from studies involving irradiation of germfree animals, "decontamination" of animals with different antimicrobial agents, and probiotic therapies[182] suggests that maintaining a properly balanced bacterial flora, rather than attempting to maximally reduce bacterial content, may be the optimal approach to minimize bowel toxicity.

Of the various intraluminal factors, pancreatic enzymes exert the most pronounced influence on acute intestinal radiation toxicity. Reducing pancreatic enzyme secretion in animals by surgical or dietary methods attenuates acute mucosal injury, as well as subsequent development of intestinal fibrosis.[52,183–185] Moreover, preclinical studies show that reducing intraluminal pancreatic secretions with a synthetic somatostatin receptor analog, octreotide, markedly ameliorates both early and delayed radiation enteropathy.[53,76] Octreotide is exceptionally well tolerated clinically and, because of its potent inhibitory effects on GI secretion and motility, it is used in patients with intractable diarrhea after cancer chemotherapy and has documented effect in patients undergoing radiation therapy.[77] Importantly, octreotide has intrinsic antitumor and antiangiogenic effects,[186–189] and there are thus no concerns about potential tumor protection. Hence, while the protective effects of octreotide are likely confined to the small intestine, this compound is a particularly promising candidate for intestinal radioprotection in the clinic.

MODULATION OF ENDOTHELIAL DYSFUNCTION

Radiation induces a plethora of changes in the microvascular endothelium. These changes play important roles in acute radiation responses, in development of radiation fibrosis, and in the mechanisms of chronicity of injury.[151,190,191]

Administration of traditional anticoagulant agents, such as heparin, warfarin, or acetyl salicylic acid, confers some, albeit inconsistent, protection against radiation injury in certain organs, including the intestine. Recent preclinical studies show that inhibition of ADP-induced platelet aggregation or direct inhibition of thrombin reduces acute and chronic intestinal radiation injury in a rat model.[192,193] The drawback of such agents is that, when administered in effective doses, they are associated with a significant risk of bleeding. Strategies aimed at restoring local endothelial anticoagulant properties, temporarily replacing the "natural anticoagulant", activated protein C, or blocking only the effects of thrombin that are mediated through its cellular receptor, proteinase-activated receptor 1, may circumvent these obstacles. Such strategies are currently under investigation.

One of the more promising endothelial-oriented protection strategies involves inhibition of the enzyme hydroxyl-methylglutaryl-coenzyme A (HMG-CoA) reductase by drugs that belong to the class of statins. Statins inhibit the rate-limiting step in cholesterol synthesis, but have been shown to exert many lipid-independent, notably vasculoprotective effects, mostly mediated by increased expression of endothelial nitric oxide synthase. The evidence supporting the use of statins to reduce the incidence and/or severity of radiation enteropathy is rather strong. Preclinical studies performed in two different laboratories have shown that statins ameliorate delayed radiation enteropathy and, albeit to a lesser extent, also the acute intestinal radiation response.[194,195] Moreover, a clinical study revealed that statin use is associated with reduced rectal toxicity in conjunction with pelvic radiation therapy.[196] It is possible that other compounds that have HMG-CoA reductase inhibitory properties, as for example, the vitamin E analog γ-tocotrienol (GT3), can be used to further enhance the efficacy of statins as an intestinal radiation response modifier. Further research in this area is clearly needed to optimize the statin dose, take advantage of differences among statins and differential regulation of downstream targets, and investigate promising combination therapies.

NEUROIMMUNOMODULATION

Interactions between the enteric nervous system and various cell types in the intestinal wall play critical roles in the intestinal response to injury. Modulation of these interactions is currently emerging as a strategy to ameliorate radiation-induced inflammation and fibrosis in the gut. The sensory (afferent) nerves of the intestine appear to be particularly important in terms of these neuroimmune interactions.

Sensory nerves were previously thought of only as conveyors of stimuli from the periphery to the central nervous system or peripheral neural circuitry. In other words, they were assumed to act in a purely unidirectional manner. It is now well established that sensory nerves serve critically important local effector functions in many organs, particularly in the intestine. Through interactions with epithelial cells and various immune cells, notably mast cells, sensory nerves are involved in maintaining the integrity of the intestinal mucosa and in mounting an appropriate response to injury. Clinical and animal studies implicate substance P, released by sensory nerves, in the intestinal radiation response,[197–200] and administration of neurokinin-1 (NK-1) receptor antagonists ameliorates some aspects of GI radiation toxicity.[201,202] Work performed in our laboratory using genetically altered animal models and pharmacological response modifiers has shown that both mast cells and sensory nerves have a protective effect against acute intestinal injury and that the two major neuropeptides released by sensory nerves have opposing effects in that substance P exacerbates, while calcitonin gene–related peptide (CGRP) ameliorates the intestinal radiation response.[203–205]

MEDICAL COUNTERMEASURES AGAINST BOWEL INJURY IN RADIATION ACCIDENTS OR RADIOLOGICAL OR NUCLEAR TERRORISM

In most radiation overexposure scenarios, injury to the bone marrow and GI tract is the primary determinant of survival because of their rapidly proliferating stem/progenitor cell compartments. Considerable progress has been made in the management of radiation-induced bone marrow injury by the use of hematopoietic cytokines, blood transfusions, antimicrobial therapy, and stem cell reconstitution. On the other hand, the management of GI radiation toxicity remains comparatively underdeveloped.

The intestinal radiation syndrome in humans occurs after total body irradiation (TBI) exposures with doses in excess of about 6 Gy. Survival is extremely unlikely with the full-blown intestinal radiation syndrome. In this situation, death occurs as a result of extensive destructive changes of epithelium and breakdown of the mucosal barrier, resulting in severe secretory diarrhea, dehydration, and electrolyte imbalance. However, injury to the GI tract also plays a major part in determining the clinical outcome after lower doses of radiation. Hence, epithelial barrier dysfunction occurs after doses as low as 0.5 to 1 Gy, and bacterial translocation with sepsis from enteric bacteria is an important, if not the major cause of lethality after radiation exposure with doses in the "hematopoietic" range. Figure 38.8 depicts the

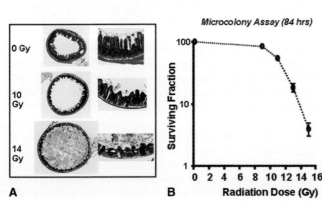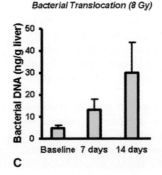

Figure 38.8. The intestinal radiation response after TBI. **A**: Dose-dependent damage of the intestinal mucosa with loss of crypts (3.5 days after TBI). **B**: Number of intestinal crypts per circumference, the so-called crypt colony assay, 3.5 days after TBI. **C**: Bacterial translocation to liver. Note that there is significant translocation after a radiation dose that does not cause appreciable decrease in the number of surviving crypts.

radiation dose-dependent decrease in the number of surviving crypts, typically counted at 3.5 days after exposure to TBI. Also shown is the bacterial translocation that occurs, usually beginning about one week after irradiation and reaching a maximum at about 2 weeks.

It is important to recognize that total body radiation exposure affects all tissues and organ systems in the body and that there are important interactions among them. While intestinal irradiation is necessary and sufficient to produce the gastrointestinal radiation syndrome"[206] and surgical removal of the exposed bowel prevents it,[207] lethality from bowel toxicity is profoundly influenced by radiation injury to other organ systems, as demonstrated by Terry and Travis in 1989.[208] In fact, reference to the gastrointestinal radiation syndrome or the hematopoietic radiation syndrome after TBI is somewhat artificial, and simply indicates that toxicity in those particular organ systems predominates clinically. In reality, the pathophysiological manifestations after radiation exposure depend heavily on interactions among multiple cell types and organ systems throughout the body and it is more appropriate to refer to radiation-induced multiple organ dysfunction syndrome or R-MODS. For an overview of GI radiation toxicity from the perspective of MODS, the reader is referred to a review by Monti et al.[209]

DEVELOPMENT OF MEDICAL COUNTERMEASURES AGAINST RADIATION

Development of medical countermeasures against radiation is focused on two distinct areas, preexposure and postexposure interventions. Preexposure countermeasures (radioprophylactic or radioprotective countermeasures) are interventions that either enhance the resistance and/or tolerance of normal tissues to radiation or interfere directly with the initial radiochemical events. In contrast, postexposure countermeasures interfere with downstream events, thus preventing or reducing the progression of radiation damage and/or facilitating the eventual resolution of or recovery from radiation injury. The first category, radioprotective or radioprophylactic countermeasures, is a critical requirement for military personnel, first responders, and rescue and cleanup workers. In contrast, in a civilian mass casualty situation, agents are needed that are effective when administered hours to days after radiation exposure.

An important difference between the development of medical countermeasures against radiation and radiation response modifiers for use in cancer patients is that the former cannot be tested in humans. As a result, the path to FDA approval for countermeasures relies more heavily on preclinical data than the development of a clinical response modifier. Another important distinction between medical countermeasures against radiation (both preexposure and postexposure) and radiation response modifiers for use in the cancer treatment situation is that potential tumor protection is much less of an issue with the former. Nevertheless, there is considerable overlap between the approaches discussed above (in the section "Preclinical and Clinical Strategies to Prevent Bowel Injury after Radiation Therapy") and the development of medical countermeasures for the radiation accident or terrorism scenario. Therefore, the following discussion of countermeasures focuses on compounds that have shown particular promise in ameliorating intestinal injury after total body radiation exposure. For a more comprehensive discussion of countermeasures against intestinal radiation injury, the reader is referred to a

recent review on the subject.[210] Finally, while the distinction is being made between preexposure and postexposure countermeasures, it should be pointed out that there is considerable overlap between these categories, that is, that some preexposure countermeasures also confer significant protection in the postexposure situation and vice versa.

PRE-EXPOSURE COUNTERMEASURES AGAINST INTESTINAL RADIATION INJURY

The list of preexposure countermeasures that have been shown to influence the level of intestinal radiation toxicity in various model systems is extensive. These countermeasures include antioxidants, free radical scavengers, and cytoprotectors on one hand, and enterotrophic strategies on the other.

Among the nutritional antioxidants, there has been strong interest in the use of vitamins A[141] and E (tocols).[142,211,212]

Tocols have been subject to particular interest because of their potent properties as radiation protectors. While there are differences in antioxidant properties among the eight naturally occurring tocols (i.e., the α, β, γ, and δ tocopherols and the α, β, γ, and δ tocotrienols), there are also major difference among them in terms of their affinity to endothelial cells and ability to inhibit the enzyme HMG-CoA reductase. The most promising tocol compounds at the present time are GT3 and δ-tocotrienol, both of which show substantial activity as HMG-CoA reductase inhibitors.[213] GT3 exhibits a dose-reduction factor around 1.3 and, in addition to protecting against hematopoietic and vascular radiation injury, also strongly protects the intestine. Moreover, because of the unique properties of GT3, the combination of GT3 with pentoxifylline (analogous to the use of vitamin E combined with pentoxifylline in the clinic) and/or with another class of HMG-CoA reductase inhibitors that exert efficacy against radiation enteropathy in preclinical and clinical studies is also being investigated.[214,215]

Free radical scavengers have also shown promise as countermeasures specifically against intestinal radiation injury after TBI. For example, gene therapy with MnSOD ameliorates some aspects of intestinal radiation toxicity.[116] Several small molecule compounds that mimic the effects of SOD and/or catalase are under development and have shown efficacy, but their ability to specifically protect from intestinal radiation lethality after TBI remains to be determined.[216–218]

Other antioxidant compounds that have been tested include, for example, probucol, an antioxidant that inhibits the formation of peroxides, confers intestinal protection in rats when given either intraluminally or systemically.[140] Melatonin reduces lethality after TBI and protects against radiation-induced intestinal injury, possibly due to its radical scavenging properties, stimulatory effects on antioxidant enzymes, and enhancement of the cellular DNA repair machinery.[219,220]

Many studies have assessed modification of COX activity or components of the arachidonic acid cascade in the context of radiation responses in normal tissues, including intestine. Inhibition of COX2, for instance, protects against intestinal radiation injury.[221] Other protective agents are PGE and its synthetic analogs, although the exact mechanisms by which these compounds confer cytoprotection are still not known. In animal studies, PGE2 is radioprotective in the intestine.[131,132] Oral administration of enprostil (a PGE2 analog) or luminal application of misoprostol (a PGE1 analog) protects against intestinal radiation toxicity.[133,134] Misoprostol and a prostacyclin analog (iloprost) were toxic when given separately, but a combination of the two compounds conferred synergistic radiation protection with considerable amelioration of toxicity.[222]

Among cytokines, growth factors, and chemokines, several have been shown to reduce intestinal injury after TBI. For example, IL-1α and IL-1β confer some radioprotection of mouse intestine.[143,144] IL-7, which plays critical roles in the development of B and T cells and also influences the function of mature NK cells and monocytes/macrophages, protects intra-epithelial lymphocytes (IELs) from undergoing apoptosis[223] and may also protect the intestinal stem cell compartment from radiation.[145] IL-15, a cytokine that is widely expressed by epithelial cells, stromal cells, and immune cells, promotes survival of IELs, inhibits expression of IL-8 and monocyte chemoattractant protein 1,[224,225] and stimulates epithelial cell proliferation.[226] While IL-15 has not been systematically studied in radiation injury, it confers an impressive degree of protection against the intestinal toxicity of irinotecan (CPT-11), a chemotherapeutic agent that is notorious for causing GI toxicity, mainly due to dose-limiting diarrhea.[227]

As mentioned above, the angiogenic growth factors, aFGF, bFGF, and VEGF, are all radioprotective in the small intestine of mice exposed to total-body irradiation.[150,151] The mechanisms of protection, however, are unclear. The many documented effects of bFGF include protection of endothelial cells from apoptosis, enhanced repair of DNA damage, and increased proliferation and enhanced restitution of intestinal epithelium. It remains to be determined whether the enteroprotective effect of bFGF is primarily a direct effect on epithelial cells,[228] secondary to reduced endothelial cell apoptosis,[151] or a combination of the two.

Direct enterotrophic growth factors, for example recombinant human KGF1, administered to mice before total-body or abdominal irradiation increased crypt survival and LD$_{50}$.[152,153] Clearly, the issues that apply to cell growth–promoting cytokines are much less important when they are used as medical countermeasures against radiation.

POST-EXPOSURE COUNTERMEASURES AGAINST INTESTINAL RADIATION INJURY

Compared to the plethora of compounds that exhibit robust protection of the intestine when applied before irradiation, the list of countermeasures with activity after radiation exposure is considerably shorter.

Breakdown of the mucosal barrier during the acute phase of radiation injury exposes subepithelial tissues to the detrimental actions of the contents of the intestinal lumen. Therefore, modifications of the intraluminal contents, particularly bacteria and pancreatic enzymes, have been explored as strategies to ameliorate intestinal radiation toxicity.

A possible role for intestinal bacteria in the development of the acute intestinal radiation response was already proposed in 1906.[229] Subsequently, the role of the bacterial flora has been extensively studied in germ-free animal models,[230–232] as well as in models involving more or less selective "decontamination" with different antimicrobial agents.[233–236] Treatment of animals with antibiotics against the aerobic gut flora after irradiation increases survival.[233] In contrast, antimicrobials that reduce the anaerobic flora may be detrimental in the TBI situation and should be avoided. Careful selection of antibiotic treatment regimen has been shown to protect lethally irradiated canines.[237]

A combination of oral and parenteral antibiotics may reduce bacterial translocation and confer considerable protection. In the clinical situation, it is likely that the proper balance in the bacterial flora is optimal in terms of minimizing radiation toxicity. Hence, there is interest in probiotic therapies as a way to enhance the resistance of the gut to irradiation and/or to minimize intestinal radiation toxicity.[182,238]

A series of dog studies from the late 1960s and early 1970s by Morgenstern and coworkers demonstrated that reducing the intraluminal content of pancreatic enzymes reduced lethality after abdominal irradiation.[183–185,239] The most promising approach to reduce intraluminal pancreatic secretions in humans may be administration of synthetic somatostatin receptor analogs. Somatostatin analogs are "universal gastrointestinal inhibitors" and are used for a number of gastroenterological indications, including intractable diarrhea, short gut syndrome, pancreatic and enterocutaneous fistulae, pancreatitis, and bleeding esophageal varices. Because of their strong inhibitory effect on secretion, somatostatin analogs result in a "pharmacological, reversible exocrine pancreatectomy." Somatostatin analogs are extremely well tolerated and the maximal tolerated dose in humans has not been reached, even though patients with neuroendocrine tumors have received doses of more than 100,000 μg/d. Based on the promising preclinical and clinical results with the somatostatin analog, octreotide, as a modifier of intestinal injury after localized irradiation, there has been interest in developing somatostatin analogs for use as countermeasures as well. Our laboratory currently investigates a novel somatostatin analog, SOM230, with superior metabolic stability and broader affinity to somatostatin receptors compared to octreotide, in the TBI model. Studies to date indicate that SOM230 ameliorates structural (mucosal) intestinal radiation injury, decreases lethality, and prolongs postradiation survival time when administered either before and after, or only after irradiation.[240]

The polypeptide compound, CBLB502, derived from Salmonella flagellin, binds to Toll-like receptor 5 to activate signaling by NF-κB. Activation of NF-κB affects p53 and induces cytoprotective cytokines and other factors, inhibitors of apoptosis, and free radical scavenging factors. CBLB502 has been reported to confer protection against both intestinal and hematopoietic lethality after TBI in mice and non–human primates. CBLB502 improves survival both when injected up to 24 hours before radiation exposure, and when injected up to 1 hour after radiation exposure.[241]

IL-11, in addition to its hematopoietic and immunomodulating activities, also serves to protect and restore the GI mucosa. Administration of IL-11 protects mice against the intestinal effects of total-body irradiation.[146–148] Despite these encouraging preclinical results, systemic administration of IL-11 to humans is hampered by severe side effects, including fluid retention and multisystem organ failure. In contrast, oral delivery of an enteric-coated formulation of recombinant human IL-11 avoids systemic uptake and is thus not associated with the toxicity seen after systemic administration.[242,243] A recent study showed significant protection against early intestinal radiation injury when human recombinant IL-11 was administered once daily directly into the intestinal lumen of rats,[149] suggesting that oral administration of an enterosoluble form of IL-11 may also be a promising radiation countermeasure. Studies with intraluminal administration of IL-11 after exposure to TBI have indeed confirmed that it is effective in ameliorating intestinal radiation toxicity (unpublished data).

FUTURE DIRECTIONS

Many early post–radiation cellular and molecular phenomena occur as part of a physiological response to injury. Hence, it is likely that cytokine overexpression is only detrimental when cellular and molecular responses are exaggerated and/or when overexpression is prolonged beyond the early phase. Post–radiation interventions should not perturb physiological (beneficial) processes, but rather target specific mechanisms responsible for exaggerating or sustaining them. To optimize interventional strategies, it is thus necessary to obtain an improved understanding of the differences between physiological and pathological responses.

Animal studies in models that involve the use of high, single doses of TBI or abdominal irradiation have limited clinical relevance in the development of intestinal radiation response modifiers. Rather, it is necessary to use animal models that allow localized irradiation, fractionated radiation schedules, and long-term observation. Structural, molecular, and functional assays that take advantage of novel imaging and other emerging technologies may enhance the ability to monitor the progression of pathology over time.

There is a glaring need for clinical, epidemiological, and outcomes studies in well-defined cohorts of cancer survivors to define the overall and organ-specific prevalence of late effects of radiation, as well as the medical, quality of life-related, social, and financial consequences of radiation-induced bowel injury. Such studies are critical for setting priorities for prophylactic and interventional clinical research, as well as for identifying optimal strategies and focus areas for future preclinical and mechanistic laboratory research. To this end, new means to objectively assess and quantify bowel injury will need to be developed.

Research is also needed to develop methods to identify patients who are more prone than others to develop delayed normal tissue toxicity after radiation therapy. To this end, efforts should be directed toward developing assays by which normal tissue toxicity can be predicted; toward developing methods to diagnose delayed radiation toxicity at the early (subclinical) stage when interventions may be more effective, as well as toward molecular epidemiology research aimed at identifying genetic or epigenetic characteristics that correlate with susceptibility to delayed radiation toxicity.

While many radiation response modifiers have shown promise in preclinical studies, few have been tested clinically. One reason for this is the lack of good clinical surrogate endpoints with sufficient specificity, sensitivity, and predictive ability. In the absence of such endpoints, clinical studies are difficult and require inordinately lengthy follow-up. In order to facilitate translation of promising preclinical results into the clinic, it is essential to develop surrogate markers that reliably predict chronic radiation-induced intestinal dysfunction. This is best done in collaboration with clinical and basic scientists who have expertise in the specific organ system of interest.

Most patients receive radiation therapy in combination with chemotherapy agents or biological response modifiers. This is intended to enhance the antitumor effect of the therapy, but there is a relative paucity of studies to address interactions among such therapies to the extent that they affect the incidence and severity of bowel injury. There is a need for basic, mechanistic studies to address the cellular and the molecular underpinnings of these interactions and for applied research to determine the best strategy to minimize side effects from normal tissues. Only through such effort will one achieve an optimal increase in the therapeutic ratio.

There is a need to engage the interest of the pharmaceutical and biotechnology industries in developing strategies to modulate intestinal radiation toxicity. Their current disinterest is largely due to an erroneous perception that the "market" is small. In fact, the "market" is the entire cohort of cancer patients receiving radiation therapy to the abdomen or pelvis, estimated at about 200,000 patients per year in the United States alone. Appropriately designed clinical and epidemiological studies should be conducted to demonstrate that effective control of intestinal radiation toxicity will increase cancer cure rates and reduce the burden of intestinal dysfunction in the large and steadily increasing cohort of cancer survivors, thus easily justifying the drug development investment.

Finally, there is a need to focus future efforts on development of preexposure and postexposure medical countermeasure against radiation. While there has been significant investment in this area during the past few years, effective countermeasures against intestinal injury remain an important capability shortfall and an unmet need.

FINANCIAL SUPPORT. Work reported here was supported by the National Institutes of Health (grants CA71382, CA83719, AI67798 [MH-J]), Defense Threat Reduction Agency (grants HDTRA1-07-C-0028 [MH-J] and H.10027-07-AR-R [KSK]) and the U.S. Veterans Administration [MH-J].

REFERENCES

1. Potten CS. Structure, function and proliferative organisation of mammalian gut. In: Potten CS, Hendry JH, eds. *Radiation and Gut*. Amsterdam: Elsevier; 1995:1–31.
2. Kellett M, Potten CS, Rew DA. A comparison of in vivo cell proliferation measurements in the intestine of mouse and man. *Epith Cell Biol*. 1992;1:147–155.
3. Bentzen SM, Dische S. Late morbidity: the Damocles sword of radiotherapy? *Radiother Oncol*. 2001; 61: 219–221.
4. Letschert JGJ, Lebesque JV, Aleman BMP, et al. The volume effect in radiation-related late small bowel complications: results of a clinical study of the EORTC Radiotherapy Cooperative Group in patients treated for rectal carcinoma. *Radiother Oncol*. 1994;32:116–123.
5. Mak AC, Rich TA, Schultheiss TE, et al. Late complications of postoperative radiation therapy for cancer of the rectum and rectosigmoid. *Int J Radiat Oncol Biol Phys*. 1994;28:597–603.
6. Eifel PJ, Levenback C, Wharton JT, et al. Time course and incidence of late complications in patients treated with radiation therapy for FIGO stage IB carcinoma of the uterine cervix. *Int J Radiat Oncol Biol Phys*. 1995;32:1289–1300.
7. Danielsson A, Nyhlin H, Stendahl U, et al. Chronic diarrhoea after radiotherapy for gynaecologic cancer: occurrence and aetiology. *Gut*. 1991;32:1180–1187.
8. Crook J, Esche B, Futter N. Effect of pelvic radiotherapy for prostate cancer on bowel, bladder, and sexual function: the patient's perspective. *Urology*. 1996;47:387–394.
9. Christie D, Denham J, Steigler A, et al. Delayed rectal urinary symptomatology in patients treated for prostate cancer by radiotherapy with or without short term neo-adjuvant androgen deprivation. *Radiother Oncol*. 2005;77:117–125.
10. Dearnaley DP, Khoo VS, Norman AR, et al. Comparison of radiation side-effects of conformal and conventional radiotherapy in prostate cancer: a randomised trial. *Lancet*. 1999;353:267–272.
11. Mundt AJ, Roeske JC, Lujan AE, et al. Initial clinical experience with intensity-modulated whole-pelvis radiation therapy in women with gynecological malignancies. *Gynecol Oncol*. 2001;82:456–463.
12. Potish RA. Factors predisposing to injury. In: Galland RB, Spencer J, eds. *Radiation Enteritis*. London: Edward Arnold; 1990:103–119.
13. LoIudice T, Baxter DOD, Balint J. Effects of abdominal surgery on the development of radiation enteropathy. *Gastroenterology*. 1977;73:1093–1097.
14. Cosset JM, Henry-Amar M, Burgers JMV, et al. Late radiation injuries of the gastrointestinal tract in the H2 and H5 EORTC Hodgkin's disease trials: Emphasis on the role of exploratory laparotomy and fractionation. *Radiother Oncol*. 1988;13:61–68.
15. Willett CG, Ooi C-J, Zietman AL, et al. Acute and late toxicity of patients with inflammatory bowel disease undergoing irradiation for abdominal and pelvic neoplasms. *Int J Radiat Oncol Biol Phys*. 2000;46:995–998.
16. Herold DM, Hanlon AL, Hanks GE. Diabetes mellitus: a predictor for late radiation morbidity. *Int J Radiat Oncol Biol Phys*. 1999;43:475–479.
17. Potish RA, Twiggs LB, Adcock LL, et al. Logistic models for prediction of enteric morbidity in the treatment of ovarian and cervical cancer. *Am J Obstet Gynecol*. 1983;147:65–72.
18. Ross JG, Hussey DH, Mayr NA, et al. Acute and late reactions to radiation therapy in patients with collagen vascular diseases. *Cancer*. 1993;71:3744–3752.

19. Lin A, Abu-Isa E, Griffith KA, et al. Toxicity of radiotherapy in patients with collagen vascular disease. *Cancer.* 2008;113:648–653.
20. Eifel PJ, Jhingran A, Badurka DC, et al. Correlation of smoking history and other patient characteristics with major complications of pelvic radiation therapy for cervical cancer. *J Clin Oncol.* 2002;20:3651–3657.
21. Gami B, Harrington K, Blake P, et al. How patients manage gastrointestinal symptoms after pelvic radiotherapy. *Aliment Pharmacol Ther.* 2003;18:987–994.
22. Trotti A, Pajak TF, Gwede CK, et al. TAME: development of a new method for summarising adverse events of cancer treatment by the Radiation Therapy Oncology Group TAME: development of a new method for summarising adverse events of cancer treatment by the Radiation Therapy Oncology Group. *Lancet Oncol.* 2007;8:613–624.
23. Khalid U, McGough C, Hackett C, et al. A modified inflammatory bowel disease questionnaire and the Vaizey Incontinence questionnaire are more sensitive measures of acute gastrointestinal toxicity during pelvic radiotherapy than RTOG grading. *Int J Radiat Oncol Biol Phys.* 2006;64:1432–1441.
24. Yeoh E, Horowitz M, Russo A, et al. Effect of pelvic irradiation on gastrointestinal function: A prospective longitudinal study. *Am J Med.* 1993;95:397–406.
25. Yeoh E, Sun WM, Russo A, et al. A retrospective study of the effects of pelvic irradiation for gynecological cancer on anorectal function. *Int J Radiat Oncol Biol Phys.* 1996;35:1003–1010.
26. Fransson P, Widmark A. Late side effects unchanged 4–8 years after radiotherapy for prostate carcinoma. *Cancer.*1999;85:678–688.
27. Kollmorgen GF, Meagher AP, Wolff BG, et al. The long-term effect of adjuvant postoperative chemoradiotherapy for rectal carcinoma on bowel function. *Ann Surg.* 1994;220: 676–682.
28. Iwamoto T, Nakahara S, Mibu R, et al. Effect of radiotherapy on anorectal function in patients with cervical cancer. *Dis Colon Rectum.* 1997;40:693–697.
29. Andreyev J. Gastrointestinal complications of pelvic radiotherapy: are they of any importance. *Gut.* 2005;54:1051–1054.
30. Capp A, Inostroza-Porta M, Bill D, et al. Is there more than one proctitis syndrome? A revisitation using data from the TROG 96.01 trial. *Radiother Oncol.* 2008; [Epub ahead of print].
31. Fajardo LF. Alimentary tract. In: Fajardo LF, ed. *Pathology of Radiation Injury.* New York, NY: Masson Publishing; 1982:47–76.
32. Fajardo LF, Berthrong M, Anderson RE. Alimentary tract. In: Fajardo LF, Berthrong M, Anderson RE, eds. *Radiation Pathology.* New York, NY: Oxford University Press; 2001: 209–247.
33. Carr KE. Effects of radiation damage on intestinal morphology. *Int Rev Cytol.* 2001;208: 1–119.
34. Hauer-Jensen M, Wang J, Denham JW. Mechanisms and modification of the radiation response of gastrointestinal organs. In: Milas L, Ang KK, Nieder C, eds. *Modification of Radiation Response: Cytokines, Growth Factors, and Other Biological Targets.* Heidelberg, Germany: Springer Verlag; 2002:49–72.
35. Denham JW, Hauer-Jensen M, Peters LJ. Is it time for a new formalism to categorise normal tissue radiation injury? *Int J Radiat Oncol Biol Phys.* 2001;50:1105–1106.
36. Denham JW, Hauer-Jensen M. The radiotherapeutic injury - a complex "wound". *Radiother Oncol.* 2002;63:129–145.
37. Hagemann RF, Sigdestad CP, Lesher S. Intestinal crypt survival and total and per crypt levels of proliferative cellularity following irradiation: single X-ray exposures. *Radiat Res.* 1971;46:533–546.
38. Hagemann RF. Intestinal cell proliferation during fractionated abdominal irradiation. *Br J Radiol.* 1976;49:56–61.
39. Lesher S, Baumann J. Cell kinetic studies of the intestinal epithelium: maintenance of the intestinal epithelium in normal and irradiated animals. *NCI Monogr.* 1969;30:185–195.
40. Carratu R, Secondulfo M, de Magistris L, et al. Assessment of small intestinal damage in patients treated with pelvic radiotherapy. *Oncol Rep.* 1998;5:635–639.
41. Hovdenak N, Fajardo LF, Hauer-Jensen M. Acute radiation proctitis: a sequential clinicopathologic study during pelvic radiotherapy. *Int J Radiat Oncol Biol Phys.* 2000;48: 1111–1117.
42. Rotolo JA, Maj JG, Feldman R, et al. Bax and bak do not exhibit functional redundancy in mediating radiation-induced endothelial apoptosis in the intestinal mucosa. *Int J Radiat Oncol Biol Phys.* 2008;70:804–815.
43. Husebye E, Hauer-Jensen M, Kjorstad K, et al. Severe late radiation enteropathy is characterized by impaired motility of proximal small intestine. *Dig Dis Sci.* 1994;39:2341–2349.
44. Husebye E, Skar V, Hoverstad T, et al. Abnormal intestinal motor patterns explain enteric colonization with gram-negative bacilli in late radiation enteropathy. *Gastroenterology.* 1995;109:1078–1089.
45. Kline JC, Buchler DA, Boone ML, et al. The relationship of reactions to complications in radiation therapy of cancer of the cervix. *Radiology.* 1972;105:413–416.
46. Bourne RB, Kearsley JH, Grove WD, et al. The relationship between early and late gastrointestinal complication of radiation therapy for carcinoma of the cervix. *Int J Radiat Oncol Biol Phys.* 1983;9:1445–1450.
47. Wang C-J, Leung SW, Chen H-C, et al. The correlation of acute toxicity and late rectal injury in radiotherapy for cervical carcinoma: evidence suggestive of consequential late effect (CQLE). *Int J Radiat Oncol Biol Phys.* 1998;40:85–91.
48. Weiss E, Hirnle P, Arnold-Bofinger H, et al. Therapeutic outcome and relation of acute and late side effects in the adjuvant radiotherapy of endometrial carcinoma stage I and II. *Radiother Oncol.* 1999;53:37–44.
49. Hauer-Jensen M, Sauer T, Devik F, et al. Effects of dose fractionation on late roentgen radiation damage of rat small intestine. *Acta Radiol Oncol.* 1983;22:381–384.
50. Travis EL, Followill D. The characterization of two types of late effects in irradiated mouse colon. In: Chapman JD, Dewey WC, Whitmore GF, eds. *Radiation Research. A Twentieth-Century Perspective.* San Diego, CA: Academic Press; 1991:154.
51. Denham JW, Hauer-Jensen M, Kron T, et al. Treatment time dependence models of early and delayed radiation injury in rat small intestine. *Int J Radiat Oncol Biol Phys.* 2000;48:887.
52. Hauer-Jensen M, Sauer T, Berstad T, et al. Influence of pancreatic secretion on late radiation enteropathy in the rat. *Acta Radiol Oncol.* 1985;24:555–560.
53. Wang J, Zheng H, Sung C-C, et al. The synthetic somatostatin analogue, octreotide, ameliorates acute and delayed intestinal radiation injury. *Int J Radiat Oncol Biol Phys.* 1999;45:1289–1296.
54. Taverner D, Talbot IC, Carr-Locke DL, et al. Massive bleeding from the ileum: a late complication of pelvic radiotherapy. *Am J Gastroenterol.* 1982;77:29–31.
55. Cox MR, Millar DM. Gastric, hepatic and small bowel infarction due to radiation aortitis in a 42 year old woman. *Aust N Z J Surg.* 1993;63:499–501.
56. Wagholikar GD, Gupta RK, Kapoor VK. Polyvisceral gangrene due to radiation enteritis. *Trop Gastroenterol.* 2002;23:104–105.
57. Lordick F, Geinitz H, Theisen J, et al. Increased risk of ischemic bowel complications during treatment with bevacizumab after pelvic irradiation: report of three cases. *Int J Radiat Oncol Biol Phys.* 2006;64:1295–1298.
58. Galland RB, Spencer J. The natural history of clinically established radiation enteritis. *Lancet.* 1985;1:1257–1258.
59. Harling H, Balslev I. Long-term prognosis of patients with severe radiation enteritis. *Am J Surg.* 1988;155:517–519.
60. Silvain C, Besson I, Ingrand P, et al. Long-term outcome of severe radiation enteritis treated by total parenteral nutrition. *Dig Dis Sci.* 1992;37:1065–1071.
61. Fischer L, Kimose HH, Spjeldnaes N, et al. Late radiation injuries of the small intestine - management and outcome. *Acta Chir Scand.* 1989;155:47–51.
62. Kimose HH, Fischer L, Spjeldnaes N, et al. Late radiation injury of the colon and rectum: Surgical management and outcome. *Dis Colon Rectum.* 1989;32:684–689.
63. Regimbeau J-M, Panis Y, Gouzi J-L, et al. Operative and long term results after surgery for chronic radiation enteritis. *Am J Surg.* 2001;182:237–242.
64. Larsen A, Reitan JB, Aase S, et al. Long-term prognosis in patients with severe late radiation enteropathy: a prospective cohort study. *World J Gastroenterol.* 2007;13:3610–3613.
65. Denham JW, O'Brien PC, Dunstan RH, et al. Is there more than one late radiation proctitis syndrome? *Radiother Oncol.* 1999;51:43–53.
66. O'Brien PC, Hamilton CS, Denham JW, et al. Spontaneous improvement in late rectal mucosal changes following radiotherapy for prostate cancer. *Int J Radiat Oncol Biol Phys.* 2003;58:75–80.
67. Cho KJ, Christie D. Rectosigmoid cancer after radiotherapy for prostate cancer can be detected early and successfully treated. *Australas Radiol.* 2006;50:228–232.
68. Andreyev J. Gastrointestinal symptoms after pelvic radiotherapy: a new understanding to improve management of symptomatic patients. *Lancet Oncol.* 2007;8:1007–1017.
69. Varma JS, Smith AN, Busuttil A. Correlation of clinical and manometric abnormalities of rectal function following chronic radiation injury. *Br J Surg.* 1985;72:875–878.
70. Heemsbergen WD, Peeters ST, Koper PC, et al. Acute and late gastrointestinal toxicity after radiotherapy in prostate cancer patients: consequential late damage. *Int J Radiat Oncol Biol Phys.* 2006;66:3–10.
71. Fenwick JD, Khoo VS, Nahum AE, et al. Correlations between dose-surface histograms and the incidence of long-term rectal bleeding following conformal or conventional radiotherapy treatment of prostate cancer. *Int J Radiat Oncol Biol Phys.* 2001;49:473–480.
72. Fiorino C, Fellin G, Rancati T, et al. Clinical and dosimetric predictors of late rectal syndrome after 3D-CRT for localized prostate cancer: Preliminary results of a multicenter prospective study. *Int J Radiat Oncol Biol Phys.* 2008;70:1130–1137.
73. van der Laan HP, van den Bergh A, Schilstra C, et al. Grading-system-dependent volume effects for late radiation-induced rectal toxicity after curative radiotherapy for prostate cancer. *Int J Radiat Oncol Biol Phys.* 2008;70:1138–1145.
74. Pollack A, Zagars GK, Starkschall G, et al. Prostate cancer radiation dose response: results of the M.D. Anderson phase III randomised trial. *Int J Radiat Oncol Biol Phys.* 2002;53: 1097–1105.
75. Litwin MS, Hays RD, Fink A, et al. Quality-of-life outcomes in men treated for localised prostate cancer. *JAMA.* 1995;273:129–135.
76. Wang J, Zheng H, Hauer-Jensen M. Influence of short-term octreotide administration on chronic tissue injury, transforming growth factor β (TGF-β) overexpression, and collagen accumulation in irradiated rat intestine. *J Pharmacol Exp Ther.* 2001;297:35–42.
77. Yavuz MN, Yavuz AA, Aydin F, et al. The efficacy of octreotide in the therapy of acute radiation-induced diarrhea: a randomized controlled study. *Int J Radiat Oncol Biol Phys* 2002;54:195–202.
78. Horiot JC. Prophylaxis versus treatment: is there a better way to manage radiotherapy-induced nausea and vomiting? *Int J Radiat Oncol Biol Phys.* 2004;60:1018–1025.
79. Maranzano E, Feyer PC, Molassiotis A, et al. Evidence-based recommendations for the use of antiemetics in radiotherapy. *Radiother Oncol.* 2005;76:227–233.
80. Zentler-Munro PL, Bessell EM. Medical management of radiation enteritis—an algorithmic guide. *Clin Radiol.*1987;38:291–294.
81. Miholic J, Vogelsang H, Schlappack O, et al. Small bowel function after surgery for chronic radiation enteritis. *Digestion.* 1989;42:30–38.
82. Dietz DW, Remzi FH, Fazio VW. Stricutreplasty for obstructing small-bowel lesions in diffuse radiation enteritis - successful outcome in five patients. *Dis Colon Rectum.* 2001;44:1772–1777.
83. Durdey P, Willimas NS. Radiation fistulae—general principles of management. In: Galland, RB, Spencer J, eds. London: Edward Arnold; 1990:215–230.
84. Denton AS, Andreyev HJN, Forbes A, et al. Systematic review of non-surgical interventions for the management of late radiation proctitis. *Br J Cancer.* 2002;87:134–143.
85. Kochhar R, Patel F, Dhar A, et al. Radiation-induced proctosigmoiditis. Prospective, randomized, double-blind controlled trial of oral sulfasalazine plus rectal steroids versus rectal sucralfate. *Dig Dis Sci.* 1991;36:103–107.
86. O'Brien PC, Franklin CI, Dear KBG, et al. A phase III double-blind randomised study of rectal sucralfate suspension in the prevention of acute radiation proctitis. *Radiother Oncol.* 1997;45:117–123.
87. Martenson JA, Bollinger JW, Sloan JA, et al. Sucralfate in the prevention of treatment-induced diarrhea in patients receiving pelvic radiation therapy: a North Central Cancer Treatment Group phase III double-blind placebo-controlled trial. *J Clin Oncol.* 2000;18:1239–1245.

88. Kneebone A, Mameghan H, Bolin T, et al. The effect of oral sucralfate on the acute proctitis associated with prostate radiotherapy: a double-blind, randomized trial. *Int J Radiat Oncol Biol Phys.* 2001;51:628–635.
89. Stellamans K, Lievens Y, Lambin P, et al. Does sucralfate reduce early side effects of pelvic radiation? A double-blind randomized trial. *Radiother Oncol.* 2003;65:105–108.
90. Pinto A, Fidalgo P, Cravo M, et al. Short chain fatty acids are effective in short-term treatment of chronic radiation proctitis. *Dis Colon Rectum.* 1999;42:788–796.
91. al-Sabbagh R, Sinicrope FA, Sellin JH, et al. Evaluation of short-chain fatty acid enemas: treatment of radiation proctitis. *Am J Gastroenterol.* 1996;91:1814–1816.
92. Vernia P, Fracasso PL, Casale V, et al. Topical butyrate for acute radiation proctitis: randomised, crossover trial. *Lancet.* 2000;356:1232–1235.
93. Talley N, Chen F, King D, et al. Short-chain fatty acids in the treatment of radiation proctitis: a randomized, double-blind, placebo-controlled, cross-over trial. *Dis Colon Rectum.* 1997;40:1046–1050.
94. Rubinstein E, Ibsen T, Rasmussen RB, et al. Formalin treatment of radiation-induced hemorrhagic proctitis. *Am J Gastroenterol.* 1986;81:44–45.
95. Saclarides TJ, King DJ, Franklin JL, et al. Formalin instillation for refractory radiation-induced hemorrhagic proctitis. *Dis Colon Rectum.* 1996;39:196–199.
96. Counter SF, Froese DP, Hart MJ. Prospective evaluation of formalin therapy for radiation proctitis. *Am J Surg.* 1999;177:396–398.
97. Jensen DM, Machicado GA, Cheng S, et al. A randomized prospective study of endoscopic bipolar electrocoagulation and heater probe treatment of chronic rectal bleeding from radiation telangiectasia. *Gastrointest Endosc.* 1997;45:20–25.
98. Leuchter RS, Petrilli ES, Dwyer RM, et al. Nd:YAG laser therapy of rectosigmoid bleeding due to radiation injury. *Obstet Gynecol.* 1982;59(S6):65–67.
99. Taylor JG, Disario JA, Buchi KN. Argon laser therapy for hemorrhagic radiation proctopathy: long term results. *Gastrointest Endosc.* 1993;39:641–644.
100. Carbatzas C, Spencer GM, Thorpe SM, et al. Nd:Yag laser treatment for bleeding from radiation proctitis. *Endoscopy.* 1996;28:497–500.
101. Taylor JG, Disario JA, Bjorkman DJ. KTP laser therapy for bleeding from chronic radiation proctopathy. *Gastrointest Endosc.* 2000;52:353–357.
102. Fantin AC, Binek J, Suter WR, et al. Argon beam coagulation for treatment of symptomatic radiation-induced proctitis. *Gastrointest Endosc.* 1999;49:515–518.
103. Tam W, Moore J, Schoeman M. Treatment of radiation proctitis with argon plasma coagulation. *Endoscopy.* 2000;32:667–672.
104. Smith S, Wallner K, Dominitz JA, et al. Argon beam coagulation for rectal bleeding after prostate brachytherapy. *Int J Radiat Oncol Biol Phys.* 2001;51:636–646.
105. Kaassis M, Oberti E, Burtin P, et al. Argon plasma coagulation for the treatment of hemorrhagic radiation proctitis. *Endoscopy.* 2002;32:673–676.
106. Zimmermann FB, Feldmann HJ. Radiation proctitis. Clinical and pathological manifestations, therapy and prophylaxis of acute and late injurious effects of radiation on the rectal mucosa. *Strahlenther Onkol.* 1998;174(S3):85–89.
107. Feldmeier JJ, Heimbach RD, Davolt DA, et al. Hyperbaric oxygen an adjunctive treatment for delayed radiation injuries of the abdomen and pelvis. *Undersea Hyperb Med.* 1996;24:215–216.
108. Moon RE, Feldmeier JJ. Hyperbaric oxygen: an evidence based approach to its application. *Undersea Hyperb Med.* 2002;29:1–3.
109. De Micheli C, Fornengo P, Bosio A, et al. Severe radiation-induced proctitis treated with botulinum anatoxin type A. *J Clin Oncol.* 2003;21:2627.
110. Kennedy M, Bruninga K, Mutlu EA, et al. Successful and sustained treatment of chronic radiation proctitis with antioxidant vitamins E and C. *Am J Gastroenterol.* 2001;96: 1080–1084.
111. Benson AB, Ajani AJ, Catalano RB, et al. Recommended guidelines for the treatment of cancer treatment-induced diarrhea. *J Clin Oncol.* 2004;22:2918–2926.
112. Rubenstein EB, Peterson DE, Schubert M, et al. Clinical practice guidelines for the prevention and treatment of cancer therapy-induced oral and gastrointestinal mucositis. *Cancer.* 2004;100:2026–2046.
113. Feyer PC, Maranzano E, Molassiotis A, et al. Radiotherapy-induced nausea and vomiting (RINV): antiemetic guidelines. *Support Care Cancer.* 2005;13:123–128.
114. Keefe DM, Schubert MM, Elting LS, et al. Updated clinical practice guidelines for the prevention and treatment of mucositis. *Cancer.* 2007;109:820–831.
115. Epperly MW, Travis EL, Sikora C, et al. Magnesium superoxide dismutase (MnSOD) plasmid/liposome pulmonary radioprotective gene therapy: modulation of irradiation-induced mRNA for IL-I, TNF-α, and TGF-β correlates with delay of organizing alveolitis/fibrosis. *Biol Blood Marrow Transplant.* 1999;5:204–214.
116. Stickle RL, Epperly MW, Klein E, et al. Prevention of irradiation-induced esophagitis by plasmid/liposome delivery of the human manganese superoxide dismutase transgene. *Radiat Oncol Invest.* 1999;7:204–217.
117. Guo H, Wolfe D, Epperly MW, et al. Gene transfer of human manganese superoxide dismutase protects small intestinal villi from radiation injury. *J Gastrointest Surg.* 2003;7: 229–236.
118. Lefaix JL, Delanian S, Leplat JJ, et al. Successful treatment of radiation-induced fibrosis using Cu/ZN-SOD and Mn-SOD: an experimental study. *Int J Radiat Oncol Biol Phys.* 1996;35:305–312.
119. Delanian S, Baillet F, Huart J, et al. Successful treatment of radiation-induced fibrosis using liposomal Cu/Zn superoxide dismutase: clinical trial. *Radiother Oncol.* 1994;32:12–20.
120. Lindegaard JC, Grau C. Has the outlook improved for amifostine as a clinical radioprotector? *Radiother Oncol.* 2000;57:113–118.
121. Ito H, Meistrich ML, Barkley T, et al. Protection of acute and late radiation damage of the gastrointestinal tract by WR-2721. *Int J Radiat Oncol Biol Phys.* 1986;12:211–219.
122. Carroll MP, Zera RT, Roberts JC, et al. Efficacy of radioprotective agents in preventing small and large bowel radiation injury. *Dis Colon Rectum.* 1995;38:716–722.
123. Kouvaris J, Kouloulias V, Malas E, et al. Amifostine as radioprotective agent for the rectal mucosa during irradiation of pelvic tumors. A phase II randomized study using various toxicity scales and rectosigmoidoscopy. *Strahlenther Onkol.* 2003;179:167–174.
124. Athanassious H, Antonadou D, Coliarakis N, et al. Protective effect of amifostine during frationated radiotherapy in patients with pelvic carcinomas: results of a randomized trial. *Int J Radiat Oncol Biol Phys.* 2003;56:1154–1160.
125. Delaney JP, Bonsack ME, Felemovicius I. Radioprotection of the rat small intestine with topical WR-2721. *Cancer.* 1994;74:2379–2384.
126. Ben-Josef E, Han S, Tobi M, et al. Intrarectal application of amifostine for the prevention of radiation-induced rectal injury. *Semin Radiat Oncol.* 2002;12:81–85.
127. Menard C, Camphausen K, Muanza T, et al. Clinical trial of endorectal amifostine for radioprotection in patients with prostate cancer: rationale and early results. *Semin Radiat. Oncol.* 2003;30:63–67.
128. Dion MW, Hussey DH, Doornbos JF, et al. Preliminary results of a pilot study of pentoxifylline in the treatment of late radiation soft tissue necrosis. *Int J Radiat Oncol Biol Phys.* 1990;19:401–407.
129. Delanian S, Balla-Mekias S, Lefaix JL. Striking regression of chronic radiotherapy damage in a clinical trial of combined pentoxifylline and tocopherol. *J Clin Oncol.* 1999;17:3283–3290.
130. Koh W, Stelzer KJ, Peterson LM, et al. Effect of pentoxifylline on radiation-induced lung and skin toxicity in rats. *Int J Radiat Oncol Biol Phys.* 1994;31:71–77.
131. Tamou S, Trott KR. Modification of late radiation damage in the rectum of rats by deproteinized calf blood serum (ActoHorm) and pentoxifylline (PTX). *Strahlenther Onkol.* 1994;170:415–420.
132. Hanson WR, Thomas C. 16,16-Dimethyl prostaglandin E2 increases survival of murine intestinal stem cells when given before photon radiation. *Radiat Res.* 1983;96:393–398.
133. Tomas-de la Vega JE, Banner BF, Hubbard M, et al. Cytoprotective effect of prostaglandin E2 in irradiated rat ileum. *Surg Gynecol Obstet.* 1984;158:39–45.
134. Keelan M, Walker K, Cheeseman CI, et al. Two weeks of oral synthetic E2 prostaglandin (enprostil) improves the intestinal morphological but not the absorptive response in the rat to abdominal irradiation. *Digestion.* 1992;53:101–107.
135. Delaney JP, Bonsack ME, Felemovicius I. Misoprostol in the intestinal lumen protects against radiation injury of the mucosa of the small bowel. *Radiat Res.* 1994;137:405–409.
136. Khan AM, Birk JW, Anderson JC, et al. A prospective randomized placebo-controlled double-blinded pilot study of misoprostol rectal suppositories in the prevention of acute and chronic radiation proctitis syndrome in prostate cancer patients. *Am J Gastroenterol.* 2000;95:1961–1966.
137. Rowe JK, Zera RT, Madoff RD, et al. Protective effect of RibCys following high-dose irradiation of the rectosigmoid. *Dis Colon Rectum.* 1993;36:681–688.
138. Delaney JP, Bonsack M, Hall P. Intestinal radioprotection by two new agents applied topically. *Ann Surg.* 1992;216:417–422.
139. Felemovicius I, Bonsack ME, Griffin RJ, et al. Radioprotection of the rat intestinal mucosa by tirilazad. *Int J Radiat Biol.* 1998;73:219–223.
140. Bonsack ME, Felemovicius I, Baptista ML, et al. Radioprotection of the intestinal mucosa of rats by probucol. *Radiat Res.* 1999;151:69–73.
141. Beyzadeoglu M, Balkan M, Demiriz M, et al. Protective effect of vitamin A on acute radiation injury in the small intestine. *Radiat Med.* 1997;15:1–5.
142. Felemovicius I, Bonsack ME, Baptista ML, et al. Intestinal radioprotection by vitamin E (alpha-tocopherol). *Ann Surg.* 1995;222:504–510.
143. Wu SG, Miyamoto T. Radioprotection of the intestinal crypts of mice by recombinant human interleukin-1 alpha. *Radiat Res.* 1990;123:112–115.
144. Hancock SL, Chung RT, Cox RS, et al. Interleukin 1 beta initially sensitizes and subsequently protects murine intestinal stem cells exposed to photon radiation. *Cancer Res.* 1991;51:2280–2285.
145. Welniak LA, Khaled AR, Anver MR, et al. Gastrointestinal cells of IL-7 receptor null mice exhibit increased sensitivity to irradiation. *J Immunol.* 2001;166:2923–2928.
146. Potten CS. Protection of the small intestinal clonogenic stem cells from radiation-induced damage by pretreatment with interleukin 11 also increases murine survival time. *Stem Cells.* 1996;14:452–459.
147. Potten CS. Interleukin-11 protects the clonogenic stem cells in murine small-intestinal crypts from impairment of their reproductive capacity by radiation. *Int J Cancer.* 1995;62:356–361.
148. Orazi A, Du X, Yang Z, et al. Interleukin-11 prevents apoptosis and accelerates recovery of small intestinal mucosa in mice treated with combined chemotherapy and radiation. *Lab Invest.* 1996;75:33–42.
149. Boerma M, Wang J, Burnett AF, et al. Local administration of interleukin-11 ameliorates intestinal radiation injury. *Cancer Res.* 2007;67:9501–9506.
150. Okunieff P, Mester M, Wang J, et al. In vivo radioprotective effects of angiogenic growth factors on the small bowel of C3H mice. *Radiat Res.* 1998;150:204–211.
151. Paris F, Fuks Z, Kang A, et al. Endothelial apoptosis as the primary lesion initiating intestinal radiation damage in mice. *Science.* 2001;293:293–297.
152. Farrell CL, Bready JV, Rex KL, et al. Keratinocyte growth factor protects mice from chemotherapy and radiation-induced gastrointestinal injury and mortality. *Cancer Res.* 1998;58:933–939.
153. Khan WB, Shui C, Ning S, et al. Enhancement of murine intestinal stem cell survival after irradiation by keratinocyte growth factor. *Radiat Res.* 1997;148:248–253.
154. Zheng H, Wang J, Koteliansky VE, et al. Recombinant soluble transforming growth factor-β type II receptor ameliorates radiation enteropathy in the mouse. *Gastroenterology.* 2000;119:1286–1296.
155. Boerma M, Wang J, Corbley MJ, Hauer-Jensen M. Targeting TGF-β as a strategy to ameliorate intestinal side effects of radiation therapy. In: *Transforming Growth Factor-beta in Cancer Therapy.* Vol 2. Totawa, NJ: Humana Press; 2008:589–608.
156. Leigh BR, Khan W, Hancock SL, et al. Stem cell factor enhances the survival of murine intestinal stem cells after photon irradiation. *Radiat Res.* 1995;142:12–15.
157. Howarth GS, Fraser R, Frisby CL, et al. Effects of insulin-like growth factor-I administration on radiation enteritis in the rat. *Scand J Gastroenterol.* 1997;32:1118–1124.
158. Vazquez I, Gomez-de-Segura IA, Grande AG, et al. Protective effect of enriched diet plus growth hormone administration on radiation-induced intestinal injury and on its evolutionary pattern in the rat. *Dig Dis Sci.* 1999;44:2350–2358.

159. Silver DF, Simon A, Dubin NH, et al. Recombinant growth hormone's effects on the strength and thickness of radiation-injured ileal anastomoses: a rat model. *J Surg Res.* 1999;85:66–70.
160. Arango V, Ettarh RR, Holden G, et al. BB-10010, an analog of macrophage inflammatory protein-1α, protects murine small intestine against radiation. *Dig Dis Sci.* 2001;46:2608–2614.
161. Brown MS, Buchanan RB, Karran SJ. Clinical observations on the effects of elemental diet supplementation during irradiation. *Clin Radiol.* 1980;31:19–20.
162. Craighead PS, Young S. Phase II study assessing the feasibility of using elemental supplements to reduce acute enteritis in patients receiving radical pelvic radiotherapy. *Am J Clin Oncol.* 1998;21:573–578.
163. Douglass HO, Milliron S, Nava H, et al. Elemental diet as an adjuvant for patients with locally advanced gastrointestinal cancer receiving radiation therapy: a prospectively randomized study. *J Parenter Enteral Nutr.* 1978;2:682–686.
164. Foster KJ, Brown MS, Alberti KG, et al. The metabolic effects of abdominal irradiation in man with and without dietary therapy with and elemental diet. *Clin Radiol.* 1980;31:13–17.
165. McArdle AH, Reid EC, Laplante MP, et al. Prophylaxis against radiation injury. The use of elemental diet prior to and during radiotherapy for invasive bladder cancer and in early postoperative feeding following radical cystectomy and ileal conduit. *Arch Surg.* 1986;121:879–885.
166. Klimberg VS, Souba WW, Olson DJ, et al. Prophylactic glutamine protects intestinal mucosa from radiation injury. *Cancer.* 1990;66:62–68.
167. Campos FG, Waitzberg DL, Mucerino DR, et al. Protective effects of glutamine enriched diets on acute actinic enteritis. *Nutricion Hospitalaria.* 1996;11:167–177.
168. McArdle AH. Elemental diets in treatment of gastrointestinal injury. *Adv Biosci.* 1994;94:201–206.
169. Hwang JM, Chan DC, Chang TM, et al. Effects of oral arginine and glutamine on radiation-induced injury in the rat. *J Surg Res.* 2003;109:149–154.
170. Kozelsky TF, Meyers GE, Sloan JA, et al. Phase III double-blind study of glutamine versus placebo for the prevention of acute diarrhea in patients receiving pelvic radiation therapy. *J Clin Oncol.* 2003;21:1669–1674.
171. Booth C, Booth D, Williamson S, et al. Teduglutide ([Gly2]GLP-2) protects small intestinal stem cells from radiation damage. *Cell Prolif.* 2004;37:385–400.
172. Torres S, Thim L, Milliat F, et al. Glucagon-like peptide-2 improves both acute and late experimental radiation enteritis in the rat. *Int J Radiat Oncol Biol Phys.* 2007;69:1583–1571.
173. Mennie AT, Dalley VM, Dinneen LC, et al. Treatment of radiation-induced gastrointestinal distress with acetylsalicylate. *Lancet.* 1975;2:942–943.
174. Stryker JA, Demers LM, Mortel R. Prophylactic ibuprofen administration during pelvic irradiation. *Int J Radiat Oncol Biol Phys.* 1979;5:2049–2052.
175. Kilic D, Egehan I, Ozenirler S, et al. Double-blinded, randomized, placebo-controlled study to evaluate the effectiveness of sulphasalazine in preventing acute gastrointestinal complications due to radiotherapy. *Radiother Oncol.* 2000;57:125–129.
176. Freund U, Scholmerich J, Siems H, et al. Unwanted side-effects in using mesalazine (5-aminosalicylic acid) during radiotherapy. *Strahlenther Onkol.* 1987;163:678–680.
177. Baughan CA, Canney PA, Buchanan RB, et al. A randomized trial to assess the efficacy of 5-aminosalicylic acid for the prevention of radiation enteritis. *Clin Oncol.* 1993;5:19–24.
178. Martenson JA, Hyland G, Moertel CG, et al. Olsalazine is contraindicated during pelvic radiation therapy: results of a double-blind randomized clinical trial. *Int J Radiat Oncol Biol Phys.* 1996;35:299–303.
179. Resbeut M, Marteau P, Cowen D, et al. A randomized double blind placebo controlled multicenter study of mesalazine for the prevention of acute radiation enteritis. *Radiother Oncol.* 1997;44:59–63.
180. Baum CA, Biddle WL, Miner PB. Failure of 5-aminosalicylic acid enemas to improve chronic radiation proctitis. *Dig Dis Sci.* 1989;34:758–760.
181. Boerma M, Wang J, Richter KK, et al. Orazipone, a locally acting immunomodulator, ameliorates intestinal radiation injury: a preclinical study in a novel rat model. *Int J Radiat Oncol Biol Phys.* 2006;66:552–559.
182. Salminen E, Elomaa I, Minkkinen J, et al. Preservation of intestinal integrity during radiotherapy using live Lactobacillus acidopheles cultures. *Clin Radiol.* 1988;39:435–437.
183. Sokol AB, Lipson LW, Morgenstern L, et al. Protection against lethal irradiation injury by pancreatic enzyme exclusion. *Surg Forum.* 1967;18:387–389.
184. Morgenstern L, Patin CS, Krohn HL, et al. Prolongation of survival in lethally irradiated dogs. *Arch Surg.* 1970;101:586–589.
185. Rachootin S, Shapiro S, Yamakawa T, et al. Potent anti-protease from Ascaris lumbricoides: Efficacy in amelioration of post-radiation enteropathy [Abstract]. *Gastroenterology.* 1972;62:796.
186. Weckbecker G, Liu R, Tolcsvai L, et al. Antiproliferative effects of the somatostatin analogue octreotide (SMS 201–995) on ZR-75–1 human breast cancer cells in vivo and in vitro. *Cancer Res.* 1992;52:4973–4978.
187. Weckbecker G, Tolcsvai L, Liu R, et al. Preclinical studies on the anticancer activity of the somatostatin analogue octreotide (SMS 201–995). *Metabolism.* 1992;41(suppl 2):99–103.
188. Weckbecker G, Tolcsvai L, Pollak M, et al. Somatostatin analogue octreotide enhances the antineoplastic effects of tamoxifen and ovariectomy on 7,12-dimethylbenz(a)anthracene-induced rat mammary carcinomas. *Cancer Res.* 1994;54:6334–6337.
189. Patel PC, Barrie R, Hill N, et al. Postreceptor signal transduction mechanisms involved in octreotide-induced inhibition of angiogenesis. *Surgery.* 1994;116:1148–1152.
190. Richter KK, Fink LM, Hughes BM, et al. Is the loss of endothelial thrombomodulin involved in the mechanism of chronicity in late radiation enteropathy? *Radiother Oncol.* 1997;44:65–71.
191. Wang J, Zheng H, Ou X, et al. Deficiency of microvascular thrombomodulin and upregulation of protease-activated receptor 1 in irradiated rat intestine: possible link between endothelial dysfunction and chronic radiation fibrosis. *Am J Pathol.* 2002;160:2063–2072.
192. Wang J, Albertson CM, Zheng H, et al. Short-term inhibition of ADP-induced platelet aggregation by clopidogrel ameliorates radiation-induced toxicity in rat small intestine. *Thromb Haemost.* 2002;87:122–128.
193. Albertson CM, Wang J, Zheng H, et al. Recombinant hirudin, a direct thrombin inhibitor, ameliorates radiation enteropathy [Abstract]. *Am J Clin Pathol.* 2000;114:300.
194. Wang J, Boerma M, Fu Q, et al. Simvastatin ameliorates radiation enteropathy development after localized, fractionated irradiation by a protein C-independent mechanism. *Int J Radiat Oncol Biol Phys.* 2007;68:1483–1490.
195. Haydont V, Bourgier C, Pocard M, et al. Pravastatin inhibits the Rho/CCN2/extracellular matrix cascade in human fibrosis explants and improves radiation-induced intestinal fibrosis in rats. *Clin Cancer Res.* 2007;13:5331–5340.
196. Irwin BC, Gupta R, Kim K, et al. Calcium channel blockers may radiosensitize patients to radiation proctitis while statins, NSAIDs may radioprotect: a case-control study (abstr.). *Gastroenterology.* 2006;130(s2):A460.
197. Christensen HD, Haley TJ. Distribution of substance P in the central nervous system and small intestine of the rat after X-irradiation. *Radiat Res.* 1968;33:588–595.
198. Esposito V, Linard C, Maubert C, et al. Modulation of gut substance P after whole-body irradiation. A new pathological feature. *Dig Dis Sci.* 1996;41:2070–2077.
199. Hockerfelt U, Franzen L, Kjorell U, et al. Parallel increase in substance P and VIP in rat duodenum in response to irradiation. *Peptides.* 2000;21:271–281.
200. Forsgren S, Hockerfelt U, Norrgard O, et al. Pronounced substance P innervation in irradiation-induced enteropathy—a study on human colon. *Regul Pept.* 2000;88:1–13.
201. Esposito V, Linard C, Wysocki J, et al. A substance P receptor antagonist (FK 888) modifies gut alterations induced by ionizing radiation. *Int J Radiat Biol.* 1998;74:625–632.
202. Alfieri AB, Gardner CJ. Effects of GR203040, an NK1 antagonist, on radiation- and cisplatin-induced tissue damage in the ferret. *Gen Pharmacol.* 1998;31:741–746.
203. Zheng H, Wang J, Hauer-Jensen M. Role of mast cells in early and delayed radiation injury in rat intestine. *Radiat Res.* 2000;153:533–539.
204. Wang J, Zheng H, Kulkarni A, et al. Regulation of early and delayed radiation responses in rat small intestine by capsaicin-sensitive nerves. *Int J Radiat Oncol Biol Phys.* 2006;64:1528–1536.
205. Wang J, Qiu X, Kulkarni A, et al. Calcitonin gene-related peptide and substance P regulate the intestinal radiation response. *Clin Cancer Res.* 2006;12:4112–4118.
206. Quastler H, Lanzl EF, Keller ME, et al. Acute intestinal radiation death. Studies on roentgen death in mice, III. *Am J Physiol.* 1951;164:546–556.
207. Osborne JW. Prevention of intestinal radiation death by removal of the irradiated intestine. *Radiat Res.* 1956;4:541–546.
208. Terry NHA, Travis EL. The influence of bone marrow depletion on intestinal radiation damage. *Int J Radiat Oncol Biol Phys.* 1989;17:569–573.
209. Monti P, Wysocki J, van der Meeren A, et al. The contribution of radiation-induced injury to the gastrointestinal tract in the development of multi-organ dysfunction syndrome or failure. *Br J Radiol.* 2005;(suppl 27):89–94.
210. Hauer-Jensen M, Kumar KS, Wang J, et al. Intestinal toxicity in radiation- and combined injury: significance, mechanisms, and countermeasures. In: Larche RA, ed. *Global Terrorism Issues and Developments.* Hauppauge, NY: Nova Science Publishers; 2008.
211. Empey LR, Papp JD, Jewell LD, et al. Mucosal protective effects of vitamin E and misoprostol during acute radiation-induced enteritis in rats. *Dig Dis Sci.* 1992;37:205–214.
212. Kumar KS, Srinivasan V, Toles R, et al. Nutritional approaches to radioprotection: Vitamin E. *Mil Med.* 2002;167:57–59.
213. Kumar KS, Ghosh SP, Hauer-Jensen M. Gamma-tocotrienol: potential as a countermeasure against radiological threat. In: Watson RR, Preedy VR, eds. *Tocotrienols: Vitamin E Beyond Tocopherols.* Boca Raton, FL: CRC Press; 2009:379–398.
214. Berbee M, Fu Q, Boerma M, et al. Gamma-tocotrienol ameliorates intestinal radiation injury and reduces vascular oxidative stress after total body irradiation by an HMG-CoA reductase-dependent mechanism. *Radiat Res.* 2009;171:596–605.
215. Ghosh SP, Kulkarni S, Hieber K, et al. Gamma-tocotrienol, a tocol antioxidant as a potent radiation countermeasure. *Int J Radiat Biol.* 2009;85:598–606.
216. Kumar KS, Vaishnav YN, Weiss JF. Radioprotection by antioxidant enzymes and enzyme mimetics. *Pharmac Ther.* 1988;39:301–309.
217. Rong Y, Doctrow SR, Tocco G, et al. EUK-134, a synthetic superoxide dismutase and catalase mimetic, prevents oxidative stress and attenuates kainate-induced neuropathology. *Proc Natl Acad Sci U S A.* 1999;96:9897–9902.
218. Vujaskovic Z, Batinic-Haberle I, Rabbani ZN, et al. A small molecular weight catalytic metalloporphyrin antioxidant with superoxide dismutase (SOD) mimetic properties protects lungs from radiation-induced injury. *Free Radical Biol Med.* 2002;33:857–863.
219. Monobe M, Hino M, Sumi M, et al. Protective effects of melatonin on gamma-ray induced intestinal damage. *Int J Radiat Biol.* 2005;81:855–860.
220. Vijayalaxmi, Meltz ML, Reiter RJ, et al. Melatonin and protection from whole-body irradiation: survival studies in mice. *Mutation Res.* 1999;425:21–27.
221. Keskek M, Gocmen E, Kilic M, et al. Increased expression of cyclooxygenase-2 (COX-2) in radiation-induced small bowel injury in rats. *J Surg Res.* 2006;135:76–84.
222. Kumar KS, Srinivasan V, Palazzolo D, et al. Synergistic protection of irradiated mice by a combination of iloprost and misoprostol. *Adv Exp Med Biol.* 1997;400B:831–839.
223. Yada S, Nukina H, Kishihara K, et al. IL-7 prevents both capsase-dependent and -independent pathways that lead to the spontaneous apoptosis of i-IEL. *Cell Immunol.* 2001;208:88–95.
224. Lai YG, Gelfanov V, Gelfanova V, et al. IL-15 promotes survival but not effector function differentiation of CD8+ TCRalphabeta+ intestinal intraepithelial lymphocytes. *J Immunol.* 1999;163:5843–5850.
225. Lugering N, Kucharzik T, Maaser C, et al. Interleukin-15 strongly inhibits interleukin-8 and monocyte chemoattractant protein-1 production in human colonic epithelial cells. *Immunology.* 1999;98:504–509.
226. Reinecker HC, MacDermott RP, Mirau S, et al. Intestinal epithelial cells both express and respond to interleukin 15. *Gastroenterology.* 1996;111:1706–1713.

227. Cao S, Black JD, Troutt AB, et al. Interleukin 15 offers selective protection from irinotecan-induced intestinal toxicity in a preclinical animal model. *Cancer Res.* 1998;58: 3270–3274.

228. Houchen CW, George RJ, Sturmoski MA, et al. FGF-2 enhances intestinal stem cell survival and its expression is induced after radiation injury. *Am J Physiol.* 1999;39:G249-G258.

229. Krause P, Ziegler K. Experimentelle Untersuchungen ueber die Einwirkung der Roentgenstrahlen auf tierische Gewebe. A. Uebersicht ueber die in der Litteratur niedergelegten Angaben ueber die Wirkung der Roentgenstrahlen auf innere Organe. *Fortschr a d Geb d Roentgenstr.* 1906;10:126–182.

230. Bealmear PM, Holtermann OA, Mirand EA. Radiation pathology and treatment. In: Coates ME, Gustafsson BE, eds. *The Germ-free Animal in Biomedical Research.* London: Laboratory Animals Ltd;1984:413–434.

231. Wilson R, Bealmear P, Matsuzawa T. Acute intestinal radiation death in germfree and conventional mice. In: Sullivan MF, ed.*Gastrointestinal Radiation Injury.* Amsterdam: Excerpta Medica Foundation: Amsterdam; 1968:148–158.

232. Mastromarino AJ, Wilson R. Increased intestinal mucosal turnover and radiosensitivity to supralethal whole-body irradiation resulting from cholic acid-induced alterations of the microecology of germfree CFW mice. *Radiat Res.* 1976;66:393–400.

233. Mastromarino AJ, Wilson R. Antibiotic radioprotection of mice exposed to supralethal whole- body irradiation independent of antibacterial activity. *Radiat Res.* 1976;68: 329–338.

234. Spratt JS, Heinbecker P, Saltzstein SL. The influence of succinylsulphathiazole (Sulfasuxidine) upon the response of canine small intestine to irradiation. *Cancer.* 1961;14: 862–874.

235. Toorop-Bouma AG, Van der Waaij D. The effect of selective decontamination of the GI-tract of mice on the survival of intestinal mucosa during X-irradiation. In: Wostmann BS, ed. *Germfree Research.* New York, NY: Alan R. Liss, Inc.; 1985:271–273.

236. Geraci JP, Jackson KL, Mariano MS. Effect of pseudomonas contamination or antibiotic decontamination of the GI tract on acute radiation lethality after neutron or gamma irradiation. *Radiat Res.* 1985;104:395–405.

237. Kumar KS, Srinivasan V, Toles RE, et al. High-dose antibiotic therapy is superior to a 3-drug combination of prostanoids and lipid A derivative in protecting irradiated canines. *J Radiat Res.* 2002;43:361–370.

238. Urbancsek H, Kazar T, Mezes I, et al. Results of a double-blind, randomized study to evaluate the efficacy and safety of antibiophilus in patients with radiation-induced diarrhoea. *Eur J Gastroenterol Hepatol.* 2001;13:391–396.

239. Morgenstern L, Hiatt N. Injurious effect of pancreatic secretions on postradiation enteropathy. *Gastroenterology.* 1967;53:923–929.

240. Fu Q, Berbee M, Boerma M, et al. The somatostatin analog SOM230 (pasireotide) ameliorates injury of the intestinal mucosa and increases survival after total body irradiation by inhibiting exocrine pancreatic secretion. *Radiat Res.* 2009;171:698–707.

241. Burdelya LG, Krivokrysenko VI, Tallant TC, et al. An agonist of Toll-like receptor 5 has radioprotective activity in mouse and primate models. *Science.* 2008;320:226–230.

242. Tseng CM, Albert L, Peterson RL, et al. In vivo absorption properties of orally administered recombinant human interleukin-11. *Pharm Res.* 2000;17:482–485.

243. Cotreau MM, Stonis L, Strahs A, et al. A multiple-dose, safety, tolerability, pharmacokinetics and pharmacodynamic study of oral recombinant human interleukin-11 (oprelvekin). *Biopharm Drug Dispos.* 2004;25:291–296.

Christopher G. Willett
Brian G. Czito

Pancreas

INTRODUCTION

With the increased use of radiation therapy in the management of upper abdominal malignancies, including neoplasms arising from the colon, liver, esophagus, stomach, pancreas, biliary tree, retroperitoneum, lymph nodes and small bowel, and the resultant prolonged survival and cures in these patients, consideration of potential complications of this treatment is required. The tolerance of the spinal cord, kidneys, small bowel, stomach, large bowel, and other GI viscera to fractionated radiation therapy has been defined and incorporated into routine treatment practice. In contrast, the potential early and late effects of fractionated radiation therapy on the normal pancreas are poorly understood, do not usually directly impact clinical practice, and remain an opportunity for further investigation and knowledge. This chapter summarizes current data regarding pathologic and physiologic changes in the pancreas induced by radiation therapy.

ANATOMY AND PHYSIOLOGY

The pancreas lies in the upper abdominal retroperitoneum at about the level of the first two lumbar vertebra. It is divided into the head (including the portion called the *uncinate process*), neck, body and tail. It has intimate contact with surrounding organs including stomach, duodenum, jejunum, kidney, and spleen, as well as major vessels (Fig. 39.1). The exocrine secretions of the pancreas enter the duodenum by the ducts of Santorini and Wirsung.[1] Pancreatic endocrine secretions enter the blood by the way of the rich capillary beds of the islets of Langerhans. A thin cover of connective tissue penetrates the pancreas, dividing it into lobules. With H&E staining, the dark cuboidal acinar cells form small glands, part of the walls of which consist of a clear cell or two from the terminal intercalated ducts.[1] The cytoplasm of the acinar cells contains protein-rich granules that release enzymes into the pancreatic duct system in response to cholecystokinin produced by the neuroendocrine cells of the duodenum. A watery, bicarbonate-rich secretion that neutralizes gastric acid/gastric chyme is produced by the intercalated duct cells, also in response to secretions from duodenal endocrine cells. Columnar cells with occasional goblet cells line the interlobular and major ducts. The islets of Langerhans, measuring about 100 mm in diameter, constituted

by cords of cuboidal cells including alpha, beta, and delta cells that secrete insulin, glucagon, somatostatin, respectively, into a rich capillary network. The acinar, duct, and islet cells have a slow turnover and are judged to be "radioresistant."[1] It is also known that following radiation therapy, bicarbonate and enzyme secretion can decrease. The acinar cells are the most radiosensitive, the duct cells less so, and the islet cells the least radiosensitive of all. In the pancreas, the vascular and connective tissues appear to have the same radiosensitivity as tissues elsewhere in the body.

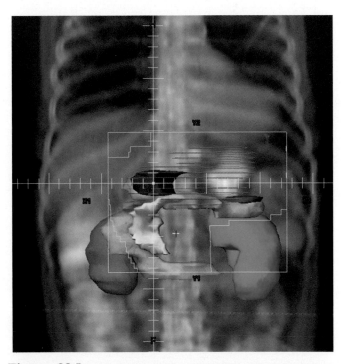

Figure 39.1. Digitally reconstructed radiograph demonstrating a radiation treatment field in a 54-year-old male with clinical T3 N1 adenocarcinoma of the distal stomach receiving preoperative chemoradiotherapy. Note relative anatomic position of the pancreas (*yellow*) in relationship to the duodenum (*light green*), stomach (*striated pink*), gross tumor (*red*), right kidney (*orange*), left kidney (*blue*), and splenic hilum (*dark green*). The entirety of the pancreas may sometimes be incidentally included in the radiation treatment fields of the upper abdominal malignancies.

EXPERIMENTAL STUDIES

Seminal studies from Colorado State University have provided invaluable data of the effects of intraoperative radiation (IORT), external beam radiation therapy (EBRT), and the combination of both on critical normal tissues including normal pancreas, using a canine model.[2,3] In one study, 24 beagle dogs underwent Billroth-II gastrojejunostomy followed by IORT with 6-MeV electrons, using a dose range from 17.5 to 40 Gy.[2] Six control dogs received Billroth-II surgery alone. Starting two weeks after surgery, dogs in the radiation group received an additional 50 Gy in 2-Gy fractions over 5 weeks using EBRT with 6-MeV x-ray to the pancreas and duodenum. Dogs were then monitored for 135 days and subsequently necropsied. Gross and histopathological changes in the pancreas and duodenum were evaluated and quantitative analysis of pancreatic lesions performed. Duodenal ulcers were found following 32.5 and 40 Gy of IORT. The pancreases were atrophic in irradiated dogs and exocrine pancreatic insufficiency occurred in one dog given 25 Gy by IORT. Gross pancreatic atrophy correlated with IORT dose. Histopathological evidence of radiation damage to the pancreas was observed in acinar cells. Islet cell injury was not apparent, although pancreatic fibrosis and damage to blood vessels and ducts were seen. Dose-response relationships were observed for the index of damage to the pancreas as a whole as measured by pancreatic fibrosis and a decrease in acinar cells. Although 25-Gy IORT plus 50-Gy EBRT was tolerated by the duodenum and pancreas up to 135 days, these doses may cause later pancreatic injury as an expression of damage to blood vessels and ducts. Exocrine pancreatic insufficiency and diabetes mellitus may thus represent potential late complications of IORT following doses of 25 Gy or higher.

In addition to the above studies, the dogs were monitored clinically and exocrine pancreatic function evaluated using an N-benzoyl-l-tyrosyl-para-aminobenzoic acid test (BT-PABA) between 3 and 135 days postoperatively.[3] As with gross pancreatic atrophy, the mean percentage of normal acinar cells correlated with IORT doses as well as with BT-PABA values ($p < 0.1$). Weight loss was significantly greater in the irradiated dogs compared to the control animals and the mean percentage of body weight correlated with mean plasma PABA values ($p < 0.01$). The use of BT-PABA to evaluate progressive exocrine pancreatic function following IORT and EBRT showed an expected trend. A progressive decrease in exocrine pancreatic function in the irradiated dogs (as determined by plasma PABA levels) may have been partly due to late radiation damage to acinar cells, secondary to vascular and ductal damage. At 135 days postoperatively, none of the dogs showed clinical signs of pancreatic insufficiency and the plasma PABA levels were within the presurgical range. The progressive decrease in plasma PABA levels indicated a potential for late development of exocrine pancreatic insufficiency. Therefore, the BT-PABA test could be useful for evaluating the progressive decrease in exocrine pancreatic function and residual radiation injury to the pancreas. Because exocrine deficiency can be well managed with replacement therapy, pancreatic injury may not be a serious complication after doses of 30-Gy IORT with 50-Gy EBRT.

In a Japanese study, the early and late effects of IORT on the exocrine and endocrine functions of the residual pancreas were assessed in patients undergoing pancreatic head resection.[4] Of 54 patients studied, 20 underwent IORT and the other 34 did not. Thirteen of 20 patients receiving IORT also received postoperative EBRT. Fasting blood sugar level, the 120-minute value following 75-g oral glucose intake (tolerance test or OGTT), BT-PABA excretion value (a pancreatic exocrine test), and the amount of postoperative pancreatic juice drainage were compared between groups A (IORT patients) and B (non-IORT patients) at preoperative, early, and late postoperative times. Fasting blood sugar levels and the OGTT showed no change at the early (<2 months) postoperative period of the two groups. At the late (>6 months) postoperative period, fasting blood sugar showed no alteration while the OGTT value increased compared to the preoperative level in both groups. In group A, the OGTT value at the late postoperative period was significantly higher than those at the preoperative and early postoperative periods. The preoperative BT-PABA excretion value was not different between the two groups, decreasing at the early postoperative period and returning to preoperative level at the late postoperative period in both groups. The decline of BT-PABA in group A was significantly larger than in group B. The total amount of postoperative pancreatic juice drainage from postoperative days 4 to 13 in group A was approximately half the level as that in group B. Univariate and multivariate regression factorial analysis showed the decline of BT-PABA values at the early postoperative period was significantly influenced by IORT. These results suggest that IORT causes significant deterioration of pancreatic exocrine function at the early postoperative period.

TOLERANCE DOSE

The exact dose of radiation that causes 5% of the patients to have radiation-induced pancreatic complications within 5 years (TD 5/5) is not known.[1] Treatment to 50 Gy may lead to pancreatic acinar atrophy and diffuse pancreatic fibrosis in some patients. Doses of 60 Gy or higher appear to result in a higher complication rate. After radiation therapy to approximately doses of 45 Gy, a pancreatic insufficiency induced malabsorption has been described.[1] A chronic pancreatitis-like syndrome has also been described at lower dose levels of 36 to 40 Gy.[5] Diabetes mellitus is not a well-established effect of pancreatic irradiation although cases have been attributed to such. Islets of Langerhans usually are well preserved after conventional doses of radiation, but altered function despite morphologic normality by light microscopy is possible. Table 39.1 shows relative radiation sensitivities of various pancreatic cell types.

MORPHOLOGY

Despite having a slow turnover rate, pancreatic acinar cells and to a lesser extent small duct cells show marked histologic change after radiation therapy.[1] The large duct epithelium and

TABLE 39.1	Radiosensitivity of Pancreatic Cell Types	
Cell Type		*Radiosensitivity*
Islets of Langerhans (alpha, beta, delta cells-endocrine cells)		+
Acinar cells (exocrine cells)		+++
Ductal cells (exocrine cells)		++

to an even greater extent the cells of the islet of Langerhans exhibit little histologic change post radiation therapy.

EARLY MORPHOLOGIC LESIONS

It is proposed that after 10 to 20 Gy of irradiation, the cytoplasmic secretory granules in the acinar cells are reduced in number or lost entirely.[1] The severity of the acinic cell injury will depend on the total dose and fraction size. Total necrosis has been reported with doses of 60 Gy. The cells of the small ducts show degenerative changes, and the ductal lumens may be distended and plugged by cellular fragments and debris. Larger ducts may show only mild cell abnormalities and lumen enlargement. The islet of Langerhans will be microscopically normal. Edema of the stroma will be present with acute inflammation present in regions of early parenchymal necrosis.

DELAYED MORPHOLOGIC LESIONS

Examination of the pancreas that was previously irradiated 6 months to years earlier may show a gray thickening of the fibrous capsule and perhaps fibrotic adhesions of the surrounding soft tissues that are also often gray and thickened.[1] The pancreas may shrink to perhaps one half of its normal size and have an indistinct lobular pattern, with the cut surface also demonstrating a gray appearance with indistinct lobules. The pancreas is even more firm than usual and infrequent calcifications may be observed. Recognizable fat necrosis is rare. Microscopically, the acinar cells are almost entirely lost or remarkably atrophic.

The irradiated pancreatic parenchyma is extremely fibrotic. Despite this severe fibrosis and loss of acinar cells, the islets of Langerhans appear normal on light microscopy. Except for the absence of active or healed fat necroses or extensive calcifications, the delayed lesions of the irradiated pancreas resemble those of chronic pancreatitis. One report described five patients 6 to 24 years after upper abdominal radiation with injuries to the pancreas that resembled chronic pancreatitis.[5] Three of these patients had pancreatitic pseudocysts, although only one had pancreatic calcifications. Another case of chronic pancreatitis following upper abdominal irradiation has also been described. As more patients receive irradiation to the upper abdomen and have long-term follow-up, other cases of postradiation chronic pancreatitis-like disease will likely be described.

PATHOGENESIS

Pathogenesis of early radiation-induced injury is that of immediate radiation-induced damage to cells, especially the acinar cells.[1] In addition, endothelial cell damage in the microcirculation adds ischemia to direct radiation cell injury. Stromal edema is the result of endothelial cell injury that causes increased capillary permeability. It is apparent that the immediate effects of ionizing radiation on fibroblasts are responsible for the progressive fibrosis of the stroma, and that the effect on myoepithelial cells and integral fibroblasts causes arterial and venous lesions resulting in ischemia during the delayed period.

Radiation damage to the duct cells is likely the source of the eventual and rare oncogenesis that develops late. Rarely, ductal cell adenocarcinomas are found in the long-term follow-up of the irradiated patient. A nearly consistent complication of irradiation of an organ is the development of neoplasm, usually after a latency of more than 5 years and sometimes after 15 to 20 years and beyond. Travis et al. reported a follow-up of a large number of men treated for possible metastases of testicular cancers in North America and Europe.[6] Among the 28,843 men observed, there were 1,406 second neoplasms observed for a ratio of observed to expected of 1.43. Among the organs that were statistically increased risk was the pancreas with an observed to expected ratio of 2.21. A case report of pancreatic cancer following radiation therapy for Hodgkin's disease has been reported.

CLINICAL MANIFESTATIONS

A chronic pancreatitis-like syndrome has been described in case reports and attributed to radiation therapy of the pancreas.[1,5] This syndrome consists of pain, steatorrhea, and the formation of pancreatic pseudocysts. Four of the five patients were diagnosed with diabetes mellitus. This is difficult to understand given the usual histological preservation of the islets of Langerhans. However, abnormal function may exist despite normal morphology by light microscopy. Malabsorption has also been reported in other case reports although it is difficult to distinguish the etiology of malabsorption syndromes because of the potential injury to the small intestine during upper abdominal irradiation.

SUMMARY

Early postirradiation pancreatic injury has been found in experimental studies. Damage to the acinar cells correlates with the reduction of bicarbonate and enzyme production that follows pancreatic irradiation. Glucose metabolism is generally not altered. The most important form of injury is delayed and observed in autopsies of irradiated humans. This consists of severe loss of pancreatic acinar cells, atrophy of small ducts and dilated large ducts with luminal cell debris combined with extensive pancreatic and stromal fibrosis. Only the islet cells of Langerhans are well preserved by light microscopy. Vascular lesions are frequently prominent and are the type found in other organs. Functional pancreatic insufficiency occurs frequently and diabetes mellitus has also been reported. Postirradiation pancreatic oncogenesis has been estimated to occur at a relative risk of 2.21.

REFERENCES

1. Fajardo L, Berthrong M, Anderson R. In: *Radiation Pathology*. New York, NY: Oxford University Press; 2001: 259–263.
2. Ahmadu-Suka F, Gillette EL, Withrow SJ, et al. Pathologic response of the pancreas and duodenum to experimental intraoperative irradiation. *Int J Radiat Oncol Biol Phys*. 1988;14: 1197–1204.
3. Ahmadu-Suka F, Gillette EL, Withrow SJ, et al. Exocrine pancreatic function following intraoperative irradiation of the canine pancreas. *Cancer*. 1988;62:1091–1095.
4. Yamaguchi K, Nakamura K, Kimura M, et al. Intraoperative radiation enhances decline of pancreatic exocrine function after pancreatic head resection. *Dig Dis Sci*. 2000;45: 1084–1090.
5. Levy P, Menzelxhiu A, Paillot B, et al. Abdominal radiotherapy is a cause for chronic pancreatitis. *Gastroenterology*. 1993;105:905–909.
6. Travis L, Curtis R, Storm H, et al. Risk of second malignant neoplasm among long-term survivors of testicular cancer. *Natl Cancer Inst*. 1997;89:1429–1439.

Stomach

INTRODUCTION

Early and late gastrointestinal (GI) injury of the stomach may occur following irradiation of lower thoracic, abdominal and pelvic malignancies of both GI and non–GI origin, only requiring that the stomach is located within the radiation field. Stomach tolerance frequently limits radiation doses that can be delivered for many tumor types. As with most other radiotherapy-associated toxicities, gastric side effects are categorized into two broad categories: early/acute reactions, such as nausea and vomiting, experienced during and soon following the completion of a course of therapy, and late/chronic reactions, such as ulceration, stricture formation, and perforation, that can arise months to years following the course of radiation therapy. The incidence and severity of radiation-induced morbidity depends on total radiation dose, radiation fraction size, treatment volume, treatment techniques, the presence or absence of other treatment modalities including systemic chemotherapy and surgery, as well as the presence of concurrent medical comorbidities. This chapter discusses the early and late responses of the stomach to radiation and combined radiochemotherapy treatment regimens.

ANATOMY

The stomach serves multiple physiologic functions in the digestive system, including that of a "mixing vat," a holding reservoir, producer of enzymes for digestion of starches, proteins and triglycerides, converter of food to a more liquefied form and even absorbs various substances. The stomach mixes saliva, food, and gastric juice (hydrochloric acid, pepsin, intrinsic factor, and gastric lipase) to form chyme. Additionally, the stomach secretes gastrin into the blood stream via G cells. Gastric epithelial cells are protected from gastric juices by a thin layer of mucus secreted by mucus surface and neck cells. Through an autocrine loop, gastrin stimulates release of hydrochloric acid and pepsinogen in the stomach, as well as stimulating contraction of the lower esophageal sphincter, increasing stomach mobility and relaxation of the pyloric sphincter.

The stomach is generally divided into anatomic regions, including the gastric cardia (region adjacent to the gastroesophageal [GE] junction), the fundus (situated superiorly), the body (mid-stomach), and the pyloric canal (distally) (Figs. 40.1 and 40.2).

The cardia surrounds the superior opening of the stomach where it connects with the GE junction (level of the lower esophageal sphincter). The rounded portion superior to the body and to the left of the cardia is the fundus. Inferior to the fundus is the large, central portion of the stomach, the body. The region of the stomach that connects to the duodenum is the pylorus, which is composed of two parts, the pyloric antrum, which connects to the body of the stomach; and the pyloric canal, which empties into the duodenum. The pylorus communicates with the duodenum of the small intestine via the pyloric sphincter (valve). This valve regulates the passage of chyme from stomach to duodenum and prevents backflow of chyme from duodenum to stomach.[1]

The stomach wall is composed of four layers: the mucosa, submucosa, muscularis, and serosa. As depicted, the muscularis layer is composed of an outer longitudinal layer, a middle circular layer, and inner oblique layer (Figs. 40.1 and 40.3).

The gastric mucosa is scattered with openings leading to mucosal pits that are lined by columnar, mucous-secreting cells. Glands containing undifferentiated progenitor cells branch from these pits and provide progenitor cells in the gland neck

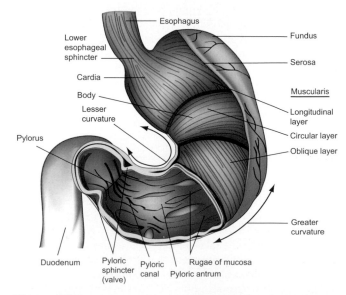

Figure 40.1. Gastric anatomy. (Courtesy of HarperCollins Publishers Inc. From Tortora GJ, Grabowski SR. *Principles of Anatomy and Physiology.* 8th ed. John Wiley & Sons, Menlo Park, CA; 1996.)

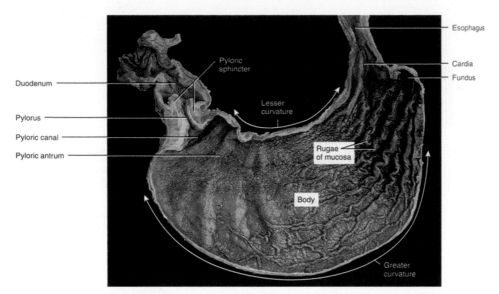

Figure 40.2. Gastric anatomy. (Courtesy of HarperCollins Publishers Inc. From Tortora GJ, Grabowski SR. *Principles of Anatomy and Physiology.* 8th ed. John Wiley & Sons, Menlo Park, CA; 1996.)

for the mucous-secreting cells (Figs. 40.3–40.5). Additionally, these progenitor cells may also differentiate into parietal (hydrochloric-acid/intrinsic factor producing), chief (pepsinogen and gastric lipase producing), and enteroendocrine (gastrin producing) cells that migrate downward into the glands. There appear to be regional anatomic differences in varying enzyme and mucus productivity, including mucous and lysozyme in the cardia: hydrochloric acid, intrinsic factor, pepsinogen, and lipase in the fundus and body; mucin and lysozyme in the pylorus; and serotonin, gastrin, and somatostatin in the fundus, body, and pylorus.

MOLECULAR MECHANISMS OF RADIATION-INDUCED GASTROINTESTINAL DAMAGE

Radiation injury is the phenotype of a complex set of interactions between multiple cytokines and molecular pathways.

Stromal injury with subsequent progressive fibrosis is the most significant component of radiation injury. The risk of fibrosis appears to increase when surgery and possibly when chemotherapy is combined with radiotherapy. In addition, the volume of tissue irradiated, total dose, and dose per fraction influence the development and severity of radiation-induced fibrosis.

APOPTOSIS

In animal studies, a rapid increase in the rate of programmed cell death (apoptosis) of GI crypts cells can be observed after exposure to low-dose radiation (1–5 cGy). The rate of apoptosis is radiation dose dependent and reaches a plateau at approximately 1 Gy. Radiation exposure also increases expression of the tumor suppressor gene *p53* in stem cell regions. Radiation-induced apoptosis is dependent on the presence of *p53*. Additionally, the rate of spontaneous and radiation-induced apoptosis is significantly increased in animals lacking *bcl-2*, suggesting a protective effect of *bcl-2* in this regard.[2] It is therefore

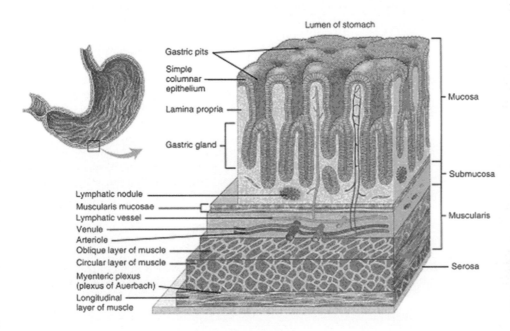

Figure 40.3. Gastric histology. (Courtesy of HarperCollins Publishers Inc. From Tortora GJ, Grabowski SR. *Principles of Anatomy and Physiology.* 8th ed. John Wiley & Sons, Menlo Park, CA; 1996.)

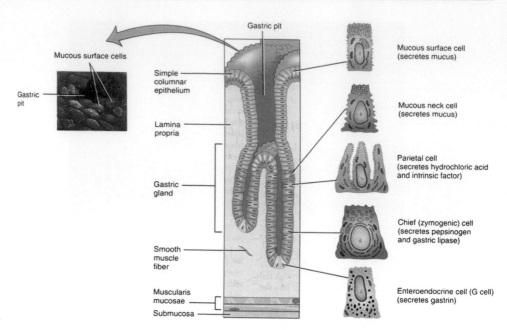

Figure 40.4. Gastric histology.

postulated that *p53* promotes apoptosis after irradiation and that *bcl-2* protects the mucosa. As an example, higher levels of *bcl-2* may explain the increased tolerance of the colorectal mucosa to radiation as compared with the small intestine.

ROLE OF CYTOKINES

Ionizing radiation activates the translation of the gene coding for transforming growth factor beta (TGF-β) in the GI tract.

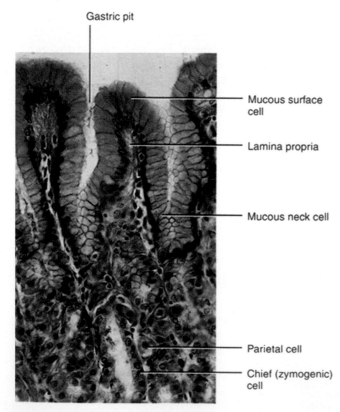

Figure 40.5. Gastric histology.

TGF-β is a potent fibrogenic and proinflammatory cytokine, leading to hyperplasia of connective tissue mast cells and leukocyte migration into the GI wall. TGF-β promotes GI fibrosis by stimulating the expression of collagen and fibronectin genes and the chemotaxis of fibroblasts. The extracellular matrix is also increased as TGF-β inhibits its degradation. The increased expression of TGF-β is especially enhanced in regions with histopathologic changes consistent with radiation damage, i.e., areas with mucosal ulceration, mucosal and serosal thickening, inflammatory cell infiltrates, and vascular sclerosis.[3,4] TGF-β exists in three isoforms: TGF-β1, TGF-β2, and TGF-β3. All three isoforms are overexpressed in the early postradiation phase. However, only isoform β1 remains elevated 6 months after radiation exposure. In the first 2 weeks after radiation, TGF-β1 messenger RNA is increased in epithelial cells, fibroblasts of the submucosa and subserosa, vascular endothelial cells, and smooth muscle cells of the GI wall. However, at 26 weeks, the expression of TGF-β1 of epithelial cells returns to baseline level but TGF-β1 expression remains elevated in vascular endothelial cells, fibroblasts, and smooth muscles cells.[5] Compared with control mouse GI tissues, TGF-β1 immunoreactivity/overexpression is substantially increased in areas of radiation-induced acute and late bowel injury.[6,7] In addition, pathologic examination of bowel specimens from patients undergoing surgery for radiation enteropathy has demonstrated increased TGF-β levels in areas demonstrating vascular sclerosis, and in fibrotic areas of the serosa and muscularis propria compared with patients who have surgery for other causes.[8] Additionally, neutralizing antibodies to TGF-β and gene therapy using decorin (a natural TGF-β inhibitor) have been shown to suppress or reverse fibrosis in preclinical models.[9]

Epidermal growth factors, interleukins, and tumor necrosis factors are also being investigated for their effects in chronic radiation injury.[10] Another cytokine implicated in the development of radiation injury is connective tissue growth factor (CTGF). CTGF expression is increased in GI radiation fibrosis associated with chronic radiation injury.[11] CTGF is commonly found in the extracellular region surrounding the area of active fibrosis or neovascularization. TGF-β1 may induce CTGF, which in turn functions as a mediator of GI radiation fibrosis by sustaining the activation of fibrogenesis in the irradiated GI tract. Mechanisms underlying the pathogenesis of radiation-induced GI damage remain an active area of investigation.

HISTOLOGIC CHANGES

Multiple factors influence radiation injury-associated pathologic changes including radiation dose, dose per fraction, length of time between therapy and tissue examination, underlying status of the irradiated alimentary segment (including vascular supply), and concurrent chemotherapy delivery. Generally speaking, higher radiation doses, shorter time periods over which radiation is delivered, and larger treatment volumes all increase the likelihood of injury. In the stomach, what has been deemed a "unique" response to radiation occurs, in that the most radiosensitive epithelial cells are the differentiated cells (parietal and chief cells) rather than the germinative cells. Studies in which serial gastric biopsies were obtained following irradiation of patients for peptic ulcer disease noted coagulation necrosis of chief and parietal cells with mucosal thinning, edema, and chronic inflammatory infiltration.[12,13] In addition, gastric acid production decreased after relatively low doses of irradiation, generally occurring quickly and in a rather patchy distribution.

Early histologic studies of low dose radiation therapy to the stomach for ulcer disease showed a loss of chief and parietal cells granules, nuclear pyknosis, and cytoplasmic darkening within 8 days following therapy initiation. Collective data from animal and human studies suggest that gastric mucosal edema, nuclear pyknosis, dilated capillaries, and endothelial swelling occur by the delivery of 20 to 25 Gy. By 50 Gy, these changes appear more severe and may include mucosal erosion and capillary thrombosis. These erosions may relate to symptomatic gastritis or even develop into gastric ulceration.[14] Shortly after treatment completion, glandular epithelial necrosis occurs with lymphocyte and plasma cell accumulation in the lamina propria. Regeneration is seen by 3 weeks following therapy, and by 4 months, histologically normal mucosa is seen, although gastric acid secretion may remain significantly decreased. Significant variations in this have been noted, including between separate areas of the stomach as well as between individual patients. Microscopically, chief (pepsinogen producing) cells show initial changes followed by parietal (acid-producing) cells. However, a decrease in acid production often precedes a decrease in pepsin production.[15] With higher radiation doses, the mucosa often demonstrates damage with the surface epithelium exhibiting a cuboidal appearance with loss of mucous, resulting in mucosal atrophy.[14]

Clinically, radiation-induced gastritis may occur within 1 week of initiating radiotherapy, with associated microscopic changes including edema, hemorrhage, and exudation. Histologic changes may also include disappearance of cytoplasmic details and granules in parietal and chief cells as early as 1 week into therapy. Cell damage and subsequent cell death are often seen, first in the depths of glands, followed by thinning of the gastric mucosa.[16] Additional mucosal changes include deepening of the glandular pits and proliferation of cells in the glandular neck. Loss of glandular architecture and thickening of the mucosa can be seen by the third week of radiotherapy. Approximately 3 weeks after completion of radiotherapy, histologic recovery may be seen, including re-epithelialization and fibrosis.

Gastric ulceration following radiation therapy is often antral due to the location of the radiation fields. Ulcers are often solitary, measuring anywhere from 0.5 to 2 cm and have been reported to be relatively refractory to dietary changes and antacid therapy.[17] Radiation-induced ulcers may heal spontaneously but can result in a moderate to marked constriction of the antral lumen due to submucosal fibrosis.[18] Radiation induced-ulceration with perforation may occur 1 to 2 months following treatment. These perforations may be walled off by bowel and adhesions, which can be mistaken for inoperable/metastatic cancer. Generally, radiation-induced ulceration requires a dose of at least 45 Gy. Ulceration often develops within 1 year following radiation delivery, although longer durations have been reported. Grossly, these ulcers often have a raised mucosal rim with a base containing fibrotic tissue, which may extend to the serosa. Histologically, ulcers may appear similar to those related to peptic acid–induced disease, with a necrotic base with underlying layers of granulation tissue, with dense fibrosis more deeply. The adjacent vasculature may show severe intimal fibrosis, causing arterial narrowing which likely, through ischemia, contributes to the ulcer itself. Compared to ulcers related to peptic acid, radiation-related ulcer perforation is believed to be more frequent, possibly because of regression of neoplastic tissue in both the acute phase and the long term.[14] The genesis of radiation-induced gastric ulceration is likely multifactorial, including related to direct injury of the mucosa leading to erosion, decreased ability to repair/regenerate the irradiated mucosal cells, as well as injury to the microvasculature including arterial (obliterate endarteritis) and venous systems, leading to ischemia/hypoxia. Clinically apparent obstructive symptoms at the pyloric level may also be more common in radiation-induced ulceration due to progressive fibrosis and vascular injury. Rare complications include gastrocutaneous fistula, arteriodigestive tract fistulas, as well as development of ulceration in the gastric conduit "neoesophagus" in patients undergoing esophagectomy.[14]

ANIMAL STUDIES

Early canine studies suggested the lining cells of the gastric gland neck and pits were more radiosensitive than parietal cells,[19] resulting in early changes likely secondary to direct mucosal cell damage.[14] Associated surface denundement resulted in lamina propria exposure and potential ulceration.

Radiation-induced canine ulcers were described as resembling human gastric peptic ulcers.[14] Early studies on rabbits in which ≥1,500 R were delivered produced gastric ulceration, manifesting in the second to fourth week post therapy. Some were associated with perforation and hemorrhage. Animals that lived 2 to 3 months following therapy showed a tendency toward healing and epitheliazation.[20] Other investigators delivered doses up to a total of 6,000 R to canine stomachs, resulting in marked weight loss, moderate-to-severe anemia, and perforating gastric ulcers within 1 month. In contrast, animals receiving a total of 4,875 R over a prolonged period did not show any significant gross or histologic abnormality of internal organs.[21]

Reports from the early 20th century described gastric mucosal atrophy with radiation therapy, leading to the hypothesis that radiation could be used to treat peptic ulcer disease.[22] Early animal studies also showed the ability of radiation therapy to decrease production of hydrochloric acid and pepsin, prompting the employment of low-dose gastric irradiation to treat peptic-ulcer disease.

Radiation to the stomach in animals using a very high, single dose of irradiation results in erosive/ulcerative gastritis. Slightly lower single doses (23 Gy) results in gastric dilatation and gastroparesis, with replacement of the normal gastric mucosa by hyperkeratinized squamous epithelium. With even lower doses, gastric obstruction occurring months following irradiation was observed, with an atrophic gastric mucosa and intestinal metaplasia observed in surviving animals.[23] In rodent models, local stomach irradiation with single doses of x-rays resulted in three distinct phases of injury (a) acute gastritis occurring within the first few weeks (b) a subchronic condition characterized by severe functional insufficiency and degenerative changes in the mucosa and submucosal, and (c) a late, chronic phase, occurring >40 weeks following radiation therapy, characterized by gastric wall fibrosis and deep ulceration, sometimes associated with stomach dilatation. Similar studies using single, high dose radiation fractions have shown a progression of gastric mucosal changes, ranging from normal at 3 days post irradiation, denundement of the fundus, and pyloric mucosa at 12 days, with complete healing at 40 days in rats; in hamsters, gastric ulceration leading to animal death was seen. Using single, high doses of radiation therapy, a proportional decrease in survival using doses from approximately 11 to 21 Gy was seen. Similarly, when radiation was delivered in two fractions, a similar proportional decrease in survival was observed when escalating dose from approximately 8 to 14 Gy/fraction. Histologic exam during the subchronic phase showed atonic dilatation of the stomach with mucosal dysplasia/atrophy and ulcerations.[24] Other rodent studies delivering 10 or 20 Gy in two fractions have described a decrease in pepsinogen levels in the pyloric mucosa beginning at 2 weeks postradiotherapy that persisted to 1 year, along with the induction of intestinal-type crypt development in the pyloric mucosa.[25]

HUMAN STUDIES

As described previously, in the early twentieth century, it was noted that radiation produced gastric mucosal atrophy. Therefore, radiation was initially used to decrease acid production in efforts to control peptic ulcer disease. It should be noted that early reports utilized radiation exposure dose or roentgens in air, which ignores the absorbed tissue dose and conversion from roentgens into cGy is not trivial; therefore, interpretation of x-ray dosages from older studies may be somewhat difficult, including the fact that dose may vary by as much as 10% to 20% from the midplane dose. Nonetheless, using low dose irradiation over ten fractions (1,500–2,000 R) for peptic ulcer disease, a large experience from the University of Chicago of nearly 3,000 patients revealed no obvious radiation-induced ulcers and no incidence of second neoplasm. Achlorhydria occurred in 10% of patients, but only lasted ≥6 months in 4%; lesser degrees of acid inhibition were also observed, with a 50% decrease in acid secretion lasting 1 year or more observed in 40% of patients. However, many patients showed only a moderate reduction in acid-producing capacity of unpredictable duration, with no effect seen in 9%.[15,26] Other experiences have also demonstrated that low dose irradiation results in a persistent reduction in gastric acid secretion in some patients, with others

normalizing within 6 months to 1 year following radiation therapy. Additional investigators have noted decreases in hydrochloric acid production preceding pepsinogen reduction, with both preceding histologic changes. However, even after resolution of radiation-induced histologic changes, secretions may still remain low.[14]

The association between higher radiation dose and chronic gastric injury has been established for many decades. An early report from Sweden described a patient receiving 55 Gy over 11 weeks to the distal stomach. The patient presented 4 months following completion of radiation with hematemesis and melena, with gastritis and edema noted on the distal stomach corresponding to the radiation field. On surgical resection, a large, necrotic area of ulceration was observed. The patient ultimately died from perioperative complications. Histologically, the gastric wall thickness was estimated at 2 cm secondary to edema. Vascular changes of endarteritis, fibrinoid necrosis of the vessels, thrombosis, and extensive interstitial hemorrhages were seen. Mucosal ulceration was associated with almost complete necrotic desquamation of the gastric lining. Glandular cells were described as heavily damaged with cytoplasmic vacuolization and loss of secretory function. Other adjacent mucosal defects with overt hemorrhage were present in the irradiated area. The severe vascular and nuclear changes were felt to distinguish it from simple ulceration.

A second patient received approximately 42 Gy over 39 days. The patient later developed chronic changes of marked gastritis and recurrent ulceration. After 4 years, the patient experienced persistent melena with anemia and underwent resection, revealing scarring due to previous ulcers with chronic gastroduodenitis, containing considerable fibrosis and inflammatory cell infiltration. These and other reports described acute gastric ulceration occurring at doses ranging from 43 to 49 Gy delivered over 5 weeks, with increased frequency observed at or above doses of 50 Gy delivered over a similar time period. These authors recommended limiting gastric dose to 43 Gy (±10%) delivered over 5 weeks using cobalt therapy.[27]

Incidental gastric irradiation for varying malignancies in the 1940s and 1950s, in particular young men with testicular neoplasms, had provided additional information on gastric tolerance. Studies from Walter Reed Army Medical Center delivering abdominal radiation using now antiquated techniques in testicular cancer patients have suggested that higher radiation doses lead to an increasing risk of late ulceration and perforation. In this series, 256 patients with testicular tumors were treated with radiation therapy (targeting the retroperitoneal lymph nodes) using orthovoltage therapy to a 10-cm wide field (extending from the pubis to the xyphoid) following radical orchiectomy. Ulceration occurred in approximately 6% of patients treated to 4,500 to 5,000 R; 10% of patients treated to 5,000 to 6,000 R; and 38% of patients treated to >6,000 R. No ulceration was seen in patients receiving <4,500 R. When doses of at least 5,000 R were delivered, approximately half of patients developed epigastric discomfort, with 35 patients noted to have a large, single ulcer on fluoroscopy. Approximately one-half of patients receiving 4,500 to 5,400 R and 63% of those receiving 5,500 to 6,400 R developed gastric injury. Symptomatic gastritis occurred approximately 2 months following radiation completion, with ulcer formation occurring at a median of 5 months. Relief by food was variable. Six (3%) required operation for significant symptoms including bleeding. At resection, significant fibrosis was seen with the stomach showing a brown, "burnt-out" appearance. An ulcer was noted on the posterior wall of the stomach near the pylorus in all cases, two of which perforated onto the pancreas, although fibrosis confined such. Clinically, at operation, affected portions of the stomach are described as displaying a "smoothed-out" appearance and "leathery" in consistency with no visible peristalsis.[28] All patients developing ulceration had a dose to the stomach of >5,000 R.[28] In this series, 5% of patients experienced perforation, all receiving doses of 6,000 to 6,400 R. Partial obstruction was noted in 9%, 11%, 5%, 13%, and 25% in patients receiving 4,000 to 4,400 R; 4,500 to 4,900 R; 5,000 to 5,400 R; 5,500 to 5,900 R; and 6,000 to 6,400 R, respectively. Similarly, radiation ulceration occurred in 7%, 0%, 15%, and 14% of patients receiving 2,500 to 3,400 R; 3,500 to 4,400 R; 4,500 to 5,400 R; and 5,500 to 6,400 R. Similarly, radiation gastritis was noted in 0%, 21%, 21%, and 32% of these patients. Radiation ulceration with perforation or obstruction was seen in 11% and 18% in the latter two groups. Overall, the total percent experiencing gastric injury, including dyspepsia, was 20%, 25%, 50%, and 63% in these groups, respectively.[18]

The introduction of megavoltage equipment (compared to earlier orthovoltage equipment) has allowed treatment of deeper-seated targets without significant skin injury, which had previously been dose limiting. More contemporary studies of patients treated with megavoltage radiation therapy for Hodgkin's lymphoma or for testicular, gastric, or cervical cancers have also established tolerance limits for gastric irradiation.[28–31] These studies delivered doses of 40 to 60 Gy. Patients who received doses above 50 Gy experienced gastric ulceration and gastric ulcer-associated perforation at rates of 15% and 10%, respectively.

In the previously described series of testicular cancers, antral ulceration was often undetected for at least 1 month with onset of symptoms sometimes delayed for up to 6 years following radiotherapy. Most of these ulcers healed poorly and even when they did, sometimes resulted in obstruction or perforation. In another series, eight patients required partial gastrectomy and three died. Another five died from hemorrhage or obstruction without surgery, felt due to radiation therapy.[15] It has been estimated that doses above 55 Gy will result in gastric mucosal injury in 50% of patients. Goldstein et al.[32] described 121 patients receiving 50 Gy to the paraaortic lymph nodes. This resulted in an ulceration rate of approximately 8%.

German investigators described 33 patients undergoing High dose rate (HDR) brachytherapy for liver malignancies adjacent to the stomach. When assessing the dose applied to 1 mL of the gastric wall, a threshold dose of 11 Gy was found for general gastric toxicity and 15.5 Gy for gastric ulceration in a single fraction. GI symptoms develop 1 to 6 months after brachytherapy with a mean time to occurrence of 6 weeks. The majority of ulcers were also detected within the first 6 weeks following treatment delivery. Endoscopy showed gastritis and ulceration in 12% and 15% of patients, respectively. Five of 13 patients receiving >15.5 Gy developed gastric ulceration.[33] A small experience evaluating body radiosurgery (using large doses per fraction) reported gastric ulceration in two patients, one of whom received incidental delivery of 20 Gy in four fractions to the distal stomach, with another developing antral ulceration after receiving 21 Gy in three fractions.[34] Similarly, a European experience evaluating the treatment of Hodgkin disease showed patients receiving higher fraction sizes were more likely to develop chronic toxicities (4% at 2 Gy/fraction, 9% at 2.5 Gy/fraction, and 22% at 3.3 Gy/fraction).[35]

SYMPTOMS

The stomach may be injured following irradiation of the upper abdomen for varying cancers, including esophageal/GE junctional, gastric and pancreatic carcinomas, as well as lymphomas. Symptoms of acute radiation injury of the stomach consist primarily of nausea and vomiting, dyspepsia, anorexia, abdominal pain, and malaise. These are more common with the concurrent administration of chemotherapy. Radiation-induced nausea and vomiting may occur within the first 24 hours following treatment. It is estimated that approximately half of patients receiving upper abdominal radiation will experience emesis within 2 to 3 weeks following initiation of irradiation.[36]

Late effects of gastric irradiation have been classified into four categories: (a) acute ulceration (occurring shortly after completion of radiation therapy), (b) gastritis with smoothened mucosal folds and mucosal atrophy on endoscopy accompanied by radiographic evidence of antral stenosis (1–12 months following irradiation), (c) dyspepsia, consisting of vague gastric symptoms without obvious clinical correlate (6 months to 4 years following irradiation), and (d) late ulceration (averaging 5 months after irradiation).[12,37] Based on the data above, the TD 5/5 (dose estimated to result in a 5% risk of complications at 5 years) for treatment of the entire stomach has been estimated at 50 Gy. Large studies of upper abdominal irradiation have suggested that prior abdominal surgery as well as using a higher dose per fraction may increase the risk of late effects.[29] If radiation is indicated, the dose to the entire stomach with conventionally administered radiation therapy is limited to 45 to 50 Gy, resulting in an estimated 5% to 10% risk of severe radiation toxicity. Where appropriate, reduced field boosts can be given to treat to doses up to 55 Gy with acceptable toxicity.

Combining chemotherapy with radiation therapy decreases the tolerance of the gastric mucosa to radiation therapy. 5-Fluorouracil (5-FU) is the most common chemotherapy agent delivered concurrently with radiation therapy in the management of GI tumors. 5-FU is a radiation sensitizer for both tumor and normal tissues, but has historically been given safely with radiation therapy at doses of 45 to 50 Gy without substantial increases in toxicity. This agent can be given in an adjuvant, neoadjuvant, or "definitive" settings for GE junction, gastric, pancreatic, and biliary cancers. Newer systemic agents have been shown to increase acute gastric toxicity when delivered with radiotherapy, including taxanes, gemcitabine, and epidermal growth factor inhibitors. These regimens remain the subject of investigation in the treatment of abdominal malignancies.

TREATMENT AND PREVENTION

The typical irradiation course for esophagogastric and pancreatic cancers consists of 45 to 54 Gy with concurrent chemotherapy. For other malignancies, including gastric lymphoma, non gastric lymphomas and testicular cancers, these doses are lower. As above, symptoms such as nausea, epigastric discomfort, or vomiting may occur, often manifesting at 20 to 25 Gy. Symptoms can occasionally be severe, particularly if higher doses are used and may result in persistent epigastric pain and possibly even hemorrhage. Acute symptoms of gastric radiation toxicity are treated with antiemetics (5-HT3 antagonists, phenothiazines, metoclopramide, glucocorticoids, benzodiazepines, antihistamines, or anticholinergics), as well as consumption of a light meal prior to delivery of radiation therapy. Randomized trials of prophylactic 5-HT3 inhibitors have shown efficacy compared to placebo in preventing radiation-induced nausea and vomiting.[38] A randomized trial of 211 patients receiving upper abdominal radiation compared the 5-HT3 inhibitor ondansetron given twice daily, with or without dexamethasone delivered daily for the first five fractions of treatment. Patients receiving dexamethasone showed a trend toward improved complete control of nausea (50% vs. 38%) and significant improvement in complete control over emesis. The authors concluded that the addition of dexamethasone resulted in modest improvement in protection against radiation-induced emesis.[39] Narcotic and nonnarcotic agents are often used for pain. Additionally, it is generally recommended that patients be placed on antacid medications, including proton pump inhibitors. Careful nutritional support along with antiemetic therapy is essential for patients undergoing radiotherapy to the abdomen. Acute symptoms generally resolve within 1 to 2 weeks following completion of radiation therapy. Rarely, symptoms can persist for months to years and may indicate chronic gastritis with associated mucosal atrophy and flattening of rugal folds (Figs. 40.6 and 40.7). Gastric ulceration may produce discomfort or pain, it may be associated with abdominal pain nausea, and even vomiting after meals if there is significant fibrosis with associated gastric outlet obstruction. Typically, radiation-induced ulcers may be relieved by food intake, although they may not respond

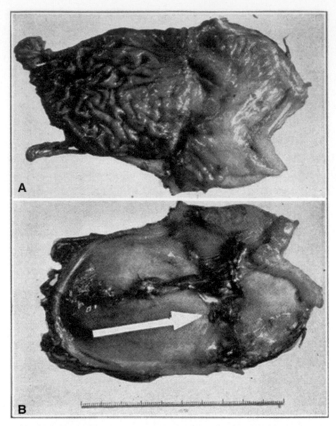

Figure 40.7. Resection specimen of patient with perforated radiation-induced ulcer. In the *upper panel*, note the similar characteristics to Figure 40.6, that is hypertrophy rugae proximally (*left*) and smoothened rugae in the irradiated region. The perforated ulcer is located centrally. On the *inferior panel* the stomach has been opened along the greater curvature, with the *arrow* pointing to the area of perforation near the edematous pylorus. (Hamilton, courtesy of the Western Surgical Association.)

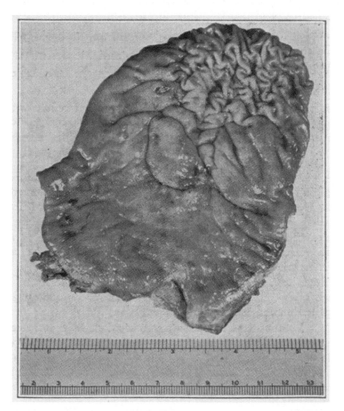

Figure 40.6. Example of gastric specimen in a patient with radiation-induced ulceration. Note hypertrophied rugae in the cardia (superiorly) and absence of rugae in the lower (irradiated) portion. A petechial mucosal hemorrhage of increasing edema was noted near the pylorus (inferiorly) with a portion of the ulcer at the inferior aspect of the specimen. (Hamilton, courtesy of the Western Surgical Association.)

to food or antacid medications (see below). Radiation gastric ulceration often presents with epigastric discomfort, which may present 2 to 3 months following completion of radiation therapy. Bleeding can occur and manifest as hematemesis, Melena, or hematochezia (Figs. 40.8–40.10). Perforation may also occur and manifest as acute pain and peritonitis. Rarely, massive hemorrhage and death may occur.

Generally, the signs and symptoms of chronic radiation injury appear within 6 to 24 months following therapy, manifested by mucosal atrophy and ulceration associated with obliterative endarteritis, which may lead to obstruction, hemorrhage, and fistula formation. Rarely, late effects may manifest up to 10 years or beyond following treatment completion. Acute effects have not definitively been correlated to the subsequent development of late effects. In contradistinction to pain associated with peptic ulceration, pain associated with radiation induced ulceration or injury and has been described as unrelenting with no relationship to meal intake. Additionally, radiation-induced ulceration has been associated with a higher likelihood of developing perforation and hemorrhage. Characteristic healing of gastric injury may be negligible despite medical management, believed secondary to underlying vascular damage rather than failure of regeneration of the epithelium, possibly requiring surgery.[32] Radiographically, prepyloric ulcers may be seen on swallowing

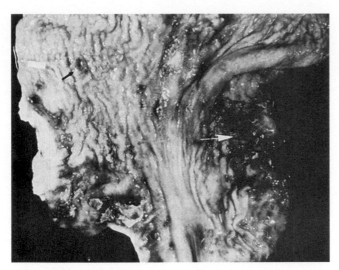

Figure 40.8. Radiation gastritis and ulceration. The stomach has been opened along the greater curvature, showing extensive hemorrhagic ulceration at the junction of the body and antral regions (*white arrow*). Note small discrete, petechial lesions distant from the ulcerated region (*black arrow*) (From Novak JM, Collins JT, Donowitz M, et al. Effects of radiation on the human gastrointestinal tract. *J Clin Gastroenterol.* 1979;1:9–39, with permission.)

studies, which may be indistinguishable from benign peptic ulceration. Historically, healing of these ulcers has been described as refractory to conservative management. Additionally, patients may develop a narrowed and deformed antrum and pylorus without obvious ulceration, along with an irregular mucosal contour and serration indicative of multiple superficial ulcerations,

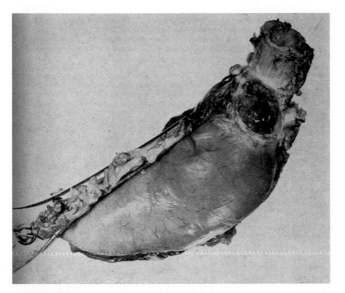

Figure 40.9. Gastric specimen from 29-year-old male receiving approximately 6,500 R for nonseminomatous germ cell tumor to the upper retroperitoneal adenopathy over 32 days. He presented approximately 5 weeks later with epigastric pain radiating to the back and later hematemesis. Upper gastrointestinal series showed constriction of the pyloric region with enlarged rugae, with ulceration. He required laparotomy for hematemesis. A posterior antral wall ulcer was noted, perforated, with considerable adjacent fibrosis and edema. Note the perforation of a 4-cm diameter ulcer in the posterior wall of the stomach. Note symptoms were refractory to conservative management (From Bowers RF, Brick IB. Surgery in radiation injury to the stomach. *Surgery* 1947;22(1):20–40, with permission.)

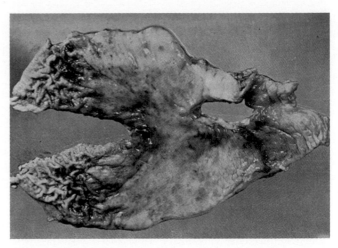

Figure 40.10. Stomach specimen from 29-year-old male receiving approximately 6,100 R over 49 days at the level of T11 for metastatic nonseminomatous germ cell tumor. The patient presented approximately 4 months following completion with epigastric burning and poor appetite. Upper GI series showed marked narrowing in the gastric antrum along with a 3-cm filling defect with a small ulceration proximal to the pyloric sphincter. At laparotomy, the stomach was edematous and vascular with an indurated area associated with crater on the posterior wall. Perforation was noted (note perforation in the posterior gastric wall). Symptoms were refractory to conservative management (From Bowers RF, Brick IB. Surgery in radiation injury to the stomach. *Surgery* 1947;22(1):20–40, with permission.)

which may be similar in appearance to a primary gastric tumor.[40] Late gastritis–related symptoms are often treated with antacids (H2 antagonist, proton pump inhibitors, sucralfate, etc.). These may be used on a long-term basis to avoid late ulceration. With more severe complications of bleeding, ulceration, gastric outlet obstruction, fistula formation, or perforation, patients may require endoscopic therapeutic approaches or rarely surgical intervention with partial gastrectomy.

Finally, it is important to note that the clinical symptoms associated with late radiation injury are often difficult to distinguish from those caused by recurrent (or new) cancer. Therefore, patients with strictures or ulcerations should also be evaluated to differentiate chronic radiation changes from cancer recurrence.

CARCINOGENESIS

Another consideration in the late effects of gastric irradiation is radiation-induced carcinogenesis. Experiments in animal models have suggested that radiation-induced gastric adenocarcinoma occurs after abdominal irradiation. A collective experience evaluating patients treated with radiation therapy for testicular cancer showed a relative risk of 2.3 for developing stomach cancer versus unirradiated controls.[41] Similarly, patients exposed to radiation from the atomic bombing in Japan showed an increase risk of gastric cancer development.[42] A study of approximately 3,700 patients treated for peptic ulcer disease with low dose irradiation (mean dose: 1,500 R) from 1936 to 1965 with an average follow-up of 25 years showed a significant increase in gastric cancer–related mortality, with an overall relative mortality risk of 2.6%.[43] Most cancers that develop following radiation therapy are adenocarcinomas, although more uncommon types including leiomyosarcomas are possible.[14]

CONCLUSION

The tolerance of the stomach to radiation therapy is limited and frequently dictates total radiation dose to many malignancies. Early radiation-induced symptoms include nausea and vomiting, with late toxicity consisting of dyspepsia, gastritis, bleeding, gastric ulceration, stricture formation, and perforation. The incidence and severity of radiation-induced stomach injury depends on total radiation dose, fraction size, volume irradiated, as well as the presence or the absence of other factors including synchronous delivery of chemotherapy, surgery, as well as medical comorbidities. Histologically, stromal injury with progressive fibrosis and microvascular injury are commonly seen, which are mediated by complex cytokine interactions. Gastric radiation tolerance is generally judged to be 45 to 50 Gy when large volumes of stomach are treated. Reduced fields may tolerate doses to 54 Gy with acceptable toxicity rates. The combination of aggressive symptomatic management and optimized modern radiation techniques should result in lower rates of acute and late radiation-induced gastric morbidity.

REFERENCES

1. Tortora G, Grabowski S. The digestive system. In: GJ Tortora and BH Derrickson, eds. *Principles of Anatomy and Physiology.* 9th ed. New York, NY: John Wiley & Sons, Inc.; 2000;818–870.
2. Potten C, Booth C. The role of radiation induced and spontaneous apoptosis in the homeostasis of the gastrointestinal epithelium. *Comp Biochem Physiol.* 1997;3:473.
3. Landberg C, Hauer-Jensen M, Sung C, et al. Expression of fibrogenic cytokines in rat small intestine after fractionated irradiation. *Radiother Oncol.* 1994;32:29.
4. Richter K, Langberg C, Sung C, et al. Increased transforming growth factor β (TGF-β) immunoreactivity is independently associated with chronic injury in both consequential and primary radiation enteropathy. *Int J Radiat Oncol Biol Phys.* 1997;19:187.
5. Wang J, Zheng H, Sung C, et al. Cellular sources of transforming grow factor-β isoforms in early and chronic radiation enteropathy. *Am J Pathol.* 1998;5:1531.
6. Wang J, Richter K, Sung C, et al. Upregulation and spatial shift in the localization of the mannose 6-phosphate/insulin-like growth factor II receptor during radiation enteropathy development in the rat. *Radiother Oncol.* 1999;50:205.
7. Skwarchuk M, Travis EL. Changes in histology and fibrogenic cytokines in irradiated colorectum of two murine strains. *Int J Radiat Oncol Biol Phys.* 1998;42:169.
8. Richter K, Fink L, Hughes B, et al. Is the loss of endothelial thrombomodulin involved in the mechanism of chronicity in late radiation enteropathy? *Radiother Oncol.* 1997;44:65.
9. Isaka Y, Brees D, Ikegaya K, et al. Gene therapy by skeletal muscle expression of decorin prevents fibrotic disease in rat kidney. *Nat Med.* 1996;2:418.
10. Herskind C, Bamberg M, Roderman H. The role of cytokines in the development of normal tissue reactions after radiotherapy. *Strahlenther Onkol.* 1998;174:12.
11. Vozenin-Brotons M-C, Fabien M, Sabourin J-C, et al. Fibrogenic signals in patients with radiation enteritis are associated with increased connective tissue growth factor expression. *Int J Radiat Oncol Biol Phys.* 2003;56:561.
12. Coia LR, Myerson RJ, Tepper JE. Late effects of radiation therapy on the gastrointestinal tract. *Int J Radiat Oncol Biol Phys.* 1995;31:1213–1236.
13. Goldgraber MB, Rubin CE, Palmer WL, et al. The early gastric response to irradiation; a serial biopsy study. *Gastroenterology.* 1954;27:1–20.
14. Fajardo L, Berthrong M, Anderson R. *Radiation Pathology.* New York, NY: Oxford University Press, Inc; 2001.
15. Novak JM, Collins JT, Donowitz M, et al. Effects of radiation on the human gastrointestinal tract. *J Clin Gastroenterol.* 1979;1:9–39.
16. Stevens K. *The Stomach and Small Intestine.* 7th ed. Mosby–Year Book, New York, NY Inc.; 1994.
17. Berthrong M, Farjardo L. Radiation injury in surgical pathology. *Am J Surg Path.* 1981;5:153–178.
18. Friedman M. Calculated risks of radiation injury of normal tissue in the treatment of cancer of the testis. Proceedings of the Second National Cancer Conference. Netherland Plaza Hotel, Cincinnati, OH: American Cancer Society, Inc., National Cancer Institute of the U.S. Public Health Service and American Association for Cancer Research; 1952:390–400.
19. Dawson A. Histologic changes in the gastric mucosa (Pavlov pouch) of the dog following irradiation. *Am J Roentgenol.* 1925;13:320–326.
20. Ingelstad R. The effect of roentgen rays on the stomach in rabbits. *Am J Roentgenol.* 1938;40:243.
21. Hueper W, DeCarvajal-Forero J. The effect of repeated irradiations of the gastric region with small doses of roentgen rays upon the stomach and blood of dogs. *Am J Roentgenol.* 1944;52:529.
22. Bruegel C. Die beeinflussing der morgenchenismus durch roentgenotrahlen. *Munchen Med Wochensehr.* 1917;64:379–380.
23. Breiter N, Trott KR, Sassy T. Effect of X-irradiation on the stomach of the rat. *Int J Radiat Oncol Biol Phys.* 1989;17:779–784.
24. Breiter N, Sassy T, Klaus-Rüdiger T. The effect of dose fractionation on radiation injury in the rat stomach. *Radiother Oncol.* 1993;27:223–228.
25. Jinn S, Furihata C, Watanabe H. The effect of x-ray irradiation on pepsinogen and on induction of intestinal-type crypts in the pyloric mucosa of the Wistar rat stomach. *Gann.* 1982;73:857–861.
26. Palmer W. *Gastric Irradiation in Peptic Ulcer.* Chicago, IL: University of Chicago Press; 1974.
27. Sylven B, Vikterlof K, Schnurer L. Gastric ulceration following cobalt teletherapy Estimation of the tolerance dose. *Acta Radiol.* 1969;8:183.
28. Hamilton CR, Horwich A, Bliss JM, et al. Gastrointestinal morbidity of adjuvant radiotherapy in stage I malignant teratoma of the testis. *Radiother Oncol.* 1987;10:85–90.
29. Cosset JM, Henry-Amar M, Burgers JM, et al. Late radiation injuries of the gastrointestinal tract in the H2 and H5 EORTC Hodgkin's disease trials: emphasis on the role of exploratory laparotomy and fractionation. *Radiother Oncol.* 1988;13:61–68.
30. Pearson JG. The present status and future potential of radiotherapy in the management of esophageal cancer. *Cancer.* 1977;39:882–890.
31. Gunderson LL, Hoskins RB, Cohen AC, et al. Combined modality treatment of gastric cancer. *Int J Radiat Oncol Biol Phys.* 1983;9:965–975.
32. Goldstein H, Rogers L, Fletcher G, et al. Radiological manifestations of radiation-induced injury to the normal upper gastrointestinal tract. *Radiology.* 1975;227:135–140.
33. Streitparth F, Pech M, Bohmig M, et al. In vivo assessment of the gastric mucosal tolerance dose after single fraction, small volume irradiation of liver malignancies by computed tomography – guided, high-dose-rate brachytherapy. *Int J Radiat Oncol Biol Phys.* 2006;65:1478–1486.
34. Blomgren H. Radiosurgery for tumors in the body: clinical experience using a new method. *J Radiosurg.* 1998;160:63–74.
35. Cosset J, Henry-Amar M, Burges J, et al. Late radiation injuries of the gastrointestinal tract in the H2 and H5 EROTC Hodgkin's disease trials: emphasis on the role of exploratory laparotomy and fractionation. *Radiother Oncol.* 1988;13:61–68.
36. Henriksson R, Bergstrom P, Franzen L, et al. Aspects on reducing gastrointestinal adverse effects associated with radiotherapy. *Acta Oncol.* 1999;38:159–164.
37. Sell A, Jensen TS. Acute gastric ulcers induced by radiation. *Acta Radiol Ther Phys Biol.* 1966;4:289–297.
38. Horiot JC, Aapro M. Treatment implications for radiation-induced nausea and vomiting in specific patient groups. *Eur J Cancer.* 2004;40:979–987.
39. Wong RK, Paul N, Ding K, et al. 5-hydroxytryptamine-3 receptor antagonist with or without short-course dexamethasone in the prophylaxis of radiation induced emesis: a placebo-controlled randomized trial of the National Cancer Institute of Canada Clinical Trials Group (SC19). *J Clin Oncol.* 2006;24:3458–3464.
40. Rogers L, Goldstein H. Roentgen manifestations of radiation injury to the gastrointestinal tract. *Gastrointest Radiol.* 1977;2:281–291.
41. Travis L, Curtis R, Storm H, et al. Risk of second malignant neoplasms among long-term survivors of testicular cancer. *J Natl Cancer Inst.* 1997;89:1429–1439.
42. Shimizu Y, Kato H, Schull W. Studies of the mortality of A-bomb survivors. Mortality, 1950–1985: part 2. Cancer mortality based on the recently revised doses (DS 86). *Radiat Res.* 1990;121:120–141.
43. Carr Z, Kleinerman R, Stovall M, et al. Malignant neoplasms after radiation therapy for peptic ulcer. *Radiat Res.* 2002;157:668–677.

Ellen Cooke
Jonathan D. Tward
Dennis C. Shrieve

Anus and Rectum

DESCRIPTION OF GROSS ANATOMY, LOCATION, AND IMAGING OF NORMAL STRUCTURE

The rectum is a tubular structure continuous with the sigmoid colon and is approximately 15 cm in length, but varies according to patient height, pelvic width, body habitus, and local pelvic anatomy, such as the specific curve of the sacral hollow. Typically, cancers located at or below the peritoneal reflection are considered rectal cancers. The rectum is divided into three segments in relation to the anal verge: the upper, middle, and lower thirds. The rectum contains the superior, middle, and inferior valves of Houston, which are not true valves but are prominent mucosal folds (Fig. 41.1). The dentate or pectinate line divides the mucosal columnar epithelium of the rectum from the squamous epithelium of the anus. The rectum is innervated by stretch nerve fibers but has no pain sensory supply.

The majority of lymphatic drainage for the superior rectum above the level of the middle rectal valve is along the superior hemorrhoidal artery, leading to the inferior mesenteric artery. Below this level at around 7 to 8 cm from the anal verge are lateral lymphatics associated with the middle hemorrhoidal artery, obturator, hypogastric and common iliac chains (Fig. 41.2). In women, lymphatics are present in the rectovaginal septum; in men, in Denonvilliers fascia. Additionally, the entire mesorectum contains lymphatics and is a common site for spread.

The anal canal is 3 to 4 cm long and extends from the anal verge to the dentate line (Fig. 41.3). It is angulated in relation to the rectum because of the pull of the sling-like puborectalis muscle creating the anorectal angle. The anal canal consists of an inner epithelial lining, a vascular subepithelium, the internal and external anal muscular sphincters, and fibromuscular supporting tissue. The internal and external anal sphincters, separated by the longitudinal layer, encircle the anal canal and have connections superior to puborectalis and the transverse perineii. The evacuation of bowel contents depends on action by the muscles of both the involuntary internal sphincter and the voluntary external sphincter. The anal canal is innervated by pain sensory nerve fibers, which end at the dentate line. The anal verge is defined as the region where the squamous epithelium that lines the lower anal canal joins with the skin of the perineum. Anal cancers can occur in the perianal skin, anal canal, or low rectum. A cancer of the low rectum that is involving the anal verge should be treated as an anal cancer.

The anal region has an extensive lymphatic system, with three main pathways. These include superior drainage along the superior hemorrhoidal vessels to the inferior mesenteric chain, along the middle and inferior hemorrhoidal vessels to the iliac chains, and inferior to the superficial inguinal nodes.

Initial imaging of the rectum is typically achieved with pelvic CT. Oral contrast helps to delineate bowel and intraluminal masses, while IV contrast is useful in distinguishing pathologic adenopathy. Pelvic MRI can be helpful in producing more detailed anatomic imaging of pelvic structures. PET/CT is not routinely indicated in rectal cancer, although it's role is evolving. The most useful imaging modality in the staging of rectal cancer is endorectal ultrasound. This test, in experienced hands, has 97% accuracy in defining the T-stage, and slightly less accuracy (80%–86%) in defining regional nodal spread of rectal cancers.[1]

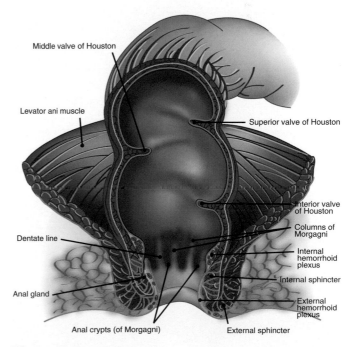

Figure 41.1. Rectal anatomy.

Middle valve of Houston

Levator ani muscle

Superior valve of Houston

Inferior valve of Houston

Columns of Morgagni

Internal hemorrhoid plexus

Internal sphincter

Dentate line

External hemorrhoid plexus

Anal gland

Anal crypts (of Morgagni)

External sphincter

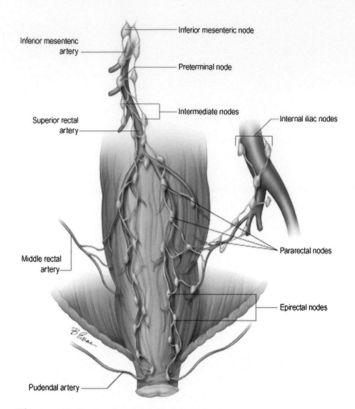

Figure 41.2. Lymphatic drainage of the rectum.

Similarly, imaging in anal cancer can be accomplished using CT and/or MRI of the pelvis. Furthermore, PET/CT scan (CAT) is indicated as a routine part of the staging workup in anal cancers, as it is more sensitive than physical exam and CT in identifying both the primary tumor and the involved inguinal lymph nodes.[2]

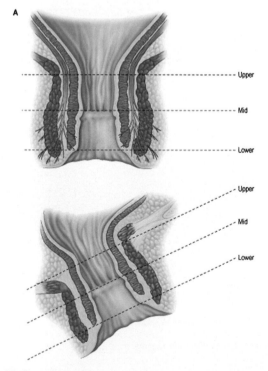

Figure 41.3. Anal anatomy.

DESCRIPTION OF HISTOLOGICAL ANATOMY OF STRUCTURE INCLUDING FUNCTIONAL UNITS IMPORTANT IN RADIATION DAMAGE

The rectal epithelium consists of simple columnar cells interspersed with goblet cells. Underlying the epithelium is the lamina propria, where crypts of Lieberkuhn (fewer but deeper than in the remainder of the colon) and lymphoid nodules reside. Deep to this, the muscularis mucosae consists of two layers, the inner circular layer and the outer longitudinal layer. The submucosa is composed of fibroelastic connective tissue. Finally, the muscularis externa is composed of an inner circular and outer longitudinal layer of muscle. The Auerbach myenteric plexus is housed between these two layers of smooth muscle.

The anal canal is lined by simple columnar/cuboidal epithelium proximally, stratified nonkeratinizing squamous epithelium distal to the anal valves, and stratified keratinizing squamous epithelium at the anus. Within the underlying lamina propria are sebaceous glands, circumanal glands, lymphoid nodules, the rectal columns of Morgagni and hair follicles at the anus. Similar to the rectum, the remaining layers consist of a muscularis mucosa (inner and outer muscle layers), submucosa composed of fibrous connective tissue and outer muscularis externa composed of the inner circular layer, which forms the internal anal sphincter and outer longitudinal layer. The external anal sphincter is composed of voluntary skeletal muscle that invests the anal canal and displays continuous tone in order to maintain a closed anal orifice. Anal adventitia attaches the anus to surrounding structures.

The tolerance of a tissue for radiation is governed by its intrinsic ability to maintain a sufficient number of clonogenic cells able to repopulate after damage to the mature functional cells of the structure following injury. Furthermore, tolerance depends on the structural organization of the tissue. Within the rectum and anus, functional subunits are structurally undefined in that clonogenic cells can migrate throughout the mucosa in order to repopulate after damage. This results in tolerance for fairly high doses of radiation.

Several mechanisms are hypothesized regarding the cause of functional radiation damage to the rectum. One theory is that damage to the vasculature caused by radiation interrupts the blood supply to the mucosa (Fig. 41.4), causing full-thickness atrophy and subsequent breakdown resulting from mechanical

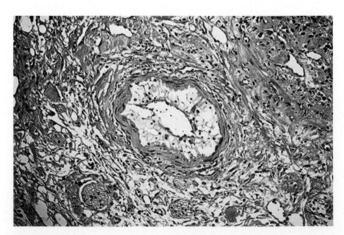

Figure 41.4. Subendothelial accumulation of foamy macrophages in a vessel in radiation colitis.

irritation and bacterial infection. These processes lead to an acute inflammatory response, which can cause fibrosis, thus leading to organ dysfunction. Prolonged expression of profibrotic cytokines, transforming growth factor beta (TGF-β1) and connective tissue growth factor (CTGF), results in fibrosis in the smooth muscle of the internal anal sphincter. Additionally, damage to the anal sphincter can result from injury of the myenteric plexus interrupting normal functioning of the musculature. Histologic analysis of rectal specimens following preoperative chemoradiotherapy (CRT) and abdominoperineal resection has revealed an increase in collagen deposition in the internal anal sphincter, as well as an increase in nerve density within the myenteric plexus.[3] Nerve density appears to increase linearly with time from radiotherapy (RT) to surgery. Overproduction of profibrogenic cytokines, such as TGF-β1, leads to deposition of collagen and smooth muscle fibrosis, likely contributing to organ dysfunction.[4–6] Similarly, chronic proctitis may be related to submucosal fibrosis and the presence of inflammatory cytokines.

DATA FOR FRACTIONATED AND SINGLE DOSE EFFECTS ON THE ANUS AND RECTUM

Various fractionation schemes have been used for anorectal cancers. In the United States and Britain, neoadjuvant or adjuvant doses in the 45 to 50 Gy range delivered over 25 to 28 fractions are considered standard for resectable rectal cancers.[7] Unresectable lesions are boosted an additional 5 to 9 Gy. Concurrent chemotherapy (CT) with 5-FU based regimens is typically employed. For most primary anal malignancies, where organ preservation is the goal, definitive doses in the 45 to 60 Gy range using conventional fractionation (1.8–2.0 Gy/d) are delivered depending on the stage and response of disease.[7] In both rectal and anal carcinomas, concomitant CT administration is considered the standard of care.

The acceptance of these regimens, and our understanding of their toxicity profiles, is largely based on randomized clinical trial data. For anal carcinomas, studies by the Wayne State University, GI Tumor Study Group (GITSG), European Organization for Research and Treatment of Cancer (EORTC), radiation therapy Oncology Group (RTOG), and United Kingdom Coordinating Committee on Cancer Research (UKCCCR) have yielded the highest level of evidence for using combined CRT with conventionally fractionated regimens in an attempt to avoid a morbid abdominoperineal resection and/or need for colostomy.[8–12].

In evaluating the isoeffectiveness of different fractionation schedules, one has to have a good estimate of the α/β ratio for rectal cancer as well as that for early and late effects on normal rectal mucosa. Unfortunately, data for anorectal cancers in this realm are sparse. Some of the most reliable estimates come from a Polish group who retrospectively evaluated three different fraction schedules: 25 Gy at 5 Gy/fraction, 30 Gy at 3 Gy/fraction, and 42 Gy at 1.5 Gy/fraction twice daily.[13] A linear-quadratic model provided an α estimate of 0.339 (SE 0.115) and β estimate of 0.067 (SE 0.027), which resulted in an α/β ratio of 5.06 Gy. According to the authors, "In all three schemes the overall radiation treatment time was short, which limits the rationales for incorporating time effect into the model. If, however, time was incorporated, the α/β ratio was 11.1 Gy and the dose increment required to compensate for repopulation was 0.15 Gy/d." The authors cautioned that due to biases they could not control in their study, their

conclusions about the rectal α/β ratio should be considered "hypothesis generating."

There are more data concerning the α/β ratio for late rectal complications. According to Fowler et al., the α/β ratio for late rectal complications is in the range of 2.5 to 5 Gy as determined by both animal and clinical data.[14,15] In spite of Fowler's assertion that the α/β ratio "might possibly be somewhat higher than 3 Gy," he specifically uses a 3 Gy value when using theoretical modeling to show a stronger enhancement of tumor effect than of late rectal complications for larger (and fewer) fractions, in prostate tumors uniquely.[14] Interestingly, Fowler has proposed a new and relatively unconfirmed method of prediction for acute rectal reactions, which he states should be considered preliminary modeling that requires further clinical data. In those predictions, the α/β ratio for early rectal complications is presumed to be 10 Gy. Given that presumption, he states that if the BED in Gy_{10} is <60 Gy, the schedule is probably safe from acute rectal complications.[14]

Long-term follow-up data from large randomized rectal cancer trials provide insight into the toxicity profiles associated with irradiation of the bowel. The published data overwhelmingly support the use of preoperative RT/CRT in the treatment of locally advanced rectal cancer. Over the last few decades, various regimens have been used in preoperative RT, including hypofractionated courses initiated by the Swedish rectal cancer trial. This trial employed 25 Gy in five fractions preoperatively. An alternative, such as the most commonly used regimen in the United States, is preoperative CRT with concurrent 5-FU and a radiation dose of 50.4 Gy in 28 fractions. The addition of CT adds toxicity, but further improves local control and pathologic complete response (pCR) rate over RT alone.[16] Most trials have shown preoperative RT improves local control and decreases toxicity compared with postoperative therapy, with a few trials showing improvement in overall survival (OS) with the addition of RT to surgery.[17,18] Although an attractive hypothesis, most data indicate that preoperative RT with or without CT does not increase the ability to perform sphincter-sparing surgery.

It is notable in considering the following literature reviews that RT for anorectal malignancies intentionally irradiates the full circumferential thicknesses of the involved parts of the anus or rectum, whereas studies in prostate cancer or gynecologic malignancies may have higher radiation doses to portions of the rectal wall adjacent to the targets of interest (cervix, prostate) that may have steep dose-gradient fall-offs over the more posterior parts of the rectum. With the advent of techniques such as three-dimensional (3D)-conformal planning, intensity-modulated radiotherapy (IMRT), and its concomitant image guidance, our understanding of rectal toxicities continues to evolve. Most of the prospective trials discussed below were performed in an era where two or four field pelvis RT techniques would have been implemented, not taking into account the anatomic detail and dose constraints that can be achieved with modern RT techniques.

CONVENTIONAL FRACTIONATION

The UKCCCR trial published in *Lancet* in 1996 was the first phase III data to show benefit to combined chemoradiation in locally advanced anal cancer, followed shortly thereafter by the EORTC trial (Bartelink et al.).[8,9] Patients in the UKCCCR trial were randomized between 45 Gy external beam alone over 4 to 5 weeks versus the same RT with concurrent 5-FU (1,000 mg/m^2 for 4 days or 750 mg/m^2 for 5 days) by continuous infusion during the first and the final weeks of RT and mitomycin (12 mg/m^2) on day 1 of the first course. Good responders, based on clinical response at 6 weeks after treatment, were treated with boost RT, and poor responders received salvage surgery. Combined modality therapy lowered the risk of local recurrence at 4 years from 59% in the RT-alone group to 36% in the combined modality group. The risk of death from anal cancer was also reduced with combined modality therapy, although overall survival (OS) was not different. Early morbidity, defined as any report of morbidity during treatment or up to 2 months following, was worse in the combined modality arm, but late complication rates were similar (Table 41.1). The authors did not specifically define a late toxicity grading system, but characterized the early toxicity as mild, moderate, or severe for skin, gastrointestinal (GI) and genitourinary domains. Fewer than 20% of patients were reported to have severe early skin or GI morbidity, and severe early genitourinary morbidity was uncommon in <2% of patients irrespective of treatment arm. For late complications, the addition of CT did not seem to increase the risk of complications. Just under 30% of the total study population had a late GI toxicity.

The EORTC trial by Bartelink et al.[9] was an additional phase III trial to show benefit in use of concurrent chemoradiation in locally advanced anal cancer. A total of 103 patients were randomized between radiation alone ($n = 52$) or concurrent CRT ($n = 51$). Radiation was 45 Gy in 1.8 Gy/fraction followed by a 6-week break, and then 15-Gy boost for complete responders and 20-Gy boost for partial responders. Chemotherapy was 5-FU (750 mg/m^2 daily 5-FU as a continuous infusion on days 1–5 and 29–33), and a single dose of mitomycin (15 mg/m^2) administered on day 1. Results indicated that combined modality therapy improved locoregional control by 18% at 5 years and improved colostomy-free rate by 32% at 5 years. The methods of the study do not describe a late toxicity grading system, but early toxicities were graded according to the WHO criteria available at the time[19]. Approximately one third of patients in each treatment arm had early grade 2 diarrhea, defined as "tolerable, but >2 days." In the RT-alone and combined modality group, 7.7% and 19.6% had early grade 3 diarrhea, defined as "Intolerable, requiring therapy." There were no significant increases in late effects between the two treatment arms, which included ulceration, fistula formation, stenosis/severe fibrosis (Table 41.2). Nevertheless, only 2 of 52 patients had a "severe" rectal ulcer in the RT-alone group, whereas 9 of 51 patients had such in the combined modality group. Fistulas, perforations, and rectal stenoses were observed, and their incidence was noted in approximately 5% of the study population.

RTOG 8704 investigated the addition of mitomycin to standard 5-FU based CRT in definitive nonsurgical treatment of anal cancer.[10] Patients received 45 to 50.4 Gy of pelvic RT with concurrent CT with 5-FU ($1,000 \text{ mg/m}^2\text{/d}$ for 4 days) and were randomized to receive mitomycin (10 mg/m^2 per dose for two doses) or no additional therapy. A statistically significant difference in the colostomy rate at 4 years (9% vs. 22% $p = 0.02$), colostomy-free survival (71% vs. 59% $p = 0.014$), and disease-free survival (73% vs. 51% $p = 0.0003$) were observed in the mitomycin arm (Fig. 41.5). Acute toxicity was defined as any toxicity occurring within 90 days of the start of treatment, and the RTOG toxicity criteria at the time were used[20] (grade 4 acute GI toxicity was defined as "acute or subacute obstruction, fistula or perforation; GI bleeding requiring transfusion; abdominal pain or tenesmus requiring tube decompression or bowel diversion"; grade 5 was death). Acute toxicity was higher

TABLE 41.1	Early and Late Morbidity as Reported in the UKCCCR Trial for Anal Cancer		
	RT	*CMT*	*p^a*
EARLY MORBIDITY	110/285	140/292	0.03
Hematological[b]			
WBC × 10^9/L			
<2.0	0	13	
<1.0	0	6	
Platelets × 10^9/L			
<50	0	7	
<25	0	7	
Skin			
Overall	76	93	
Severe	39	50	
GI			
Overall	39	46	
Severe	5	14	
Genitourinary			
Overall	13	20	
Severe	1	3	
LATE MORBIDITY[c]	106/285	122/292	0.39
Skin	47	59	
GI	77	84	
Genitourinary	19	18	
Other	14	23	
MORBIDITY AFTER SURGICAL SALVAGE	63/114	37/67	1.00
Wound[d]	22 (35%)	12 (32%)	
Colostomy	6 (10%)	2 (5%)	
Other	51 (81%	27 (73%)	

[a]χ^2 with Yate correction, 1 degree of freedom.
[b]No reduced hemoglobin concentrations were recorded.
[c]Excludes reports after residual/recurrent disease.
[d]Includes abdominal and perineal wounds.
WBC, white blood cells.
CMT, combined modality therapy.

TABLE 41.2	Late Morbidity as Reported by Bartelink et al.[9]	
Severe Late Side Effects		
Side Effect	*XRT*	*XRT + CT*
Anal damage		
Ulcer	2	9
Fistula	3	2
Perforation	2	2
Rectal stenosis requiring surgery	2	3
Skin ulceration	2	3
Severe fibrosis	4	3

Note: 52 patients were treated in the XRT-alone group, 51 patients in the combined modality arm.
CT, chemotherapy; XRT, radiotherapy..

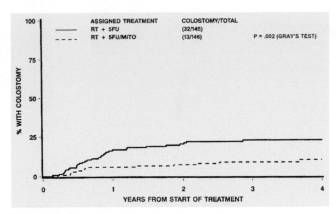

Figure 41.5. Time to colostomy as reported in RTOG 8704.

in the mitomycin arm (23% vs. 7% grade 4 or 5 toxicity p = 0.001); however, this toxicity was primarily hematologic. Only 4% of patients in the 5-FU arm and 7% of patients in the 5-FU plus Mitomycin C arm developed an early non-hematologic grade 4 or 5 toxicity. Furthermore, this trial revealed that salvage for persistent disease after neoadjuvant chemoradiation with additional nonsurgical treatment is feasible. For residual disease, a boost of 9 Gy given with 5-FU and cisplatin resulted in a 50% salvage rate (12/24 patients rendered disease free without radical surgery).

A small series (34 patients) from the Central California Research Group evaluated long-term morbidity (defined as occurring >90 days after commencement of treatment) in patients with anal cancer treated with RT (36–50.4 Gy in 1.8 Gy/fraction) and concurrent 5-FU (1,000 mg/m² /d for 4 days) and mitomycin (15 mg/m²) given during weeks 1 and 4. They reported excellent 10-year colostomy-free survival and low rates of late morbidity using the RTOG/EORTC late toxicity grading system.[11] There were no late toxicities reported in 30% of the patients, whereas 60% of patients reported a grade 1 or 2 toxicity (mild to moderate diarrhea, cramping, excessive rectal mucous, or intermittent bleeding). Chronic diarrhea (grade 1 or 2) was the most frequently observed late complication in 17 patients (50%). There were no grade 4 (necrosis/perforation or fistula) complications noted of the small/large intestines or anal canal (Table 41.3).[11] In addition, only one patient (3%) was noted to have a grade 3 (obstruction or bleeding, requiring surgery) complication for the bowels or anal canal. No patient required surgery/colostomy due to a recurrence at 10 years of follow-up.

RTOG 92-08 began as a phase II single arm study for patients with anal cancer evaluating split course RT to a total dose higher than past standards (59.6 Gy) with concurrent 5-FU (two cycles of 1,000 mg/m² over 24 hours for 4 days) and mitomycin (10 mg/m² bolus) over 8.5 weeks with a mandatory treatment break of 2 weeks.[12] The study closed and reopened with a single arm schema with no mandatory treatment break. Survivals were estimated using the Kaplan-Meier method, and results were compared with the mitomycin arm of RTOG 87-04. With median follow-up of 12 years in the split course group and 8.8 years in the continuous RT group, there was no significant difference in Local Regional Failure (LRF) or OS when compared with RTOG 87-04.[21] No patient in either treatment group experienced a grade 3 or higher late toxicity. Overall this trial indicated very low toxicity rates, with only 5% of patients experiencing grade 2 late complications. Five-year estimates of colostomy-free survival rates were 58% in the mandatory break group and 75% in the continuous RT group. This compares with 75% at 4 years in RTOG 87-04. Thus, the conclusion was drawn that although dose escalation had not been adequately tested in this trial, treatment breaks should be minimized as they resulted in more patients having to undergo salvage radical surgery while having little effect on decreasing late toxicity.

Several retrospective series including patients with anal cancer of various stages treated with RT with or without CT report local failures on the order of 5% to 30%.[22-30] Additionally, colostomy-free survival is generally good, ranging from 55% to 90%. Late toxicity is on the order of 12% to 30% grade 3 and 4 RTOG/EORTC toxicity in these series, with trends toward lower toxicity in patients treated after the mid-1980s with improved RT delivery.

A meta-analysis of preoperative RT versus surgery alone for resectable rectal cancer including data from 6,426 patients indicated a reduction in 5-year overall mortality (OR: 0.84, 95% CI: 0.72–0.98, p = 0.03), cancer-related mortality (OR: 0.71, 95% CI: 0.61–0.85, $p < 0.001$), and a reduction in local recurrence (OR: 0.49, 95% CI: 0.38–0.62, $p < 0.001$) with the addition of preoperative RT to surgery.[18] There was a large variation in RT regimens, with doses ranging from 5 to 45 Gy, daily dose from 1.75 to 5 Gy, and fraction number from 1 to 25. The most frequent complications were sepsis (18.3%), anastomotic leak (5.2%), and bowel obstruction (5.2%). The RT group had statistically higher rates of sepsis (21% vs. 15% $p < 0.001$) and total postoperative complications (21% vs. 17.8% p = 0.03), although postoperative mortality was not different between the two groups. There was an indication that patients who received an RT regimen with a BED higher than 30 Gy did worse in regard

TABLE 41.3	Incidence of Late Morbidity After CRT for Anal Cancer as Reported by John et al.[11]				
Incidence of Late Morbidity from Chemoradiation in 34 Patients with Anal Cancer					
Toxicity	*Grade 0*	*Grade 1*	*Grade 2*	*Grade 3*	*Grade 4*
Small/large intestine	17 (50%)	9 (26%)	7 (20%)	1 (3%)	0
Skin	24 (70%)	4 (12%)	3 (9%)	1 (3%)	2 (6%)
Anal cancer	18 (53%	5 (15%)	10 (29%)	1 (3%)	0
Worst toxicity per patient	10 (29%)	10 (29%)	10 (29%)	2 (6%)	2 (6%)

Note: In addition to above, one patient each developed ureteral stenosis and uterine prolapse.

TABLE 41.4	Comparison of Side Effect Profiles in Preoperative Versus Postoperative CRT

Grade 3 or 4 Toxic Effects of CRT, According to Actual Treatment Given[a]

Type of Toxic Effect	Preoperative CRT (n = 339)	Postoperative CRT (n = 237)	p Value
	% of Patients		
ACUTE			
Diarrhea	12	18	0.04
Hematologic effects	6	8	0.27
Dermatologic effects	11	15	0.09
Any grade 3 or 4 toxic effect	27	40	0.001
LONG TERM			
GI effects[b]	9	15	0.07
Strictures at anastomotic site	4	12	0.003
Bladder problems	2	4	0.21
Any grade 3 or 4 toxic effect	14	24	0.01

[a]All patients who received any preoperative or postoperative RT according to protocol were included in this analysis. Some patients had more than one toxic effect.

[b]The GI effects were chronic diarrhea and small-bowel obstruction. The incidence of small-bowel obstruction requiring reoperation was 2% in the preoperative-treatment group and 1% in the postoperative-treatment group ($p = 0.70$).

to postoperative mortality. The authors conclude that there is a slightly higher risk of postoperative complications with preoperative RT, but this does not translate into a survival detriment. Additionally, preoperative RT improves Local Control (LC), cause specific survival (CSS), and OS.

A landmark German study using conventionally fractionated RT of 421 patients looking at preoperative CRT versus postoperative CRT indicated improved local control and toxicity profiles in the preoperative group.[31] Acute and long-term toxic effects were graded according to a German classification system that corresponds to the World Health Organization criteria for assessing the toxicity of CT and that is compatible with the criteria of the RTOG and the European Organization for Research and Treatment of Cancer with respect to the acute and late adverse effects of RT.[32] Patients received 50.4 Gy in 1.8 Gy/fraction to the tumor and pelvic nodes with concurrent 5-FU (1,000 mg/m^2/d) during the first and fifth weeks of radiation as a continuous 120-hour infusion. Subsequent to completion of concurrent therapy, four additional cycles of bolus 5-FU were applied (500 mg/m^2). Radiation was identical in the pre-op and post-op arms except for an additional 5.4-Gy boost given in the postoperative setting. Overall grade 3 and 4 acute toxic effects occurred in 27% in the preoperative group versus 40% in the postoperative group ($p = 0.001$). Late toxicity was 14% and 24%, respectively ($p = 0.01$). The most overwhelming difference in the profile of late toxic effects was significantly less chronic diarrhea and anastomotic stricture in the preoperative group (Table 41.4).

In a French trial FFCD 9,203 ($n = 733$) comparing preoperative RT (45 Gy in 25 fractions) ± CT with 5-FU (350 mg/m^2/d for the first and fifth weeks of RT), CRT decreased local recurrence at 5 years (8.1% vs. 16.5%), as well as pCR rates (11.4% vs. 3.6%).[16] Acute toxicity was worse in the CRT group (grades 3 and 4 14% vs. 2.7% $p < 0.05$). There was no difference in sphincter preservation rates or OS between groups.

In one of the few studies designed specifically to assess RT toxicities following pelvic RT, Haddock et al.[33] reported prospectively collected data on patient-reported bowel function at baseline and over a period of 1 year. Eligible patients received whole pelvic RT to a total dose of 45 to 53.5 Gy in 1.7- to 2.1-Gy fractions. All measures of bowel function worsened during RT, with measures of increased urgency, clustering of bowel movements, and incontinence persisting at 1 year (Table 41.5).

HYPOFRACTIONATION

There are few data on the potential effects of altered fractionation schedules in reducing anorectal injury. MD Anderson published their experience with sphincter-sparing local excision and adjuvant radiation for anal-rectal melanomas using a hypofractionated regimen of 30 Gy in five fractions over 2.5 weeks.[34] Treatment was well tolerated, aside from the development of acute radiation-related dermatitis, particularly in the inguinal folds, which was usually a self-limited toxicity. Of 23 patients treated, six developed a chronic radiation-related toxicity: mild scrotal edema (grade 1) occurred in two patients and moderate proctitis requiring prolonged medical management (grade 2) occurred in four patients. The actuarial 5-year complication-free survival rate was 71%. The median time to development of these complications was 8 months (range, 1–12 months). No patient- or treatment-related factor was associated with the development of a complication.

The Swedish Rectal Cancer trial investigated the use of preoperative RT (25 Gy in five fractions) versus surgery alone. The trial indicated improvement in local control and OS in the RT group.[17] Patients were treated between 1987 to 1990, and long-term follow-up regarding late toxicity has been reported.[35,36] In a recently published report by Birgisson et al.,[36] Swedish

TABLE 41.5	Bowel Function at Baseline Compared with 12 months Postradiotherapy									

Patient-Reported Measures of Bowel Function at Baseline (week 0) and Up to 12 Months After Radiation

	Week (%)									
Measure	*0*	*1*	*2*	*3*	*4*	*5*	*6*	*7*	*8*	*12 Months (%)*
Nocturnal bowel movements	5	8	19	21	25	23	19	22	3	9
Fecal incontinence	2	5	10	7	9	10	18	16	3	20
Clustering	26	32	40	50	51	50	53	45	38	39
Need for protective clothing	2	7	10	9	8	6	7	7	0	6
Gas-stool discrimination problem	23	30	32	44	38	32	42	33	38	41
Occasional liquid stools	18	19	41	44	49	52	38	29	38	28
Urgency	33	38	46	51	57	57	62	54	49	53
Cramping	15	15	25	31	38	36	38	28	28	18
Blood in stool	12	5	8	24	23	21	28	22	25	16

Values are percentage of patients reporting.

hospital records for patients admitted with GI diagnoses were reviewed and patients treated on the Swedish Rectal Cancer Trial were identified. Patients who received RT had increased relative risk (RR) of small bowel obstruction (2.49; 95% CI: 1.48–4.19) and abdominal pain (2.09; 95% CI: 1.03–4.24). The risk of small bowel obstruction requiring surgery was greatly increased in the radiation group (RR: 7.42; 95% CI: 2.23–24.66). Other late toxicities were not significantly increased in the RT group (Table 41.6). Although irradiated patients were at a higher risk for hospital admission during the first 6 months after primary treatment, there was no difference between the irradiated and nonirradiated groups after 6 months, suggesting that significant late toxicities were not occurring at a higher rate in the RT group.[35] Two-hundred and three patients of 220 total on the trial completed a questionnaire at 5 years regarding late bowel function.[37] A total of 171 were included in the analysis, exclusions being made for presence of a stoma or significant dementia. Median bowel frequency per week, incontinence of loose stool, urgency, and incomplete emptying were all more common in the group that had received RT. Additionally, 30% of the RT group compared with 10% of the surgery-alone group reported impairment in social life because of bowel dysfunction.

In a Dutch trial, the efficacy of 25 Gy in five fractions in conjunction with total mesorectal excision (TME) was evaluated, and long-term morbidity reported.[38] Although RT improved local control compared to TME alone, patients reported similar symptoms as the patients treated on the Swedish Rectal Trial.

TABLE 41.6	Hospital Admissions Following Pelvic Radiation Therapy					
	Early Admission		Late Admission		All Admissions	
	RT: No RT	*RR*	*RT: No RT*	*RR*	*RT: No RT*	*RR*
Small bowel obstruction[a]	12:5	2.34 (0/82, 6.67)	51:20	2.49 (1.48, 4.19)	63:25	2.47 (1.55, 3.92)
Surgical treatment	7:4	1.70 (0.49, 5.82)	24:3	7.42 (2.23, 24.66)	31:7	4.12 (1.81, 9.37)
Conservative treatment	5:1	4.04 (0.47, 34.88)	33:17	1.82 (1.01, 3.26)	38:18	1.96 (1.12, 3.45)
Constipation	6:5	1/36 (0.43, 4.28)	27:12	1.89 (0.95, 3.77)	33:17	1.75 (0.97, 3.15)
Abdominal pain	6:1	5.88 (0.71, 49.01)	25:11	2.09 (1.03, 4.24)	31:12	2.40 (1.23, 4.68)
Stoma disorder[b]	3:3	1.04 (0.21, 5.14)	12:8	1.31 (0.54, 3.21)	15:11	1.24 (0.57, 2.70)
GI bleeding	4:0	[c]	10:7	1 16 (0.43, 3.11)	14:7	1.70 (0.68, 4.28)
Fistula	3:1	[c]	10:7	1.22 (0.46, 3.11)	12:7	1/48 (0.58, 3.97)
Stenotic anastomosis[d]	3:6	0.45 (0.11, 1.79)	5:3	1.68 (0.40, 7.11)	8:9	0.82 (0.32, 2.14)
Abscess	6:0	[c]	5:3	1.62 (0.39, 6.81)	11:3	3.64 (1.01, 13.09)
Nausea	0:0	[c]	9:1	7.94 (1.00, 62.68)	9:1	7.94 (1.00, 62.68)

Values in parentheses are 95% confidence intervals.

[a]Number of first admissions; some patients were admitted on more than one occasion and have been counted in both surgical and conservative treatment groups.

[b]Analyzed only in patients undergoing abdominoperineal resection (radiation therapy [RT] , 243; no RT, 256).

[c]RR could not be calculated because of the low numbers involved.

[d]Analyzed only in patients treated with low anterior resection (RT, 205; no RT, 194).

Number of first admissions; some patients were admitted on more than one occasion and have been counted in both early and late admission groups.

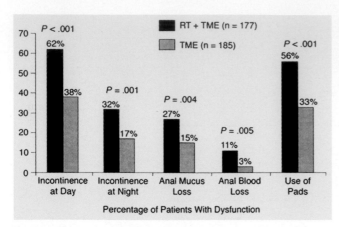

Figure 41.6. Comparison of bowel function in patients receiving surgery alone or surgery with RT.

There were higher rates of fecal incontinence (56% vs. 33%; $p < 0.001$), bleeding (11% vs. 3%; $p = 0.004$), and mucous loss (27% vs. 15%; $p < 0.001$) in the RT group (Fig. 41.6). There was no significant difference in patients requiring hospital treatment for complications (Fig. 41.7).

After follow-up of 5 to 10 years on patients treated on the Uppsala trial comparing 25 Gy in five fractions given preoperatively versus 60 Gy over 7 to 8 weeks given postoperatively, late side effects were reviewed revealing an increase in the incidence of small bowel obstruction after postoperative therapy (11%) versus preoperative RT (5%).[39] Eleven of 98 patients noted significant late bowel morbidity in the preoperative RT group compared with 5 of 34 in the postoperative RT group, and 5 of 44 in a surgery-alone comparison group, but these differences were not statistically significant. The authors conclude that there is no indication of significantly increased long-term toxicity with preoperative RT, and improved local control is achieved with this regimen.

In the prostate cancer literature, a hypofractionation trial for 97 patients with localized prostate cancer was performed comparing 70 Gy in 28 fractions using IMRT with 78 Gy in 39 fractions using 3D-conformal therapy (3D-CRT). The actuarial RTOG grade 2 and 3 rectal toxicity at 30 months was 5% in the hypofractionated group compared with 12% in the standard arm ($p = $ NS).[40,41]

DOSE ESCALATION

Patients undergoing definitive, adjuvant, or salvage RT for prostate cancer routinely receive doses exceeding 60 Gy to portions of the rectum. In a randomized dose escalation study comparing 70 Gy ($n = 150$) versus 78 Gy ($n = 151$) external beam RT using a 3D-conformal technique at MD Anderson Cancer center, at 10 years 13% of patients had grade ≥ 2 rectal toxicity versus 26% of patients in the higher dose arm.[42] Dose escalation trials performed at Massachusetts General Hospital of 393 total patients using mixed conformal proton/photon plans (70.2 Gy-8% vs. 79.2 GyE-17%), a Dutch multicenter trial of 669 patients (68 Gy-25% vs. 78 Gy-36%), and a Medical Research Council of 843 patients (64 Gy-24% vs. 74 Gy-33%) showed similar results.[43–45]

Rectal toxicity at high dose prescriptions to the prostate can be abrogated by the use of IMRT over 3D-CRT. At Memorial Sloan Kettering, a series of 61 patients were treated to 81 Gy to the prostate using either a 3D-CRT or IMRT technique. The combined rates of acute grade 1 and 2 rectal toxicities and the risk of late grade 2 rectal bleeding were significantly lower in the IMRT patients. The 2-year actuarial risk of grade 2 bleeding was 2% for IMRT and 10% for 3D-CRT.[46] This experience prompted this group to compare 81 Gy to 86.4 Gy using the IMRT technique in 772 patients. 1.5% of the patients experienced moderate (grade 2) rectal toxicity (usually rectal bleeding and pain) and 0.5% experienced grade 3 rectal toxicity (ulceration). The 3-year actuarial rate of $\geq$ grade 2 rectal bleeding was 4%. They found no difference in the rate of toxicity between the two treatment groups. Of note, the 3-year actuarial prostate specific antigen (PSA) relapse-free survival rates among patients with low, medium, and high risk for biochemical relapse treated with 81 Gy were 93%, 84%, and 81%, respectively.[47] The decrease in late toxicity is felt to be due to volumetric sparing of the rectum relative to the prostate gland, which will be discussed later in the chapter.

EXTREMELY HYPOFRACTIONATED EXTERNAL BEAM RADIOTHERAPY

For optimal tumor control, the fractionation schedule of RT should coincide with the fractionation sensitivity of the specific tumor relative to nearby normal tissues. A number of recent publications have suggested that the α/β ratio for prostate tumors is low, in the range of 1 to 3 Gy prompting examination of extreme hypofractionation regimens in this disease site

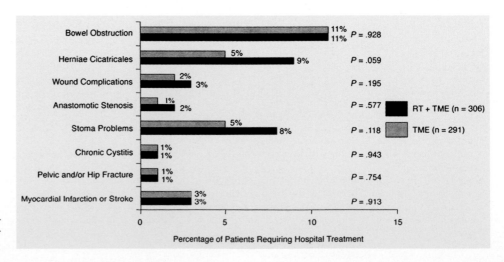

Figure 41.7. Rates of hospital admission in patients receiving surgery or surgery and RT.

in order to increase the therapeutic ratio. One of the greatest concerns regarding this approach is the effect on surrounding normal tissue late effects, which could be increased with large dose per fraction. Using a fractionation scheme of 33.5 Gy in five fractions, 40 patients were treated at Virginia Mason Medical Center for low-risk prostate cancer.[48] They reported no incidence of >grade 2 acute GI toxicity. Additionally, at a median follow-up of 41 months, no late grade 3 or higher toxicity was observed. Stanford also reported their experience with extreme hypofractionation in the treatment of prostate cancer. In a prospective phase II trial, 41 patients were treated with 36.25 Gy in five fractions using image-guided stereotactic body radiation therapy with a CyberKnife device.[49] With a median follow-up of 33 months, there were no RTOG grade 3, 4, or 5 acute or late rectal toxicities. Two patients experienced grade 3 late urinary toxicity. Additionally, a reduced rate of rectal side effects was observed with every other day treatment versus 5 consecutive days (0% vs. 38%, $p = 0.035$). Although these results are promising, longer follow-up is necessary before conclusions are drawn regarding late toxicities when employing very large doses per fraction with stereotactic body RT techniques.

PROSTATE BRACHYTHERAPY

The experience with low dose rate (LDR) brachytherapy for prostate cancer also sheds light on the issue of late rectal toxicity as it relates to dose and volume. Mount Sinai reported on 212 patients who were treated with 160 Gy iodine-125 prostate implants with median follow-up of 28 months.[50] In total, 22 patients developed grade 2 proctitis, defined as rectal bleeding occurring at least once per week for at least 1 month. The development of proctitis was significantly volume dependent for a given dose. They reported <5% incidence of grade 2 proctitis given the following parameters: 3 cc rectal volume < 100 Gy, 2 cc < 140 Gy, 1.2 cc < 180 Gy, and 0.5 cc < 220 Gy. With a median follow-up of 32 months, Waterman and Dicker[51] reported on 98 patients treated with iodine-125 brachytherapy, of which 10 developed grade 2 proctitis, and noted <5% incidence of grade 2 proctitis when doses to the rectal surface area were limited to 31% of surface to 100 Gy, 19% of surface to 150 Gy, 9% of surface to 200 Gy. The Harvard University experience is similar, reporting on 91 total patients, no patients with <8 cc of rectal volume at 100 Gy required medical intervention with argon plasma coagulation (grade 3 toxicity), while 20% of patients with >8 cc at 100 Gy required intervention.[52] The Columbia University conducted a study to evaluate the Common Terminology Criteria for Adverse Events (version 3) in which they analyzed 135 postimplant patients' scores on acute and late rectal morbidity.[53] The volume of rectum receiving 25% of the prescription dose ($\%V_{25}$) of >25% predicted for grade 1 diarrhea, and the percentage of rectal volume receiving 10% of the prescription dose ($\%V_{10}$) of > 40% predicted for maximum GI toxicity.

High dose rate (HDR) brachytherapy data for treatment of prostate cancer are relatively sparse, with shorter length of follow-up. Various regimens are used in the reported series, to include 48 to 54 Gy/8 to 9 fractions/5 days and 38 Gy/4 fractions/2 days. The trials range in size from 52 to 111 patients. In regard to acute toxicity, series report 0% to 3% grade 2 acute GI toxicity with no grade 3 or higher events.[54–56] One series of 149 patients out of William Beaumont reports decreased rectal pain with HDR versus LDR (6% vs. 20%, $p = 0.017$).[55] Grade 2 or higher late toxicity rates vary from

0% to 9%.[54,55] The most severe late toxicity reported was a grade 4 toxicity, perforation requiring colostomy, and occurred in a patient treated with the 48 to 54 Gy/8 to 9 fractions over 5-day regimen. A recent dosimetric study from Japan with 83 patients and median follow-up of 35 months reports that rectal V_{40} < 8 cc and D5 cc < 27 Gy significantly predict for decreased late rectal complications.[57] Grade 1 and 3 rectal bleeding occurred in 42% with V_{40} > 8 cc compared with 8% when V_{40} limited to <8 cc ($p < 0.001$). Those with D5 cc < 27 Gy experienced a late complication rate of 11% versus D5 cc > 27 Gy complication rate of 50% ($p < 0.001$).

GYNECOLOGIC MALIGNANCIES

Both external beam RT and brachytherapy techniques have long been used in the management of gynecologic malignancies. For both uterine and cervical malignancies, conventionally fractionated pelvic RT regimens are often employed, usually combined with CT, often platinum based, in dose ranges of 45 to 60 Gy. The toxicity to the anorectal structures is therefore similar to those toxicities observed for similar regimens used in non–IMRT-based GI malignancy treatment protocols as described above. However, various brachytherapy techniques are also used in adjunct to, or instead of, pelvic external beam therapies. MD Anderson Cancer Center retrospectively published comprehensive late complication data for 1,784 patients treated at their institution for FIGO stage IB cervical cancer treated between 1960 and 1989.[58] Almost all patients were treated with 40 Gy of RT at 2-Gy fractions per day to a pelvic field using an AP:PA field technique with a 25-MV Betatron or an 18 to 25 MV linear accelerator. This was followed by low-dose rate intracavitary brachytherapy using a Fletcher-Suit applicator loaded with standard radium or cesium tubes/pellets. When used, the cesium source strength was arranged in the tandem and ovoids to mimic standard radium loading (typically 15-10-10 mgRaEq in the tandem, and 15 mgRaEq in the ovoids).[59] These would then dwell for a period typically of around 48 to 72 hours to deliver 6,000 to 6,500 mgRaEq to the prescription point A. The Fletcher system prescription rules were designed to deliver approximately 70 to 75 Gy to the rectal wall (approximately 54% of the prescription dose to "point A," most commonly defined as 2 cm superior to the lowest end of the intrauterine source, and 2 cm lateral to the tandem, equivalent to approximately 31 cGy/h at the rectal wall[60]). The authors developed their own rectal toxicity grading system as follows: grade 1-transient pain, urgency, grade 2-persistent intermittent mild pain; transient ulcer; mild stricture minimal symptoms, grade 3-severe persistent pain; severe stricture managed medically, grade 4-colostomy or fistula. The risk of developing grade 3 or worse rectal complications was 1%/y for the first 2 years, then a sharp decline to 0.06%/y for years 2 through 25. Rates of fistula formations were doubled for patients who had adjuvant extrafascial hysterectomies (5.3% vs. 2.6% at 20 years, $p = 0.04$), similar to rates observed for patients who had pretreatment laparotomies (5.2% vs. 2.9%, $p = 0.07$). In all 45 patients had major rectal complications: 14 cases of severe bleeding, 20 cases of stricture, and 16 cases of rectovaginal fistula. In another large study from Mallinkrodt, combined external beam and brachytherapy doses <75 Gy to the rectal point were associated with a 4% rate of severe rectal complications, whereas doses exceeding 75 Gy had a 9% rectal complication rate.[61] In the same study, it was noted that when doses were < 80% of the point A dose to the rectal point, there was only a 2.5% incidence of severe late rectal complication, whereas after 80% the complication rate was 7.3%. However, when MD Anderson tried to apply the Mallinkrodt findings to their own dataset, they could not confirm that the rectal dose/point A ratio was an important predictor of toxicity.[60] Translating LDR dosimetric constraints to HDR brachytherapy techniques remains a controversial topic. Both the Mallinkrodt and MD Anderson experiences have shown that adding CT to definitive pelvic external beam radiation therapy (EBRT) + cervical LDR brachytherapy does not seem to add to rectal complications.[60,61] This has also been evaluated prospectively in RTOG 90-01, which randomized women to extended field (pelvic + paraortic) EBRT and brachytherapy or definitive CRT (concurrent cisplatin and 5-FU) for cervical cancer. The conclusion was that the addition of CT did not result in increased late treatment side effects.[62]

RTOG 92-10 investigated a twice-daily RT regimen with external beam to the pelvis and paraortic lymph nodes going to 48 to 58 Gy at 1.2 Gy/fraction, followed by 1 to 2 LDR intracavitary implants as described above.[63] The therapy was combined with cisplatin (75 mg/m^2 on days 1, 22, and 43) and 5-FU (1,000 mg/m^2/24 hours on days 1, 22, and 43) CT. Using the RTOG toxicity criteria, of 29 evaluable patients, 3, 2, 0, and 3 patients had grade 1, 2, 3, and 4 late rectal toxicities, respectively. With a 10% late rectal grade 4 complication rate (life threatening) and a 17% any grade 4 (hematologic, urinary, rectal, etc.) late toxicity rate, this treatment regimen was abandoned.

As a result of the Mallinkrodt experience, many institutions using HDR cervical brachytherapy attempt to keep the rectal dose to under 80% of the prescription dose to point A. HDR brachytherapy has been quickly adopted by practicing gynecologic specialists due to its ease of use, lack of in-patient hospitalization, and nursing training requirements in the setting of toxicity profiles that seem similar to LDR therapy. Like prostate cancer HDR toxicity outcomes, data evaluating late rectal complications for cervical HDR brachytherapy are also scant. McGill University in Montreal evaluated late rectal toxicities in 50 patients with bulky, locally advanced cervical cancer treated with 46 Gy to the pelvis with a four-field box technique at 2 Gy/fraction with concomitant weekly cisplatinum at 320 mg/m^2 and three HDR intracavitary treatments (tandem and colpostats 78%, tandem and cylinder 12%, tandem and ring 10%) given on a weekly basis to a total dose of 30 Gy (10 Gy/fraction) to point A. Although they showed excellent complete response rates in the 84% to 100% range depending on stage, some substantial toxicities were noted. Using the RTOG late toxicity grading criteria, 12% of patients had a grade 3 rectal ulcer, whereas 8% had a grade 4. Of the people who developed grade 3 or higher rectal ulcer, 40% went on to require permanent colostomy due to persistent and uncontrolled rectal bleeding. Sixteen percent of the patients had complete resolution of rectal ulcers with repeated cortisone enemas. One patient in the study developed a rectal-vaginal fistula after repeated rectal biopsies of the ulcer. The authors concluded that there were significantly more rectal complications with total prescription doses exceeding 76 Gy.

A Taiwanese group performed a controlled cohort analysis of combined cisplatinum CRT with HDR brachytherapy versus the same RT treatment without the cisplatinum[64]. RT consisted of 45 Gy in 25 fractions to the whole pelvis, followed by a 12.6-Gy boost to the parametrium. Four courses of intracavitary HDR using 6.0 Gy to point A were performed. Chemotherapy consisted of weekly cisplatin at a dose of 40 mg/m^2 for five to six cycles. Their analysis revealed no toxicity differences between the combined CT and radiation-alone cohorts. In addition, they did not observe a survival benefit with the CT. Only 2.9% of patients developed a late grade 3 or 4 radiation proctitis in the combined therapy group, whereas there was 2% rate within the RT-alone cohort. The median duration of symptoms lasted approximately 12 months. Late radiation proctitis of any grade was noted in approximately 25% of both groups.

REIRRADIATION

Data from reirradiation of recurrent rectal cancer contribute to our understanding of the toxicity of pelvic RT and the relative tolerance of bowel for high doses of radiation. Lingareddy et al. reported on 52 patients with recurrent rectal cancer who were treated with reirradiation.[65] Previous pelvic RT with a median dose of 50.4 Gy had been given, and dose on retreatment was median of 30.6 Gy. They employed a technique with opposed laterals with 25 MV photons, treating the presacral region and gross disease plus 2-cm margin. When possible, they used hyperfractionation at 1.2 Gy bid. Total dose ranged from 66.6 to 104.9 Gy (median: 84.4 Gy). Late grade 3 toxicity was 23% and grade 4 was 10%. Patients treated with hyperfractionation had decreased late toxicity of 18% versus 47% for doses given once daily. Toxicity for the whole cohort is shown in Table 41.7.

Mohiuddin et al.[66] from the same institution reported on 103 patients with recurrent rectal cancer who had received a median previous dose of 50.4 Gy. Median time to retreatment was 19 months, and the median dose was 34.8 Gy. Hyperfractionation was used when possible. Total doses ranged from 70.6 to 100.8 with median 85.8 Gy. With a median follow-up of 2 years, rates of late complications were acceptable (Table 41.8). Again, hyperfractionation improved the incidence of late toxicity. Some patients were able to undergo surgical resection after RT and had better survival than those patients not undergoing resection. Overall, reirradiation to cumulative doses of 70 to 100 Gy has resulted in late toxicity rates of 2% to 15%, with proctitis and chronic diarrhea being most common, and more serious complications requiring surgical intervention ranging from 2% to 8%.[65–68]

No significant difference has been shown in the incidence of late complications in relation to cumulative radiation dose.[65,66,68]

TABLE 41.7	Late Toxicity After Reirradiation of the Bowel
Late Toxicity	
RTOG grade 3 toxicity	12/52 (23%)
Small bowel obstruction	9/52 (17%)
Cystistis	3/52 (6%)
RTOG grade 4 toxicity	5/52 (10%)
Fistula	4/52 (8%)
Skin ulceration	1/52 (2%)

TABLE 41.8	Late Complications After Reirradiation of the Bowel

Late Complications	
Chronic severe diarrhea (grade 3)	18/103 (17%)[a]
Small bowel	15/103 (15%)
Fistula	4/103 (4%)
Skin ulceration	2/103 (2%)

[a]Of these patients, ten required parenteral nutrition.

Mohiuddin et al.[68] report data that suggest increased cumulative dose is associated with higher late morbidity, and very limited patient numbers likely explain why these differences were not statistically significant (Fig. 41.8).

In conclusion, our understanding of the effects of fractionated RT on the rectum and anus is formed mainly from close examination of clinical trials and reported toxicity. Clinically, acute effects tend to resolve shortly after RT and therefore weigh less on the treatment planning process than the prospect of late effects, which can be long lasting or permanent and often require surgical intervention, and can permanently affect quality of life. Up to 75% of patients undergoing pelvic RT will experience acute anorectal symptoms. Late effects, including radiation proctitis and chronic diarrhea, vary in incidence in published series from 5% to 20%.[69,70] About 5% of patients develop other serious late complications such as fistula formation, stricture, ulceration, or fecal incontinence.[70] The prostate cancer literature, including data from dose escalation and brachytherapy, indicates that anorectal tolerance for RT may not be as simple as once assumed; there appears to be significant volume effects that play a significant role in determining outcome. Additionally, data from reirradiation in rectal cancer reveal the fairly high tolerance of the rectum and anus for high doses of RT, with cumulative doses of 70 to 100 Gy resulting in late toxicity of <20%.

TESTING OF FUNCTION FOLLOWING IRRADIATION, DEFINITION OF TOXICITY (ACUTE AND LATE EFFECTS)

Tissue damage is mediated by the inherent cellular radiosensitivity of the tissue, the tissue kinetics, and the organization of cells within the tissue. Damage is usually divided into acute and late effects. There can also be development of consequential late effects that result from persistent severe early reactions. Up to 75% of patients undergoing pelvic RT will experience acute side effects.[69] These manifestations include diarrhea, colitis, frequency, urgency, mucous discharge, rectal pain, bleeding, tenesmus, and fecal incontinence. Acute effects can be graded according to the RTOG scoring criteria as illustrated in Table 41.9.

Late bowel effects are generally more dose limiting than acute effects, as they tend to be longer lasting, even permanent, and can be severe, producing significant morbidity and/ or requiring surgical intervention. They involve all tissue layers and can result from vascular injury, predisposing to mechanical irritation and bacterial infection. This leads to an acute inflammatory response. Additionally, in the presence of profibrotic cytokines, overgrowth of fibromuscular tissue can lead to stenosis, adhesions, and serosal breakdown. The median time to onset of late effects has been reported to be 8 to 12 months, but they can occur many years after RT. The most commonly reported late effects after radiation of the bowel are frequent bowel movements and urgency.[33] Other potential late effects include incontinence of stool, rectal bleeding (Fig. 41.9), fibrosis, stenosis, fistulas, ulceration (Fig. 41.10), and secondary cancers. The incidence of secondary cancers is very low, with radiation-induced rectal cancers being slightly more common than anal cancers.[71,72] There are occasional radiation-induced anal cancers reported in the literature.[73,74] Late effects can be graded in a similar manner to early effects according to the RTOG criteria, as illustrated in Table 41.10. Additionally, the EORTC and RTOG formed a committee to update the late injury to normal tissue classification systems in 1992, the Late Effects of Normal Tissue, leading to the introduction of the Subjective Objective Management Analytic classification system for late toxicity. This takes into account both subjective patient assessed data with objective measures such as physical exam

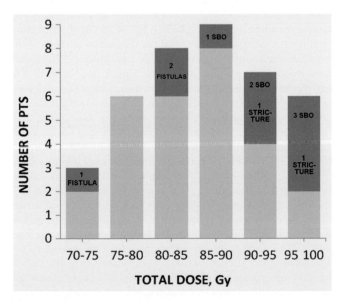

Figure 41.8. Late complications as a function of dose after reirradiation.

TABLE 41.9	RTOG Acute Radiation Morbidity Scoring Criteria

Grade	Criteria
0	No change
1	Increased frequency or change in quality of bowel habit not requiring medication/rectal discomfort not requiring analgesics
2	Diarrhea requiring parasympatholytic drugs (e.g., lomotil)/mucous discharge not necessitating sanitary pads/rectal or abdominal pain requiring analgesics
3	Diarrhea requiring parenteral support/severe mucous or bloody discharge necessitating sanitary pads/abdominal distension (distended loops of bowel on radiograph)
4	Acute or subacute obstruction, fistula or perforation, GI bleeding requiring transfusion, abdominal pain or tenesmus requiring tube decompression or bowel diversion

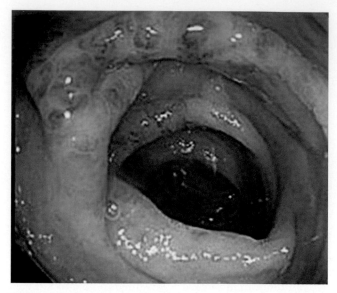

Figure 41.9. Colonoscopic view of an RTOG grade II lesion. Resulting in radiation proctitis. The patient is a 69-year-old man treated with 5,040 cGy in 28 fractions to the whole pelvis with a four-field plan, and a 2,520-cGy boost to the prostate and seminal vesicles using a seven-field IMRT technique. The lesion appeared 1 year after completing definitive therapy.

TABLE 41.10		**RTOG Late Radiation Morbidity Scoring Criteria**

Grade	Criteria
0	None
1	Mild diarrhea, mild cramping, bowel movement five times daily, slight rectal discharge, or bleeding
2	Moderate diarrhea and colic, bowel movement more than five times daily, excessive rectal mucus, or intermittent bleeding
3	Obstruction or bleeding requiring surgery
4	Necrosis/perforation/fistula
5	Death directly related to radiation late effects

findings, active steps taken to ameliorate symptoms and analytic quantifiable findings on imaging or laboratory testing.

Analysis of function following radiation is most commonly assessed with regular history and physical examination in follow-up. Some series have reported using anorectal manometry in order to evaluate anorectal function following RT. In one series of ten patients experiencing chronic radiation proctitis manifesting as urgency, frequency, and incontinence, anorectal manometry was performed and compared to age-matched controls. In the patients who had been radiated, the maximum resting anal canal pressure and the physiologic sphincter length were significantly lower. The squeeze pressure of the external anal sphincter was not significantly different. These results indicate that the internal anal sphincter may play a role in chronic radiation proctitis.[75] Histological findings in surgical specimens reveal abnormalities in the myenteric plexus, which may be responsible for functional abnormalities.[75,76] A similar

study utilizing anal manometry tested all patients before and after a course of 45-Gy pelvic RT, regardless of whether they were symptomatic.[77] Twenty patients were tested initially, with only ten available for follow-up after treatment at an average of 35 months. Nine out of ten patients reported no bowel dysfunction, and one patient who was incontinent before treatment remained incontinent. There were no differences in mean maximum squeeze or resting pressures found after RT in these ten patients.

TIME, DOSE, VOLUME RECOMMENDATIONS BASED ON BEST AVAILABLE DATA INCLUDING RISK ASSESSMENT

Emami et al.[78] report no volume effect for the rectum, and based mainly on clinical judgment report a TD 5/5 for the rectum of 60 Gy, and a TD 50/5 of 80 Gy for the endpoints of severe proctitis, necrosis, fistula formation, and stenosis.

Other data suggest that at low doses a volume effect is not exhibited, but that at high doses a clinical volume effect is observed, in that a larger area of damage produces a more severe clinical result. The prostate cancer literature indicates that patients treated with high dose RT of 70 Gy or more show a significant increase in late rectal complications if >25% of the rectal volume receives high dose.[79,80] Numerous series have indicated that in treating the prostate to higher doses and thus at least a portion of rectum to a higher dose, late rectal toxicity is increased.[44,46,80–82] In a series looking at dosimetric parameters and their correlation with various toxicities, late grade 2 or higher GI complications were associated with anal wall volumes exposed to low and intermediate doses, and with the mean dose to the anal wall.[83] Rectal bleeding was strongly associated with the anorectal wall V_{55}, V_{60}, and V_{65}. The toxicity rate at 4 years was 1% when the V_{65} was kept below 23%, and was 10% when the V_{65} was above 28%.[83] The incidence of rectal incontinence was correlated with nearly all dosimetric parameters of the anal wall; if the D-mean was limited to <46 Gy, the incidence of incontinence requiring pads did not exceed 10%.[83] Heemsbergen et al.[84] examined GI complaints as a function of the dose-area parameters to different regions of the rectum and anus in a group of men treated for prostate cancer to a total dose of 66 Gy and found that for bleeding and mucous loss, there was a correlation between the dose received by the upper

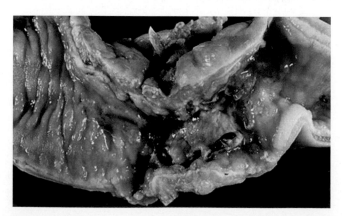

Figure 41.10. Radiation ulceration/perforation.

70% to 80% of the rectum, and for fecal incontinence, there was a correlation with the dose to the lower 40% to 50% suggesting dose-location interaction.

In the treatment of anal cancer, doses ≥54 Gy given with concurrent 5-FU and mitomycin have been associated with improved local control (77% vs. 61% $p = 0.04$), disease-free survival (74% vs. 56% $p = 0.09$) and OS (84% vs. 47%, $p = 0.02$) compared with regimens delivering doses <54 Gy.[85] A trend toward improved survival was observed for patients whose overall treatment time totaled <40 days. As discussed previously, in RTOG 92-08 a planned treatment break of 2 weeks resulted in a lower 5-year colostomy free survival rate than the group that received continuous RT with no break, suggesting that treatment breaks should be minimized. In general, available data suggest that treatment should be delivered in a timely manner, with treatment breaks avoided if possible.

STRATEGIES FOR AVOIDING TOXICITY

OPTIMIZATION OF RADIATION DOSE FRACTIONATION AND TIMING OF DELIVERY

One of the most widely employed strategies for improving toxicity associated with RT is the use of dose fractionation. Fractionation of RT is an important aspect of treatment delivery—it allows normal tissue to repopulate, as well as the repair of DNA damage in injured cells. Tumor cells become more susceptible to radiation as they proliferate and are less effective at repairing DNA damage when compared to normal cells. Conventional fractionation of RT has been 1.8 to 2.0 Gy/d, five fractions per week. Different fractionation schemes have been investigated in various cancer sites with the hope of limiting normal tissue toxicity while improving tumor control. Hyperfractionation is the increase in total dose of radiation by increasing the number of fractions, while reducing the size of the dose per fraction. The aim is to reduce or maintain late complications while increasing tumor control through dose escalation. Accelerated fractionation allows a reduction in overall treatment duration while increasing the number of fractions to more than five per week. Hypofractionation reduces the overall treatment time and number of fractions while increasing the dose per fraction.

The effects of altered fractionation on rectal and anal complications have not been well studied, and some have been previously discussed in the section entitled "Data for fractionated and single dose effects on structure." A hyperfractionation trial in bladder cancer comparing three daily fractions of 1 Gy every 4 hours to a total dose of 84 Gy was compared to conventional fractionation 2 Gy/d to 64 Gy, both given as split course, resulted in better tumor control and improved OS at 10 years in the hyperfractionation group. There were more bowel complications necessitating surgery in the hyperfractionated group; however, this was not statistically significant as more patients were alive and at risk in this group.[86]

As discussed previously, hypofractionation has become a popular method of treatment for prostate cancer, preliminarily demonstrating acceptable rates of late rectal toxicity. An ongoing RTOG study (0415) hopes to confirm these findings in a phase III setting. Additionally, as detailed in the "Brachytherapy" and "Extremely Hypofractionated External Beam Radiotherapy" sections, there are recent data in these realms preliminarily indicating acceptable rectal toxicity, but longer follow-up will be essential in making more definitive conclusions regarding late toxicity.

Timing of RT can also affect long-term complication rates and can therefore be another factor to consider when developing strategies to avoid toxicity. In a series from Memorial Sloan Kettering, patients receiving RT in combination with low anterior resection for rectal cancer were evaluated 2 to 8 years after completion of their treatment.[87] Thirty-nine patients had preoperative RT, eleven had postoperative, and fifty-nine had no RT. There was a statistically significant difference in the number of patients experiencing greater numbers of bowel movements per day and more episodes of clustered bowel movements, with better results in the preoperative and no RT groups. Furthermore, there was no difference in anal continence or satisfaction with bowel function between the three groups. It is generally accepted that preoperative RT is less morbid because of smaller treatment volumes. Furthermore, preoperative treatment does not necessitate radiation of the neorectum.

USE OF RADIOPROTECTIVE AGENTS

Pharmacologic radioprotectant agents ideally work by protecting normal tissue without conferring tumor protection, theoretically produced both through inhibition of indirect DNA damage by inhibition of free radicals and through facilitation of DNA repair allowing recovery of injured cells. For an overwhelming majority of agents showing promise in animal models, clinical human data have been disappointing. Amifostine applied intrarectally in clinical trials has shown mixed results; in prostate cancer reduced severity of symptoms with intrarectal amifostine was demonstrated, whereas no benefit was demonstrated in a gynecologic cancer trial.[88,89] A promising randomized trial in 205 patients undergoing pelvic RT indicated reduction in acute intestinal toxicity with systemic amifostine compared with no treatment.[90] Other radioprotectants in clinical trials attempting to reduce rectal toxicity include misoprostol, sucralfate, aminosalicylates, methylxanthines, and glutamine show mixed, but mostly disappointing results.

IMPROVEMENTS IN RADIATION DELIVERY: 3D CONFORMAL, IMRT

Advances in radiation delivery have been abundant in the last several decades, providing strategies for avoiding toxicity. 3D-CRT introduced in the early 1990s has allowed more conformal treatment plans, thereby reducing normal tissue toxicity. Several series have reported reduced incidence of acute toxicity with 3D-CRT compared to conventional treatments, by a magnitude of close to 50%.[20,91,92] The incidence of late toxicity has also decreased with 3D-CRT. In a randomized trial, late radiation proctitis has been shown to be reduced with 3D-CRT compared with conventional therapy without effect on local control of prostate cancer. At 64 Gy, incidence of grade 1 or higher and grade 2 or higher toxicity with 3D-CRT was 37% and 5%, respectively, compared with 56% and 15% with conventional treatment.[93] 3D-CRT also reduces fecal incontinence and perianal skin toxicity.[69] 3D-CRT allows sparing of both the anterior and the posterior regions of the skin by two to ten times compared with conventional treatments, as well as sparing of the perineal region.[94] Using 3D-CRT, the 85% isodose line covers 25% of the perineal surface, compared with 65% with conventional techniques.[94] The data align with clinical observation of decreased dermatitis when using conformal techniques.

Building on the successes of 3D-CRT, IMRT allows further refinement of RT delivery. By modulating the radiation beam fluence of each treatment field, a variation of dose delivered across the field is created allowing radiation dose to be conformed to the target while sparing normal structures. Several trials have shown the benefit of IMRT in reducing the volume of normal tissue structures exposed to high doses of radiation. Zelefsky et al.[95] reported reduction in 3-year actuarial grade 3 or higher rectal toxicity from historic controls of 14% to 4%, with no grade 4 complications in patients treated to 81 to 86.4 Gy using IMRT. Similarly, in 2008, data from Memorial Sloan Kettering with a median of 10-years of follow-up indicated the use of IMRT significantly reduced the risk of late GI toxicities (≥grade 2) compared with 3D-CRT (13% to 5%; $p < 0.001$).[96] In a series out of Finland, 20 patients treated for anal cancer with CRT using IMRT and 39 patients treated with CRT using 3D-CRT were evaluated for differences in acute and late morbidity.[97] IMRT resulted in a significant reduction in acute skin and mucosal reactions, acute > grade 2 diarrhea, and resulted in a decreased number of treatment breaks. Twenty-nine patients in this study received their boost via high dose rate brachytherapy, resulting in a trend toward lower incidence of late radiation-induced proctitis in these patients.

TREATMENT OF INJURY

Treatment of radiation injury to the rectum and anus is highly dependent on the type of injury. In general, management of late complications is challenging, often requiring invasive surgical intervention.

There is a fairly large body of data examining various treatment strategies of hemorrhagic radiation proctitis. Conservative management options include topical treatments, such as steroid and sucralfate enemas. Historically, these methods have been successful initially, but have produced a short-lived response in many patients. An evaluation of 14 patients at a Malaysian University revealed 2/5 patients treated with hydrocortisone enemas continued to bleed through the treatment.[98] Sucralfate enemas effectively alleviated symptoms in 11/11 patients. One patient who received hydrocortisone and one who received sucralfate had recurrent bleeding at mean of 6 months and both were managed with formalin injection. Conservative management should be attempted initially, with invasive options reserved for refractory patients.

A second-line treatment after failure of topical treatment includes formalin instillation. In a series of 16 patients with hemorrhagic proctitis refractory to topical methods of therapy, formalin solution was instilled into the rectum, mainly under local anesthesia, and produced cessation of bleeding in 12 patients, reduced to sporadic bleeding in 3, and 1 patient required three treatments before bleeding stopped.[99] A minority of patients developed short-term anal pain and tenesmus after the procedure. The Methodist Hospital experience is similar, as they report 100 patients treated with rectal instillation of 10% formalin, an office-based procedure, producing 93% success rate after an average of 3.5 administrations.[100] Complications were minor and only occurred in 1.1%. At median follow-up of 18 months, eight patients had re-bled and all responded to further formalin instillation. The use of Botulinum anatoxin type A injection has been reported in refractory cases as well.[101]

Other options for treatment of refractory radiation-induced proctitis include endoscopic therapy utilizing argon plasma coagulation. A probe passed through the scope delivers a field of argon gas to the mucosal surface where it is ionized by a high-voltage filament, resulting in superficial mucosal heating and coagulation of friable blood vessels. In an Italian study out of Milan, 27 patients were followed prospectively after treatment with argon plasma coagulation.[102] A mean of two procedures per patient were performed, with an average of 72 days between sessions. The treatment reduced the mean bleeding severity score from 2.8 to 0.5 ($p < 0.0001$). Complications were high, with rectal ulceration occurring in 52%, and fever and anal pain in 7%, although patients who developed ulcers were asymptomatic, and thus no discontinuation of treatment or further monitoring was required. Healing was examined in half the patients who developed an ulcer at a mean of 141 days and no strictures were observed. Other series report an expected reduction in bleeding in 80% to 90% of cases.[103]

Hyperbaric oxygen has been reported to be an effective management strategy in refractory radiation proctitis.[104,105] In a blinded, randomized controlled trial, Clarke et al. showed an absolute risk reduction in the healing response of patients treated with 30 treatments of hyperbaric oxygen compared to regular atmospheric air. Furthermore, the hyperbaric group had improvement in symptoms and better quality of life. Unfortunately, a crossover design following the initial 30 treatments does not allow for assessment of the durability of the results.

Management of radiation-induced fistulas can be challenging and morbid. The Cleveland Clinic reported their experience with rectourethral fistulas following prostate RT, indicating that management is mainly surgical.[106] They report 22 patients with development of fistulas, presenting 6 months to 20 years following RT. Surgical management included permanent fecal and urinary diversion in four patients, repair and preservation of fecal and urinary function in five patients, and in six patients who were candidates for reconstruction with preservation, five underwent proctectomy and coloanal pull-through with BMG repair of the urethra and the sixth underwent primary closure of the rectum and BMG repair of the urethra with gracilis muscle interposition. Their experience indicates that most patients can be treated initially with fecal and urinary diversion, and in properly selected patients function can be restored using BMG urethral repair and coloanal pull-through, or primary repair with gracilis muscle interposition. In a series out of France, although coloanal sleeve anastamosis (also known as the *Soave procedure*) can be an effective treatment for fistula initially, all patients required temporary ileostomy, which was successfully reversed in 7/8. Two of eight patients in their series developed recurrent fistulas.[107]

CONCLUSION

The utilization of RT in the treatment of rectal and anal malignancies has contributed significantly to the local control and survival of patients with these diagnoses. Acute toxicity from radiation of the bowel is common, but is usually managed medically and in most cases resolves after completion of treatment. Late toxicity poses a bigger challenge, in that complications are often morbid, affecting quality of life, and often require surgical management. Clinicians are well aware of the observed variations in the severity of toxicity from patient to patient, despite relatively similar delivered radiation doses. Individual heterogeneity in the response to RT has been experimentally displayed in animal models. Skwarchuk and Travis[108] used mouse models to demonstrate that the same dose of 30 Gy given to two different lineage of mice produce strikingly different rate of bowel complications. This leads to the conclusion that individual thresholds for developing a complication may vary based on genetic and/or environmental factors. Care must be taken to deliver a treatment within the therapeutic window, in order to achieve the highest possible rate of cure while limiting long-term toxicity.

ACKNOWLEDGEMENTS. The authors gratefully acknowledge Jakob Rinderknecht who was invaluable in assisting with the preparation of this chapter.

REFERENCES

1. Snady H, Merrick MA. Improving the treatment of colorectal cancer: the role of EUS. *Cancer Invest.* 1998;16:572–581.
2. Cotter SE, Grigsby PW, Siegel BA, et al. FDG-PET/CT in the evaluation of anal carcinoma. *Int J Radiat Oncol Biol Phys.* 2006;65:720–725.
3. Da Silva GM, Berho M, Wexner SD, et al. Histologic analysis of the irradiated anal sphincter. *Dis Colon Rectum.* 2003;46:1492–1497.
4. Martin M, Lefaix J, Delanian S. TGF-beta1 and radiation fibrosis: a master switch and a specific therapeutic target? *Int J Radiat Oncol Biol Phys.* 2000;47:277–290.
5. Wang J, Zheng H, Sung CC, et al. Cellular sources of transforming growth factor-beta isoforms in early and chronic radiation enteropathy. *Am J Pathol.* 1998;153:1531–1540.
6. Richter KK, Langberg CW, Sung CC, et al. Increased transforming growth factor beta (TGF-beta) immunoreactivity is independently associated with chronic injury in both consequential and primary radiation enteropathy. *Int J Radiat Oncol Biol Phys.* 1997;39:187–195.
7. The NCCN Anal Clinical Practice Guidelines in Oncology (Version 2.2008). National Comprehensive Cancer Network Inc., 2010
8. Epidermoid anal cancer: results from the UKCCCR randomised trial of radiotherapy alone versus radiotherapy, 5-fluorouracil, and mitomycin. UKCCCR Anal Cancer Trial Working Party. UK Co-ordinating Committee on Cancer Research. *Lancet.* 1996;348:1049–1054.
9. Bartelink H, Roelofsen F, Eschwege F, et al. Concomitant radiotherapy and chemotherapy is superior to radiotherapy alone in the treatment of locally advanced anal cancer: results of a phase III randomized trial of the European Organization for Research and Treatment of Cancer Radiotherapy and Gastrointestinal Cooperative Groups. *J Clin Oncol.* 1997;15:2040–2049.
10. Flam M, John M, Pajak TF, et al. Role of mitomycin in combination with fluorouracil and radiotherapy, and of salvage chemoradiation in the definitive nonsurgical treatment of epidermoid carcinoma of the anal canal: results of a phase III randomized intergroup study. *J Clin Oncol.* 1996;14:2527–2539.
11. John M, Flam M, Palma N. Ten-year results of chemoradiation for anal cancer: focus on late morbidity. *Int J Radiat Oncol Biol Phys.* 1996;34:65–69.
12. John M, Pajak T, Flam M, et al. Dose escalation in chemoradiation for anal cancer: preliminary results of RTOG 92-08. *Cancer J Sci Am.* 1996;2:205–211.
13. Suwinski R, Wzietek I, Tarnawski R, et al. Moderately low alpha/beta ratio for rectal cancer may best explain the outcome of three fractionation schedules of preoperative radiotherapy. *Int J Radiat Oncol Biol Phys.* 2007;69:793–799.
14. Fowler JF: The radiobiology of prostate cancer including new aspects of fractionated radiotherapy. *Acta Oncol.* 2005;44:265–76.
15. Fowler JF, Ritter MA, Chappell RJ, et al. What hypofractionated protocols should be tested for prostate cancer? *Int J Radiat Oncol Biol Phys.* 2003;56:1093–1104.
16. Gerard JP, Conroy T, Bonnetain F, et al. Preoperative radiotherapy with or without concurrent fluorouracil and leucovorin in T3–4 rectal cancers: results of FFCD 9203. *J Clin Oncol.* 2006;24:4620–4625.
17. Improved survival with preoperative radiotherapy in resectable rectal cancer. Swedish Rectal Cancer Trial. *N Engl J Med.* 1997;336:980–987.
18. Camma C, Giunta M, Fiorica F, et al. Preoperative radiotherapy for resectable rectal cancer: A meta-analysis. *JAMA.* 2000;284:1008–1015.
19. WHO Handbook for Reporting Results of Cancer Treatment. Geneva: World Health Organization; 1979.
20. Cox JD, Stetz J, Pajak TF. Toxicity criteria of the Radiation Therapy Oncology Group (RTOG) and the European Organization for Research and Treatment of Cancer (EORTC). *Int J Radiat Oncol Biol Phys.* 1995;31:1341–1346.
21. Konski A, Garcia M, Jr, John M, et al. Evaluation of planned treatment breaks during radiation therapy for anal cancer: update of RTOG 92-08. *Int J Radiat Oncol Biol Phys.* 2008;72:114–118.
22. Lagrange JL, Chauvel P, Francois E, et al. Conservative treatment of epidermoid cancer of the anal canal combining radiotherapy and curietherapy. Experience at the Antoine-Lacassagne Center. *Ann Gastroenterol Hepatol (Paris).* 1990;26:45–49.
23. Sommer K, Brockmann WP, Wiegel T, et al. The therapeutic results and early and late toxicities of the treatment of anal canal carcinoma by radiotherapy or chemoradiotherapy. *Strahlenther Onkol.* 1991;167:445–451.
24. Allal AS, Mermillod B, Roth AD, et al. Impact of clinical and therapeutic factors on major late complications after radiotherapy with or without concomitant chemotherapy for anal carcinoma. *Int J Radiat Oncol Biol Phys.* 1997;39:1099–1105.
25. Gerard JP, Mauro F, Thomas L, et al. Treatment of squamous cell anal canal carcinoma with pulsed dose rate brachytherapy. Feasibility study of a French cooperative group. *Radiother Oncol.* 1999;51:129–131.
26. Mai SK, Grieger J, Lachmann R, et al. Radiochemotherapy for anal carcinoma—effectivity and late toxicity. *Onkologie.* 2002;25:55–59.
27. Dubois JB, Azria D, Ychou M. External beam radiation therapy and interstitial brachytherapy in the treatment of anal canal carcinomas: a series of 70 patients. *Bull Cancer.* 2003;90:1107–1110.
28. Nguyen WD, Mitchell KM, Beck DE. Risk factors associated with requiring a stoma for the management of anal cancer. *Dis Colon Rectum.* 2004;47:843–846.
29. Dwyer MK, Gebski VJ, Jayamohan J. The bottom line: outcomes after conservation treatment in anal cancer. *Australas Radiol.* 2006;50:46–51.
30. de Bree E, van Ruth S, Dewit LG, et al. High risk of colostomy with primary radiotherapy for anal cancer. *Ann Surg Oncol.* 2007;14:100–108.
31. Sauer R, Becker H, Hohenberger W, et al. Preoperative versus postoperative chemoradiotherapy for rectal cancer. *N Engl J Med.* 2004;351:1731–1740.
32. Seegenschmiedt MH, Sauer R. The systematics of acute and chronic radiation sequelae. *Strahlenther Onkol.* 1993;169:83–95.
33. Haddock MG, Sloan JA, Bollinger JW, et al. Patient assessment of bowel function during and after pelvic radiotherapy: results of a prospective phase III North Central Cancer Treatment Group clinical trial. *J Clin Oncol.* 2007;25:1255–1259.
34. Ballo MT, Gershenwald JE, Zagars GK, et al. Sphincter-sparing local excision and adjuvant radiation for anal-rectal melanoma. *J Clin Oncol.* 2002;20:4555–4558.
35. Birgisson H, Pahlman L, Gunnarsson U, et al. Adverse effects of preoperative radiation therapy for rectal cancer: long-term follow-up of the Swedish Rectal Cancer Trial. *J Clin Oncol.* 2005;23:8697–8705.
36. Birgisson H, Pahlman L, Gunnarsson U, et al. Late gastrointestinal disorders after rectal cancer surgery with and without preoperative radiation therapy. *Br J Surg.* 2008;95:206–213.
37. Dahlberg M, Glimelius B, Graf W, et al. Preoperative irradiation affects functional results after surgery for rectal cancer: results from a randomized study. *Dis Colon Rectum.* 1998;41:543–9; discussion 549–551
38. Peeters KC, van de Velde CJ, Leer JW, et al. Late side effects of short-course preoperative radiotherapy combined with total mesorectal excision for rectal cancer: increased bowel dysfunction in irradiated patients—a Dutch colorectal cancer group study. *J Clin Oncol.* 2005;23:6199–6206.
39. Frykholm GJ, Glimelius B, Pahlman L. Preoperative or postoperative irradiation in adenocarcinoma of the rectum: final treatment results of a randomized trial and an evaluation of late secondary effects. *Dis Colon Rectum.* 1993;36:564–572.
40. Kupelian PA, Reddy CA, Klein EA, et al. Short-course intensity-modulated radiotherapy (70 Gy at 2.5 Gy per fraction) for localized prostate cancer: preliminary results on late toxicity and quality of life. *Int J Radiat Oncol Biol Phys.* 2001; 51:988–993.
41. Kupelian PA, Reddy CA, Carlson TP, et al. Preliminary observations on biochemical relapse-free survival rates after short-course intensity-modulated radiotherapy (70 Gy at 2.5 Gy/fraction) for localized prostate cancer. *Int J Radiat Oncol Biol Phys.* 2002;53:904–912.
42. Pollack A, Zagars GK, Starkschall G, et al. Prostate cancer radiation dose response: results of the M. D. Anderson phase III randomized trial. *Int J Radiat Oncol Biol Phys.* 2002;53:1097–1105.
43. Zietman AL, DeSilvio ML, Slater JD, et al. Comparison of conventional-dose vs. high-dose conformal radiation therapy in clinically localized adenocarcinoma of the prostate: a randomized controlled trial. *JAMA.* 2005;294:1233–1239.
44. Peeters ST, Heemsbergen WD, van Putten WL, et al. Acute and late complications after radiotherapy for prostate cancer: results of a multicenter randomized trial comparing 68 Gy to 78 Gy. *Int J Radiat Oncol Biol Phys.* 2005;61:1019–1034.
45. Dearnaley DP, Sydes MR, Graham JD, et al. Escalated-dose versus standard-dose conformal radiotherapy in prostate cancer: first results from the MRC RT01 randomised controlled trial. *Lancet Oncol.* 2007;8:475–487.
46. Zelefsky MJ, Fuks Z, Happersett L, et al. Clinical experience with intensity modulated radiation therapy (IMRT) in prostate cancer. *Radiother Oncol.* 2000;55:241–249.
47. Zelefsky MJ, Fuks Z, Leibel SA. Intensity-modulated radiation therapy for prostate cancer. *Semin Radiat Oncol.* 2002;12:229–237.
48. Madsen BL, Hsi RA, Pham HT, et al. Stereotactic hypofractionated accurate radiotherapy of the prostate (SHARP), 33.5 Gy in five fractions for localized disease: first clinical trial results. *Int J Radiat Oncol Biol Phys.* 2007;67:1099–1105.
49. King CR, Brooks JD, Gill H, et al. Stereotactic body radiotherapy for localized prostate cancer: interim results of a prospective phase II clinical trial. *Int J Radiat Oncol Biol Phys.* 2009;73:1043–1048.
50. Snyder KM, Stock RG, Hong SM, et al. Defining the risk of developing grade 2 proctitis following 125I prostate brachytherapy using a rectal dose-volume histogram analysis. *Int J Radiat Oncol Biol Phys.* 2001;50:335–341.
51. Waterman FM, Dicker AP. Probability of late rectal morbidity in 125I prostate brachytherapy. *Int J Radiat Oncol Biol Phys.* 2003;55:342–353.
52. Albert M, Song JS, Schultz D, et al. Defining the rectal dose constraint for permanent radioactive seed implantation of the prostate. *Urol Oncol.* 2008;26:147–152.
53. Shah JN, Ennis RD. Rectal toxicity profile after transperineal interstitial permanent prostate brachytherapy: use of a comprehensive toxicity scoring system and identification of rectal dosimetric toxicity predictors. *Int J Radiat Oncol Biol Phys.* 2006;64:817–824.
54. Yoshioka Y, Konishi K, Oh RJ, et al. High-dose-rate brachytherapy without external beam irradiation for locally advanced prostate cancer. *Radiother Oncol.* 2006;80:62–68.
55. Grills IS, Martinez AA, Hollander M, et al. High dose rate brachytherapy as prostate cancer monotherapy reduces toxicity compared to low dose rate palladium seeds. *J Urol.* 2004;171:1098–1104.
56. Martin T, Baltas D, Kurek R, et al: 3-D conformal HDR brachytherapy as monotherapy for localized prostate cancer. A pilot study. *Strahlenther Onkol.* 2004;180:225–232.

57. Konishi K, Yoshioka Y, Isohashi F, et al. Correlation between dosimetric parameters and late rectal and urinary toxicities in patients treated with high-dose-rate brachytherapy used as monotherapy for prostate cancer. *Int J Radiat Oncol Biol Phys*, 2009;75:1003–1007.

58. Eifel PJ, Levenback C, Wharton JT, et al. Time course and incidence of late complications in patients treated with radiation therapy for FIGO stage IB carcinoma of the uterine cervix. *Int J Radiat Oncol Biol Phys*. 1995;32:1289–1300.

59. Fyles A, Keane TJ, Barton M, et al. The effect of treatment duration in the local control of cervix cancer. *Radiother Oncol*. 1992;25:273–279.

60. Katz A, Eifel PJ. Quantification of intracavitary brachytherapy parameters and correlation with outcome in patients with carcinoma of the cervix. *Int J Radiat Oncol Biol Phys*. 200048:1417–1425.

61. Perez CA, Grigsby PW, Lockett MA, et al. Radiation therapy morbidity in carcinoma of the uterine cervix: dosimetric and clinical correlation. *Int J Radiat Oncol Biol Phys*. 1999;44:855–866.

62. Eifel PJ, Winter K, Morris M, et al. Pelvic irradiation with concurrent chemotherapy versus pelvic and para-aortic irradiation for high-risk cervical cancer: an update of radiation therapy oncology group trial (RTOG) 90-01. *J Clin Oncol*. 2004;22:872–880.

63. Grigsby PW, Heydon K, Mutch DG, et al. Long-term follow-up of RTOG 92-10: cervical cancer with positive para-aortic lymph nodes. *Int J Radiat Oncol Biol Phys*. 2001;51:982–987.

64. Chen SW, Liang JA, Hung YC, et al. Concurrent weekly cisplatin plus external beam radiotherapy and high-dose rate brachytherapy for advanced cervical cancer: a control cohort comparison with radiation alone on treatment outcome and complications. *Int J Radiat Oncol Biol Phys*. 2006;66:1370–1377.

65. Lingareddy V, Ahmad NR, Mohiuddin M. Palliative reirradiation for recurrent rectal cancer. *Int J Radiat Oncol Biol Phys*. 199738:785–790.

66. Mohiuddin M, Marks G, Marks J. Long-term results of reirradiation for patients with recurrent rectal carcinoma. *Cancer*. 200295:1144–1150.

67. Morris DE. Clinical experience with retreatment for palliation. *Semin Radiat Oncol*. 2000;10:210–221.

68. Mohiuddin M, Marks GM, Lingareddy V, et al. Curative surgical resection following reirradiation for recurrent rectal cancer. *Int J Radiat Oncol Biol Phys*. 1997;39:643–649.

69. Abbasakoor F, Vaizey CJ, Boulos PB. Improving the morbidity of anorectal injury from pelvic radiotherapy. *Colorectal Dis*. 2006;8:2–10.

70. Hayne D, Vaizey CJ, Boulos PB. Anorectal injury following pelvic radiotherapy. *Br J Surg*. 2001;88:1037–1048.

71. Caporale A, Angelico F, Cosenza MU, et al. A late complication of pelvic radiotherapy: leiomyosarcoma of the rectum. Report of a case and review of the literature. *Hepatogastroenterology*. 2003;50:1933–1936.

72. Kimura T, Iwagaki H, Hizuta A, et al. Colorectal cancer after irradiation for cervical cancer—case reports. *Anticancer Res*. 1995;15:557–558.

73. LaFerla GA, MacKay C. Radiation induced carcinoma of the anus. *Scott Med J*. 1987;32:88–89.

74. Birgisson H, Pahlman L, Gunnarsson U, et al. Occurrence of second cancers in patients treated with radiotherapy for rectal cancer. *J Clin Oncol*. 2005;23:6126–6131.

75. Varma JS, Smith AN, Busuttil A. Function of the anal sphincters after chronic radiation injury. *Gut*. 1986;27:528–533.

76. Varma JS, Smith AN. Anorectal function following colo-anal sleeve anastomosis for chronic radiation injury to the rectum. *Br J Surg*. 1986;73:285–289.

77. Birnbaum EH, Myerson RJ, Fry RD, et al. Chronic effects of pelvic radiation therapy on anorectal function. *Dis Colon Rectum*. 1994;37:909–915.

78. Emami B, Lyman J, Brown A, et al. Tolerance of normal tissue to therapeutic irradiation. *Int J Radiat Oncol Biol Phys*. 1991;21:109–122.

79. Storey MR, Pollack A, Zagars G, et al. Complications from radiotherapy dose escalation in prostate cancer: preliminary results of a randomized trial. *Int J Radiat Oncol Biol Phys*. 2000;48:635–642.

80. Pollack A, Zagars GK, Smith LG, et al. Preliminary results of a randomized radiotherapy dose-escalation study comparing 70 Gy with 78 Gy for prostate cancer. *J Clin Oncol*. 2000;18:3904–3911.

81. Zelefsky MJ, Fuks Z, Hunt M, et al. High dose radiation delivered by intensity modulated conformal radiotherapy improves the outcome of localized prostate cancer. *J Urol*. 2001;166:876–881.

82. Lee CM, Lee RJ, Handrahan DL, et al. Comparison of late rectal toxicity from conventional versus three-dimensional conformal radiotherapy for prostate cancer: analysis of clinical and dosimetric factors. *Urology*. 2005;65:114–119.

83. Peeters ST, Lebesque JV, Heemsbergen WD, et al. Localized volume effects for late rectal and anal toxicity after radiotherapy for prostate cancer. *Int J Radiat Oncol Biol Phys*. 2006;64:1151–1161.

84. Heemsbergen WD, Hoogeman MS, Hart GA, et al. Gastrointestinal toxicity and its relation to dose distributions in the anorectal region of prostate cancer patients treated with radiotherapy. *Int J Radiat Oncol Biol Phys*. 2005;61:1011–1018.

85. Constantinou EC, Daly W, Fung CY, et al. Time-dose considerations in the treatment of anal cancer. *Int J Radiat Oncol Biol Phys*. 1997;39:651–657.

86. Naslund I, Nilsson B, Littbrand B. Hyperfractionated radiotherapy of bladder cancer. A ten-year follow-up of a randomized clinical trial. *Acta Oncol*. 1994;33:397–402.

87. Nathanson DR, Espat NJ, Nash GM, et al. Evaluation of preoperative and postoperative radiotherapy on long-term functional results of straight coloanal anastomosis. *Dis Colon. Rectum* 46:888–894.

88. Ben-Josef E, Han S, Tobi M, et al. Intrarectal application of amifostine for the prevention of radiation-induced rectal injury. *Semin Radiat Oncol*. 2002;12:81–85.

89. Montana GS, Anscher MS, Mansbach CM II, et al. Topical application of WR-2721;to prevent radiation-induced proctosigmoiditis. A phase I/II trial. *Cancer*. 1992;69:2826–2830.

90. Kouvaris J, Kouloulias V, Malas E, et al. Amifostine as radioprotective agent for the rectal mucosa during irradiation of pelvic tumors. A phase II randomized study using various toxicity scales and rectosigmoidoscopy. *Strahlenther Onkol*. 2003;179:167–174.

91. Hanks GE, Schultheiss TE, Hunt MA, et al. Factors influencing incidence of acute grade 2 morbidity in conformal and standard radiation treatment of prostate cancer. *Int J Radiat Oncol Biol Phys*. 1995;31:25–29.

92. Koper PC, Stroom JC, van Putten WL, et al. Acute morbidity reduction using 3DCRT for prostate carcinoma: a randomized study. *Int J Radiat Oncol Biol Phys*. 1999;43:727–734.

93. Dearnaley DP, Khoo VS, Norman AR, et al. Comparison of radiation side-effects of conformal and conventional radiotherapy in prostate cancer: a randomised trial. *Lancet*. 1999;353:267–272.

94. Devic S, Hegyi G, Vuong T, et al. Comparative skin dose measurement in the treatment of anal canal cancer: conventional versus conformal therapy. *Med Phys*. 2004;31:1316–1321.

95. Zelefsky MJ, Fuks Z, Hunt M, et al. High-dose intensity modulated radiation therapy for prostate cancer: early toxicity and biochemical outcome in 772 patients. *Int J Radiat Oncol Biol Phys*. 2002;53:1111–1116.

96. Zelefsky MJ, Levin EJ, Hunt M, et al. Incidence of late rectal and urinary toxicities after three-dimensional conformal radiotherapy and intensity-modulated radiotherapy for localized prostate cancer. *Int J Radiat Oncol Biol Phys*. 2008;70:1124–1129.

97. Saarilahti K, Arponen P, Vaalavirta L, et al. The effect of intensity-modulated radiotherapy and high dose rate brachytherapy on acute and late radiotherapy-related adverse events following chemoradiotherapy of anal cancer. *Radiother Oncol*. 2008;87:383–390.

98. Gul YA, Prasannan S, Jabar FM, et al. Pharmacotherapy for chronic hemorrhagic radiation proctitis. *World J Surg*. 2002;26:1499–1502.

99. Saclarides TJ, King DG, Franklin JL, et al. Formalin instillation for refractory radiation-induced hemorrhagic proctitis. Report of 16 patients. *Dis Colon Rectum*. 1996;39:196–199.

100. Haas EM, Bailey HR, Farragher I. Application of 10 percent formalin for the treatment of radiation-induced hemorrhagic proctitis. *Dis Colon Rectum*. 2007;50:213–217.

101. De Micheli C, Fornengo P, Bosio A, et al. Severe radiation-induced proctitis treated with botulinum anatoxin type A. *J Clin Oncol*. 2003;21:2627

102. Ravizza D, Fiori G, Trovato C, et al. Frequency and outcomes of rectal ulcers during argon plasma coagulation for chronic radiation-induced proctopathy. *Gastrointest Endosc*. 2003;57:519–525.

103. Postgate A, Saunders B, Tjandra J, et al. Argon plasma coagulation in chronic radiation proctitis. *Endoscopy*. 2007;39:361–365.

104. Bem J, Bem S, Singh A. Use of hyperbaric oxygen chamber in the management of radiation-related complications of the anorectal region: report of two cases and review of the literature. *Dis Colon Rectum*, , 2000;43:1435–1438.

105. Clarke RE, Tenorio LM, Hussey JR, et al. Hyperbaric oxygen treatment of chronic refractory radiation proctitis: a randomized and controlled double-blind crossover trial with long-term follow-up. *Int J Radiat Oncol Biol Phys*. 2008;72:134–143.

106. Lane BR, Stein DE, Remzi FH, et al. Management of radiotherapy induced rectourethral fistula. *J Urol*. 2006;175:1382–1387; discussion 1387–1388.

107. Chirica M, Parc Y, Tiret E, et al. Coloanal sleeve anastomosis (Soave procedure): the ultimate treatment option for complex rectourinary fistulas. *Dis Colon Rectum*. 2006;49:1379–1383.

108. Skwarchuk MW, Travis EL. Murine strain differences in the volume effect and incidence of radiation-induced colorectal obstruction. *Int J Radiat Oncol Biol Phys*. 1998;41:889–895.

Breast

INTRODUCTION

The female breasts are organs with important physiological as well as psychosocial functions. When the breast is irradiated intentionally, as it often is as part of the standard clinical target volume after breast-conserving surgery for breast cancer, a number of acute and late changes may develop in the breast parenchyma and overlying skin. These changes may lead to significant distress. Furthermore, both when radiation is delivered intentionally and when it is received incidentally, as during the course of radiation therapy (RT) for other diseases, such as Hodgkin lymphoma, radiation-induced carcinogenesis is also a concern.

This chapter reviews the potential injurious effects of radiation, both when delivered intentionally and when delivered incidentally, on normal breast tissue. Other chapters in this book address the additional side effects of radiotherapy that intends to target the breast and regional nodes upon adjacent organs, such as lung, heart, bone, and brachial plexus.

FUNCTION AND ANATOMY

Mammary glands in female mammals allow for nursing the young,[1] with a number of benefits to both newborn and mother.[2-7] In human society, in addition to this physiologic function, the female breast also plays an important psychological role and is, for many women, related to their sexuality, gender identity, and social functioning.[8,9] As Millsted and Frith[10] note, "Women's breasts are invested with social, cultural and political meanings which shape the ways in which we make sense of and experience our embodied selves." As a result, cosmesis is an important endpoint of any procedure affecting the breast, including cancer therapy.

The human breast originates embryologically from the ectodermal primitive milk streak or galactic band in the fifth week of fetal development. The thoracic portion of this band eventually develops to form the mammary ridge, which then thickens, invaginates into the chest wall mesenchyme, and grows. The nipple and areola form from the differentiation of mesenchymal cells into smooth muscle, and epithelial buds branch to form future secretory alveoli. After exposure to placental sex hormones in the third trimester, the branched epithelial tissues canalize to form mammary ducts. The breast parenchyma differentiates near the end of gestation with the development of lobuloalveolar structures that contain colostrum. Further canalization and

ductal development occurs in early childhood. During puberty, exposure to hormones further promotes breast development in girls, with estrogens leading to the stimulation of the longitudinal growth of ductal epithelium and progesterone contributing to the full development of the mammary tissues.[1,11]

The adult breasts are located bilaterally on the chest wall between the second and sixth ribs, between sternum and axilla, with projection of breast tissue into the axillary region as the axillary tail of Spence.[1] The breast is enveloped by fascia and supported by the suspensory ligaments of Cooper. As Osborne describes, "The contour of the breast varies but is usually dome-like, with a conical configuration in the nulliparous woman and a pendulous contour in the parous woman. The breast comprises three major structures: skin, subcutaneous tissue, and breast tissue, with the last comprising both parenchyma and stroma. The parenchyma is divided into 15 to 20 segments that converge at the nipple in a radial arrangement."[11]

The internal mammary and lateral thoracic arteries provide the major blood supply of the breast, with a more minor contribution from the intercostal arteries and minimal participation of branches of the axillary and subclavian arteries. As Vorherr[1] describes, "The lymphatics of the breast originate in the lymph capillaries of the mammary connective tissue grid, which surrounds parenchymal mammary structures." Lymph capillaries are abundant in the breast. Somatic sensory and autonomous nerves innervate the breast (Fig. 42.1).

NATURE OF RADIATION-INDUCED TOXICITY

When the breast is irradiated intentionally, as part of the standard clinical target volume in the adjuvant treatment of breast cancer after breast-conserving surgery, a number of acute and late changes may develop in the breast parenchyma and overlying skin and may lead to significant pain and psychological distress. These changes are related to time, dose, and volume, as in other organs. Given the unique form and function of the female human breast, no useful animal models are available to study the acute and late effects of radiotherapy.

The injurious effects of radiation upon the breast are generally divided into two groups of effects: acute toxicities and late radiation effects. Acute toxicities include breast edema and skin erythema, sometimes accompanied by dry or even moist desquamation of the treated skin. Late effects include

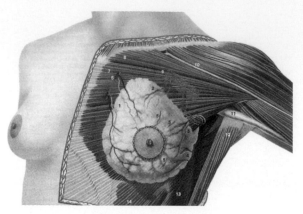

Figure 42.1. Normal anatomy of the breast and pectoralis major muscle. 1. Perforating branches from internal mammary artery and vein; 2. Pectoral branches from thoracoacromial artery and vein; 3. External mammary branch from lateral thoracic artery and vein; 4. Branches from subscapular and thoracodorsal arteries and veins; 5. Lateral branches of third, fourth, and fifth intercostals arteries and veins; 6. Internal mammary artery and veins; 7. Sternocostal head of pectoralis major muscle; 8. Clevicular head of pectoralis major muscle; 9. Axillary artery and vein; 10. Cephalic vein; 11. Axillary sheath; 12. Latissimus dorsi muscle; 13. Serratus anterior muscle; 14. External abdominal oblique muscle. (From Osborne MP. Breast anatomy and development. In: Harris JR, Lippman ME, Morrow M, et al., eds. *Diseases of the Breast.* 3rd ed. Philadelphia, PA: Lippincott Williams & Wilkins; 2004:3–14, with permission.)

persistent skin changes and fibrosis that can lead to contour deformities.

ACUTE TOXICITY

The Radiation Therapy Oncology Group (RTOG) has provided a useful scoring system to evaluate radiation-related acute skin toxicity (Table 42.1).[12]

Skin changes develop during radiotherapy in over 90% of women receiving radiation for breast cancer,[13] but these changes are infrequently severe by RTOG criteria. Skin changes during radiotherapy are primarily the result of injury to the epidermis.[14,15] Erythema results from changes in the permeability of capillaries. Desquamation results from damage to the actively dividing basal cell layer of the epidermis, from which cells differentiate and then migrate into more superficial layers of the stratum spinosum, stratum granulosum, and ultimately the outermost stratum corneum. After a dose of 20 to 25 Gy in 2-Gy fractions, there is a reduction in the number of mitotic cells in the basal cell layer. If the reduction in the number of mitotic cells is such that repopulation is sustained, dry desquamation occurs; if the number of cells in the clonogenic population is insufficient to sustain repopulation, moist desquamation occurs, with attendant exposure of the dermal layer and serous drainage.[16]

Breast edema is another acute to subacute reaction, thought to result from disruption of lymphatic drainage, and appears to be related not only to the use of radiotherapy but also to the surgery performed. Clarke et al.[17] noted breast edema after radiation in 6% of patients who had no axillary surgery, 25% of those having axillary sampling, and 79% having axillary dissection. Breast edema is sometimes quite pronounced and bothersome, but it tends to resolve over time in the majority of patients.[18] Indeed, while 33% of 733 women with early-stage breast cancer treated with breast conservation at the Joint Center for Radiation Therapy between 1968 and 1981 demonstrated mild edema and 6% exhibited moderate or severe edema in the first year, only 20% of patients continued to have edema beyond 3 years that tended to resolve slowly between the fourth and eighth years.[19] The risk of breast edema also appears to be related to breast size. Pezner et al.[20] found that breast edema occurred in 3 of 20 breasts with bra cup size A or B (15%), but in 13 of 27 breasts (48%) with larger cup sizes ($p < 0.03$).

LATE EFFECTS

Whereas early skin toxicity is related to reaction in the epidermis, late effects are primarily related to changes in the dermis and the vasculature that lies therein.[21] Persistent late changes in the skin may include hyperpigmentation; depigmentation has also been documented, particularly in patients with vitiligo.[22,23] Telangiectasias tend to form after a relatively long latency time[24–26] in areas of particularly high surface dose, such as those in skin folds and junctions between fields, and tend to be highly technique dependent. Patient factors, such as smoking, may also increase risk.[27]

Fibrosis is perhaps the predominant mechanism by which breast radiotherapy impacts upon overall cosmesis in the long term. Fibrosis tends to manifest 6 to 18 months after radiotherapy and may be progressive over time.[18] However, it is often difficult to disaggregate the effects of breast radiation from those of breast surgery, as the two modalities are commonly utilized together, and the resulting outcome is often assessed only with a global score for overall cosmesis that incorporates the injurious effects of both. For example, the commonly used "Harvard criteria" rely upon comparison of the treated breast to the contralateral breast.[28] As Kurtz notes, "[I]t is often difficult, without prior comparison, to distinguish radiation-related distortion and retraction from postoperative changes. Moreover, volume loss resulting from resolution of breast oedema may unmask surgically-related defects which may be interpreted as radiation-induced shrinkage." Quantitative cosmesis scores, based upon objective measurements of retraction and/or deformation (assessed by determining the displacement of the nipple or external breast contour), have been proposed by some groups in an attempt to facilitate sequential, standardized assessment

TABLE 42.1	RTOG Acute Toxicity Scoring Criteria for Skin[12]				
Toxicity Score	0	1	2	3	4
Description	No change over baseline	Follicular, faint, or dull erythema, dry desquamation, epilation, decreased sweating	Tender or bright erythema, patchy moist desquamation, moderate edema	Confluent moist desquamation, other than skin folds, pitting edema	Ulceration, hemorrhage, necrosis

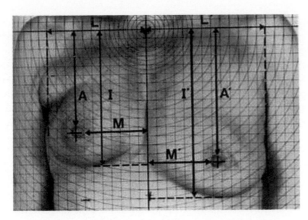

Figure 42.2. Scoring system for measurement of breast contour and nipple asymmetries. Differences (A´–A) and (I´–I) qualify upward retraction of the nipple position and the inferior breast contour, whereas (M´–M) and (L´–L) measure asymmetry in the mediolateral sense. (Reprinted from van Limbergen E, van der Schueren E, van Tongelen K. Cosmetic evaluation of breast-conserving treatment for mammary cancer. 1. Proposal of a quantitative scoring system. *Radiother Oncol.* 1989;16:159–167, with permission.)

(Figs. 42.2 and 42.3).[29] Other, more complex systems have also been proposed.[30–32]

In an attempt to quantify the marginal effect of radiotherapy after breast-conserving surgery, Liljegren et al. compared cosmetic outcomes among patients randomized to receive sector resection and axillary dissection alone versus those assigned to the same surgery plus 54 Gy of breast radiation. They evaluated patients at 3, 12, 24, and 36 months after treatment, finding that good to excellent results were reported by 84% to 90% of the irradiated patients and 91% to 95% of those receiving surgery alone. Other observers reported 81% to 86% good to excellent cosmesis in the irradiated patients and 87% to 93% of the patients undergoing surgery alone. Thus, they concluded that "doses to 54 Gy of radiotherapy influence the result negatively, but from a clinical standpoint to a moderate extent".[33]

Cosmetic assessments performed by patients tend to be more positive than those performed by health care professionals. Kurtz and Miralbell[34] estimate from the published literature that overall, 55% to 65% of patients have excellent cosmesis, 25% to 35% good cosmesis, 5% to 10% fair cosmesis, and <5% poor cosmesis after breast-conserving surgery and RT.

EVIDENCE REGARDING EFFECTS OF FRACTIONATION AND TIME, DOSE, VOLUME RECOMMENDATIONS

STANDARD WHOLE BREAST IRRADIATION

As with other organs, radiation-induced toxicity in the breast is strongly dependent upon time, dose, and volume. The most commonly employed fractionation scheme for whole breast

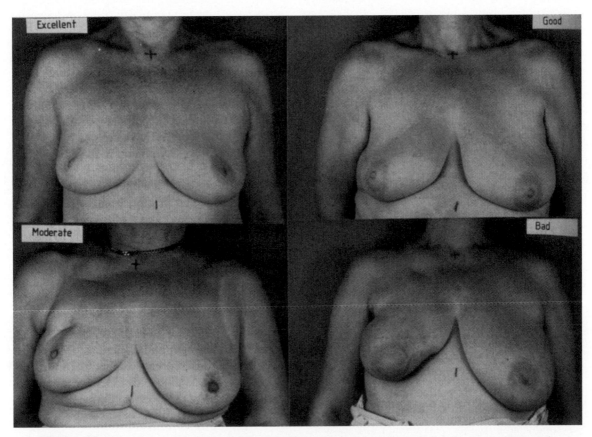

Figure 42.3. Examples of qualitative assessment of breast cosmesis following radiotherapy by a scoring panel. (Reprinted from van Limbergen E, van der Schueren E, van Tongelen K. Cosmetic evaluation of breast-conserving treatment for mammary cancer. 1. Proposal of a quantitative scoring system. *Radiother Oncol.* 1989;16:159–167, with permission.)

radiotherapy in the United States in recent years has been 50 Gy in 2 Gy/fraction.[35] Administering a similar total dose with larger fraction sizes, as administered in the early 1960s at several centers facing resource constraints,[36] has been shown to lead to increased toxicity.[37,38] With standard fractionation, whole breast doses higher than 50 Gy have also been shown to lead to substantial rates of late effects.[39]

BOOST TREATMENT

The administration of an additional boost dose to the region of the tumor bed has now been shown to reduce local recurrence in all patients with invasive breast cancer treated by breast conservation, with the greatest absolute benefit in younger patients, who are at higher risk of recurrence.[40] This has led many practitioners to incorporate a boost into their standard treatment regimens for breast cancer.

However, administration of a boost may lead to complications within the high-dose region. The EORTC 22881-10882 randomized trial of a 16-Gy boost or no boost after whole breast radiotherapy of 50 Gy in conventional 2-Gy fractions revealed a significant difference in incidence of fibrosis between the two arms. Boost was accomplished with external beam radiation (electrons or a tangential technique) in 90% of boosted patients; 10% received a low-dose-rate interstitial implant. Cumulative incidence of moderate fibrosis at 10 years was 28.1% in patients receiving the boost, compared with 13.2% of those not receiving the boost ($p < 0.001$). Cumulative incidence of severe fibrosis at 10 years was 4.4% in the boosted patients and 1.6% in those not receiving a boost ($p < 0.001$). In the Lyon study of a 10-Gy electron boost after 50 Gy in 20 fractions to the whole breast, at 2 years the boost group was found to have a higher rate of grade 1 and 2 telangiectasia (12.4% vs. 5.9%, although no difference in self-assessed overall cosmesis score (with 90% reporting good to excellent results).[41]

HYPOFRACTIONATED WHOLE BREAST IRRADIATION

In recent years, interest in hypofractionated whole breast irradiation (WBI) has increased, largely due to a desire to minimize costs and improve access to adjuvant radiation, which has clearly been established as an integral component of the care of many patients with breast cancer.[42] In light of the toxicity observed in the 1960s with the use of larger fractions when total dose was maintained, adoption of hypofractionation in recent years has involved the use of a larger dose per fraction along with a reduced total dose, in order to maintain normal tissue tolerance. As Whelan et al.[43] notes, there may be potential radiobiological advantages from hypofractionation that may compensate for the reduction in total dose. Indeed, if breast cancer cells have a lower α/β ratio than previously believed,[44,45] it may be possible to maintain equivalent tumor control with shorter hypofractionated schedules delivering lower total doses.

Several recently published trials have investigated the use of hypofractionated regimens of irradiation to the whole breast. Whelan et al. conducted a trial in 1,234 women with invasive, node-negative breast cancer treated by lumpectomy with negative pathologic margins.

Patient accrual was limited to women of small to moderate breast size (breast separation ≤ 25 cm) and few patients received adjuvant systemic chemotherapy. The trial randomized women to receive hypofractionated WBI of 42.5 Gy in 16 fractions over 22 days or standard WBI of 50 Gy in 25 fractions over 35 days. In an initial report published in 2002 after 5 years of follow-up, local recurrence-free survival was excellent in both groups, and there was no difference in cosmetic outcome. The percentage of patients with good or excellent global cosmetic outcome at 5 years was 76.8% in the hypofractionated arm and 77.4% in the standard arm.[46] At 5 years, the percentage of patients with moderate or severe late toxicity of the skin or subcutaneous tissue was low. Grade 2 or 3 radiation skin toxicity was seen in 3% of patients in each arm. Five percent of standard arm patients developed subcutaneous fibrosis compared to 7% of patients in the hypofractionated arm. Overall, 87% of patients in the hypofractionated arm and 82% of the patients in the standard arm developed no skin toxicity; 66% of patients in the hypofractionated arm and 60% of patients in the standard arm developed no subcutaneous toxicity. Two cases of radiation pneumonitis developed in each arm, and one rib fracture developed in the standard arm. In recent updates, the 10-year rate of good or excellent cosmesis was 70% in the hypofractionated arm and 71% in the standard arm, for an absolute difference of 1.5% (95% CI, 6.9%–9.8%).[47] Thus, it seems possible to accomplish hypofractionated WBI with this schedule and achieve similar cosmetic outcomes to those observed with standard fractionation in patients with characteristics similar to those entered on study. However, it is important to note that a boost was not utilized in this study, the overall rate of good to excellent cosmesis is somewhat lower than that observed in many US institutional series,[48] and long-term results regarding potential late effects in adjacent organs (such as the heart, which may considerably longer to demonstrate late toxicity) have yet to mature.

In 2005, British investigators published the results of a randomized trial assigning 1,410 patients to standard fractionated WBI or one of two nonaccelerated but hypofractionated schedules of 42.9 or 39 Gy in 13 fractions over 5 weeks.[49] t 5 years, the risk of scoring any change in breast appearance was 39.6% after 50 Gy, 45.7% after 42.9 Gy, and 30.3% after 39 Gy, from which an α/β ratio of 3.6 Gy was estimated. The risk of developing any radiation effect was much lower for patients allocated to 39 Gy in 13 fractions than those allocated to 42.9 Gy in 13 fractions. There was also a significant difference between the 50 and 39 Gy arms of the trial ($p = 0.01$), with weaker evidence for a difference between 50 and 42.9 Gy ($p = 0.05$). The percent remaining free from moderate or marked palpable breast induration at 5 years was 76.9% after 50 Gy, 64.4 after 42.9 Gy, and 84.0% after 39 Gy. After 10 years, these percentages were 63.7%, 48.9%, and 72.3%. A subset of patients (723) were randomly assigned to boost irradiation of 14 Gy delivered by electrons to the tumor bed or no boost; an additional 687 patients received boost as part of their standard treatment. There was a significantly lower rate of induration and telangiectasia among patients randomized to no boost.

The recently reported UK Standardization of Radiotherapy A (START A) trial attempted to build upon these findings by comparing 50 Gy in 25 fractions over 5 weeks with 41.6 or 39 Gy in 13 fractions over 5 weeks in 2,236 patients. Photographic assessments were similar between the 50- and 41.6-Gy arms, but there were lower rates of change in breast appearance after 39 Gy than 50 Gy, with a hazard ratio of 0.69 ($p = 0.01$). The START B trial, also recently reported, compared 50 Gy in 25 fractions over 5 weeks to 40 Gy in 15 fractions over 3 weeks in 2,215 women. In that study, reported at a median follow-up of 6 years, photographic and patient assessments suggested lower rates of late adverse effects in the accelerated hypofractionated arm ($p = 0.06$ for photographic change in breast appearance).

Further studies are underway to build upon these findings. In the British FAST trial, women received even higher doses per fraction: 50 Gy in 25 fractions, 30 Gy in 5 fractions, or 28.5 Gy in 5 fractions, all over 5 weeks, and maturation of these results will provide further interesting information on these issues.[50] Others are investigating the incorporation of a concurrent boost with the use of intensity-modulated radiotherapy (IMRT).[51]

ACCELERATED PARTIAL BREAST IRRADIATION

Even when hypofractionated, most whole breast treatments require several weeks for administration. Furthermore, whole breast radiation exposes adjacent normal tissues to potential radiation-associated toxicity. If treatment of only a portion of the breast were to yield equivalent efficacy, exposure of adjacent tissues might be more limited, and an even more accelerated and hypofractionated schedule might be tolerable. Because the majority of in-breast tumor recurrences after breast-conserving surgery occur in the vicinity of the lumpectomy cavity,[52–54] it has been hypothesized that radiation treatment targeting a smaller volume of tissue may yield an equivalent benefit to WBI. However, other studies have shown that recurrences may occur outside even a generous volume beyond the primary tumor[55] and that microscopic disease may extend far from the original primary site.[56–58] Thus, both the toxicity and the effectiveness of accelerated partial breast irradiation (APBI) are the subjects of considerable ongoing investigation.

A number of techniques have been employed to administer APBI. Early studies primarily utilized multicatheter interstitial implants. The largest reported series of patients treated with multicatheter brachytherapy to date is from the William Beaumont Hospital,[54,59,60] where investigators have reported in detail the long-term cosmetic results in 199 patients after a median follow-up of 6.4 years. Long-term cosmesis was found to be good to excellent in 95% to 99% of patients over time, with stabilization at 2 years. Breast pain, edema, erythema, and hyperpigmentation were all found to diminish over time. Fibrosis and hypopigmentation increased until 2 years and then stabilized. The rate of fat necrosis was 11% at 5 years and the rate of telangiectasia 34% at 5 years (predominantly grade 1).[61] The extremely high rates of good to excellent cosmesis have been confirmed with even longer follow-up by the same group.[62] Several other institutions have also reported their experiences with multicatheter brachytherapy, generally with similarly high rates of local control and good to excellent cosmesis, with limited follow-up, as summarized in Table 42.2.

TABLE 42.2			Toxicity in Large Clinical Series of Patients Treated with Multicatheter Interstitial Brachytherapy for APBI	
Institution	*Cases*	*Follow-up*	*Technique*	*Complications and Cosmesis*
Guy's Hospital (second pilot)[172]	50	6.3 y	MDR (45 Gy in 4–6 h/fraction for 4 d)	Among 26 cases evaluated at 3 y post-RT, 81% excellent or good patient-assessed cosmesis; 65% assessed to have altered texture of breast on physician assessment
Oschner Clinic[173]	51	75 mo	LDR (45 Gy over 4 d: 25 cases) or HDR (32 Gy in 8 fractions bid: 26 cases)	22% grade 1 and 2 complications, 8% grade 3 (including two cases fat necrosis); 75% excellent/good cosmesis at median follow-up 20 mo
London Regional Cancer Clinic[174–176]	39	91 mo	HDR 37.2 Gy in 10 fractions, 5–7 days	10.3% fat necrosis; cosmesis at 12 mo rated a mean of 78.5 on scale of 50–100; 16/27 patients assessed at 5 years had fibrosis
William Beaumont f Hospital[54,60,61,62,177]	199	8.6 y	LDR (50 Gy over 4 d: 120 cases) or HDR (32 Gy in 8 fractions or 34 Gy in 10 fractions bid: 79 cases)	Good to excellent cosmesis in 99% long term
RTOG[178–180]	99	44 mo	LDR (45 Gy over 3.5–5 d: 33 cases) or HDR (34 Gy in 10 fractions bid: 66 cases)	Grade 3 toxicity (at any follow-up) in 10%, at last follow-up grade 3 toxicity in 4%
Tufts/Brown University[181,182]	75	73 mo	HDR (34 Gy in 10 fractions bid)	Excellent cosmesis in 67% and good in 24% at last follow-up; late skin toxicity grade 1 in 19% and grade 2 in 4%; late subcutaneous toxicity grade 1 in 15%, 2 in 12%, 3 in 5%, and 4 in 13%; use of adriamycin-based chemotherapy associated with increased incidence of higher grade skin toxicity, fat necrosis, and suboptimal cosmesis
National Institute of Oncology, Hungary[183,184]	45	81 mo	HDR (30.3 Gy or 36.4 Gy in 7 fractions bid)	Excellent/good cosmesis in 84.4%, 26.7% late grade 2 or worse radiation effects; 2.2% symptomatic fat necrosis
Massachusetts General Hospital[185]	48	23 mo	LDR 50–60 Gy in 0.5 Gy/h	Very good to excellent cosmesis in 91.8%
University of Kansas[186]	25	47 mo	LDR 20–25 Gy in 1–2 d	All very good to-excellent cosmesis
Virginia Commonwealth University[187]	44	42 mo	LDR (45 Gy in 90 h) or HDR (34 Gy in 10 fractions bid)	79.6% good/excellent cosmesis

Other techniques for APBI that have developed more recently include intracavitary brachytherapy using a balloon-based catheter. With this device, concerns include the potential for fibrosis and tissue necrosis related to placement of the balloon (and source) too close to the skin or rupture of the balloon by surgical clips. A registry study initiated by the manufacturer of the device, for which management was later transferred to the American Society of Breast Surgeons, has shown 93% of patients with good or excellent cosmetic outcome at 36 months among 1,440 selected patients treated with the device.[63] However, the study design allows a substantial potential for selection bias, as well as potential under-reporting of toxicity, to affect the results. Delay of catheter insertion may be important in reducing what otherwise may be a substantial risk of persistent seroma formation.[64]

Another technique under investigation is the localized administration of a single fraction of RT while the patient is still on the operating table, before the surgical wound is closed.[65,66] Veronesi et al.[67] have reported on a series of patients treated with single-fraction intraoperative electron doses of 17 to 21 Gy. With a median of 20 months of follow-up (range: 4–57 months), of 590 patients treated, 19 patients (3.2%) had developed breast fibrosis (severe in 1, but which resolved within 24 months). Fat necrosis was observed in 15 patients (2.5%) 1 to 4 weeks after surgery and subsequently resolved. Investigators at University College, London, have administered radiation utilizing the INTRABEAM, a miniature electron-beam-driven source of low-energy x-rays (50 kV).[68] This allows delivery of 20 Gy to a depth of 2 mm and 5 Gy at a depth of 1.0 cm when the spherical applicator is inserted into the tumor bed. Tungsten-impregnated rubber shielding is used to protect the heart and lungs and to stop stray irradiation. In British patients treated with this technique, with median follow-up of 42 months, mean provider-assessment scores (on a scale with 5 being best) were 3.5 for appearance, 2.7 for texture, and 3.7 for comfort.[69] Investigators at Memorial Sloan-Kettering have reported on the feasibility and early cosmetic results of an approach involving high-dose-rate iridium therapy delivered intraoperatively to deliver a dose of 20 Gy at 1 cm from the surface of the applicator (0.5 cm from the deep surface).[70] After treating 18 patients, the investigators constrained dose at the lateral aspect of the breast applicator to 18 Gy at 1 cm after observing considerable retraction and fibrosis in 5 of the first 18 patients. Clearly, further follow-up is necessary to monitor the evolution of cosmetic outcomes with intraoperative techniques.

With improvements in target localization and dosimetric planning, there has also been an increasing interest in the possibility of accomplishing partial breast irradiation utilizing more commonly available methods of external beam RT. Potential advantages of external beam treatment include the ability to offer the treatment after full pathologic information is available without subjecting the patient to a second invasive procedure or anesthesia, decreased operator dependence, and less financial expense.[71]

While increased homogeneity of dose with external beam therapy might also reduce certain complications seen in brachytherapy series, such as fat necrosis, determining appropriate dose for tumor control by extrapolating from doses used in the brachytherapy studies has been difficult precisely because of the large differences in dose homogeneity between these techniques.[72] Moreover, improved target coverage with external beam techniques comes at the cost of a higher integral dose to the remaining normal breast.[73] Only a few studies to date have reported the clinical outcomes of APBI using external beam techniques, and the limited existing evidence has involved regimens of varying dose and fractionation. In an early study, Christie Hospital's Holt Radium Institute randomly assigned 708 patients to wide field RT with 4 MV photons to a dose of 40 Gy in 15 fractions over 21 days, or to limited field radiation with 8 to 14 MeV electrons to a dose of 40 to 42.5 Gy in 8 fractions over 10 days.[74] After a median of 65 months of follow-up,[75] a larger percentage of patients treated with limited versus wide fields had marked telangiectasias (33% vs. 12%) or marked fibrosis (14% vs. 5%).

Subsequent single institutional studies have generally used more cautious dosing schedules and more advanced planning techniques. Formenti et al.[76,77] at NYU have developed a technique of three-dimensional (3D) conformal external beam APBI in the prone position, administering 30 Gy to the tumor bed plus a 1.5 to 2 cm margin in five fractions within 10 days, noting that a biologically effective dose calculation for tumor effect with an α/β ratio of 4 (derived from several studies on irradiation of breast cancer cell lines)[78–80] suggests equivalence of this dose to a regimen of 50 Gy in 25 fractions, while a calculation for fibrosis using an α/β of 2 suggests equivalence to a dose of 60 Gy in 30 fractions.[81] In their early experience with the first 47 patients, with a median of 18 months of follow-up, they report limited acute toxicity, mainly grade 1 and 2 erythema, with 21 late toxicities occurring in 14 patients (all grade 1). Cosmetic results were rated as fair in two patients at 12 and 18 months of follow-up. In an update including 35 patients followed at least 28 months, reported thus far in only preliminary form, good to excellent cosmesis was reported by 92% of these patients, although 26% had detectable radiation-related toxicities.[82]

Investigators at the William Beaumont Hospital have described their experience with a technique of 3D conformal external beam APBI performed in the supine position.[83] In contrast to the parallel-opposed minitangents generally utilized by the NYU group, the Beaumont group has utilized four to five non-coplanar photon beams. The dose prescribed was 34 Gy to the tumor bed plus expansion in the first six patients and 38.5 Gy in the remainder, all in ten fractions. The investigators note that the latter fractionation yields a radiobiologically equivalent tumor dose of approximately 45 Gy in 25 fractions, assuming a typical tumor-associated α/β ratio of 10. In an initial report considering the experience of the first 31 patients, with a median follow-up of only 10 months, acute toxicities were minimal.[84] In a recent update, among 21 patients with a cosmetic assessment with a minimum follow-up of 24 months, 91% received a rating of excellent or good.[85] In light of these promising preliminary results, the Beaumont fractionation scheme is being utilized for patients receiving conformal external radiation for partial breast irradiation on the ongoing RTOG 0413/NSABP B-39 randomized trial seeking to explore both the efficacy and the toxicity of partial breast irradiation further.[86]

Although the early results of a small randomized trial from Hungary have hearteningly not shown large or significant differences in 5-year local recurrence and have shown improved cosmesis with PBI (7 fractions of 5.2 Gy each using HDR multicatheter brachytherapy or a nonaccelerated external beam regimen of 25 fractions of 2 Gy using electrons) when compared to 50-Gy WBI in selected patients,[87,88] the long-term results of the large RTOG/NSABP randomized study must mature before APBI is likely to be considered a safe and effective technique for general application in the United States. After all, two institutions have recently reported in preliminary form cautionary findings regarding high rates of fair and poor cosmetic outcomes with external beam PBI utilizing the same fractionation schedule as the RTOG/NSABP trial.[89,90] Therefore, we caution the reader that the ideal techniques, dose, and fractionation schedules for partial breast irradiation are still being defined. For the time being, it is prudent to administer partial breast irradiation in the context of a formal protocol whenever possible.

STRATEGIES FOR AVOIDING AND MANAGING INJURY

RADIATION TECHNIQUE AND ENSURING DOSE HOMOGENEITY

Radiation technique is important when targeting the breast or chest wall, and care must be taken to ensure dose homogeneity. Commonly accepted standards for dose homogeneity include the requirement that the maximum dose not exceed 110% of the prescription dose and that minimum dose exceed 95%.[18,91] Higher energy megavoltage beams (usually 6 MVp) are preferred over cobalt because of the greater homogeneity allowed, and when the separation is particularly large, even higher energy beams (10–18 MVp) should be considered. It has also been known for many years that inserting wedges into the treatment field may be useful in providing tissue compensation to improve homogeneity. In our practice, we have found lateral wedges to be useful in the treatment of breast cancer patients, but we believe medial wedges are best avoided due to concerns of scattered dose to the contralateral breast potentially leading to secondary malignancies.[92]

A simple, two-dimensional (2D) wedged technique is limited by the fact that the breast contour varies considerably from the superior-most to inferior-most aspect of the breast. Thus, while a simple wedge may achieve excellent homogeneity along the central axis of the breast, substantial areas of dose higher than that prescribed (so-called hot spots) may exist at other levels. With the development of 3D treatment planning systems and now widespread availability of linear accelerators with multileaf collimation capabilities, it is now possible to provide differential segmental blocking of the radiation beam through the treatment field. This has led to an interest in administering radiation to the breast using several segmented fields, using either forward planning or inverse planning to determine beam weighting. This technique has commonly been called "breast IMRT," but it is important to note that this is a relatively simple technique that aims primarily to improve dose homogeneity and differs from the inverse-planned beamlet intensity modulation that is usually employed in other treatment sites with the aim of improving dose conformality.[93] Figure 42.4 illustrates the impact of different techniques upon dose homogeneity in an example patient case.

Investigators from William Beaumont Hospital found decreased rates of dermatitis and edema in patients treated with a forward-planned IMRT technique utilizing multiple segments than among patients treated with 2D planning in an earlier era (36).[94–99] Researchers at Fox-Chase also compared patients treated with IMRT to patients treated in an earlier era with 2D plans, finding a decrease in acute desquamation.[100]

More recently, a Canadian study randomizing 358 patients to breast IMRT versus 2D wedged treatment has reported a reduction in acute moist desquamation from 47.8% to 31.2% with the use of an IMRT technique consisting of a mean of four to six segments.[101] Also recently, researchers of the British Breast Technology Group reported improvements in long-term cosmesis in patients randomized to IMRT compared with those randomized to standard 2D wedge-compensated treatment.[102] Although it is clear that intensity modulation leads to decreased toxicity compared with 2D planning, the question of how many segments are actually necessary to achieve the observed benefit and whether this treatment merits being billed at the substantially higher IMRT charge code remains hotly debated.[109]

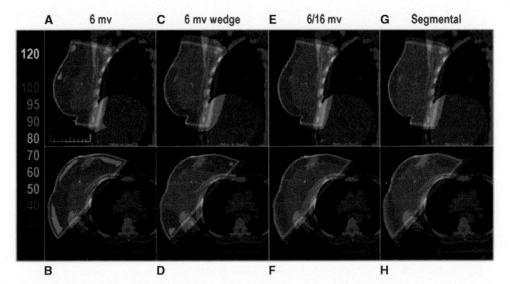

Figure 42.4. Dosimetric effects of various changes in technique on the scan of a patient with relatively large body habitus. **A,B**: Open 6 MV tangent fields. Note significant dose inhomogeneity. **C,D**: 6 MV with the addition of a 30-degree wedge in the path of the lateral tangent beam. **E,F**: Mixed beam energy (6 MV for the medial tangent and 16 MV for the lateral tangent). **G,H**: Several forward planned, intensity-modulated segments (two 6-MV beam segments and four 16-MV beam segments in total), resulting in improvement of overall dose homogeneity.

Boost doses to the tumor bed may be delivered using a variety of techniques, including external beam radiotherapy and brachytherapy.[103,104] 3D planning of external beam boost treatment based on CT imaging of the operative cavity appears to provide better target coverage and less irradiation of non-target tissue than clinical planning based upon palpation and inspection of the breast and scar.[105,106]

TOPICAL AND SYSTEMIC AGENTS TO PREVENT INJURY OR PROMOTE HEALING

A large number of studies have attempted to identify topical agents that might defend against the cutaneous toxicity associated with RT,[16] with interest in this subject emerging soon after the potential therapeutic benefits of radiotherapy were first identified.[107] Agents studied most recently in breast cancer patients have included aloe vera,[108–110] dexpanthenol cream,[111] chamomile cream and almond ointment,[112] sucralfate cream,[113] hyaluronic acid cream,[114] topical steroids,[115–117] Biafine,[118–120] and calendula.[121] Most studies have been small and failed to demonstrate substantial or significant benefits, although there may be some prophylactic benefit from hyaluronic acid or calendula, as well as benefit in terms of symptomatic relief from the application of topical steroids. In a small randomized study of skin washing, no detrimental effect of skin washing was observed, and nonsignificant trends favored the washing group, and skin washing should not be avoided during treatment.[122]

At the University of Michigan, patients are generally counseled to utilize calendula or Alra creams twice a day during the early weeks of their treatment. Topical steroids are generally reserved for follicular eruptions with symptomatic pruritis. Should skin toxicity progress to moist desquamation, Silvadene or domeboro compresses can provide symptomatic relief and expedite skin healing.

Systemic therapy with radioprotectants to prevent radiation-induced fibrosis is another subject of active investigation,[123] as is the appropriate treatment once it develops. Strategies for treatment include anti-inflammatory medications such as interferon gamma or steroids, vascular therapy with hyperbaric oxygen or pentoxifylline, and antioxidant therapies such as superoxide dismutase or tocopherol (vitamin E).[124] Delanian and colleagues have reported a randomized trial in patients with superficial radiation-induced fibrosis of the breast, revealing that patients receiving a combination of pentoxifylline and tocopherol had improved regression of fibrosis than patients treated with placebo (60% vs. 43%, $p = 0.04$).[125] The same group has reported an exponential regression of fibrosis with this combination treatment, with a two third maximum response after a mean of 2 years of treatment and a risk of rebound if treatment duration was too short. They recommend long treatment (≥3 years) in patients with severe fibrosis.[126]

SPECIAL PATIENT SITUATIONS

OBESITY

In general, it has been observed that radiation toxicity is most pronounced in patients with larger breasts.[30] Acute toxicity is pronounced in areas of higher skin doses due to the bolus effects of skin folds; late effects are influenced by the greater dose inhomogeneity involved in the treatment of larger

breasts.[127] Indeed, in the Canadian study of whole breast hypofractionation described above, women with "breast deemed too large to permit satisfactory RT (i.e., the maximum width of breast tissue >25 cm)" were excluded from participation. Moreover, in the Canadian study of IMRT described above, breast size was the only factor other than treatment technique with an independently significant association with moist desquamation. Thus, particular caution is warranted in this patient population, and IMRT may be a particularly beneficial consideration. Prone techniques that minimize the effects of skin folds may also be particularly useful in this patient population.[128–132] A combination of these two methods may also be employed.[133] Novel approaches to immobilization of the large or pendulous breast have also been described.[134–136]

CHEMOTHERAPY

Concurrent chemotherapy may increase the risk of radiation-related complications. A number of studies have examined the tolerability of concurrent radiotherapy and cytoxan, methotrexate and 5-FU (CMF)[137] or taxanes.[138–140] Caution appears to be warranted in light of substantial rates of severe acute skin reactions that may occur.[141] Toxicity associated with concurrent anthracycline-based therapy has been particularly concerning, and this approach is generally avoided.[142] Regarding long-term effects on cosmesis, investigators at the University of Pennsylvania have shown in a retrospective study that while patients receiving chemotherapy (the majority of whom received concurrent cytoxan and 5-FU) had slightly lower rates of good or excellent cosmesis at 3 years, by 5 years there was no significant difference.[143]

While a recent French study reported promising results with concurrent mitoxantrone-based treatment, and while interest in exploring concurrent treatment continues, especially in light of the promising findings of the recent trials of IMRT, further investigation is clearly necessary. For now, the most common approach in the USA is to treat breast cancer patients requiring both chemotherapy and radiation with a sequential rather than concurrent administration schedule, and studies from the Joint Center for Radiation Therapy have suggested that patients treated with sequential CMF or doxorubicin-based chemotherapy and radiation had only a slight decrement in cosmesis compared to patients treated with radiation alone.[144]

Whether hormonal therapy with tamoxifen might contribute to decrements in cosmesis after radiotherapy has also been the subject of concern and investigation.[145] Retrospective studies from the University of Pennsylvania have suggested no adverse cosmetic effects with the use of hormonal therapy[159] and no significant difference in complications related to concurrent versus sequential administration of tamoxifen.[146]

COLLAGEN VASCULAR DISEASE

Patients with active connective tissue disease have been documented to experience severe toxicity even with conventional dose and fractionation.[147–151] The mechanism by which this increased radiosensitivity occurs has not been well characterized, but it has been hypothesized that radiation-induced small vessel damage is accentuated by the coexisting vascular disease in these patients or that radiation may predispose these patients to an auto-immune response to their own breast tissue. Active connective tissue disease is considered a relative contraindication to RT, and patients with a history of connective tissue disease should be informed of the additional risks of radiation. (See Chapter 6 for further discussion.)

BREAST RECONSTRUCTION

Substantial evidence now supports the integral role of RT after mastectomy in selected patients at substantial risk of harboring a locoregional reservoir of disease.[42,152–155] Because of the important psychosocial functions of the breast, breast reconstruction is often pursued by patients undergoing mastectomy. The effects of radiation upon the outcomes of breast reconstruction are therefore also critically important to understand.

The best approach to integrating radiotherapy and reconstruction has yet to be defined. Limited evidence from retrospective series suggests that complication rates are substantial in women undergoing implant-expander reconstruction, regardless of sequencing with radiation, and a number of series suggest that these rates are higher than among patients receiving implants without radiation.[156–159] Complications include scarring at the interface between implant and tissue, capsular contracture, and impaired healing. Women undergoing radiation after autologous reconstruction also face higher rates of complications than women undergoing autologous reconstruction without radiation.[160,161] Complications for which risks are increased include fat necrosis, fibrosis, atrophy, and flap contracture.

As Wilkins and Atisha[162] conclude, "In general, for patients who need postmastectomy RT, delayed autologous flap reconstruction is thought to provide the best cosmetic result with the fewest complications." In patients who do decide upon implant reconstruction, a delay of at least 2 months after completion of radiation before commencing reconstruction is felt to be prudent. A delayed-immediate approach is another alternative that merits further study.[163]

RADIATION-INDUCED CARCINOGENESIS

Radiation-induced carcinogenesis is a concern in all irradiated tissues, as described in detail in a previous chapter in this book. For the purposes of this discussion, it is important to note that considerable study has been conducted to determine the actual risks of breast cancer after incidental radiation exposure to the breast.[164–169] The Oxford meta-analysis has shown an increased incidence of a number of secondary malignancies, including contralateral breast cancer, lung cancer, esophageal cancer, leukemia, and soft tissue sarcoma after the treatment of breast cancer with radiotherapy.[42] Potential methods of reducing these important risks, including reduction in the irradiated volume as with partial breast irradiation, continue to be the subject of ongoing investigation.[170,171]

CONCLUSION

The acute and late toxicities associated with radiation exposure to the breast may cause considerable distress to patients. Strategies to minimize these effects continue to be an important subject for ongoing investigation. Furthermore, as new radiation techniques, doses, and fractionation continue to be explored for the treatment of breast cancer, detailed and standardized analyses of impact upon treatment-related toxicity are essential.

REFERENCES

1. Vorherr H. *The Breast: Morphology, Physiology, and Lactation*. New York, NY: Academic Press, Inc.; 1974.
2. Gartner LM, Morton J, Lawrence RA, et al. Breastfeeding and the use of human milk. *Pediatrics*. 2005;115:496–506.
3. Mortensen EL, Michaelsen KF, Sanders SA, et al. The association between duration of breastfeeding and adult intelligence. *JAMA*. 2002;287:2365–2371.
4. Newcomb PA, Storer BE, Longnecker MP, et al. Lactation and a reduced risk of premenopausal breast cancer. *N Engl J Med*. 1994;330:81–87.
5. Jernstrom H, Lubinski J, Lynch HT, et al. Breast-feeding and the risk of breast cancer in BRCA1 and BRCA2 mutation carriers. *J Natl Cancer Inst*. 2004;96:1094–1098.
6. Howie PW, Forsyth JS, Ogston SA, et al. Protective effect of breast feeding against infection. *Br Med J*. 1990;300:11–16.
7. Armstrong J, Reilly JJ. Breastfeeding and lowering the risk of childhood obesity. *Lancet*. 2002;359:2003–2004.
8. Yalom M. *A History of the Breast*. New York, NY: Alfred A. Knopf; 1997.
9. Latteier C. *Breasts: The Woman's Perspective on an American Obsession*. New York, NY: The Haworth Press; 1998.
10. Millsted R, Frith H. Being large-breasted: women negotiating embodiment. *Women Stud Int Forum*. 2003;26:455–465.
11. Osborne MP. Breast anatomy and development. In: Harris JR, Lippman ME, Morrow M, et al., eds. *Diseases of the Breast*. 3rd ed. Philadelphia, PA: Lippincott Williams & Wilkins; 2004:3–14.
12. Cox JD, Stetz J, Pajak TF. Toxicity criteria of the Radiation Therapy Oncology Group (RTOG) and the European Organization for Research and Treatment of Cancer (EORTC). *Int J Radiat Oncol Biol Phys*. 1995;31:1341–1346.
13. Porock D, Kristjanson L. Skin reactions during radiotherapy for breast cancer: the use and impact of topical agents and dressings. *Eur J Cancer Care*. 1999;8:143–153.
14. Hall EJ. *Radiobiology for the Radiologist*. Philadelphia, PA: Lippincott Williams & Wilkins; 2000:215.
15. Hall EJ. *Radiobiology for the Radiologist*. Philadelphia, PA: Lippincott Williams & Wilkins; 2000:346.
16. White J, Joiner MC. Toxicity from Radiation in Breast Cancer. In: Small JW, Woloschak GE, eds. *Radiation Toxicity: A Practical Guide*. New York, NY: Springer; 2005:65–109.
17. Clarke D, Martinez A, Cox RS, et al. Breast edema following staging axillary node dissection in patients with breast carcinoma treated by radical radiotherapy. *Cancer*. 1982;49:2295–2299.
18. Kurtz JM. Impact of radiotherapy on breast cosmesis. *Breast*. 1995;4:163–169.
19. Rose MA, Olivotto I, Cady B, et al. Conservative surgery and radiation therapy for early breast cancer: long-term cosmetic results. *Arch Surg*. 1989;124:153–157.
20. Pezner RD, Patterson MP, Hill LR, et al. Breast edema in patients treated conservatively for Stage I and II breast cancer. *Int J Radiation Oncol Biol Phys*. 1985;11:1765–1768.
21. Hall EJ. *Radiobiology for the Radiologist*. Philadelphia, PA: Lippincott Williams & Wilkins; 2000:345.
22. Weitzen R, Pfeffer R, Mandel M. Case 3. Vitiligo after radiotherapy for breast cancer in a woman with depigmentation disorder. *J Clin Oncol*. 2005;23:644–644.
23. Munshi A, Jain S, Budrukkar A, et al. Radiotherapy-induced depigmentation in a patient with breast cancer. *Indian J Cancer*. 2007;44:157–158.
24. Bentzen SM, Thames HD, Overgaard M. Latent-time estimation for late cutaneous and subcutaneous radiation reactions in a single-follow-up clinical study. *Radiother Oncol*. 1989;15:267–274.
25. Bentzen SM, Turesson I, Thames HD. Fractionation sensitivity and latency of telangiectasia after postmastectomy radiotherapy: a graded response analysis. *Radiother Oncol*. 1990;18:95–106.
26. Turesson I. The progression rate of late radiation effects in normal tissue and its impact on dose-response relationships. *Radiother Oncol*. 1989;15:217–226.
27. Lilla C, Ambrosone CB, Kropp S, et al. Predictive factors for late normal tissue complications following radiotherapy for breast cancer. *Breast Cancer Res Treat*. 2007;106:143–150.
28. Harris JR, Levene MB, Svensson G, et al. Analysis of cosmetic results following primary radiation therapy for stage 1 and stage 2 carcinoma of the breast. *Int J Radiat Oncol Biol Phys*. 1979;5:257–261.
29. van Limbergen E, van der Schueren E, van Tongelen K. Cosmetic evaluation of breast-conserving treatment for mammary cancer. 1. Proposal of a quantitative scoring system. *Radiother Oncol*. 1989;16:159–167.
30. Gray JR, McCormick B, Cox L, et al. Primary breast irradiation in large-breasted or heavy women: analysis of cosmetic outcome. 32nd Annual Meeting of the American Society for Therapeutic Radiology and Oncology. Miami Beach, FL, 1990. *Int J Radiat Oncol Biol Phys*. 1991;21:347–354.
31. Sacchini V, Luini A, Tana S, et al. Quantitative and qualitative cosmetic evaluation after conservative treatment for breast cancer. *Eur J Cancer*. 1991;27:1395–1400.
32. Amalric R, Spitalier JM. *La Césiumthérapie Curative des Cancers du Sein*. Paris, France: Masson et Cie; 1973.
33. Liljegren G, Holmberg L, Westman G. The cosmetic outcome in early breast cancer treated with sector resection with or without radiotherapy. *Eur J Cancer*. 1993;29A:2083–2089.
34. Kurtz JM, Miralbell R. Radiation therapy and breast conservation: cosmetic results and complications. *Semin Radiat Oncol*. 1992;2:125–131.
35. Ceilley E, Jagsi R, Goldberg S, et al. Radiotherapy for invasive breast cancer in North America and Europe: results of a survey. 44th Annual Meeting of the American Society for

Therapeutic Radiology and Oncology. New Orleans, LA, 2002. *Int J Radiat Oncol Biol Phys.* 2005;61:365–373.

36. Fletcher GH. Hypofractionation: lessons from complications. *Radiother Oncol.* 1991;20:10–15.
37. Johansson S, Svensson H, Denekamp J. Dose response and latency for radiation-induced fibrosis, edema, and neuropathy in breast cancer patients. *Int J Radiat Oncol Biol Phys.* 2002;52:1207–1219.
38. Fehlauer F, Tribius S, Alberti W, et al. Late effects and cosmetic results of conventional versus hypofractionated irradiation in breast-conserving therapy. *Strahlenther Onkol.* 2005;181:625–631.
39. Delouche G, Bachelot F, Premont M, et al. Conservation treatment of early breast cancer: long-term results and complications. *Int J Radiat Oncol Biol Phys.* 1987;13:29–34.
40. Bijker N, Meijnen P, Peterse JL, et al. Breast-conserving treatment with or without radiotherapy in ductal carcinoma-in-situ: ten-year results of European Organisation for Research and Treatment of Cancer randomized phase III trial 10853—A study by the EORTC Breast Cancer Cooperative Group and EORTC Radiotherapy Group. *J Clin Oncol.* 2006;24: 3381–3387.
41. Romestaing P, Lehingue Y, Carrie C, et al. Role of a 10-Gy boost in the conservative treatment of early breast cancer: results of a randomized clinical trial in Lyon, France. *J Clin Oncol.* 1997;15:963–968.
42. Early Breast Cancer Trialists Collaborative Group (EBCTCG). Effects of radiotherapy and of differences in the extent of surgery for early breast cancer on local recurrence and 15-year survival: an overview of the randomised trials. *Lancet.* 2005;366:2087–2106.
43. Whelan TJ, Kim DH, Sussman J. Clinical experience using hypofractionated radiation schedules in breast cancer. *Semin Radiat Oncol.* 2008;18:257–264.
44. Cohen L. Radiotherapy in breast cancer I: the dose-time relationship—theoretical considerations. *Br J Radiol.* 1952;25:636–642.
45. Douglas BG, Castro JR. Novel fractionation schemes and high linear energy transfer. *Prog Exp Tumor Res.* 1984;28:152–165.
46. Whelan T, MacKenzie R, Julian J, et al. Randomized trial of breast irradiation schedules after lumpectomy for women with lymph node-negative breast cancer. *J Natl Cancer Inst.* 2002;94:1143–1150.
47. Whelan TJ, Pignol J, Julian I, et al. Long-term results of a randomized trial of accelerated hypofractionated whole breast irradiation following breast conserving surgery in women with node-negative breast cancer. 50th Annual Meeting of the American Society for Therapeutic Radiology and Oncology. Boston, MA, 2008. *Int J Radiat Oncol Biol Phys.* 2008;72:S28
48. Ben-David MA, Sturtz DE, Griffith KA, et al. Long-term results of conservative surgery and radiotherapy for ductal carcinoma in situ using lung density correction: the University of Michigan experience. *Breast J.* 2007;13:392–400.
49. Yarnold J, Ashton A, Bliss J, et al. Fractionation sensitivity and dose response of late adverse effects in the breast after radiotherapy for early breast cancer: long-term results of a randomised trial. *Radiother Oncol.* 2005;75:9–17.
50. Yarnold J, Bloomfield D, LeVay J, et al. Prospective randomized trial testing 5.7 Gy and 6.0 Gy fractions of whole breast radiotherapy in women with early breast cancer (FAST) trial. *Clin Oncol.* 2004;16:S30.
51. Freedman GM, Anderson PR, Goldstein LJ, et al. Four-week course of radiation for breast cancer using hypofractionated intensity modulated radiation therapy with an incorporated boost. *Int J Radiat Oncol Biol Phys.* 2007;68:347–353.
52. Clark RM, McCulloch PB, Levine MN, et al. Randomized clinical trial to assess the effectiveness of breast irradiation following lumpectomy and axillary dissection for node-negative breast cancer. *J Natl Cancer Inst.* 1992;84:683–689.
53. Vicini FA, Kestin LL, Goldstein NS. Defining the clinical target volume for patients with early-stage breast cancer treated with lumpectomy and accelerated partial breast irradiation: a pathologic analysis. *Int J Radiat Oncol Biol Phys.* 2004;60:722–730.
54. Vicini FA, Kestin L, Chen P, et al. Limited-field radiation therapy in the management of early-stage breast cancer. *J Natl Cancer Inst.* 2003;95:1205–1211.
55. Veronesi U, Marubini E, Mariani L, et al. Radiotherapy after breast-conserving surgery in small breast carcinoma: long-term results of a randomized trial. *Ann Oncol.* 2001;12: 997–1003.
56. Holland R, Veling SHJ, Mravunac M, et al. Histologic multifocality of T-is, T1–2 breast carcinomas: implications for clinical trials of breast-conserving surgery. *Cancer.* 1985;56: 979–990.
57. Vaidya JS, Vyas JJ, Chinoy RF, et al. Multicentricity of breast cancer: whole-organ analysis and clinical implications. *Br J Cancer.* 1996;74:820–824.
58. Morimoto T, Okazaki K, Komaki K, et al. Cancerous residue in breast-conserving surgery. *J Surg Oncol.* 1993;52:71–76.
59. Vicini FA, Baglan KL, Kestin LL, et al. Accelerated treatment of breast cancer. *J Clin Oncol.* 2001;19:1993–2001.
60. Benitez PR, Chen PY, Vicini FA, et al. Partial breast irradiation in breast-conserving therapy by way of interstitial brachytherapy. 5th Annual Meeting of the American Society of Breast Surgeons. Las Vegas, NV, 2004. *Am J Surg.* 2004;188:355–364.
61. Chen PY, Vicini FA, Benitez P, et al. Long-term cosmetic results and toxicity after accelerated partial-breast irradiation—A method of radiation delivery by interstitial Brachytherapy for the treatment of early-stage breast carcinoma. *Cancer.* 2006;106:991–999.
62. Vicini FA, Antonucci JV, Wallace M, et al. Long-term efficacy and patterns of failure after accelerated partial breast irradiation: a molecular assay-based clonality evaluation. *Int J Radiat Oncol Biol Phys.* 2007;68:341–346.
63. Vicini F, Beitsch PD, Quiet CA, et al. Three-year analysis of treatment efficacy, cosmesis, and toxicity by the American Society of Breast Surgeons MammoSite Breast Brachytherapy Registry Trial in patients treated with accelerated partial breast irradiation (APBI). 49th Annual Meeting of the American Society for Therapeutic Radiology and Oncology. Los Angeles, CA, 2007. *Cancer.* 2008;112:758–766.
64. Evans SB, Kaufman SA, Price LL, et al. Persistent seroma after intraoperative placement of mammosite for accelerated partial breast irradiation: incidence, pathologic anatomy, and contributing factors. *Int J Radiat Oncol Biol Phys.* 2006;65:333–339.
65. Veronesi U, Orecchia R, Luini A, et al. A preliminary report of intraoperative radiotherapy (IORT) in limited-stage breast cancers that are conservatively treated. *Eur J Cancer.* 2001;37:2178–2183.
66. Orecchia R, Ciocca M, Lazzari R, et al. Intraoperative radiation therapy with electrons (ELIOT) in early-stage breast cancer. 8th International Conference on Primary Therapy of Early Breast Cancer. St Gallen, Switzerland, 2003. *Breast.* 2003;12:483–490.
67. Veronesi U, Gatti G, Luini A, et al. Full-dose intraoperative radiotherapy with electrons during breast-conserving surgery. *Arch Surg.* 2003;138:1253–1256.
68. Vaidya JS, Baum M, Tobias JS, et al. The novel technique of delivering targeted intraoperative radiotherapy (Targit) for early breast cancer. *Eur J Surg Oncol.* 2002;28:447–454.
69. Vaidya JS, Tobias JS, Baum M, et al. Intraoperative radiotherapy for breast cancer. *Lancet Oncol.* 2004;5:165–173.
70. Beal K, McCormick B, Zelefsky MJ, et al. Single-fraction intraoperative radiotherapy for breast cancer: early cosmetic results. *Int J Radiat Oncol Biol Phys.* 2007;69:19–24.
71. Formenti SC. External-beam partial-breast irradiation. *Semin Radiat Oncol.* 2005;15:92–99.
72. Cuttino LW, Todor D, Pacyna L, et al. Three-dimensional conformal external beam radiotherapy (3D-CRT) for accelerated partial breast irradiation (APBI)—What is the correct prescription dose? 46th Annual Meeting of the American Society for Therapeutic Radiology and Oncology. Atlanta, GA, 2004. *Am J Clin Oncol-Cancer Clin Trials.* 2006;29:474–478.
73. Weed DW, Edmundson GK, Vicini FA, et al. Accelerated partial breast irradiation: a dosimetric comparison of three different techniques. *Brachytherapy.* 2005;4:121–129.
74. Ribeiro GG, Dunn G, Swindell R, et al. Conservation of the breast using two different radiotherapy techniques: interim report of a clinical trial. *Clin Oncol.* 1990;2:27–34.
75. Ribeiro GG, Magee B, Swindell R, et al. The Christie Hospital breast conservation trial: an update at 8 years from inception. *Clin Oncol.* 1993;5:278–283.
76. Formenti SC, Rosenstein B, Skinner KA, et al. T1 stage breast cancer: adjuvant hypofractionated conformal radiation therapy to tumor bed in selected postmenopausal breast cancer patients—Pilot feasibility study. *Radiology.* 2002;222:171–178.
77. Truong MT, Hirsch AE, Formenti SC. Novel approaches to postoperative radiation therapy as part of breast-conserving therapy for early-stage breast cancer. *Clinical Breast Cancer.* 2003;4:253–263.
78. Barendsen GW. Dose fractionation, dose rate and iso-effect relationships for normal tissue responses. *Int J Radiat Oncol Biol Phys.* 1982;8:1982–97.
79. Steel G, Deacon J, Duchesne GM, et al. The dose rate effect in human tumour cells. *Radiother Oncol.* 1987;9:299–310.
80. Yamada Y, Ackerman I, Franssen R, et al. Does the dose fractionation schedule influence local control of adjuvant radiotherapy for early stage breast cancer? *Int J Radiat Oncol Biol Phys.* 1999;44:99–104.
81. Formenti SC, Truong MT, Goldberg JD, et al. Prone accelerated partial breast irradiation after breast-conserving surgery: preliminary clinical results and dose-volume histogram analysis. *Int J Radiat Oncol Biol Phys.* 2004;60:493–504.
82. Wernicke AG, Gidea-Addeo D, Magnolfi C, et al. External beam partial breast irradiation following breast-conserving surgery: preliminary results of cosmetic outcome of NYU 00-23. 48th Annual Meeting of the American Society for Therapeutic Radiology and Oncology. Philadelphia, PA, 2006. *Int J Radiat Oncol Biol Phys.* 2006;66:S32.
83. Baglan KL, Sharpe MB, Jaffray D, et al. Accelerated partial breast irradiation using 3D conformal radiation therapy (3D-CRT). *Int J Radiat Oncol Biol Phys.* 2003;55:302–311.
84. Vicini FA, Remouchamps V, Wallace M, et al. Ongoing clinical experience utilizing 3D conformal external beam radiotherapy to deliver partial-breast irradiation in patients with early-stage breast cancer treated with breast-conserving therapy. *Int J Radiat Oncol Biol Phys.* 2003;57:1247–1253.
85. Vicini FA, Chen P, Wallace M, et al. Interim cosmetic results and toxicity using 3D conformal external beam radiotherapy to deliver accelerated partial breast irradiation in patients with early-stage breast cancer treated with breast-conserving therapy. *Int J Radiat Oncol Biol Phys.* 2007;69:1124–1130.
86. (RTOG) RTOG. A randomized phase III study of conventional whole breast irradiation (WBI) versus partial breast irradiation (PBI) for women with stage 0, I, or II breast cancer. NSABP Protocol B-39; RTOG Protocol 0413. 2007. <http://www.rtog.org/members/protocols/0413/0413.pdf>
87. Lovey K, Fodor J, Major T, et al. Fat necrosis after partial-breast irradiation with brachytherapy or electron irradiation versus standard whole-breast radiotherapy—4-year results of a randomized trial. *Int J Radiat Oncol Biol Phys.* 2007;69:724–731.
88. Polgar C, Fodor J, Major T, et al. Breast-conserving treatment with partial or whole breast irradiation for low-risk invasive breast carcinoma-5-year results of a randomized trial. *Int J Radiat Oncol Biol Phys.* 2007;69:694–702.
89. Jagsi R, Ben-David M, Moran J, et al. Adverse cosmesis in a protocol investigating IMRT with active breathing control for accelerated partial breast irradiation (APBI). 50th Annual Meeting of the American Society for Therapeutic Radiology and Oncology. Boston, MA, 2008. *Int J Radiat Oncol Biol Phys.* 2008;72:S153.
90. Hepel JT, Tokita M, MacAusland SG, et al. Toxicity of 3D-CRT for accelerated partial breast irradiation. 50th Annual Meeting of the American Society for Therapeutic Radiology and Oncology. Boston, MA, 2008. *Int J Radiat Oncol Biol Phys.* 2008;72:S5–S5.
91. Bartelink H, Garavaglia G, Johansson KA, et al. Quality assurance in conservative treatment of early breast cancer. Report on a consensus meeting of the EORTC radiotherapy and breast cancer cooperative groups and the EUSOMA (European Society of Mastology). *Radiother Oncol.* 1991;22:323–326.
92. Fraass BA, Roberson PL, Lichter AS. Dose to the contralateral breast due to primary breast irradiation. *Int J Radiat Oncol Biol Phys.* 1985;11:485–497.
93. Haffty BG, Buchholz TA, McCormick B. Should intensity-modulated radiation therapy be the standard of care in the conservatively managed breast cancer patient? *J Clin Oncol.* 2008;26:2072–2074.
94. Harsolia A, Kestin L, Grills I, et al. In clinical toxicities compared with conventional wedge-based breast radiotherapy. *Int J Radiat Oncol Biol Phys.* 2007;68:1375–1380.
95. Vicini FA, Sharpe M, Kestin L, et al. Optimizing breast cancer treatment efficacy with intensity-modulated radiotherapy. *Int J Radiat Oncol Biol Phys.* 2002;54:1336–1344.

96. Lo YC, Yasuda G, Fitzgerald TJ, et al. Intensity modulation for breast treatment using static multi-leaf collimators. *Int J Radiat Oncol Biol Phys.* 2000;46:187–194.

97. Kestin LL, Sharpe MB, Frazier RC, et al. Intensity modulation to improve dose uniformity with tangential breast radiotherapy: initial clinical experience. *Int J Radiat Oncol Biol Phys.* 2000;48:1559–1568.

98. Chui CS, Hong L, Hunt M, et al. A simplified intensity modulated radiation therapy technique for the breast. *Med Phys.* 2002;29:522–529.

99. van Asselen B, Schwarz M, van Vliet-Vroegindeweij C, et al. Intensity-modulated radiotherapy of breast cancer using direct aperture optimization. *Radiother Oncol.* 2006;79: 162–169.

100. Freedman GM, Anderson PR, Li JS, et al. Intensity modulated radiation therapy (IMRT) decreases acute skin toxicity for women receiving radiation for breast cancer. *Am J Clin Oncol.* 2006;29:66–70.

101. Pignol JP, Olivotto I, Rakovitch E, et al. A multicenter randomized trial of breast intensity-modulated radiation therapy to reduce acute radiation dermatitis. Joint Annual Meeting of the Canadian Association of Radiation Oncology/Canadian Organization of Medical Physicists. Toronto, Canada, 2007. *J Clin Oncol.* 2008;26:2085–2092.

102. Donovan E, Bleakley N, Denholm E, et al. Randomised trial of standard 2D radiotherapy (RT) versus intensity modulated radiotherapy (IMRT) in patients prescribed breast radiotherapy. *Radiother Oncol.* 2007;82:254–264.

103. Touboul E, Belkacemi Y, Lefranc JP, et al. Early breast cancer: influence of type of boost (electrons vs. iridium-192 implant) on local control and cosmesis after conservative surgery and radiation therapy. *Radiother Oncol.* 1995;34:105–113.

104. Budrukkar AN, Sarin R, Shrivastava SK, et al. Cosmesis, late sequelae and local control after breast-conserving therapy: influence of type of tumour bed boost and adjuvant chemotherapy. *Clin Oncol.* 2007;19:596–603.

105. Benda RK, Yasuda G, Sethi A, et al. Breast boost: are we missing the target? A dosimetric comparison of two boost techniques. 88th Scientific Assembly and Annual Meeting of the Radiological Society of North America. Chicago, IL, 2002. *Cancer.* 2003;97: 905–909.

106. Kovner F, Agay R, Merimsky O, et al. Clips and scar as the guidelines for breast radiation boost after lumpectomy. *Eur J Surg Oncol.* 1999;25:483–486.

107. Collins E, Collins C. Roentgen dermatitis treated with fresh whole leaf of aloe vera. *Am J Roentgenol.* 1935;33:396–397.

108. Williams MS, Burk M, Loprinzi CL, et al. Phase III double-blind evaluation of an aloe vera gel as a prophylactic agent for radiation-induced skin toxicity. *Int J Radiat Oncol Biol Phys.* 1996;36:345–349.

109. Heggie S, Bryant GP, Tripcony L, et al. A phase III study on the efficacy of topical aloe vera gel on irradiated breast tissue. *Cancer Nurs.* 2002;25:442–451.

110. Olsen DL, Raub W Jr, Bradley C, et al. The effect of aloe vera gel/mild soap versus mild soap alone in preventing skin reactions in patients undergoing radiation therapy. *Oncol Nurs Forum.* 2001;28:543–547.

111. Lokkevik E, Skovlund E, Reitan JB, et al. Skin treatment with Bepanthen cream versus no cream during radiotherapy—A randomized controlled trial. *Acta Oncol.* 1996;35: 1021–1026.

112. Maiche AG, Grohn P, Makihokkonen H. Effect of chamomile cream and almond ointment on acute radiation skin reaction. *Acta Oncol.* 1991;30:395–396.

113. Maiche A, Isokangas OP, Grohn P. Skin protection by sucralfate cream during electron beam therapy. *Acta Oncol.* 1994;33:201–203.

114. Liguori V, Guillemin C, Pesce GF, et al. Double-blind, randomized clinical study comparing hyaluronic acid cream to placebo in patients treated with radiotherapy. *Radiother Oncol.* 1997;42:155–161.

115. Bostrom A, Lindman H, Swartling C, et al. Potent corticosteroid cream (mometasone furoate) significantly reduces acute radiation dermatitis: results from a double-blind, randomized study. *Radiother Oncol.* 2001;59:257–265.

116. Schmuth M, Wimmer MA, Hofer S, et al. Topical corticosteroid therapy for acute radiation dermatitis: a prospective, randomized, double-blind study. *Br J Dermatol.* 2002;146:983–991.

117. Potera ME, Lookingbill DP, Stryker JA. Prophylaxis of radiation dermatitis with a topical cortisone cream. *Radiology.* 1982;143:775–777.

118. Fisher J, Scott C, Stevens R, et al. Randomized phase III study comparing Best Supportive Care to Biafine as a prophylactic agent for radiation-induced skin toxicity for women undergoing breast irradiation: Radiation Therapy Oncology Group (RTOG) 97-13. *Int J Radiat Oncol Biol Phys.* 2000;48:1307–1310.

119. Szumacher E, Wighton A, Franssen E, et al. Phase II study assessing the effectiveness of biafine cream as a prophylactic agent for radiation-induced acute skin toxicity to the breast in women undergoing radiotherapy with concomitant CMF chemotherapy. Annual Meeting of the Canadian Association of Radiologists. Toronto, Canada, 2001. *Int J Radiat Oncol Biol Phys.* 2001;51:81–86.

120. Fenig E, Brenner B, Katz A, et al. Topical Biafine and Lipiderm for the prevention of radiation dermatitis: a randomized prospective trial. *Oncol Rep.* 2001;8:305–309.

121. Pommier P, Gomez F, Sunyach MP, et al. Phase III randomized trial of *Calendula officinalis* compared with trolamine for the prevention of acute dermatitis during irradiation for breast cancer. *J Clin Oncol.* 2004;22:1447–1453.

122. Roy I, Fortin A, Larochelle M. The impact of skin washing with water and soap during breast irradiation: a randomized study. *Radiother Oncol.* 2001;58:333–339.

123. Koukourakis MI, Yannakakis D. High dose daily amifostine and hypofractionated intensively accelerated radiotherapy for locally advanced breast cancer. A phase I/II study and report on early and late sequelae. *Anticancer Res.* 2001;21(4B):2973–2978.

124. Delanian S, Lefaix J-L. Current management for late normal tissue injury: radiation-induced fibrosis and necrosis. *Semin Radiat Oncol.* 2007;17(2):99–107.

125. Delanian S, Porcher R, Balla-Mekias S, et al. Randomized, placebo-controlled trial of combined pentoxifylline and tocopherol for regression of superficial radiation-induced fibrosis. *J Clin Oncol.* 2003;21(13):2545–2550.

126. Delanian S, Porcher R, Rudant J, et al. Kinetics of response to long-term treatment combining pentoxifylline and tocopherol in patients with superficial radiation-induced fibrosis. *J Clin Oncol.* 2005;23(34):8570–8579.

127. Moody AM, Mayles WPM, Bliss JM, et al. The influence of breast size on late radiation effects and association with radiotherapy dose inhomogeneity. *Radiother Oncol.* 1994;33:106–112.

128. Merchant TE, McCormick B. Prone position breast irradiation. *Int J Radiat Oncol Biol Phys.* 1994;30:197–203.

129. Mahe MA, Classe JM, Dravet F, et al. Preliminary results for prone-position breast irradiation. 86th Scientific Assembly and Annual Meeting of the Radiological Society of North America (RSNA). Chicago, IL, 2000. *Int J Radiat Oncol Biol Phys.* 2002;52:156–160.

130. Algan O, Fowble B, McNeeley S, et al. Use of the prone position in radiation treatment for women with early stage breast cancer. *Int J Radiat Oncol Biol Phys.* 1998;40:1137–1140.

131. Grann A, McCormick B, Chabner ES, et al. Prone breast radiotherapy in early-stage breast cancer: a preliminary analysis. *Int J Radiat Oncol Biol Phys.* 2000;47:319–325.

132. Stegman LD, Beal KP, Hunt MA, et al. Long-term clinical outcomes of whole-breast irradiation delivered in the prone position. 47th Annual Meeting of the American Society for Therapeutic Radiology and Oncology. Denver, CO, 2005. *Int J Radiat Oncol Biol Phys.* 2007;68:73–81.

133. Goodman KA, Hong L, Wagman R, et al. Dosimetric analysis of a simplified intensity modulation technique for prone breast radiotherapy. 44th Annual Meeting of the American Society for Therapeutic Radiology and Oncology. New Orleans, LA, 2002. *Int J Radiat Oncol Biol Phys.* 2004;60:95–102.

134. Bentel GC, Marks LB, Whiddon CS, et al. Acute and late morbidity of using a breast positioning ring in women with large/pendulous breasts. *Radiother Oncol.* 1999;50:277–281.

135. Bentel GC, Marks LB. A simple device to position large/flaccid breasts during tangential breast irradiation. *Int J Radiat Oncol Biol Phys.* 1994;29:879–882.

136. Zierhut D, Flentje M, Frank C, et al. Conservative treatment of breast cancer: modified irradiation technique for women with large breasts. *Radiother Oncol.* 1994;31:256–261.

137. Isaac N, Panzarella T, Lau A, et al. Concurrent cyclophosphamide, methotrexate, and 5-fluorouracil chemotherapy and radiotherapy for breast carcinoma—A well tolerated adjuvant regimen. Annual Meeting of the Canadian Association of Radiation Oncologists. Edmonton, Canada, 2000. *Cancer.* 2002;95:696–703.

138. Ellerbroek N, Martino S, Mautner B, et al. Breast-conserving therapy with adjuvant paclitaxel and radiation therapy: feasibility of concurrent treatment. *Breast J.* 2003;9:74–78.

139. Formenti SC, Volm M, Skinner KA, et al. Preoperative twice-weekly paclitaxel with concurrent radiation therapy followed by surgery and postoperative doxorubicin-based chemotherapy in locally advanced breast cancer: a phase I/II trial. *J Clin Oncol.* 2003;21: 864–870.

140. Bellon JR, Lindsley KL, Ellis GK, et al. Concurrent radiation therapy and paclitaxel or docetaxel chemotherapy in high-rise breast cancer. *Int J Radiat Oncol Biol Phys.* 2000;48: 393–397.

141. Hanna YM, Baglan KL, Stromberg JS, et al. Acute and subacute toxicity associated with concurrent adjuvant radiation therapy and paclitaxel in primary breast cancer therapy. *Breast J.* 2002;8:149–153.

142. Fiets WE, van Helvoirt RP, Nortier JWR, et al. Acute toxicity of concurrent adjuvant radiotherapy and chemotherapy (CMF or AC) in breast cancer patients: a prospective, comparative, non-randomised study. *Eur J Cancer.* 2003;39:1081–1088.

143. Markiewicz DA, Schultz DJ, Haas JA, et al. The effects of sequence and type of chemotherapy and radiation therapy on cosmesis and complications after breast conservation therapy. *Int J Radiation Oncol Biol Phys.* 1996;35(4):661–668.

144. Abner AL, Recht A, Vicini FA, et al. Cosmetic results after surgery, chemotherapy, and radiation therapy for early breast cancer. *Int J Radiation Oncol Biol Phys.* 1991;21(3): 331–338.

145. Wazer DE, DiPetrillo T, Schmidt-Ulrich R, et al. Factors influencing cosmetic outcome and complication risk after conservative surgery and radiotherapy for early-stage breast carcinoma. *J Clin Oncol.* 1992;10:356–363.

146. Harris EE, Christensen VJ, Hwang WT, et al. Impact of concurrent versus sequential tamoxifen with radiation therapy in early-stage breast cancer patients undergoing breast conservation treatment. *J Clin Oncol.* 2005;23:11–16.

147. Wo J, Taghian A. Radiotherapy in setting of collagen vascular disease. *Int J Radiat Oncol Biol Phys.* 2007;69:1347–1353.

148. Morris MM, Powell SN. Irradiation in the setting of collagen vascular disease: acute and late complications. *J Clin Oncol.* 1997;15:2728–2735.

149. Lin A, Abu-Isa E, Griffith KA, et al. Toxicity of radiotherapy in patients with collagen vascular disease. *Cancer.* 2008;113:648–653.

150. Fleck R, McNeese MD, Ellerbroek NA, et al. Consequences of breast irradiation in patients with preexisting collagen vascular diseases. *Int J Radiat Oncol Biol Phys.* 1989;17:829–833.

151. Robertson JM, Clarke DH, Pevzner MM, et al. Breast conservation therapy: severe breast fibrosis after radiation therapy in patients with collagen vascular disease. *Cancer.* 1991;68:502–508.

152. Pierce LJ. The use of radiotherapy after mastectomy: a review of the literature. *J Clin Oncol.* 2005;23:1706–1717.

153. Overgaard M, Hansen PS, Overgaard J, et al. Postoperative radiotherapy in high-risk premenopausal women with breast cancer who receive adjuvant chemotherapy. *N Engl J Med.* 1997;337:949–955.

154. Overgaard M, Jensen MB, Overgaard J, et al. Postoperative radiotherapy in high-risk postmenopausal breast cancer patients given adjuvant tamoxifen: Danish Breast Cancer Cooperative Group DBCG 82c randomised trial. *Lancet.* 1999;353:1641–1648.

155. Ragaz J, Olivotto IA, Spinelli JJ, et al. Locoregional radiation therapy in patients with high-risk breast cancer receiving adjuvant chemotherapy: 20-year results of the British Columbia randomized trial. *J Natl Cancer Inst.* 2005;97:116–126.

156. Krueger EA, Wilkins EG, Strawderman M, et al. Complications and patient satisfaction following expander/implant breast reconstruction with and without radiotherapy.

41st Annual Meeting of the American Society for Therapeutic Radiology and Oncology. San Antonio, TX, 1999. *Int J Radiat Oncol Biol Phys.* 2001;49:713–721.

157. Contant CME, van Geel AN, van der Holt B, et al. Morbidity of immediate breast reconstruction (IBR) after mastectomy by a subpectorally placed silicone prosthesis: the adverse effect of radiotherapy. *Eur J Surg Oncol.* 2000;26:344–350.

158. Tallet AV, Salem N, Moutardier V, et al. Radiotherapy and immediate two-stage breast reconstruction with a tissue expander and implant: complications and esthetic results. *Int J Radiat Oncol Biol Phys.* 2003;57:136–142.

159. Ascherman JA, Hanasono MM, Newman MI, et al. Implant reconstruction in breast cancer patients treated with radiation therapy. 73rd Annual Meeting of the American Society of Plastic Surgeons. Philadelphia, PA, 2004. *Plast Reconstr Surg.* 2006;117:359–365.

160. Williams JK, Carlson GW, Bostwick J, et al. The effects of radiation treatment after TRAM flap breast reconstruction. 75th Annual Meeting of the American Association of Plastic and Reconstructive Surgeons. Hilton Head Island, SC, 1996. *Plast Reconstr Surg.* 1997;100:1153–1160.

161. Rogers NE, Allen RJ. Radiation effects on breast reconstruction with the deep inferior epigastric perforator flap. Meeting of the Louisiana Society for Plastic and Reconstructive Surgery. Baton Rouge, LA, 2000. *Plast Reconstr Surg.* 2002;109:1919–1924.

162. Wilkins EG, Atisha DM. Breast reconstruction in women with breast cancer. In: Hayes DF, Wazer DE, eds. UpToDate.com. 2008. <http://www.utdol.com/online/content/topic.do?topicKey=breastcn/13517&view=print>

163. Kronowitz SJ, Hunt KK, Kuerer HM, et al. Delayed-immediate breast reconstruction. 82nd Annual Meeting of the American Association of Plastic Surgeons. Baltimore, MD, 2003. *Plast Reconstr Surg.* 2004;113:1617–1628.

164. Ng AK, Bernardo MVP, Weller E, et al. Second malignancy after Hodgkin disease treated with radiation therapy with or without chemotherapy: long-term risks and risk factors. *Blood.* 2002;100:1989–1996.

165. Preston DL, Mattsson A, Holmberg E, et al. Radiation effects on breast cancer risk: a pooled analysis of eight cohorts. *Radiat Res.* 2002;158:220–235.

166. Thompson DE, Mabuchi K, Ron E, et al. Cancer incidence in atomic bomb survivors. 2. Solid tumors, 1958–1987. *Radiat Res.* 1994;137:S17–S67.

167. Boice JD, Preston D, Davis FG, et al. Frequent chest X-ray fluoroscopy and breast cancer incidence among tuberculosis patients in Massachusetts. *Radiat Res.* 1991;125:214–222.

168. Shore RE, Hildreth N, Woodard E, et al. Breast cancer among women given X-ray therapy for acute postpartum mastitis. *J Natl Cancer Inst.* 1986;77:689–696.

169. Mattsson A, Leitz W, Rutqvist LE. Radiation risk and mammographic screening of women from 40 to 49 years of age: effect on breast cancer rates and years of life. *Br J Cancer.* 2000;82:220–226.

170. Woo TCS, Pignol JP, Rakovitch E, et al. Body radiation exposure in breast cancer radiotherapy: impact of breast IMRT and virtual wedge compensation techniques. *Int J Radiat Oncol Biol Phys.* 2006;65:52–58.

171. Sohn JW, Macklis R, Suh JH, et al. A mobile shield to reduce scatter radiation to the contralateral breast during radiotherapy for breast cancer: preclinical results. *Int J Radiat Oncol Biol Phys.* 1999;43:1037–1041.

172. Fentiman IS, Deshmane V, Tong D, et al. Caesium(137) implant as sole radiation therapy for operable breast cancer: a phase II trial. *Radiother Oncol.* 2004;71:281–285.

173. King TA, Bolton JS, Kuske RR, et al. Long-term results of wide field brachytherapy as the sole method of radiation therapy after segmental mastectomy for T-is,T-1,T-2 breast cancer. Annual Meeting of the American Society of Breast Surgeons. Charleston, South Carolina, 2000. *Am J Surg.* 2000;180:299–304.

174. Perera F, Engel J, Holliday R, et al. Local resection and brachytherapy confined to the lumpectomy site for early breast cancer: a pilot study. *J Surg Oncol.* 1997;65:263–267.

175. Perera F, Yu E, Engel J, et al. Patterns of breast recurrence in a pilot study of brachytherapy confined to the lumpectomy site for early breast cancer with six years' minimum follow-up. *Int J Radiat Oncol Biol Phys.* 2003;57:1239–1246.

176. Perera F, Chisela F, Stitt L, et al. TLD skin dose measurements and acute and late effects after lumpectomy and high-dose-rate brachytherapy only for early breast cancer. *Int J Radiat Oncol Biol Phys.* 2005;62:1283–1290.

177. Vicini FA, Baglan KL, Kestin LL, et al. Accelerated treatment of breast cancer. *J Clin Oncol.* 2001;19:1993–2001.

178. Kuske RR, Winter K, Arthur D, et al. A phase I/II trial of brachytherapy alone following lumpectomy for select breast cancer: toxicity analysis of Radiation Therapy Oncology Group 95-17. *Int J Radiat Oncol Biol Phys.* 2002;54:S87.

179. Kuske RR, Winter K, Arthur DW, et al. A phase II trial of brachytherapy alone following lumpectomy for stage I or II breast cancer: initial outcomes of RTOG 95-17. 40th Annual Meeting of the American Society of Clinical Oncology. New Orleans, LA, 2004. *J Clin Oncol.* 2004;22:18S.

180. Kuske RR, Winter K, Arthur DW, et al. Phase II trial of brachytherapy alone after lumpectomy for select breast cancer: toxicity analysis of RTOG 95-17. *Int J Radiat Oncol Biol Phys.* 2006;65:45–51.

181. Wazer DE, Berle L, Graham R, et al. Preliminary results of a phase I/II study of HDR brachytherapy alone for T1/T2 breast cancer. 43rd Annual Meeting of the American Society for Therapeutic Radiology and Oncology. San Francisco, CA, 2001. *Int J Radiat Oncol Biol Phys.* 2002;53:889–897.

182. Wazer DE, Kaufman S, Cuttino L, et al. Accelerated partial breast irradiation: an analysis of variables associated with late toxicity and long-term cosmetic outcome after high-dose-rate interstitial brachytherapy. *Int J Radiat Oncol Biol Phys.* 2006;64:489–495.

183. Polgar C, Sulyok Z, Fodor J, et al. Sole brachytherapy of the tumor bed after conservative surgery for T1 breast cancer: five-year results of a phase I–II study and initial findings of a randomized phase III trial. *J Surg Oncol.* 2002;80:121–128.

184. Polgar C, Major T, Fodor J, et al. High-dose-rate brachytherapy alone versus whole breast radiotherapy with or without tumor bed boost after breast-conserving surgery: seven-year results of a comparative study. *Int J Radiat Oncol Biol Phys.* 2004;60:1173–1181.

185. Lawenda BD, Taghian AG, Kachnic LA, et al. Dose-volume analysis of radiotherapy for T1N0 invasive breast cancer treated by local excision and partial breast irradiation by low-dose-rate interstitial implant. *Int J Radiat Oncol Biol Phys.* 2003;56:671–680.

186. Krishnan L, Jewell WR, Tawfik OW, et al. Breast conservation therapy with tumor bed irradiation alone in a selected group of patients with stage I breast cancer. *Breast J.* 2001;7:91–96.

187. Arthur DW, Koo D, Zwicker RD, et al. Partial breast brachytherapy after lumpectomy: low-dose-rate and high-dose-rate experience. 43rd Annual Meeting of the American Society for Therapeutic Radiology and Oncology. San Francisco, CA, 2001. *Int J Radiat Oncol Biol Phys.* 2003;56:681–689.

Frank J.P. Hoebers
Peter C. Ferguson
Brian O'Sullivan

Bone

INTRODUCTION

Radiation-associated bone complications may affect patients of any age and gender and are associated with potential lifelong risks of occurrence. The consequences can be serious and include pathologic fractures, deformity, osteoradionecrosis (ORN), and the induction of secondary bone tumors. In addition to pure radiation treatment factors (i.e., total dose and fractionation), their development is also influenced by the deleterious effects of other treatments such as surgery and chemotherapy, as well as by several host factors. The latter include genetic abnormalities, age, gender, and menopausal status as well as the vascular and structural integrity of associated tissues. Due to the long latency of bone complications that may manifest over many years, the literature is biased toward reporting outcome of more favorable prognosis patients with longer-term survival. Consequently breast cancer, prostate cancer, cervical cancer, lymphoma/Hodgkins disease, and certain types of childhood malignancy predominate in our understanding of the risk, manifestations, and treatment of these complications.

NORMAL ANATOMY AND PHYSIOLOGY OF BONE

During early fetal development, the skeleton is initially composed largely of hyaline cartilage, which serves as the scaffold on which bone eventually develops. In the skull, maxilla and mandible primitive mesenchymal cells develop directly into osteoblasts, which form bone via a process called membranous ossification. The remainder of the skeleton is converted from cartilage to bone by endochondral ossification. During fetal and early postnatal life, poorly understood signals result in the development of primary (in central bone) and secondary (at the epiphyses of long bones) ossification centers. Some bones have single ossification centers (e.g., zygomatic, carpal, and tarsal bones), while multiple ossification centers arise and contribute to longitudinal growth of long bones. The primary and secondary ossification centers are separated by the epiphyseal growth plate, which is essential for longitudinal bone growth and which is the most radiation-sensitive region of the growing bone. The growth plate is composed of highly organized layers of cartilage. Adjacent to the secondary ossification center lies the reserve zone where immature chondrocytes contribute to the subjacent proliferative zone. Cells in this layer rapidly proliferate and

manifest histologically as columns of cells parallel to the long axis of the bone. Juxtaposed to the proliferation zone, chondrocytes enlarge and contribute to ossification of the matrix in the zone of provisional calcification and cartilage is converted to bone. This process of sequential growth of new bone away from the epiphysis contributes to longitudinal bone growth, with the most active sites being the distal femur, proximal tibia, and proximal femur. The growth plate ceases to exist when the individual reaches skeletal maturity, usually in midteenage years.

Despite its inert appearance, bone is a dynamic tissue the function of which depends on both its cellular components and extracellular matrix and exists in two forms. Cortical bone consists largely of long parallel cylinders of extracellular matrix called osteons, which are closed packed together in the Haversian system and provide maximal resistance to bending and compression in the diaphyses of long bones. Cancellous bone is more porous, consisting of branching trabeculae around irregular spaces and oriented to resist forces in multiple directions. It is found in the metaphyses of long bones and in the skull, vertebrae, and pelvis. The extracellular matrix of bone has both organic and inorganic elements. The organic component is largely (94%) type I collagen[1] arranged in highly crosslinked parallel bundles that provide maximal resistance to bending. The inorganic component is a crystallized compound of calcium phosphate referred to as hydroxyapatite.[1]

Three specialized cellular populations exist: the osteoblasts, osteoclasts, and osteocytes. During bone synthesis, a proportion of osteoblasts become embedded in the extracellular matrix and develops into osteocytes, which compose up to 90% of the cellular component of mature bone. Osteoclasts are mobile multinucleated cells responsible for bone resorption.[2] Extensive intercellular cytoplasmic connections between osteocytes, osteoclasts, and osteoblasts are likely responsible for the spatial organization of the cellular component of bone that regulates formation and breakdown.

Normal bone development and maintenance is a process of precisely regulated bone absorption and synthesis in response to mechanical, chemical, and metabolic stimuli. The outer surface of bone comprises the periosteum containing an outer layer of cells resembling fibroblasts that serve as the site of attachments of muscles. The inner layer contains osteoprogenitor cells that develop into osteoblasts, which in turn contribute to axial bone growth and are also responsible for fracture healing. Following fracture, osteoblasts develop into chondroblasts that synthesize a cartilaginous matrix that is then resorbed by osteoclasts and replaced by new bone by trailing osteoblasts. The periosteum also contains numerous blood vessels, which enter the cortex via the Haversian system to supply nutrients to osteocytes embedded within the bony trabeculae.

BIOLOGICAL EFFECTS OF RADIATION ON BONE

EFFECTS OF RADIATION ON GROWING IMMATURE BONE

The physeal plate is responsible for longitudinal bone growth in the skeletally immature individual and is most susceptible to the effects of radiation.[3–5] Consequently, the most common skeletal effect of radiation in children is longitudinal growth arrest with a resulting shortened or angulated limb.

The rapidly proliferating cells of the proliferative zone appear to be the most sensitive region of the growth plate.[6] Within only days of exposure, a single dose of radiation can decrease cell proliferation and cell number, and decrease overall epiphyseal growth.[4] With lower doses, the proliferative zone may be repopulated from progenitor cells in the reserve zone, and growth restored at a reduced and less well organized level. With higher doses, the effects can be permanent, with an inability for the proliferative zone to be repopulated.

Chondrocytes in the zone of provisional calcification may also be depleted in numbers following radiation so that newly calcified bone becomes absorbed by the unopposed action of osteoclasts, leading to thickening of the growth plate. Recovery of chondrocyte function can occur after a period of several months, and longitudinal growth can resume.[5,7]

EFFECTS OF RADIATION ON MATURE BONE

Radiation leads to obliterative endarteritis and endothelial cell cytoplasmic vacuolization in early stages.[8] Subsequently, intimal fibrosis and hypertrophy of the media layer of the blood vessel can lead to luminal narrowing in the Haversian system. As a result, bone blood flow has been shown to be decreased after radiation,[9] and, in a rat model, vascularized bone grafts also fail to heal to recipient tibias that have been irradiated to 50 Gy.[10]

Osteoblast proliferation is affected by radiation resulting in fewer cells to synthesize bone matrix, and bone atrophy may result especially in response to injury or mechanical loading.[5,11] The end result of the radiation effects on osteoblasts is that bone absorption can continue in a relatively unopposed fashion. Osteoclast bone resorption can continue but without concomitant bone formation, decreased bone density develops that is predisposed to fracture. Radiographically cortical osteopenia and coarse trabeculation are often evident.[3] The reduction in bone vascularity, combined with impaired bone formation from irradiated osteoblasts, results in alteration of the fracture-healing environment, often resulting in nonunion.

CLINICAL CONSEQUENCES OF RADIATION TO GROWING IMMATURE BONE

The clinical consequences of radiation on growing bone are variable and may be dramatic and are summarized below. Despite the significance of the clinical problem, robust estimates of the

TABLE 43.1	Factors Associated with the Severity of Radiation-Induced Growth Abnormalities of Bone
Total radiation dose	
Dose per fraction?	
Volume of bone treated	
Partial or inhomogeneous irradiation of bone	
Anatomical site of radiation exposure	
Age at time of radiation exposure	
Use of chemotherapy	

causative dose effects remain uncertain. Data from several studies indicate that the steep part of the dose-response curve for radiation injury to growing immature bone may lie between 15 and 35 Gy.[12–15] There are no good data on the effects of radiation fraction size on the risk of growth abnormalities. In addition to the dose parameters, the volume treated, age at time of radiation,[14–17] use of chemotherapy,[18,19] and also the growth activity of the bone at time and site of radiation exposure are additional important variables (Table 43.1).

CRANIOFACIAL GROWTH ABNORMALITIES FOLLOWING RADIATION

Craniofacial growth retardation in children can lead to serious consequences including facial asymmetry, which may have significant cosmetic and functional consequences. The observed abnormalities can be quantified by established radiologic metrics (Fig. 43.1)[20] and may include skull/facial bone hypoplasia, micrognathia, malocclusion, reduced mobility of temporomandibular joint and trismus, and/or velopharyngeal incompetence. The effects of radiation on dental development include reduced mineralization, reduced tooth size and/or agenesis of teeth.[21] These various craniofacial deformities can have serious psychosocial impacts for childhood cancer survivors.[22–24]

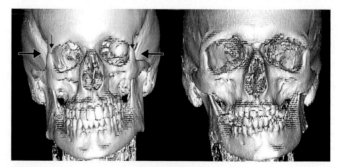

Figure 43.1. The left 3D reconstructed CT image depicts a craniofacial growth deformity in a 41-year-old female who survived bilateral retinoblastoma. At the age of 1 year, she underwent left-sided enucleation, followed by external beam radiation to a dose of 5,000 roentgens to the left orbit and intra-arterial administration of triethylene melamine. The right-sided tumor was treated by primary radiation to a dose of 3,500 roentgens. Note a bilateral decreased orbital volume, a reduced lateral orbital distance (distance between the most anterior tip of each lateral orbital wall, *small arrows*), and a reduced intertemporal distance (distance between the most medial aspect of each temporalis groove, *large arrows*).[20] For reference, on the right side a 3D reconstruction CT-scan of an unaffected, normal individual is shown.

Incidence and Effect of Radiation Dose

Most young children treated with radiation therapy (RT) for craniofacial rhabdomyosarcoma experience clinical or radiological dentofacial abnormalities after a minimal prescribed dose of 50 Gy. [25] Guyuron et al.[26] demonstrated a threshold dose of 30 Gy for adverse effects on craniofacial bone in childhood cancer survivors treated at a mean age of 4.7 years (range: 1–17). An important factor contributing to damage to the growing craniofacial skeleton is age below 5 to 6 years when the growing bones undergo rapid proliferation.[14,16] Sonis et al.[14] showed that the incidence of craniofacial abnormalities (mainly micrognathia) was 90% in patients receiving 24 Gy of cranial irradiation before the age of 5, compared with no craniofacial abnormalities in patients receiving 0 or 18 Gy and/or patients receiving 24 Gy at the age of 5 or older. The combination of cyclophosphamide and total body irradiation (TBI) doses of 10 Gy are associated with reduced craniofacial growth, especially in children 6 years or younger.[16] Thus, lower doses of radiation combined with chemotherapy also affect bone growth. Jaffe et al.[27] analyzed 68 children by disease treated and showed that the incidence of deformities was highest among patients treated for rhabdomyosarcoma (median doses of 55 Gy) compared with patients treated for Hodgkin disease and leukemia (median dose 35 Gy). This suggests that even after doses above 30 to 35 Gy additional damage to growing bone may be expected.

BONE GROWTH ABNORMALITIES OF THE SPINE, PELVIS, AND EXTREMITIES

Radiation treatment to the vertebral column is associated with short stature. Partial irradiation of the vertebra can cause focal growth arrest resulting in scoliosis and kyphosis. Irradiation to the extremities may result in significant discrepancies in limb length. The severity of these effects depends on radiation dose and on the rate of bone growth at time of radiation treatment. Infants, young children, and adolescents during their growth spurts are most susceptible.

Short Stature

The main detriment to bone growth in children treated to the entire spine is a disproportionate alteration in sitting as compared to standing height, especially in patients who had received 35 Gy or more to the axial skeleton.[13] Willman et al.[15] measured height impairment in 124 survivors of pediatric Hodgkin disease and found it to be most severe among children treated in prepubertal age and given radiation to a dose of at least 33 Gy to the whole spine. The average height impairment was 7.7%, corresponding to a height loss of 13 cm. Less height impairment was evident with lower radiation dose, partial spine treatment, or older aged children. Data from the Dutch Late effects Study Group on 285 childhood cancer survivors showed that both craniospinal irradiation and cranial irradiation resulted in impaired adult height with the largest effect seen below the age of 8 years.[17]

In an analysis on stature loss in over 2,700 children treated on National Wilms Tumor Study Group protocol 1 to 4, younger patients had a higher risk of growth deficit and higher doses of radiation resulted in more stature reduction.[28] For patients <1 year at diagnosis and who received 10 Gy or more of flank RT, the predicted adult height impairment was 7.7 cm compared to the no-RT group. An RT-dose dependency was observed with an average reduction in height among all patients of about 4 to 7 cm following doses of 15 Gy or more.

Observations suggest that chemotherapy probably has an additional effect on the growth reduction following radiation compared to radiation alone, but reports are inconsistent.

Scoliosis and Kyphosis

Scoliosis following radiation is predominantly related to partial irradiation of the spine or to inhomogeneous dose distribution to the vertebral column as can occur in the treatment of Wilms tumor.[29,30] Paulino et al.[12] reported a 43% incidence of scoliosis in 42 patients with Wilms tumor treated with radiation between 1968 to 1994. Median time to development of scoliosis was 102 months, with a range of 16 to 146 months. The actuarial incidence of scoliosis at 5, 10, and 15 years after RT was 5%, 52%, and 57%, respectively The incidence was significantly lower (26%) in patients treated to a dose lower than 24 Gy compared with those receiving a dose of 24 Gy or higher (63%). Only one patient required surgical intervention for stabilization of the spine.

Limb Shortening

Radiation to long bones can interfere with growth and ultimately lead to discrepancies in length of the involved extremities.[31] About 80% of the growth from the humerus comes from the proximal growth center, 70% of femoral growth from the distal epiphysis, and 60% of tibial growth comes from proximal growth center. Therefore, irradiation of an entire knee including the adjacent femoral and tibial epiphyses may cause severe shortening in limb length,[12,32,33] necessitating surgical corrective interventions (see section 7.3.2).

Slipped Femoral Capital Epiphysis

Radiation-induced slippage of the epiphysis may occur without other risk factors after irradiation of the femoral head [34–38] with a threshold dose of about 25 to 30 Gy.[36,37] Young age seemed to be critical as it was observed in 47% of children irradiated before 4 years of age compared with only 5% of older patients.[37]

CLINICAL CONSEQUENCES OF RADIATION TO MATURE BONE

Radiation doses in ordinary clinical use do not ordinarily result in profound acute injury to bony structures. Therefore, late effects characterize the clinically relevant radiation-induced changes of mature bone. A long latent period before the changes are detected clinically is characteristic due to the slow metabolic turnover rate of bone. The late effects include damage to osteoblasts, decreased matrix formation, and osteopenia and are typically seen one year after radiation.[39] Repair of bone may occur with deposition of bone on unresorbed trabeculae. This can initially be asymptomatic and demonstrable on radiographs as focal areas of increased opacity in close proximity to areas of mottled bone with osteopenia [40] and referred to as radiation-induced osteitis. Ultimately, depending on the anatomical site of the involved bone and the severity of the injury,

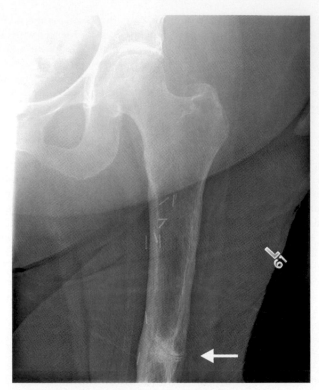

Figure 43.2. AP radiograph of proximal femur of 72-year-old woman, 12 years after resection and postoperative radiation of soft-tissue sarcoma of the thigh. The radiograph shows irregular cortices, cortical lucencies, and an undisplaced insufficiency fracture (*arrow*). The patient was asymptomatic at the time of presentation.

this may manifest symptoms due to osteonecrosis or stress/insufficiency fractures (Fig. 43.2), or may present as a pathological fracture due to the structural weakness (Fig. 43.3). These conditions are described below.

OSTEORADIONECROSIS OF MANDIBLE

The mandible is one of the more frequently damaged bones following radiotherapy and ORN of this bone is one of the more devastating sequelae of curative radiotherapy for head-and-neck malignancy. A recent comprehensive review is available.[41] The combination of cellular depletion, poor vascularity, insufficient oxygenation (potentially related to vascular compromise or the influence of continued cigarette smoking), and infection appears to contribute to this syndrome. Typically, it manifests 6 months to several years following radiotherapy though the risk is lifelong at a lower rate subsequently. Radiographic criteria include osteoporosis, mottling of bone due to resorption, bone sclerosis and a thickened periosteum. Bone lysis (Fig. 43.4) and fracture (Fig. 43.5) may eventually result. The most common clinical hallmark is bone exposure with necrotic bone apparent within chronically ulcerated mucosa or less commonly through ulcerated skin with sinus formation. This has led to the classic definition of ORN as the presence of devitalized exposed bone in an irradiated field that fails to heal for three months.[41] A continued conduit for infection established in this way may contribute to the sustained and propagating nature of the process in atrophic bone with diminished vascularity and poor defense against infection. Several predictable scenarios are seen and have spawned a number of classification systems based around the themes of disability, symptomatology, and the nature of the treatment required for management. Thus, lower grades can generally be classified according to whether ulceration with bone exposure heals spontaneously, while higher grades, including fracture of the mandible, generally require surgical repair.

Predisposing factors include total dose delivered to the mandible and is therefore especially linked to the use of brachytherapy applied close to the mandible. External beam may also be causative but ORN is almost never seen below 60 Gy with conventionally fractionated radiotherapy (i.e., 2 Gy/fraction).

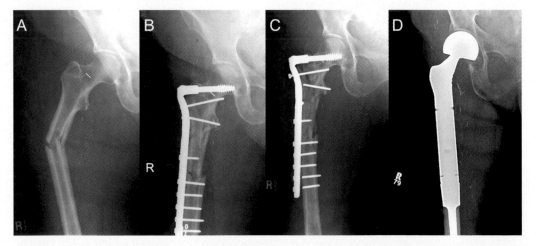

Figure 43.3. **A**: Radiograph of proximal femur of 78-year-old woman, 6 years after preoperative radiation and resection of soft-tissue sarcoma of thigh. This patient developed a sudden onset of pain with minimal trauma. Radiograph shows comminuted transverse fracture, usually associated with high-energy injury, suggesting poor bone quality as a result of radiation. **B**: Radiograph after stabilization of fracture using plate fixation. The fracture is well aligned. **C**: Radiograph taken 9 months after fixation of fracture. The fracture has displaced and there is evidence of fracture of multiple screws, suggesting nonunion. **D**: Radiograph after resection of proximal femur and insertion of tumor prosthesis. It was felt that any further attempt at fixation of the fracture in this elderly woman would be unlikely to result in union and that prosthetic insertion would allow for immediate weight bearing.

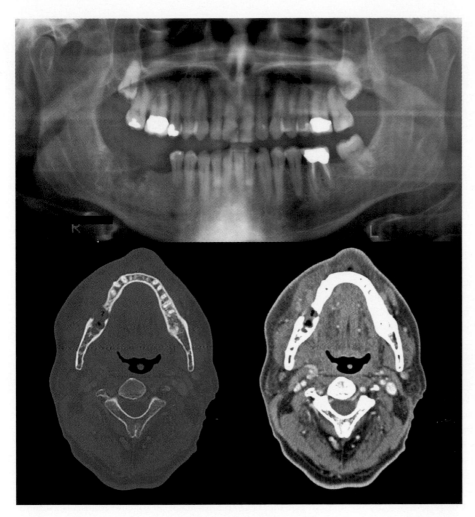

Figure 43.4. ORN of the right mandible in a 52-year-old male, who was treated 7 years earlier for squamous cell carcinoma of the left tonsillar region, by external beam radiation to a dose of 60 Gy in 30 fractions directed to the primary and lymph nodes in the left neck and a dose of 50 Gy in 25 fractions to the uninvolved right neck. The upper panel shows a panoramic radiography on which an abnormal sclerosis of the body of right mandible, resorption of bone, and indication of a small sequester was identified. The corresponding CT-scan (lower two panels) demonstrates the destructive lytic osseous process but also shows associated soft-tissue swelling in the buccal space, consistent with an inflammatory process. A biopsy of the lesion was performed and this did not show evidence for recurrent disease.

Higher intensities of radiotherapy delivery increase the risk and can reach an incidence of 20% with intensive fractionation approaches if the mandible is not excluded from the target volume. Obviously, avoidance of radiotherapy approaches that preferentially deposit dose in bone is advisable. For example, orthovoltage radiotherapy for adjacent skin or lip cancers should be applied judiciously and perhaps limited to small volume boosts to augment more usual radiotherapy approaches. Conversely, bone avoidance with intensity modulated RT (IMRT) strategies seems to have virtually reduced the inci-

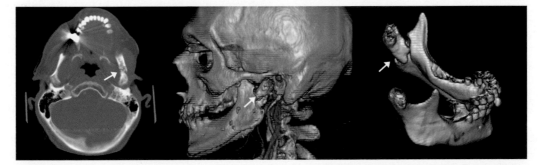

Figure 43.5. Axial CT scan (left panel), full 3-D reconstruction of CT scan (middle panel), and 3-D reconstruction of mandible only (right panel) of a 49-year-old male showing fragmentation and fracture of the left mandible (*arrows*). The condylar process of the ascending ramus of the mandible is fractured off the body of the mandible and rotated anteriorly and medially. On the axial CT, the bone appears sclerotic and thickened. No soft-tissue mass is identified. On intraoral examination, no bone exposure was observed. Seven years earlier, the patient received radiation to a dose of 60 Gy in 30 fractions to the parotid bed and left neck, following a left parotidectomy because of extensive adenoid cystic carcinoma. His other risk factor was sustained heavy cigarette smoking. As the patient was asymptomatic, he was managed conservatively without intervention. The presentation is atypical for ORN of the mandible, because of absence of the following findings: bone exposure, soft-tissue mass, and symptoms (pain and infection).

dence of ORN to a historic phenomenon in expert hands.[42,43] Attention to oral hygiene and dentition is critical. In general, dental management should focus proactively on decayed or broken teeth as well as gingival problems prior to commencing radiotherapy especially since postradiotherapy extraction is a strong predisposing factor. Very decayed teeth may need careful extraction, ensuring the socket edges are smooth, and then closure by suturing the overflying mucosa. Healing for a period of at least 1 to 2 weeks is then advisable if the site is to be included in the radiotherapy target volume.

OSTEORADIONECROSIS OF OTHER BONES

Avascular necrosis of the femoral or humeral heads has been reported 2 to 3 years after irradiation.[44] Libshitz and Edeiken[45] described necrosis after receiving 30 to 60 Gy to the femoral heads in 16 of 44 children. This complication occurred bilaterally in four of five patients who received irradiation to both hips but is lower when the femoral and humeral heads are shielded and when lower doses are used.[46] In 15 leukemia survivors diagnosed with avascular femoral head necrosis, both steroids and RT appeared to be implicated in the pathogenesis of avascular necrosis.[47]

ORN has been described in numerous other anatomical sites, including the head-and-neck region,[48,49] sternum and ribs,[50] vertebra,[51] and pelvis.[52] However, these are generally case report series and do not provide information about predisposing risk factors or radiation dose effects. However, in the setting of head-and-neck reirradiation, ORN has been identified as a well-documented complication[53,54] and may even be life threatening if complicated by hemorrhage from associated vascular injury in the head and neck or chest.[49]

RADIATION-INDUCED FRACTURES OF BONES OF THE TRUNK AND EXTREMITIES

Pathologic Fractures of Long Bones

Pathologic fractures are defined as fractures occurring in irradiated bone that develops after no or minimal trauma. Most data on pathologic fractures in long bones are derived from experience in the treatment of soft-tissue sarcoma, pelvic tumors, and pediatric sarcoma with most studies focusing on fractures in the femur as these are common and immediately disabling. The neck and the shaft are the most common femoral sites.[55,56]

SOFT-TISSUE SARCOMA RT. Crude incidences of fracture rates in patient series treated with surgery and (in most series postoperative) radiation for soft-tissue sarcoma of extremities (see Figs. 43.2 and 43.3) range from 1.2% to 7.3%.[55–61] Overall the 5-year actuarial risk of fracture ranges from 3% to 8.6%.[55–58] These fractures are often sustained after no or minimal trauma,[57,60] and an absence of antecedent symptoms or pain in the affected limb is common (see Fig. 43.3).[60] The mean interval between radiation treatment and fracture development is generally between 2 and 5 years,[55–58,60,61] although fractures may occur as early as within 1 year[56,61] or more than 10 years after RT.[55,57,60]

FRACTURE RATE AND RADIATION DOSE. In only one study has an effect of the radiation dose and the sequence of surgery and radiation on the occurrence of pathologic fractures

of the lower limbs after treatment for soft-tissue sarcoma been reported,[55] while other studies were unable to demonstrate a dose-effect relationship.[56,58,61] This may be due to low number of patients in clinical settings who require long follow-up to assess this complication. Only recently, with the development of complex radiotherapy treatment planning applications that include image acquisition and registration, and formal anatomic digital segmentation have routine radiotherapy dose volume measurements relevant to actual bone irradiation been readily available. For example, in a study reported for patients treated over a long period of time at the Princess Margaret Hospital, we defined radiation dose according to the prescription used because we were unable to relate it to the actual bone irradiated as the majority of patients were treated in the two-dimensional radiotherapy planning era.[55] Dose was classified as "low" if the prescribed dose was 50 Gy and "high" if 60 to 66 Gy. The timing of radiation was preoperative, postoperative, or preoperative followed by postoperative boost. In this series of 364 patients, 27 fractures occurred in 23 patients, resulting in a fracture rate of 6.3%. In the high-dose group, 24 fractures were seen in 20 patients, whereas only three fractures occurred in three patients in the low-dose group, resulting in a fracture rate of 10% and 2%, respectively. The overall actuarial 5-year estimate of fracture frequency was 4%, and it was 7% and 0.6% for the high- and the low-dose group, respectively ($p = 0.007$). This factor remained significant on multivariate analysis. In the analysis of the effect of postoperative versus preoperative RT, the same 5-year frequency rate was found (7% and 0.6%, $p = 0.008$), due to the fact that radiation dose and timing were closely related. Thus, 60 to 66 Gy is usually delivered in the postoperative setting, whereas 50 Gy is a standard dose for preoperative radiation. These reported fracture risks are lower than the risk suggested by Emami et al.[62] who estimated that the TD 5/5 and TD 5/50 for late femoral/humeral toxicity (necrosis) were 52 and 65 Gy, respectively. The explanation may be that the data from Emami addressed treatment of the entire femoral volume, whereas in other analyses, such as those from our center, the dose volume parameters are more selective and consequently less well characterized.[55,63]

In a more recent report from the Princess Margaret Hospital, a very detailed dose-volume analysis was performed in matched patients with or without fractures following limb sparing surgery and RT.[64] The fracture incidence was lower when the mean dose to the bone was <37 Gy or the maximum dose was <59 Gy. There was a trend toward a lower mean field size for nonfracture patients compared to the patients that did develop a fracture.

RISK FACTORS FOR PATHOLOGICAL FRACTURES. In addition to RT dose, certain other factors are relevant (Table 43.2). Thus, full course inclusion of the entire circumference of the femur within the radiation fields (as often occurs in parallel-opposing treatment techniques) is not advisable.[57] Periosteal stripping leads to disruption of nutrient vessels and therefore affects the vascularity of the outer cortex.[65,66] Because the stripping process also leads to removal of the osteoprogenitor cells in the periosteum, it results in decreased potential for healing and regeneration.[67] The impact of periosteal stripping of the femur is to increase the 5-year rate of fracture to 29% ($p < 0.0001$). An increased risk of fracture associated with surgical exposure of the bone has also been demonstrated in other studies[57,58] including partial cortical bone resection.[68] Other

TABLE 43.2	**Risk Factors for Pathologic Fractures of Long Bones**

Total radiation dose
Dose per fraction
Inclusion of the entire circumference of bone within the radiation
 portals
Periosteal stripping of bone
Partial resection of bone
Female gender
Older age
Postmenopausal status
Use of chemotherapy

risk factors include osteoporosis, which is linked to female gender,[55,60] older age or postmenopausal status,[56,61] and the use of chemotherapy.[56,57]

Pelvic RT

Generally, fractures have been identified in pelvic diseases requiring relatively high doses of radiotherapy including gynecological, rectal, and anal canal cancers. The studies have been undertaken in the different settings, including institutional series, data emanating from clinical trials, and population-based analyses.[69–71] The majority suffer from absence of robust analyses of risk factors or control of confounding factors, but they portray a picture that is consistent with the femoral bone situation, and specifically that dose administered and volume treated are important. In contrast, the risk of fracture is low after radiation treatment doses generally used in the treatment for lymphoma or testicular cancer (30–40 Gy),[62] where fracture seem exceptionally rare after RT for these malignancies.[72–74]

RT for Pediatric Malignancy

The pediatric literature is confounded by the fact that most of the data pertain to sarcoma management where multiple factors may play a role.[75] Frequently, the original tumor itself arose within the bone that was irradiated (e.g., Ewings sarcoma). Causation is therefore difficult to study since RT directly, tumor recurrence, or second primary in the bone can all be relevant.[33,76] An informative observation from the University of Florida concerns the role of fractionation for Ewing sarcoma of the extremities where patients who received once-daily radiation (to a dose of 47–61 Gy at 1.8–2 Gy/fraction) had a significantly higher rate of fracture (36%) compared to its virtual complete disappearance in a later cohort treated with hyperfractionated twice-daily radiation (to a dose of 50.4–60 Gy at 1.2 Gy/fraction) while maintaining similar local control.[77,78]

Pelvic Insufficiency Fractures

After pelvic radiation for gynecological, genitourinary, or gastrointestinal cancer, patients may develop radiation-induced fractures of the pelvic bones especially adjacent to the weight-bearing sacroiliac joints.[79–82] These often present as pelvic insufficiency fractures (PIF), also called hair fractures or stress fractures. Up to 50% are bilateral, 10% to 20% occur in the pubic bone, and 5% in the acetabulum. Multiple fractures are seen in over 60% of cases.

The incidence of PIF after pelvic RT shows a large variation in incidence from 1.7% to 4.7% in older series[83–85] to more recent frequencies of 40% or greater.[81,82,86,87] Modern imaging such as MRI and bone scintigraphy with higher sensitivity for detecting asymptomatic bone abnormalities is the likely explanation, especially if evaluated prospectively. Indeed, the 5-year rate of incidence of PIF was usually found to be lower (2.1%–13%) when confined to symptomatic patients only.[81,82,85] It is also important to distinguish bone metastases from PIF.[88]

Symptomatic PIF typically presents as a mild-to-moderately painful lesion that may persist for some months to over 1 year.[81–83,88] In a minority (13%) of cases, symptoms of PIF are severe and may require narcotic treatment and/or hospitalization.[82]

RISK FACTORS FOR PIF. Analysis of risk factors for PIF has been performed in only a minority of studies.[82,86] In an older clinical series of 244 cervical carcinoma patients treated with radiation, the incidence of pelvic bone injury was 8.5% after x-ray treatment and 0.6% after Cobalt-treatment,[89] probably related to the increased bone absorption of low-energy radiation. Generally, the risk seems to center around factors that include corticosteroid use, older age, and the presence of osteopenia.[90] Not surprisingly radiation dose, especially when it exceeds 50 Gy, seems particularly important (5-year incidence of PIF of 2% versus 23% for doses < or > 50.4 Gy, respectively).[87] A recent multivariate analysis on 83 cases with PIF demonstrated that older age, low body weight, and radiation dose were significantly associated with increased risk of PIF.[82] Associated factors such as multiple deliveries may further complicate the risk estimate.[86]

Pathologic Fractures of Ribs

RIB FRACTURES AFTER BREAST CANCER TREATMENT. The reported incidence of rib fracture following radiation for breast cancer ranges from <1% to 19%.[91–101] Interpretation and comparison of these figures is difficult since some series reported on asymptomatic rib fractures detected on standard follow-up chest films,[95,98] while others reported on clinically detected rib fractures only.[97,99] Modern radiation techniques with avoidance of normal structures improved matching of separate radiation treatment fields (and hence less overdosage), and the use of linear accelerators with higher photon energies appears to be associated with lower rib fracture rates (e.g., <2%)[92,93,97,101] compared to traditional radiotherapy approaches in the 1960s to 1980s where rates approaching 19% existed.[94,95,98,100] Tangential radiation fields, the most commonly used technique, need to be applied meticulously since focal areas of overdose with higher dose per fraction regions delivered to the chest wall may potentially result (Fig. 43.6), especially with lower-energy techniques.[102]

RADIATION-RELATED RISK FACTORS. Some radiation-related risk factors have been established (Table 43.3). These include large dose per fraction as illustrated by the study of Overgaard. Mainly asymptomatic, radiologically detected rib fractures were detected in patients treated with postmastectomy radiation between 1978 and 1980 using either standard dose per fraction (approximately 2.3 Gy/fraction), five times per week to a total dose of 51.3 Gy in 22 fractions or high dose per fraction (approximately 3.9 Gy/fraction), two times per week to a total dose of 46.4 Gy in 12 fractions. The incidence of rib

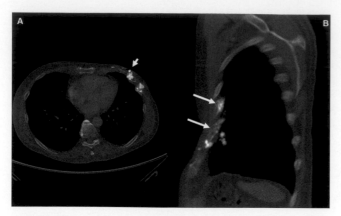

Figure 43.6. Axial (**A**) and sagittal (**B**) computerized tomography depiction of long-term rib damage in a 64-year-old male treated 40 years previously for Ewings sarcoma of the left mid chest. In recent years, he has presented with multiple fractures in the treated ribs (left 4, 5, and 6 ribs). Disorganized fracture healing (*long arrows*) is evident with hypertrophic changes and heterotopic bone in soft tissues due to the impaired bone quality and osteitis. The possibility of radiation-induced malignancy is less likely due to the number of bones involved that correspond to the ribs that were treated. Ulceration is also evident where the relatively protruberant foci of disorganized bone growth are eroding the areas of significant soft-tissue atrophy (short arrow). This patient had received cyclosphosphamide and 3-Gy TBI as microscopic systemic adjuvants plus 45 Gy in 16 daily treatments by two tangential cobalt beams to the chest wall (administered by alternate fields per day). Because each field was not treated, each day the resulting applied dose from the individual fields was necessarily higher at their entry points (approximately 3.7 Gy) to deliver the required daily dose (approximately 2.8 Gy) at the prescription area on each alternate day and probably contributed to the problem. (See also Figure 43.7.)

fracture in the high dose per fraction group was 19% as opposed to 6% in the low-dose group ($p < 0.05$).[98]

More recently performed moderate hypofractionation randomized phase 3 trials did not show an increased risk of late toxicity including rib fractures following radiation treatment using doses per fraction of 2.7 to 3.2 Gy to a total dose of 39 to 41.6 Gy in 13 to 16 fractions as compared to the standard fractionation scheme of 50 Gy in 25 fractions.[92,93,101] In the Canadian study of Whelan et al.,[101] only one rib fracture was reported (in the standard fractionation arm). In the two U.K. trials (START A and START B), identical incidences of rib fractures were reported.[92,93] The reported incidence of rib fracture was 1.5% and the confirmed incidence of rib fracture was 0.2% with no differences between the standard and the experimental treatment arms. So, it appears that the dose per fraction is a factor in the development of bone injury above a certain threshold (somewhere above 3.2–3.9 Gy/fraction) even when the total dose administered is modest (e.g., 46.4 Gy).

TABLE 43.3	Risk Factors for Radiation-Induced Rib Fractures

High total radiation dose
Dose per fraction (hypofractionation)
Low machine energy
Large volume of rib/chest wall included in radiation fields
Peripheral lung cancer treated with stereotactic body radiotherapy

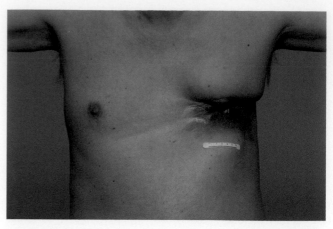

Figure 43.7. Clinical photograph of the patient whose images are shown in Figure 43.6. Note the significant soft-tissue atrophy, ulceration, tethering, and deformity of superficial tissues overlying the site of fractures due to radiotherapy effects and consequent migration of heterotopic bone through subcutaneous tissues.

Other potential factors include a minimal effect of radiation beam energy (i.e., 4 vs. 6–8 MV beams) in a very large retrospective study[99] and an association with the dose and volume of breast irradiated and with the use of adjuvant chemotherapy, although the latter is not a consistent observation.[94]

CLINICAL FINDINGS OF RADIATION-INDUCED RIB FRACTURES. The clinical characteristics of radiation-induced rib fractures range from radiological findings alone to clinical findings of pain and swelling.[95,98,99] They can occur between 1 month and 5 years (median time of 12–27 months).[94,99] Usually more than 1 rib is involved and fortunately most will heal without intervention.[99] Chronic sequelae may include dysfunctional reactive healing and secondary soft-tissue manifestations related to soft-tissue atrophy in the irradiated region (Fig. 43.7).

APBI AND RIB FRACTURES. There has been an emerging interest in the use of accelerated partial breast irradiation (APBI) with either brachytherapy or external beam radiation. The results in terms of risk of rib fractures seem to be favorable with no reported fractures in the series using ten fraction schedules.[103,104] In contrast, a Japanese series reported that 2 of 45 patients (4.4%) presented with rib fractures following 36 Gy in 6 fractions with median follow-up of 31 months.[105]

Recent phase 1 to 2 studies of APBI using 3D-conformal external beam radiotherapy (EBRT) have reported favorable control rates and low toxicity profiles with no rib fractures reported after delivery of 34 to 38.5 Gy in ten fractions[106,107] or 30 Gy in five fractions.[108] Follow-up remains short and no data from randomized phase 3 trials are available. In the series from Massachusetts General Hospital, 1 out of 99 patients presented with a rib fractures after APBI by EBRT to a dose of 32 Gy in 8 fractions.[109]

Limited data are available for ORN, as opposed to rib fractures, of the chest wall after treatment with radiation, although it can include sternum and/or multiple ribs and is often accompanied by soft-tissue necrosis.[110]

RIB FRACTURES AFTER LUNG CANCER TREATMENT. Stereotactic body radiation therapy (SBRT) has emerged as a curative treatment for early stage non–small-cell lung cancer (NSCLC). The incidences of rib fractures have not been reported in all studies,[111,112] but some series have observed fractures in 0.8% to 5% of cases.[113–115] Recently, several reports of SBRT for peripheral lung tumors have analyzed the risk of rib fracture in detail. At the Princess Margaret Hospital, 42 patients with peripheral T1-2 NSCLC received SBRT to a dose of 54 to 60 Gy in 3 fractions.[116] The crude incidence of rib fracture was 21% and the 2-year estimated incidence was 48%. The median distance of the tumor to the chest wall was 0.4 cm. The median dose (without heterogeneity correction) to the fractured ribs was 43 Gy (26–74), indicating that a significant proportion of rib fractures may develop in areas receiving less than the prescribed dose. In a combined experience of SBRT for 60 patients with peripheral primary or metastatic lung lesions from the Universities of Virginia and Colorado, 17 (28%) experienced Grade 3 chest wall pain and five rib fractures.[117] The median interval to the onset of severe pain and/or fracture was 7.1 months. The chest wall volume receiving 30 Gy best predicted the risk of severe pain and/or rib fracture ($R^2 = 0.9552$). A volume threshold of 30 cm^3 was observed before severe pain and/or rib fracture was reported. A 30% risk of developing severe chest wall toxicity correlated with a volume of 35 cm^3 receiving 30 Gy prompting the authors to suggest the chest wall should be considered an organ at risk in radiotherapy treatment planning. Based on the data observed, they have suggested that the volume receiving 30 Gy in three to five fractions should be limited to <30 cm^3.[117]

Pathologic Fractures of Clavicles and Vertebra

Radiation-induced fractures and/or ORN of the clavicles have been mainly seen after treatment for breast cancer[118] and/or head-and-neck cancer.[49,118–120] Radiation-induced fractures and ORN of vertebra involving the cervical,[121–123] thoracic,[89,124,125] or lumbar spine,[51,126] may also occur but are uncommon. The injury includes signs of osteoporosis, sclerosis, and compression fracture, but there is no information on risk related to radiation dose parameters and/or other risk factors.

RADIATION-INDUCED TUMORS

The induction of tumors by therapeutic or accidental irradiation is one of the most severe late effects of radiation exposure. Benign and malignant tumors can develop in bone tissues and the risk population is enlarging with the ever increasing proportion of long-term cancer survivors.

BENIGN TUMORS

The most common radiation-induced benign bone tumors are radiation-induced osteochondromata (RIO) typically as a response to epiphysial injury from radiation.[127] They are seen exclusively in childhood after a wide range of radiation doses varying from 12 to 60 Gy, including localized EBRT and TBI.[127–132] Several series have reported incidence rates of 4.8% to 14% after local external beam radiation.[12,29,127,130,131] Series analyzing the risk of RIO after TBI often report higher rates ranging from 9% to 23%.[129,132,133] Comparing these heterogeneous series is difficult since different patient groups with varying radiation treatment doses and different follow-up strategies exist. The latency time is highly variable with onset intervals spanning 17 months to 9 years, and they are often discovered incidentally. They may be single or multiple and in any anatomical location

TABLE 43.4	Diagnostic Criteria for Radiation-Induced Sarcoma of Bone Defined by Arlen et al.[136]

Microscopic or radiological evidence of a benign condition or a malignancy of a different histological type, for which the radiation was given.

Administration of a course of RT and a sarcoma subsequently developing in the path of the radiation beam.

A relatively long asymptomatic period between irradiation of the primary tumor and the diagnosis of the secondary sarcoma of at least 3–4 y.

The diagnosis of the secondary sarcoma established by histology.

including long bones, pelvis, chest wall, clavicle and scapula, or vertebral bodies.[130,132,134,135] Although usually asymptomatic, pain may be present[130,132] or less commonly compressive syndromes may result (e.g., on the spinal cord with neurological deficits) requiring surgical intervention.[134,135]

MALIGNANT TUMORS

The development of malignant tumors, including bone sarcoma, is a long-recognized, feared, and devastating complication following exposure to radiation. They occur in patients treated for benign diseases and in long-term survivors of malignancy. Some formalization of the definition of radiation-induced sarcoma (RIS) exists to assist in interpretation, reporting, and management (Table 43.4).[136] Most authors have used the term RIS[136–139] which implies that radiation would be the only etiological factor. When assessing the risk of RIS of bone, it is important to relate this to the baseline risk. An important factor is the inherent risk of secondary cancer in cancer patients not treated with RT that may also be elevated compared to the general population (GP),[140,141] although this is not confirmed in all studies.[142,143] Accurate estimation of second cancer risk in general, and bone sarcoma in particular, after radiation treatment is therefore difficult and some reservation should be applied when interpreting results.

The series on second primary bone cancers in childhood survivors generally show higher relative risks (RRs) when compared to adult series, due to the rapid proliferation of bone during childhood. The risk for second primary cancer can increase up to decades after exposure.[144]

Bone Sarcoma after Accidental Irradiation or Internal Radiation Exposure

This chapter will not provide a detailed discussion of the induction of bone sarcoma following accidental irradiation or internal exposure. However, an increased incidence of bone sarcoma has been reported among workers in nuclear energy facilities using radioactive plutonium,[145,146] atomic bomb survivors,[147] patients exposed to radium-224 by intravenous administration (for diseases like ankylosing spondylitis or tuberculosis),[148] and dial painters who used radium paint for luminescence of watch dials.[149,150]

Radiation-Induced Bone Tumors in Adults

In patients treated with radiation during adulthood, the information regarding a dose-effect relationship for radiation-induced bone cancer is limited and less detailed than the data

TABLE 43.5	$RR_{RT/GP}$ of Second Primary Bone Cancer After Radiation (RT) by Disease Site for Adult Cancer Survivors, Compared to the GP

First Author and Reference	Disease Site	No. of Patients	Study Period	Mean Follow-up in Years (Range)	Endpoint	RR (95% CI)	Remarks
Rubino[152]	Breast	6,597	1954–1983	7.9 (1–37)	STS and bone sarcoma	10.5 (5.6–17.6)	Including angiosarcoma
Brenner[142]	Prostate	~	1973–1993	4.2	STS and bone sarcoma	1.8	Significantly increased RR for in-field sarcoma
Storm[141]	Cervix	24,970	1943–1982	n.r.	Bone sarcoma	2.1 (n.s.)	RR of 2.3 for patients not treated with RT (n.s.)
Kleinerman[140]	Cervix	86,193	1935–1990	10.4	Bone sarcoma	3.0 (1.7–4.8)	RR of 1.2 for patients not treated with RT (n.s.)
Chaturvedi[154]	Cervix	104,760	1943–2001	12.2 (1–55)	Bone sarcoma	3.0 (1.81–4.7)	RR of 1.2 for patients not treated with RT (n.s.)
Travis[156]	Testicular	28,843	1935–1993	10.2	Bone sarcoma	2.4 (0.89–5.31)	Quoted RR is for total group (RT and no-RT)

CI, confidence interval; No., number; n.r., not reported; n.s. not significant; RR, relative risk; STS, soft-tissue sarcoma.

on childhood cancer survivors discussed later. In general, the overall incidence of RIS of bone is low and has been estimated to be 0.03% of all patients receiving RT, to about 0.2% of patients receiving radiation treatment who achieve 5-year survival.[139]

Large databases, including population-based cancer registries, have addressed the risk of second primary bone cancers in large cohorts after treatment of breast,[151–153] prostate,[142] and cervical cancer (Table 43.5).[140,141,154]

TABLE 43.6	RR of Secondary Sarcoma in Survivors of Childhood Cancer, Compared to the GP

First Author and Reference	Disease Site	No. of Patients	Study Period and Pt. Selected	Mean Follow-up in Years (Range)	Endpoint	RR (95% CI)	RR by Treatment (95% CI)	20-y Cum. Incidence
Tucker[144]	Miscellaneous solid childhood cancers	9,170	1936–1979 2-y survivors	n.r.	Sarcoma of bone	133 (98–176)		2.8%
Le Vu[158]	Miscellaneous solid childhood cancers	4,257	1942–1986 3-y survivors	15 (3–48)	Sarcoma of bone	100 (68–141)	RT: 30 (6–88) Chemo: 25 (0.3–139) RT+Chemo: 200 (133–289)	1.03%
Hawkins[159]	Miscellaneous childhood cancers, incl. leukemia	13,175	1940–1983 3-y survivors	10.7	Sarcoma of bone	43 (32–56)		0.9%
Jenkinson[162]	Miscellaneous childhood cancers, incl. leukemia	16,541	1926–1987 3-y survivors	10	Sarcoma of bone	41 (31–54)	RT: 32 Chemo: 32 RT+chemo: 34	3.1% (for all second cancers, incl. bone)
Henderson[161]	Miscellaneous childhood cancers, incl. leukemia	14,372	1970–1986 5-y survivors	Median 20 (5–34)	All sarcoma	9 (7–11)	RT: 11.3 (9–14) No-RT: 2.7 (2–6.6)	RT: 0.89% No-RT: 0.24%
Wong[160]	Retinoblastoma	1,604	1914–1984 1-y survivors	Median 4.2	Sarcoma of bone	255 (198–328)		At 50 y, for all 2nd cancers: Hereditary Rb: 51% Nonhereditary: 5% RT: 58% No-RT: 27%

CI, confidence interval; Cum., cumulative; No., number; n.r., not reported; Pt., patient; Rb, retinoblastoma; RR, relative risk; RT, radiotherapy; S., surgery.

Kuttesch et al.[155] analyzed the incidence of secondary cancer in 266 Ewing sarcoma survivors. The patients were survivors of childhood and early adulthood cancers. 16 patients developed a second malignancy. In the patients treated with radiation doses <48 Gy, the 20-year incidence of secondary sarcoma was 0% as compared to an incidence of about 5% in cases treated with doses between 48 and 59 Gy and about 20% after radiation doses of 60 Gy or higher ($p = 0.002$).

Rubino et al. reported on 12 patients who developed a chest wall sarcoma after breast cancer treatment.[152] This included both bone sarcoma and soft-tissue sarcoma (including angiosarcoma and Stewart Treves syndrome). The risk of sarcoma appeared to be dose dependent, with an increasing RR being associated with increasing radiation dose. Due to the low numbers of cases, the patients were analyzed in three dose cohorts (14 Gy or less, between 14 and 44 Gy, and 45 Gy or more). The associated RR for each of the three dose intervals was 1, 1.6, and 30.6, respectively. The risk was best described by a quadratic model ($p < 0.001$).

Although increased risks for a variety of cancers are present in long-term survivors of testicular cancer or lymphoma, large cohort studies have not been able to demonstrated significantly increased risks of bone sarcoma after treatment with radiation for these cancers.[156,157]

Radiation-Induced Bone Tumors after Childhood Cancer

Because both chemotherapy and radiation are often used in the management of pediatric malignancies, it is important to appreciate the contribution of both modalities in assessing the risk of secondary cancer in this vulnerable population (and see Table 43.6 for a summary of the reported series). For example in a study of 4,257 survivors of solid childhood cancers treated in France and United Kingdom, Le Vu et al.[158] showed that the 20-year cumulative incidence of osteosarcoma as a second cancer was 1.03% for all patients and the RR was 100 (95% CI: 68–141) compared to the GP. The RR of bone sarcoma for patients treated with radiation was 30 (95% CI: 6–88), when compared to the population, but increased to 200 (95% CI: 133–289) after both chemotherapy and radiation. Also, the RR for chemotherapy alone was 25. The highest risk for osteosarcoma was found after treatment for bilateral retinoblastoma (20-year cumulative incidence: 12.1% [95% CI: 1.04–23.0]).

After adjustment for RT, the risk associated with alkylating agents increases further with cumulative drug exposure.[159] Another modifier of risk includes young age at diagnosis

<table>
<tr><td>**TABLE 43.7**</td><td>Factors Contributing to Second Primary Cancer of Bone After Childhood Malignancy</td></tr>
</table>

Radiation treatment
(Alkylating) Chemotherapy
Genetic predisposition, e.g., retinoblastoma
Age at time of radiation exposure
Gender
Environmental

(treatment) of retinoblastoma.[160–162] Female gender was associated with an increased risk of second cancer, in a cohort of childhood Hodgkin disease survivors.[163]

These studies demonstrate that the risk of second primary bone tumors among survivors of childhood cancer is increased compared to the GP, although the absolute risk may not be very high, except among certain specific tumor types (e.g., retinoblastoma). The risk is associated with the use of RT and (alkylating) chemotherapy agents. Generally, the factors contributing to second primary bone cancers following childhood malignancy can be summarized as shown (see Table 43.7). This provides a rationale for active surveillance as well as studies focusing on modification of therapeutic protocols in certain high-risk groups.

As evident in Table 43.8 and Figure 43.8, with increasing dose, there was an increasing RR for (bone) sarcoma with relatively low RRs up to 10 to 30 Gy and considerable increase in RR for doses of 50 Gy and over. In two series, the RR decreased for doses higher than 50 Gy,[158,159] but in the other two[144,160] the RR showed an increase over the total dose range analyzed, including doses over 60 Gy. The observed decrease in RR for the highest doses analyzed may be explained by the fact that at these dose levels the balance between radiation-related cancer induction and cell death may have been shifted toward increased cell death rather than cancer induction. In a combined analysis of published reports on 109 radiation-induced osteosarcomas,[138] it appeared that 35% of these occurred in cases with radiation doses of <45 Gy, indicating that doses considered to be relatively low may contribute to a large proportion of RIS.

Clinical Aspects of Radiation-Induced Bone Cancer

There are two peaks in distribution of the age of development of the RIS. One exists in the second decade of life and the

<table>
<tr><td>**TABLE 43.8**</td><td colspan="11">RR for Radiation-Induced Sarcoma in Survivors of Childhood Cancer, by Radiation Dose Compared to Patients not Treated with RT</td></tr>
<tr><td>*First Author and Reference*</td><td>*First Cancer*</td><td>*Second Cancer, Sarcoma*</td><td colspan="8">*Dose Intervals (Gy)*</td><td>*RR Adjusted for Chemo*</td><td>*Model*</td></tr>
<tr><td></td><td></td><td></td><td>0</td><td><5</td><td><10</td><td>10–30</td><td>30–40
RR</td><td>30–50</td><td>30/40–60</td><td>>50 or 60 Gy</td><td></td><td></td></tr>
<tr><td>Tucker[144]</td><td>All</td><td>Bone</td><td>1</td><td>0.6</td><td>6</td><td>16.9</td><td></td><td>21.2</td><td>38.3</td><td></td><td>Yes</td><td></td></tr>
<tr><td>Hawkins[159]</td><td>All</td><td>Bone</td><td>1</td><td>0.7</td><td>12.4</td><td></td><td>93.8</td><td></td><td>64.7</td><td></td><td>Yes</td><td>Linear trend</td></tr>
<tr><td>Le Vu[158]</td><td>All</td><td>Bone</td><td>1</td><td>7.8</td><td>24.2</td><td></td><td>183.7</td><td></td><td>48.4</td><td></td><td>Yes</td><td>Linear trend</td></tr>
<tr><td>Wong[160]</td><td>Retinoblastoma</td><td>Soft tissue and bone</td><td>1</td><td>1.9</td><td>3.7</td><td></td><td></td><td>4.5</td><td>10.7</td><td></td><td></td><td></td></tr>
</table>

Last column provides information on the model used to describe the dose-response relation.

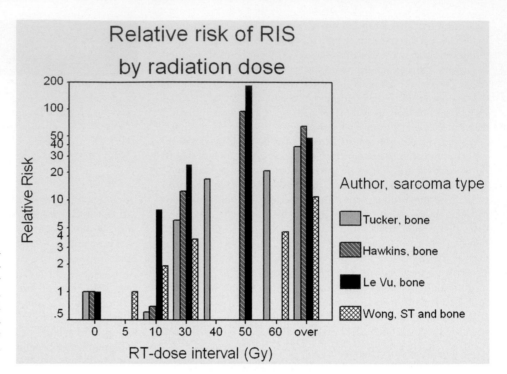

Figure 43.8. The RR for the development of radiation-induced sarcoma following the treatment of childhood cancer is radiation-dose dependent. Data derived from Tucker,[144] Le Vu,[158] Hawkins,[159] and Wong.[160] The bars represent the RR for a given dose interval as indicated in Table 43.8. The RR on the *Y*-axis is depicted on a logarithmic scale.

other is in the age group over 50 years, the former comprising patients treated for childhood cancer (Fig. 43.9) and the latter are survivors of solid tumors in adulthood.[164] It has been suggested that higher radiation doses are associated with shorter latency periods,[165] although this has not been confirmed in all studies.[137,138] The latency period appears shorter for patients with bilateral compared to unilateral retinoblastoma (69.5 vs. 135 mo, $p = 0.04$).[138] Additional contradictory information concerns the use of anthracyclins, which are associated with a shortened latent period in one report[166] but not in another.[167]

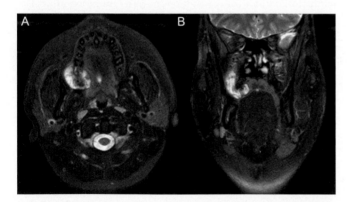

Figure 43.9. Axial (**A**) and coronal (**B**) T2-weighted MRI scan of 23-year-old male who presented with a mass involving the right maxillary and retromolar trigone region. The patient was treated at the age of 2 for acute lymphatic leukemia by chemotherapy (vincristine, methotrexate, and prednisone) and cranial irradiation to a dose of 18 Gy in ten fractions. The large mass extends onto the soft palate, into the posterior right buccal space onto the right lateral pterygoid muscle and into the infratemporal pterygoid region. An initial biopsy suggested a chondrosarcoma. Due to rapid progression, it was decided to proceed with surgical resection. Final pathology after maxillectomy revealed the diagnosis of a radiation-induced chondroblastic osteosarcoma and he subsequently received adjuvant chemotherapy (methotrexate, cisplatin, and doxorubicin).

The most common anatomic sites for radiation-induced bone cancer are the head/neck, trunk/chest, and the pelvis (Fig. 43.10). This is consistent with the location of the preceding cancers both in childhood and adult cancer survivors.[168] In women, RIS usually occur around the shoulder and pelvis because of the frequent use of radiotherapy for breast and gynecologic cancers and the expected long-term survival of these patients.

Usually, a RIS of bone occurs within or in the periphery of the radiation field.[144] Histologically, osteosarcoma accounts for the majority of RIS in most series, with percentages ranging from 49% to 85% of cases.[144,164,166,168–173]

Optimal treatment of localized RIS of bone is similar to the treatment of bone sarcomas that are not radiation-related. Historically, secondary bone sarcoma has been characterized by a very poor prognosis with 5 year survival rates of <30%.[165,174] In part these series overrepresented advanced stage disease, often in poorly accessible (central) locations that were not readily amenable to surgery.[175] More recent studies have demonstrated improved outcome in suitable patients selected for optimal therapy including modern chemotherapy and surgery. Contemporary series that apply these principles report 5-year survival rates following treatment for RIS of 41% to 68%,[138,169,176] as compared to patients treated by surgery only (50%) or chemotherapy only (17%).

TREATMENT OF RADIATION INJURY TO BONE

MEDICAL TREATMENT

Osteoradionecrosis

Pentoxifylline is a methylxanthine derivative that has hemorrheologic and vasodilatory effects; it also lowers blood viscosity, improves erythrocyte flexibility, inhibits proliferation of

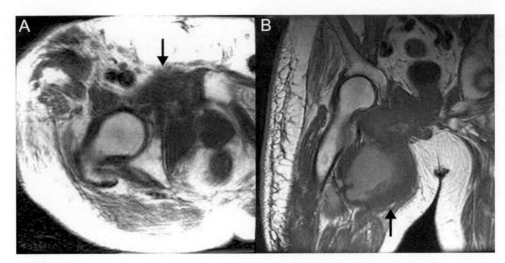

Figure 43.10. **A**: Axial T1-weighted MRI scan of right hip and pelvis in 74-year-old man with history of radiation for prostate cancer. There is marrow replacement in the superior pubic ramus and a large soft-tissue mass (*arrow*). **B**: Coronal T1 weighted MRI of right hip with radiation associated bone sarcoma of the anterior pelvis. There is a large soft-tissue mass in the adductor compartment (*arrow*). Histology showed an osteosarcoma. The interval between the osteosarcoma and previous radiation was 3 years.

human dermal fibroblasts, and increases tissue oxygen levels and appeared to improve outcome in soft-tissue necrosis resulting from radiotherapy.[177] It also appeared to ameliorate the clinical situation in a case report of radiation-induced pelvic fractures.[178]

Delanian and Lefaix[110] developed a protocol for the treatment of ORN combining pentoxifylline with tocopherol and the bisphosphonate clodronate. The rationale for this combined approach is that tocopherol (vitamin E) scavenges the reactive oxygen species and contributes to the reduction of fibrosis. Clodronate is a new-generation bisphosphonate that inhibits bone resorption by reducing the number and activity of osteoclasts.[179] Improvement in a small cohort has been reported,[180] but randomized trial data are needed to draw firm conclusions about the value of this treatment.

Growth Impairment

Administration of exogenous growth hormone (GH) to patients with established growth disturbances following cranial radiation treatment[181] or TBI[133,182–184] has been applied in order to treat radiation-induced growth delay. It has been used in the setting of documented GH deficiency or in case of impaired growth, without GH deficiency. In multiple regression analysis, GH treatment appeared to result in a significant increase in final height in children undergoing bone marrow transplantation prior to the age of 10 years, whereas no significant effect of GH therapy was found in childhood bone marrow transplantation recipients after the age of 10 years.[184]

GH administration also appeared to have a positive effect on height even in the absence of GH deficiency. Although GH appears to be able to decrease the height loss induced by radiation, ultimate growth recovery remains incomplete compared to normal values.[181]

Administration of GH has also been studied in the management of craniofacial growth reduction following TBI with GH starting at a mean age of 12 years for a mean duration of 3.6 years. It appeared that GH only had minor effects on cranial base dimensions, probably due to the fact that growth in this area is complete at a relative early age.[182] However, the effects of GH on mandibular dimensions were considerable with values equivalent or sometimes exceeding those of controls. Others have also confirmed this differential effect of GH on the craniofacial skeleton in patients with idiopathic GH deficiency.[185]

HYPERBARIC OXYGEN THERAPY

Hyperbaric oxygen (HBO) has enjoyed a tradition of wide usage in the treatment of ORN of the mandible based on the theoretical premise that persistent hypoxia is a major factor in propagating this chronic nonhealing wound and that HBO encourages angiogenesis, fibroblast proliferation, and collagen synthesis.[41] Marx et al.[186] compared HBO with penicillin alone following dental extraction and found a lower incidence of ORN in the HBO arm of this randomized trial. However, numerous subsequent studies of careful application of dental extraction and radiotherapy principles have shown the risk to be extremely low in the absence of HBO.[41] Despite this, the use of HBO for the management of established ORN became generally accepted, presumably because of the severe nature of the complication and the wish to address it by all means possible. Nevertheless, an undercurrent of concern existed that this expensive modality may not be as effective as hoped. For example, surgical treatment with removal of devitalized bone and grafting seems to be more important than HBO and, moreover, there seemed to be a contrary view about whether HBO had value beyond the results of surgery itself.[187,188] Suspicion also existed that it may even contribute to complications.[189] In this milieu of controversy, investigators in France conducted a randomized placebo-controlled double-blind trial for patients with established ORN but excluding fracture or bone reabsorption to the lower mandibular border. The trial was stopped early because of lack of benefit of HBO in preventing progression, relieving pain, or inducing recovery.[190] It also appeared that those treated with HBO actually had a less favorable outcome than the patients treated with placebo. The study was also complicated by a crossover design for some patients who progressed to requiring surgery, and some were stratified at the outset according to whether they needed surgery or not. For these reasons, the primary value of HBO as normally applied as an adjunct to surgery is blurred. Additional methodological issues have also been discussed.[191] It is also generally recognized that the study reported by Annane and colleagues has problems of wide applicability since it excluded severe ORN cases where HBO is most often used. Not surprisingly with this state of the evidence, a Cochrane Collaboration review was unable to provide strong supportive evidence for the use of HBO though there seemed to be a signal of effect, including reduction of ORN following dental extracton.[192] The authors also contacted the author of the French study to confirm the conclusion that the findings of their study could not be used to decide optimal treatment for severe forms of mandibular ORN. The eventual conclusion was that the application of HBO to selected patients and tissues may still be justified.[192]

HBO has also been used in the treatment of ORN in sites other than the mandible. No randomized data are available and studies consist of case reports or small retrospective series.

Interpretation is more complex due to the frequent use of additional interventions such as antibiotics and surgery (e.g., debridement and sequestrectomy). The sites mainly include other head-and-neck sites such as the external auditory canal, temporal/mastoid bone, facial bones or skull.[122,193-196] Other sites in which ORN was treated with HBO include chest wall [197,198] and pelvis.[194,199]

SURGICAL TREATMENT

Procedures to Treat Fractures

By far the greatest proportion of radiation associated fractures occur in the weight-bearing bones of the pelvis and lower extremity. Understandably, fractures of the pelvis usually relate to treatment of genitourinary, colorectal, and gynecological cancers,[69] whereas fractures of the femur and tibia are generally seen in association with combined radiation and surgical resection of extremity sarcomas. Vascular compromise, including periosteal stripping and vascular ligation that may accompany sarcoma resections, may render the bone avascular and impair bone healing.[200-202] Prophylactic intramedullary nailing at the time of a sarcoma resection in susceptible patients may be considered, but this may not be cost effective, may lead to other complications, and does not always guarantee that fractures will not develop.

The rare radiation-associated fracture in the non–weight-bearing bones of the upper extremity and nonarticular fractures of the pelvis can often be managed nonoperatively. Painful nonunions, displaced intra-articular fractures, and fractures in weight-bearing bones (especially in the lower extremity), almost always require surgical management to restore function and ambulation. Internal fixation with plates or arthroplasty components is augmented with cement injected into osteoporotic bone to provide initial maximal better stability and fixation and does not rely on bone ingrowth into a prosthesis, which is deficient in irradiated bone. Conventional surgical fixation, such as insertion of an intramedullary nail, requires augmentation with autologous iliac crest bone grafting to provide an osteoinductive stimulus. Selected patients with recalcitrant femoral diaphysis nonunion fractures may benefit from vasularized fibular grafting if they can tolerate the procedure

(e.g., patients without peripheral vascular disease).[203] Selected fractures of the femoral shaft may also be managed with resection and a cemented intercalary prosthesis that may permit early weightbearing and thereby quickly restore independence for these patients. These principles also apply to the management of proximal femoral fractures. Prosthetic insertion can provide immediate weight bearing especially where prior attempts with plate fixation have been unsuccessful (see Fig. 43.3).

Procedures to Treat Growth Deformities

Growth disturbance of an irradiated limb occurs due to radiation-induced injury to the growth plate. Although the best treatment is always avoidance, should irradiation of an immature epiphyseal plate be necessary, it is preferable to treat the entire growth plate to avoid continued growth of the remaining unirradiated growth plate with consequent angular deformity.[3] The latter is more difficult to correct surgically than a discrepancy in extremity length. Treatment of symmetrical altered growth due to irradiation of the physis depends on the bone affected and the anticipated discrepancy at skeletal maturity. To a large extent, the anticipated discrepancy depends on the age of the child. The younger the child at the time of radiation physeal injury, the greater the impact on the growth of the extremity and the larger the expected discrepancy. Growth arrest in upper extremity bones is more readily tolerated compared to the lower extremity.

Significant alterations in leg lengths can lead to pelvic obliquity, hip dysplasia, and degenerative disease of the lumbar spine.[204] For this reason, it is important to accurately anticipate the expected leg length discrepancy at skeletal maturity. Older children, and especially teenagers, generally tolerate this disability and no treatment is needed. If the patient is symptomatic, shoe lifts are usually prescribed for a small discrepancy.[204] For large differences (e.g., 2 and 6 cm), an epiphysiodesis of the contralateral unaffected physis is often undertaken to ensure that leg lengths that are close to equal. Any minor discrepancies can be overcome with shoe lifts.

In a very young child, the differences may be very severe and are usually overcome with a combination of surgical lengthening of the affected bone and shortening of the contralateral unaffected bone.[204] In a lengthening procedure, an external fixator device is applied with fixation through the proximal and distal aspects of the affected femur or tibia. The bone is then osteotomized in the middle and over the next several weeks, the external fixator is lengthened by the patient by approximately 1 to 1.5 mm each day.[205] In this way, the periosteum, which remains intact, becomes stretched out and lays down new bone, called the "regenerate." When the desired amount of lengthening is obtained, the procedure is stopped, but the external fixator remains in place for several more weeks while the regenerate matures. For anticipated leg length discrepancies of >20 cm, a severely deformed and dysfunctional leg is usually the result and is probably best addressed by extremity amputation and early prosthetic fitting.[206] Very young children, in whom this significant discrepancy is expected, usually adapt well to prosthetic rehabilitation.

Procedures to Treat Osteoradionecrosis of the Mandible

Advanced symptomatic cases of mandibular ORN that remain refractory to conservative measures will usually require relatively radical surgery ordinarily reserved for the patient who is fit and cancer-free. Generally, wide resection of necrotic bone with immediate free flap reconstruction is the best option for treatment of advanced ORN. The fundamental goal is removal of all devitalized bone including complete sequestrectomy and replacement with healthy vascularized tissue pedicled outside the radiotherapy volume. Generally, HBO is employed bearing in mind the caveats discussed earlier regarding the available evidence for this modality (section 7.2).

STRATEGIES TO AVOID RADIATION INJURY TO BONE

RADIATION TECHNIQUES

Avoiding the late effects of radiation on bone can be accomplished by reducing the dose of radiation delivered to bone. In the event that the bone in itself is not a designated target structure of the radiation treatment, this can be accomplished through the use of conformal or intensity modulated RT (IMRT) to avoid application of extraneous high radiation doses on bone. The beneficial use of IMRT in reducing radiation dose exposure of bone was described earlier for mandibular ORN prevention [42,43] and likely also applies to several other situations, including the pelvis,[207,208] and soft-tissue sarcoma.[209]

In pediatric oncology, radiation to growing bone results in the development of skeletal deformation (e.g., asymmetry, scoliosis) due to locally impaired bone growth. To prevent this, standard radiation techniques achieving uniform radiation doses and avoiding steep dose gradients over growing bone are sometimes chosen over IMRT. An example of this is the inclusion of the whole vertebral column within the radiation portals in case of treatment for a paraspinal neuroblastoma or intra-abdominal tumors of childhood.[131] However, the potential benefits of this must be weighed against the increased radiation exposure of other organs, for example, the kidneys.

Other ways to avoid radiation-induced bone damage include reducing the dose per fraction, as discussed earlier in the reduction of pathological fracture incidence due to radiation in children treated for Ewing sarcoma.[77] Recently, it has been suggested that the use of protons instead of photon may result in a decreased risk second cancers after radiation treatment in adults,[210] especially when using a scanning beam instead of a scattering foil.[211] However, clinical data are very limited and final conclusions on this topic cannot be made yet.

CYTOPROTECTIVE AGENTS

The cytoprotective drug Amifostine has been studied as a potential agent to protect bone and conserve bone growth after radiation.[212] In an animal model, Damron et al. showed that treatment with amifostine before fractionated radiation treatment resulted in a dose-dependent decrease in longitudinal bone growth loss when compared to radiation alone.[213,214] Bone mineral density (BMD) analysis and histological examination of irradiated bone revealed that amifostine treatment increased the BMD[215] and increased the number of surviving osteogenic cells.[216]

In addition to preservation of longitudinal bone growth, the protective effects of amifostine have also been studied in the context of radiation-induced craniofacial growth impairment, again in an animal model.[217,218] However, no useful clinical data are available yet regarding the radioprotective effects of amifostine on bone.[219]

CONCLUSION

Although typically considered calcified and inert, the osseous skeleton is one of the most active and important organ systems. It is also one of the largest and therefore is exposed to the effects of radiotherapy in all anatomic regions and for any indication. The skeleton is also critical to maintaining activities independently and efficiently and has substantial impact on external appearance and body habitus. Therefore, damage to bone is detrimental to numerous domains spanning the physiological, the physical, and the psychological. This is especially so if bone injury results in deformity, mechanical instability of important anatomic structure, or pain. Most devastating is the potential for malignant tumor induction. All may manifest many years following radiation exposure. As discussed earlier, the occurrence of these problems is often multifactorial and may be profoundly influenced by host factors. Sadly, the latter is most evident in the circumstances surrounding the treatment of young children who are at greatest risk due to ongoing skeletal development and their expected long prognosis. However, no group is safe from these effects. Minimization of damage must commence with careful consideration of the indications for radiotherapy in different settings and particularly taking account of host vulnerabilities. Biological and anatomic issues must be considered and the interplay between dose, fractionation, volume to be irradiated, and the use of other treatments understood. A careful approach that addresses these issues should be able to mitigate the risk of adverse outcome in the future.

REFERENCES

1. Sommerfeldt DW, Rubin CT. Biology of bone and how it orchestrates the form and function of the skeleton. *Eur Spine J.* 2001;10(suppl 2):S86–S95.
2. Fujikawa Y, Quinn JM, Sabokbar A, et al. The human osteoclast precursor circulates in the monocyte fraction. *Endocrinology.* 1996;137(9):4058–4060.
3. Bluemke DA, Fishman EK, Scott WW Jr. Skeletal complications of radiation therapy. *Radiographics.* 1994;14(1):111–121.
4. Eifel PJ, Donaldson SS, Thomas PR. Response of growing bone to irradiation: a proposed late effects scoring system. *Int J Radiat Oncol Biol Phys.* 30 1995;31(5):1301–1307.
5. Williams HJ, Davies AM. The effect of X-rays on bone: a pictorial review. *Eur Radiol.* 2006;16(3):619–633.
6. Schecter N, Lewis V. The bone. In: Cox J, Ang K, eds. *Radiation Oncology—Rationale Techniques Results.* 8th ed. St. Louis, MO: Mosby, 2003:857–883.
7. Dawson WB. Growth impairment following radiotherapy in childhood. *Clin Radiol.* 1968;19(3):241–256.
8. Hopewell JW. Radiation-therapy effects on bone density. *Med Pediatr Oncol.* 2003;41(3):208–211.
9. Pitkanen MA, Hopewell JW. Functional changes in the vascularity of the irradiated rat femur. Implications for late effects. *Acta Radiol Oncol.* 1983;22(3):253–256.
10. Lehner B, Bauer J, Rodel F, et al. Radiation-induced impairment of osseous healing with vascularized bone transfer: experimental model using a pedicled tibia flap in rat. *Int J Oral Maxillofac Surg.* 2004;33(5):486–492.
11. Ahmad M, Sampair C, Nazmul-Hossain AN, et al. Therapeutic doses of radiation alter proliferation and attachment of osteoblasts to implant surfaces. *J Biomed Mater Res A.* 2008;86(4):926–934.
12. Paulino AC, Wen BC, Brown CK, et al. Late effects in children treated with radiation therapy for Wilms' tumor. *Int J Radiat Oncol Biol Phys.* 2000;46(5):1239–1246.
13. Probert JC, Parker BR. The effects of radiation therapy on bone growth. *Radiology.* Jan 1975;114(1):155–162.
14. Sonis AL, Tarbell N, Valachovic RW. Dentofacial development in long-term survivors of acute lymphoblastic leukemia. A comparison of three treatment modalities. *Cancer.* 1990;66(12):2645–2652.
15. Willman KY, Cox RS, Donaldson SS. Radiation induced height impairment in pediatric Hodgkin's disease. *Int J Radiat Oncol Biol Phys.* 1994;28(1):85–92.
16. Dahllof G, Forsberg CM, Ringden O, et al. Facial growth and morphology in long-term survivors after bone marrow transplantation. *Eur J Orthod.* 1989;11(4):332–340.

17. Noorda EM, Somers R, van Leeuwen FE, et al. Adult height and age at menarche in childhood cancer survivors. *Eur J Cancer.* 2001;37(5):605–612.
18. Olshan JS, Gubernick J, Packer RJ, et al. The effects of adjuvant chemotherapy on growth in children with medulloblastoma. *Cancer.* 1992;70(7):2013–2017.
19. Wallace WH, Shalet SM. Chemotherapy with actinomycin D influences the growth of the spine following abdominal irradiation. *Med Pediatr Oncol.* 1992;20(2):177.
20. Waitzman AA, Posnick JC, Armstrong DC, et al. Craniofacial skeletal measurements based on computed tomography: part II. Normal values and growth trends. *Cleft Palate Craniofac J.* 1992;29(2):118–128.
21. Dahllof G. Craniofacial growth in children treated for malignant diseases. *Acta Odontol Scand.* 1998;56(6):378–382.
22. Pertschuk MJ, Whitaker LA. Psychosocial adjustment and craniofacial malformations in childhood. *Plast Reconstr Surg.* 1985;75(2):177–184.
23. Pertschuk MJ, Whitaker LA. Psychosocial outcome of craniofacial surgery in children. *Plast Reconstr Surg.* 1988;82(5):741–746.
24. Pope AW, Snyder HT. Psychosocial adjustment in children and adolescents with a craniofacial anomaly: age and sex patterns. *Cleft Palate Craniofac J.* 2005;42(4):349–354.
25. Estilo CL, Huryn JM, Kraus DH, et al. Effects of therapy on dentofacial development in long-term survivors of head and neck rhabdomyosarcoma: the Memorial Sloan-Kettering Cancer Center experience. *J Pediatr Hematol Oncol.* 2003;25(3):215–222.
26. Guyuron B, Dagys AP, Munro IR, et al. Effect of irradiation on facial growth: a 7- to 25-year follow-up. *Ann Plast Surg.* 1983;11(5):423–427.
27. Jaffe N, Toth BB, Hoar RE, et al. Dental and maxillofacial abnormalities in long-term survivors of childhood cancer: effects of treatment with chemotherapy and radiation to the head and neck. *Pediatrics.* 1984;73(6):816–823.
28. Hogeboom CJ, Grosser SC, Guthrie KA, et al. Stature loss following treatment for Wilms tumor. *Med Pediatr Oncol.* 2001;36(2):295–304.
29. Riseborough EJ, Grabias SL, Burton RI, et al. Skeletal alterations following irradiation for Wilms' tumor: with particular reference to scoliosis and kyphosis. *J Bone Joint Surg Am.* 1976;58(4):526–536.
30. Willich E, Kuttig H, Pfeil G, et al. Vertebral changes after irradiation for Wilms' tumor in early childhood. A retrospective interdisciplinary long-term study of 82 children. *Strahlenther Onkol.* 1990;166(12):815–821.
31. Anderson M, Green WT, Messner MB. Growth and predictions of growth in the lower extremities. *J Bone Joint Surg Am.* 1963;45-A:1–14.
32. Gonzalez DG, Breur K. Clinical data from irradiated growing long bones in children. *Int J Radiat Oncol Biol Phys.* Jun 1983;9(6):841–846.
33. Paulino AC. Late effects of radiotherapy for pediatric extremity sarcomas. *Int J Radiat Oncol Biol Phys.* 2004;60(1):265–274.
34. Chapman JA, Deakin DP, Green JH. Slipped upper femoral epiphysis after radiotherapy. *J Bone Joint Surg Br.* 1980;62(3):337–339.
35. Fletcher BD, Crom DB, Krance RA, et al. Radiation-induced bone abnormalities after bone marrow transplantation for childhood leukemia. *Radiology.* 1994;191(1):231–235.
36. Liu SC, Tsai CC, Huang CH. Atypical slipped capital femoral epiphysis after radiotherapy and chemotherapy. *Clin Orthop Relat Res.* 2004(426):212–218.
37. Silverman CL, Thomas PR, McAlister WH, et al. Slipped femoral capital epiphyses in irradiated children: dose, volume and age relationships. *Int J Radiat Oncol Biol Phys.* 1981;7(10):1357–1363.
38. Wolf EL, Berdon WE, Cassady JR, et al. Slipped femoral capital epiphysis as a sequela to childhood irradiation for malignant tumors. *Radiology.* 1977;125(3):781–784.
39. Howland WJ, Loeffler RK, Starchman DE, et al. Postirradiation atrophic changes of bone and related complications. *Radiology.* 1975;117(3 pt 1):677–685.
40. Paling MR, Herdt JR. Radiation osteitis: a problem of recognition. *Radiology.* 1980;137(2):339–342.
41. Lyons A, Ghazali N. Osteoradionecrosis of the jaws: current understanding of its pathophysiology and treatment. *Br J Oral Maxillofac Surg.* 2008;46(8):653–660.
42. Ben-David MA, Diamante M, Radawski JD, et al. Lack of osteoradionecrosis of the mandible after intensity-modulated radiotherapy for head and neck cancer: likely contributions of both dental care and improved dose distributions. *Int J Radiat Oncol Biol Phys.* 2007;68(2):396–402.
43. Studer G, Studer SP, Zwahlen RA, et al. Osteoradionecrosis of the mandible: minimized risk profile following intensity-modulated radiation therapy (IMRT). *Strahlenther Onkol.* 2006;182(5):283–288.
44. Prosnitz LR, Lawson JP, Friedlaender GE, et al. Avascular necrosis of bone in Hodgkin's disease patients treated with combined modality therapy. *Cancer.* 1981;47(12):2793–2797.
45. Libshitz HI, Edeiken BS. Radiotherapy changes of the pediatric hip. *Am J Roentgenol.* 1981;137(3):585–588.
46. Dalinka MK, Mazzeo VP Jr. Complications of radiation therapy. *Crit Rev Diagn Imaging.* 1985;23(3):235–267.
47. Hanif I, Mahmoud H, Pui CH. Avascular femoral head necrosis in pediatric cancer patients. *Med Pediatr Oncol.* 1993;21(9):655–660.
48. Cooper JS, Fu K, Marks J, et al. Late effects of radiation therapy in the head and neck region. *Int J Radiat Oncol Biol Phys.* 1995;31(5):1141–1164.
49. Syed MI, Clark LJ, Adams C. Life threatening hemorrhage from osteoradionecrosis of the ribs and clavicle. *Laryngoscope.* 2007;117(9):1594–1595.
50. Blijham GH, Vermeulen A, Mendes de Leon DE. Osteonecrosis of sternum and rib in a patient treated for Hodgkin's disease. *Cancer.* 1985;56(9):2292–2294.
51. Sato Y, Uematsu H, Yoshida M, et al. Osteonecrosis induced by intraoperative radiotherapy for pancreatic cancer. *Eur Radiol.* 2006;16(1):242–243.
52. Micha JP, Goldstein BH, Rettenmaier MA, et al. Pelvic radiation necrosis and osteomyelitis following chemoradiation for advanced stage vulvar and cervical carcinoma. *Gynecol Oncol.* 2006;101(2):349–352.
53. De Crevoisier R, Bourhis J, Domenge C, et al. Full-dose reirradiation for unresectable head and neck carcinoma: experience at the Gustave-Roussy Institute in a series of 169 patients. *J Clin Oncol.* 1998;16(11):3556–3562.
54. Kasperts N, Slotman B, Leemans CR, et al. A review on re-irradiation for recurrent and second primary head and neck cancer. *Oral Oncol.* 2005;41(3):225–243.
55. Holt GE, Griffin AM, Pintilie M, et al. Fractures following radiotherapy and limb-salvage surgery for lower extremity soft-tissue sarcomas. A comparison of high-dose and low-dose radiotherapy. *J Bone Joint Surg Am.* 2005;87(2):315–319.
56. Lin PP, Schupak KD, Boland PJ, et al. Pathologic femoral fracture after periosteal excision and radiation for the treatment of soft tissue sarcoma. *Cancer.* 1998;82(12):2356–2365.
57. Cannon CP, Ballo MT, Zagars GK, et al. Complications of combined modality treatment of primary lower extremity soft-tissue sarcomas. *Cancer.* 2006;107(10):2455–2461.
58. Helmstedter CS, Goebel M, Zlotecki R. Pathologic fractures after surgery and radiation for soft tissue tumors. *Clin Orthop Relat Res.* 2001(389):165–172.
59. Keus RB, Rutgers EJ, Ho GH, et al. Limb-sparing therapy of extremity soft tissue sarcomas: treatment outcome and long-term functional results. *Eur J Cancer.* 1994;30A(10):1459–1463.
60. Lin PP, Boland PJ, Healey JH. Treatment of femoral fractures after irradiation. *Clin Orthop Relat Res.* 1998(352):168–178.
61. Livi L, Santoni R, Paiar F, et al. Late treatment-related complications in 214 patients with extremity soft-tissue sarcoma treated by surgery and postoperative radiation therapy. *Am J Surg.* 2006;191(2):230–234.
62. Emami B, Lyman J, Brown A, et al. Tolerance of normal tissue to therapeutic irradiation. *Int J Radiat Oncol Biol Phys.* 15 1991;21(1):109–122.
63. Gortzak Y, Lockwood GA, Mahendra A, et al. Prediction of pathologic fracture risk of the femur after combined modality treatment of soft tissue sarcoma of the thigh. *Cancer.* 2010;116(6):1553–1559.
64. Dickie CI, Parent AL, Griffin AM, et al. Bone fractures following external beam radiotherapy and limb-preservation surgery for lower extremity soft tissue sarcoma: relationship to irradiated bone length, volume, tumor location and dose. *Int J Radiat Oncol Biol Phys.* 2009;75(4):1119–1124.
65. Kowalski MJ, Schemitsch EH, Kregor PJ, et al. Effect of periosteal stripping on cortical bone perfusion: a laser doppler study in sheep. *Calcif Tissue Int.* 1996;59(1):24–26.
66. Whiteside LA, Ogata K, Lesker P, et al. The acute effects of periosteal stripping and medullary reaming on regional bone blood flow. *Clin Orthop Relat Res.* 1978(131):266–272.
67. Buckwalter JA, Cooper RR. Bone structure and function. *Instr Course Lect.* 1987;36:27–48.
68. Bell RS, O'Sullivan B, Nguyen C, et al. Fractures following limb-salvage surgery and adjuvant irradiation for soft-tissue sarcoma. *Clin Orthop Relat Res.* 1991(271):265–271.
69. Baxter NN, Habermann EB, Tepper JE, et al. Risk of pelvic fractures in older women following pelvic irradiation. *JAMA.* 2005;294(20):2587–2593.
70. Holm T, Singnomklao T, Rutqvist LE, et al. Adjuvant preoperative radiotherapy in patients with rectal carcinoma. Adverse effects during long term follow-up of two randomized trials. *Cancer.* 1996;78(5):968–976.
71. Grigsby PW, Roberts HL, Perez CA. Femoral neck fracture following groin irradiation. *Int J Radiat Oncol Biol Phys.* 1995;32(1):63–67.
72. Gospodarowicz M. Testicular cancer patients: considerations in long-term follow-up. *Hematol Oncol Clin North Am.* 2008;22(2):245–255, vi.
73. Hodgson DC, Hudson MM, Constine LS. Pediatric Hodgkin lymphoma: maximizing efficacy and minimizing toxicity. *Semin Radiat Oncol.* 2007;17(3):230–242.
74. Noordijk EM, Carde P, Dupouy N, et al. Combined-modality therapy for clinical stage I or II Hodgkin's lymphoma: long-term results of the European Organisation for Research and Treatment of Cancer H7 randomized controlled trials. *J Clin Oncol.* 2006;24(19):3128–3135.
75. Wall JE, Kaste SC, Greenwald CA, et al. Fractures in children treated with radiotherapy for soft tissue sarcoma. *Orthopedics.* 1996;19(8):657–664.
76. Wagner LM, Neel MD, Pappo AS, et al. Fractures in pediatric Ewing sarcoma. *J Pediatr Hematol Oncol.* 2001;23(9):568–571.
77. Bolek TW, Marcus RB Jr, Mendenhall NP, et al. Local control and functional results after twice-daily radiotherapy for Ewing's sarcoma of the extremities. *Int J Radiat Oncol Biol Phys.* 1996;35(4):687–692.
78. Indelicato DJ, Keole SR, Shahlaee AH, et al. Definitive radiotherapy for Ewing tumors of extremities and pelvis: long-term disease control, limb function, and treatment toxicity. *Int J Radiat Oncol Biol Phys.* 2008;72(3):871–877.
79. Cooper KL, Beabout JW, Swee RG. Insufficiency fractures of the sacrum. *Radiology.* 1985;156(1):15–20.
80. Abe H, Nakamura M, Takahashi S, et al. Radiation-induced insufficiency fractures of the pelvis: evaluation with 99mTc-methylene diphosphonate scintigraphy. *Am J Roentgenol.* 1992;158(3):599–602.
81. Ikushima H, Osaki K, Furutani S, et al. Pelvic bone complications following radiation therapy of gynecologic malignancies: clinical evaluation of radiation-induced pelvic insufficiency fractures. *Gynecol Oncol.* 2006;103(3):1100–1104.
82. Oh D, Huh SJ, Nam H, et al. Pelvic insufficiency fracture after pelvic radiotherapy for cervical cancer: analysis of risk factors. *Int J Radiat Oncol Biol Phys.* 2008;70(4):1183–1188.
83. Huh SJ, Kim B, Kang MK, et al. Pelvic insufficiency fracture after pelvic irradiation in uterine cervix cancer. *Gynecol Oncol.* 2002;86(3):264–268.
84. Konski A, Sowers M. Pelvic fractures following irradiation for endometrial carcinoma. *Int J Radiat Oncol Biol Phys.* 1996;35(2):361–367.
85. Tai P, Hammond A, Dyk JV, et al. Pelvic fractures following irradiation of endometrial and vaginal cancers-a case series and review of literature. *Radiother Oncol.* 2000;56(1):23–28.
86. Ogino I, Okamoto N, Ono Y, et al. Pelvic insufficiency fractures in postmenopausal woman with advanced cervical cancer treated by radiotherapy. *Radiother Oncol.* 2003;68(1):61–67.
87. Blomlie V, Rofstad EK, Talle K, et al. Incidence of radiation-induced insufficiency fractures of the female pelvis: evaluation with MR imaging. *Am J Roentgenol.* 1996;167(5):1205–1210.
88. Moreno A, Clemente J, Crespo C, et al. Pelvic insufficiency fractures in patients with pelvic irradiation. *Int J Radiat Oncol Biol Phys.* 1999;44(1):61–66.
89. Shimanovskaya K, Shiman AD. *Radiation Injury of Bone.* New York, NY: Pergamon Press; 1983.

90. Bliss P, Parsons CA, Blake PR. Incidence and possible aetiological factors in the development of pelvic insufficiency fractures following radical radiotherapy. *Br J Radiol.* 1996;69(822):548–554.

91. Bates TD. A prospective clinical trial of post-operative radiotherapy delivered in three fractions per week versus two fractions per week in breast carcinoma. *Clin Radiol.* 1975;26(3):297–304.

92. Bentzen SM, Agrawal RK, Aird EG, et al. The UK Standardisation of Breast Radiotherapy (START) Trial A of radiotherapy hypofractionation for treatment of early breast cancer: a randomised trial. *Lancet Oncol.* 2008;9(4):331–341.

93. Bentzen SM, Agrawal RK, Aird EG, et al. The UK Standardisation of Breast Radiotherapy (START) Trial B of radiotherapy hypofractionation for treatment of early breast cancer: a randomised trial. *Lancet.* 2008;371(9618):1098–1107.

94. Boyages J, Bosch C, Langlands AO, et al. Breast conservation: long-term Australian data. *Int J Radiat Oncol Biol Phys.* 1992;24(2):253–260.

95. Clarke D, Martinez A, Cox RS. Analysis of cosmetic results and complications in patients with stage I and II breast cancer treated by biopsy and irradiation. *Int J Radiat Oncol Biol Phys.* 1983;9(12):1807–1813.

96. Danoff BF, Pajak TF, Solin LJ, et al. Excisional biopsy, axillary node dissection and definitive radiotherapy for Stages I and II breast cancer. *Int J Radiat Oncol Biol Phys.* 1985;11(3):479–483.

97. Meric F, Buchholz TA, Mirza NQ, et al. Long-term complications associated with breast-conservation surgery and radiotherapy. *Ann Surg Oncol.* 2002;9(6):543–549.

98. Overgaard M. Spontaneous radiation-induced rib fractures in breast cancer patients treated with postmastectomy irradiation. A clinical radiobiological analysis of the influence of fraction size and dose-response relationships on late bone damage. *Acta Oncol.* 1988;27(2):117–122.

99. Pierce SM, Recht A, Lingos TI, et al. Long-term radiation complications following conservative surgery (CS) and radiation therapy (RT) in patients with early stage breast cancer. *Int J Radiat Oncol Biol Phys.* 1992;23(5):915–923.

100. Stotter AT, McNeese MD, Ames FC, et al. Predicting the rate and extent of locoregional failure after breast conservation therapy for early breast cancer. *Cancer.* 1989;64(11):2217–2225.

101. Whelan T, MacKenzie R, Julian J, et al. Randomized trial of breast irradiation schedules after lumpectomy for women with lymph node-negative breast cancer. *J Natl Cancer Inst.* 2002;94(15):1143–1150.

102. Chin LM, Cheng CW, Siddon RL, et al. Three-dimensional photon dose distributions with and without lung corrections for tangential breast intact treatments. *Int J Radiat Oncol Biol Phys.* 1989;17(6):1327–1335.

103. Dragun AE, Aguero EG, Harmon JF, et al. Chest wall dose in MammoSite breast brachytherapy: radiobiologic estimations of late complication risk based on dose-volume considerations. *Brachytherapy.* 2005;4(4):259–263.

104. Vicini F, Beitsch PD, Quiet CA, et al. Three-year analysis of treatment efficacy, cosmesis, and toxicity by the American Society of Breast Surgeons MammoSite Breast Brachytherapy Registry Trial in patients treated with accelerated partial breast irradiation (APBI). *Cancer.* 2008;112(4):758–766.

105. Yoshida K, Nose T, Masuda N, et al. Preliminary result of accelerated partial breast irradiation after breast-conserving surgery. *Breast Cancer.* 2009;16(2):105–112.

106. Leonard C, Carter D, Kercher J, et al. Prospective trial of accelerated partial breast intensity-modulated radiotherapy. *Int J Radiat Oncol Biol Phys.* 2007;67(5):1291–1298.

107. Vicini FA, Chen P, Wallace M, et al. Interim cosmetic results and toxicity using 3D conformal external beam radiotherapy to deliver accelerated partial breast irradiation in patients with early-stage breast cancer treated with breast-conserving therapy. *Int J Radiat Oncol Biol Phys.* 2007;69(4):1124–1130.

108. Formenti SC, Truong MT, Goldberg JD, et al. Prone accelerated partial breast irradiation after breast-conserving surgery: preliminary clinical results and dose-volume histogram analysis. *Int J Radiat Oncol Biol Phys.* 2004;60(2):493–504.

109. Taghian AG, AlmEl-Din M, Smith BL, et al. Interim results of a phase I/II trial of 3D-conformal external beam accelerated partial breast irradiation in patients with early breast cancer. *Int J Radiat Oncol Biol Phys.* 2008;72 (1 suppl 1):S4.

110. Delanian S, Lefaix JL. Complete healing of severe osteoradionecrosis with treatment combining pentoxifylline, tocopherol and clodronate. *Br J Radiol.* 2002;75(893):467–469.

111. Nagata Y, Takayama K, Matsuo Y, et al. Clinical outcomes of a phase I/II study of 48 Gy of stereotactic body radiotherapy in 4 fractions for primary lung cancer using a stereotactic body frame. *Int J Radiat Oncol Biol Phys.* 1 2005;63(5):1427–1431.

112. Timmerman R, Papiez L, McGarry R, et al. Extracranial stereotactic radioablation: results of a phase I study in medically inoperable stage I non-small cell lung cancer. *Chest.* 2003;124(5):1946–1955.

113. Fritz P, Kraus HJ, Blaschke T, et al. Stereotactic, high single-dose irradiation of stage I non-small cell lung cancer (NSCLC) using four-dimensional CT scans for treatment planning. *Lung Cancer.* 2008;60(2):193–199.

114. Onishi H, Araki T, Shirato H, et al. Stereotactic hypofractionated high-dose irradiation for stage I nonsmall cell lung carcinoma: clinical outcomes in 245 subjects in a Japanese multiinstitutional study. *Cancer.* 2004;101(7):1623–1631.

115. Zimmermann FB, Geinitz H, Schill S, et al. Stereotactic hypofractionated radiotherapy in stage I (T1–2 N0 M0) non-small-cell lung cancer (NSCLC). *Acta Oncol.* 2006;45(7):796–801.

116. Voroney JPJ, Hope A, Dahele MR, et al. Pain and rib fracture after stereotactic radiotherapy for peripheral non-small cell lung cancer. *Int J Radiat Oncol Biol Phys.* 2008; 72 suppl 1):S35–S36

117. Dunlap NE, Cai J, Biedermann GB, et al. Chest wall volume receiving >30 Gy predicts risk of severe pain and/or rib fracture after lung stereotactic body radiotherapy. *Int J Radiat Oncol Biol Phys.* 2010;76(3):796–801.

118. Wang EH, Sekyi-Otu A, O'Sullivan B, et al. Management of long-term postirradiation periclavicular complications. *J Surg Oncol.* 1992;51(4):259–265.

119. Pellard S, Moss L, Boyce JM, et al. Diagnostic dilemma of an atraumatic clavicle fracture following radical treatment for laryngeal carcinoma. *J Laryngol Otol.* 2005;119(12):1013–1014.

120. Stofman GM, Lowry LD, Cohn JR, et al. Osteoradionecrosis of the head and neck: a case of a clavicular-tracheal fistula secondary to osteoradionecrosis of the sternoclavicular joint. *Ann Otol Rhinol Laryngol.* 1988;97(5 pt 1):545–549.

121. Donovan DJ, Huynh TV, Purdom EB, et al. Osteoradionecrosis of the cervical spine resulting from radiotherapy for primary head and neck malignancies: operative and nonoperative management. Case report. *J Neurosurg Spine.* 2005;3(2):159–164.

122. Lim AA, Karakla DW, Watkins DV. Osteoradionecrosis of the cervical vertebrae and occipital bone: a case report and brief review of the literature. *Am J Otolaryngol.* 1999;20(6):408–411.

123. Mut M, Schiff D, Miller B, et al. Osteoradionecrosis mimicking metastatic epidural spinal cord compression. *Neurology.* 2005;64(2):396–397.

124. von Rottkay P. Two cases of radiation-induced osteonecroses of the thoracic vertebral bodies after accelerated irradiation of bronchial carcinoma. *Strahlentherapie.* 1985;161(11):704–705.

125. Warscotte L, Duprez T, Lonneux M, et al. Concurrent spinal cord and vertebral bone marrow radionecrosis 8 years after therapeutic irradiation. *Neuroradiology.* 2002;44(3):245–248.

126. Candardjis G. 20-year survival of seminoma after repeated radiation treatment at 200 kV for abdominal metastases of seminoma: renal and vertebral sequelae. *Radiol Clin (Basel).* 1976;45(5):388–391.

127. Cole AR, Darte JM. Osteochondromata following irradiation in children. *Pediatrics.* 1963;32:285–288.

128. Chew FS, Weissleder R. Radiation-induced osteochondroma. *AJR Am J Roentgenol.* 1991;157(4):792.

129. Harper GD, Dicks-Mireaux C, Leiper AD. Total body irradiation-induced osteochondromata. *J Pediatr Orthop.* 1998;18(3):356–358.

130. Libshitz HI, Cohen MA. Radiation-induced osteochondromas. *Radiology.* 1982;142(3):643–647.

131. Neuhauser EB, Wittenborg MH, Berman CZ, et al. Irradiation effects of roentgen therapy on the growing spine. *Radiology.* 1952;59(5):637–650.

132. Taitz J, Cohn RJ, White L, et al. Osteochondroma after total body irradiation: an age-related complication. *Pediatr Blood Cancer.* 2004;42(3):225–229.

133. Bakker B, Oostdijk W, Geskus RB, et al. Growth hormone (GH) secretion and response to GH therapy after total body irradiation and haematopoietic stem cell transplantation during childhood. *Clin Endocrinol (Oxf).* 2007;67(4):589–597.

134. Blamoutier A, Guigui P, Rillardon L, et al. Thoracic spinal cord compression by radiation-induced exostosis: a case report and review of the literature. *Rev Chir Orthop Reparatrice Appar Mot.* 2002;88(5):514–517.

135. Gorospe L, Madrid-Muniz C, Royo A, et al. Radiation-induced osteochondroma of the T4 vertebra causing spinal cord compression. *Eur Radiol.* 2002;12(4):844–848.

136. Arlen M, Higinbotham NL, Huvos AG, et al. Radiation-induced sarcoma of bone. *Cancer.* 1971;28(5):1087–1099.

137. Kim JH, Chu FC, Woodward HQ, et al. Radiation induced sarcomas of bone following therapeutic radiation. *Int J Radiat Oncol Biol Phys.* 1983;9(1):107–110.

138. Koshy M, Paulino AC, Mai WY, et al. Radiation-induced osteosarcomas in the pediatric population. *Int J Radiat Oncol Biol Phys.* 15 2005;63(4):1169–1174.

139. Patel SR. Radiation-induced sarcoma. *Curr Treat Options Oncol.* 2000;1(3):258–261.

140. Kleinerman RA, Boice JD Jr, Storm HH, et al. Second primary cancer after treatment for cervical cancer. An international cancer registries study. *Cancer.* 1995;76(3):442–452.

141. Storm HH. Second primary cancer after treatment for cervical cancer. Late effects after radiotherapy. *Cancer.* 1988;61(4):679–688.

142. Brenner DJ, Curtis RE, Hall EJ, et al. Second malignancies in prostate carcinoma patients after radiotherapy compared with surgery. *Cancer.* 2000;88(2):398–406.

143. Suit H, Goldberg S, Niemierko A, et al. Secondary carcinogenesis in patients treated with radiation: a review of data on radiation-induced cancers in human, non-human primate, canine and rodent subjects. *Radiat Res.* 2007;167(1):12–42.

144. Tucker MA, D'Angio GJ, Boice JD Jr, et al. Bone sarcomas linked to radiotherapy and chemotherapy in children. *N Engl J Med.* 1987;317(10):588–593.

145. Koshurnikova NA, Gilbert ES, Sokolnikov M, et al. Bone cancers in Mayak workers. *Radiat Res.* 2000;154(3):237–245.

146. Sokolnikov ME, Gilbert ES, Preston DL, et al. Lung, liver and bone cancer mortality in Mayak workers. *Int J Cancer.* 2008;123(4):905–911.

147. Samartzis D, Nishi N, Hayashi M, et al. Bone Sarcomas in Atomic Bomb Survivors of Hiroshima and Nagasaki. *Int J Radiat Oncol Biol Phys.* 2008;72(1 suppl 1):S120.

148. Nekolla EA, Kreisheimer M, Kellerer AM, et al. Induction of malignant bone tumors in radium-224 patients: risk estimates based on the improved dosimetry. *Radiat Res.* 2000;153(1):93–103.

149. Carnes BA, Groer PG, Kotek TJ. Radium dial workers: issues concerning dose response and modeling. *Radiat Res.* 1997;147(6):707–714.

150. Rowland RE, Stehney AF, Lucas HF. Dose-response relationships for radium-induced bone sarcomas. *Health Phys.* 1983;44(suppl 1):15–31.

151. Yap J, Chuba PJ, Thomas R, et al. Sarcoma as a second malignancy after treatment for breast cancer. *Int J Radiat Oncol Biol Phys.* 2002;52(5):1231–1237.

152. Rubino C, Shamsaldin A, Le MG, et al. Radiation dose and risk of soft tissue and bone sarcoma after breast cancer treatment. *Breast Cancer Res Treat.* 2005;89(3):277–288.

153. Hatfield PM, Schulz MD. Postirradiation sarcoma. Including 5 cases after X-ray therapy of breast carcinoma. *Radiology.* 1970;96(3):593–602.

154. Chaturvedi AK, Engels EA, Gilbert ES, et al. Second cancers among 104,760 survivors of cervical cancer: evaluation of long-term risk. *J Natl Cancer Inst.* 2007;99(21):1634–1643.

155. Kuttesch JF Jr, Wexler LH, Marcus RB, et al. Second malignancies after Ewing's sarcoma: radiation dose-dependency of secondary sarcomas. *J Clin Oncol.* 1996;14(10):2818–2825.

156. Travis LB, Curtis RE, Storm H, et al. Risk of second malignant neoplasms among long-term survivors of testicular cancer. *J Natl Cancer Inst.* 1997;89(19):1429–1439.

157. van Leeuwen FE, Klokman WJ, Hagenbeek A, et al. Second cancer risk following Hodgkin's disease: a 20-year follow-up study. *J Clin Oncol.* 1994;12(2):312–325.

158. Le Vu B, de Vathaire F, Shamsaldin A, et al. Radiation dose, chemotherapy and risk of osteosarcoma after solid tumours during childhood. *Int J Cancer.* 1998;77(3):370–377.

159. Hawkins MM, Wilson LM, Burton HS, et al. Radiotherapy, alkylating agents, and risk of bone cancer after childhood cancer. *J Natl Cancer Inst.* Mar 6 1996;88(5):270–278.

160. Wong FL, Boice JD Jr, Abramson DH, et al. Cancer incidence after retinoblastoma. Radiation dose and sarcoma risk. *JAMA.* 1997;278(15):1262–1267.

161. Henderson TO, Whitton J, Stovall M, et al. Secondary sarcomas in childhood cancer survivors: a report from the Childhood Cancer Survivor Study. *J Natl Cancer Inst.* 2007;99(4):300–308.

162. Jenkinson HC, Hawkins MM, Stiller CA, et al. Long-term population-based risks of second malignant neoplasms after childhood cancer in Britain. *Br J Cancer.* 2004;91(11):1905–1910.

163. Constine LS, Tarbell N, Hudson MM, et al. Subsequent malignancies in children treated for Hodgkin's disease: associations with gender and radiation dose. *Int J Radiat Oncol Biol Phys.* 2008;72(1):24–33.

164. Sheppard DG, Libshitz HI. Post-radiation sarcomas: a review of the clinical and imaging features in 63 cases. *Clin Radiol.* 2001;56(1):22–29.

165. Wiklund TA, Blomqvist CP, Raty J, et al. Postirradiation sarcoma. Analysis of a nationwide cancer registry material. *Cancer.* 1991;68(3):524–531.

166. Newton WA Jr, Meadows AT, Shimada H, et al. Bone sarcomas as second malignant neoplasms following childhood cancer. *Cancer.* 1991;67(1):193–201.

167. Meadows AT, Strong LC, Li FP, et al. Bone sarcoma as a second malignant neoplasm in children: influence of radiation and genetic predisposition for the Late Effects Study Group. *Cancer.* 1980;46(12):2603–2606.

168. Brady MS, Gaynor JJ, Brennan MF. Radiation-associated sarcoma of bone and soft tissue. *Arch Surg.* 1992;127(12):1379–1385.

169. Kalra S, Grimer RJ, Spooner D, et al. Radiation-induced sarcomas of bone: factors that affect outcome. *J Bone Joint Surg Br.* 2007;89(6):808–813.

170. Lee YY, Van Tassel P, Nauert C, et al. Craniofacial osteosarcomas: plain film, CT, and MR findings in 46 cases. *Am J Roentgenol.* 1988;150(6):1397–1402.

171. Lorigan JG, Libshitz HI, Peuchot M. Radiation-induced sarcoma of bone: CT findings in 19 cases. *Am J Roentgenol.* 1989;153(4):791–794.

172. Smith J. Radiation-induced sarcoma of bone: clinical and radiographic findings in 43 patients irradiated for soft tissue neoplasms. *Clin Radiol.* 1982;33(2):205–221.

173. Tountas AA, Fornasier VL, Harwood AR, Leung PM. Postirradiation sarcoma of bone: a perspective. *Cancer.* 1979;43(1):182–187.

174. Huvos AG, Woodard HQ, Cahan WG, et al. Postradiation osteogenic sarcoma of bone and soft tissues. A clinicopathologic study of 66 patients. *Cancer.* 1985;55(6):1244–1255.

175. Robinson E, Neugut AI, Wylie P. Clinical aspects of postirradiation sarcomas. *J Natl Cancer Inst.* 1988;80(4):233–240.

176. Tabone MD, Terrier P, Pacquement H, et al. Outcome of radiation-related osteosarcoma after treatment of childhood and adolescent cancer: a study of 23 cases. *J Clin Oncol.* 1999;17(9):2789–2795.

177. Futran ND, Trotti A, Gwede C. Pentoxifylline in the treatment of radiation-related soft tissue injury: preliminary observations. *Laryngoscope.* 1997;107(3):391–395.

178. Bese NS, Ozguroglu M, Kamberoglu K, et al. Pentoxifylline in the treatment of radiation-related pelvic insufficiency fractures of bone. *Radiat Med.* 2003;21(5):223–227.

179. Rodan GA, Fleisch HA. Bisphosphonates: mechanisms of action. *J Clin Invest.* 1996;97(12):2692–2696.

180. Delanian S, Depondt J, Lefaix JL. Major healing of refractory mandible osteoradionecrosis after treatment combining pentoxifylline and tocopherol: a phase II trial. *Head Neck.* 2005;27(2):114–123.

181. Adan L, Sainte-Rose C, Souberbielle JC, et al. Adult height after growth hormone (GH) treatment for GH deficiency due to cranial irradiation. *Med Pediatr Oncol.* 2000;34(1):14–19.

182. Forsberg CM, Krekmanova L, Dahllof G. The effect of growth hormone therapy on mandibular and cranial base development in children treated with total body irradiation. *Eur J Orthod.* 2002;24(3):285–292.

183. Frisk P, Arvidson J, Gustafsson J, et al. Pubertal development and final height after autologous bone marrow transplantation for acute lymphoblastic leukemia. *Bone Marrow Transplant.* 2004;33(2):205–210.

184. Sanders JE, Guthrie KA, Hoffmeister PA, et al. Final adult height of patients who received hematopoietic cell transplantation in childhood. *Blood.* 2005;105(3):1348–1354.

185. Funatsu M, Sato K, Mitani H. Effects of growth hormone on craniofacial growth. *Angle Orthod.* 2006;76(6):970–977.

186. Marx RE, Johnson RP, Kline SN. Prevention of osteoradionecrosis: a randomized prospective clinical trial of hyperbaric oxygen versus penicillin. *J Am Dent Assoc.* 1985;111(1):49–54.

187. Maier A, Gaggl A, Klemen H, et al. Review of severe osteoradionecrosis treated by surgery alone or surgery with postoperative hyperbaric oxygenation. *Br J Oral Maxillofac Surg.* 2000;38(3):173–176.

188. Teng MS, Futran ND. Osteoradionecrosis of the mandible. *Curr Opin Otolaryngol Head Neck Surg.* 2005;13(4):217–221.

189. Gal TJ, Yueh B, Futran ND. Influence of prior hyperbaric oxygen therapy in complications following microvascular reconstruction for advanced osteoradionecrosis. *Arch Otolaryngol Head Neck Surg.* 2003;129(1):72–76.

190. Annane D, Depondt J, Aubert P, et al. Hyperbaric oxygen therapy for radionecrosis of the jaw: a randomized, placebo-controlled, double-blind trial from the ORN96 study group. *J Clin Oncol.* 2004;22(24):4893–4900.

191. Feldmeier JJ, Hampson NB, Bennett M. In response to the negative randomized controlled hyperbaric trial by Annane et al in the treatment of mandibular ORN. *Undersea Hyperb Med.* 2005;32(3):141–143.

192. Bennett MH, Feldmeier J, Hampson N, et al. Hyperbaric oxygen therapy for late radiation tissue injury. *Cochrane Database Syst Rev.* 2005;(3):CD005005.

193. Wang PC, Tu TY, Liu KD. Cystic brain necrosis and temporal bone osteoradionecrosis after radiotherapy and surgery in a patient of ear carcinoma. *J Chin Med Assoc.* 2004;67(9):487–491.

194. Ashamalla HL, Thom SR, Goldwein JW. Hyperbaric oxygen therapy for the treatment of radiation-induced sequelae in children. The University of Pennsylvania experience. *Cancer.* 1996;77(11):2407–2412.

195. Hao SP, Tsang NM, Chang KP, e tal. Osteoradionecrosis of external auditory canal in nasopharyngeal carcinoma. *Chang Gung Med J.* 2007;30(2):116–121.

196. Vudiniabola S, Pirone C, Williamson J, et al. Hyperbaric oxygen in the therapeutic management of osteoradionecrosis of the facial bones. *Int J Oral Maxillofac Surg.* 2000;29(6):435–438.

197. Feldmeier JJ, Heimbach RD, Davolt DA, et al. Hyperbaric oxygen as an adjunctive treatment for delayed radiation injury of the chest wall: a retrospective review of twenty-three cases. *Undersea Hyperb Med.* 1995;22(4):383–393.

198. Vriens BH, Klaase JM, Schornagel JH, et al. A solitary sternal lesion found by skeletal scintigraphy following treatment for breast carcinoma. *Ned Tijdschr Geneeskd.* 2007;151(35):1909–1914.

199. Videtic GM, Venkatesan VM. Hyperbaric oxygen corrects sacral plexopathy due to osteoradionecrosis appearing 15 years after pelvic irradiation. *Clin Oncol (R Coll Radiol).* 1999;11(3):198–199.

200. Farouk O, Krettek C, Miclau T, et al. The topography of the perforating vessels of the deep femoral artery. *Clin Orthop Relat Res.* 1999(368):255–259.

201. Utvag SE, Grundnes O, Reikeraos O. Effects of periosteal stripping on healing of segmental fractures in rats. *J Orthop Trauma.* 1996;10(4):279–284.

202. Zhang L, Bail H, Mittlmeier T, et al. Immediate microcirculatory derangements in skeletal muscle and periosteum after closed tibial fracture. *J Trauma.* 2003;54(5):979–985.

203. Duffy GP, Wood MB, Rock MG, et al. Vascularized free fibular transfer combined with autografting for the management of fracture nonunions associated with radiation therapy. *J Bone Joint Surg Am.* 2000;82(4):544–554.

204. Moseley C. Leg Length Discrepancy and angular deformity of the lower limbs. In: Morrissy R, Weinstein S, eds. *Lovell and Winter's Pediatric Orthopaedics.* Vol 2. 4th Ed. Philadelphia, PA: Lippincott-Raven, 1996:849–901.

205. Ilizarov GA, Deviatov AA. Surgical elongation of the leg. *Ortop Travmatol Protez.* 1971;32(8):20–25.

206. Gillespie R, Torode IP. Classification and management of congenital abnormalities of the femur. *J Bone Joint Surg Br.* 1983;65(5):557–568.

207. Al-Mamgani A, Heemsbergen WD, Peeters ST, et al. Role of intensity-modulated radiotherapy in reducing toxicity in dose escalation for localized prostate cancer. *Int J Radiat Oncol Biol Phys.* 2009;73(3):685–691.

208. Mell LK, Tiryaki H, Ahn KH, et al. Dosimetric comparison of bone marrow-sparing intensity-modulated radiotherapy versus conventional techniques for treatment of cervical cancer. *Int J Radiat Oncol Biol Phys.* 2008;71(5):1504–1510.

209. Griffin AM, Euler CI, Sharpe MB, et al. Radiation planning comparison for superficial tissue avoidance in radiotherapy for soft tissue sarcoma of the lower extremity. *Int J Radiat Oncol Biol Phys.* 2007;67(3):847–856.

210. Chung CSK, Keating N, Yock T, et al. Comparative analysis of second malignancy risk in patients treated with proton therapy versus conventional photon therapy. *Int J Radiat Oncol Biol Phys.* 2008;72 (1 suppl 1):S8.

211. Hall EJ. Intensity-modulated radiation therapy, protons, and the risk of second cancers. *Int J Radiat Oncol Biol Phys.* 2006;65(1):1–7.

212. Mell LK, Movsas B. Pharmacologic normal tissue protection in clinical radiation oncology: focus on amifostine. *Expert Opin Drug Metab Toxicol.* 2008;4(10):1341–1350.

213. Damron TA, Spadaro JA, Margulies B, et al. Dose response of amifostine in protection of growth plate function from irradiation effects. *Int J Cancer.* 20 2000;90(2):73–79.

214. Damron TA, Spadaro JA, Tamurian RM, et al. Sparing of radiation-induced damage to the physis: fractionation alone compared to amifostine pretreatment. *Int J Radiat Oncol Biol Phys.* 2000;47(4):1067–1071.

215. Margulies B, Morgan H, Allen M, et al. Transiently increased bone density after irradiation and the radioprotectant drug amifostine in a rat model. *Am J Clin Oncol.* 2003;26(4):106–114.

216. Gevorgyan AM, La Scala GC, Sukhu B, et al. Radiation-induced craniofacial bone growth inhibition: in vitro cytotoxicity in the rabbit orbitozygomatic complex periosteum-derived cell culture. *Plast Reconstr Surg.* 2008;121(3):763–771.

217. Forrest CR, O'Donovan DA, Yeung I, et al. Efficacy of radioprotection in the prevention of radiation-induced craniofacial bone growth inhibition. *Plast Reconstr Surg.* 2002;109(4):1311–1323; discussion 1324.

218. La Scala GC, O'Donovan DA, Yeung I, et al. Radiation-induced craniofacial bone growth inhibition: efficacy of cytoprotection following a fractionated dose regimen. *Plast Reconstr Surg.* 2005;115(7):1973–1985.

219. Gevorgyan A, La Scala GC, Neligan PC, et al. Radioprotection of craniofacial bone growth. *J Craniofac Surg.* 2007;18(5):995–1000.

Brian D. Lawenda
Peter A.S. Johnstone

Skin

ACUTE AND LATE EFFECTS OF RADIATION ON SKIN AND HAIR

BACKGROUND

Among the earliest experiments in radiation biology were those that were conducted on skin, and they continue to serve as the foundation of our understanding of radiation-induced skin effects as they relate to dose, volume, fractionation, and treatment time. In these experiments, a variety of isoeffect curves, cell survival curves, and formulas were established from the clinical findings (i.e., erythema, desquamation, necrosis, skin regrowth) as they related to the total radiation dose, dose per fraction, and overall treatment time.[1] Radiation-induced skin changes typically follow well-defined stages of progression and have been subdivided into various classifications systems (e.g., Tessmer[2]: early, intermediate and late; Rubin and Casarett[3]: acute, subacute, chronic and late; Fajardo[4]: early and delayed; Radiation Therapy Oncology Group/European Organisation for Research and Treatment of Cancer (RTOG/EORTC): acute and late,[5,6] acute, late and consequential,[7] etc.) Radiation-induced skin effects may be the most significant factor impacting the quality of life of patients treated with radiation therapy, and in some extreme cases, these effects can be life threatening.[8-10] It is therefore important to understand the pathophysiology of radiation effects on these tissues, and be aware of therapeutic approaches to minimize and manage skin toxicity. It is also crucial to remember that most of the early data collected on the effects of radiation on skin relate to radiation applications that were non–skin sparing: orthovoltage and kilovoltage radiation.

PATHOLOGIC SKIN CHANGES COMMENCING AFTER INITIATION OF IRRADIATION

The epidermis is composed of a basal layer of dividing stem cells (the target of early radiation effects) and 10 to 20 superficial layers of nondividing, differentiating, keratinizing epithelial cells.[1] The dermis is a dense, amorphous network of fibroblasts, capillaries, lymphatics, nerves, glands, hair follicles, and proteins. Late radiation effects predominantly affect the fibroblasts and blood vessels of the dermal layer.[1]

Unless otherwise specified, we will describe the classic radiation effects of 40 to 50 Gy on skin using once-daily fractionation, in 2-Gy fractions, over 4 to 5 weeks. These are considered either early (0–6 months after initiating radiation) or late effects (>6 months after initiating radiation).[3,4] Our discussion refers to changes induced by specific doses at the level of the epidermis and dermis (Fig. 44.1).

EARLY EFFECTS

Early radiation effects typically result from the loss of the rapidly proliferating cellular components in the irradiated skin (basal epithelial stem cells). Within the first week of radiation, some patients may develop a transient erythema, caused by an inflammatory response leading to capillary vasodilation, increased vascular permeability and edema.[1,11] This can develop within the first few hours after a single dose 5 Gy or greater and may subside within 24 to 48 hours.[1,12,13] Mitotic inhibition occurs in germinal cells of the epidermis, hair follicles, and sebaceous glands following doses of 2 to 4 Gy.[4] This leads to a loss of the epidermal basal cells, which produce the more superficial layers of keratinizing epithelial cells.[12,13] In general, erythema demarcating the radiation field starts in the second or third week of fractionated radiation (10–20 Gy).[14] Epilation usually develops by the second or third week of treatment and, based on estimates from data on atomic bomb survivors, may develop with doses as low as 0.75 Gy.[1,4,15,16] Sebaceous glands are as radiosensitive as hair follicles; therefore, skin dryness often occurs at the same time as the development of hair loss.[1,4] Prior to the development of dry skin and epilation, various histologic changes occur within the epidermal skin cells and skin appendages (i.e., sebaceous glands, sweat glands, and hair follicles) including cytoplasmic swelling, nuclear shrinkage, condensation of chromatin, and intercellular edema in the lower epidermis.[4] If the threshold dose for permanent alopecia is not exceeded, regrowth of hair typically begins within 2 to 3 months after the radiation course and continues for up to a year.[4,17]

Erythema becomes progressively more evident by the third and fourth week of treatment.[4] At this point, the erythema is often sharply demarcated by the edges of the radiation field, and the skin may be warm and edematous.[4,14] The predominant histologic changes in the erythema phase include dilation of blood vessels, expansion of papillae from edema in the upper dermis, swollen endothelial cells, arteriole obstruction with fibrin thrombi, lymphocytic infiltrate, and small foci of hemorrhage in the upper dermis.[4] Inflammatory changes in the tissues are characterized by the initial influx of neutrophils

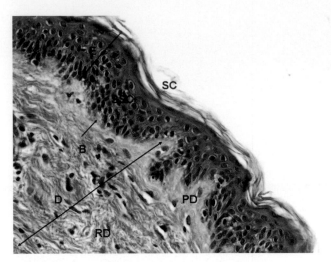

Figure 44.1. Histology of normal skin. The epidermis (*E*) is a two layered structure made up of the stratum corneum (*SC*) composed of flattened remnants of stratified squamous cells (SCC) that arise from basal cells at the basement membrane (*B*) and mature as they migrate toward the skin surface to eventually be lost through sloughing. The dermis (*D*) is composed of the more superficial papillary dermis (*PD*) and the deeper reticular dermis (*RD*). The epidermis is attached to the dermis by the basement membrane. (Photomicrograph courtesy of Dr. Ting Liu, Dept of Pathology, University of Utah, School of Medicine.)

within the first week of radiation. This is then followed by the migration of other inflammatory cells into the dermis (inflammatory exudate), including macrophages, eosinophils, plasma cells, lymphocytes, and mast cells.[2,4]

If the total delivered dose to the skin does not exceed 30 Gy, the erythema phase will typically be followed by the "dry desquamation phase" in the fourth or fifth week of radiation.[3] This phase is characterized by pruritis, scaling, and hyperpigmentation due to increased melanin production in the basal layer.[4] Additionally, there is flattening of the dermal papillae and thinning of the epidermis.[14] The inflammatory changes

generally resolve within the next few weeks, leaving an area of hyperpigmentation by 2 months.[4] If the total delivered dose is >40 Gy, the erythema phase may be followed by the "moist desquamation phase," which has similar histologic features to a second-degree burn.[4,18] Early in this phase, bullae form in the suprabasal and subepidermal layers. Ultimately, the irradiated epidermis and roofs of the bullae are shed. A fibrinous layer covers the denuded surface.[14] Dermal and subepidermal edema persists along with the development of stromal fibrin formation and an epidermal inflammatory infiltrate.[4] Unless larger doses per fraction are used, re-epithelialization typically occurs within 10 days of the development of moist desquamation, and is complete by the sixth to eighth week of radiation.[4] Re-epithelialization occurs from islands of less affected basal cells.[14] The early phases of erythema and desquamation are also referred to as *radiation dermatitis*.[4] Desquamation typically develops after 3 to 6 weeks, as the typical transit time for the epidermal basal cells is 12 to 48 days.[12,13] Depending on the level of depletion of the proliferating basal cells, desquamation will either progress to dry or moist desquamation.[14] At radiation doses that are sufficiently high to cause complete depletion of the basal layer stem cells, healing occurs by migration of cells from outside the irradiated area.[1]

Among the more commonly referenced morbidity grading systems in the literature is that of the RTOG/EORTC cooperative groups, who have developed both acute and late toxicity grading systems to standardize clinical findings based on severity (Table 44.1).[5,6] Another commonly cited morbidity grading system is that of the US National Cancer Institute (NCI); however, the latest update of the NCI Common Terminology Criteria for Adverse Events grading system (NCI-CTCAE-v3.0) no longer separates acute and late adverse effects[19]; "…The era of complex multimodality integration, use of predetermined time-based limits [i.e., 'late effects' occur after 90 days] for designating acute vs. late in individual patient is no longer applicable."[20]

In humans, the α/β ratios for the early effects of erythema and desquamation have been reported as 12 and 11 Gy, respectively, when overall treatment time is <29 days.[21]

TABLE 44.1	RTOG/EORTC Skin and Subcutaneous Tissue Morbidity Scoring Criteria					
System	*Grade 0*	*Grade 1*	*Grade 2*	*Grade 3*	*Grade 4*	*Grade 5*
RTOG/EORTC (acute)[5] Day 1–90 from the commencement of radiation therapy	No change over baseline	Follicular, faint or dull erythema/epilation/ dry desquamation/ decreased sweating	Tender or bright erythema, patchy moist desquamation/ moderate edema	Confluent, moist desquamation other than skin folds, pitting edema	Ulceration, hemorrhage, necrosis	Death
RTOG/EORTC (late-skin)[6] After 90 days from the commencement of radiation therapy	None	Slight atrophy Pigmentation change Some hair loss	Patch atrophy; Moderate telangiectasia; Total hair loss	Marked atrophy; Gross telangiectasia	Ulceration	Death
RTOG/EORTC (late-subcutaneous tissues)[6] After 90 days from the commencement of radiation therapy	None	Slight induration (fibrosis) and loss of subcutaneous fat	Moderate fibrosis but asymptomatic Slight field contracture <10% linear reduction	Severe induration and loss of subcutaneous tissue Field contracture >10% linear measurement	Necrosis	Death

LATE EFFECTS

Late radiation effects typically manifest in the slowly proliferating cell populations in the skin (e.g., endothelial cells, fibroblasts). These cells are generally more sensitive to increasing fraction sizes than rapidly proliferating cells, that is, they are characterized by a lower α/β ratio. If the early-responding stem cells become depleted below a threshold number sufficient to repair the injured skin, the early/acute skin injury may persist as a chronic injury (also known as a *consequential late effect*).[1]

Various clinical and subclinical effects develop in the months to years after initiating radiation, including hyper and/or hypopigmentation, epidermal and/or dermal atrophy, skin dryness (due to the loss of sebaceous glands), loss of sweat glands and ducts, alopecia, telangiectasia, nuclear atypia of basal keratinocytes and melanocytes, dyskeratosis, loss of rete ridges, disappearance of the epidermal basement membrane, fibrin formation along the dermoepidermal junction, and decreased numbers of upper dermal blood capillaries.[4,13,18,22] Additionally, there may be myointimal proliferation of the arterioles and arteries at the dermal-subcutaneous junction and hyalinization and thickening of the media.[4,23] Radiation-induced damage to endothelial cells appears to contribute significantly to late toxicity in a dose-dependent manner.[7,24,25] These changes may lead to thrombosis or luminal obliteration. Rarely, vascular wall necrosis develops, but when this occurs, it may be associated with thrombosis, necrosis, ulceration, and hemorrhage.[4,13]

Fibrosis progressively develops in the papillary dermis, reticular dermis, and subcutaneous adipose tissues. Fibrinous exudate is one of the most characteristic features of soft tissue radiation injury, and is evident within the stroma of the dermis and epidermis.[4,26] Histologically, it appears as a progressive process with deposition of fibrillary and elastic fibers and collagen.[4] Initially, the deposits are delicate, irregular, and patchy. Later, these deposits become more dense and amorphous, often with collagen formation around the capillaries, nerves, and glands.[27] The associated fibroblasts are prominent and have large, hyperchromatic nuclei.[27,28] As the developmental stages of fibrosis progress, fibroblasts undergo differentiation into postmitotic fibrocytes.[29–31]

There are numerous cytokines, growth factors, and other proteins that have been associated with the complex cascade of events involved in the development of fibrosis, vascular changes, and other late radiation effects[23,31–37] (Table 44.2). This process begins during or shortly after radiation exposure, and may continue for years. We are only beginning to understand the interplay of agents in this process. It is clear that this is potentially a progressive process over time, which emphasizes the importance of long follow-up in clinical trials reporting skin toxicity. The authors of a small phase I/II trial of accelerated partial breast irradiation (APBI), using a high dose-rate (HDR) interstitial brachytherapy technique (34 Gy in ten fractions, Bid), reported increasing rates of moderate to severe subcutaneous fibrosis in patients up to 5 years after treatment; 15.2%, 18.2%, 18.8%, and 35.7% at follow-up intervals of ≤6 months, >6 but ≤24 months, >24 but ≤60 months, and >60 months, respectively.[47]

The risk of developing late effects of radiation on the skin may be independent of severity of the acute effects. For example, Bentzen and Overgaard[48] demonstrated that late development of telangiectasias was more likely to occur in patients who had experienced moist desquamation during radiotherapy (RT), whereas subcutaneous fibrosis was not. They also reported that early phase erythema was not associated with the subsequent development of telangiectasias or fibrosis. Other studies have reported that there is a significant correlation between the development of acute skin reactions (dose dependent) and the subsequent development of late skin toxicity (i.e., telangiectasias and/or changes in pigmentation).[49]

TABLE 44.2	Cytokines and Growth Factors Implicated as Mediators for the Development of Late Radiation Effects on Skin
Cytokines, Growth Factors, and Other Proteins	**Potential Mechanisms of Actions**
IL-1 beta	Stimulates proliferation of keratinocytes and fibroblasts[38,39]
	Stimulates metallomatrix proteases[38,39]
	Increases dermal angiogenesis[40]
	Inflammatory mediator[31,35,36]
IL-6	Inflammatory mediator[31,35,36]
IL-8	Chemokine[41]
Eotaxin	Chemokine[41]
TGF-B1	Enhances collagen production in response to radiation[33,36,42]
	Accelerates the terminal differentiation of progenitor fibroblasts to postmitotic functional fibrocytes[43]
	Stimulates the synthesis of extracellular matrix proteins and MMPs[44]
PDGF	Induces fibroblast differentiation[43]
	Stimulates the synthesis of extracellular matrix proteins and MMPs[38,39]
CCN2	Involved with TGF-B1 in stimulating fibrosis[45]
TNF-α	Inflammatory mediator[31,35,36]
CTGF	Promotes fibrosis and secreted by fibroblasts and endothelial cells[37]
Smad3	Transduces signaling effects through TGF-B1 (increases chemoattraction and elaboration of extracellular matrix by fibroblasts, inhibitory effects of keratinocyte proliferation and migration)[46]

CTGF, connective tissue growth factor; IL, interleukin; MMPs, matrix metalloproteinases; PDGF, platelet derived growth factor; TGF, transforming growth factor; TNF, tumor necrosis factor.

Ulcers can develop at any time interval after radiation. Early ulcer formation (weeks to months after radiation) is due to radiation necrosis of the epidermis with sloughing, and can occur as early as 2 weeks after receiving high skin doses.[4] These ulcers typically heal, but they can recur over time.[4] Chronic radiation changes to areas of the skin exposed to high radiation doses can lead to epidermal and dermal atrophy and hypovascularity, making it susceptible to injury by trauma, infection, and further radiation exposure.[4] Delayed ulcer formation (months to years after radiation) occurs more commonly than early ulcer formation, and is predominantly due to dermal ischemia and necrosis in an area of hypovascularized skin.[4,13,50] These ulcers are frequently caused by trauma to areas of skin with a severely impaired wound-healing capacity.[12] These ulcers often heal slowly over months or years, and are typically covered with a fibrinopurulent exudate with minimal granulation tissue formation at the base.[4]

Hyperplasia of the epidermis and/or dermis, although uncommon, can develop years after radiation exposure.[4] The associated hyperkeratosis can lead to foci of irregular acanthosis and dysplasia, which are very similar in appearance to solar keratosis.[4] Carcinoma can develop in some of these keratoses, with a reported average latency period after therapeutic radiation of 23 years.[22,51,52] Squamous and basal cell carcinomas are the most common therapeutic radiation-induced malignancies of the epidermis, with squamous cell carcinomas being more frequent.[4,22,52–54] Mesenchymal spindle-cell tumors, benign and malignant, are less common but do occur.[4,55]

The development of temporary and permanent alopecia is dose dependent.[15] Temporary alopecia occurs within 2 to 3 weeks after irradiation and, if the permanent alopecia dose threshold has not been exceeded, recovers within 2 to 3 months after completion of treatment.[17] Single doses as low as 0.75 to 2 Gy have been recorded to induce temporary alopecia.[16,17,56] Permanent alopecia may develop after single doses of 7 Gy,[57] and there is a reported 50% risk of developing permanent alopecia (i.e., using 2 Gy/fraction/d) with a fractionated dose of 43 Gy.[15] Dermal atrophy and permanent loss of hair follicles continue to progress beyond 12 months after irradiation; therefore, the determination of whether permanent alopecia will develop may not be obvious for some time.[50] There is a dose-dependent reduction in hair shaft diameter and length (2.3%/Gy) that results from damage to germinal cells and other radiation-associated changes in the tissue microenviroment.[1,58] Other factors may increase the risk of developing permanent radiation-induced alopecia: concurrent administration of radiosensitizing chemotherapy, administration of chemotherapeutic agents that can cause alopecia, and a personal history of preexisting alopecia.[15]

The late radiation effects on capillaries occur at approximately 40 Gy with conventionally fractionated doses, while arterial damage does not occur until fractionated doses of 50 to 70 Gy.[1] Endothelial cells and smooth muscle cells are the target of late radiation effects.[1]

RADIATION EFFECTS ON WOUND HEALING

Radiation therapy appears to interrupt normal wound-healing mechanisms by changes in vasculature, effects on fibroblasts, and varying levels of regulatory growth factors.[33,59,60] These effects are important to consider when determining the timing of RT with respect to surgery. Studies of preoperative radiation therapy have demonstrated an increased risk of wound-healing complications when compared to postoperative radiation therapy.[61,62] However, late effects associated with preoperative irradiation appear to be less significant than those following postoperative radiation therapy. This has been attributed to the relatively larger irradiated volumes irradiated in the postoperative setting. The late tensile strength of irradiated wounds does not appear to be diminished months to years following radiation therapy.[7]

Fibroblasts are frequently considered to be the predominant target cell for delayed wound healing associated with radiation therapy; however, recent clinical data demonstrate that the degree of radiation injury to fibroblasts does not directly correlate with the risk of surgical wound-healing complications following preoperative radiation therapy.[63] This suggests that other factors likely play a more dominant role in wound healing, such as alteration of vasculature and growth factor modulation.

Within hours to days following irradiation, the hyperplastic response seen in keloid formation, pterygia, and the myointimal hyperplasia in blood vessels can be diminished.[7] It has been postulated that this effect may be due to the inhibition of the contractile phase of wound healing mediated by myofibroblasts.[7] Radiation therapy has been employed successfully in the management of each of these conditions.[64–66]

Adjuvant radiation therapy following immediate plastic surgical flap reconstructions has been demonstrated in some studies to lead to higher rates of surgical revisions and poorer cosmesis than in unirradiated flaps.[67,68] This may be due to the impaired microvasculature and enhanced fibrotic response that occurs following surgery.[69] Other groups have reported no significant differences in functional or cosmetic outcomes following flap irradiation.[70] Breast implant reconstructions have been associated with the highest risk of post–irradiation complications, requiring major revisions.[71] Employing a staged approach (surgery followed by radiation therapy followed by reconstruction), whenever possible, avoids unnecessary irradiation of flaps and breast implants and is suggested by some groups as the safest approach.[72] Using new software technology to avoid high radiation doses to future flaps may be an alternative strategy to reduce flap complications.[73]

EFFECT OF TOTAL SKIN DOSE, FRACTIONATION, AND VOLUME

TOTAL DOSE

In general, as the total skin dose increases, the incidence of both acute and late effects increases.[49,74] In a large EORTC trial, late cosmetic outcome in patients randomized to receive a breast boost (16 Gy) after breast-conserving surgery and whole-breast radiation (50 Gy) has been reported to be inferior to woman who did not receive a boost.[75] At a median follow-up of 10.8 years, moderate to severe fibrosis was higher in the boost arm compared to the no boost arm (28% and 13%, respectively). Numerous APBI trials have demonstrated increased acute and late skin and subcutaneous tissue toxicities and worse cosmesis with increasing skin dose.[76–78] A large study of 1,149 cases of skin cancer treated with superficial x-rays demonstrated that total dose, field size, and dose per fraction were significantly related to the frequency of late cosmetic changes (i.e., hypo/hyperpigmentation, telangiectasias, and erythema).[74]

DOSE PER FRACTION

Radiation-induced skin toxicity becomes progressively more significant with increasing dose per fraction. Late-responding tissues (fibroblasts and endothelial cells) are more affected by increasing dose per fraction than early-responding tissues such as skin basal cells and are proportionally more spared with reduction in the dose per fraction.[7] Hypofractionated regimens are becoming more prevalent in the practice of radiation therapy; therefore, understanding the effects of such treatments on skin toxicity is increasingly important.

Stereotactic body radiation therapy (SBRT) employs hypofractionated regimens with large fraction sizes. Determining dose-response data from SBRT studies with reported skin toxicities is difficult for numerous reasons: dose prescriptions and fractionation regimens are variable, lack of consistent and standardized reporting of skin toxicity assessments post treatment, variability in numbers of beams, variability in the volume of skin irradiated in each beam, calculated skin isodose values are infrequently reported, skin toxicity assessments may not be reported or are reported using different criteria.[79] Using the linear-quadratic model, which is based on biologically equivalent dose from conventionally fractionated treatments to the skin, to establish skin dose limits may or not apply to large fraction sizes (i.e., >8 Gy/fraction).[79,80] Above this dose range, cells may have significantly less ability to repair DNA damage. Daily fractionation at doses in this range is considered ablative, whereas lower doses (i.e., 2.25–8 Gy/fraction) are still used in hypofractionated regimens but are nonablative.[10]

Dose/volume constraints have recently been proposed by investigators at the University of Texas Southwestern for the use in SBRT treatment planning (Table 44.3). It is important to note that these constraints are only proposed guidelines, and they are constantly being updated as new data are collected. The RTOG is prospectively collecting patient dosimetry information and clinical toxicity data for all patients enrolled to SBRT trials, which will eventually be used to establish formal dose/volume constraints.[10] It may be relevant to reexamine the historical data collected during the early experiments in radiation biology on skin effects (i.e., pig skin), in order to help establish dose-response limits in SBRT treatment planning.

Skin toxicity has been reported in only a minority of SBRT cases, which is likely due to the relatively low total dose delivered at the skin surface from any one of the high-energy, skin-sparing, beams. Nonetheless, it is important to recognize that skin toxicities have occurred using SBRT and radiation planning techniques should attempt to minimize the entrance and exit skin doses. In a report of 15 extracranial cases treated with SBRT to varying doses (median dose per fraction: 7 Gy; median number of fractions: 6; planning treatment volume (PTV) prescribed to the 75%–85% isodose line), the authors reported that only one patient developed acute grade 1 radiation dermatitis.[81] At 18 months median follow-up, they observed late grade 2 painful subcutaneous fibrosis and grade 2 pain in a surgical scar. Another group reported two cases of skin ulcers and one case of subcutaneous emphysema among 237 patients treated for lung cancer using SBRT (dose range: 40–60 Gy, in four or five fractions).[82] In another (n = 27 patients) of SBRT for lung cancer (median follow-up: 17 months; dose range: 40–50 Gy, in four fractions), the authors reported an 11.1% rate of grade 2 to 3 radiation dermatitis and chest wall pain. These effects occurred only in patients who received >35 Gy to the skin and rib.[83] In a prospective phase I/II study of SBRT for liver metastases, the authors reported a single case of grade 3 skin toxicity (necrosis and painful subcutaneous fibrosis) among a total of 21 patients with >6 months of follow-up.[79] The patients in this study received 60 Gy in three fractions, and the patient with the grade 3 skin toxicity was treated to a posterior lobe lesion using five static noncoplanar beams; on analysis, the center of the involved skin area had a hotspot located 1 cm deep to the skin surface that was "more than 48 Gy."

Interestingly, the results of recently reported phase three trials of hypofractionated whole-breast irradiation have demonstrated equivalency in respect to cosmetic outcomes and late skin effects compared to conventional fractionation schedules.[84] Explanations for this could simply be that the overall dose in the hypofractionated arms has not been sufficiently high to cause significantly increased late effects or that the length of follow-up in these early reports has not been long enough to observe the full development of late effects.

In a phase three trial of 1,234 breast cancer patients, which compared an accelerated hypofractionated radiation course (42.5 Gy in 16 fractions, over 22 days) to a standard fractionation course (50 Gy in 25 fractions, over 35 days), no differences in cosmetic outcomes were found between the two groups; good to excellent in 77% of patients in each arm at 5-year median follow-up[85] and 70% (accelerated hypofractionation arm) versus 71% (conventional fractionation arm), at 10 years.[86] At 10 years, there were no differences in the rates of moderate (6%) and late severe radiation (3%) skin morbidity, and no differences in moderate (8%) and late severe radiation (4%) subcutaneous tissue morbidity.[86]

TABLE 44.3	University of Texas Southwestern Skin Dose Constraints (SBRT)			
No. of Fractions	*Volume (cc)*	*Volume Max (Gy)*	*Max Point Dose (Gy)*	*Endpoint (≥ Grade 3)*
1	<10	14.4[10]	16[10]	Ulceration
		23[a]	26[a]	
3	<10	22.5 (7.5 Gy/fx)[10]	24 (8 Gy/fx)[10]	Ulceration
		30 (10 Gy/fx)[a]	33 (11 Gy/fx)[a]	
4	<10	33.2 (8.3 Gy/fx)[a]	36 (9 Gy/fx)[a]	Ulceration
5	<10	30 (6 Gy/fx)[10]	32 (6.4 Gy/fx)[10]	Ulceration

[a]Timmerman RD, *personal communication*, SBRT Constraints (June 2008)-UT Southwestern; 2008.

In another large randomized controlled trial ($n = 1,410$), patients received one of three external beam fractionation regimens (all given over 5 weeks: 50 Gy in 25 fractions, 42.9 Gy in 13 fractions, or 39 Gy in 13 fractions) and were assessed for late changes in breast appearance.[87] At 5 years minimum follow-up, the risk of having any changes in breast appearance was 39.6% (50 Gy), 45.7% (42.9 Gy), and 30.3% (39 Gy); an α/β ratio for changes in breast appearance was estimated to be 3.6 Gy. An α/β ratio for palpable breast induration (fibrosis) was estimated to be 3.1 Gy.

In the START (Standardization of Breast Radiotherapy) trials, cosmetic outcomes were superior in the lower dose regimens.[88,89] The START A trial ($n = 2,236$ patients) consisted of a three-arm randomization, each delivered over 5 weeks (50 Gy in 25 fractions, 41.6 Gy in 13 fractions of 3.2 Gy each, and 39 Gy in 13 fractions).[89] At 5.1-year median follow-up, patients in the 39 Gy arm had a lower hazard ratio for development of breast changes (i.e., skin and breast appearance and swelling) than those patients in the 50-Gy arm; HR = 0.69 and estimated α/β ratio for late breast changes was 3.4 Gy.

The START B trial ($n = 2,215$ patients) was a randomization between two arms, 50 Gy in 25 fractions versus 40 Gy in 15 fractions (over 3 weeks).[88] At a 6-year median follow-up, the authors reported a trend toward lower rates of late changes in breast appearance in the 40-Gy arm compared to the 50-Gy arm.[88]

In a small prospective study, comparing patients ($n = 45$) who underwent APBI with HDR interstitial implant (30.3 or 36.4 Gy, in seven fractions, over 4 days) versus patients ($n = 80$) who underwent whole-breast external beam radiotherapy (EBRT) (50 Gy ± 10–16 Gy EBRT boost), the authors reported good-to-excellent late (7 year) cosmetic results in 84.4% and 68.3% of patients, respectively.[90]

The authors of an early report on a prospective phase I/II trial ($n = 99$), comparing HDR (34 Gy in 10 Bid fractions) to low dose-rate (LDR) (45 Gy over 3.5–6 days) multicatheter implants after breast-conserving surgery, reported poor cosmetic results in 0% to 2% (HDR cases) and 8% to 14% (LDR cases) at 2 years follow-up (rated by patients and physicians).[91,92] As rated by the radiation oncologists at 2 years follow-up, telangiectasias, atrophy, pockmarks, hyperpigmentation, erythema, fibrosis, and dimpling were noted in 23%/27% (HDR/LDR), 0%/9%, 63%/68%, 3%/23%, 8%/5%, 23%/50%, and 20%/32% of patients.[92]

VOLUME

In general, the ability of skin to repair increasing doses of radiation is inversely proportional to the volume of irradiated skin.[1] Clinical studies demonstrate that treatment of large volumes, with either brachytherapy or external beam radiation therapy, is associated with increased rates fibrosis and worse cosmetic outcomes.[74,93–95]

In a randomized trial of 129 patients who received either preoperative radiation therapy (50 Gy) or postoperative radiation therapy (66 Gy) for the treatment of extremity soft tissue sarcoma, the authors reported that larger treatment volumes were associated with greater rates of fibrosis ($p = 0.002$), joint stiffness ($p = 0.006$), and edema ($p = 0.06$).[61] Volume of breast tissue irradiated directly correlates with cosmetic outcome. In a report of 75 patients who underwent HDR APBI (using interstitial implants), those who had a higher volume of tissue encompassed by the 150% and 200% isodose lines (V_{150} and V_{200}, respectively) developed greater skin toxicity and worse cosmetic results.[95]

EFFECT OF RADIATION TYPE AND ENERGY

The degree of skin sparing for any particular radiation therapy modality is one of the primary factors in the development of skin toxicity. The depth of the maximum dose (D_{max}) deposited in irradiated tissues increases with increasing photon energy. Radiation planning techniques can take advantage of the use of this property when target tissues do not involve the skin and other superficial structures. Obviously, when target tissues involve the skin, choosing a modality or technique that delivers maximum dose to the skin is optimal (i.e., superficial x-ray therapy, electrons, tangential beams, use of tissue compensator bolus materials, etc.) With the early use of low-energy x-rays in RT, skin toxicity was typically dose limiting since the maximum dose was deposited close to the skin surface, leading to significant acute toxicity. The advent of higher energy x-rays (i.e., megavoltage) allowed for the maximum dose to be delivered below the skin surface, which can lead to mild/moderate acute skin toxicity but increasing late skin toxicity (i.e., fibrosis, telangiectasias).[1]

Particle-based radiation therapy (i.e., neutrons, protons, carbon ions, electrons, etc.) techniques are associated with increased skin toxicity due to their inherently less favorable skin-sparing dose distributions, as compared to high-energy photons.[96]

Passively scattered proton fields have a higher entrance dose at the skin (75%–90%) compared to megavoltage photon beams (30%–60%).[97,98] Patients treated with a single proton field, in the phase I/II APBI trial, developed acute moist desquamation at the treatment site. This effect was reduced when employing more than one beam.[99] It is important to consider the different relative biological effectiveness (RBE) of the radiation modality employed, as this may need to be factored into the dose/fractionation regimen to minimize both acute and late skin toxicity (i.e., higher RBEs are associated with decreased sublethal damage repair with fractionation).[1]

EFFECT OF REIRRADIATION

The tolerance of the skin to the effects of reirradiation has been described in many reports. Based on tolerance data (predominantly from rodent models) to recover from the acute effects of radiation, the skin is able to tolerate reirradiation with 90% to 100% of the full-tolerance dose 2 to 6 months after initial treatment.[100–108] Following doses that were less than full tolerance, the skin can tolerate full-tolerance doses of reirradiation after only 4 to 6 weeks of recovery.[108] Repeatedly irradiating the skin with large single doses (at 6- or 9-week intervals) leads to diminishing retreatment tolerance (for recovery from acute effects) with successive doses.[101,107]

The mechanism implicated in the inability to recover from acute radiation effects to full-tolerance doses with reirradiation appears to be due to the loss of skin stem cells (epidermal crypt cells).[101,102] Data on skin tolerance of reirradiation for late effects (late necrosis) are less consistent. The data for late effects (late necrosis) on pig skin do not demonstrate any appreciable reduction in the full-tolerance doses for reirradiation.[105] This contrasts with data on mouse skin, in which reductions in the tolerance to reirradiation has been reported for late necrosis.[100,107] Importantly, the mouse studies induced severe acute radiation reactions (moist desquamation), whereas the pig skin study did not use doses sufficiently high to induce severe effects. The degree of severity of the acute effects may explain the differences in the ability to recover full tolerance to reirradiation.[109]

RISK FACTORS THAT MAY EXACERBATE RADIATION-INDUCED SKIN TOXICITY

Some groups have reported that advanced age, diabetes, smoking, compromised tissue perfusion secondary to surgery and/or prior radiation therapy, and concurrent chemotherapy may be associated with an increased risk in the development of skin toxicity with radiation therapy.[110–114] These risk factors are likely related to effects on decreasing wound healing and tissue ischemia: decreased angiogenesis, endothelial cell damage, microvascular fibrosis/occlusion, fibroblast injury, etc.

Age is less consistently agreed upon as a risk factor for increased skin toxicity. One study reported that young age (i.e., ≤30 years old) was associated with increased risk of late effects, possibly due to the duration of time for late effects to develop.[115] Another group reported a significantly decreased rate of acute skin erythema in women over the age of 70 years, compared to younger women, who received conventional EBRT whole-breast irradiation.[116]

CONGENITAL FACTORS THAT MAY EXACERBATE RADIATION-INDUCED SKIN TOXICITY

Some patients are more likely to develop specific radiation late effects (i.e., telangiectasias and/or subcutaneous fibrosis), but determining this does not always correlate with other acute or late effects.[81–83] Genetic differences between individuals have been hypothesized as the predominant explanation for the large variation observed in the development of radiation-induced telangiectasias among patients treated with breast irradiation, as only 10% to 20% of the variation could be explained by the random nature of radiation-induced cell killing and random variations in dosimetry and dose delivery.[117] It appears that there is likely individual variability in one's risk of developing late radiation reactions that is associated with certain genetic phenotypes (e.g., genetic variants of: ATM, TGFB1, XRCC1, XRCC3, SOD2, hHR21).[48,118,119] These specific genetic variations are not well understood and are an active area of research.

Some groups have demonstrated that inherent radiosensitivity of an individual's fibroblasts, using an in vitro assay (i.e., surviving fraction), may correlate with the development of telangiectasias and fibrosis.[118,120–122] Other groups have suggested that factors other than the radiosensitivity of the skin fibroblasts likely also play a role in the development of late effects and delayed wound healing.[63]

Connective tissue disorders (CTD) such as systemic lupus erythematosis (SLE) and scleroderma have traditionally been considered relative contraindications to radiation therapy due to the possibility of enhanced skin toxicity in these patients.[123] The role of radiation therapy in these patients remains an area of controversy and is discussed in detail in Chapter 6.[124]

POTENTIAL EFFECT OF RACIAL DIFFERENCES ON RADIATION-INDUCED SKIN REACTIONS

In a study of 308 cancer patients who completed a local symptom inventory questionnaire, significantly more black patients (20%) reported severe skin reactions at the treatment site than white patients (8%).[125] A direct correlation was observed between severity of skin problems and pain at the treatment site ($r = 0.541$, $p < 0.001$). Total radiation exposure did not significantly correlate with the report of skin problems at the treatment site for white or black patients. In a study of 1,614 patients ($n = 101$ African American, $n = 1,513$ white) treated with lumpectomy and radiation therapy, the authors reported that African American patients had poorer cosmetic results (edema, fibrosis, and pigmentation); overall cosmesis was good to excellent in 55% of African Americans versus 90% of whites.[126]

Mechanisms that might explain these reported differences in skin toxicities require further study.

THE CUTANEOUS SYNDROME

Radiation injury to the skin has been referred to as *the cutaneous syndrome* when in reference to industrial, accidental, or nontherapeutic radiation exposures.[127,128] This syndrome is attributed to more than 50% of all the radiation-related deaths from the Chernobyl nuclear accident.[129] The skin dose and the type of radiation exposure are important variables in predicting the eventual skin lesions that may develop. As with any radiation-induced skin reaction, they may occur within days to years following exposure. A severity grading system has been proposed by Waselenko et al.[127] (Table 44.4).

TABLE 44.4	Cutaneous Syndrome Severity Scale
Severity	*Symptoms or Findings*
Degree 1	Minimal and/or transient erythema, pruritis, no or rare skin blistering and/or desquamation, epidermal ulceration and/or necrosis, no onycholysis
Degree 2	Moderate erythema, 10% body surface area affected, mild intermittent pain, rare hemorrhages, dry desquamation, dermal ulceration and/or necrosis, partial onycholysis
Degree 3	Marked erythema, 10%–40% body surface area affected, moderate-persistent pain, bullae, moist-patchy desquamation, subcutaneous ulceration and/or necrosis, partial onycholysis
Degree 4	Severe erythema, >40% body surface area affected, severe-persistent pain, bullae and hemorrhage, moist-confluent desquamation, muscle/bone ulceration and/or necrosis, complete onycholysis

Source: Waselenko JK, MacVittie TJ, Blakely WF, et al. Medical management of the acute radiation syndrome: Recommendations of the Strategic National Stockpile Radiation Working Group [see comment]. *Ann Intern Med.* 2004;140:1037–1051.

RADIATION-INDUCED SKIN TOXICITY FOLLOWING FLUOROSCOPY

Prolonged skin exposure during fluoroscopically guided procedures (i.e., percutaneous intravascular procedures, etc.) is fraught with the potential for causing radiation-induced skin reactions. It is imperative that careful attention to dose rate, exposure time, and prior radiation exposure is taken into account with each procedure.[130,131] Skin reactions can range from none/minimal erythema to severe ulcerations and/or necrosis, requiring plastic surgical soft tissue coverage.[132,133] Although real-time monitoring of maximum skin dose is not possible in most cardiac intervention procedures, angiographic x-ray units display the patient's total entrance skin dose in real time. One can estimate maximum skin dose as approximately 50% of the total entrance skin dose for each target vessel.[134]

ENHANCEMENT OF RADIATION-INDUCED SKIN REACTIONS BY SYSTEMIC AGENTS

Numerous systemic agents (Table 44.5) have been described to enhance the effects of radiation on skin (radiosensitizers) and/or lead to the development of an inflammatory reaction called *radiation recall dermatitis* (RRD). A drug is typically considered a radiation-sensitizing agent when it causes enhanced skin reactions within a short interval of its administration and irradiation (i.e., <7 days).[196,197] The severity and risk of developing an enhanced radiation skin reaction decreases over time as the interval between drug administration and irradiation increases.[196,197] Long-term sequelae may include skin atrophy, fibrosis, and telangiectasias. Proposed mechanisms for radiation sensitization include diminished sublethal damage repair,

changes in cell cycle kinetics (i.e., increasing percentage of cells in the radiosensitive G2 and M phases), increased blood supply, and reoxygenation of the irradiated tissues.[196–201]

RRD is an inflammatory reaction that occurs following the administration of certain systemic agents in areas of skin that have been previously irradiated.[189,196,197] Similar to the skin reaction seen in radiation enhancement, the eruption of RRD is usually a well-demarcated, erythematous, macular-papular skin eruption that may be painful and exhibit desquamation and/or ulceration.[197,202] Generally, skin reactions occurring after longer time intervals (i.e., >7 days), between administration of the drug and the development of the skin reaction, are classified as RRD.[196,197] Additionally, RRD may occur after exposure to ultraviolet light.[203–205]

Histological findings in the epidermis and dermis can include epidermal dysplasia, necrosis, increased nuclear atypia, a mixed inflammatory infiltrate, dermal fibrosis, vasodilatation, atypical fibroblasts, solar elastosis, and pigmentation of the basal layer.[178,202] Although the exact mechanisms involved in the development of RRD are not known, multiple hypotheses have been suggested including radiation-induced vascular injury and increased permeability,[206] depleted and/or damaged epithelial stem cell populations,[207,208] sensitization of epithelial stem cells,[187] and idiosyncratic drug hypersensitivity reactions.[197,209,210]

RRD can occur within minutes to months after the administration of an inciting agent, and the route of administration may modify the kinetics of the presentation and resolution of this response (i.e., RRD seems to present and resolve more rapidly with intravenous vs. with oral administration).[171,176,206] The time interval between the radiation and the administration of the agent, which caused RRD, can be days or many years after radiation.[196,197] Some groups have suggested a dose-response relationship, where administration of higher doses of an agent may increase the risk of developing this reaction.[139] Additionally,

TABLE 44.5	Drugs Implicated in Radiation Sensitization and/or Radiation Recall Dermatitis		
Drug	*Radiation-Induced Reactions*	*Drug*	*Radiation-Induced Reactions*
Dactinomycin	Radiation sensitization[135,136] Radiation "recall reaction"[24,137]	Docetaxel/Paclitaxel	Radiation sensitization[163–166] Radiation "recall reaction"[167–169]
Dacarbazine	Radiation "recall reaction"[138]	Gemcitibine	Radiation sensitization[170]
Doxorubicin/Daunorubicin/ Idarubicin	Radiation sensitization[135,136] Radiation "recall reaction"[24,139,140]	Tamoxifen	Radiation "recall reaction"[171] Radiation "recall reaction"[172–174]
		Capecitabine	Radiation sensitization[175]
Bleomycin	Radiation sensitization[141–143] Radiation "recall reaction"[144]	6-Mercaptopurine	Radiation "recall reaction"[176] Radiation sensitization[177]
Oxaliplatin	Radiation "recall reaction"[145]	Cyclophosphamide	Radiation "recall reaction"[178–180]
Cisplatin	Radiation sensitization[146–148]	Lomustine	Radiation "recall reaction"[181]
Lantreotide	Radiation "recall reaction"[149]	Edatrexate/Trimetrexate	Radiation "recall reaction"[182,183]
Cetuximab	Radiation sensitization[150–152]	Etoposide	Radiation "recall reaction"[184]
Pemetrexed	Radiation "recall reaction"[153]	Cytarabine	Radiation "recall reaction"[181]
Hydroxyurea	Radiation sensitization[154] Radiation "recall reaction"[155]	Vinblastine Carmustine	Radiation "recall reaction"[185] Radiation sensitization[186]
Methotrexate	Radiation sensitization[141,154] Radiation "recall reaction"[156]	Simvastatin Tuberculosis medications (rifampin,	Radiation "recall reaction"[187] Radiation "recall reaction"[188]
Melphalan	Radiation "recall reaction"[157]	isoniazide, pyrazinamide)	
Arsenic trioxide	Radiation "recall reaction"[158]	Gatifloxacin/Levofloxacin	Radiation "recall reaction"[189–191]
Mitomycin-C	Radiation sensitization[141,159]	Interferon α-2b	Radiation "recall reaction"[192]
Fluorouracil	Radiation sensitization[148,160,161] Radiation "recall reaction"[162]	Phenteramine Cefazolin/Cefotetan	Radiation "recall reaction"[193] Radiation "recall reaction"[194,195]

there are reports of a radiation dose-response relationship in which the risk of developing a recall reaction may be contingent upon exceeding a threshold dose.[144,196,197,211]

Management of RRD frequently involves the administration of corticosteroids, non–steroidal anti-inflammatory agents, antihistamines, and withdrawal of the inciting drug.[196,197] Mild cases of RRD can be managed conservatively, without anti-inflammatory medications, as they typically resolve spontaneously within days to weeks.[196,197]

Tamoxifen has been reported by some groups to increase the risk of developing radiation fibrosis when administered following[212] or concurrently with radiation therapy[213–215]; however, this has not been observed in all studies.[216–218] Although the mechanisms of action are not understood, Tamoxifen is reported to be an effective first-line treatment for reducing fibrosis in patients with idiopathic retroperitoneal fibrosis.[219,220] The conflicting data and the variable profibrogenic and antifibrogenic responses of Tamoxifen must be clarified in future studies to better understand the mechanisms of action on the potential fibrogenic pathway when administered with radiation.

STRATEGIES FOR REDUCING RADIATION-INDUCED SKIN TOXICITY

BEAM ENERGY

Decreasing dose to the skin with external beam radiation may be able to reduce the risk of developing permanent alopecia and other radiation-induced skin changes.[15] The use of higher energy photons (i.e., 10 MV vs. 6 MV, Fig. 44.2), presumably due to greater "skin-sparing" effects, has been correlated with a lower risk of permanent alopecia.[15] Higher beam energies

are associated with decreased acute skin reactions in patients undergoing EBRT after breast-conserving surgery.[221] In addition to beam energy, employing multiple, non–coplanar beams (i.e., rotational arcs, intensity-modulated radiation therapy (IMRT), and non–coplanar conventional radiation therapy techniques) can reduce the higher skin doses associated with overlapping fields.[15,222,223]

INTENSITY-MODULATED RADIATION THERAPY

IMRT and helical therapy have been reported to be able to deliver lower doses to normal non–target breast tissue compared to 3D conformal techniques, without compromising dose to the target volume.[224–226] In a single institution study of 281 patients treated with breast-conserving surgery and IMRT to the whole breast, the authors reported good to excellent cosmetic results in 99% of patients, at 12 months follow-up; additionally no patients developed telangiectasias or significant fibrosis.[227] In a multicenter, double-blind, prospective, randomized controlled trial, 358 patients were allocated to receive either whole-breast IMRT or standard whole-breast radiation (tangent beams using wedges).[228] The authors reported significantly less acute radiation skin toxicity (i.e., moist desquamation) in patients who received IMRT versus standard radiation therapy; 31.2% and 47.8%, respectively. These favorable, albeit early, results were credited to tight dose-volume constraints and uniform dose homogeneity throughout the breast with the use of IMRT.

In another study, the authors compared the results of 93 patients who underwent breast-conserving surgery followed by whole-breast IMRT (median dose, 45 Gy followed by a boost to 61 Gy) to that of a control cohort of 79 patients who were treated with wedge-based conventional radiation therapy.[94]

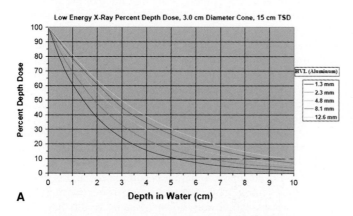

A

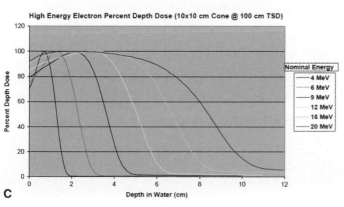

C

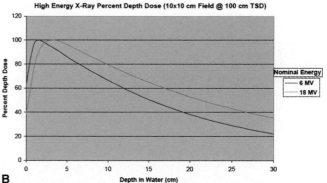

B

Figure 44.2. Depth dose curves for various energies of photons and electrons. **A**: The surface (skin) dose for low-energy x-ray beams (≤150 kVp) is 100% (maximum dose, D_{max}). To achieve significant dose at depth, extremely high surface doses are required. This situation is improved somewhat by "filters" that preferentially absorb lower-energy, less penetrating photons. **B**: Megavoltage photons are more penetrating than kilovoltage and have important skin-sparing properties. Surface dose *decreases* with increasing photon energy. 6-MV photons have a surface dose 60% of D_{max} compared to 40% for 18 MV. D_{max} is reached at a depth of 1.5 cm for the 6-MV compared to 3.5 cm for 18 MV. There is then comparable attenuation of the two beams at subsequent depths. **C**: Megavoltage electrons demonstrate less skin sparing and are less penetrating than photons of comparable energies. Surface dose *increases* with increasing electron energy, D_{max} is reached at a depth dependent on electron energy and beam attenuation (dose fall off with depth) is much more rapid than in the case of photons.

They reported a significant reduction in acute grade 2 or higher radiation dermatitis, edema, and hyperpigmentation in favor of treatment with IMRT. Chronic grade 2 or higher breast edema was also significantly reduced with IMRT, although there was no significant difference in cosmesis scores between the two groups. In a small study ($n = 24$ patients), three types of preoperative RT plans (conventional plan, 3D-CRT plan, and IMRT plan) for extremity soft tissue sarcoma was compared to determine the amount of dose reduction possible to the planned surgical skin flaps required for tumor resection and wound closure, without compromising target coverage.[73] The authors reported that the IMRT plans substantially lowered the dose to the future surgical skin flaps, sparing a greater percentage of this structure's volume without compromising target (tumor) coverage; an average of 86.4% of the planned skin flaps received ≥30 Gy in the original plans compared with 83.4% in the conformal plans and only 34.0% in the IMRT plans ($p = 0.0001$). IMRT improved target conformality compared with the original and conformal plans (1.27, 2.34, and 1.76, respectively, $p = 0.0001$).

Longer follow-up will be necessary to confirm whether these results will translate to improved late radiation-induced skin effects.

STEREOTACTIC BODY RADIATION THERAPY

It is important when planning SBRT treatments, which employ large fraction sizes, that careful attention be paid to the calculated skin and subcutaneous tissue doses. Increased acute (i.e., acute radiation dermatitis and desquamation) and late effects (i.e., necrosis, painful subcutaneous fibrosis) have been reported with high skin doses.[79,81,82,229,230] Precise dose/volume constraints are not currently available; however, some groups have proposed guidelines based on case reports of toxicity, historical data, and mathematical models (see Table 44.3).

PARTIAL BREAST IRRADIATION

As previously mentioned, late fibrosis and worse cosmetic outcomes are more common with larger treatment volumes.[93] Partial breast radiation therapy techniques significantly reduce the volume of skin receiving higher doses of radiation compared to whole-breast radiation.[231] With proper patient selection and technique, cosmetic outcomes have been reported to be good to excellent in the vast majority of cases.[232–234] Partial breast irradiation (PBI) can be accomplished with 3D conformal EBRT (i.e., conventional 3D conformal radiation therapy, IMRT, helical tomotherapy, etc.), intraoperative radiation therapy (IORT) (electrons or kilovoltage x-rays), various LDR and HDR brachytherapy techniques (i.e., multiplanar/multicatheter implants, MammoSite, SAVI, Contura, etc.), or proton beam radiation therapy.[235–238] The American Society of Breast Surgeons recommends APBI only in patients with tumors <3 cm in size.[239] Additionally, careful attention of the distance from the high-dose treatment volume to the skin surface is crucial in dosimetric planning.[90,240]

In a large prospective study ($n = 1,449$ cases) of patients who underwent HDR APBI, using the MammoSite device, good-to-excellent cosmetic results were recorded in 93% of patients, at a median follow-up of 30.1 months.[237] A preliminary report of the same trial, at 36 months median follow-up, notes that 9.7% of the treated breasts have developed telangiectasias at last follow-up.[78] Bra cup sizes A or B, smaller balloon-to-skin distances, and smaller balloon fill volumes (≤50 mL) were all associated with increased telangiectasia formation.

Skin dose can be minimized with careful dosimetric planning of APBI treatments by either increasing the source to skin distance or by modified loading/dwell position timing. The authors of a retrospective study of 483 patients who were treated with APBI (using the MammoSite device) reported that skin spacing of <6 mm from the balloon surface to the skin was associated with an increased risk of severe acute skin reaction ($p = 0.0178$) and telangiectasia ($p = 0.0280$).[76] In a study of 191 patients, the use of margins of 7 mm or greater from the surface of the MammoSite balloon to the skin was associated with significantly improved cosmetic results and a lower incidence of acute radiation dermatitis.[77] Preliminary reports of multicatheter devices (SAVI and Contura) demonstrate that significantly lower skin doses are achievable, than with the single lumen MammoSite device, in the treatment of tumor cavities within 7 to 10 mm of the skin surface.[241–243]

IORT, performed at the time of breast-conserving surgery, can been similarly used to deliver either a boost or a definitive adjuvant radiation dose following breast-conserving surgery. In a study of 50 patients who underwent lumpectomy and a single 10-Gy intraoperative electron radiation therapy (IOERT) boost followed by 50-Gy EBRT, good to excellent long-term (9.1-year median follow-up) cosmetic results were recorded in all patients; only 12% patients developed grade 2 late subcutaneous fibrosis.[244] Ivaldi et al.[245] published their results on the use of a single 12-Gy IOERT boost, in 211 patients at the time of breast-conserving surgery. This was then followed by a hypofractionated whole-breast EBRT regimen (13 daily fractions of 2.85 Gy). The authors reported the following maximal acute skin toxicity (1 month after treatment): 3.8% grade 3, 28.6% grade 2, 67.6% grade 1, and no grade 0 or grade 4 cases. The recorded late skin toxicity was grade 4 in 1 patient (0.9%), grade 3 in 1 patient, and grade 2 or less in 106 patients (98.2%). Veronesi et al.[246] reported their preliminary findings on 590 patients who underwent breast-conserving surgery followed by a single 21-Gy IOERT dose (biologically equivalent to 58–60 Gy in 1.8–2.0 Gy fractions). At a median follow-up of 20 months, only 3.2% of patients developed fibrosis (with only one patient developing severe fibrosis).

Dose homogeneity throughout the irradiated tissue volume is directly correlated with cosmetic outcomes. Patients who have brachytherapy implants with a lower dose homogeneity index (DHI) have been shown to have less skin toxicity and better cosmetic results.[95] Additionally, as the volume of tissue receiving higher doses increases, significantly worse cosmetic results have been reported.[95,247] These dosimetric factors are important in designing implants with less toxicity and superior cosmetic results.

PARTICLE BEAM RADIATION THERAPY

High linear energy transfer (LET) particle therapies (i.e., carbon ions, neutrons, pions, etc.) are associated with significantly increased late normal tissue toxicities when compared to photon therapy.[248–250] In one study of 232 radiation sites treated for soft tissue sarcomas (6.2 MeV, fast neutrons, 6–12 Gy total dose), severe fibrosis of the subcutaneous tissues occurred in 40% after 2 years.[251] In another study of 83 radiation sites treated for soft tissue sarcomas (STSs), the authors reported moderate or severe fibrosis in 13% of the cases who received

<13.4 Gy and in 54% of the cases who received a higher total dose.[252] The authors of a small feasibility study, of 20 patients who received proton beam APBI (using two to four separate beams, ten daily fractions of 4 cobalt Gray equivalents), reported only occasional RTOG grade 1 to 2 acute skin toxicity following treatment.[238] Compared to two methods of photon PBI (including reduced tangential fields and five-field conformal techniques), dose-volume histogram analysis revealed that the use of proton beams provided a significant reduction in doses to the ipsilateral breast and skin. A variety of treatment planning techniques can be employed to reduce the skin dose including using mixed-photon/particle treatment plans, increasing the number of non–overlapping beams, and employing scanning particle beam technology.[97,253]

BODY FIXATION DEVICES AND PATIENT-POSITIONING TECHNIQUES

The use of fixation devices in a radiation beam may act as bolus when in contact with the underlying skin and should be taken into account when attempting to minimize higher skin doses.[254] The use of repositioning devices (i.e., plastic ring/tube) can be employed in patients with large or flaccid breasts during simulation and treatment in order to prevent the breast from lying directly on the abdominal wall.[255] These devices have been reported to decrease the risk of developing significant skin reactions (acute: moist desquamation; late: fibrosis and telangiectasias) in the inframammary fold. Prone positioning is another method that has been shown to reduce the inhomogeneities in the inframammary skin fold in these patients.[256–258] Treatment of the tumor bed boost volume in breast cancer patients using a lateral decubitus positioning for the electron boost allows for a decrease in the distance from the skin to the deepest area of the target volume. This improves electron coverage of the tumor bed and reduces the entrance dose to the skin.[259]

SURFACE DOSIMETRY CALCULATIONS AND MEASUREMENTS

Careful attention to skin dose, during radiation planning, may lead to decreased skin toxicities. Accurate surface dosimetric measurements may allow for adjustments in radiation dose and treatment volumes, particularly when the skin is not considered target tissue. The use of 3D image-guided brachytherapy (i.e., CT imaging with implant in place) and in vivo skin surface dosimetry (i.e., metal-oxide-semiconductor field-effect transistor (MOSFET) and film dosimetry) permits adjustments to be made in the brachytherapy treatment plan to account for the actual source to skin distances.[260]

TOPICAL AND SYSTEMIC AGENTS MAY REDUCE RADIATION-INDUCED SKIN EFFECTS

Radioprotection of hair follicles and skin using topical or systemic agents has been explored in both animal and human models. Animal experiments have demonstrated significant reductions in temporary alopecia and acute skin reactions with some agents including prostaglandin E_2, WR-2721, nitroxide, keratinocyte growth factor, Panax ginseng, caffeine, circumin, celecoxib, vitamin C, ergotein, allopurinol gel, growth hormone, esculentoside A.[261–274]

Pentoxifylline (with or without alpha-tocopherol) has been reported to decrease radiation-induced subcutaneous fibrosis.[30,275] Pentoxifylline is a xanthine derivative that appears to inhibit platelet aggregation and enhance microvascular blood flow; however, the exact mechanisms explaining how this agent reduces fibrosis is not known. The optimal doses and duration of treatment with pentoxifylline are also not known, but some data suggest that long-term (>2–3 years) use may be necessary to obtain and maintain the best results.[30]

Aloe vera has been proposed to exhibit anti-inflammatory properties and is commonly applied to the skin by patients undergoing radiation to reduce the severity of radiation dermatitis.[276] Most groups have not shown a significant reduction or prevention of radiation dermatitis with the application of topical aloe vera.[277–280]

In a small prospective randomized clinical trial of 45 pediatric patients who underwent radiation therapy and were randomized to either topical application of an anionic polar phospholipid (APP)–based cream or an aloe vera–based gel, the authors reported significantly improved variables favoring APP cream use; dryness ($p = 0.002$) and erythema ($p = 0.002$).[281]

Topical steroids appear to delay the time to development of acute radiation dermatitis, but do not prevent it.[282] Topical trolamine (a salicylate cream) has not been shown to reduce acute radiation dermatitis in a large prospective randomized controlled trial.[283]

A phase three, double-blind trial of 100 patients undergoing radiation therapy for treatment of head and neck cancers demonstrated a significant reduction in acute grade 3 radiation dermatitis in patients randomized to an oral zinc supplement compared to a placebo-controlled cohort.[284] Additionally, the patients receiving the zinc supplement had a delayed onset of grade 2 dermatitis compared to the control patients.

Human studies have demonstrated reductions in the acute skin reactions using topical superoxide dismutase or orgotein (a metalloprotein form of superoxide dismutase).[285,286] In a study by Halperin et al.,[287] topical vitamin C applied to the scalp of patients undergoing whole-brain radiation therapy did not reduce the incidence of acute radiation dermatitis.

In a small, randomized controlled study of 61 patients who were undergoing radiation therapy for vulvar cancer, the authors reported a significant reduction in severity and duration of acute radiation dermatitis in patients who received a topical application of granulocyte-macrophage colony-stimulating factor (GM-CSF) and steroid cream compared to those who received a steroid cream alone.[288]

The nitroxide agent, Tempol, has been reported to have radioprotective effects on hair follicles when applied topical to the scalp prior to whole-brain radiation therapy. A small phase one study demonstrated that the application of a topical solution of Tempol, 15 minutes before each fraction of radiation treatment, appeared to reduce the degree of acute alopecia in short-term follow-up.[289]

Long-term follow-up data for the efficacy of these agents in preventing permanent alopecia and other late radiation effects remain unknown.[15]

PHOTOBIOMODULATION AND LASER THERAPY

Low-energy lasers (also known as *cold lasers*) and light-emitting diodes (LEDs) have been reported to reduce the acute effects of radiation on skin and mucous membranes.[290,291] Proposed mechanisms of action of low-energy lasers and LEDs encompass a vast area of research called *photobiomodulation*. The basic science research on low-level light therapy (LLLT) demonstrates that it promotes wound healing, reduces inflammation and pain, through effects on multiple mechanisms (Table 44.6).

In a small study, LED photomodulation has been reported to reduce acute skin reactions in patients undergoing whole-breast IMRT after breast-conserving surgery.[290] The authors compared the acute skin reactions in 19 patients who received LED exposure to the irradiated breast (following each treatment) to an age-matched control cohort; LED cohort: 94.7% grade 0 or 1 reaction and 5.3% grade 2 reaction, control cohort: 14.3% grade 1 reaction, 85.7% grade 2 or 3 reaction.[290] Treatment interruptions were required in 67.9% of patients in the control cohort, compared to only 5.3% in the LED-treated cohort. These results were not confirmed in a preliminary report of a small phase three trial comparing whole-breast irradiation with and without daily LED photomodulation; no difference in the incidence or degree of radiation dermatitis was noted between the two arms.[306]

Radiation-induced mucositis was significantly reduced in a double-blind study, of 30 patients treated with radiation therapy for cancers of the head and neck.[307] Patients were randomized to receive daily, low-energy helium-neon laser therapy (25–60 mW, He–Ne, wavelength 632.8 nm) or placebo laser treatment throughout their course of radiation therapy. The patients in the true laser arm had significant reductions in grade 3 mucositis (8% vs. 35%) and severe pain (2% vs. 24%).

In a report by Schindl et al.,[308] low-intensity (power: 30 mW, wavelength: 632.8 nm, intensity: 3 mW/cm^2) helium-neon laser irradiation was shown to be effective in the induction of wound healing of chronic radiation-induced skin ulcers after radiation therapy. Patients were treated three times weekly with a dose of 30 J/cm^2. Complete wound closure was achieved within 5 to 8 weeks in the three patients described in this report.

Telangiectasias, which occur in areas of skin that receive high radiation doses, have been effectively treated using high-energy lasers (i.e., pulsed-dye laser).[309] High-energy lasers are ablative and work through thermal reactions with the tissues.

TABLE 44.6	**Proposed Mechanisms of Action for Stimulating Wound Healing with LLLT**

Mechanisms of Action

Enhanced wound healing (i.e., increased tensile strength, reduced wound-healing time, reduced inflammatory cell migration, increased mitochondrial activity, increases fibroblast cell migration, increases angiogenesis, reduction of edema)[292–297]

Increased cellular metabolism (i.e., increased ATP production, increased mitochondrial activity)[293,298]

Increases blood perfusion (i.e., increases nitric oxide synthase)[299]

Increases angiogenesis (i.e., increases VEGF, endothelial cell proliferation)[299,300]

Reduces inflammation (i.e., reduces COX-2 mRNA, reduces myeloperoxide activity, reduces NF-kappa B activation, reduction of reactive oxygen species)[301–304]

Non–opioid-dependent mechanisms responsible for pain control (i.e., pain control involves hyperalgesic mediators instead of peripheral opioid receptors)[305]

THERAPEUTIC APPROACHES FOR MANAGING RADIATION-INDUCED SKIN MORBIDITY

SKIN CARE

Prior to initiating RT, patients should be instructed about appropriate skin care. To avoid excessive irritation and dryness, the skin should be gently cleaned using a neutral pH, moisturizing soap or cleanser.[310] Friction to the irradiated skin should be minimized.[311]

To help protect against excessive skin dryness (which occurs as a result of the loss of sweat and sebaceous gland function), hydrophilic moisturizing products, which absorb water and act as mild lubricants, are often recommended.[312] Products containing alcohol or menthol should be avoided, as they remove natural lipids and are drying to the skin.[310]

The use of underarm deodorants during radiation therapy for breast cancer is often discouraged; however, there was no evidence of an increase in acute skin toxicity in a small phase three trial that investigated this question (radiation therapy with and without deodorant).[313]

Pruritis can be treated with colloidal oatmeal baths, cornstarch, and/or mild topical steroids (i.e., hydrocortisone cream 1%).[310] Topical corticosteroids have been shown to reduce the inflammation associated with acute radiation dermatitis; however, they should be used with caution as they may delay skin healing and cause atrophy of dermal collagen, increasing the susceptibility to infection.[310,314–316]

Areas of moist desquamation can be kept clean using astringent soaks and mild cleansers (i.e., diluted hydrogen peroxide). Antibiotic creams (i.e., silver sulfadiazine 1%) may be used to prevent infection from Gram-positive and Gram-negative bacteria and *Candida albicans*.[310] If cellulitis is suspected clinically, topical and/or systemic antibiotics should be started. Hydrocolloidal wound dressings (i.e., DuoDERM; ConvaTec, a Bristol-Meyers Squibb Company, Princeton, NJ) and/or non–adherent films (i.e., Tegaderm; 3M Health Care, St Paul, MN) may be placed on areas of moist desquamation to promote enzymatic lysis of necrotic tissue, thereby enhancing inflammatory phagocytosis of necrotic debris and bacteria.[317] Wound dressings, additionally, serve as a barrier from external debris and bacteria, prevent soiling of clothing, and decrease friction to the underlying skin.[310] The authors of a prospective randomized controlled trial, comparing dry dressings to hydrogel dressings in 357 patients with moist desquamation, recently reported that hydrogel dressings failed to improve pain symptoms and actually delayed healing.[318]

Irradiated skin is more sensitive to UV light; therefore, patients should also be instructed to limit the exposure of the irradiated skin (during and after treatment) to sunlight or other sources of UV light (i.e., tanning beds, etc.). Sunscreen with an SPF of 15 or greater is recommended to any areas of previously irradiated skin.[310] To help prevent further dryness and irritation, fragrances and perfumes should not be applied to the irradiated skin. Frequently, irradiated skin remains permanently dry (xerosis) after a course of treatment. A moisturizing skin cleanser with neutral-pH detergents is useful to keep the skin clean and moisturized.[310]

To date, there is insufficient evidence to support or refute specific topical or oral agents for the prevention or management of acute skin reaction.[319]

HYPERBARIC OXYGEN THERAPY

Clinical studies have suggested that hyperbaric oxygen therapy (HBOT) is effective in mitigating various radiation-induced toxicities, particularly osteoradionecrosis, radiation cystitis, radiation proctitis, and chronic non–healing ulcers.[320,321] Multiple mechanisms of action have been proposed that may explain the effects of HBOT on the stimulation of wound healing and the repair of late radiation effects: eradication of anaerobic bacteria (i.e., through the temporary increase in tissue oxygenation, augmentation of neutrophil bactericidal activity), enhanced angiogenesis (stimulated by high oxygen tension in the tissue), and fibroblast proliferation.[320,322,323] HBOT protocols, for the treatment/prevention of osteoradionecrosis and soft tissue radionecrosis, may employ 20 to 30 sessions at 2.4 to 2.8 atmospheres of pressure (atm) delivered over approximately 90 minutes.[321]

SUMMARY

In this chapter, we identified many of the endogenous and exogenous factors that may lead to radiation-induced skin injury. The underlying mechanisms involved in this complex process continue to be the subject of ongoing research. As we develop a greater understanding of these mechanisms and the variables that increase the potential for radiation injury, it is conceivable that with the addition of specific biological modifiers and/or skin-sparing radiation therapy techniques, skin toxicity will be able to be minimized without compromising treatment efficacy.

The views expressed in this article are those of the authors and do not reflect the official policy or position of the Department of the Navy, Department of Defense, or the US Government.

REFERENCES

1. Hall EJ. *Radiobiology for the Radiologist.* 5th ed. Philadelphia, PA: Lippincott Williams & Wilkins; 2000.
2. Tessmer CF. Radiation effects in skin. In: Berdjis CC, ed. *Pathology of Irradiation.* Baltimore, MD: Williams & Wilkins; 1971:146–170.
3. Rubin P, Casarett GW. *Clinical Radiation Pathology.* Vol 2. Philadelphia, PA: W.B Saunders; 1968.
4. Fajardo LF. *Skin Pathology of Radiation Injury.* New York, NY: Masson Publishing; 1982: 186–200.
5. Radiation Therapy Oncology Group, European Organisation for Research and Treatment of Cancer. Acute radiation morbidity scoring criteria. Available at: http://www.rtog.org/members/toxicity/acute.html. Accessed 9/13/08.
6. Radiation Therapy Oncology Group, European Organisation for Research and Treatment of Cancer. RTOG/EORTC late radiation morbidity scoring schema. Available at: http://www.rtog.org/members/toxicity/late.html. Accessed 9/13/08.
7. Withers HR, McBride WH. Radiation effects on normal tissues. In: Meyer JL, ed. *Radiation Injury. Advances in Management and Prevention.* Vol 32. Basel: Karger; 1999:1–8.
8. Travis EL. Genetic susceptibility to late normal tissue injury. *Semin Radiat Oncol.* 2007;17:149 155.
9. Schreiber D, Bell RS, Wunder JS, et al. Evaluating function and health related quality of life in patients treated for extremity soft tissue sarcoma. *Qual Life Res.* 2006;15:1439–1446.
10. Timmerman RD. An overview of hypofractionation and introduction to this issue of seminars in radiation oncology. *Semin Radiat Oncol.* 2008;18:215–222.
11. Jolles B, Harrison RG. Enzymic processes and vascular changes in the skin radiation reaction. *Br J Radiol.* 1966;39:12–18.
12. Brush J, Lipnick SL, Phillips T, et al. Molecular mechanisms of late normal tissue injury. *Semin Radiat Oncol.* 2007;17:121–130.
13. Archambeau JO, Pezner R, Wasserman T. Pathophysiology of irradiated skin and breast. *Int J Radiat Oncol Biol Phys.* 1995;31:1171–1185.
14. Kaanders JH, Ang KK. Early reactions as dose-limiting factors in radiotherapy. *Semin Radiat Oncol.* 1994;4:55–67.
15. Lawenda BD, Gagne HM, Gierga DP, et al. Permanent alopecia after cranial irradiation: Dose-response relationship [see comment]. *Int J Radiat Oncol Biol Phys.* 2004;60:879–887.
16. Stram DO, Mizuno S. Analysis of the DS86 atomic bomb radiation dosimetry methods using data on severe epilation. *Radiat Res.* 1989;117:93–113.
17. Olsen EA. Anagen hair loss: Radiation. In: Olsen EA, ed. *Disorders of Hair Growth: Diagnosis and Treatment.* New York, NY: McGraw Hill; 1994:225–226.
18. Ackerman AB. *Histologic Diagnosis of Inflammatory Skin Diseases.* Philadelphia, PA: Lea & Febiger; 1978:201–202, 765–767.
19. National Cancer Institute CTC Development Team. Common terminology criteria for adverse events v3.0. Available at: http://ctep.cancer.gov/forms/CTCAEv3.pdf. Accessed 9/17/08.
20. National Cancer Institute CTC Development Team. Common terminology criteria for adverse events – Frequently asked questions. Available at: https://webapps.ctep.nci.nih.gov/webobjs/ctc/webhelpfaq/Welcome_to_CTCAE.htm. Accessed 9/17/08.
21. Turesson I, Thames HD. Repair capacity and kinetics of human skin during fractionated radiotherapy: Erythema, desquamation, and telangiectasia after 3 and 5 year's follow-up. *Radiother Oncol.* 1989;15:169–188.
22. Warren S. Radiation effects on the skin. In: Helwig EB, Mostofi FK, eds. *The Skin.* Baltimore, MD: Williams & Wilkins; 1971:261–278.
23. Herrmann T, Baumann M, Dörr W. *Clinical Radiation Biology.* Munich, Germany: Elsevier; 2006.
24. Phillips TL, Fu KK. Quantification of combined radiation therapy and chemotherapy effects on critical normal tissues. *Cancer.* 1976;37:1186–1200.
25. Remy J, Wegrowski J, Crechet F, et al. Long-term overproduction of collagen in radiation-induced fibrosis. *Radiat Res.* 1991;125:14–19.
26. Stewart JR, Fajardo LF. Radiation-induced heart disease. Clinical and experimental aspects. *Radiol Clin North Am.* 1971;9:511–531.
27. Fajardo LF. *General Morphology. Pathology of Radiation Injury.* New York, NY: Masson Publishing; 1982:6–14.
28. Fajardo LF, Berthrong M. Radiation injury in surgical pathology. Part I. *Am J Surg Pathol.* 1978;2:159–199.
29. Delanian S, Lefaix JL. Current management for late normal tissue injury: Radiation-induced fibrosis and necrosis. *Semin Radiat Oncol.* 2007;17:99–107.
30. Delanian S, Porcher R, Rudant J, et al. Kinetics of response to long-term treatment combining pentoxifylline and tocopherol in patients with superficial radiation-induced fibrosis [see comment]. *J Clin Oncol.* 2005;23:8570–8579.
31. Haase O, Rodemann HP. Fibrosis and cytokine mechanisms: Relevant in hadron therapy? *Radiother Oncol.* 2004;73(suppl 2):S144–S147.
32. Barcellos-Hoff MH. How do tissues respond to damage at the cellular level? The role of cytokines in irradiated tissues. *Radiat Res.* 1998;150:S109–S120.
33. Devalia HL, Mansfield L. Radiotherapy and wound healing. *Int Wound J.* 2008;5:40–44.
34. Autio P, Saarto T, Tenhunen M, et al. Demonstration of increased collagen synthesis in irradiated human skin in vivo. *Br J Cancer.* 1998;77:2331–2335.
35. Bentzen SM. Preventing or reducing late side effects of radiation therapy: Radiobiology meets molecular pathology. *Nat Rev Cancer.* 2006;6:702–713.
36. Martin M, Lefaix J, Delanian S. TGF-beta1 and radiation fibrosis: A master switch and a specific therapeutic target? *Int J Radiat Oncol Biol Phys.* 2000;47:277–290.
37. Vozenin-Brotons MC, Milliat F, Sabourin JC, et al. Fibrogenic signals in patients with radiation enteritis are associated with increased connective tissue growth factor expression. *Int J Radiat Oncol Biol Phys.* 2003;56:561–572.
38. Yamamoto T, Eckes B, Mauch C, et al. Monocyte chemoattractant protein-1 enhances gene expression and synthesis of matrix metalloproteinase-1 in human fibroblasts by an autocrine IL-1 alpha loop. *J Immunol.* 2000;164:6174–6179.
39. Liu W, Ding I, Chen K, et al. Interleukin 1beta (IL1B) signaling is a critical component of radiation-induced skin fibrosis. *Radiat Res.* 2006;165:181–191.
40. Romero LI, Zhang DN, Herron GS, et al. Interleukin-1 induces major phenotypic changes in human skin microvascular endothelial cells. *J Cell Physiol.* 1997;173:84–92.
41. Muller K, Meineke V. Radiation-induced alterations in cytokine production by skin cells. *Exp Hematol.* 2007;35:96–104.
42. Rodemann HP, Bamberg M. Cellular basis of radiation-induced fibrosis. *Radiother Oncol.* 1995;35:83–90.
43. Burger A, Loffler H, Bamberg M, et al. Molecular and cellular basis of radiation fibrosis. *Int J Radiat Biol.* 1998;73:401–408.
44. Riedel K, Kremer T, Ryssel H, et al. TGF-beta antisense oligonucleotides modulate expression of matrix metalloproteinases in isolated fibroblasts from radiated skin. *In Vivo.* 2008;22:1–7.
45. Haydont V, Riser BL, Aigueperse J, et al. Specific signals involved in the long-term maintenance of radiation-induced fibrogenic differentiation: A role for CCN2 and low concentration of TGF-beta1. *Am J Physiol Cell Physiol.* 2008;294:C1332–C1341.
46. Roberts AB, Russo A, Felici A, et al. Smad3: a key player in pathogenetic mechanisms dependent on TGF-beta. *Ann N Y Acad Sci.* 2003;995:1–10.
47. Kaufman SA, DiPetrillo TA, Price LL, et al. Long-term outcome and toxicity in a Phase I/II trial using high-dose-rate multicatheter interstitial brachytherapy for T1/T2 breast cancer. *Brachytherapy.* 2007;6:286–292.
48. Bentzen SM, Overgaard M. Relationship between early and late normal-tissue injury after postmastectomy radiotherapy. *Radiother Oncol.* 1991;20:159–165.
49. Perera F, Chisela F, Stitt L, et al. TLD skin dose measurements and acute and late effects after lumpectomy and high-dose-rate brachytherapy only for early breast cancer. *Int J Radiat Oncol Biol Phys.* 2005;62:1283–1290.
50. Hopewell JW. The skin: Its structure and response to ionizing radiation. *Int J Radiat Biol.* 1990;57:751–773.
51. Pack GT, Davis J. Radiation cancer of the skin. *Radiology.* 1965;84:436–442.
52. Martin H, Strong E, Spiro RH. Radiation-induced skin cancer of the head and neck. *Cancer.* 1970;25:61–71.
53. Cannon B, Randolph JG, Murry JE. Malignant irradiation for benign conditions. *N Engl J Med.* 1959;260:197–202.
54. Glucksman A, Lamerton LF, Mayneord WV. Carcinogenic effects of radiation. *Cancer.* 1957;1:497–539.
55. Rachmaninoff N, McDonald JR, Cook JC. Tumors of skin following irradiations. *Am J Clin Pathol.* 1961;36:427–437.

56. Kyoizumi S, Suzuki T, Teraoka S, et al. Radiation sensitivity of human hair follicles in SCID-hu mice. *Radiat Res.* 1998;149:11–18.

57. Valentin J. Avoidance of radiation injuries from medical interventional procedures. *Ann ICRP.* 2000;30:7–67.

58. Sieber VK, Sugden EM, Alcock CJ, et al. Reduction in the diameter of human hairs following irradiation. *Br J Radiol.* 1992;65:148–151.

59. Tibbs MK. Wound healing following radiation therapy: a review. *Radiother Oncol.* 1997;42:99–106.

60. Cannon CP, Ballo MT, Zagars GK, et al. Complications of combined modality treatment of primary lower extremity soft-tissue sarcomas. *Cancer.* 2006;107:2455–2461.

61. Davis AM, O'Sullivan B, Turcotte R, et al. Late radiation morbidity following randomization to preoperative versus postoperative radiotherapy in extremity soft tissue sarcoma. *Radiother Oncol.* 2005;75:48–53.

62. O'Sullivan B, Gullane P, Irish J, et al. Preoperative radiotherapy for adult head and neck soft tissue sarcoma: Assessment of wound complication rates and cancer outcome in a prospective series. *World J Surg.* 2003;27:875–883.

63. Hill RP, Kaspler P, Griffin AM, et al. Studies of the in vivo radiosensitivity of human skin fibroblasts. *Radiother Oncol.* 2007;84:75–83.

64. Ogawa R, Miyashita T, Hyakusoku H, et al. Postoperative radiation protocol for keloids and hypertrophic scars: Statistical analysis of 370 sites followed for over 18 months. *Ann Plast Surg.* 2007;59:688–691.

65. Isohashi F, Inoue T, Xing S, et al. Postoperative irradiation for pterygium: Retrospective analysis of 1,253 patients from the Osaka University Hospital. *Strahlenther Onkol.* 2006;182:437–442.

66. Ulutin HC, Pak Y. Endovascular radiotherapy for stenosis after percutaneous transluminal coronary angioplasty. *Radiat Med.* 2001;19:175–179.

67. Stralman K, Mollerup CL, Kristoffersen US, et al. Long-term outcome after mastectomy with immediate breast reconstruction. *Acta Oncol.* 2008;47:704–708.

68. Carlson GW, Page AL, Peters K, et al. Effects of radiation therapy on pedicled transverse rectus abdominis myocutaneous flap breast reconstruction. *Ann Plast Surg.* 2008;60:568–572.

69. Jugenburg M, Disa JJ, Pusic AL, et al. Impact of radiotherapy on breast reconstruction. *Clin Plast Surg.* 2007;34:29–37; abstract v–vi.

70. Most MD, Allori AC, Hu K, et al. Feasibility of flap reconstruction in conjunction with intraoperative radiation therapy for advanced and recurrent head and neck cancer. *Laryngoscope.* 2008;118:69–74.

71. Wong JS, Ho AY, Kaelin CM, et al. Incidence of major corrective surgery after post-mastectomy breast reconstruction and radiation therapy. *Breast J.* 2008;14:49–54.

72. Heller L, Ballo MT, Cormier JN, et al. Staged reconstruction for resection wounds in sarcoma patients treated with brachytherapy. *Ann Plast Surg.* 2008;60:58–63.

73. Griffin AM, Euler CI, Sharpe MB, et al. Radiation planning comparison for superficial tissue avoidance in radiotherapy for soft tissue sarcoma of the lower extremity. *Int J Radiat Oncol Biol Phys.* 2007;67:847–856.

74. Rupprecht R, Lippold A, Auras C, et al. Late side-effects with cosmetic relevance following soft X-ray therapy of cutaneous neoplasias. *J Eur Acad Dermatol Venereol.* 2007;21:178–185.

75. Bartelink H, Horiot JC, Poortmans PM, et al. Impact of a higher radiation dose on local control and survival in breast-conserving therapy of early breast cancer: 10-year results of the randomized boost versus no boost EORTC 22881-10882 trial. *J Clin Oncol.* 2007;25:3259–3265.

76. Cuttino LW, Keisch M, Jenrette JM, et al. Multi-institutional experience using the MammoSite radiation therapy system in the treatment of early-stage breast cancer: 2-year results. *Int J Radiat Oncol Biol Phys.* 2008;71:107–114.

77. Jeruss JS, Vicini FA, Beitsch PD, et al. Initial outcomes for patients treated on the American Society of Breast Surgeons MammoSite clinical trial for ductal carcinoma-in-situ of the breast. *Ann Surg Oncol.* 2006;13:967–976.

78. Keisch ME, Vicini FA, Beitsch PD, et al. Factors associated with skin telangiectasias and cosmetic outcomes in patients treated on the American Society of Breast Surgeons MammoSite registry trial. *Int J Radiat Oncol Biol Phys.* 2008;72:S180.

79. Kavanagh BD, Schefter TE, Cardenes HR, et al. Interim analysis of a prospective phase I/II trial of SBRT for liver metastases. *Acta Oncol.* 2006;45:848–855.

80. Guerrero M, Li XA. Extending the linear-quadratic model for large fraction doses pertinent to stereotactic radiotherapy. *Phys Med Biol.* 2004;49:4825–4835.

81. Nuyttens JJ, Prevost JB, Van der Voort van Zijp NC, et al. Curative stereotactic robotic radiotherapy treatment for extracranial, extrapulmonary, extrahepatic, and extraspinal tumors: Technique, early results, and toxicity. *Technol Cancer Res Treat.* 2007;6:605–610.

82. Nagata Y, Matsuo Y, Norihisa Y, et al. Clinical outcomes of stereotactic body radiotherapy for primary and secondary lung cancer. *Int J Radiat Oncol Biol Phys.* 2008;72:S431–S432.

83. Chang JY, Balter P, Dong L, et al. Early results of stereotactic body radiation therapy (SBRT) in centrally/superiorly located stage I or isolated recurrent NSCLC. *Int J Radiat Oncol Biol Phys.* 2008;72:967–971.

84. Whelan TJ, Kim DH, Sussman J. Clinical experience using hypofractionated radiation schedules in breast cancer. *Semin Radiat Oncol.* 2008;18:257–264.

85. Whelan T, MacKenzie R, Julian J, et al. Randomized trial of breast irradiation schedules after lumpectomy for women with lymph node-negative breast cancer [see comment]. *J Natl Cancer Inst.* 2002;94:1143–1150.

86. Whelan TJ, Pignol JP, Julian J, et al. Long-term results of a randomized trial of accelerated hypofractionated whole breast irradiation following breast conserving surgery in women with node negative breast cancer. *Int J Radiat Oncol Biol Phys.* 2008;72:S28.

87. Yarnold J, Ashton A, Bliss J, et al. Fractionation sensitivity and dose response of late adverse effects in the breast after radiotherapy for early breast cancer: Long-term results of a randomised trial [see comment]. *Radiother Oncol.* 2005;75:9–17.

88. Start Trialists' Group, Bentzen SM, Agrawal RK, et al. The UK standardisation of breast radiotherapy (START) trial B of radiotherapy hypofractionation for treatment of early breast cancer: A randomised trial [see comment]. *Lancet.* 2008;371:1098–1107.

89. Bentzen SM, Agrawal RK, Aird EG, et al. The UK standardisation of breast radiotherapy (START) trial A of radiotherapy hypofractionation for treatment of early breast cancer: A randomised trial. *Lancet Oncol.* 2008;9:331–341.

90. Polgar C, Major T, Fodor J, et al. High-dose-rate brachytherapy alone versus whole breast radiotherapy with or without tumor bed boost after breast-conserving surgery: Seven-year results of a comparative study. *Int J Radiat Oncol Biol Phys.* 2004;60:1173–1181.

91. Kuske RR, Winter K, Arthur DW, et al. Phase II trial of brachytherapy alone after lumpectomy for select breast cancer: Toxicity analysis of RTOG 95-17. *Int J Radiat Oncol Biol Phys.* 2006;65:45–51.

92. Rabinovitch R, Winter K, Taylor M, et al. Toxicity and cosmesis from RTOG 95-17: A phase I/II trial to evaluate brachytherapy as the sole method of radiation therapy for stage I and II breast carcinoma. San Antonio Breast Cancer Symposium, San Antonio, TX; 2007.

93. Budrukkar AN, Sarin R, Shrivastava SK, et al. Cosmesis, late sequelae and local control after breast-conserving therapy: Influence of type of tumour bed boost and adjuvant chemotherapy. *Clin Oncol (R Coll Radiol).* 2007;19:596–603.

94. Harsolia A, Kestin L, Grills I, et al. Intensity-modulated radiotherapy results in significant decrease in clinical toxicities compared with conventional wedge-based breast radiotherapy. *Int J Radiat Oncol Biol Phys.* 2007;68:1375–1380.

95. Wazer DE, Kaufman S, Cuttino L, et al. Accelerated partial breast irradiation: An analysis of variables associated with late toxicity and long-term cosmetic outcome after high-dose-rate interstitial brachytherapy. *Int J Radiat Oncol Biol Phys.* 2006;64:489–495.

96. Jereczek-Fossa BA, Krengli M, Orecchia R. Particle beam radiotherapy for head and neck tumors: Radiobiological basis and clinical experience. *Head Neck.* 2006;28:750–760.

97. Levin WP, Kooy H, Loeffler JS, et al. Proton beam therapy. *Br J Cancer.* 2005;93:849–854.

98. Weber DC, Ares C, Lomax AJ, et al. Radiation therapy planning with photons and protons for early and advanced breast cancer: An overview. *Radiat Oncol.* 2006;1:22.

99. Taghian AG, Kozak KR, Katz A, et al. Accelerated partial breast irradiation using proton beams: Initial dosimetric experience. *Int J Radiat Oncol Biol Phys.* 2006;65:1404–1410.

100. Brown JM, Probert JC. Early and late radiation changes following a second course of irradiation. *Radiology.* 1975;115:711–716.

101. Chen FD, Hendry JH. Residual skin injury after repeated irradiation: Differences observed using healing, macrocolony, and microcolony endpoints. *Int J Radiat Oncol Biol Phys.* 1988;15:943–948.

102. Chen FD, Hendry JH. Re-irradiation of mouse skin: similarity of dose reductions for healing and macrocolony endpoints. *Radiother Oncol.* 1988;11:153–159.

103. Denekamp J. Residual radiation damage in mouse skin 5 to 8 months after irradiation. *Radiology.* 1975;115:191–195.

104. Masuda K, Matsuura K, Withers HR, et al. Response of previously irradiated mouse skin to a second course of irradiation: Early skin reaction and skin shrinkage. *Int J Radiat Oncol Biol Phys.* 1986;12:1645–1651.

105. Simmonds RH, Hopewell JW, Robbins ME. Residual radiation-induced injury in dermal tissue: Implications for retreatment. *Br J Radiol.* 1989;62:915–920.

106. Leith JT, McDonald M, Howard J. Residual skin damage in rats 1 year after exposure to X rays or accelerated heavy ions. *Radiat Res.* 1982;89:209–213.

107. Hendry JH. The tolerance of mouse tails to necrosis after repeated irradiation with X rays. *Br J Radiol.* 1978;51:808–813.

108. Terry NH, Tucker SL, Travis EL. Time course of loss of residual radiation damage in murine skin assessed by retreatment. *Int J Radiat Biol.* 1989;55:271–283.

109. Stewart FA, Van der Kogel AJ. Retreatment tolerance of normal tissues. *Semin Radiat Oncol.* 1994;4:103–111.

110. Lilla C, Ambrosone CB, Kropp S, et al. Predictive factors for late normal tissue complications following radiotherapy for breast cancer. *Breast Cancer Res Treat.* 2007;106:143–150.

111. Tho LM, McIntyre A, Rosst A, et al. Acute supraclavicular skin toxicity in patients undergoing radiotherapy for breast cancer: an evaluation of the 'T'-grip method of patient positioning. *Clin Oncol (R Coll Radiol).* 2006;18:133–138.

112. Palazzi M, Tomatis S, Orlandi E, et al. Effects of treatment intensification on acute local toxicity during radiotherapy for head and neck cancer: Prospective observational study validating CTCAE, version 3.0, scoring system. *Int J Radiat Oncol Biol Phys.* 2008;70:330–337.

113. Toledano A, Garaud P, Serin D, et al. Concurrent administration of adjuvant chemotherapy and radiotherapy after breast-conserving surgery enhances late toxicities: Long-term results of the ARCOSEIN multicenter randomized study. *Int J Radiat Oncol Biol Phys.* 2006;65:324–332.

114. Herold DM, Hanlon AL, Hanks GE. Diabetes mellitus: a predictor for late radiation morbidity. *Int J Radiat Oncol Biol Phys.* 1999;43:475–479.

115. Guadagnolo BA, Zagars GK, Ballo MT. Long-term outcomes for desmoid tumors treated with radiation therapy. *Int J Radiat Oncol Biol Phys.* 2008;71:441–447.

116. Lim KHC, Earnest A. Risk factors affecting acute toxicity following radiotherapy for breast cancer in an Asian population. *Int J Radiat Oncol Biol Phys.* 2008;72:S190.

117. Safwat A, Bentzen SM, Turesson I, et al. Deterministic rather than stochastic factors explain most of the variation in the expression of skin telangiectasia after radiotherapy. *Int J Radiat Oncol Biol Phys.* 2002;52:198–204.

118. Loeffler JS, Harris JR, Dahlberg WK, et al. In vitro radiosensitivity of human diploid fibroblasts derived from women with unusually sensitive clinical responses to definitive radiation therapy for breast cancer. *Radiat Res.* 1990;121:227–231.

119. Andreassen CN, Overgaard J, Alsner J, et al. ATM sequence variants and risk of radiation-induced subcutaneous fibrosis after postmastectomy radiotherapy. *Int J Radiat Oncol Biol Phys.* 2006;64:776–783.

120. Brock WA, Tucker SL, Geara FB, et al. Fibroblast radiosensitivity versus acute and late normal skin responses in patients treated for breast cancer. *Int J Radiat Oncol Biol Phys.* 1995;32:1371–1379.

121. Geara FB, Peters LJ, Ang KK, et al. Prospective comparison of in vitro normal cell radiosensitivity and normal tissue reactions in radiotherapy patients. *Int J Radiat Oncol Biol Phys.* 1993;27:1173–1179.

Chapter 44 • Skin 513

122. Johansen J, Bentzen SM, Overgaard J, et al. Evidence for a positive correlation between in vitro radiosensitivity of normal human skin fibroblasts and the occurrence of subcutaneous fibrosis after radiotherapy. *Int J Radiat Biol.* 1994;66:407–412.
123. Gold DG, Miller RC, Petersen IA, et al. Radiotherapy for malignancy in patients with scleroderma: The Mayo Clinic experience. *Int J Radiat Oncol Biol Phys.* 2007;67:559–567.
124. Wo J, Taghian A. Radiotherapy in setting of collagen vascular disease. *Int J Radiat Oncol Biol Phys.* 2007;69:1347–1353.
125. Ryan JL, Bole C, Hickok JT, et al. Post-treatment skin reactions reported by cancer patients differ by race, not by treatment or expectations. *Br J Cancer.* 2007;97:14–21.
126. Tuamokumo NL, Haffty BG. Clinical outcome and cosmesis in African-American patients treated with conservative surgery and radiation therapy. *Cancer J.* 2003;9:313–320.
127. Waselenko JK, MacVittie TJ, Blakely WF, et al. Medical management of the acute radiation syndrome: Recommendations of the Strategic National Stockpile Radiation Working Group [see comment]. *Ann Intern Med.* 2004;140:1037–1051.
128. Gottlober P, Bezold G, Weber L, et al. The radiation accident in Georgia: Clinical appearance and diagnosis of cutaneous radiation syndrome. *J Am Acad Dermatol.* 2000;42: 453–458.
129. Barabanova AV. Acute radiation syndrome with cutaneous syndrome. In: RC Ricks, ME Berger and MO' Hara Jr, *The Medical Basis for Radiation Accident Preparedness*; Elsevier, NY; 2002. pp. 217–230.
130. Balter S, Detorie NA, Mahesh M. Federal regulations (effective June 2006) require dose monitors on all new fluoroscopes: How will this help clinicians keep track of patient dose? *J Am Coll Radiol.* 2007;4:130–132.
131. Balter S, Moses J. Managing patient dose in interventional cardiology. *Catheter Cardiovasc Interv.* 2007;70:244–249.
132. Frazier TH, Richardson JB, Fabre VC, et al. Fluoroscopy-induced chronic radiation skin injury: A disease perhaps often overlooked. *Arch Dermatol.* 2007;143:637–640.
133. Hashimoto I, Sedo H, Inatsugi K, et al. Severe radiation-induced injury after cardiac catheter ablation: A case requiring free anterolateral thigh flap and vastus lateralis muscle flap reconstruction on the upper arm. *J Plast Reconstr Aesthet Surg.* 2008;61:704–708.
134. Chida K, Kagaya Y, Saito H, et al. Total entrance skin dose: An effective indicator of maximum radiation dose to the skin during percutaneous coronary intervention. *Am J Roentgenol.* 2007;189:W224–W227.
135. Redpath JL, Colman M. The effect of adriamycin and actinomycin D on radiation-induced skin reactions in mouse feet. *Int J Radiat Oncol Biol Phys.* 1979;5:483–486.
136. Lelieveld P, Scoles MA, Brown JM, et al. The effect of treatment in fractionated schedules with the combination of X-irradiation and six cytotoxic drugs on the RIF-1 tumor and normal mouse skin. *Int J Radiat Oncol Biol Phys.* 1985;11:111–121.
137. Coppes MJ, Jorgenson K, Arlette JP. Cutaneous toxicity following the administration of dactinomycin. *Med Pediatr Oncol.* 1997;29:226–227.
138. Kennedy RD, McAleer JJ. Radiation recall dermatitis in a patient treated with dacarbazine. *Clin Oncol (R Coll Radiol).* 2001;13:470–472.
139. Cassady JR, Richter MP, Piro AJ, et al. Radiation-adriamycin interactions: Preliminary clinical observations. *Cancer.* 1975;36:946–949.
140. Aristizabal SA, Miller RC, Schlichtemeier AL, et al. Adriamycin-irradiation cutaneous complications. *Int J Radiat Oncol Biol Phys.* 1977;2:325–331.
141. von der Maase H. Experimental studies on interactions of radiation and cancer chemotherapeutic drugs in normal tissues and a solid tumour. *Radiother Oncol.* 1986;7:47–68.
142. Molin J, Sogaard PE, Overgaard J. Experimental studies on the radiation-modifying effect of bleomycin in malignant and normal mouse tissue in vivo. *Cancer Treat Rep.* 1981;65:583–589.
143. Forastiere AA, Vikram B, Spiro RH, et al. Radiotherapy and bleomycin-containing chemotherapy in the treatment of advanced head and neck cancer: Report of six patients and review of the literature. *Int J Radiat Oncol Biol Phys.* 1981;7:1441–1450.
144. Stelzer KJ, Griffin TW, Koh WJ. Radiation recall skin toxicity with bleomycin in a patient with Kaposi sarcoma related to acquired immune deficiency syndrome. *Cancer.* 1993;71:1322–1325.
145. Chan RT, Au GK, Ho JW, et al. Radiation recall with oxaliplatin: Report of a case and a review of the literature. *Clin Oncol (R Coll Radiol).* 2001;13:55–57.
146. Fu KK, Lam KN. Early and late effects of cisplatin and radiation at acute and low dose rates on the mouse skin and soft tissues of the leg. *Int J Radiat Oncol Biol Phys.* 1991;20: 327–332.
147. Bartelink H, Kallman RF, Rapacchietta D, et al. Therapeutic enhancement in mice by clinically relevant dose and fractionation schedules of cis-diamminedichloroplatinum (II) and irradiation. *Radiother Oncol.* 1986;6:61–74.
148. Adelstein DJ, Saxton JP, Lavertu P, et al. A phase III randomized trial comparing concurrent chemotherapy and radiotherapy with radiotherapy alone in resectable stage III and IV squamous cell head and neck cancer: Preliminary results. *Head Neck.* 1997;19: 567–575.
149. Bauza A, Del Pozo LJ, Escalas J, et al. Radiation recall dermatitis in a patient affected with pheochromocytoma after treatment with lanreotide. *Br J Dermatol.* 2007;157:1061–1063.
150. Bolke E, Gerber PA, Lammering G, et al. Development and management of severe cutaneous side effects in head-and-neck cancer patients during concurrent radiotherapy and cetuximab. *Strahlenther Onkol.* 2008;184:105–110.
151. Billan S, Abdah-Bortnyak R, Kuten A. Severe desquamation with skin necrosis: a distinct pattern of skin toxicity secondary to head and neck irradiation with concomitant cetuximab. *Isr Med Assoc J.* 2008;10:247.
152. Berger B, Belka C. Severe skin reaction secondary to concomitant radiotherapy plus cetuximab. *Radiat Oncol.* 2008;3:5.
153. Khanfir K, Anchisi S. Pemetrexed-associated radiation recall dermatitis. *Acta Oncol.* 2008;47:1–2.
154. Guigon M, Frindel E, Tubiana M. Effects of the association of chemotherapy and radiotherapy on normal mouse skin. *Int J Radiat Oncol Biol Phys.* 1978;4:233–238.
155. Sears ME. Erythema in areas of previous irradiation in patients treated with hydroxyurea (Nsc-32065). *Cancer Chemother Rep.* 1964;40:31–32.
156. Jaffe N, Paed D, Farber S, et al. Favorable response of metastatic osteogenic sarcoma to pulse high-dose methotrexate with citrovorum rescue and radiation therapy. *Cancer.* 1973;31:1367–1373.
157. Kellie SJ, Plowman PN, Malpas JS. Radiation recall and radiosensitization with alkylating agents. *Lancet.* 1987;1:1149–1150.
158. Keung YK, Lyerly ES, Powell BL. Radiation recall phenomenon associated with arsenic trioxide. *Leukemia.* 2003;17:1417–1418.
159. Plasswilm L, Seegenschmiedt MH, Ganssauge F, et al. Simultaneous radiochemotherapy for recurrent and metastatic breast carcinoma: Evaluation of two treatment concepts. *Am J Clin Oncol.* 1996;19:403–407.
160. Susser WS, Whitaker-Worth DL, Grant-Kels JM. Mucocutaneous reactions to chemotherapy. *J Am Acad Dermatol.* 1999;40:367–398; quiz 399–400.
161. Alley E, Green R, Schuchter L. Cutaneous toxicities of cancer therapy. *Curr Opin Oncol.* 2002;14:212–216.
162. Vonessen CF, Kligerman MM, Calabresi P. Radiation and 5-Fluorouracil: a controlled clinical study. *Radiology.* 1963;81:1018–1027.
163. Biete Sola A, Marruecos Querol J, Calvo Manuel FA, et al. Phase II trial: Concurrent radiochemotherapy with weekly docetaxel for advanced squamous cell carcinoma of head and neck. *Clin Transl Oncol.* 2007;9:244–250.
164. Hanna YM, Baglan KL, Stromberg JS, et al. Acute and subacute toxicity associated with concurrent adjuvant radiation therapy and paclitaxel in primary breast cancer therapy. *Breast J.* 2002;8:149–153.
165. Feher O, Martins SJ, Lima CA, et al. Pilot trial of concomitant chemotherapy with paclitaxel and split-course radiotherapy for very advanced squamous cell carcinoma of head and neck. *Head Neck.* 2002;24:228–235.
166. Rosenthal DI, Okani O, Truelson JM, et al. Intensive radiation therapy concurrent with up to 7-week continuous-infusion paclitaxel for locally advanced solid tumors: Phase I studies. *Semin Oncol.* 1997;24:S2-81–S2-84.
167. Bokemeyer C, Lampe C, Heneka M, et al. Paclitaxel-induced radiation recall dermatitis. *Ann Oncol.* 1996;7:755–756.
168. Raghavan VT, Bloomer WD, Merkel DE. Taxol and radiation recall dermatitis. *Lancet.* 1993;341:1354.
169. Piroth MD, Krempien R, Wannenmacher M, et al. Radiation recall dermatitis from docetaxel. *Onkologie.* 2002;25:438–440.
170. Benasso M, Merlano M, Sanguineti G, et al. Gemcitabine, cisplatin, and radiation in advanced, unrespectable squamous cell carcinoma of the head and neck: a feasibility study. *Am J Clin Oncol.* 2001;24:618–622.
171. Burstein HJ. Side effects of chemotherapy. Case 1. Radiation recall dermatitis from gemcitabine. *J Clin Oncol.* 2000;18:693–694.
172. Kundranda MN, Daw HA. Tamoxifen-induced radiation recall dermatitis. *Am J Clin Oncol.* 2006;29:637–638.
173. Singer EA, Warren RD, Pennanen MF, et al. Tamoxifen-induced radiation recall dermatitis. *Breast J.* 2004;10:170–171.
174. Parry BR. Radiation recall induced by tamoxifen. *Lancet.* 1992;340:49.
175. McGinn CJ, Lawrence TS. Recent advances in the use of radiosensitizing nucleosides. *Semin Radiat Oncol.* 2001;11:270–280.
176. Ortmann E, Hohenberg G. Treatment side effects. Case 1. Radiation recall phenomenon after administration of capecitabine. *J Clin Oncol.* 2002;20:3029–3030.
177. McMeekin TO, Moschella SL. Iatrogenic complications of dermatologic therapy. Primum non nocere. *Med Clin North Am.* 1979;63:441–452.
178. Borroni G, Vassallo C, Brazzelli V, et al. Radiation recall dermatitis, panniculitis, and myositis following cyclophosphamide therapy: Histopathologic findings of a patient affected by multiple myeloma. *Am J Dermatopathol.* 2004;26:213–216.
179. Looney WB, Ritenour ER, Hopkins HA. Solid tumor models for the assessment of different treatment modalities: XVI. Sequential combined modality (Cyclophosphamide-Radiation) therapy. *Cancer.* 1981;47:860–869.
180. Holoye PY, Byers RM, Gard DA, et al. Combination chemotherapy of head and neck cancer. *Cancer.* 1978;42:1661–1669.
181. Wallenborn PA 3rd, Postma DS. Radiation recall supraglottitis. A hazard in head and neck chemotherapy. *Arch Otolaryngol.* 1984;110:614–617.
182. Weiss RB, James WD, Major WB, et al. Skin reactions induced by trimetrexate, an analog of methotrexate. *Invest New Drugs.* 1986;4:159–163.
183. Perez EA, Campbell DL, Ryu JK. Radiation recall dermatitis induced by edatrexate in a patient with breast cancer. *Cancer Invest.* 1995;13:604–607.
184. Fontana JA. Radiation recall associated with VP-16-213 therapy. *Cancer Treat Rep.* 1979;63:224–225.
185. Lampkin BC. Skin reaction to vinblastine. *Lancet.* 1969;1:891.
186. Lelieveld P, Brown JM, Goffinet DR, et al. The effect of BCNU on mouse skin and spinal cord in single drug and radiation exposures. *Int J Radiat Oncol Biol Phys.* 1979;5:1565–1568.
187. Abadir R, Liebmann J. Radiation reaction recall following simvastatin therapy: a new observation. *Clin Oncol (R Coll Radiol).* 1995;7:325–326.
188. Extermann M, Vogt N, Forni M, et al. Radiation recall in a patient with breast cancer treated for tuberculosis. *Eur J Clin Pharmacol.* 1995;48:77–78.
189. Kang SK. Images in clinical medicine. Radiation recall reaction after antimicrobial therapy. *N Engl J Med.* 2006;354:622.
190. Jain S, Agarwal J, Laskar S, et al. Radiation recall dermatitis with gatifloxacin: a review of literature. *J Med Imaging Radiat Oncol.* 2008;52:191–193.
191. Cho S, Breedlove JJ, Gunning ST. Radiation recall reaction induced by levofloxacin. *J Drugs Dermatol.* 2008;7:64–67.
192. Thomas R, Stea B. Radiation recall dermatitis from high-dose interferon alfa-2b. *J Clin Oncol.* 2002;20:355–357.
193. Ash RB, Videtic GM. Radiation recall dermatitis after the use of the anorexiant phentermine in a patient with breast cancer. *Breast J.* 2006;12:186–187.

194. Garza LA, Yoo EK, Junkins-Hopkins JM, et al. Photo recall effect in association with cefazolin. *Cutis.* 2004;73:79–80, 85.

195. Ayoola A, Lee YJ. Radiation recall dermatitis with cefotetan: a case study. *Oncologist.* 2006;11:1118–1120.

196. Azria D, Magne N, Zouhair A, et al. Radiation recall: a well recognized but neglected phenomenon. *Cancer Treat Rev.* 2005;31:555–570.

197. Camidge R, Price A. Characterizing the phenomenon of radiation recall dermatitis. *Radiother Oncol.* 2001;59:237–245.

198. Stewart FA. Keynote address: Modulation of normal tissue toxicity by combined modality therapy: Considerations for improving the therapeutic gain. *Int J Radiat Oncol Biol Phys.* 1991;20:319–325.

199. Fu KK, Phillips TL. Biologic rationale of combined radiotherapy and chemotherapy. *Hematol Oncol Clin North Am.* 1991;5:737–751.

200. O'Rourke ME. Enhanced cutaneous effects in combined modality therapy. *Oncol Nurs Forum.* 1987;14:31–35.

201. Tishler RB, Schiff PB, Geard CR, et al. Taxol: A novel radiation sensitizer. *Int J Radiat Oncol Biol Phys.* 1992;22:613–617.

202. Smith KJ, Germain M, Skelton H. Histopathologic features seen with radiation recall or enhancement eruptions. *J Cutan Med Surg.* 2002;6:535–540.

203. Del Guidice SM, Gerstley JK. Sunlight-induced radiation recall. *Int J Dermatol.* 1988;27:415–416.

204. Halliday GM, Byrne SN, Kuchel JM, et al. The suppression of immunity by ultraviolet radiation: UVA, nitric oxide and DNA damage. *Photochem Photobiol Sci.* 2004;3:736–740.

205. Le Scodan R, Wyplosz B, Couchon S, et al. UV-light induced radiation recall dermatitis after a chemoradiotherapy organ preservation protocol. *Eur Arch Otorhinolaryngol.* 2007;264:1099–1102.

206. Bostrom A, Sjolin-Forsberg G, Wilking N, et al. Radiation recall—Another call with tamoxifen. *Acta Oncol.* 1999;38:955–959.

207. Hellman S, Botnick LE. Stem cell depletion: an explanation of the late effects of cytotoxins. *Int J Radiat Oncol Biol Phys.* 1977;2:181–184.

208. Seymour CB, Mothersill C, Alper T. High yields of lethal mutations in somatic mammalian cells that survive ionizing radiation. *Int J Radiat Biol Relat Stud Phys Chem Med.* 1986;50:167–179.

209. Wintroub BU, Stern R. Cutaneous drug reactions: pathogenesis and clinical classification. *J Am Acad Dermatol.* 1985;13:167–179.

210. Camidge R, Price A. Radiation recall dermatitis may represent the Koebner phenomenon. *J Clin Oncol.* 2002;20:4130; author reply 4130.

211. Yeo W, Leung SF, Johnson PJ. Radiation-recall dermatitis with docetaxel: establishment of a requisite radiation threshold. *Eur J Cancer.* 1997;33:698–699.

212. Dorr W, Bertmann S, Herrmann T. Radiation induced lung reactions in breast cancer therapy. Modulating factors and consequential effects. *Strahlenther Onkol.* 2005;181:567–573.

213. Johansen J, Overgaard J, Overgaard M. Effect of adjuvant systemic treatment on cosmetic outcome and late normal-tissue reactions after breast conservation. *Acta Oncol.* 2007;46:525–533.

214. Hughes KS, Schnaper LA, Berry D, et al. Lumpectomy plus tamoxifen with or without irradiation in women 70 years of age or older with early breast cancer. *N Engl J Med.* 2004;351:971–977.

215. Azria D, Lemanski C, Zouhair A, et al. Adjuvant treatment of breast cancer by concomitant hormonotherapy and radiotherapy: state of the art. *Cancer Radiother.* 2004;8:188–196.

216. Bollet MA, Kirova YM, Antoni G, et al. Responses to concurrent radiotherapy and hormone-therapy and outcome for large breast cancers in post-menopausal women. *Radiother Oncol.* 2007;85:336–345.

217. McClay EF, Bogart J, Herndon JE 2nd, et al. A phase III trial evaluating the combination of cisplatin, etoposide, and radiation therapy with or without tamoxifen in patients with limited-stage small cell lung cancer: Cancer and Leukemia Group B Study (9235). *Am J Clin Oncol.* 2005;28:81–90.

218. Fodor J. Interactions between radiation and hormonal therapy in breast cancer: simultaneous or sequential treatment. *Orv Hetil.* 2006;147:121–125.

219. Moroni G, Gallelli B, Banfi G, et al. Long-term outcome of idiopathic retroperitoneal fibrosis treated with surgical and/or medical approaches. *Nephrol Dial Transplant.* 2006;21:2485–2490.

220. Vaglio A, Salvarani C, Buzio C. Retroperitoneal fibrosis. *Lancet.* 2006;367:241–251.

221. Iwakawa M, Noda S, Yamada S, et al. Analysis of non-genetic risk factors for adverse skin reactions to radiotherapy among 284 breast cancer patients. *Breast Cancer.* 2006;13:300–307.

222. Dunbar SF, Tarbell NJ, Kooy HM, et al. Stereotactic radiotherapy for pediatric and adult brain tumors: Preliminary report [see comment]. *Int J Radiat Oncol Biol Phys.* 1994;30:531–539.

223. Loeffler JS, Siddon RL, Wen PY, et al. Stereotactic radiosurgery of the brain using a standard linear accelerator: a study of early and late effects. *Radiother Oncol.* 1990;17:311–321.

224. Rusthoven KE, Carter DL, Howell K, et al. Accelerated partial-breast intensity-modulated radiotherapy results in improved dose distribution when compared with three-dimensional treatment-planning techniques. *Int J Radiat Oncol Biol Phys.* 2008;70:296–302.

225. McIntosh A, Read PW, Khandelwal SR, et al. Evaluation of coplanar partial left breast irradiation using tomotherapy-based topotherapy. *Int J Radiat Oncol Biol Phys.* 2008;71:603–610.

226. Freedman GM, Anderson PR, Li J, et al. Intensity modulated radiation therapy (IMRT) decreases acute skin toxicity for women receiving radiation for breast cancer. *Am J Clin Oncol.* 2006;29:66–70.

227. Vicini FA, Sharpe M, Kestin L, et al. Optimizing breast cancer treatment efficacy with intensity-modulated radiotherapy. *Int J Radiat Oncol Biol Phys.* 2002;54:1336–1344.

228. Pignol JP, Olivotto I, Rakovitch E, et al. A multicenter randomized trial of breast intensity-modulated radiation therapy to reduce acute radiation dermatitis. *J Clin Oncol.* 2008;26:2085–2092.

229. Voroney JPJ, Hope A, Dahele MR, et al. Pain and rib fracture after stereotactic radiotherapy for peripheral non-small cell lung cancer. *Int J Radiat Oncol Biol Phys.* 2008;72:S35–S36.

230. Dunlap NE, Biedermann GB, Yang W, et al. Chest wall volume receiving more than 30 Gy predicts risk of severe pain and/or rib fracture following lung SBRT. *Int J Radiat Oncol Biol Phys.* 2008;72:S36.

231. Sauer R, Sautter-Bihl ML, Budach W, et al. Accelerated partial breast irradiation: consensus statement of 3 German Oncology societies. *Cancer.* 2007;110:1187–1194.

232. Swanson TA, Vicini FA. Overview of accelerated partial breast irradiation. *Curr Oncol Rep.* 2008;10:54–60.

233. Arthur DW, Vicini FA, Kuske RR, et al. Accelerated partial breast irradiation: an updated report from the American Brachytherapy Society [see comment][republished from *Brachytherapy.* 2002;1(4):184–190; PMID: 15062164]. *Brachytherapy.* 2003;2:124–130.

234. Wallner P, Arthur D, Bartelink H, et al. Workshop on partial breast irradiation: State of the art and the science, Bethesda, MD, December 8–10, 2002. *J Natl Cancer Inst.* 2004;96:175–184.

235. Cormack RA, Devlin PM. Brachytherapy partial breast irradiation: analyzing effect of source configurations on dose metrics relevant to toxicity. *Int J Radiat Oncol Biol Phys.* 2008;71:940–944.

236. Belkacemi Y, Chauvet MP, Giard S, et al. Partial breast irradiation as sole therapy for low risk breast carcinoma: early toxicity, cosmesis and quality of life results of a MammoSite brachytherapy phase II study. *Radiother Oncol.* 2009;90:23–29.

237. Vicini F, Beitsch PD, Quiet CA, et al. Three-year analysis of treatment efficacy, cosmesis, and toxicity by the American Society of Breast Surgeons MammoSite Breast Brachytherapy Registry Trial in patients treated with accelerated partial breast irradiation (APBI). *Cancer.* 2008;112:758–766.

238. Bush DA, Slater JD, Garberoglio C, et al. A technique of partial breast irradiation utilizing proton beam radiotherapy: Comparison with conformal x-ray therapy. *Cancer J.* 2007;13:114–118.

239. The American Society of Breast Surgeons. Revised consensus statement for accelerated partial breast irradiation. 12/8/2005. Available at: http://www.breastsurgeons.org/apbi.shtml. Accessed 9/7/2008.

240. Dickler A, Kirk MC, Chu J, et al. The MammoSite breast brachytherapy applicator: A review of technique and outcomes. *Brachytherapy.* 2005;4:130–136.

241. Cross C, Brown A, Escobar P, et al. Partial breast brachytherapy utilizing the single-entry, multicatheter SAVI device in patients with less than 7 mm skin-to-cavity distance: Favorable acute skin toxicity outcomes from a phase II trial. *Int J Radiat Oncol Biol Phys.* 2008;72:S182.

242. Gao M, Albuquerque K. Dosimetric comparison between single-lumen balloon (MammoSite) and multi-lumen balloon (Contura) in partial breast brachytherapy. *Int J Radiat Oncol Biol Phys.* 2008;72:S511.

243. Foo M, Rogers K, Raulerson S, et al. Comparative dosimetry of 3 single-entry, afterloading brachytherapy applicators for partial breast irradiation: SAVI, Contura and Mammosite. *Int J Radiat Oncol Biol Phys.* 2008;72:S512.

244. Lemanski C, Azria D, Thezenas S, et al. Intraoperative radiotherapy given as a boost for early breast cancer: Long-term clinical and cosmetic results. *Int J Radiat Oncol Biol Phys.* 2006;64:1410–1415.

245. Ivaldi GB, Leonardi MC, Orecchia R, et al. Preliminary results of electron intraoperative therapy boost and hypofractionated external beam radiotherapy after breast-conserving surgery in premenopausal women. *Int J Radiat Oncol Biol Phys.* 2008;72:485–493.

246. Veronesi U, Orecchia R, Luini A, et al. Full-dose intraoperative radiotherapy with electrons during breast-conserving surgery: experience with 590 cases. *Ann Surg.* 2005;242:101–106.

247. Jagsi R, Ben-David M, Moran J, et al. Adverse cosmesis in a protocol investigating IMRT with active breathing control for accelerated partial breast irradiation (APBI). *Int J Radiat Oncol Biol Phys.* 2008;72:S153.

248. Balosso J. Radiation tolerance of healthy tissues, high-LET beam particularities. *Radiother Oncol.* 2004;73(suppl 2):S141–S143.

249. Kimmig B, Engenhart R, Muller M, et al. Quantification of subcutaneous fibrosis after combined photon neutron therapy. *Strahlenther Onkol.* 1990;166:76–77.

250. Cohen L, Schultheiss TE, Hendrickson FR, et al. Normal tissue reactions and complications following high-energy neutron beam therapy: I. Crude response rates. *Int J Radiat Oncol Biol Phys.* 1989;16:73–78.

251. Steingraber M, Lessel A, Jahn U. Fast neutron therapy in treatment of soft tissue sarcoma – the Berlin-Buch study. *Bull Cancer Radiother.* 1996;83(suppl):122s–124s.

252. Hubener KH, Schwarz R, Gleisberg H. Neutron therapy of soft tissue sarcomas and status report from the Radiotherapy Department of the Hamburg University Hospital. *Strahlenther Onkol.* 1989;165:309–310.

253. Schwartz M, Herrup D, Safai S, et al. Reduction of skin dose by pencil beam scanning and IMPT in partial breast irradiation. *Int J Radiat Oncol Biol Phys.* 2008;72:S520.

254. Carl J, Vestergaard A. Skin damage probabilities using fixation materials in high-energy photon beams. *Radiother Oncol.* 2000;55:191–198.

255. Bentel GC, Marks LB. A simple device to position large/flaccid breasts during tangential breast irradiation. *Int J Radiat Oncol Biol Phys.* 1994;29:879–882.

256. Mahe MA, Classe JM, Dravet F, et al. Preliminary results for prone-position breast irradiation. *Int J Radiat Oncol Biol Phys.* 2002;52:156–160.

257. Merchant TE, McCormick B. Prone position breast irradiation. *Int J Radiat Oncol Biol Phys.* 1994;30:197–203.

258. Stegman LD, Beal KP, Hunt MA, et al. Long-term clinical outcomes of whole-breast irradiation delivered in the prone position. *Int J Radiat Oncol Biol Phys.* 2007;68:73–81.

259. Ludwig MS, Strom EA, McNeese MD, et al. The lateral decubitus breast boost: Description, rationale and efficacy. *Int J Radiat Oncol Biol Phys.* 2008;72:S171.

260. Kim S, Oh S, Gale A, et al. In vivo dosimetry of skin dose during HDR breast brachytherapy using balloon catheter. *Int J Radiat Oncol Biol Phys.* 2008;72:S524.

261. Cuscela D, Coffin D, Lupton GP, et al. Protection from radiation-induced alopecia with topical application of nitroxides: Fractionated studies. *Cancer J Sci Am.* 1996;2:273–278.

262. Goffman T, Cuscela D, Glass J, et al. Topical application of nitroxide protects radiation-induced alopecia in guinea pigs. *Int J Radiat Oncol Biol Phys.* 1992;22:803–806.

263. Hebbar SA, Mitra AK, George KC, et al. Caffeine ameliorates radiation-induced skin reactions in mice but does not influence tumour radiation response. *J Radiol Prot.* 2002;22:63–69.

264. Malkinson FD, Geng L, Hanson WR. Prostaglandins protect against murine hair injury produced by ionizing radiation or doxorubicin. *J Invest Dermatol.* 1993;101:135S–137S.

265. Geng L, Hanson WR, Malkinson FD. Topical or systemic 16, 16 dm prostaglandin E₂ or WR-2721 (WR-1065) protects mice from alopecia after fractionated irradiation. *Int J Radiat Biol.* 1992;61:533–537.

266. Hanson WR, Pelka AE, Nelson AK, et al. Subcutaneous or topical administration of 16,16 dimethyl prostaglandin E₂ protects from radiation-induced alopecia in mice. *Int J Radiat Oncol Biol Phys.* 1992;23:333–337.

267. Kim SH, Jeong KS, Ryu SY, et al. Panax ginseng prevents apoptosis in hair follicles and accelerates recovery of hair medullary cells in irradiated mice. *In Vivo.* 1998;12:219–222.

268. Booth C, Potten CS. Keratinocyte growth factor increases hair follicle survival following cytotoxic insult. *J Invest Dermatol.* 2000;114:667–673.

269. Okunieff P, Xu J, Hu D, et al. Curcumin protects against radiation-induced acute and chronic cutaneous toxicity in mice and decreases mRNA expression of inflammatory and fibrogenic cytokines. *Int J Radiat Oncol Biol Phys.* 2006;65:890–898.

270. Liang L, Hu D, Liu W, et al. Celecoxib reduces skin damage after radiation: Selective reduction of chemokine and receptor mRNA expression in irradiated skin but not in irradiated mammary tumor. *Am J Clin Oncol.* 2003;26:S114–S121.

271. Kitagawa J, Nasu M, Okumura H, et al. Allopurinol gel mitigates radiation-induced mucositis and dermatitis. *J Radiat Res (Tokyo).* 2008;49:49–54.

272. Tekin SB, Ertekin MV, Erdogan F, et al. Is growth hormone a radioprotective agent? *J Eur Acad Dermatol Venereol.* 2006;20:293–298.

273. Xiao Z, Su Y, Yang S, et al. Protective effect of esculentoside A on radiation-induced dermatitis and fibrosis. *Int J Radiat Oncol Biol Phys.* 2006;65:882–889.

274. Okunieff P. Interactions between ascorbic acid and the radiation of bone marrow, skin, and tumor. *Am J Clin Nutr.* 1991;54:1281S–1283S.

275. Delanian S, Porcher R, Balla-Mekias S, et al. Randomized, placebo-controlled trial of combined pentoxifylline and tocopherol for regression of superficial radiation-induced fibrosis. *J Clin Oncol.* 2003;21:2545–2550.

276. Vogler BK, Ernst E. Aloe vera: a systematic review of its clinical effectiveness. *Br J Gen Pract.* 1999;49:823–828.

277. Nystrom J, Svensk AC, Lindholm-Sethson B, et al. Comparison of three instrumental methods for the objective evaluation of radiotherapy induced erythema in breast cancer patients and a study of the effect of skin lotions. *Acta Oncol.* 2007;46:893–899.

278. Richardson J, Smith JE, McIntyre M, et al. Aloe vera for preventing radiation-induced skin reactions: A systematic literature review. *Clin Oncol (R Coll Radiol).* 2005;17:478–484.

279. Heggie S, Bryant GP, Tripcony L, et al. A phase III study on the efficacy of topical aloe vera gel on irradiated breast tissue. *Cancer Nurs.* 2002;25:442–451.

280. Olsen DL, Raub W Jr, Bradley C, et al. The effect of aloe vera gel/mild soap versus mild soap alone in preventing skin reactions in patients undergoing radiation therapy. *Oncol Nurs Forum.* 2001;28:543–547.

281. Merchant TE, Bosley C, Smith J, et al. A phase III trial comparing an anionic phospholipid-based cream and aloe vera-based gel in the prevention of radiation dermatitis in pediatric patients. *Radiat Oncol.* 2007;2:45.

282. Omidvari S, Saboori H, Mohammadianpanah M, et al. Topical betamethasone for prevention of radiation dermatitis. *Indian J Dermatol Venereol Leprol.* 2007;73:209.

283. Elliott EA, Wright JR, Swann RS, et al. Phase III trial of an emulsion containing trolamine for the prevention of radiation dermatitis in patients with advanced squamous cell carcinoma of the head and neck: Results of Radiation Therapy Oncology Group Trial 99-13. *J Clin Oncol.* 2006;24:2092–2097.

284. Lin LC, Que J, Lin LK, et al. Zinc supplementation to improve mucositis and dermatitis in patients after radiotherapy for head-and-neck cancers: a double-blind, randomized study. *Int J Radiat Oncol Biol Phys.* 2006;65:745–750.

285. Valencia J, Velilla C, Urpegui A, et al. The efficacy of orgotein in the treatment of acute toxicity due to radiotherapy on head and neck tumors. *Tumori.* 2002;88:385–389.

286. Manzanas Garcia A, Lopez Carrizosa MC, Vallejo Ocana C, et al. Superoxidase dismutase (SOD) topical use in oncologic patients: treatment of acute cutaneous toxicity secondary to radiotherapy. *Clin Transl Oncol.* 2008;10:163–167.

287. Halperin EC, Gaspar L, George S, et al. A double-blind, randomized, prospective trial to evaluate topical vitamin C solution for the prevention of radiation dermatitis. CNS cancer consortium. *Int J Radiat Oncol Biol Phys.* 1993;26:413–416.

288. Kouvaris JR, Kouloulias VE, Plataniotis GA, et al. Dermatitis during radiation for vulvar carcinoma. Prevention and treatment with granulocyte-macrophage colony-stimulating factor impregnated gauze. *Wound Repair Regen.* 2001;9:187–193.

289. Metz JM, Smith D, Mick R, et al. A phase I study of topical Tempol for the prevention of alopecia induced by whole brain radiotherapy. *Clin Cancer Res.* 2004;10:6411–6417.

290. DeLand MM, Weiss RA, McDaniel DH, et al. Treatment of radiation-induced dermatitis with light-emitting diode (LED) photomodulation. *Lasers Surg Med.* 2007;39:164–168.

291. Schubert MM, Eduardo FP, Guthrie KA, et al. A phase III randomized double-blind placebo-controlled clinical trial to determine the efficacy of low level laser therapy for the prevention of oral mucositis in patients undergoing hematopoietic cell transplantation. *Support Care Cancer.* 2007;15:1145–1154.

292. Woodruff LD, Bounkeo JM, Brannon WM, et al. The efficacy of laser therapy in wound repair: A meta-analysis of the literature. *Photomed Laser Surg.* 2004;22:241–247.

293. Silveira PC, Streck EL, Pinho RA. Evaluation of mitochondrial respiratory chain activity in wound healing by low-level laser therapy. *J Photochem Photobiol B Biol.* 2007;86:279–282.

294. Houreld N, Abrahamse H. In vitro exposure of wounded diabetic fibroblast cells to a helium-neon laser at 5 and 16 J/cm². *Photomed Laser Surg.* 2007;25:78–84.

295. Correa F, Martins RA, Correa JC, et al. Low-level laser therapy (GaAs lambda = 904 nm) reduces inflammatory cell migration in mice with lipopolysaccharide-induced peritonitis. *Photomed Laser Surg.* 2007;25:245–249.

296. Corazza AV, Jorge J, Kurachi C, et al. Photobiomodulation on the angiogenesis of skin wounds in rats using different light sources. *Photomed Laser Surg.* 2007;25:102–106.

297. Albertini R, Villaverde AB, Aimbire F, et al. Anti-inflammatory effects of low-level laser therapy (LLLT) with two different red wavelengths (660 nm and 684 nm) in carrageenan-induced rat paw edema. *J Photochem Photobiol B Biol.* 2007;89:50–55.

298. Oron U, Ilic S, De Taboada L, et al. Ga-As (808 nm) laser irradiation enhances ATP production in human neuronal cells in culture. *Photomed Laser Surg.* 2007;25:180–182.

299. Tuby H, Maltz L, Oron U. Modulations of VEGF and iNOS in the rat heart by low level laser therapy are associated with cardioprotection and enhanced angiogenesis. *Lasers Surg Med.* 2006;38:682–688.

300. Agaiby AD, Ghali LR, Wilson R, et al. Laser modulation of angiogenic factor production by T-lymphocytes. *Lasers Surg Med.* 2000;26:357–363.

301. Rizzi CF, Mauriz JL, Freitas Correa DS, et al. Effects of low-level laser therapy (LLLT) on the nuclear factor (NF)-kappaB signaling pathway in traumatized muscle. *Lasers Surg Med.* 2006;38:704–713.

302. Aimbire F, Lopes-Martins RA, Albertini R, et al. Effect of low-level laser therapy on hemorrhagic lesions induced by immune complex in rat lungs. *Photomed Laser Surg.* 2007;25:112–117.

303. Albertini R, Aimbire F, Villaverde AB, et al. COX-2 mRNA expression decreases in the subplantar muscle of rat paw subjected to carrageenan-induced inflammation after low level laser therapy. *Inflamm Res.* 2007;56:228–229.

304. Fujimaki Y, Shimoyama T, Liu Q, et al. Low-level laser irradiation attenuates production of reactive oxygen species by human neutrophils [see comment]. *J Clin Laser Med Surg.* 2003;21:165–170.

305. Ferreira DM, Zangaro RA, Villaverde AB, et al. Analgesic effect of He–Ne (632.8 nm) low-level laser therapy on acute inflammatory pain [erratum appears in *Photomed Laser Surg.* 2007;25(1):63 Note: Piccolo, G [corrected to Picolo, G]]. *Photomed Laser Surg.* 2005;23:177–181.

306. Cheng JC, Fife D, Behnam S, et al. Prevention of radiation dermatitis using light-emitting diode (LED) photomodulation: a prospective, randomized, and controlled study. *Int J Radiat Oncol Biol Phys.* 2008;72:S181.

307. Bensadoun RJ, Franquin JC, Ciais G, et al. Low-energy He/Ne laser in the prevention of radiation-induced mucositis. A multicenter phase III randomized study in patients with head and neck cancer. *Support Care Cancer.* 1999;7:244–252.

308. Schindl A, Schindl M, Pernerstorfer-Schon H, et al. Low intensity laser irradiation in the treatment of recalcitrant radiation ulcers in patients with breast cancer – long-term results of 3 cases. *Photodermatol Photoimmunol Photomed.* 2000;16:34–37.

309. Ruiz-Genao DP, Cordoba S, Garcia FVMJ, et al. Post-radiotherapy telangiectasias. Treatment with pulsed-dye laser. Sequential histological studies. *Actas Dermosifiliogr.* 2006;97:345–347.

310. Mendelsohn FA, Divino CM, Reis ED, et al. Wound care after radiation therapy. *Adv Skin Wound Care.* 2002;15:216–224.

311. Dunne-Daly CF. Skin and wound care in radiation oncology. *Cancer Nurs.* 1995;18:144–160; quiz 161–142.

312. Ratliff C. Impaired skin integrity related to radiation therapy. *J Enterostomal Ther.* 1990;17:193–198.

313. Theberge V, Dagnault A, Harel F. Use of axillary deodorant and the impact on acute skin toxicity during radiation therapy for breast cancer: A randomized trial. *Int J Radiat Oncol Biol Phys.* 2008;72:S178.

314. Michalowski AS. On radiation damage to normal tissues and its treatment. II. Anti-inflammatory drugs. *Acta Oncol.* 1994;33:139–157.

315. Glees JP, Mameghan-Zadeh H, Sparkes CG. Effectiveness of topical steroids in the control of radiation dermatitis: A randomised trial using 1% hydrocortisone cream and 0.05% clobetasone butyrate (Eumovate). *Clin Radiol.* 1979;30:397–403.

316. Jungersted JM, Hellgren LI, Jemec GB, et al. Lipids and skin barrier function—A clinical perspective. *Contact Dermatitis.* 2008;58:255–262.

317. Varghese MC, Balin AK, Carter DM, et al. Local environment of chronic wounds under synthetic dressings. *Arch Dermatol.* 1986;122:52–57.

318. Macmillan MS, Wells M, MacBride S, et al. Randomized comparison of dry dressings versus hydrogel in management of radiation-induced moist desquamation. *Int J Radiat Oncol Biol Phys.* 2007;68:864–872.

319. Bolderston A, Lloyd NS, Wong RK, et al. The prevention and management of acute skin reactions related to radiation therapy: a systematic review and practice guideline. *Support Care Cancer.* 2006;14:802–817.

320. Bui QC, Lieber M, Withers HR, et al. The efficacy of hyperbaric oxygen therapy in the treatment of radiation-induced late side effects. *Int J Radiat Oncol Biol Phys.* 2004;60:871–878.

321. Bennett MH, Feldmeier J, Hampson N, et al. Hyperbaric oxygen therapy for late radiation tissue injury. *Cochrane Database Syst Rev.* 2005;CD005005.

322. Marx RE, Ehler WJ, Tayapongsak P, et al. Relationship of oxygen dose to angiogenesis induction in irradiated tissue. *Am J Surg.* 1990;160:519–524.

323. Mader JT, Adams KR, Wallace WR, et al. Hyperbaric oxygen as adjunctive therapy for osteomyelitis. *Infect Dis Clin North Am.* 1990;4:433–440.

CHAPTER

45

Paul Okunieff
Amy K. Huser

Treatment Approaches to Late Radiation Injury

INTRODUCTION

Numerous radiation exposure scenarios exist, including cancer therapy, industrial and nuclear accidents, as well as intentionally harmful exposures such as use of a radiological dispersion device or other nefarious action. Indeed, humans receive small amounts of natural background radiation from the Earth, while NASA and other space agency researchers are working to prevent or ameliorate the effects of solar and cosmic exposures. In this chapter, we focus on the more common and concerning exposures.

In the realm of cancer treatment, radiation-induced toxicity (dose limiting or otherwise) is of primary concern. However, as treatments have become more efficacious and sparing of normal tissues, more patients are long-term survivors of treatment; therefore, secondary malignancies and noncancerous disease remain the long-term focus. The hope of researchers and physicians faced with the problem of radiation-induced toxicity, no matter its source, lies in the notion that early intervention can affect, ameliorate, or obviate the development of late effects.

OVERVIEW OF CANCER SURVIVORSHIP RESEARCH

Half of the population in the United States can expect to develop a malignancy sometime in their lives and one in six can expect to die from cancer-related sequellae.[1] The majority of those who develop cancer can expect to be cured but, in the process, they will have received aggressive treatments including surgery, radiation, and chemotherapy. At the present time, over

10 million Americans (e.g., 1 in 30 adults) are survivors of cancer therapy and could therefore be at higher risk for developing illnesses hastened or caused by treatment.[2–5] The side effects of treatment, which occur during the course of therapy but usually have largely subsided within a few months of completing therapy, have been studied and interventions are available. Long-term sequella, occurring months, years, or decades after treatment, however, have most usually been studied only in the pediatric population. There is increasing interest and need to better understand the types of clinical studies that should be emphasized in the broader population, the mechanism of the toxicity, and therefore potential interventions.[6]

Regarding radiation toxicity, interventions used before or during treatment have been termed "protectors,"[7] those that are given during the asymptomatic period following irradiation are termed "mitigators," and those that are used to treat presenting clinical symptoms are in the "treatment" category. Toxicity scoring has moved forward over the years, beginning with RTOG and related semiquantitative scales, followed by the addition of quantitative biological assays in the LENT/SOMA scales.[8] More recently, the National Cancer Institute has recommended that all scoring of adverse events be accomplished using a common system, termed the CTCAE, to evaluate toxicity related to combined modality therapy comprehensively. The CTCAE is currently on version 3 and is attempting to be flexible so that it can grow along with the sciences associated with adverse event measurement and therapy.[9,10] There is clearly great need for standardization of measurements of adverse events, since the current state of the literature is very inconsistent and therefore it is nearly impossible to compare different studies.

MECHANISMS OF TOXICITY FROM SINGLE AND COMBINED MODALITY TREATMENTS, INCLUDING RADIATION

The classical mechanism presumed to account for both early and late adverse effects of radiation involves depopulation of clonogenic cells. These proliferating cells originate in either vascular or epithelial compartments, and their rate of regeneration dictates the time at which the toxicity is experienced. The classical concept involves rapidly renewing cells that have earlier toxicity than slowly renewing cells because they mortalize after a finite number of doublings, after which the tissue stagnates and dies. In this model, inflammation augments toxicity through its unsuccessful attempts to heal the poorly renewing tissues. Early mucositis, dermatitis, and marrow depopulation are quite consistent with this hypothesis, as is the lower alpha/beta (and thus greater dose-fraction response) of tissues in most slowly renewing organs. The model, however, falls short when it attempts to define the number of stem cells in these tissues and/or the number of regenerating units. The model also tends to be inconsistent when considering the extremely sensitive vascular endothelial cell, which has little or no capacity for DNA repair.[11,12]

More modern approaches attempt to improve on the classical understanding, suggesting that endothelial cell apoptosis signals epithelial cell apoptosis, and the cell loss that occurs through apoptosis primarily accounts for the toxicity. This model, like the classical model, not only does not solve the inconsistencies with regard to responses seen late in animal models and humans, but also adds some new inconsistencies to our understanding of early toxicity. This model, however, has led to the discovery of some interventions that appear to be effective at reducing early toxicities. A final and more satisfactory addition to the classical model with regard to late consequences of therapy includes the role that inflammatory cytokines and inflammation might play in the process.[10,13–15] The hypothesis that aberrant expression of inflammatory cytokines engages in a dynamic and often self-amplifying process that causes progression of toxicity has been studied in great detail over the past 15 years. Research in this area has allowed for examination of many types of interventions, some of which appear successful. The roles that apoptosis and inflammatory factors play in the progress of adverse effects of radiation exposure will be discussed in this chapter.

OVERVIEW OF RANGE OF USUAL TREATMENT APPROACHES

The current standard treatment approaches for adverse late effects associated with radiation exposure are limited in number. Most include procedures that augment tissue oxygenation or reduce tissue inflammation.[16] This includes surgical excision of necrotic, avascular tissue, repair using vascularized tissue grafts for ulcerated or perforated organs, hyperbaric oxygen treatment, or use of vascular active agents to improve tissue perfusion (e.g., pentoxifylline and others).

SURGERY

Surgery for radiation sequella includes surgical removal of necrotic material, replacement of lost function using prostheses, vascularized grafts for nonhealing wounds, or resection and reconstruction of redundant necrotic organs such as a loop of bowel.[17–19] In general, dilation procedures for stenotic organs are of limited benefit if stents are not also employed. Foreign bodies likewise are generally poorly tolerated if the tissue is not revascularized, due to poor healing.

HYPERBARIC OXYGEN

Hyperbaric oxygen treatment typically includes one to three dives of 0.5 to 3 hours at 2 to 3 ATA, given daily for 2 to 6 weeks.[20] In most treatment series, approximately 30% of patients experience wound healing and tissue recovery. Hyperbaric oxygen does not appear to benefit patients with CNS toxicity, and this treatment appears most effective for ischemic tissue damage including bone necrosis. In animal studies, bone growth was preserved in young treated animals up to a higher radiation dose limit than animals not receiving hyperbaric oxygen treatment. This improved bone growth preservation included better periosteal blood flow in the treated animals.[21,22] The mechanism of healing is unknown but probably includes a combination of improved cellular recovery during the hyperbaric period, reduced inflammation, and perhaps reactive upregulation of antioxidants like superoxide dismutase.

PENTOXIFYLLINE (WITH OR WITHOUT ADJUVANT DRUGS)

Recently, pentoxifylline with or without tocopherol has been used as a treatment for fibrovascular toxicity after irradiation.[16,23–26] Pentoxifylline is normally used to improve red blood cell flexibility, since these cells can become very rigid in a hypoxic environment. The improved flexibility of red blood cells allows better flow through tortuous vessels in patients with chronic vascular insufficiency syndromes. Pentoxifylline appears to function only as a therapeutic; it does not appear to function as a mitigator and may even sensitize tumors (and normal tissues) when used concurrently with radiation exposure. Some studies suggest that tocopherol is needed to achieve maximum benefit from pentoxifylline, though not all studies agree.[23,25] There are many explanations for the benefit of these agents. Perhaps most importantly, they both improve vascular function, making hypoxic and chaotic neoangiogenic tissues function more efficiently, improving the micromilieu and allowing for normalized healing. Benefits in some cases can be very impressive and include regression of fibrosis.[23] Treatment requires several weeks to reach maximum benefit. The drug can be discontinued in many patients without recurrence of side effects, which is important because many patients report nausea and other gastrointestinal side effects as a result of treatment. However, even a small improvement in a patient's fibrosis- and inflammation-related symptoms can have a profound impact on the quality of their daily living.

NEW UNDERSTANDING OF MECHANISMS

TARGET VOLUME

The adverse effects associated with radiation exposure occur with a very sharp dose response. Below a critical dose, there are almost no measurable consequences of treatment.[27–33] A 10%

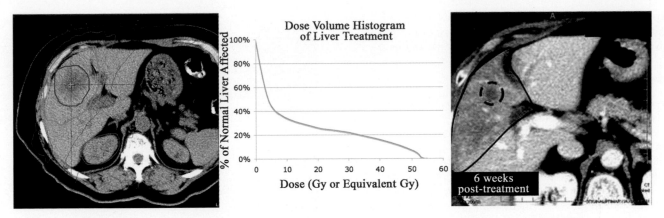

Figure 45.1. Normal tissue responses to partial liver irradiation. The liver metastasis was treated to 50 Gy at 5 Gy/fraction. The tumor volume is outlined in pink. The green isodose line is at ≈37 Gy. The dose volume histogram demonstrates that approximately 20% of the liver (excluding the tumor) was over 37 Gy. Six weeks following radiation, there is hypoperfusion in the shape of the 37-Gy isodose line (*solid black line*) with compensatory enlargement of the left lobe of the liver. The tumor is the necrotic region within the hatched line.

increase in dose or fraction size near the critical dose, however, can steeply raise the rate of complication to 50%, and a second 10% increase can lead to near certain tissue lethality. The severity of clinical illness experienced by the patient is, with few exceptions, powerfully related to the volume of the organ exposed to a dose above a critical level. As with localized surgery, the survivability of the damage is related to the plasticity of the organ and its ability to heal after partial organ damage (Fig. 45.1). Estimates of tolerance dose have been established empirically for most organs,[34] and these estimates were recently updated in the literature.[35] Stereotactic techniques tend to treat only small volumes of normal tissue and therefore are expected to cause severe local histological toxicity, but that toxicity is often subclinical or minimally asymptomatic.[36–38] Indeed, improvements in imaging and targeting technologies make many side effects of radiation much less severe even as doses and dose per fraction increases to the tumor.[39–41]

INFLAMMATORY CYTOKINES

The cytokines expressed by epithelial cells or macrophages most commonly associated with early and late toxicity include those that activate inflammatory pathways.[13,42–45] Among these, the IL-1 signaling cascade appears to be very important[46–48] (Fig. 45.2). IL-1α and IL-1β are differentially expressed in different tissues and vary among different murine models and humans.[47,49–52] The overexpression of either isoform is associated with a higher rate of susceptibility to complications. Indeed, mice transgenic for these molecules suffer spontaneous fibrosis even without radiation exposure. IL-1Ra, like the alpha and beta forms, binds to the IL-1R1 receptor but does not activate the kinase cascade and therefore blocks receptor activation. IL-1Ra seems to increase during a fractionated course of radiation, and mice overexpressing IL-1Ra tend to be resistant to fibrosis of many types. IL-1R2 is a decoy receptor. It binds both the alpha and the beta forms but does not initiate the signaling cascade. The TGF-β pathway appears more complicated than the IL-1 pathway, but like the IL-1 pathway, aberrant expression of this cytokine family appears sufficient (though probably not necessary) for production of fibrovascular toxicity after irradiation in mouse and humans.[39,53–56] Impressively, circulating levels of

TGF-β1 seem to powerfully predict liver and lung fibrosis after chemotherapy or bone marrow transplant for breast cancer patients.[57] Other cytokines have also been implicated in radiation toxicity and many provide powerful markers of risk for a predisposition to late treatment-related toxicity.[46,47,52,53,58,59] It is not yet clear whether interventions aimed at reducing cytokine

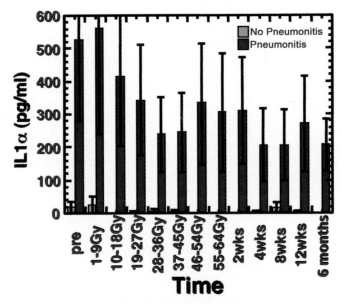

Figure 45.2. Circulating plasma levels of IL-1α in patients undergoing thoracic radiation. Specimens were collected before beginning irradiation, weekly during the course of radiation therapy, and then at follow-up visits up to 6 months. Circulating plasma levels of IL-1α in patients who eventually developed symptomatic or radiographic pneumonitis are indicated by red bars. Levels for those who did not develop pneumonitis are indicated in *green* (most of these levels are very low). Individuals with a predisposition to have increased IL-1α invariably developed some degree of pneumonitis, indicating that this cytokine might be sufficient (though not necessary) to produce this radiation complication. (Modified from Chen Y, Williams J, Ding I, et al. Radiation pneumonitis and early circulatory cytokine markers. *Semin Radiat Oncol.* 2002;12(1 suppl 1):26–33, with the kind permission of Dr. Yuhchyau Chen.)

expression or blocking the signal cascades associated with these cytokines can reduce the severity, frequency, or progression of adverse effects of radiation.[13] Research is active in this area.

APOPTOSIS FACTORS

Premature loss of cells clearly decreases organ function and can lead to increased toxicity after irradiation.[60,61] This is especially true for early toxicity wherein depopulation effects dominate over fibrovascular effects. Cascades involved in apoptosis including p53, TNF, TRAIL, caspases, and so forth have all been associated with more severe side effects of radiation,[62,63] particularly when the bone marrow compartment is the organ of investigation.[59,64] Inhibition of apoptosis as a method for protecting organs against radiation toxicity is controversial.[65–67] Some studies support this approach, often with compelling results. In a recent, elegant animal study, mice unable to apoptose gut epithelium due to genetically defined alterations in the apoptosis pathways appear to have no intrinsic resistance to acute radiation toxicity.[68] The role that apoptosis might play in late radiation sequellae is less clear. However, many of the same factors that induce apoptosis are also causally related to necrosis and inflammation (e.g., TNF). Thus, inhibition of apoptotic pathways has proven in some models to have potential benefit and deserves further study.[68]

OXIDATIVE STRESS

Chronic oxidative stress, a physiochemical process, may, more than any other factor, influence the severity and rate of progression of the toxic response set up by the initial treatment event.[69,70] Most treatments, whether surgical, chemical, or radiological, involve damage to the vascular system. During vascular recovery, inflammation and abnormal healing processes can create fibrosis, aberrant angiogenesis, and areas of ischemia and inflammation. Oxidative stress, radiation exposure, and probably some chemotherapeutic agents damage cellular DNA, including mitochondrial DNA, leading to abnormal mitochondrial function.[71–74] These processes all lead to increased cellular oxidative stress. Abnormal vascular function can also lead to cycles of ischemia and reperfusion in microregions that causes a chronic oxidative injury process. The importance of this process in the progression of toxicity is great since interventions to prevent chronic reperfusion injury are easily incorporated into a mitigation or therapeutic program. For example, the chain of mitochondrial electron transport might be augmented by a combination of ascorbic acid and tocopherol, an easily created nutritional supplement.[73,75,76]

PREMATURE MATURATION OF STEM AND PROGENITOR CELLS

Stem and progenitor cells appear to proliferate and differentiate based on external signals including components of the cytokine micromilieu.[77,78] Stem cell biology is a very active and immature field, but the eventual promise of stem cell biology for preservation and more rapid and comprehensive recovery of irradiated tissues is substantial. For example, it appears that TGF-β signaling pathways can cause proliferation and then premature differentiation of fibroblast progenitors to mature fibroblasts that elaborate collagen.[77] Likewise, some bone marrow progenitors appear to differentiate into solid organ epithelium when needed, allowing for more complete recovery

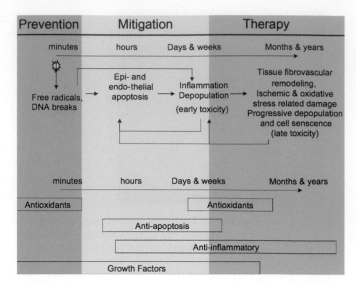

Figure 45.3. Most interventions against deleterious effects of radiation are of four different categories. Antioxidants are most useful if present during the irradiation but might also play a role in reducing the chronic oxidative stress that progresses at late times following radiation exposure. Growth factors can be beneficial at any time before, during, or after irradiation. Antiapoptotic factors prevent toxicity during the hours or days after the exposure, during which time there is a peak loss of cells due to apoptosis. Anti-inflammatory agents appear to be of greatest benefit at intermediate and late times where tissue damage precipitates a deleterious inflammatory response that worsens the injury.

of liver and perhaps gastrointestinal epithelium.[77,78] Learning which components of the cytokine signal after irradiation augment beneficial growth and differentiation and which are deleterious might some day allow patient-specific therapies.[77,78]

AGENTS UNDER INVESTIGATION

The agents that appear to have benefit for alleviation of adverse effects of treatment include agents that fall generally into the category of antioxidants, growth factors, vascular active agents, anti-inflammatory agents, and antiapoptotic agents. There is obvious overlap among the categories (i.e., some agents have multiple actions). Since some of these interventions are expected to selectively benefit specific organs when given at specific times after irradiation, most agents appear to be organ- and time specific (Fig. 45.3). In this section, we review the various categories of agents in development for alleviation of radiation-induced toxicity. The NIH/NIAID (in the United States of America) is currently funding the Centers for Medical Countermeasures against Radiation (CMCR) program. Table 45.1 and Figure 45.4 include an overview of all agents currently under investigation in the CMCR program (Table 45.1) (Fig. 45.4).

ANTIOXIDANTS

Antioxidant agents that reduce mitochondrial- and reperfusion-related chronic cellular oxidative stress have had some benefit and remain of great interest.[73] To date, we do not yet know the oxidative potentials that are most efficacious and whether more than one antioxidant should be used in combination to achieve the best oxidative damage protection. Cardiolipin,

TABLE 45.1	Candidate Radiation-Related Compounds Under Investigation in the Centers for Medical Countermeasures Against Radiation Program (CMCR—NIAID/NIH)

Category	Mechanism	Compound	Manufacturer	FDA Approved[a]
Antioxidant	MnSOD-catalase mimetic (salenMn)	EUK-134	Atrium (IP—Tyrian Diagnostics)	N
	MnSOD-catalase mimetic (salenMn)	EUK-189	Boston University (IP—Tyrian Diagnostics)	N
	MnSOD-catalase mimetic (cyclic salenMn)	EUK-207	Boston University (IP—Tyrian Diagnostics)	N
	MnSOD-catalase mimetic (orally available, porphyrinMn)	EUK-400 series	Boston University (IP—Tyrian Diagnostics)	N
	MnSOD mimetics/liposomes	MnSOD-PL	IP—Tyrian Diagnostics	N
	Mn porphyrin	MnTE-2-PyP5+	Novel	N
	MnSOD mimetics	MnTnHex-2-PyP5+	Novel	N
	Antioxidant	Pentoxifylline (Trental)	Aventis	Y
	Antioxidant	Vitamin C (ascorbic acid)	Various	Y (nutr suppl)
	Antioxidant	WW85	Inotek	N
	ROS scavenger/hemigramicidin–TEMPO conjugates	XJB-5-131	U Pittsburgh	N
	Anti-inflammatory—COX-2 inhibitor	Celecoxcib (Celebrex)	Pfizer	Y
	Anti-inflammatory—spicy food supplement, IL-1 and TNF pathways, inhibits NF-κB	Curcumin (diferuloylmethane)	Calbiochem	N (nutr suppl)
	Anti-inflammatory	Esculentoside A (EsA & h-EsA)	Eva Pharma	N
Anti-inflammatory	Anti-inflammatory/inhibits NF-κB	Ethyl pyruvate	Various	N
	Protein tyrosine kinase inhibitor	Genistein (Solaray)	Various	N (nutr suppl)
	Anti-inflammatory—blocks early, late IR toxicity	IL-1Ra	Biovitrum	Y
	Statin shown to lower cholesterol	Lovastatin (Mevacor, Altocor)	Merck	Y
	Anti-inflammatory—Chinese herb	Triptolide	Various	N
Antiapoptotic	Small molecule FAS antagonist	SF	Various	N
	Fibroblast growth factors	bFGF derivatives	Various	N
	Endothelial progenitor cells	Endothelial progenitor cells	Duke University	N
	Growth factor/tyrosine kinase receptor	Flt-3 ligand	Amgen	N
Growth factor	Growth colony stimulating factor	G-CSF	Amgen	Y
	growth hormone	Human growth hormone	Genentech (*Research use*)	Y
	Keratinocyte growth factor	KGF	Amgen	Y
	Somatostatin analog	Octreotide (Sandostatin)	Novartis	Y
	Somatostatin analog	SOM230	Novartis	N

[a]FDA approved for other applications; not yet FDA approved as radiation countermeasures.
Source: The information in this table was kindly provided by Dr. Andrea DiCarlo-Cohen (NIAID) and the CMCR Center Leadership.

which is involved in caspase activation and apoptosis, has been suggested as an important mitochondrial target precipitating oxidative cellular damage.[72,79] Priority agents under investigation in this class include enzymatic antioxidants (e.g., superoxide dismutase gene therapy[80,81]), sulfhydryl molecules (e.g., glutathione[82,83]), chemical antioxidants (e.g., amifostine[84,85]), and vitamins (e.g., ascorbic acid and tocopherol[86,87]). An antioxidant and anti-inflammatory nutrient in food, curcumin, shows promise as a cutaneous radiation protector.[88,89]

GROWTH FACTORS

Most growth factors are also antiapoptotic agents. Because growth factor receptors are typically cell type specific, the benefit is expected to be organ specific as well. Agents that appear to be of benefit include the fibroblast growth factor family, many of which are also powerfully angiogenic but usually do not produce a vascular leak syndrome as part of the angiogenic process. Among these, basic FGF (FGF2) is probably the most advantageous with regard to the range of organs it benefits.[90–93] Keratinocyte growth factors 1 and 2 (FGF7 and FGF10) appear to also benefit the gastrointestinal and probably the hematopoietic system, and are of additive benefit with FGF2.[91,94–97] Enthusiasm for exogenous FGF2 (as opposed to the KGFs) will be tempered by the role that it plays in tumor progression and thus the concern that it might encourage tumor recurrence. Many patients with fibrovascular complications of radiation already have high levels of endogenous FGF2 and thus may not need exogenous agents.[23,98] Formerly very popular, EPO, another growth factor, does seem to promote metastases and is now used less frequently to manage chemotherapy-related fatigue.[99,100] Many hematopoietic growth factors are under investigation including those that stimulate erythrocytes and megakaryocytes in addition to G-CSF, which is already commonly used for hematopoietic toxicity due to either radiation or chemotherapy. Research regarding the optimal combinations of growth factors is active.

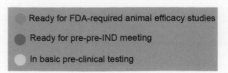

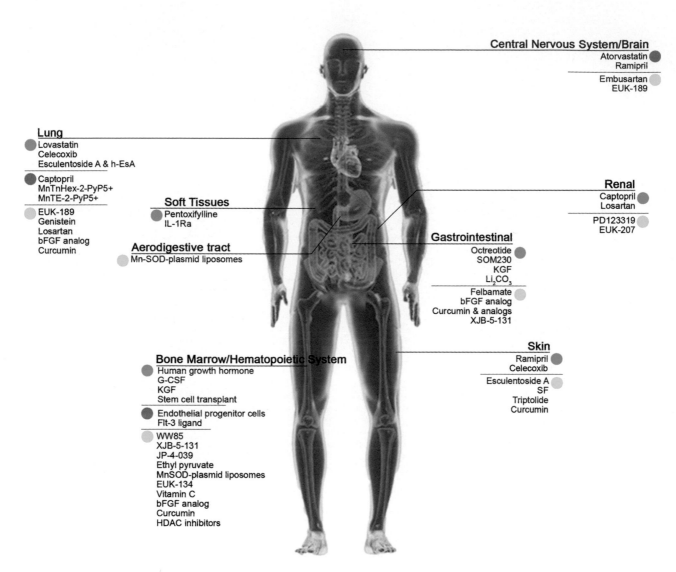

Figure 45.4. Current list of priority agents being tested by the CMCR as interventions for a radiological event. Agents are listed in combination with the organ wherein their action is expected to be most significant. Different agents will be needed for different organs. Because the benefit of many agents is organ specific, it is expected that optimal combinations of agents will be needed for most victims.

VASCULAR ACTIVE AGENTS

The mechanism by which rheological agents such as pentoxifylline reduce soft tissue fibrosis and by which the angiotensin-blocking antihypertensive agents achieve prevention and mitigation of lung and kidney damage is uncertain.[101–104] Clinical studies using these agents have been stalled in part due to the low frequency of symptomatic disease created by modern therapy (and the high rate of tumor progression for some of the relevant diseases). These agents appear to have benefits when given long after cancer treatment and are therefore of great interest since they have known minimal chronic toxicity profiles.[103,105,106] Pentoxifylline is commonly prescribed for late fibrovascular changes after radiation or combined radiation and surgery and durable improvements are seen in at about 30% of patients.[23] Randomized trials testing efficacy of angiotensin-converting enzyme inhibitors have been opened, but none has yet been completed. It is reasonable to predict that patients taking these agents for other clinical indications should have renal and pulmonary benefits as well.[107]

ANTI-INFLAMMATORY AGENTS

Inflammatory cytokines including KC, MCP1, IL-1, IL-6, TNF, and others have all been shown to powerfully impact radiation-induced reactions at both early and late time points in animal models.[108,109] Many including IL-1, IL-6, TGF-β have also been associated with similar syndromes in humans.[46,57] Anti-inflammatory agents aimed at COX-2, including celecoxib, have significant effects on animals and newer agents appear even more promising.[110–112] For this reason, agents aimed at reduction of inflammation present an exciting opportunity. Agents under investigation in the category include approved anti-inflammatory agents such as COX-2 inhibitors, and statins that reduce macrophage recruitment such as atorvastatin (Lipitor) and lovastatin. No anti-inflammatory agents have yet been proven fully satisfactory, and the most commonly employed are corticosteroid agents such as prednisone (commonly used for pulmonary toxicity) and dexamethasone (Decadron) for brain edema. Exciting potential agents in this class are targeted agents for rheumatoid arthritis, such as IL-1Ra (Anakinra).

ANTIAPOPTOTIC AGENTS

The role of antiapoptotic agents in management of radiation-related toxicity is controversial.[45,65,67] While some animal studies have indicated that early intervention following normally lethal exposures can extend survival,[113] others believe that organs involved in late effects are unlikely to benefit from these agents since, contrary to dogma, they are not prone to apoptotic death. For example, when the chest is irradiated for tumor, or chemotherapy is infused systemically, the malignancy apoptoses, while the heart and lungs do not. Nevertheless, there are categories of cells in normal tissues that do apoptose in response to therapy and that can benefit from antiapoptotic agents. These include the hematopoietic system, and probably the mucosa and skin. Both the extrinsic and the intrinsic apoptotic pathways are involved in treatment-induced apoptosis; hence, approaches to reduce apoptosis through specific signaling pathways have not always succeeded even in animal models. It is likely that combination agents will be required. Another interesting approach to development of an antiapoptotic response has been to develop innate antiapoptosis through exposure to a mild irritant. Experimental approaches of this sort include lightly scratching or brushing a tar mixture on the mucosa before irradiation, or pretreating cells with a sublethal dose of chemotherapy before irradiation. Animal studies are currently underway using agents that stimulate systemic responses that emulate bacteremia. The belief is that these agents, like growth factors, induce survival proteins such as NF-κB through TRAIL-like receptor signaling.[63,114,115] Agents in this category include CBLB502, a minimally immune-reactive fragment of bacterial flagellan. Others are under investigation including antibodies and other agents that block the TNF pathway. Other agents in this class deserving investigation are etanercept (Embrel), infliximab (Remicade), and adalimumab (Humira).

LONG-TERM EFFECTS OF NEW TECHNOLOGIES

New technologies are increasing our exposures to ionizing radiation. Improvements in computerized tomography (CT), thinner slice thickness of noninvasive imaging, and more frequent physician orders for this procedure are of public health interest. This is particularly true for young children. New radiation techniques including advanced targeting systems employ increased use of cone beam CT and megavoltage CT. Increased use of noncoaxial fields for cancer therapy also increases integral dose to nontarget tissues (even if it also reduces the peak doses given to the most sensitive tissues). Finally, the various space agencies interested in extending space exploration have funded studies that focus on the role that different radiation doses play in producing more subtle radiation side effects.

Very low doses of radiation may have much greater effects than previously assumed.[116,117] For example, there is evidence of decreased cognitive function after even low doses of radiation, with alteration in the cytokine expression profiles, and possible delayed (low level) demyelination.[118–120] These low-dose exposures may have long-term effects on a number of neurological functions. Low doses probably induce occasional secondary cancer, a very severe consequence if the originating medicinal exposure was for a very benign situation.[117] Indeed, while many of these side effects are nearly undetectable, the methods to evaluate these toxicities are growing and are of great interest. Most of the pathways involved in this low-level toxicity appear similar to those that cause the more severe toxicities.[121] Specifically, the mechanisms commonly include alterations in growth factor and growth factor receptor expression, chronically altered redox state, and low-grade chronic inflammation. It is reasonable to speculate that recovery from this more mild level of damage may be easier to achieve than will be possible for severe, clinically evident, tissue damage.[7,122]

RADIATION EXPOSURE RESEARCH: BIOTERROR AND ACCIDENTS

The scenarios in which accidental or malevolent radiation exposure may occur are many.[123–125] They include use of a conventional or improvised nuclear device, which will produce mass casualties, a radiological dispersal device (RDD or "dirty bomb"), which will inflict a smaller number of casualties,[126–127] and experimental/industrial exposure accidents and incidents that tend to involve relatively few individuals.[123] All can produce late consequences of varying degrees of severity.

INTENTIONAL EXPOSURE

Although there are many problems inherent with data from the Hiroshima and Nagasaki atomic bomb survivors, such as ongoing low-dose exposure that complicates the issue, many long-term studies indicate late disease development in survivors. Indeed, many investigators have noted increased cardiovascular disease experienced by survivors,[128–132] and recently Kusunoki and Hayashi[132] theorized that long-term inflammation experienced by atomic bomb survivors could have contributed significantly to their cardiovascular disease. The focus of this research is beginning to turn toward the progeny of survivors.

NUCLEAR AND INDUSTRIAL ACCIDENTS

The Chernobyl nuclear power plant accidental release of iodine-131, cesium-134, and cesium-137 in 1986 remains the largest and most well-known radiation exposure accident. In the immediate aftermath, 1,000 people on-site and first responders received considerable doses between 2 and 20 Gy, 134 people were diagnosed with acute radiation syndrome, and 28 died within the first few weeks and months following exposure. During the following year, 350,000 people received prolonged exposure (100 mSv: equivalent to 40 years of background exposure in just 1 year). These exposed workers now have a twofold increase in incidence of non-CLL leukemia, and an increase of 100,000 cancer deaths is expected for this population.[133] While we have methods for measurement of radiation-induced chronic chromosomal alterations in these patients, it remains unclear how relevant these alterations are to future cancer risk. Similarly, it is not yet known whether interventions aimed at reduction of these genetic alterations will increase or lower future risk of disease.

An industrial accident of much smaller scale occurred a few years after Chernobyl, in 1989, in Tokaimura, Japan, at a nuclear fuel processing facility. This event is an example of initial, successful treatment of the acute syndromes only to lose the patients to profound late effects. Three workers handling Uranium-235 were critically exposed, and 96 people on-site and first responders received <1 Gy. The two workers who received the largest dose died: one had received 18 Gy (died at day 82) and the other had received 6 to 10 Gy (died at 7 months). Both had been rescued from bone marrow crisis (with peripheral blood stem cell transplant and cord blood cell infusion, respectively) and GI crisis, only to succumb to lung toxicity.[134] The lesson here is that preparing for radiological emergencies must include attention to organs other than those acutely affected by radiation.

The very real potential of radiological terror and large-scale industrial accidents contaminating the environment has escalated the demand for research and product development for mitigation of toxicity. Agents in all four classes are in development, including agents that reduce vascular damage and oxidative stress, agents that inhibit apoptosis, agents that reduce radiation and combined injury-related chronic inflammation, and agents that augment beneficial replication and maturation of stem cells. The agents in development primarily focus on aspects of the bone marrow, gastrointestinal tract, lung, and integumental system. Most agents in development seem to benefit defined organs and must be given at specific times following exposure. Some are very specific for certain side effects (Fig. 45.4). Agents for prevention, mitigation, and therapy are in development, and some should find their way to approval over the next decade.

FDA APPROVAL PROCESS

New agents that target important pathways involved in normal tissue toxicity are being developed by pharmaceutical companies at a rate never before achieved in human medicine. The process by which these targeted agents become drugs approved by the US Federal Drug Administration (FDA) as protectors, mitigators, or therapeutics for adverse reactions of radiation exposure is demanding and difficult. For example, there must be evidence that a preventive agent reduces the severity or frequency of an uncommon toxicity at a satisfactory rate.

Protectors in particular must not also increase the frequency of treatment failure due to "inactivation" of other possibly concurrent therapies such as chemotherapy. For late effects of treatment, the duration of a randomized trial might make these studies technically impossible. Mitigative agents pose some of the same problems in the attempt to gain FDA approval. Until satisfactory molecular or subclinical imaging markers become available that are validated by the FDA for following the response to treatments, it is unlikely that many mitigation or prevention agents will be approved. This is unfortunate since many of the best targeted agents are likely to be of most benefit as prevention or mitigation agents.

Therapeutic agents, those given to treat a manifest toxicity, have the easiest route to approval because placebo treatments are easily implemented, patients can be tested in a blind-crossover design that allows each subject to serve as their matched control, and toxicity can be scored as a composite endpoint that includes area under the curve. As noted above, there are few if any agents approved as therapeutics for radiation or combined modality-induced adverse events. The use of this approach to agent approval is likely to produce new agents over the next decade.

CONCLUSION

There are presently very few interventions for toxicity after radiation exposure. In the oncologic treatment arena, single modality localized irradiation or combined treatment toxicity that includes localized very high-dose radiation treatment causes what is sometimes dose-limiting toxicity. Thankfully, severe local toxicity is usually well tolerated due to the small volume of normal tissue exposed to irradiation and the plasticity of the organ being irradiated. Some organs, however, do not tolerate even partial organ treatment and therefore decreasing volume does not reduce risk of symptomatic complications.

To date, the most accepted therapies for treatment-related toxicity remain hyperbaric oxygen (which likely works through both the antioxidant and the anti-inflammatory pathways) and pentoxifylline ± tocopherol (likely working through reduction of oxidative stress and other antioxidant mechanisms). Surgery for removal or repair of necrotic or nonhealing ischemic tissue is also commonly employed for difficult cases.

Drug treatments aimed at altering the incidence, severity, or progression of adverse events after radiation exposure come in four general categories. These include antioxidants, antiapoptotic agents, anti-inflammatory agents, and growth factors. Few agents in any of these categories are commonly used, and some of the most effective are likely to overlap several mechanisms of action. It is clear that different agents have utility that can be organ specific, and many will have greatest benefit when given at specific times, before or after the onset of symptoms.

In part fueled by the national need to develop agents in case of bioterror, there is a great deal of exciting research interest in developing new and better mitigators of radiation toxicity. The growing frequency of cancer survivors has also stimulated greater interest in understanding the long-term implications of otherwise successful but necessarily toxic therapy. New agents aimed specifically at the cancer survivor population may have substantial hurdles to overcome in the approval process; however, many agents are currently under investigation and are likely to become available, including some that are already approved for other purposes. Thus, the future is bright regarding availability of agents to reduce the sequellae of both high-dose radiation oncology treatments, thereby allowing better and increased application of this life-saving therapy, and whole- or partial-body exposure due to radiation accidents or incidents.

REFERENCES

1. Ries LAG, Melbert D, Krapcho M, et al. SEER Cancer Statistics Review, 1975–2005. Bethesda, MD: National Cancer Institute, Available at: http://seer.cancer.gov/csr/1975_2005/, based on November 2007 SEER data submission, posted to the SEER web site, 2008.
2. Ng AK, Travis LB. Subsequent malignant neoplasms in cancer survivors. *Cancer J.* 2008;14(6):429–434.
3. Travis LB, Yahalom J. Cancer survivorship: facing forward. *Hematol Oncol Clin North Am.* 2008;22(2):365–371.
4. Constine LS, Tarbell N, Hudson MM, et al. Subsequent malignancies in children treated for Hodgkin's disease: associations with gender and radiation dose. *Int J Radiat Oncol Biol Phys.* 2008;72(1):24–33.
5. Basu SK, Schwartz C, Fisher SG, et al. Unilateral and bilateral breast cancer in women surviving pediatric Hodgkin's disease. *Int J Radiat Oncol Biol Phys.* 2008;72(1):34–40.
6. NCI—The Nation's investment in cancer research: Connecting the Cancer Community. *An Annual Plan and Budget Proposal for Fiscal Year 2009.* Washington, DC: US Department of Health and Human Services; 2007.
7. Stone HB, Moulder JE, Coleman CN, et al. Models for evaluating agents intended for the prophylaxis, mitigation and treatment of radiation injuries. Report of an NCI Workshop, December 3–4, 2003. *Radiat Res.* 2004;162(6):711–728.
8. Rubin P, Constine LS, Fajardo LF, et al. RTOG Late Effects Working Group. Overview: late effects of normal tissues (LENT) scoring system. *Int J Radiat Oncol Biol Phys.* 1995;31(5):1041–1042.
9. Trotti A, Colevas AD, Setser A, et al. CTCAE v3.0: development of a comprehensive grading system for the adverse effects of cancer treatment. *Semin Radiat Oncol.* 2003;13(3): 176–181.
10. Williams J, Chen Y, Rubin P, et al. The biological basis of a comprehensive grading system for the adverse effects of cancer treatment. *Semin Radiat Oncol.* 2003;13(3):182–188.
11. Thames HD. Repair kinetics in tissues: alternative models. *Radiother Oncol.* 1989;14(4): 321–327.
12. Kwa SL, Theuws JC, Wagenaar A, et al. Evaluation of two dose-volume histogram reduction models for the prediction of radiation pneumonitis. *Radiother Oncol.* 1998;48(1):61–69.
13. Rubin P, Johnston CJ, Williams JP, et al. A perpetual cascade of cytokines postirradiation leads to pulmonary fibrosis. *Int J Radiat Oncol Biol Phys.* 1995;33(1):99–109.
14. Okunieff P, Cornelison T, Mester M, et al. Mechanism and modification of gastrointestinal soft tissue response to radiation: role of growth factors. *Int J Radiat Oncol Biol Phys.* 2005;62(1):273–278.
15. Kim JH, Brown SL, Jenrow KA, et al. Mechanisms of radiation-induced brain toxicity and implications for future clinical trials. *J Neurooncol.* 2008;87(3):279–286.
16. Delanian S, Lefaix JL. Current management for late normal tissue injury: radiation-induced fibrosis and necrosis. *Semin Radiat Oncol.* 2007;17(2):99–107.
17. Hoffman KE, Horowitz NS, Russell AH. Healing of vulvo-vaginal radionecrosis following revascularization. *Gynecol Oncol.* 2007;106(1):262–264.
18. Deganello A, Gallo O, De Cesare JM, et al. Surgical management of surgery and radiation induced peristomal neck ulcerations. *B-ENT.* 2008;4(3):169–174.
19. Hirsch DL, Bell RB, Dierks EJ, et al. Analysis of microvascular free flaps for reconstruction of advanced mandibular osteoradionecrosis: a retrospective cohort study. *J Oral Maxillofac Surg.* 2008;66(12):2545–2556.
20. Gothard L, Stanton A, MacLaren L, et al. Non-randomised phase II trial of hyperbaric oxygen therapy in patients with chronic arm lymphoedema and tissue fibrosis after radiotherapy for early breast cancer. *Radiother Oncol.* 2004;70(3):217–224.
21. Okunieff P, Wang X, Rubin P, et al. Radiation-induced changes in bone perfusion and angiogenesis. *Int J Radiat Oncol Biol Phys.* 1998;42(4):885–889.
22. Okunieff P, Wang X, Li M, et al. Chronic radiation bone toxicity is associated with decreased perfusion without elevation of circulating or soft tissue TGF beta or TNF alpha. *Adv Exp Med Biol.* 1998;454:325–333.
23. Okunieff P, Augustine E, Hicks JE, et al. Pentoxifylline in the treatment of radiation-induced fibrosis. *J Clin Oncol.* 2004;22(11):2207–2213.
24. Boerma M, Roberto KA, Hauer-Jensen M. Prevention and treatment of functional and structural radiation injury in the rat heart by pentoxifylline and alpha-tocopherol. *Int J Radiat Oncol Biol Phys.* 2008;72(1):170–177.
25. Delanian S, Porcher R, Balla-Mekias S, et al. Randomized, placebo-controlled trial of combined pentoxifylline and tocopherol for regression of superficial radiation-induced fibrosis. *J Clin Oncol.* 2003;21(13):2545–2550.
26. Nieder C, Zimmermann FB, Adam M, et al. The role of pentoxifylline as a modifier of radiation therapy. *Cancer Treat Rev.* 2005;31(6):448–455
27. Hall EJ. Weiss lecture. The dose-rate factor in radiation biology. *Int J Radiat Biol.* 1991;59(3):595–610.
28. Thames HD, Bentzen SM, Turesson I, et al. Fractionation parameters for human tissues and tumors. *Int J Radiat Biol.* 1989;56(5):701–710.
29. Thames HD, Ang KK. Altered fractionation: radiobiological principles, clinical results, and potential for dose escalation. *Cancer Treat Res.* 1998;93:101–128.
30. Flickinger JC, Lunsford LD, Kondziolka D. Dose prescription and dose-volume effects in radiosurgery. *Neurosurg Clin N Am.* 1992;3(1):51–59
31. Flickinger JC, Kondziolka D, Niranjan A, et al. Dose selection in stereotactic radiosurgery. *Prog Neurol Surg.* 2007;20:28–42.
32. Bentzen SM. Steepness of the radiation dose-response curve for dose-per-fraction escalation keeping the number of fractions fixed. *Acta Oncol.* 2005;44(8):825–828.
33. Lindegaard JC, Overgaard J, Bentzen SM, et al. Is there a radiobiologic basis for improving the treatment of advanced stage cervical cancer? *J Natl Cancer Inst Monogr.* 1996;(21): 105–112.
34. Emami B, Lyman J, Brown A, et al. Tolerance of normal tissue to therapeutic irradiation. *Int J Radiat Oncol Biol Phys.* 1991;21(1):109–122.
35. Milano MT, Constine LS, Okunieff P. Normal tissue tolerance dose metrics for radiation therapy of major organs. *Semin Radiat Oncol.* 2007;17(2):131–140.
36. Chang BK, Timmerman RD. Stereotactic body radiation therapy: a comprehensive review. *Am J Clin Oncol.* 2007;30(6):637–644.
37. Niranjan A, Flickinger JC. Radiobiology, principle and technique of radiosurgery. *Prog Neurol Surg.* 2008;21:32–42.
38. Milano MT, Constine LS, Okunieff P. Normal tissue toxicity after small field hypofractionated stereotactic body radiation. *Radiat Oncol.* 2008;3:36–45.
39. Marks LB, Munley MT, Bentel GC, et al. Physical and biological predictors of changes in whole-lung function following thoracic irradiation. *Int J Radiat Oncol Biol Phys.* 1997;39(3):563–570.
40. Marks LB, Yu X, Vujaskovic Z, et al. Radiation-induced lung injury. *Semin Radiat Oncol.* 2003;13(3):333–345.
41. Brock KK. Image registration in intensity- modulated, image-guided and stereotactic body radiation therapy. *Front Radiat Ther Oncol.* 2007;40:94–115.
42. Neta R, Oppenheim JJ. Radioprotection with cytokines–learning from nature to cope with radiation damage. *Cancer Cells.* 1991;3(10):391–396.
43. Morgan GW, Breit SN. Radiation and the lung: a reevaluation of the mechanisms mediating pulmonary injury. *Int J Radiat Oncol Biol Phys.* 1995;31(2):361–369.
44. Herskind C, Bamberg M, Rodemann HP. The role of cytokines in the development of normal-tissue reactions after radiotherapy. *Strahlenther Onkol.* 1998;174(suppl 3):12–15.
45. Hill RP, Rodemann HP, Hendry JH, et al. Normal tissue radiobiology: from the laboratory to the clinic. *Int J Radiat Oncol Biol Phys.* 2001;49(2):353–365.
46. Chen Y, Williams J, Ding I, et al. Radiation pneumonitis and early circulatory cytokine markers. *Semin Radiat Oncol.* 2002;12(1 suppl 1):26–33.
47. Liu W, Ding I, Chen K, et al. Interleukin 1beta (IL1B) signaling is a critical component of radiation-induced skin fibrosis. *Radiat Res.* 2006;165(2):181–191.
48. Müller K, Meineke V. Radiation-induced alterations in cytokine production by skin cells. *Exp Hematol.* 2007;35(4 suppl 1):96–104.
49. Neta R, Okunieff P. Cytokine-induced radiation protection and sensitization. *Semin Radiat Oncol.* 1996;6(4):306–320.
50. Vegesna V, McBride WH, Taylor JM, et al. The effect of interleukin-1 beta or transforming growth factor-beta on radiation-impaired murine skin wound healing. *J Surg Res.* 1995;59(6):699–704.
51. Johnston CJ, Piedboeuf B, Rubin P, et al. Early and persistent alterations in the expression of interleukin-1 alpha, interleukin-1 beta and tumor necrosis factor alpha mRNA levels in fibrosis-resistant and sensitive mice after thoracic irradiation. *Radiat Res.* 1996;145(6):762–767.
52. Chen Y, Hyrien O, Williams J, et al. Interleukin (IL)-1A and IL-6: applications to the predictive diagnostic testing of radiation pneumonitis. *Int J Radiat Oncol Biol Phys.* 2005;62(1): 260–266.
53. Nishioka A, Ogawa Y, Hamada N, et al. Analysis of radiation pneumonitis and radiation-induced lung fibrosis in breast cancer patients after breast conservation treatment. *Oncol Rep.* 1999;6(3):513–517.
54. Quarmby S, Fakhoury H, Levine E, et al. Association of transforming growth factor beta-1 single nucleotide polymorphisms with radiation-induced damage to normal tissues in breast cancer patients. *Int J Radiat Biol.* 2003;79(2):137–143.
55. Kahán Z, Csenki M, Varga Z, et al. The risk of early and late lung sequelae after conformal radiotherapy in breast cancer patients. *Int J Radiat Oncol Biol Phys.* 2007;68(3):673–681
56. Alsner J, Rødningen OK, Overgaard J. Differential gene expression before and after ionizing radiation of subcutaneous fibroblasts identifies breast cancer patients resistant to radiation-induced fibrosis. *Radiother Oncol.* 2007;83(3):261–266.
57. Anscher MS, Peters WP, Reisenbichler H, et al. Transforming growth factor beta as a predictor of liver and lung fibrosis after autologous bone marrow transplantation for advanced breast cancer. *N Engl J Med.* 1993;328(22):1592–1598.
58. Finkelstein JN, Horowitz S, Sinkin RA, et al. Cellular and molecular responses to lung injury in relation to induction of tissue repair and fibrosis. *Clin Perinatol.* 1992;19(3): 603–620.
59. Neta R. Modulation with cytokines of radiation injury: suggested mechanisms of action. *Environ Health Perspect.* 1997;105(suppl 6):1463–1465.
60. Fuks Z, Persaud RS, Alfieri A, et al. Basic fibroblast growth factor protects endothelial cells against radiation-induced programmed cell death in vitro and in vivo. *Cancer Res.* 1994;54(10):2582–2590.
61. Haimovitz-Friedman A, Kolesnick RN, Fuks Z. Differential inhibition of radiation-induced apoptosis. *Stem Cells.* 1997;15(suppl 2):43–47.
62. Belka C, Jendrossek V, Pruschy M, et al. Apoptosis-modulating agents in combination with radiotherapy-current status and outlook. *Int J Radiat Oncol Biol Phys.* 2004;58(2):542–554.
63. Gudkov AV, Komarova EA. Prospective therapeutic applications of p53 inhibitors. *Biochem Biophys Res Commun.* 2005;331(3):726–736.
64. Strom E, Sathe S, Komarov PG, et al. Small-molecule inhibitor of p53 binding to mitochondria protects mice from gamma radiation. *Nat Chem Biol.* 2006;2(9):474–479.
65. Bristow RG, Benchimol S, Hill RP. The p53 gene as a modifier of intrinsic radiosensitivity: implications for radiotherapy. *Radiother Oncol.* 1996;40(3):197–223.
66. Hu Q, Hill RP. Radiosensitivity, apoptosis and repair of DNA double-strand breaks in radiation-sensitive Chinese hamster ovary cell mutants treated at different dose rates. *Radiat Res.* 1996;146(6):636–645.
67. Brush J, Lipnick SL, Phillips T, et al. Molecular mechanisms of late normal tissue injury. *Semin Radiat Oncol.* 2007;17(2):121–130.
68. Kirsch DG, Santiago PM, Haigis KM, et al. Utilizing mouse genetics to dissect the cellular target and molecular mechanism of acute and late toxicity of abdominal radiation therapy [Abstract]. *Int J Radiat Oncol Biol Phys.* 2006;66(suppl):590.

69. Epperly MW, Osipov AN, Martin I, et al. Ascorbate as a "redox sensor" and protector against irradiation-induced oxidative stress in 32D CL 3 hematopoietic cells and subclones overexpressing human manganese superoxide dismutase. *Int J Radiat Oncol Biol Phys.* 2004;58(3):851–861.

70. Ryter SW, Kim HP, Hoetzel A, et al. Mechanisms of cell death in oxidative stress. *Antioxid Redox Signal.* 2007;9(1):49–89.

71. Cardoso SM, Pereira C, Oliveira R. Mitochondrial function is differentially affected upon oxidative stress. *Free Radic Biol Med.* 1999;26(1–2):3–13.

72. Hoye AT, Davoren JE, Wipf P, et al. Targeting mitochondria. *Acc Chem Res.* 2008;41(1):87–97.

73. Okunieff P, Swarts S, Keng P, et al. Antioxidants reduce consequences of radiation exposure. *Adv Exp Med Biol.* 2008;614:165–178.

74. Jiang J, Belikova NA, Hoye AT, et al. A mitochondria-targeted nitroxide/hemigramicidin S conjugate protects mouse embryonic cells against gamma irradiation. *Int J Radiat Oncol Biol Phys.* 2008;70(3):816–825.

75. Chaudière J, Ferrari-Iliou R. Intracellular antioxidants: from chemical to biochemical mechanisms. *Food Chem Toxicol.* 1999;37(9–10):949–962.

76. Weiss JF, Landauer MR. Protection against ionizing radiation by antioxidant nutrients and phytochemicals. *Toxicology.* 2003;189(1–2):1–20.

77. Robb L. Cytokine receptors and hematopoietic differentiation. *Oncogene.* 2007;26(47):6715–6723.

78. Metcalf D. Hematopoietic cytokines. *Blood.* 2008;111(2):485–491.

79. Gonzalvez F, Gottlieb E. Cardiolipin: setting the beat of apoptosis. *Apoptosis.* 2007;12(5):877–885.

80. Greenberger JS, Epperly MW. Antioxidant gene therapeutic approaches to normal tissue radioprotection and tumor radiosensitization. *In Vivo.* 2007;21(2):141–146.

81. Greenberger JS. Gene therapy approaches for stem cell protection. *Gene Ther.* 2008;15(2):100–108.

82. Moran LK, Gutteridge JM, Quinlan GJ. Thiols in cellular redox signalling and control. *Curr Med Chem.* 2001;8(7):763–772.

83. Wojtczak L, Slyshenkov VS. Protection by pantothenic acid against apoptosis and cell damage by oxygen free radicals—the role of glutathione. *Biofactors.* 2003;17(1–4):61–73.

84. Block KI, Gyllenhaal C. Commentary: the pharmacological antioxidant amifostine—implications of recent research for integrative cancer care. *Integr Cancer Ther.* 2005;4(4):329–351.

85. Garden AS, Lewin JS, Chambers MS. How to reduce radiation-related toxicity in patients with cancer of the head and neck. *Curr Oncol Rep.* 2006;8(2):140–145.

86. Packer L, Valacchi G. Antioxidants and the response of skin to oxidative stress: vitamin E as a key indicator. *Skin Pharmacol Appl Skin Physiol.* 2002;15(5):282–290.

87. Koch CJ, Biaglow JE. Toxicity, radiation sensitivity modification, and metabolic effects of dehydroascorbate and ascorbate in mammalian cells. *J Cell Physiol.* 1978;94(3):299–306.

88. Jagetia GC, Rajanikant GK. Curcumin treatment enhances the repair and regeneration of wounds in mice exposed to hemibody gamma-irradiation. *Plast Reconstr Surg.* 2005;115(2):515–528.

89. Okunieff P, Xu J, Hu D, et al. Curcumin protects against radiation-induced acute and chronic cutaneous toxicity in mice and decreases mRNA expression of inflammatory and fibrogenic cytokines. *Int J Radiat Oncol Biol Phys.* 2006;65(3):890–898.

90. Okunieff P, Wu T, Huang K, et al. Differential radioprotection of three mouse strains by basic or acidic fibroblast growth factor. *Br J Cancer.* 1996;27:S105–S108.

91. Kennedy SH, Rouda S, Qin H, et al. Basic FGF regulates interstitial collagenase gene expression in human smooth muscle cells. *J Cell Biochem.* 1997;65(1):32–41.

92. Ding I, Huang K, Wang X, et al. Radioprotection of hematopoietic tissue by fibroblast growth factors in fractionated radiation experiments. *Acta Oncol.* 1997;36(3):337–340.

93. Okunieff P, Fenton BM, Zhang L, et al. Fibroblast growth factors (FGFS) increase breast tumor growth rate, metastases, blood flow, and oxygenation without significant change in vascular density. *Adv Exp Med Biol.* 2003;530:593–601.

94. Khan WB, Shui C, Ning S, et al. Enhancement of murine intestinal stem cell survival after irradiation by keratinocyte growth factor. *Radiat Res.* 1997;148(3):248–253.

95. Okunieff P, Li M, Liu W, et al. Keratinocyte growth factors radioprotect bowel and bone marrow but not KHT sarcoma. *Am J Clin Oncol.* 2001;24(5):491–495.

96. Hérodin F, Grenier N, Drouet M. Revisiting therapeutic strategies in radiation casualties. *Exp Hematol.* 2007;35(4 suppl 1):28–33.

97. McDonnell AM, Lenz KL. Palifermin: role in the prevention of chemotherapy- and radiation-induced mucositis. *Ann Pharmacother.* 2007;41(1):86–94.

98. Okunieff P, Barrett AJ, Phang SE, et al. Circulating basic fibroblast growth factor declines during Cy/TBI bone marrow transplantation. *Bone Marrow Transplant.* 1999;23(11):1117–1121.

99. Blackwell K, Gascón P, Sigounas G, et al. rHuEPO and improved treatment outcomes: potential modes of action. *Oncologist.* 2004;9(suppl 5):41–47.

100. Lai SY, Childs EE, Xi S, et al. Erythropoietin-mediated activation of JAK-STAT signaling contributes to cellular invasion in head and neck squamous cell carcinoma. *Oncogene.* 2005;24(27):4442–4449.

101. Cohen EP, Robbins ME. Radiation nephropathy. *Semin Nephrol.* 2003;23(5):486–499.

102. Robbins ME, Diz DI. Pathogenic role of the renin-angiotensin system in modulating radiation-induced late effects. *Int J Radiat Oncol Biol Phys.* 2006;64(1):6–12.

103. Moulder JE, Fish BL, Cohen EP. Treatment of radiation nephropathy with ACE inhibitors and AII type-1 and type-2 receptor antagonists. *Curr Pharm Des.* 2007;13(13):1317–1325.

104. Moulder JE, Cohen EP. Future strategies for mitigation and treatment of chronic radiation-induced normal tissue injury. *Semin Radiat Oncol.* 2007;17(2):141–148.

105. Molteni A, Wolfe LF, Ward WF, et al. Effect of an angiotensin II receptor blocker and two angiotensin converting enzyme inhibitors on transforming growth factor-beta (TGF-beta) and alpha-actomyosin (alpha SMA), important mediators of radiation-induced pneumopathy and lung fibrosis. *Curr Pharm Des.* 2007;13(13):1307–1316.

106. Cohen EP, Irving AA, Drobyski WR, et al. Captopril to mitigate chronic renal failure after hematopoietic stem cell transplantation: a randomized controlled trial. *Int J Radiat Oncol Biol Phys.* 2008;70(5):1546–1551.

107. Zhao W, Robbins ME. Inflammation and chronic oxidative stress in radiation-induced late normal tissue injury: therapeutic implications. *Curr Med Chem.* 2009;16(2):130–143.

108. Williams JP, Hernady E, Johnston CJ, et al. Effect of administration of lovastatin on the development of late pulmonary effects after whole-lung irradiation in a murine model. *Radiat Res.* 2004;161(5):560–567.

109. Haydont V, Gilliot O, Rivera S, et al. Successful mitigation of delayed intestinal radiation injury using pravastatin is not associated with acute injury improvement or tumor protection. *Int J Radiat Oncol Biol Phys.* 2007;68(5):1471–1482.

110. Dicker AP. COX-2 inhibitors and cancer therapeutics: potential roles for inhibitors of COX-2 in combination with cytotoxic therapy: reports from a symposium held in conjunction with the Radiation Therapy Oncology Group June 2001 Meeting. *Am J Clin Oncol.* 2003;26(4):S46–S47.

111. Liang L, Hu D, Liu W, et al. Celecoxib reduces skin damage after radiation: selective reduction of chemokine and receptor mRNA expression in irradiated skin but not in irradiated mammary tumor. *Am J Clin Oncol.* 2003;26(4):S114–S121.

112. Xiao Z, Su Y, Yang S, et al. Protective effect of esculentoside A on radiation-induced dermatitis and fibrosis. *Int J Radiat Oncol Biol Phys.* 2006;65(3):882–889.

113. Hérodin F, Bourin P, Mayol JF, et al. Short-term injection of antiapoptotic cytokine combinations soon after lethal gamma -irradiation promotes survival. *Blood.* 2003;101(7):2609–2616.

114. Gudkov AV, Komarova EA. The role of p53 in determining sensitivity to radiotherapy. *Nat Rev Cancer.* 2003;3(2):117–129.

115. Shankar S, Singh G, Srivastava RK. Chemoprevention by resveratrol: molecular mechanisms and therapeutic potential. *Front Biosci.* 2007;12:4839–4854.

116. Hall EJ, Brenner DJ. Cancer risks from diagnostic radiology. *Br J Radiol.* 2008;81(965):362–378.

117. Brenner DJ, Hall EJ. Computed tomography—an increasing source of radiation exposure. *N Engl J Med.* 2007;357(22):2277–2284.

118. Crang AJ, Franklin RJ, Blakemore WF, et al. The differentiation of glial cell progenitor populations following transplantation into non-repairing central nervous system glial lesions in adult animals. *J Neuroimmunol.* 1992;40(2–3):243–253.

119. Bögler O, Wren D, Barnett SC, et al. Cooperation between two growth factors promotes extended self-renewal and inhibits differentiation of oligodendrocyte-type-2 astrocyte (O-2A) progenitor cells. *Proc Natl Acad Sci USA.* 1990;87(16):6368–6372.

120. Moore AH, Olschowka JA, Williams JP, et al. Regulation of prostaglandin E2 synthesis after brain irradiation. *Int J Radiat Oncol Biol Phys.* 2005;62(1):267–272.

121. Mayer M, Noble M. N-acetyl-L-cysteine is a pluripotent protector against cell death and enhancer of trophic factor-mediated cell survival in vitro. *Proc Natl Acad Sci USA.* 1994;91(16):7496–7500.

122. Verbaeys C, Hoebeke P, Oosterlinck W. Complicated postirradiation vesicovaginal fistula in young women: keep off or try reconstruction? *Eur Urol.* 2007;51(1):243–246.

123. González AJ, Lauriston S. Taylor Lecture: Radiation protection in the aftermath of a terrorist attack involving exposure to ionizing radiation. *Health Phys.* 2005;89(5):418–446.

124. Turai I, Veress K, Günalp B, et al. Medical response to radiation incidents and radionuclear threats. *BMJ.* 2004;328(7439):568–572.

125. Goans RE, Waselenko JK. Medical management of radiological casualties. *Health Phys.* 2005;89(5):505–512.

126. Harper FT, Musolino SV, Wente WB. Realistic radiological dispersal device hazard boundaries and ramifications for early consequence management decisions. *Health Phys.* 2007;93(1):1–16.

127. Musolino SV, Harper FT. Emergency response guidance for the first 48 hours after the outdoor detonation of an explosive radiological dispersal device. *Health Phys.* 2006;90(4):377–385.

128. Preston DL, Shimizu Y, Pierce DA, et al. Studies of mortality of atomic bomb survivors. Report 13: solid cancer and noncancer disease mortality: 1950–1997. *Radiat Res.* 2003;160(4):381–407.

129. Yamada M, Wong FL, Fujiwara S, et al. Noncancer disease incidence in atomic bomb survivors, 1958–1998. *Radiat Res.* 2004;161(6):622–632.

130. Preston DL, Ron E, Tokuoka S, et al. Solid cancer incidence in atomic bomb survivors: 1958–1998. *Radiat Res.* 2007;168(1):1–64.

131. Schultz-Hector S, Trott KR. Radiation-induced cardiovascular diseases: is the epidemiologic evidence compatible with the radiobiologic data? *Int J Radiat Oncol Biol Phys.* 2007;67(1):10–18.

132. Kusunoki Y, Hayashi T. Long-lasting alterations of the immune system by ionizing radiation exposure: implications for disease development among atomic bomb survivors. *Int J Radiat Biol.* 2008;84(1):1–14.

133. Kinley D III, ed. Chernobyl's Legacy: Health, Environmental and Socio-Economic Impacts and Recommendations to the Governments of Belarus, the Russian Federation and Ukraine. *The Chernobyl Forum: 2003–2005.* 2nd rev. ed. Vienna, Austria: IAEA; 2006.

134. Report on the Preliminary Fact Finding Mission Following the Accident at the Nuclear Fuel Processing Facility in Tokaimura, Japan. Vienna, Austria: IAEA; 1999.

Index